The 5-Minute Herb and Dietary Supplement Consult

ABOUT THE EDITOR

Adriane Fugh-Berman, MD, is Assistant Clinical Professor in the departments of Medicine and Health Care Sciences, George Washington University School of Medicine. She consults on herbs and dietary supplements for the Federal Trade Commission, the National Institutes of Health (NIH), and other federal and state agencies.

Dr. Fugh-Berman is the author of *Alternative Medicine: What Works* and is co-author of *The National Women's Health Network's The Truth about Hormone Replacement Therapy* (Prima/Random House, 2002). She authored the first chapter on alternative medicine in *Harrison's Principles of Internal Medicine* and serves on the editorial boards of *Pharmacotherapy, Focus on Alternative and Complementary Therapies* (U.K.), and *HerbalGram*. She is an internationally known speaker, addressing both professional and consumer audiences.

Dr. Fugh-Berman is a member of the Institute of the US Pharmacopoeia Dietary Supplements Expert Committee; the Physician Data Query (PDQ) Adult Treatment Advisory Editorial Board, and the American Botanical Council Advisory Board. She also is a medical advisor to the National Women's Health Network, a science-based, independent consumer advocacy group that takes no money from pharmaceutical, medical device, or dietary supplement companies.

Former positions include medical officer, Contraception and Reproductive Health Branch, National Institute of Child Health and Human Development, NIH; coordinator of field investigations, Office of Alternative Medicine, NIH; and medical director, Green Cross Clinic and Taoist Health Institute, Washington, D.C.

Dr. Fugh-Berman graduated from Georgetown University School of Medicine and did postgraduate training in the Residency Program in Social Medicine at Montefiore Hospital in the Bronx. Her work has appeared in the *Lancet, JAMA, Annals of Internal Medicine, British Journal of Clinical Pharmacology, Menopause, Preventive Cardiology, Economic Botany, and Primary Care*, as well as many consumer publications.

The 5-Minute Herb and Dietary Supplement Consult

ADRIANE FUGH-BERMAN, MD

ASSISTANT CLINICAL PROFESSOR

DEPARTMENT OF HEALTH CARE SCIENCES

AND DEPARTMENT OF MEDICINE

GEORGE WASHINGTON UNIVERSITY SCHOOL OF MEDICINE

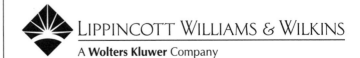

LIPPINCOTT WILLIAMS & WILKINS
A **Wolters Kluwer** Company

Philadelphia · Baltimore · New York · London
Buenos Aires · Hong Kong · Sydney · Tokyo

Acquisitions Editor: Timothy Y. Hiscock
Developmental Editor: Stacey L. Baze
Production Editor: Allison L. Risko
Manufacturing Manager: Colin Warnock
Cover Designer: LWW Desktop Division, NY
Compositor: Techbooks, PA; LWW Desktop Division, NY
Printer: R.R. Donnelly

Printed in the USA

Library of Congress Cataloging-in-Publication Data
The 5-minute herb and dietary supplement consult. Adriane Fugh-Berman—1st ed.
　　p. ;　cm
　　Includes bibliographic references and index.
　　ISBN 0-683-30273-6 (alk. paper)
　　1. Herb and dietary supplements, manuals, etc.　I. Title: Five-minute herb and dietary supplement consult.　II. Fugh-Berman, Adriane.
　　[DNLM: 1. Herb and dietary supplement manuals.　WS 39 Z99 2003]
RJ48.A15 2003
618.92-dc21
DNLM/DLC
　　　　　　　　　　　　　　　　　　　　2002030018

Care has been taken to confirm the accuracy of the information presented and to describe generally accepted practices. However, the author and publisher are not responsible for errors or omissions or for any consequences from application of the information in this book and make no warranty, expressed or implied, with respect to currency, completeness, or accuracy of the contents of the publication. Application of this information in a particular situation remains the responsibility of the practitioner.

The author and publisher have exerted every effort to ensure that the product selection and dosage set forth in this text are in accordance with current recommendations and practice at the time of publication. However, knowledge regarding the proper use of herbs and dietary supplements is ever changing. As new research and clinical experience broaden our understanding, changes in use may be necessary or appropriate. Readers are advised to check the most current medical literature and product information provided by the manufacturer of each product and to verify the recommended dose, the method and duration of administration, and contraindications.

To the memory of my maternal grandparents,
Sarah Fugh 傅劉倬漢 *and Philip Fugh* 傅涇波.

Acknowledgments

I am grateful first and always to my mother, Aline Fugh Berman, who acknowledges no limits and takes courage to formidable and sometimes life-threatening extremes. Both my mother and my late father, Daniel M. Berman, taught me to question everything and to consider convention only an option. Without my adopted aunt Liling Li's 李景秋 loving and devoted care of my mother, this book could not have been written. Liling Li is the best cook in the world, and her dumplings, noodles, and other fabulous dishes have been a source of unspeakable joy in my life. Many thanks also to my aunts Seyere 傅好玲 and Ooyere 傅莉, wonderful cooks as well, who also cared for my mother and in doing so, cared for me.

Many friends and colleagues were of assistance to me in this project, but my deepest gratitude is reserved for the following people:

Ted Kaptchuk and Tony Scialli, who understand and support me in innumerable ways.

My painstaking reviewers, Dennis Awang, Maria Linder, and Jerry Cott, who corrected many errors; any remaining errors are of course my responsibility.

Judy Davis, who spent more work hours in the same room with me than anyone, for her tactful help and friendship, and for bringing order, beauty, and homemade wonderful pies to my office.

My wonderful research assistants, Brooke Grandle, who handled near-impossible tasks with aplomb, Mark Devenport, whose conscientiousness knew no bounds, and Pragyna Seetharam and Mahesh Seetharam, who dealt with unreasonable requests graciously, even while studying for medical exams. Also Nancy Morgan, who stayed with my aged cat Roo while I traveled.

Thea Lee, Cindy Pearson, Fran Pollner, Amy Allina, Vickie Leonard, and Mieke Meurs, who made me keep a semblance of a social life; our monthly dinners, in which no one is polite and everyone is funny, are vital to my mental health. Charlea Massion, in whose Santa Cruz abode I wrote part of this book, for support, respite, the beautiful notes, and for reminding me to include flowers, poetry, and massages in my life. Arthur Naiman, my first publisher (one always remembers the first) and fast friend, who gave me great advice and told great jokes.

Most of my relatives, but especially my cousins, April Lee, for computer support, and comedic riffs on family dynamics, and Sarah Lee and Dave Stanke, for many kinds of support, especially the New York respites. My aunt Dora Fugh Lee, for calligraphy. Mary Leckie, who has been in my life since childhood, and along with my mother has taught me always to be an activist, and to keep a sense of humor. Thanks also to my brother, Stuart Chang Berman, and my sister-in-law, Eileen Berman.

Many friends and colleagues have given me gifts of knowledge and aid. I thank all of them, but especially Jim Duke, Mark Blumenthal, Roy Upton, Tieraona Low Dog, Steve Bratman, Edzard Ernst, James Dillard, John McPartland, Elizabeth Jeffery and Dominique Piot–Gourneau.

Adriane Fugh-Berman
Washington, D.C.

Contents

CONTENTS

SECTION II: REFERENCES / 353–426

SECTION III: REFERENCE TABLES

CONTENTS

Introduction

This is a personal book. These are not systematic reviews, nor are they random. MEDLINE, TOXLINE, and other databases were searched for every entry, references were dredged, friends and colleagues queried, and my own voluminous files searched. An attempt has been made to be thorough, but I make no claim of having included every source. I included all randomized controlled trials with relevant endpoints from reliable sources; I rarely included studies from alternative medical journals and Chinese medical literature, as their quality is not yet up to Western methodological standards.

Full studies were obtained and analyzed in almost all cases. I occasionally threw out studies because I couldn't find them, or interpret them. I have limited translation resources but have cited a few key articles in other languages when I could piece together enough information to be reassured as to study reliability. Trustworthy secondary sources that include European studies include the *ESCOP Monographs* (European Scientific Cooperative on Phytotherapy, Exeter, U.K.; fascicules published in 1997 and 1999); the *Expanded Commission E Monographs* (Blumenthal M, Goldberg A, Brinckmann J, Integrative Medicine Communications, Newton, MA, 2000); *Rational Phytotherapy* (Schulz V, Hänsel R, Tyler VE, Springer-Verlag, Berlin, 1998); *Principles and Practice of Phytotherapy* (Mills S, Bone K, Churchill Livingstone, Edinburgh, 2000); *Herbal Drugs and Phytopharmaceuticals* (Wichtl M, Bisset NM (ed) Medpharm Scientific publishers, Stuttgart 1994), *Adverse Effects of Herbal Drugs,* Vols.1-3 (De Smet PAGM, Keller K, Hänsel R, Chandler RF, Springer-Verlag, Berlin, 1992,1993, 1997); *Handbook on Medicinal Herbs* (Duke JA, CRC Press, Boca Raton FL, 2001); *WHO monographs on selected medicinal plants*, vol. 1,World Health Organization, Geneva, 1999); *Tyler's Honest Herbal* (Foster S, Tyler VE, 4th ed., Haworth Press, New York, 1999) and any other books by Tip Tyler, who died in 2001; his knowledge, spirit, and manners will be missed.

Constraints of space and tolerance have limited animal and *in vitro* information. In some cases, subjects worthy of a book on their own have been condensed to near-telegraphic brevity in order to fit the two-page format. Other entries contain much non-human data and bizarre ramblings. Entries include relevant animal studies on efficacy, safety, and pharmacology, unless superseded by relevant human studies.

There are no randomized controlled trials for many supplements; under these circumstances, I adopted a strategy that goes by the authoritative-sounding name, best evidence, emphasizing human studies if available, animal studies in a pinch, and *in vitro* studies in desperation. In general, *in vitro* mutagenicity or carcinogenicity studies were not included because of their lack of predictive value. Information on pregnancy and lactation has been included where available; where the subheading is missing, no information was identified.

Because this book is personal I've occasionally left things out in a fit of pique, or dragged in completely tangential material because it was too interesting not to mention. I beg the reader's indulgence.

If you wonder why I am bothering clinicians with botanist names appended to Latin binomials, it is because some of my friends are botanists. I fear their wrath. *World Economic Plants* (Wiersema JH, León B, CRC Press, Boca Raton, 1999) was the primary source for names.

Readers are invited to pick and choose the material that interests them and ignore the rest. I have striven for accuracy, but I hope that the book is entertaining as well as educational.

Adriane Fugh-Berman

Abbreviations

A, B, C

ABR auditory brainstem responses
ACE angiotensin converting enzyme
ACF aberrant crypt foci
ACTH adrenocorticotropic hormone
ADL activities of daily living
ADP adenosine diphosphate
AHRQ Agency for Health Care Research and Quality
ALT alanine transaminase
ALS amyotrophic lateral sclerosis
ANA antinuclear antibody
APTT activated partial thromboplastin time
ASR acoustic startle response
AST aspartate transaminase
ATP adenosine triphosphate
A-V atrioventricular
AVED ataxia with vitamin E deficiency
BAL dimercaprol
BCAA branched-chain amino acid
BHS breath-holding spells
b.i.d. *bis in die*, twice a day
BMD bone mineral density
BMI body mass index
BP blood pressure
BPH benign prostatic hyperplasia
BUN blood urea nitrogen
BV bacterial vaginosis
CABG coronary artery bypass graft
CAD coronary artery disease
CAH chronic active hepatitis
CAPB cocamidopropyl betaine
CBC complete blood count
CEE conjugated equine estrogens
CFU colony forming unit
CGI Clinical Global Impression
CHD coronary heart disease
CHF congestive heart failure
cGMP cyclic guanosine monophosphate
CI confidence interval
CIN cervical intraepithelial neoplasia
CNM certified nurse-midwife
CNS central nervous system
COPD chronic obstructive pulmonary disease
CPB competitive protein binding
CPK creatine phosphokinase
CRF chronic renal failure
CT computed tomography

D, E, F

DBP vitamin D binding protein
DBP diastolic blood pressure
D&C dilation and curettage
deet diethyltoluamide
DGL deglycyrrhizinated licorice
DGLA dihomo-γ-linolenic acid
DHA docosahexaenoic acid
DHEA dehydroepiandrosterone
DHEA-S DHEA-sulfate
DHT dihydrotestosterone
DIT diiodothyronine
DMSO dimethyl sulfoxide
DPA dual photon absorptiometry
DTPA diethylenetriamine pentaacetic acid
DXA dual-energy x-ray absorptiometry
ECT electroconvulsive treatment
EDTA ethylenediaminetetraacetic acid
EEG electroencephalogram
EF ejection fraction

EGOT erythrocyte glutamate-oxaloacetate transaminase
EGPT erythrocyte glutamate-pyruvate transaminase
EGR erythrocyte glutathione reductase
EKG electrocardiogram
EMG electromyogram
EMS eosinophilia-myalgia syndrome
EPA Environmental Protection Agency
EPA eicosapentaenoic acid
EPO evening primrose oil
ER estrogen receptor
ESR erythrocyte sedimentation rate
ESRD end-stage renal disease
ESRS Extrapyramidal Symptom Rating Scale
FAA Federal Aviation Administration
FAD flavin adenine dinucleotide
5-FU 5-fluorouracil
5-HTP 5-hydroxytryptophan
FDA Food and Drug Administration
FMN flavin mononucleotide
FSH follicle stimulating hormone
FSP familial spastic paraparesis
FVC forced vital capacity

G, H, I

GA glycyrrhetinic acid
GABA γ-aminobutyric acid
GAG glucosaminoglycan
GC-MS gas chromatography-mass spectrometry
GH growth hormone
GL glycyrrhizinic acid, glycyrrhizin
GnRH gonadotropin-releasing hormone
GRAS generally recognized as safe
G6PD glucose-6-phosphate dehydrogenase
HCC hepatocellular cancer
HCSE horse chestnut seed extract
HDL high-density lipoprotein
HGP hepatic glucose production
HPLC high-pressure liquid chromatography
HR heart rate
HRT hormone replacement therapy
HSV herpes simplex virus
IBS irritable bowel syndrome
IBW ideal body weight
ICC Indian childhood cirrhosis
IDDM insulin-dependent diabetes mellitus
IFN interferon
IIH iodine-induced hyperthyroidism
IL interleukin
INR international normalized ratio
IP ipriflavone
IPSS International Prostate Symptom Score
IUGR intrauterine growth retardation

J, K, L

KOH potassium hydroxide
LAK lymphokine activated killer
LDH lactate dehydrogenase
LDL low-density lipoprotein
LES lower esophageal sphincter
LFT liver function tests
LH luteinizing hormone
LMH lysine monohydrochloride
LOAEL lowest observable adverse event level
LT leukotriene
LV left ventricular

M, N, O

MAO monoamine oxidase
MAOI monoamine oxidase inhibitor
MBC minimum bactericidal concentration
MBC_{90} minimum bactericidal concentration for 90% of organisms
MCV mean corpuscular volume
MDMA methylenedioxymethamphetamine
MED minimal erythemal dose
MI myocardial infarction
MIC minimum inhibitory concentration
MIC_{90} minimum inhibitory concentration for 90% of organisms
MIDD maternally inherited diabetes mellitus and deafness
MIT monoiodothyronine
MOPP mechlorethamine, vincristine (Oncovin), procarbazine, and prednisone
MRI magnetic resonance imaging
MSUD maple syrup urine disease
NA nicotinic acid
NAC N-acetylcysteine
NAE N-acylethanolamine
NAG N-acetylglucosaminidase
NADH reduced form of nicotinamide adenine dinucleotide
NCI National Cancer Institute
NDGA nordihydroguaiaretic acid
NE niacin equivalent
NIDDM noninsulin-dependent diabetes mellitus
NMDA N-methyl-D-aspartate
NOAEL no observed adverse effect level
NSAID nonsteroidal antiinflammatory drug
OCD obsessive-compulsive disorder
ORAC oxygen radicals absorbance capacity
ORS oral rehydration solutions
OSHA Occupational Safety and Health Administration
OTC over-the-counter

P, Q, R

PA pyrrolizidine alkaloid
PAA poly-L-aspartic acid
PAS para-aminosalicylic acid
PALA N-phosonactyl-L-aspartic acid
PANSS Positive and Negative Syndrome Scales
PD panic disorder
PEL-TWA permissible exposure limit-time weighted average
PEP-CK phosphoenol pyruvate carboxykinase
PET positron emission tomography
PFT pulmonary function tests
PG prostaglandin
PIH pregnancy-induced hypertension
PKU phenylketonuria
PLE polymorphous light eruption
PLP pyridoxal 5′phosphate
PMN polymorphonuclear neutrophil
PMS premenstrual syndrome
p.o. *per os*, by mouth
POMS profile of mood states
PSA prostate-specific antigen
PT prothrombin time
PUFA polyunsaturated fatty acid
q.d. *quaque die*, evey day
q.i.d. *quater in die*, four times a day
RA rheumatoid arthritis
RDA recommended daily allowance
RDS respiratory distress syndrome

RIA radioimmunoassay
RLS restless legs syndrome
ROP retinopathy of prematurity
RR relative risk
RSD reflex sympathetic dystrophy
RSV respiratory syncytial virus

S, T, U
SAD seasonal affective disorder
SAMe S-adenosyl-L-methionine
SBP systolic blood pressure
SDS sodium dodecyl sulfate
SHBG sex hormone binding globulin
SIDS sudden infant death syndrome
SJW St. John's wort
SLE systemic lupus erythematosus
SLS sodium lauryl sulfate

SOD superoxide dismutase
SRI serotonin reuptake inhibitor
SSRI selective serotonin reuptake inhibitor
10-HDA trans-10-hydroxy-2-decenoic acid
T3 triiodothyronine
T4 thyroxine
TC total cholesterol
TCM traditional Chinese medicine
TD tardive dyskinesia
TDI tolerable daily intake
THC tetrahydrocannabinol
TIBC total iron-binding capacity
t.i.d. *ter in die*, three times a day
TNF tumor necrosis factor
TPN total parenteral nutrition
TRH thyrotropin-releasing hormone
TSH thyroid-stimulating hormone

TTFCA total triterpenic fraction of *Centella asiatica*
TTP thiamin pyrophosphate
TURP transurethral resection of prostate
UDA *Urtica dioica* agglutinin
UDCA ursodeoxycholic acid
UTI urinary tract infection
UV ultraviolet

V, W, X, Y, Z
VLDL very-low-density lipoprotein
VPC ventricular premature complex
WBC white blood cell
WHO World Health Organization
WKS Wernicke-Korsakoff syndrome
XGVHR xenogeneic graft-versus-host reaction

SECTION I
Herbs and Nutritional Supplements A to Z

Aconite

 10 Second Take

An extremely toxic herb, aconite can result in poisoning even from small amounts found in traditional Chinese or Indian herbal mixtures.

 Basics

LATIN NAME

Aconitum napellus, A. carmichaeli, A. coreanum, A. kusnezoffii

FAMILY

Rananculaceae

OTHER COMMON NAMES

Monkshood, wolfsbane, leopard killer

DESCRIPTION

• *Aconitum* species are used medicinally in traditional Chinese and Ayurvedic medicine.
• Common ingredient in herbal mixtures purchased in or imported from Hong Kong, China, Japan, and India. In Hong Kong, "chuanwu" (the main root of *A. carmichaeli*), and "caowu" (the root of *A. kusnezoffii*) are the most commonly used forms. "Fuzi" (the lateral root-tuber of *A. carmichaeli*) is more commonly used in mainland China (1).

PART USED

Tuber

KNOWN ACTIVE CONSTITUENTS

• Aconitine and other C_{19} diterpenoid alkaloids, including mesaconitine and hypaconitine.
• Other cardiotonic substances include coryneine chloride (dopamine methochloride), which has α-adrenergic qualities, and higenamine, a β-agonist.
• Dopamine, noradrenaline, and tyramine found in some *Aconitum* species (1).

MECHANISM/PHARMACOKINETICS

• *Aconitum* affects the voltage-sensitive sodium channels of excitable membranes and is toxic to both neurons and cardiac cells. Persistent activation of sodium channels results in increased sodium uptake, prolonged depolarization, and delayed repolarization. In cardiac cells, aconite has both negative inotropic effects (apparently vagal as they can be blocked with atropine) and positive inotropic effects (caused by prolongation of sodium influx during the action potential). Sodium-calcium exchange results in increased intracellular calcium levels: increased automaticity combined with increased vagal activity and slowed atrioventricular (A-V) conduction leads to arrhythmias (1). In nerve cells, prolonged depolarization preventing repolarization results in conduction block and muscle paralysis.
• Aconite alkaloids were quantified in the body fluids of a 40-year-old woman who committed suicide by ingesting aconite (2). Levels of the alkaloid jesaconitine were 69.1 ng/mL in blood and 237.8 ng/mL in urine. The highest levels of jesaconitine were seen in the kidneys, liver, and bile; significant amounts were also seen in the gastrointestinal tract, especially in the ileal contents. The authors suggested that aconite alkaloids are eliminated by the liver and kidneys and also in feces.

 Evidence

CLINICAL TRIALS

• No clinical trials identified.

ANIMAL/IN VITRO

• Intraperitoneal administration of aconite extract (3 mg/kg q.d. × 7 days) or aconitine (3 μg/kg q.d. × 7 days) increased plasma corticosterone levels significantly in mice (3). Aconitine has analgesic effects in mice and antiinflammatory effects in rats (4). Aconite alkaloids can be grouped into compounds that activate or block Na^+ channels, but the high-affinity alkaloids with antinociceptive properties were also the most toxic compounds (5). The authors of this report concluded that aconite compounds are unsuitable as analgesics because the lethal dose is too close to the effective dose.
• Aconitine applied to cat atria causes fibrillation that can be suppressed by amiodarone or atropine (6).

OTHER CLAIMED BENEFITS/ACTIONS

• Antiinflammatory
• Analgesic
• Cardiotonic
• Musculoskeletal problems

Aconite

Risks

WARNING

• Ingestion of any amount of aconite may result in potentially fatal cardiac arrhythmias.
• Severe poisoning has been observed following ingestion of preparations containing as little as 6 g of cured rootstocks (7).

ADVERSE REACTIONS

• Aconite poisoning

—Mild poisoning cases may result in nausea, vomiting, and paresthesias (8). Initial symptoms usually appear within 90 minutes of ingestion (1). Most patients present with neurologic symptoms, most commonly oral numbness or burning progressing to peripheral paraesthesias and generalized muscle weakness. Nausea and vomiting are also common; other symptoms may include chest pain, abdominal pain, diarrhea, hyperventilation, respiratory distress, dizziness, sweating, confusion, headache, and excessive lacrimation (1).
—Cardiovascular effects include bradycardia, hypotension, and a range of arrhythmias similar to that caused by cardiac glycoside toxicity (ventricular or supraventricular tachycardia, sinus bradycardia with first degree heart block, bundle branch block with junctional escape rhythm, or *torsades de pointes*) (1). Bidirectional tachycardia has been reported (9). In one series of 17 cases of aconite poisoning, 11 patients required high-dose inotropic support, 8 required mechanical ventilation, and 7 required cardiopulmonary resuscitation (7).
—Several deaths have been associated with herbal medicines containing aconite (7,10); the herb has also been successfully used for suicide (2) and homicide (11). Autopsy of a homicide victim poisoned by aconite revealed hemorrhagic pulmonary edema and diffuse contraction-band necrosis in the myocardium, findings similar to that seen in epinephrine administration or release of endogenous catecholamines (11).

• Treatment of aconite poisoning

—Patients with suspected aconite poisoning should be hospitalized and placed on cardiac monitors for at least 24 hours, the period within which ventricular arrhythmias are most likely to occur (1). Although patients with aconite poisoning are sometimes given activated charcoal, it is not known whether this treatment is effective in preventing absorption of aconitine (8). There is no specific antidote for aconite, and treatment is mainly supportive. Atropine may be given if symptoms of cholinergic excess are apparent (1).
—Antiarrhythmics are often helpful, but cardioversion appears to be markedly unsuccessful in converting arrhythmias. In a case series of 17 cases of aconite poisoning, repeated direct-current cardioversion was unsuccessful in 10 patients (apparently all patients for whom cardioversion was attempted) (7). No single antiarrhythmic was uniformly effective. Suppression of ventricular tachycardia was eventually achieved in 5 patients receiving amiodarone, 2 patients on flecainide, and 1 each on procainamide or mexiletine. Arrhythmias resolved spontaneously in 6 patients, and 2 patients died from refractory ventricular tachycardia. The 15 other patients were stabilized within 24 hours and discharged; no sequelae were observed at a median of 15 months follow-up (7).
—In a case report of bidirectional tachycardia, the arrhythmia was finally suppressed by 0.7 mg/kg of flecainide by slow intravenous infusion; junctional rhythm persisted for 4 hours before normal sinus rhythm was restored (9). Before administration of flecainide, other failed measures included vagotonic maneuvers or intravenous adenosine triphosphate with edrophonium hydrochloride (each suppressed the arrhythmia transiently). Neither intravenous lignocaine (lidocaine) nor synchronized direct current cardioversion (200 J) had any effect.
—More recently, individual case reports of successful reversal of aconite-induced arrhythmias include amiodarone suppression of polymorphic ventricular tachycardia (12) and a case of magnesium treatment of long QT syndrome with *torsades de pointes* (13).

DRUG INTERACTIONS

• None reported. The incidence and severity of adverse events would be expected to increase if aconite were combined with digoxin or other cardiac glycosides.

Dose

COMMON DOSAGE FORMS

• *Decoction* or *infusion* as part of a mixture of herbs.
• Recommended doses have traditionally been 8 to 12 g, but reports of toxicity have resulted in many practitioners recommending lower doses of 1.5 to 3.0 g (7).

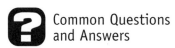

Common Questions and Answers

Q: Doesn't the processing done in preparing aconite for use in traditional Asian medicines reduce its toxicity?
A: Yes. Raw aconite tubers are always processed by soaking or boiling the tubers (with or without lime or other chemicals) before slicing and drying them (1). This processing, by hydrolyzing alkaloids into less toxic benzylaconine derivatives, may reduce the alkaloid content to 10% of its original level (1). However, alkaloid types and amounts may vary with the species, where the herb was grown, time of harvest, and method of processing. In addition, dosage and preparation instructions may not be followed correctly. Poisonings are much more common when aconite is self-prescribed than when it is prescribed by a traditional Chinese medicine practitioner.
Aconite is an important and versatile herb in traditional Chinese medicine. Given that the conditions for which aconite is used are either minor conditions (musculoskeletal problems) or conditions (pain, heart failure) for which there are other effective medications, the question remains whether there is reason to use this quite toxic herb at all.

Q: What is the incidence of aconite poisoning?
A: The incidence is unknown. The diagnosis of aconite poisoning may be missed in mild cases or in areas where this sort of poisoning is rare. In one hospital in Hong Kong, at least 18 cases of known aconite poisoning were observed in a 4-year period (1).

Q: What is the origin of the names monkshood and wolfsbane?
A: The hooded flower resembles a monk's cowl, hence the name monkshood. Aconite was a widely used arrow poison in Asia and medieval Europe and was used for both hunting and warfare (14). In ancient Rome, it was so widely used by professional poisoners that simply cultivating the plant was considered a capital offense. On the Greek island of Chios it was used for euthanasia of the old and infirm. The term wolfsbane comes from its use to poison meat laid out for wolves.

3

Alanine

 ## 10 Second Take

Alanine is a safe amino acid that may help prevent nocturnal hypoglycemia in diabetics and possibly treat diarrhea.

 ## Basics

DESCRIPTION

An abundant nonessential amino acid

FOOD SOURCES

Protein-containing foods

MAIN FUNCTIONS/PHARMACOKINETICS

• A glucagon-releasing amino acid; it also functions as a carrier of nitrogen from peripheral tissues to the liver for excretion. It can be transaminated to form aspartate. Alanine plays an important role in hepatic gluconeogenesis and ureagenesis (1). The splanchnic bed extracts and metabolizes most alanine from muscle (2).
• Free alanine concentration in venous plasma is 213 to 472 μmol/L, in arterial plasma it is 249 μmol/L (1). Urinary output is 240 μmol/24 hours.

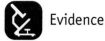 ## Evidence

CLINICAL TRIALS

• Diabetes

—In patients with insulin-dependent diabetes mellitus (IDDM), alanine raises glucagon and plasma glucose but not C-peptide or insulin. In normal subjects, alanine increases plasma glucagon, C-peptide, and insulin but not plasma glucose (3). Both alanine (40 g) and terbutaline (5 mg p.o. or 0.25 mg s.c.) produced sustained glucose recovery after hypoglycemia was induced in patients with IDDM (4).

• Prevention of nocturnal hypoglycemia

—Alanine is more effective than a snack but less effective than terbutaline in preventing nocturnal hypoglycemia. A crossover study of 15 patients with IDDM tested the effects of an individualized dose of NPH insulin given alone or (on three separate occasions) in combination with a 200 kcal snack, alanine (40 g plus 10 g glucose, providing about 200 kcal), or terbutaline (5 mg) (5). Compared with insulin alone, all treatments significantly increased mean plasma glucose levels during the first half of the night. During the second half of the night, mean plasma glucose levels were equivalent among the control group, those receiving a snack, and those receiving alanine; the terbutaline-treated group had significantly higher glucose levels than the other groups. Low nocturnal glucose levels ≤40 mg/dL (2.2 mmol/L) occurred less often in groups treated with terbutaline or alanine. Low glucose levels occurred on only one occasion each in the terbutaline and alanine groups but occurred on 13 occasions (seven patients) in the control arm and 10 occasions (six patients) in the snack arm of the trial.

• Diarrhea

—Studies are mixed on whether alanine-enriched oral rehydration solutions (ORS) are any better than solutions without alanine. One study of 97 males, aged 6 to 59 years, admitted with dehydration associated with *Vibrio cholerae* or enterotoxigenic *Escherichia coli* found that ORS containing L-alanine are better than standard oral rehydration formulas in treating diarrhea (6).
—A randomized controlled clinical trial in 55 children compared hypoosmolar ORS with L-alanine and glucose (osmolality 255 mosmol/L) with standard ORS (osmolality 311 mosmol/L) and intravenous polyelectro-lyte solutions (osmolality 293 mosmol/l) and found that the alanine-containing oral formula was equivalent to the intravenous solution; both were superior to standard ORS (7).
—However, another randomized double-blind trial in 129 male children aged 3 to 48 months with acute noncholera diarrhea found no significant difference between ORS with or without alanine (8).
—A randomized, apparently single-blind study of 20 male infants with acute diarrhea and dehydration found no advantage of alanine-enriched (30 mmol/L) ORS solution over standard ORS in vomiting, fluids needed to correct dehydration, or serum electrolytes (9).

ANIMAL/IN VITRO

• Hepatoprotective effect

—High-dose alanine increased survival and liver function in rats with acute liver failure caused by D-galactosamine (10).
—Intracerebroventricular injection of D-alanine (200 to 600 mcg) but not L-alanine (600 mcg) in rats antagonized the effects of methamphetamine on stimulating locomotion (11).

 Risks

No risks identified.

Alfalfa

 10 Second Take

Alfalfa may lower cholesterol levels but raw seeds and sprouts contain a toxin, canavanine. Canavanine has been associated with systemic lupus erythematosus (SLE) and pancytopenia.

 Basics

LATIN NAME

Medicago sativa

FAMILY

Leguminosae (Fabaceae)

OTHER COMMON NAMES

Chilean clover, lucerne, buffalo grass

DESCRIPTION

- A deep-rooted, perennial fodder plant; its sprouts are used as food.
- Whole herb or leaves are most used medicinally.

PART USED

Seed, sprouts, stem, leaves

KNOWN ACTIVE CONSTITUENTS

- Canavanine, a nonprotein amino acid, is found mainly in the raw seed and sprouts. Phenolic compounds include coumestrol; alfalfa seeds are reported to contain stachydrine and L-homostachydrine (1).
- Alfalfa also contains saponins (glycosides of soya sapogenols) and esterified bidesmosides and tridesmosides of acidic oleanenes (medicagenic acid, 16α-hydroxymedicagenic acid, and hederagenin) (2).

MECHANISM/PHARMACOKINETICS

- Alfalfa appears to inhibit the gastrointestinal absorption of cholesterol.
- Pharmacokinetics have not been delineated.
- Canavanine, a toxin, is structurally similar to arginine; by competing for receptors, it may inactivate arginine-containing enzymes (3). Canaline, a metabolite of the ornithine analog canavaline, may inhibit pyridoxal phosphate and associated enzymes. It is possible that the substitution of L-canavanine for arginine in proteins results in targeting of abnormal proteins by the immune system, resulting in autoantibody production (4). L-canavanine abrogates concanavalin A-induced suppressor cell function in vivo in a dose-dependent manner; in immunoregulatory cells from normal subjects and those with SLE, L-canavanine increased release of IgG and DNA-binding activity (5); it also decreased mitogenic response to phytohemagglutinin and concanavalin A (but not pokeweed mitogen).

 Evidence

CLINICAL TRIALS

- Hypercholesterolemia

—Fifteen patients with type II hyperlipoproteinemia were given 40 g of heat-treated alfalfa seeds t.i.d. with meals for 8 weeks. Total cholesterol fell 17%, from 9.58 to 8.0 mmol/L ($p < 0.001$) and low density lipoprotein (LDL) cholesterol fell 18% from 7.69 to 6.33 mmol/L ($p < 0.01$). Apolipoprotein B decreased 34%, from 2.17 to 1.43 g/L ($p < 0.05$); there was no change in apolipoprotein A-1 (6).

ANIMAL/IN VITRO

- Hypercholesterolemia

—Alfalfa hay in the diet or partially hydrolyzed saponins from alfalfa hay prevented hypercholesterolemia and atherosclerosis in cholesterol-fed monkeys; alfalfa seeds decreased hypercholesterolemia and atherosclerosis in cholesterol-fed rabbits (1,7).

- Antifungal effect

—Alfalfa root saponins have specific antifungal effects and are active against various forms of Candida, Torulopsis, (8) and Cryptococcus neoformans (9) in vitro. A liposomal dosage form of compound G2 (the gluco derivative of medicagenic acid) conferred a survival advantage in mice infected with Cryptococcus neoformans (9). A topical preparation of the gluco derivative of medicagenic acid was effective in curing skin lesions of guinea pigs infected with Trichophyton mentagrophytes (9).

OTHER CLAIMED BENEFITS/ACTIONS

- Diabetes
- Arthritis
- Cancer
- Boils
- Urinary problems
- Bowel problems
- Ulcers
- Vitamin deficiency
- Debility
- Menses induction
- Heart disease
- Halitosis
- Hypothrombinemic purpura

Risks

ADVERSE REACTIONS

• Pancytopenia

—Pancytopenia has been observed in a 59-year-old man who was ingesting large amounts of alfalfa saponins (up to 160 g daily) as part of a cholesterol-lowering study (10).

• SLE

—Two women with quiescent SLE experienced reactivation after long-term consumption of alfalfa tablets (11). In the first case, a 40-year-old woman with a 26-year history of SLE developed symptoms 9 months after consuming 15 alfalfa tablets daily (her disease had been clinically inactive for at least 4 years). In the second case, a 50-year-old woman with a 25-year history of mild SLE associated with membranous glomerulonephritis (she had been in remission for an unspecified period) developed rising antinuclear antibody (ANA) and cryoglobulins and progressive hypocomplementemia; renal biopsy showed diffuse proliferative glomerulonephritis. She had been ingesting eight tablets daily for 2 1/2 years. Although these cases are scantily documented, they are plausible, given other clinical reports and animal studies (12).
—Four patients developed a reversible SLE-like syndrome (symptoms included arthralgias, myalgias, and rash) with positive ANA (solid pattern) after consuming 12 to 24 alfalfa tablets daily for 3 weeks to 7 months.

• Uric acid effects

—Serum urate levels increased from 296 to 336 μmol/L in patients receiving 120 g heat-treated alfalfa seeds per day in a cholesterol-lowering trial (6). Alfalfa may contain purines that can precipitate a gout attack in susceptible individuals.

• Dermatologic reactions

—Six cases of pruritic, patchy, erythematous eruptions have been reported associated with the use of alfalfa seeds in capsules or teas (1).

• Other symptoms

—Ingestion of more than 120 g seeds/day can cause gastrointestinal symptoms (flatulence, diarrhea, abdominal discomfort, and anorexia) (1).

ANIMAL TOXICITY

• L-canavanine sulfate reactivated SLE-like symptoms in cynomolgus monkeys previously exposed to alfalfa seeds (4).
• L-canavanine is toxic in rats, mice, and lower organisms. Long-term consumption of partially hydrolyzed dietary alfalfa hay saponins (1% to 1.2% of diet) was not toxic to monkeys (1).
• Estrogenic effects have been reported in cattle consuming large amounts of alfalfa as fodder (1).

 Dose

COMMON DOSAGE FORMS

• *Dried herb:* 5 to 10 g t.i.d. in capsules or as infusion.
• *Liquid extract:* [1:1 in 25% ethanol (EtOH)] 5 to 10 mL t.i.d.

 Common Questions and Answers

Q: Is the consumption of alfalfa sprouts safe?
A: Limited consumption of alfalfa sprouts in salads and sandwiches is probably nothing to worry about, but daily ingestion should be avoided. Patients with autoimmune diseases should avoid alfalfa sprouts altogether.

Q: Can alfalfa toxins be rendered safe?
A: Yes, by cooking; avoiding raw seed and sprouts is key. Heat appears to denature toxic components of alfalfa while preserving antihypercholesterolemic effects (13). Although there is certainly a case to be made for further study of alfalfa's lipid-lowering effects, other components of alfalfa may also be problematic (the mechanism behind the single case of pancytopenia is unclear).

Aloe

 10 Second Take

Aloe leaf contains a strong anthraquinone laxative. The inner leaf gel, used externally for minor wounds or burns, is harmless and may promote healing; however, it should not be applied to deep wounds or third-degree burns.

 Basics

LATIN NAME

Aloe vera (L.) Burm.f. = *Aloe barbadensis* Miller

FAMILY

Aloeaceae

OTHER COMMON NAMES

Aloes, Barbadoes aloe, Curacao aloe (*Aloe vera*), Cape aloe (*Aloe ferox* Miller and hybrids)

DESCRIPTION

• Desert-dwelling succulents; aloe vera gel refers to the mucilaginous gel within the leaves; aloes refers to the dried leaf juice.

PART USED

• The mucilaginous gel inside the leaves and extracts of the secretory glands from the leaves are used for distinctly different purposes.

KNOWN ACTIVE CONSTITUENTS

• Leaf gel

—Polysaccharides, (pectins, hemicelluloses, glucomannan, acemannan, and mannose derivatives), amino acids, sterols (lupeol, campesterol, and β-sitosterol), tannins, and enzymes (1). In *A. ferox* arabinogalactans and rhamnogalacturonans are more prominent than glucomannans (2). Minerals (including aluminium, boron, barium, calcium, iron, magnesium, sodium, phosphorous, silicon, and strontium) have also been reported in the gel (2).

• Leaf extract

—*A. barbadensis* contains the *C*-glucoside anthrones aloin A (barbaloin, 15% to 40%) and aloin B and two 5-methyl chromone *C*-glucosides, aloeresin A and aloesin (formerly aloeresin B). Free anthraquinone, aloe-emodin–anthrone and several new *C*-glycosyl-chromones were recently isolated (3). Cape aloes (*A. ferox* Miller and other species) contains the anthrone-*C*-glycosides aloin A, aloin B, and 5-hydroxyaloin A; the anthrone *C*- and *O*-glycosides aloinoside A and aloinoside B, aloeresins, aloe-emodin, cinnamic acid, and 1-methyl-tetralin derivatives (4).

MECHANISM/PHARMACOKINETICS

• Anthraquinone glycosides in aloe leaves are strong purgatives that pass to the colon unmodified. Intestinal flora break down *O*-glycosides and (to a lesser extent) *C*-glycosides, to active metabolites, especially aloe-emodin-9-anthrone. These metabolites act as a stimulant laxative, accelerating colonic transport through inhibition of the Na^+/K^+ pump and stimulation of mucus and chloride secretion (4).
• Aloe contains a carboxypeptidase that inhibits bradykinin (5). Aloe vera gel or extract inhibits arachidonic acid. Salicylic acid is present in aloe (also, emodin, aloin, and aloe-emodin can be broken down into salicylates); these are known to reduce prostaglandin production. Magnesium lactate in aloe can inhibit the conversion of histidine to histamine in mast cells (6).
• In a pharmacokinetic study, the equivalent of 16.4 mg hydroxyanthracene derivatives p.o. × 7 days found aloe-emodin in plasma only sporadically (maximum concentrations of less than 2 ng/mL). The metabolite rhein was present in concentrations of 6 to 28 ng/mL after a single dose; no accumulation was seen (4).

 Evidence

CLINICAL TRIALS

Leaf gel (internal)

• Diabetes

—A controlled trial in Thailand of 72 adult diabetics not receiving hypoglycemics found that ingesting a tablespoonful of aloe vera gel twice daily for 42 days resulted in significant reductions in blood sugar and triglycerides (7). Mean blood glucose decreased from 250 to 142 mg/dL and triglycerides from 220 to 123 mg/dL; there was no change in total cholesterol. Another trial, by the same investigators, of aloe vera gel in diabetics treated with glibenclamide, found similar results (8).

Leaf gel (topical)

• Wound healing

—Eighteen patients with facial acne scars were treated with dermabrasion, after which one side of each patient's face was treated with polyethylene oxide dressings soaked in stabilized aloe vera gel; the other side was treated with polyethylene oxide dressings (9). Dressings were changed twice daily for 4 or 5 days. Intense vasoconstriction and reduced edema was noted on the aloe-treated sites at 24 to 48 hours, and the aloe-treated sites healed more rapidly in every case. By the fifth or sixth day, new epidermis often covered twice as much of the aloe-treated sites as the control sites. Patients reported slight initial burning with the aloe gel, an effect that could be reduced by chilling the gel.
—A trial of aloe vera gel in 21 women with surgical wound complications requiring healing by second intention found that aloe significantly increased healing time compared with women who were not treated with the gel (10) (see question and answer section).

• Burns

—A non-blinded study in 27 patients admitted to a burn unit tested the effect of 85% aloe vera gel against Vaseline gauze dressing on each half of a partial-thickness burn (11). Dressings were changed twice daily; wounds were inspected and photographed weekly until complete reepithelialization. The aloe-treated burns healed in 11.89 days [standard deviation (SD) 4.39] and the Vaseline gauze-treated area healed in 18.18 days (SD 8.87), a significant difference ($p < 0.002$). Histologically, more rapid growth of squamous epithelium, development of dermal tissue, and less inflammatory cell infiltration were seen in the aloe-treated side. Minimal transient pain was noted on gel application.

• Radiation burn prophylaxis

—A double-blind trial of aloe vera gel as a prophylactic for radiation-induced dermatitis found no difference between aloe and placebo gel or between aloe and no treatment (12).

- Aphthous ulcers

—A component of aloe gel, acemannan, has been shown to be effective in treating aphthous stomatitis (13). A double-blind randomized trial of 60 patients with a history of recurrent aphthous ulcers assigned patients to acemannan hydrogel or an over-the counter product as an active control. Lesions treated with acemannan hydrogel healed in 5.89 days, whereas those treated with the active control healed in 7.8 days. Freeze-dried acemannan hydrogel appeared to be equivalent to acemannan hydrogel in an open-label arm of this trial.

Leaf extract

- Psoriasis

—A double-blind, placebo-controlled trial of 60 patients with slight to moderate chronic psoriasis found that topically applied 0.5% aloe vera extract cured 83.3% of patients versus 6.6% of those on placebo cream (14). Treatment was for a maximum of 4 weeks, but patients were followed for a year.

ANIMAL/IN VITRO

- Dermatologic effects

—In animal models, aloe vera gel has shown beneficial effects in wound healing and inflammation. Increased fibroblast proliferation and new capillary growth has been noted in *in vitro* wound healing models (2). Beneficial effects have also been demonstrated in frostbite (15).

- Cancer

—Several fractions of aloe, or whole freeze-dried leaves, have shown antitumor properties in animals (2). Aloe-emodin appears to have specific activity against neuroectodermal tumor activity *in vitro* and *in vivo*. A study in immunocompromised mice revealed inhibition of human neuroectodermal tumor growth; no toxic effects on animals were noted and proliferation of normal fibroblasts or hemopoietic progenitor cells was not affected (16).

- Other effects

—Aloe-emodin mitigated the hepatotoxic effect of carbon tetrachloride in rats (17).
—Injected anthraquinones from aloe reduced adjuvant-induced arthritis in rats (18).
—Polysaccharide fractions from aqueous whole leaf extracts decreased blood glucose in alloxan-treated mice (2).
—Studies of antibacterial effects of aloe have been mixed (2). Acemannan, an acetylated polymannan isolated from aloe gel, has shown antiviral effects against several viruses including HIV (2).
—Aloe gel fed to rats lowered calcitonin and parathyroid hormone (2).

OTHER CLAIMED BENEFITS/ACTIONS

- *Gel:* Burns, eczema, acne, dry skin
- *Leaf extract:* Abortifacient; induction of menses, "inner cleansing"

 Risks

ADVERSE REACTIONS

Leaf Extract

- As with all stimulant purgatives, in large doses aloe can cause gastrointestinal irritation, abdominal pain, bloody diarrhea, dehydration, and electrolyte imbalance.
- Aloe may color urine brown or red, a harmless pH-dependent phenomenon.
- Chronic use of aloe can result in a harmless and reversible pigmentation of the colon called pseudomelanosis coli.

Gel

- Hypersensitivity has been reported (18).

DRUG INTERACTIONS

- Anthraquinone laxatives can decrease absorption of intestinally absorbed drugs.
- Urine discoloration my cause false-positive results for urinary urobilinogen or urinary estrogens by Kaber procedure (1).
- Laxatives

—Aloe leaf extract should not be used with other laxatives, especially cascara or senna, which also contain anthraquinones.

- Diuretics

—Concurrent use of non-potassium-sparing diuretics with aloe leaf extract could precipitate hypokalemia.

PREGNANCY AND LACTATION

- Aloe leaf extract may cause uterine contractions and/or abortion. Anthraquinones may be secreted into breast milk.
- Aloe leaf extract should not be used in the presence of nausea, vomiting, diarrhea, dehydration, ileus, inflammatory bowel disease, intestinal obstruction, abdominal pain, or kidney disease.

ANIMAL TOXICITY

- Mice fed 50 mg/kg/day dry aloe extract showed no severe pathology; colonic mucosa was slightly inflamed and sorbitol-dehydrogenase levels were increased (indicating possible liver dysfunction) (19).

 Dose

COMMON DOSAGE FORMS

- *Aloe vera gel:* gel, cream, lotion, component of cosmetics, shampoos, and so forth. The most common use is topical, although it is sometimes orally ingested.
- *Aloe leaf extract* (aloes): dried juice or liquid extract.
- Adults and children older than 10 years: For constipation, the appropriate dose is the smallest effective amount. The usual dose is the equivalent of 10 to 30 mg of hydroxyanthracene derivatives (calculated as barbaloin) p.o. q.h.s. (4), 0.04–0.11 g *A. vera* or 0.06 to 0.17 g *A. ferox* (1). The effect may take 6 to 24 hours. Not recommended for children younger than 10 years. Not recommended for use for more than 2 weeks.
- Whole leaf extract may contain both gel and leaf extract.

 Common Questions and Answers

Q: Does aloe help or hurt wound healing?
A: Aloe vera gel should not be used in deep wounds requiring healing by secondary intention (see clinical trials). For cuts, scratches, and abrasions, aloe is helpful. Its effects are primarily in promoting re-epithelialization: an advantage in a superficial wound but exactly what you do not want in a deep wound.

Q: Is aloe vera gel helpful in burns?
A: For minor burns, yes. It should not be used in third-degree burns. One animal study found that it promoted healing in first- and second-degree burns but appeared to increase infection rates in third-degree burns (8).

Q: Does aloe vera gel taken internally have a laxative effect?
A: It should not, if it is really just the gel. The anthraquinone glycosides responsible for the purgative effect are only in leaf exudate, not the gel. However, I have had patients report significant diarrhea after consuming gel: a sign that the gel was contaminated with the leaf.

Angelica

 10 Second Take

Angelica is a benign herb used for flavoring and medicinally; however, it may cause photosensitivity and should not be used in patients on anticoagulants.

 Basics

LATIN NAME

Angelica sinensis (Oliv.) Diels, *A. archangelica, A. atropurpurea, A. dahurica*

FAMILY

Apiaceae/Umbelliferae

OTHER COMMON NAMES

- Dong quai, *danggui, tang-kwei, tang-kuei,* or Chinese angelica (*A. sinensis*); European angelica (*A. archangelica*)

DESCRIPTION

- Angelica species are biennial or perennial plants that may grow to 7 feet in height, with umbels of greenish-white flowers.
- It grows wild on mountainsides, in damp meadows, or near water and is also cultivated both for flavoring and for medicinal use.

PART USED

- Dried root and rhizomes (*A. sinensis,* others); leaf (*A. atropurpurea,* others)

KNOWN ACTIVE CONSTITUENTS

- Coumarins are thought to be the active constituents. These include furocoumarins, bergapten, imperatorin, psoralens, angelicone, angelol, osthol, and oxypeucedanin.
- *A. sinensis* also contains the lactones angelicide, butylidenephthalide, butylphthalide and ligustilide; safrole and isosafrole; ferulic acid; and β-sitosterol (1).
- *A. angelica* contains more than 20 furanocoumarins including angelicin, archangelicin (kwannin), osthol, bergapten, isoimperatorin, umbelliferone, and xanthotoxin. The essential oil contains 80% to 90% monoterpene hydrocarbons, predominately β-phellandrene (13% to 28%) and α-pinene (14% to 31%). Also present are sesquiterpenes, phenolic carboxylic acids, archangelenone, sitosterol, fatty acids, tannins, and saccharoses (2).

 Evidence

CLINICAL TRIALS

- Menopausal symptoms

—A randomized, double-blind, placebo-controlled clinical trial of 71 postmenopausal women with hot flashes found that 24 weeks of treatment with dong quai (*A. sinensis*) was no more effective than placebo in alleviating hot flashes or improving the Kupperman index (which assesses the incidence and severity of 11 menopausal symptoms). The number of hot flashes decreased from an average of 47 to 35 per week in the dong quai group and from 33 to 27.5 in the placebo group; there was no significant difference between groups. Both groups experienced an approximately 25% reduction in symptoms according to the Kupperman index (3). There were no significant differences between the two groups in endometrial thickness (measured by ultrasound), vaginal maturation index, or any clinical measure.

CASE REPORT

- Increased hematocrit

—A 56-year-old male patient with end-stage renal disease, iron-deficiency anemia, and mild secondary hyperparathyroidism was receiving dialysis three times weekly and had been receiving approximately 620 units/kg/week recombinant human erythropoietin (rHuEPO) for 5 months, with only moderate effects (4). One month after initiating weekly use of an herbal tea containing roots of *A. sinensis* (about 12 g) and about 52 g of *"Radix paeoniae alba"* (probably white peony, *Radix Paeoniae Lactiflorae* or *Paeonia lactiflora* Pall) his hematocrit rose from 29.7% to 34.4% (no change in iron or rHuEPO were made during this time nor were any blood transfusions given). During the previous 5 months his hematocrit had been stable in the mid to low 20s. During the 5 months of herbal therapy the mean hematocrit increased from 26.5% to 32.6% and the dose of rHuEPO was reduced by more than 90% (from 620 to 54 units/kg/wk). The patient also reported an increase in appetite and food intake within 2 weeks of starting the herbs. Approximately 1 month after that, the patient experienced two episodes of hypotension during dialysis, after which nifedipine was discontinued. During the 5 months of the herbal therapy the serum albumin rose from 3.6 to 4.4 g/dL.

ANIMAL/IN VITRO

- Angelica appeared to have antioxidant effects, protecting human umbilical vein endothelial cells against oxidized low density lipoprotein (LDL)-induced damage and inhibited intercellular adhesion molecule-1 expression of endothelial cells (5).
- A 70% methanol extract of Japanese angelica root, administered intraduodenally in a dose of 3 g/kg, induced uterine contractions in rabbits (6). However, studies in rats showed neither an anti-implantation nor an abortifacient effect of *A. sinensis* root extracts (1).
- Aqueous root extract of *A. sinensis* administered orally or intraperitoneally to mice suppressed serum titers of IgE but had no effect on IgG (1).
- Several coumarins isolated from *A. edulis* inhibit human platelet aggregation and exhibit antitumor-promoting activity, as measured by TPA-stimulated ^{32}Pi incorporation into phospholipids of cultured cells (7).
- Volatile constituents of *A. sinensis* are associated with transient blood pressure elevation; a nonvolatile water-soluble fraction of root extract, the essential oil, has hypotensive and vasodilatory effects (1).

OTHER CLAIMED BENEFITS/ACTIONS

- *A. sinensis* (root): Dysmenorrhea, irregular menses, amenorrhea, premenstrual syndrome, and metrorrhagia.
- *A. archangelica* (root): Respiratory problems, dyspepsia, flatulence, bloating, diuretic, appetite stimulant, antiinflammatory, induction of menses, insomnia, neuralgia (topical), arthritis (topical).
- *A. atropurpurea* (leaf): Antiinflammatory, dyspepsia, flatulence, pleuritic pain.

Risks

ADVERSE REACTIONS

• Phytodermatitis has been reported in three members of the same family who worked in an angelica garden (8) (photosensitivity can occur with any plant containing furocoumarins).

DRUG INTERACTIONS

• Warfarin

—Two cases of increased international normalized ratio (INR) have been reported in patients on warfarin (9,10). *A. sinensis* may affect the pharmacodynamics but not the pharmacokinetics of warfarin. Six rabbits were treated with a single dose of subcutaneous warfarin (2 mg/kg); half the rabbits also received 3 days of treatment with *A. sinensis* (2 g/kg, administered orally) (11). No significant variations in single-dose pharmacokinetics of warfarin were seen. However, *A. sinensis* significantly lowered prothrombin time (PT) 3 days after concurrent treatment with warfarin. There was no effect of *A. sinensis* alone on PT.
—A separate group of six rabbits received daily doses of warfarin (0.6 mg/kg) until steady state levels were reached; 3 days of treatment with *A. sinensis* did not affect PT or steady state concentrations significantly (this study is difficult to interpret because two rabbits died on the seventh day).

• Tolbutamide

—No clinical cases of interactions have been reported. In rats, an extract of *A. dahurica*, intravenously administered (10 mg/kg), delayed elimination of tolbutamide (12).

• Diazepam

—No clinical cases of interactions have been reported. In rats, an extract of *A. dahurica*, intravenously administered (10 mg/kg), did not affect pharmacokinetic parameters of intravenous diazepam (10 mg/kg); however, after oral administration of diazepam (5 mg/kg) with *A. dahurica* extract (1 g/kg p.o.), C_{max} of diazepam was four times the levels reached with diazepam alone (12). This indicates a possible effect on first-pass metabolism. Cytochrome P450 isoenzymes (especially CYP2C11) were inhibited in an *in vitro* rat liver microsomal assay.

PREGNANCY/LACTATION

Aqueous extracts of angelica root are reputed to be abortifacient; however, studies in rats showed neither an anti-implantation nor an abortifacient effect (1).

ANIMAL TOXICITY

• The essential oil of *A. archangelica* root and seed is considered nontoxic in rodents in doses up to 5 g/kg.
• The essential oil of the root and seed is classified as a mild skin irritant.
• Topical application of the oil of root (but not the oil of seed) causes photosensitivity (13).

 Dose

COMMON DOSAGE FORMS

• *Dried root:* slices up to 3 to 10 g per day, or 0.5 to 2 g as infusion or decoction up to t.i.d.

• *Liquid extract:* (1:1, 25% ethanol) 0.5 to 2 mL t.i.d.

Tincture, oils, or *spirits* may be used externally for neuralgic and rheumatic complaints.

 Common Questions and Answers

Q: What is angelica used to flavor?
A: It can be used to flavor candies or cakes but is most popular for this use in Europe. Perhaps the most familiar form in which North Americans consume angelica is in liqueurs such as Benedictine or Chartreuse.

Anise, Aniseed

 10 Second Take

Anise is a very safe herb used as a flavoring and medicinally in children and adults for coughs and gastrointestinal complaints; clinical trial data are lacking.

 Basics

LATIN NAME

Pimpinella anisum

FAMILY

Umbelliferae/Apiaceae

DESCRIPTION

• Anise is a fragrant plant with white flowers that is native to western Asia and the Mediterranean.
• It is cultivated in southern Europe, the Mediterranean, the Middle East, India, Mexico, Chile, Egypt, and the former USSR.

PART USED

Seed (fruit)

KNOWN ACTIVE CONSTITUENTS

• The essential oil contains 80% to 95% *E*-anethole, *Z*-anethole, estragole, anisaldehyde, and pseudoisoeugenyl-2-methylbutyrate; sesquiterpene hydrocarbons; monoterpene hydrocarbons; flavonol glycosides; phenolic acids; a phenolic glycoside; and coumarins.

MECHANISM/PHARMACOKINETICS

• No data is available on anise seed. An elimination study of *E*-anethole found that 70% to 85% is absorbed after oral administration. It is excreted via the kidney and lung.
• Orally administered radioactively labeled *E*-anethole was metabolized by an oxidative pathway to 4-methoxyhippuric acid. It was 54% to 69% renally excreted, and at least 13% to 17% was exhaled. Excretion was almost complete in 8 hours (1).

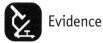 Evidence

CLINICAL TRIALS

• No clinical trials identified.

ANIMAL/IN VITRO

• The essential oil has antimicrobial and antifungal effects and has antispasmodic effects in isolated guinea pig tracheal muscle.
• An aniseed infusion caused a small increase in transport velocity in isolated ciliated frog epithelium.
• Essential oils administered orally or by gavage increased respiratory secretions in anesthetized guinea pigs and rats. Vapor inhalation of the essential oil in anesthetized rabbits also increased respiratory secretions by 19% to 82% in a dose-dependent manner; however, the highest doses of inhaled vapor caused tissue damage and, in 20% of rabbits, death (1). In anesthetized cats, an emulsion containing two drops of essential oil administered by gavage reversed the inhibitory effects of opium on expectoration (1).
• Subcutaneous administration of 100 mg per day essential oil stimulated liver regeneration after partial hepatectomy in rats (2).

OTHER CLAIMED BENEFITS/ACTIONS

• Dyspepsia
• Bloating
• Flatulence
• Bronchitis
• Aphrodisiac
• Menses induction
• Colic
• Expectorant

Risks

ADVERSE REACTIONS

• Maternal ingestion of a lactation tea that contained extracts of licorice (*Glycyrrhiza glabra*), fennel (*Foeniculum vulgare*), anise, and goat's rue (*Galega officinalis*) was linked to drowsiness, hypotonia, lethargy, emesis, and poor suckling in two breast-fed neonates; an infection workup was negative and symptoms and signs resolved on discontinuation of the tea (and a 2-day break from breast feeding) (3).
• Nonspecific symptoms (drowsiness and weakness) were also reported by one of the mothers. Anise is widely used in children and considered safe; the adverse effect reported here is most likely due to licorice or goat's rue.

PREGNANCY/LACTATION

• This herb is safe for use in pregnancy and lactation and is reputed to increase milk production.

 Dose

COMMON DOSAGE FORMS

• *Dried fruit:* 0.5 to 1 g t.i.d.
• *Infusion:* made from 0.5 to 5 g crushed or coarsely powdered fruit q.d. to t.i.d.
• Children may be given 1 to 2 g daily as infusion; infants may have a teaspoon of infusion in their bottle.

 Common Questions and Answers

Q: Does anise have the same adverse effects as licorice?
A: No. Although both of these herbs have the typical licorice flavor, they are unrelated plants. Both contain anethole, which gives each its licorice flavor, but only licorice contains glycyrrhizin and its derivatives, which can cause hypertension and hypokalemia in heavy consumers of licorice (see licorice). Anise is completely safe. Most, but not all, "licorice" candies manufactured in North America are actually flavored with anise rather than licorice. Labeling is uninformative here, because either flavoring falls under the category "natural flavorings."

Q: Are licorice-flavored liqueurs made from licorice or anise?
A: Almost all are made from anise. Anise flavors Greek ouzo and French anisette. Pastis, a French liqueur, may be made with either anise or licorice. Anise is one of a number of herbs in Benedictine, Danziger Goldwasser, and other herbal liqueurs.

Arginine

10 Second Take

Arginine, a benign amino acid, increases nitric oxide; in high doses it acts as a vasodilator.

Basics

DESCRIPTION

• Although arginine is a nonessential amino acid, dietary intake is important (especially in catabolic states).
• Diet largely determines plasma levels because arginine synthesis rates do not increase in response to inadequate supply (synthesis increases in response to high amino acid intake, which leads to high urea formation). Formed mainly by the liver, arginine can also be formed by the kidney.

FOOD SOURCES

• Meats, seafood, eggs, dairy products, nuts, beans, whole grains, and gelatin.

MAIN FUNCTIONS/PHARMACOKINETICS

• Integral to protein synthesis, nitrogen metabolism (as an intermediate in the urea cycle), and ammonia detoxification. It is an important precursor to creatine phosphate and nitric oxide (a relaxation factor).
• In the urea cycle, arginase hydrolyzes arginine to urea and ornithine in the cytoplasm; ornithine is converted to citrulline in mitochondria. Citrulline combines first with carbamoyl phosphate and then with aspartic acid to form arginosuccinate, which is cleaved to arginine and succinate. During this process two nitrogen atoms (one from mitochondrial ammonia and one from cytosolic aspartate) plus carbon dioxide are shuttled into urea and excreted. Endocrine effects include stimulation of secretion of catecholamines, insulin, glucagon, growth hormone, and prolactin (1).

Evidence

CLINICAL TRIALS

• Heart failure

—A randomized, double-blind, crossover study in 15 participants with moderate to severe heart failure found that oral L-arginine hydrochloride (5.6 to 12.6 g daily) increased 6-minute walking distance from 390 to 422 meters, and lowered scores on the Living with Heart Failure questionnaire from 55 to 42 (2). It also increased forearm blood flow during exercise, improved arterial compliance, and reduced circulating endothelin levels.

• Angina

—A crossover study in 25 participants with stable angina found that L-arginine (6 g/day × 3 days) significantly increased exercise tolerance (from 604 ± 146 seconds to 647 ± 159 seconds) but had no effect on exercise-induced EKG changes (3).
—Another randomized, double-blind, placebo-controlled crossover study in 36 patients with stable class II or III angina found that an L-arginine supplement (6.6 g/day) improved flow-mediated vasodilation, treadmill exercise time, and quality-of-life scores (4).

• Other cardiovascular risk factors

—A placebo-controlled crossover study found no benefit of adjunctive arginine (9 g arginine/day for 1 month) on markers of nitric oxide release or bioactivity in 30 patients with coronary artery disease (CAD) (5).
—A randomized double-blind crossover trial in 10 men with CAD found that L-arginine (7 g t.i.d.) improved endothelium-dependent brachial artery dilation. No difference was seen in blood pressure, heart rate, fasting lipids, or endothelium-independent dilation of the brachial artery (6).
—A controlled trial of 50 patients undergoing coronary artery bypass grafting found no benefit of 1 g L-arginine intravenously during the first 30 minutes of cardioplegic arrest on serum troponin I levels (7).
—A controlled trial in 10 healthy men found that L-arginine (500 mg/kg intravenously over 30 minutes) significantly decreased mean blood pressure (from 81.2 to 74.0 mm Hg), increased heart rate (from 60.3 to 69.7 beats/minute), (8) decreased renal vascular resistance, and increased renal plasma flow (from 616.6 to 701.0 mL/minute). L-Arginine significantly decreased angiotensin converting enzyme (ACE) activity (from 10.4 to 8.9 nmol/mL/minute) and plasma angiotensin II (from 19.3 to 12.7 pg/mL).
—In a randomized double-blind placebo-controlled crossover study in 27 hypercholesterolemic subjects, arginine 7 g t.i.d. significantly improved endothelium-dependent dilation over placebo; lipid levels were unaffected (9).

—A placebo-controlled trial compared infused placebo to arginine (16 g i.v.) in nine hypercholesterolemic patients; no changes occurred in maximal working capacity or indices of myocardial ischemia (10).
—A double-blind trial in hypercholesterolemic subjects found that 8.4 g arginine daily reduced excessive platelet aggregation (11).

• Peripheral vascular disease

—In patients with critical limb ischemia (peripheral arterial occlusive disease stages Fontaine III or IV), intravenous arginine (30 g over 60 minutes) significantly increased femoral blood flow; urinary nitric oxide and cGMP excretion also increased (12). Prostaglandin E1 increased only femoral blood flow; placebo had no effect.
—A double-blind, placebo-controlled study of 39 patients with intermittent claudication found that 8 g L-arginine b.i.d. or 40 μg prostaglandin E$_1$ (PGE$_1$) b.i.d. for 3 weeks both significantly improved pain-free walking distance and absolute walking distance (13). L-arginine, but not PGE$_1$, improved endothelium-dependent vasodilation in the femoral artery and increased urinary nitrate and cyclic guanosine monophosphate (cGMP) excretion.

• Erectile dysfunction

—A randomized crossover trial found no benefit of arginine (500 mg t.i.d. × 17 days) over placebo in 32 patients with mixed-type impotence (14).
—Another randomized, double-blind study in 50 men with organic erectile dysfunction tested 5 g/day arginine against placebo for 6 weeks (15). Objective measures did not improve, but 9/29 arginine-treated patients compared with 2/17 controls reported significant subjective improvement in sexual function. Only men with initially low levels of nitric oxide metabolites benefited.

• Interstitial cystitis

—Randomized, placebo-controlled trials of arginine in the treatment of interstitial cystitis have not found a benefit (16–18).

• Assisted reproduction

—A study of 34 women undergoing assisted reproduction with poor ovarian response to gonadotrophin tested oral arginine (16 g/day) beginning on day one of menses, until at least one follicle greater than 17 mm in diameter was identified (19) as an adjunct to flare-up gonadotrophin-releasing hormone analogue and elevated follicle stimulating hormone (FSH) in 17 women. Compared with controls, the arginine-treated group had a lower cancellation rate (2/17 vs. 13/17), more collected oocytes, significantly improved uterine and perifollicular arterial flow, and more pregnancies (3 vs. 0, however, all pregnancies were lost).

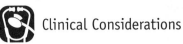

- Raynaud's phenomenon

—A double-blind crossover study found no significant effect on cutaneous vascular responses of L-arginine (8 g/day × 4 weeks) in control subjects or patients with primary Raynaud's phenomenon (20).

- Diabetes

—In a study comparing nine obese subjects, nine noninsulin-dependent diabetes mellitus (NIDDM) patients, and seven healthy subjects, intravenous arginine (0.52 mg kg^{-1} minute^{-1}) increased insulin sensitivity significantly in all groups (21). Impaired insulin-mediated vasodilation improved in obese and diabetic subjects; no change was noted in normal volunteers. No effect was noted on insulin levels, IGF-1, free fatty acids, or C-peptide levels.

—A placebo-controlled crossover trial in 30 diabetic subjects found that L-arginine (free base 1 g b.i.d. × 3 months) significantly reduced the lipid peroxidation product malondialdehyde (22). Malondialdehyde levels returned to baseline after 3 months. Reducing lipid peroxidation may reduce long-term microangiopathic complications.

- Cancer

—Nine of 18 patients with colorectal cancer were given L-arginine 30 g/day for 3 days before surgery (23). Tumors from arginine-supplemented patients contained increased numbers of lymphocyte subsets expressing CD16 and CD56 surface markers. There were no differences in total numbers of T cells or B cells.

- Primary ciliary dyskinesia

—A randomized double-blind placebo-controlled trial tested nebulized arginine (3 g) in 10 patients with primary ciliary dyskinesia (a genetic disease characterized by defective motility of cilia and low nasal nitric oxide levels) and 10 normal volunteers (24). Compared with placebo, arginine significantly increased nasal nitric oxide levels and ciliary beat frequency in both groups.

- Esophageal motility and gallbladder dynamics

—An 8-day randomized crossover study in 10 healthy male volunteers tested L-arginine (30 g/day) against placebo (glycine 13 g/day) (25). L-arginine significantly reduced postprandial lower esophageal pressure and suppressed physiologic late postprandial rise in lower esophageal pressure. Fasting and residual gallbladder volumes were significantly greater after L-arginine ingestion. There was no effect on esophageal motility or reflux.

—A randomized, double-blind placebo-controlled crossover trial tested arginine in eight patients (five women) with noncardiac chest pain and esophageal motor disorders without gastroesophageal reflux (26). Intravenous L-arginine (100 mL of a 10% arginine solution) did not substantially inhibit lower esophageal sphincter (LES) tone or amplitude or duration of pressure waves, but chronic oral intake (30 mL of a solution containing 10% L-arginine t.i.d. × 6 weeks) significantly decreased the frequency and intensity of chest pain attacks and reduced medication use.

- Asthma

—Aerosolized NG-monomethyl-L-arginine reduced bronchoconstriction after bradykinin challenge in a randomized, double-blind, placebo-controlled crossover study of 10 asthmatic patients (27).

- Immune enhancement

—Several recent studies tested supplemental diets containing arginine or arginine plus omega-3 fatty acids in cancer patients undergoing surgery (28), burn patients (29), and HIV-infected patients (30); these studies found no significant changes in immunologic parameters.

- Sperm motility

—Compared with sperm incubated with culture medium, sperm incubated with NG-monomethyl-L-arginine showed a higher percentage total motility and percentage of rapidly motile sperm at 24 hours (31); no significant differences were seen at 6 hours.

 ## Clinical Considerations

DEFICIENCY SIGNS AND SYMPTOMS

- Arginine deficiency increases plasma ammonia levels and urinary orotic acid excretion.

FACTORS DECREASING AVAILABILITY/ABSORPTION

- Catabolic states may cause arginine to become conditionally essential. Mechanisms may include reduced dietary intake, reduced absorption, increased degradation, and reduced intestinal citrulline synthesis.

FACTORS INCREASING AVAILABILITY/ABSORPTION

- Arginase deficiency, an inborn error of metabolism, causes neurologic symptoms after the neonatal period. A highly synthetic, arginine-free diet should be administered for the first several months (32).

LABORATORY TESTS

Normal plasma concentrations are 40 to 140 μmol/L (32).

 ## Risks

ADVERSE REACTIONS

- Hyperkalemia in renal failure patients can result from intravenous administration of arginine. A 15-year-old male hemodialysis patient who accidentally ingested 1.5 g L-arginine orally was asymptomatic, but serum potassium rose from 5.4 mmol, 1 hour after ingestion, to 6.1 mmol (normal 3.5 to 5.5 mmol/L), 2-hours postingestion; sodium polystyrene sulfonate normalized potassium levels (33).
- A 21-month-old died following an accidental overdose of arginine (34).

Dose

CORRECTING DEFICIENCY

Patients with urea cycle enzyme defects (except arginase deficiency) should receive arginine (100 to 500 mg/kg body weight/day).

Arnica

 10 Second Take

Arnica is poisonous, but homeopathic forms or topical herbal preparations, mainly used for trauma, are safe. The herb should never be used internally except in homeopathic form.

 Basics

LATIN NAME

Arnica montana L.

FAMILY

Compositae/Asteraceae

OTHER COMMON NAMES

Wolf's bane, leopard's bane, mountain tobacco

DESCRIPTION

- A perennial herb with yellow daisy-like flowers.
- It grows wild in several parts of Europe, including Spain, Italy, Switzerland, former Yugoslavia, and southern Russia. Other *Arnica* species grow wild in North America.
- Most preparations of *Arnica* used in North America are homeopathic, not herbal preparations (see questions and answers). Both are discussed here.

PART USED

Flower

KNOWN ACTIVE CONSTITUENTS

- Sesquiterpene lactones including helenalin and 11α,13-dihydrohelenalin and their esters.
- Other constituents include carboxylic acids, diterpenes, flavonols, pyrrolizidine alkaloids (tussilagin and isotussilagin), polyacetylenes, caffeic acid, coumarins, and fatty acids (1).
- Homeopathic preparations may reveal none of the previous ingredients by analysis.

MECHANISM/PHARMACOKINETICS

- Sesquiterpene lactones appear to interact with proteins containing thiol groups. They are known to have antiinflammatory properties and act at multiple receptor sites, suppressing prostaglandin synthesis and uncoupling oxidative phosphorylation of human polymorphonuclear neutrophils (PMNs) (1).
- Helenalin slows the recovery kinetics of calcium, perhaps through membrane stabilization, which may account for its toxic effects (2). Little is known about how other constituents of arnica contribute to its actions.

 Evidence

CLINICAL TRIALS

Homeopathic arnica

- A systematic review of placebo-controlled trials of orally administered homeopathic arnica found eight trials: two for delayed-onset muscle soreness, two for experimentally inflicted mechanical bruising, two for prevention of postsurgical complications after tooth extraction, one for acute orthopedic trauma, and one for stroke (3). Only two trials showed a statistically significant positive result: a study of delayed-onset muscle soreness in 42 healthy women (4) and a study of 59 patients after tooth extraction, which found less pain in the arnica group but no difference in bleeding (5). Four studies showed no difference between groups: these included a study on delayed-onset muscle soreness in 36 marathoners (6), a study of prevention of postsurgical complications after tooth extraction in 118 patients (7), a study of 20 orthopedic patients who had suffered acute trauma (8), and a study of 40 stroke patients (9). Both studies of bruising reported in the same article (10) were "numerically positive" (meaning that they did not include formal statistical analysis but an advantage for the arnica group was claimed). Most trials were methodologically poor.
- Delayed-onset muscle soreness

—A systematic review of homeopathic remedies (mainly *Arnica* and *Rhus tox*) for delayed-onset muscle soreness found eight placebo-controlled trials with a total of 311 patients (11). Most trials were methodologically poor. Only three trials were randomized (none of which showed a significant difference between groups). The authors conclude that published evidence does not support the hypothesis that homeopathic remedies are more effective than placebo.

—A randomized, placebo-controlled trial of 50 volunteers tested a combination of homeopathic arnica and *Rhus toxicodendron* (poison ivy) for delayed-onset muscle soreness; no statistically significant difference was seen between the two groups (12).

- Postoperative symptoms and complications

—A randomized, double-blind, placebo-controlled trial of homeopathic arnica for pain and infection after total abdominal hysterectomy found no significant differences between the two groups (13).
—A study reported in abstract form of three randomized double-blind placebo-controlled trials of homeopathic arnica after knee surgery found significantly reduced knee swelling after cruciate ligament surgery but not after arthroscopy or artificial knee joint implantation (14).

Herbal arnica

- Myalgia

—In a small placebo-controlled study of 12 male volunteers with muscle aches, a topical arnica flower gel was more effective than placebo in treating muscle aches in all 12 male volunteers (15).

ANIMAL/IN VITRO

- Antimicrobial effects

—Isolated constituents have shown activity against many bacteria (including *Staphylococcus aureus, Bacillus subtilis, Mycobacterium phlei,* and *Proteus vulgaris*). Antifungal activity against *Botrytis cinerea* has also been shown (1).

- Cytotoxic effects

—Sesquiterpene lactones have demonstrated activity against GLC4 and COLO 320 tumor cell lines.
—Arnica sesquiterpenes inhibited tumor growth of Ehrlich ascites in mice and Walker 256 carcinosarcoma in rats (1).

- Antiinflammatory effects

—In rats, helenalin injected intraperitoneally has been shown to inhibit carrageenan-induced edema of the paw and adjuvant-induced arthritis. Intraperitoneally injected helenalin at a dose of 20 mg/kg body weight reduced the writhing reflex in mice by 93% (1).
—Several inflammation parameters were suppressed by helenalin and dihydrohelenalin in enzyme assays performed on rodent liver homogenates and human PMNs (1).

- Other

—Helenalin demonstrates a concentration-dependent inotropic effect on the guinea pig auricle and the cat papillary muscle. Antihistamine effect has been demonstrated in a smooth muscle cell preparation (1).

OTHER CLAIMED BENEFITS/ACTIONS

- Wounds
- Injuries
- Bruises
- Phlebitis
- Arthralgia
- Mucositis
- Abortifacient
- Cardiac tonic

Risks

WARNING

Arnica is poisonous and should not be taken internally except in homeopathic preparations.

ADVERSE REACTIONS

—A 19-year-old male who consumed tea made from arnica leaves and flowers developed myalgias, headache, and shaking chills within 2 hours (16). On examination, the patient was hyperthermic, hypotensive, and tachycardic, and was treated with fluids and dopamine. Symptoms slowly improved over 6 days; over time, liver function tests normalized and the 25 pounds the patient had lost were regained.
—Children have experienced severe gastroenteritis and bradycardia from ingesting species of arnica (17). There is a case reported in which ingestion of 30 mL of a 20% arnica tincture caused serious but nonfatal symptoms (18).
—At very high doses cardiac arrhythmia and death may result. Helenolides are known to be toxic to the heart (2).
—Arnica has also been reported to cause miscarriage (19).

• Dermatologic

—Topical arnica is sensitizing in some people and can cause allergic reactions. Arnica contact allergy is common; exposure may be from tincture, cosmetics, soaps, moisturizers, or shampoos.
—The sesquiterpene lactone helenalin, helenalin methacrylate, helenalin isovalerate, helenalin acetate, carabrone, arnicolide A, and xanthalongin have all been shown to be contact sensitizers, and those sensitive to arnica should avoid all sesquiterpene lactone-containing plants (19).

ANIMAL TOXICITY

Median LD_{50} of helenalin ranges from 85 mg/kg in hamsters to 150 mg/kg in mice.

 Dose

COMMON DOSAGE FORMS

• *Arnica is mainly available in oral and topical homeopathic preparations, but herbal topical creams and gels also exist.*
• *Topical cream, gel, poultice, diluted tincture, or arnica oil (1 part herb extract to 5 parts vegetable oil)*
• *Mouthwash* [diluted tincture or infusion made from 2 g drug and 100 mL water (not to be swallowed)]

 Common Questions and Answers

Q: What is the difference between herbal arnica and homeopathic arnica?
A: It is vitally important to know which is which, because for oral ingestion one is dangerous and the other is safe. In North America most arnica preparations sold (both oral and topical) are homeopathic; in Europe about half of all arnica products sold are homeopathic. Homeopathy is a form of "energy medicine" that does not require the actual physical presence of the substance a remedy contains; the preparation is said to contain a "memory" of the substance from which it is prepared. Homeopathic preparations contain somewhere between a dilute and nonexistent amount of arnica and, thus, are harmless. There is also no need to worry about topical preparations, whether they are homeopathic or herbal; both are harmless (although neither should be used on broken skin).
Herbal arnica for internal use is poisonous and should be avoided completely. Arnica would be likely to be particularly dangerous in patients with cardiac disease. A traditional use of the herb is to treat cardiac disease, and some would argue that the herb can be safely used by competent herbalists. I do not agree. Titrating a safe dose of a poisonous herb is always tricky, and arnica does not occupy a unique therapeutic niche. There are more benign herbs (and drugs) that can be used for cardiac disease or any other condition treated by arnica.

Ashwagandha

 10 Second Take

Ashwagandha is benign. *In vivo* studies indicate antistress, antiinflammatory, and anticancer activities; however, relevant clinical studies are lacking.

 Basics

LATIN NAME

Withania somnifera (L.) Dunal

FAMILY

Solanaceae

OTHER COMMON NAMES

Winter cherry, Indian ginseng, Asgandh (Hindi), Aasoganda (Nepalese), Bahman (Persian), Ba-dzi-gandha (Tibetan)

DESCRIPTION

• An evergreen shrub up to 1.5 m high that grows throughout the subtropical parts of India. It also grows wild in Pakistan, Spain, Afghanistan, and many parts of Africa.
• Its orange-red berries are enclosed within its calyx. Ashwagandha, in Sanskrit, means sweat of the horse, which describes its smell.

PART USED

• Seeds, shoots, juice, leaves, and roots have all been used.
• The root is most commonly used.

KNOWN ACTIVE CONSTITUENTS

• The roots contain anahygrine, meso-anaferine, cuscohygrine, isopelletierine, hygrine, tropine, pseudotropine, choline, withasomnine, somniferine, withaninine, nicotine, scopeletin, withanolide, and other compounds.
• The leaf contains withaferin A, withanolide glycosides, reducing sugars, somnitol, withanone, glycine, cystine, glutamic acid, alpha-alanine, proline, tryptophane, tannins, and flavonoids (1). Withanolides are steroidal lactones, of which withaferin A and withaferin D have been most studied.

MECHANISM/PHARMACOKINETICS

• Withaferin A appears to act as a spindle poison in mouse sarcoma tumor cells, affecting spindle microtubules in metaphase (2). At low doses (10.5 μg/mL) withaferin A affects cell cycle progression of Chinese hamster V79 cells by blocking cells in G2 + M phase.
• No information on pharmacokinetics is available.

 Evidence

CLINICAL TRIALS

• No relevant published clinical trials were identified.
• A review article published in 1996 states that crude extract has been administered to advanced oral carcinoma patients as an adjunct to radiation therapy; no side effects were noted, and response was said to be "encouraging" (3).

ANIMAL/IN VITRO

• Antitumor effects

—Withaferin A, derived from the leaf, appears to have cancer inhibitory effects *in vitro* and *in vivo*.
—Mice inoculated intraperitoneally with Ehrlich ascites carcinoma were given 10 to 60 mg/kg withaferin A intraperitoneally 24 hours later (4). Compared with saline control, doses of 10 to 40 mg/kg significantly increased mean survival time (however, doses of 50 and 60 mg did not affect mean survival time). The percentage of survivors at 120 days increased in a dose-dependent manner. (The table and text state that 85% of rats given 60 mg survived 120 days. Because there were 10 rats per group, 85% seems a peculiar number; perhaps one rat was moribund?)
—In another experiment in the same report, intraperitoneal withaferin A with or without radiation treatment was administered to mice 1, 3, or 5 days after inoculation with Ehrlich ascites carcinoma. The combined treatment synergistically increased 120-day survival but also increased toxicity. Apparently the most effective dose was 30 mg/kg (it is stated, but not explained, that doses above 40 mg/kg were "not tolerated in combination with radiation").

—In a later study by the same investigators, different dose schedules were tested (5). A combination of radiotherapy with two doses (30 mg/kg withaferin A per dose) was the most effective treatment, resulting in 100% survivors on day 120 (radiation alone resulted in 0 survivors, while withaferin A 30 mg/kg resulted in 80% survivors). *In vitro*, withaferin A had a strong radiosensitizing effect on Chinese hamster V79 cells (6).
—In older studies, withaferin inhibited the growth of Sarcoma 180 (2) and Ehrlich ascites carcinoma in mice. In a controlled study in mice, withanolide D in doses of 15 to 30 mg/kg significantly reduced "average tumor weight" in mice inoculated with Sarcoma 180; doses of 15 mg/kg significantly reduced average tumor weight in mice inoculated with Ehrlich ascites carcinoma (7).
—An alcoholic extract of root injected intraperitoneally in mice inoculated with Sarcoma 180 found a dose-dependent increase in complete responses with doses more than 400 mg/kg; doses of 1,000 mg/kg were toxic (8). Aqueous extract was much less effective.
—A crude alcohol extract of the whole plant (200 mg/kg) protected mice against urethane-induced lung adenomas; mortality was significantly reduced, and the incidence of lung adenoma was reduced 75% compared with controls (9).

• Antistress effects

—Antistress activity of ashwagandha has been demonstrated in several animal studies, including forced swimming tests in rats and reduction in stress-induced reactions in mice and rats (10).

• Antiinflammatory effects

—In rats, three of five fractions of an extract of *Withania* (administered peritoneally) inhibited inflammation and cotton-pellet-induced granuloma tissue formation significantly more than controls in rats; the effect was equivalent to 5 mg/kg hydrocortisone sodium succinate (11). Numerous other studies have shown significant antiinflammatory and antiarthritic effects of ashwagandha root powder in mice and rats (10).

- Antifungal effects

—Two withanolides were found to have antifungal effects (12). Ashwagandha given orally (100 mg/kg × 7 days) prolonged the survival of mice infected with *Aspergillus fumigatus* (13).

- Endocrine effects

—In mice, 1.4 g/kg/day by gastric intubation increased serum triiodothyronine (T_3) and thyroxin (T_4) concentrations and hepatic glucose-6-phosphate dehydrogenase (G6PD) activity; hepatic levels of iodothyronine 5′-monodeiodinease activity did not change (14).

- Antioxidant and other effects

—Ashwagandha root powder decreased lipid peroxidation and increased superoxide dismutase and catalase activity in mice after 30 days of treatment; no effect was seen with 15 days of treatment (0.7 and 1.4 g/kg body weight/day) (15). Oral administration of ashwagandha (100 mg/kg) prevents stress-induced elevation of lipid peroxidation in rabbits and mice (16).

—In rat brain slices, a *Withania* extract slightly enhanced acetylcholinesterase activity in basal forebrain nuclei and slightly enhanced acetylcholinesterase activity in lateral septum and globus pallidus (17).

OTHER CLAIMED BENEFITS/ACTIONS

- Cancer
- Debility
- Rheumatism
- Pain
- Diuretic
- Arthritis, analgesia
- Sedative
- Asthma
- Neurologic diseases
- Tuberculosis
- Aphrodisiac
- Tonic
- Abortion/contraceptive
- Toothache (inhaled smoke)

 Risks

PREGNANCY/LACTATION

This herb is reputed to have abortifacient properties and should not be used during pregnancy.

ANIMAL TOXICITY

- An acute toxicity study in mice found that the LD_{50} was 1,260 mg/kg body weight when injected intraperitoneally (no mortality was observed in doses up to 1,100 mg/kg). Intraperitoneal injections of extract in a dose of 100 mg/kg body weight for 30 days did not result in mortality or changes in blood counts but did increase acid phosphatase content and reduce the weights of spleen, thymus, and adrenals in male rats (18). For withaferin A, no deaths occurred after a single injection of up to 40 mg. There was a sharp increase in mortality with doses greater than 70 mg; LD_{50} was 80 mg/kg (5).

 Dose

COMMON DOSAGE FORMS

- *Dried root:* 3 to 6 g daily.
- Decoction with milk or ghee (clarified butter). Also taken as medicated wine, ghee, jam, or oil.
- Also available in liquid extracts, capsules, tablets, standardized extracts, Ayurvedic herb mixtures, and topical preparations.

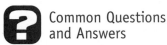 Common Questions and Answers

Q: Are there nonmedicinal uses of ashwagandha?
A: Yes, twigs of *Withania* are chewed for cleaning teeth, and the fruits of *Withania coagulans* are used as a vegetable rennet to coagulate milk.

Aspartate/Aspartic acid

 10 Second Take

Aspartic acid is a benign, nonessential amino acid helpful in wound healing; it may have other therapeutic indications.

 Basics

DESCRIPTION

• A nonessential amino acid that can be formed from alanine or asparagine.
• Concentration in plasma is 1 to 11 μmol/L; 24 hour urinary output is 60 μmol/24 hours and plasma clearance (half-life) is 3 hours (1).

FOOD SOURCES

Aspartic acid is present in almost all proteins; in addition, it can be synthesized endogenously.

MAIN FUNCTIONS/PHARMACOKINETICS

• Incorporated into purines and pyrimidines, it is also important in urea biosynthesis and as a glucogenic precursor.
• Asparagine is converted into aspartate by asparaginase.

 Evidence

CLINICAL TRIALS

• Adjuvant cancer treatment

—N-phosonacetyl-L-aspartic acid (PALA) may augment the cytotoxic effects of 5-fluorouracil (5-FU) by inhibiting pyrimidine biosynthesis. PALA 5-FU combinations have been tested in advanced gastric adenocarcinoma (2), with radiation in pancreatic cancer (3), with interferon in head and neck cancers (4), with methotrexate in advanced colorectal cancer (5), with methotrexate in advanced pancreatic cancer (6), and with folinic acid in advanced colorectal cancer (7). Of the preceding trials, only the Kohne trial (a Phase II trial in 26 patients with advanced colorectal cancer) and the Ardalan trial (a Phase I trial of 10 patients with pancreatic cancers) concluded that the combination treatments had any beneficial activity. A crossover pharmacokinetic study in six patients failed to find a significant effect of PALA on 5-FU pharmacokinetics (8).

• Leg ulcers

—Diabetic ulcers appear to heal faster with application of arginine-glycine-aspartic acid (Argidine Gel, or RGD) peptide matrix. A study in 65 diabetic patients with full-thickness neurotrophic foot ulcers compared RGD topical gel to topical saline (each applied twice weekly for up to 10 weeks) (9). There was a significant difference between the two groups; 14/40 (35%) of patients in the RGD group experienced complete ulcer healing compared with 2/25 (8%) in the placebo group. RGD peptide matrix also significantly increased the rate of ulcer closure over 10 weeks. The contribution of arginine to this effect is unclear.

• Burns

—In pediatric patients with partial-thickness scald burns, RGD peptide matrix was compared with silver sulfadiazine in matched burn sites for up to 21 days (10). RGD treatment resulted in significantly faster healing (2.5 days faster than control), a higher healing rate, a greater (37%) extent of burn closure, and fewer grafting procedures (control sites were grafted at a rate four times higher than treated sites).

• Opiate withdrawal

—L-aspartic acid has been investigated as a treatment to help addicts through withdrawal. Thirty-one opiate addicts given 8 g L-aspartic acid for 7 days after withdrawal of opiates were compared with 12 opiate addicts who received chlorpromazine (50 mg) and diazepam (60 mg). The intensity and duration of 13/16 abstinence syndrome signs were significantly better in the aspartic acid group than the chlorpromazine and diazepam group (11).
—A prior uncontrolled trial in eight opiate addicts administered 2 g L-aspartic acid four times daily for up to 5 days while opiates were tapered. Mild abstinence signs and symptoms were observed during the treatment; none of the subjects experienced abstinence signs or drug craving during a 2-week follow-up (12).

- Hepatic encephalopathy

—Oral or intravenous L-ornithine-L-aspartate may benefit cirrhotic patients with hepatic encephalopathy. A randomized, placebo-controlled, double-blind trial in 126 subjects with subclinical hepatic encephalopathy tested 20 g/day L-ornithine-L-aspartate (infused intravenously over 4 hours) for 7 days (13). Compared with the placebo group, fasting and postprandial venous ammonia concentrations, mental state gradation, Number Connection Test performance times, and the Portal Systemic Encephalopathy Index improved significantly more in the treated group.

—L-ornithine-L-aspartate (6 g p.o. t.i.d. × 14 days) was tested in a randomized, placebo-controlled, double-blind trial in 66 participants with stable overt or subclinical hepatic encephalopathy (14). Fasting and postprandial blood ammonia concentrations, mental state grades, Number Connection Test performance times, and the Portal Systemic Encephalopathy Index improved significantly more in the treated group compared with placebo.

CASE REPORT

- Pyruvate carboxylase deficiency

—A 7-year-old girl with severe hepatic pyruvate carboxylase deficiency, progressive motor neurologic impairment, and high serum levels of lactate and pyruvate was treated with thiamin and aspartic acid for 7 years (15). During this time her neurologic condition remained stable and lactate and pyruvate levels stabilized. On withdrawal of aspartic acid, lactate and pyruvate concentrations increased markedly, returning to normal when aspartic acid was resumed.

ANIMAL/IN VITRO

- Wound healing/burns

—In pigs with second-degree burns, RGD protein matrix results in faster healing (16). Epithelialization of skin grafts on athymic mice is enhanced by a matrix containing arginine-glycine-aspartic acid peptide and hyaluronic acid, compared with a matrix of hyaluronic acid alone (17).

- Reducing aminoglycoside toxicity

—Poly-L-aspartic acid (PAA) protects human proximal tubule cells in vitro from aminoglycoside-induced electrophysiologic alterations (18). In rats, PAA blocks the nephrotoxic effects of aminoglycosides (without reducing antibiotic effectiveness); a study in guinea pigs found a protective effect of PAA on cochlear ototoxicity (19). Arginine-glycine-aspartic acid peptides may prevent tubular obstruction in the ischemic model of acute renal failure; in rats, RGD peptides attenuate renal injury and accelerate recovery of renal function (20).

- Drug delivery

—PAA has also been studied as a drug carrier for drugs targeted at the colon (21).

 Risks

ANIMAL TOXICITY

- In rats fed 50 mg/kg D-aspartic acid or L-aspartic acid for 28 days, no pathologic changes in organs or signs of subacute toxicity in liver or kidney were found (22).
- Very large quantities of aspartate cause neuronal necrosis in newborn mice; however, at least four studies in nonhuman primates have failed to produce this effect (23).

Astragalus

 10 Second Take

Astragalus is a relatively safe Chinese herb that has interesting immunostimulating effects; however, reliable clinical trial data are lacking.

 Basics

LATIN NAME

Astragalus membranaceus (Fisch.) Bge.

FAMILY

Fabaceae/Leguminosae

OTHER COMMON NAMES

Huang qi, bei qi (Mandarin); *beg kei, buck qi* (Cantonese); *ogi* (Japanese); *Hwanggi* (Korean)

DESCRIPTION

• A perennial herb up to 80 cm tall with pinnate compound leaves, astragalus has taproots and yellow flowers.
• It favors mountainsides, sunny grasslands, and forest margins and is found in northeastern China, Siberia, and central Mongolia.
• Roots are harvested when the plant is 4 or 5 years old.

PART USED

Dried roots

KNOWN ACTIVE CONSTITUENTS

• Astragalus contains polysaccharides (including astragaloglucans termed polysaccharides A–D or astragalans I–IV), triterpene glycosides (including unique astragalosides I–VIII), flavonoids, and isoflavonoids.
• Also phenolic acids (including ferulic and caffeic acid) and sitosterol.

 Evidence

CLINICAL TRIALS

• Although clinical trials of astragalus exist, most are uncontrolled and/or published in the Chinese medical literature (see questions and answers).
• Cancer/immune stimulation

—A study in 16 hemodialysis patients tested the addition of 30 mL astragalus to an intravenous drip given during dialysis visits (2 to 3 times weekly) for 2 months (1). Lymphocyte cultures from the treated group were compared with lymphocyte cultures from 15 controls (who received intravenous infusion without astragalus). In the treated group but not in the control group, serum interleukin (IL)-2 increased significantly and serum levels of sIL-2R (which has immunosuppressive activity, decreasing IL-2 activity) decreased significantly.
—A Chinese placebo-controlled study in which 14 volunteers ingested 8 g of dried astragalus root daily found that, compared with controls, blood samples from the treated group (drawn 2 weeks and 2 months after treatment) indicated increased interferon production by leukocytes (2).
—Chinese studies of a combination of astragalus and ligustrum (*Ligustrum lucidum*) as an adjunct treatment to radiation reportedly reduced mortality in patients with breast cancer or non-small-cell lung cancer but had no effect on cervical cancer (2).

• Human sperm motility

—Of 18 aqueous extracts of Chinese herbs tested in a sperm motility test, only astragalus had a beneficial effect; at 10 mg/mL, an aqueous extract of astragalus increased motility of sperm in semen 46.6% and washed sperm 38.2%, compared with control (3).

• Radiation exposure

—In one study published in a U.S. journal, a mixed herb preparation containing astragalus and eleuthero (*Eleutherococcus senticosis,* also *Acanthopanax senticosis*) was tested in subjects with chronic radiation exposure or who were undergoing radiation therapy (4). Although significant increases in white blood cells and platelets are claimed, the data in this report are too sketchy to interpret, with results apparently reported only on a subset of those treated.

ANIMAL/IN VITRO

• Cancer/immune stimulation

—A combination of astragalus and ligustrum, compared with saline, reduced tumor load in BALB/c mice implanted intraperitoneally with renal carcinoma cells (5).
—Aqueous extracts of crude root obtained from pharmacies in Canada, Hong Kong, and the United States were found to have a wide range of potency in stimulating macrophage activity. Honey-baked astragalus [a traditional Chinese medicine (TCM) preparation] did not stimulate phagocytic activity in murine macrophage cell lines. One study indicates that astragalus potentiates the stimulatory effect of IL-2 on the tumor-cell killing activity of lymphokine-activated killer (LAK) cells *in vitro* (6). An astragalus decoction protected mice from infection by parainfluenza virus.
—An aqueous extract of astragalus increased the immune response of T cells from cancer patients, as assessed by xenogeneic graft-versus-host reaction (XGVHR); several active immunostimulating fractions of this extract were isolated (7). A partially purified fraction prevented cyclophosphamide-induced immunosuppression in rats (8).

• Miscellaneous

—A mixed herb preparation containing astragalus and eleuthero (*Eleutherococcus senticosis*) (30 mg q.d. × 10 days) reduced mortality in mice exposed to lethal doses of radiation (800 rads) from 100% to 65% (4). In mice exposed to 400 rads, white blood cell counts decreased to a lesser extent than in a control group and recovered more rapidly (4).
—An ethanol extract of astragalus (3 g/kg/day × 11 days) prevented induced hepatic injury in mice. Fractionated saponins from two species of astragalus reduced liver damage induced by various agents in mice (2).
—A glucoside from astragalus mitigated arrhythmias and increased the survival time of guinea pigs exposed to the cholinesterase inhibitor dimethoate (9).
—Saponin fractions of astragalus have shown dose-dependent negative inotropic effects (2).
—In rats, a combination of astragalus and ligustrum (240 mg crude extract × 12 days) was ineffective in preventing cyclophosphamide-induced myelosuppression (10).
—Astragalus appears to have antioxidant effects and antibacterial effects against a broad range of organisms (2).

OTHER CLAIMED BENEFITS/ACTIONS

• Tonic
• Immune stimulant
• Cancer
• Chronic degenerative diseases

Risks

 Dose

 Common Questions and Answers

DRUG INTERACTIONS

• None reported.
• However, if this herb actually acts as an immunostimulant, it may interact with immunosuppressive drugs.

ANIMAL TOXICITY

• In rats, a crude aqueous extract of astragalus administered by lavage had no toxicity in doses up to 100 g/kg; the LD_{50} in mice is approximately 40 g/kg intraperitoneally.

COMMON DOSAGE FORMS

• *Powdered, dried root*: 10 to 30 g per day (up to 60 g daily for serious conditions).
• *Decoction*: made from 10 to 30 g dried root in 0.5 to 1 L water. Larger doses may be used.
• *Fluid extract*: (1:2) 4 to 8 mL per day.
• *In TCM formulas*: 1.5 to 9 g.
• *Soup*: 30 g/3.5 L soup.

Q: What have you got against the Chinese medical literature?
A: The scientific literature from China is not up to international scientific standards. A systematic review found an extremely high percentage of positive outcomes in trials reported from China; 100% (36/36) acupuncture trials done in China were positive, and 99% (108/109) of nonacupuncture controlled trials from China reported positive outcomes for the treatment (the one exception found the treatments equivalent) (11). Although publication bias is a problem in every country, it is worse in some countries than others. This review also found a high rate of positive trials in controlled acupuncture trials from Russia/USSR (10/11), Taiwan (6/6), Japan (5/5), Austria (8/9), Italy (8/9), and France (5/6). In contrast, 50% to 60% of controlled acupuncture trials in the United States, Sweden, United Kingdom, Denmark, and Germany reported favorable responses for the treatment. The second part of this review retrieved all controlled clinical trials of treatments besides acupuncture from five countries; studies reported as positive were China 99% (108/109), Russia/USSR 97% (28/29), Taiwan 95% (38/40), Japan 89% (107/120), and England 75% (80/107). Although publication standards are improving in China, they are not yet up to par.

Q: Aren't there *Astragalus* species that grow in the United States?
A: Yes. There are more than 1,700 species within the *Astragalus* genus. One species, *Astragalus mollissimus*, common in New Mexico and Texas, contains swainsonine, which can cause locoism (bizarre behavior, apparently caused by neurologic damage) in horses, cattle, prairie dogs, and even bees (12).

Bearberry

 10 Second Take

Bearberry exerts antimicrobial activity in alkalinized urine, but there are no clinical trials of this herb for urinary tract infection (UTI) treatment. Bearberry is not benign and should not be used for more than a few days.

 Basics

LATIN NAME

Arctostaphylos uva-ursi (L.) Spreng.

FAMILY

Ericaceae

OTHER COMMON NAMES

Uva ursi, kinnikinnick, upland cranberry

DESCRIPTION

• Bearberry is a small, evergreen shrub common in open forest clearings in northern United States and Canada.
• It has woody trailing stems; leathery leaves; pink, urn-shaped flowers; and red mealy berries.

PART USED

Leaf

KNOWN ACTIVE CONSTITUENTS

• The active components of bearberry are hydroquinone derivatives that include arbutin (between 5% to 15%), methylarbutin (up to 4%), and small amounts of the free aglycones hydroquinone and methylhydroquinone.
• Other constituents include tannins (up to 20% gallotannins), gallic acid, galloylarbutin, flavonoids, and triterpenes (ursolic acid and uvaol).

MECHANISM/PHARMACOKINETICS

• Arbutin is rapidly absorbed after oral administration of bearberry extract or arbutin (1). Hydrolytic cleavage of arbutin by intestinal flora creates hydroquinone, which is then probably conjugated in the intestine or liver before renal excretion (2). Phenolic metabolites are excreted in the urine beginning several hours after administration and peaking within 6 hours. Within 24 hours, 70% to 75% of the administered dose is excreted (3). Hydroquinone, which reforms in alkaline urine, is thought to account for the herb's antibacterial effects in the urinary tract (2).
• Coated arbutin tablets, available in Germany, retard absorption for 3 to 24 hours without affecting bioavailability (1).

 Evidence

CLINICAL TRIALS

• No relevant treatment trials were identified. A thinly reported, double-blind, placebo-controlled prophylaxis trial tested a product called UVA-E, containing hydroalcoholic extracts of bearberry (standardized for arbutin and methylarbutin) and dandelion (*Taraxacum officinale*) root and leaf for the prevention of recurrent cystitis (4). Fifty-seven women (age 32 to 63 years) who had at least three episodes of antibiotic-responsive cystitis in the past year and at least one episode within the past 6 months were given placebo or UVA-E (three tablets t.i.d.) for 1 month. Participants were then followed for 1 year. Five of 27 placebo-treated patients and none of the 30 UVA-E-treated patients experienced an episode of cystitis by the end of the 12-month follow-up. The difference was significant. This report contains no data beyond the previous summary and contains no bacteriologic information. Although it is stated that tests for bacteruria were performed at 6 and 12 months, these and other relevant data are not presented.
• Urinary antiseptic

—Bearberry appears to exert antibacterial effects only in alkalinized urine. Urine samples from healthy volunteers collected 3 hours after administration of 1.0 or 0.1 g arbutin were tested against 74 strains of bacteria, including *Escherichia coli*, *Proteus mirabilis*, *Pseudomonas aeruginosa*, and *Staphylococcus aureus*. Twenty synthetic antibiotics were also tested. Only gentamicin, nalidixic acid, and urine collected after administration of 1.0 g bearberry (adjusted to pH 8) were effective against all strains tested (3).
—A similar experiment using urine samples collected from healthy volunteers following consumption of 800 mg of pure arbutin (or bearberry tea containing the equivalent amount of arbutin) showed marked antibacterial properties *in vitro* only if the urine was adjusted to pH 8. Urine of pH 6 was ineffective (3).
—Alkalinization of urine may be difficult to maintain. In one experiment, 10 g of sodium hydrogen carbonate was administered with a coated tablet containing 50 mg of arbutin. Participants did not attain sufficiently alkalinized urine even with this intervention (only one participant attained a urinary pH of 8 and that was only for 1 hour). Not surprisingly, given insufficient alkalinization, no free hydroquinone (detection limit 1 μg/mL) was found in the urine of treated volunteers (1).

ANIMAL/IN VITRO

• Several studies of bearberry extracts in animal models of inflammation have shown an antiinflammatory effect; it appears to have synergistic effects with steroidal and nonsteroidal pharmaceutical antiinflammatory agents (5).
• Antimicrobial effects have been demonstrated for bearberry against a variety of microorganisms, including *E. coli*, *Proteus vulgaris*, *S. aureus*, *Enterobacter aerogenes*, *Streptococcus faecalis*, *Salmonella typhi*, and *Candida albicans* (5). Arbutin and hydroquinone are active against *Ureaplasma urealyticum* and *Mycoplasma hominis in vitro* (5).
• Aqueous extract of bearberry decreased cell surface hydrophobicity, enhanced cell aggregation of 10 *Helicobacter pylori* strains, and had a marked bacteriostatic activity (apparently resulting from tannins; tannic acid had a similar effect) (6).

OTHER CLAIMED BENEFITS/ACTIONS

• Diuretic
• Cystitis, urethritis, dysuria
• Nephrolithiasis
• Hemorrhoids (topical)
• Postpartum swelling (topical)

Risks

ADVERSE REACTIONS

• Nausea, vomiting, and stomach irritation can occur because of the high tannin content of bearberry leaf. Although the amount of free hydroquinone is small, it is of some concern. Hydroquinone is a topical irritant and hepatotoxin (3). Oral ingestion of one gram of hydroquinone has caused tinnitus, nausea, vomiting, dyspnea, delirium, cyanosis, seizures, and collapse; 2 to 5 g may be lethal (7). It is extremely unlikely that a toxic level of hydroquinone could be achieved with bearberry ingestion (see questions and answers).
• Bearberry should not be used in those with hepatic or renal disease.
• Bearberry should not be taken for longer than 1 to 2 weeks or more frequently than five times per year.
• Other effects

—Discolored urine

Hydroquinone may cause urine to appear greenish brown. Exposure to air will further darken the urine because of oxidation of the hydroquinone (8).

DRUG INTERACTIONS

• A water extract of bearberry augmented the effect of dexamethasone on allergic and inflammatory models (picryl chloride-induced contact dermatitis and carrageenan-induced paw edema); no effect was noted with the bearberry extract alone (9).
• Drugs or food that acidify urine would be expected to decrease the efficacy of bearberry in treating UTIs.

PREGNANCY/LACTATION

Pregnant or lactating women should not use this herb. Arbutin is teratogenic (3).

ANIMAL TOXICITY

• No data for bearberry leaf has been reported. Large doses of hydroquinone are toxic. The oral LD_{50} for a single dose of hydroquinone in 2% aqueous solution is 320 mg/kg in rats, 400 mg/kg in mice, 550 mg/kg in guinea pigs, 70 mg/kg in cats, and 200 mg/kg in dogs (3).

 Dose

COMMON DOSAGE FORMS

• *Dried leaves*, finely cut or coarsely powdered, as infusion, decoction, or cold water macerate t.i.d. to q.i.d. (the cold water macerate, in which the herb is placed in cold water for 6 to 12 hours, is preferred, because this method extracts arbutin but extracts much less of the tannins, which cause gastrointestinal discomfort).
• *Coated tablets*, available in Germany, would be expected to decrease the incidence of stomach irritation or nausea.
• The daily dose is the equivalent of 400 to 800 mg arbutin daily, divided into 2 to 3 doses.
• *Liquid extract:* (1:1 in 25% alcohol) 1.5 to 4 mL t.i.d.
• Children: Not recommended.

 Common Questions and Answers

Q: Is this herb dangerous?
A: Bearberry is not highly toxic, and no human poisonings with bearberry were identified. Although use for up to a week is probably safe, longer use should be avoided. There are several toxic components to this herb. Tannins in bearberry can cause gastrointestinal side effects, including nausea and constipation. Hydroquinone is much more toxic than tannins, but the level of free hydroquinones in bearberry is small. Arbutin is not well absorbed but can be converted to hydroquinone by intestinal flora. Hydroquinone is easily absorbed but is probably conjugated and excreted renally as a conjugate (2). Hydroquinone then reforms from conjugates only under alkaline conditions in the urinary tract. In summary, the amount of free, bioavailable hydroquinone from bearberry ingestion is unlikely to reach toxic levels.

Q: Is this herb useful clinically?
A: It is unclear how easy it is to achieve clinical benefits with bearberry, because maintaining alkalinized urine is necessary for the generation of hydroquinone and the subsequent antimicrobial effect in the urinary tract. It would be difficult to maintain a consistent urinary pH of 8 through diet alone, and even simultaneous administration of an alkalinizing agent may be insufficient (see clinical trials). Bearberry is not a benign herb and should not be used regularly or for more than a week at a time. Although it may have antibacterial effects in alkalinized urine, the lack of clinical trial data and the potential side effects of this herb make this a poor first-line choice for cystitis treatment.

Q: Have adverse effects been reported from smoking bearberry?
A: Some American Indians use the dried leaves of several species of bearberry as the primary ingredient in ceremonial smoking mixtures. Kinnikinnick means "smoking mixture" (10). No toxic effects from smoking bearberry have been reported.

Betaine

 10 Second Take

Betaines (including glycine betaine, betaine hydrochloride, cocamidopropyl betaine) are harmless dietary constituents; betaine glycine is important as a renal osmolyte.

 Basics

DESCRIPTION

• Betaine or glycine betaine (*N,N,N*-trimethylglycine) is a sweet, crystalline alkaloid, originally derived from beets.
• The term betaine is also used generically to refer to compounds having a quaternary amine or analogous function that is cationic at all pH values, with a net charge of zero at neutral pH (1).
• Glycine betaine is the most common dietary betaine found in many plants; trigonelline and proline betaine are also common, whereas homarine, dimethylsulfoniopropionate, and arsenobetaine are minor dietary constituents mainly found in seafood.
• Carnitine, a metabolite, is also considered a betaine.

MECHANISM/PHARMACOKINETICS

• Important functions of betaine include its role as an important renal osmolyte (osmolytes maintain cellular integrity by stabilizing the hydration layer of proteins and by counteracting intracellular dehydration and, thus, helping to protect macromolecules against denaturation by heat, urea, or solvents).
• Betaine is also important as a methyl donor. Choline is converted to betaine, primarily in the liver and kidney (betaine cannot be converted back to choline). The enzyme choline dehydrogenase (found in mitochondrial membranes) oxidizes choline to betaine aldehyde, which is then oxidized by an aldehyde dehydrogenase to betaine.

 Evidence

CLINICAL TRIALS

• Steatohepatitis

—A randomized, double-blind placebo-controlled trial of 191 patients with nonalcoholic steatohepatitis tested betaine glucuronate (combined with diethanolamine glucuronate and nicotinamide ascorbate) p.o. b.i.d. for 8 weeks (2). The combination significantly decreased hepatic steatosis by 25% ($p < 0.01$) and hepatomegaly by 6% ($p < 0.05$); there was no significant effect of the placebo. The treatment also decreased abdominal discomfort and reduced liver transaminases. Fifty-two percent of patients rated the treatment "very good" or "good", compared with 34% of those receiving placebo (a significant difference). There was no difference in adverse events between the treated group and the placebo group.

• Hypochlorhydria

—Betaine hydrochloride contains 23% hydrochloric acid by weight; it is used in conventional medicine to treat hypochlorhydria (3).

• Homocysteinemia in cystathionine β-synthase deficiency

—Betaine may be used as adjunctive treatment in patients with inborn errors of transsulfuration (as a methyl donor, betaine can activate alternative pathways for removing homocysteine) (4). Betaine may be most effective in lowering homocysteine levels in pyridoxine-responsive homocystinemia (5) but can also be effective in nonpyridoxine sensitive cystathionine β-synthase deficiency (4).

• Homocysteinemia in hemodialysis patients

—Betaine does not appear to add any benefit to folic acid in lowering homocysteine levels in hemodialysis patients. One study randomized 29 hemodialysis patients (26 completed the study) to folic acid 5 mg q.d. with or without betaine 4 g daily. Total plasma homocysteine and methionine levels were measured after an overnight fast and then 6 and 24 hours after a methionine load. Patients were then re-randomized to 1 or 5 mg of folic acid daily. Although folate significantly decreased homocysteine, betaine did not have additional homocysteine-lowering effects (6). A very small open study of three hemodialysis patients with persistent hyperhomo-cysteinemia (>22 μmol/L) despite supplemental folic acid found that 1 week of betaine supplementation resulted in no significant change in total plasma homocysteine (7).

ANIMAL/IN VITRO

• Hepatoprotective effects

—Betaine increases levels of S-adenosylmethionine (SAMe), which has low bioavailability both orally or parenterally. Supplemental dietary betaine at the 0.5% level doubles SAMe in animals and can increase levels fivefold in ethanol-fed rats (8). Increase of hepatic SAMe protects rats against ethanol-induced steatosis (9). An experiment designed to determine the minimum betaine dose that would protect the liver from fatty infiltration (the early stage of alcoholic liver injury) found that only the highest dose tested (0.5% of diet) generated enough SAMe to protect against ethanol-induced steatosis (8). Betaine and taurine (also a hepatic osmolyte) attenuate hyperosmolarity-aggravated ischemia-reoxygenation injury in rat liver (10).
—In rats injected four times daily with carbon tetrachloride, supplementation with oral betaine reduced centrilobular hepatic lipidosis and hepatic triglyceride levels (11). In mice, decreased serum alanine transaminase (ALT) was observed after oral (15 mg/kg) or intraperitoneal (3 mg/kg) administration of betaine 24 hours after carbon tetrachloride-induced injury (12). In addition, orally administered betaine reduced liver necrosis.
—*In vitro,* glycine betaines in urine contribute to aminoglycoside resistance found in hypertonic urine (13). Bacteria also use betaines as osmolytes; because betaines are in urine and may be accumulated by infecting bacteria, betaines have a role in urinary tract infection.

Risks

ADVERSE REACTIONS

• A case of esophagitis in a 40-year-old woman was attributed to the use of digestive enzymes and betaine HCL (2,124 mg daily) in much higher doses than recommended (14).
• Cocamidopropyl betaine (CAPB) has been linked to allergic contact dermatitis (15) (see questions and answers).

 Dose

COMMON DOSAGE FORMS

• In cystathionine β-synthase deficiency

—Adults: 6 g/day (5)
—Children: 100 to 600 mg/kg/day (5)

 Common Questions and Answers

Q: Isn't betaine in toothpaste?
A: CAPB is an amphoteric surfactant common in shampoos, body shampoos, and many oral hygiene products. It can cause contact dermatitis (15) but appears to be less irritating to oral mucosa than another common detergent, sodium dodecyl sulfate (SDS), also called sodium lauryl sulfate (SLS) (16). A crossover study of 30 patients with recurrent aphthous ulcers found a significantly higher frequency of aphthous ulcers when patients brushed with SLS toothpaste than when they used a CAPB-containing or detergent-free toothpaste (17).
In a double-blind placebo-controlled crossover study of 13 subjects with chronic dry mouth, a 4% betaine toothpaste was associated with a significant decrease in several subjective symptoms of dry mouth. No changes were observed in oral flora or in the appearance of the oral mucosa (18).

Q: What are normal serum levels of betaine?
A: Betaine has low renal clearance and a narrow range of concentrations in blood. In normal human plasma the concentration of glycine betaine is usually between 20 and 70 μmol/L and is often higher in adult males (median 44 μmol/L) than females (34 μmol/L). Concentrations are lower in renal disease (median 28 μmol/L), and urinary excretion is often elevated. Although plasma concentrations are normal in diabetics, urinary excretion is often elevated (19); poor glycemic control may be associated with increased urinary betaine in diabetics (20).

Betel

 10 Second Take

Betel nuts are a commonly used psychoactive masticatory in South Asia and the western Pacific Basin. Usually combined with other ingredients in a "quid," betel nut chewing is linked to oral cancers.

 Basics

LATIN NAME

Areca catechu (information on betel leaf, *Piper betle*, in questions and answers)

FAMILY

Palmae

OTHER COMMON NAMES

Betel nut, areca nut

DESCRIPTION

• Betel nuts are the seeds of fruits produced by the areca palm, a tall, erect palm that can reach 90 feet in height.
• The areca palm has a slender, ringed stem topped with a whorl of feather-like leaves.
• The betel palm is cultivated in India, throughout southeast Asia, the Philippines, Malaysia, Fiji, Guam, and the rest of the Pacific Islands.

PART USED

• Seed

KNOWN ACTIVE CONSTITUENTS

• Betel contains several pyridine alkaloids, predominately arecoline, a central nervous system stimulant.
• Betel is high in tannins. The immature nut (considered superior) may contain up to 47% tannins, primarily polymerized leucocyanidins. The tannin levels decrease as the nut matures. Processing also decreases tannin levels, which are 8% to 15% in the processed nut (1).
• Betel nut is very high in copper (dry weight 205 to 535 nmol/g) (2).

MECHANISM/PHARMACOKINETICS

• Arecoline, the main psychoactive ingredient in betel nut, is a parasympathomimetic agent, acting primarily at muscarinic receptor sites. Paradoxically, arecoline increases heart rate, thus, sympathetic stimulation also occurs (3). In humans, heart rate increases begin within 2 minutes, peak at 4 to 6 minutes, and last 16.8 minutes.

• Betel elevates plasma epinephrine and norepinephrine levels. Betel quid chewing also causes hyperthermia (atropine abolishes the effect) and widespread cortical desynchronization on electroencephalogram (EEG) (4). Lime hydrolyzes arecoline and guvacoline into arecaidine (a less potent cholinergic agonist than arecoline) and guvacine, both of which strongly inhibit γ-aminobutyric acid (GABA) uptake (3).

 Evidence

CLINICAL TRIALS

• An uncontrolled trial of 28 male machine operators tested the effect of betel nut chewing on psychophysiologic variables (5). The only statistically significant effect was an increase in pulse rate. There were no significant changes in blood pressure, visual choice-reaction time, digit span, or hand-eye coordination. Betel quid chewing did not change simple reaction time but did decrease choice reaction time (4).

Schizophrenia

• A cross-sectional study of 70 people with schizophrenia in the Republic of Palau, Micronesia, found that betel-chewers ($n = 40$) scored significantly lower than nonusers (including 18 nonusers and "12 casual users" who used two or fewer betel nuts a day) on the positive and negative scales of the Positive and Negative Syndrome Scales (PANSS) (6). There were no differences in the Extrapyramidal Symptom Rating Scale (ESRS). Among those not receiving antipsychotic medication (10 chewers and 6 nonchewers), chewers scored lower on positive symptoms and total scores, but there was no difference in negative symptoms.

ANIMAL/IN VITRO

• Cancers

—An extract of cured betel nuts produced malignant mesenchymal tumors in all 30 rats tested in one experiment (7). Uncured betel nut extracts, tannin-containing fractions, and arecoline have also been associated with tumors in animals (1,7).

OTHER CLAIMED BENEFITS/ACTIONS

• Antihelminthic
• Aphrodisiac
• Breath freshener
• Fatigue
• Menses induction
• Dentifrice
• Laxative
• Urinary tract disorders
• Appetite stimulant
• Cardiac tonic
• Skin diseases
• Diarrhea
• Antibiotic
• Antifungal

 Risks

ADVERSE REACTIONS

• Acute poisoning/myocardial infarction

—A review of betel poisonings reported to the Taiwan Poison Control Center between 1988 to 1998 identified 17 cases. The most common acute symptoms were tachycardia/palpitations, tachypnea/dyspnea, hypotension, sweating, vomiting, dizziness, and chest discomfort. Three cases of coma (two coingested alcohol, one coingested sedatives) and two myocardial infarctions (one fatal) were reported (8). Both myocardial infarctions occurred in men in their 40s who were habitual betel users and who coingested alcohol (8).
—In Taiwan, a 47-year-old smoker with no known history of cardiovascular disease experienced a myocardial infarction within minutes of chewing his first betel quid, containing "pinang-wang," considered a choice, stronger type of betel nut (9).
—Arecoline has bronchoconstrictive effects and can precipitate acute asthma attacks (10).

• Cancer

—A case-control study of 263 age- and sex-matched pairs of patients with hepatocellular cancer and controls found that betel quid chewing increased the risk of hepatocellular carcinoma (OR 3.49, 95% CI 1.74 to 6.96) in a dose- and duration-dependent manner; an interactive effect was seen with chronic infection with either hepatitis B or C (11).
—Oral cancers have been linked to betel chewing since 1928; esophageal cancers are also linked with betel use (1). Oral squamous cell carcinoma caused by betel quid occurs primarily in the midbuccal mucosa and the lateral borders of the tongue (parts of the mouth directly contacted by the quid) (12). Tannins appear to be the main carcinogen in betel; the presence of tobacco in quids increases the risk of cancer (1). Safrole, found in *Piper betel* flowers (an unusual quid component used in Taiwan) is a known carcinogen, and safrole-like DNA adducts have been identified in betel quid-associated oral squamous cell carcinoma (13).
Tannins may be the prime carcinogen in betel (1), but alkaloids in the nut and nitrosamines arising from various ingredients in the quid may also be factors. Also, the addition of lime increases cell turnover and alkalinizes betel quids to pH 10, possibly increasing the generation of reactive oxygen species. Oral squamous cell cancers were noted to correspond to the site of lime application in 77% of 169 cases in Papua New Guinea (12).

• Precancerous oral lesions

—Betel use causes oral submucous fibrositis, a progressive sclerosing condition characterized by atrophy and dysplasia of the mucosal epithelium, often accompanied by mucosal leukoplakia and loss of lingual papillae (14). Copper released by betel nut when chewed has been proposed as a possible factor in the pathogenesis of oral submucous fibrositis (2).

• Addiction

—Betel appears to be psychologically and physiologically addictive.

• Effects on teeth and gingiva

—Betel stains the saliva a reddish color and stains the teeth, gingiva, and oral mucosa red or black. There is some evidence to suggest that chewing betel helps prevent dental caries, possibly via mechanical cleansing or altering salivary pH. It is also possible that the darkened layer on the teeth forms a barrier to cariogenic agents (14). Although betel is traditionally thought of as beneficial to the teeth and gums, it is difficult to assess possible benefits because there is a high rate of tooth decay and periodontal disease in populations that chew betel.

• Other effects

—Betel chewing causes facial flushing, sweating, a feeling of warmth, and objective increases in skin temperature as well (mean increase of 2°C on the ear and 0.5°C on the forehead) (15). This response was almost completely abolished by atropine and partially inhibited by propranolol, indicating that both sympathetic and parasympathetic mechanisms are involved in the skin thermal response.
—Theoretical concerns include possible exacerbation of Parkinson's disease symptoms [extrapyramidal effects are exacerbated in patients on neuroleptics (see drug interactions)]; its sympathomimetic effects could be a concern for those with cardiovascular disease.

DRUG INTERACTIONS

• Central nervous system (CNS) depressants may increase toxicity.
• Neuroleptics

—Two cases have been reported of schizophrenic patients treated with neuroleptics (flupenthixol and fluphenazine) who developed major exacerbation of extrapyramidal effects after chewing betel nuts on a regular basis (16).

Dose

MODE OF ADMINISTRATION

Masticated in a manner similar to chewing tobacco (complete with spitting)

COMMON DOSAGE FORMS

• Betel nut is used recreationally.
• Doses may be as high as 30 nuts a day, with up to 200 leaves of betel leaf (1).

Common Questions and Answers

Q: How common is the use of betel?
A: Between 10% and 20% of the world's population uses betel (17); its use is common throughout south Asia, the western Pacific basin, and West Africa. Only nicotine, alcohol, and caffeine are more commonly used psychoactive drugs than betel (14).

Q: How is the nut processed?
A: There are diverse ways of preparing betel nut, which may be harvested at the tannin-rich, green, immature stage or after the nut has ripened and turned red. In the Solomon Islands, the raw nut is simply chewed. However, most betel is dried, cured, and/or flavored. Elaborate curing processes—and sometimes serving rituals—are typical of other psychoactive substances used socially, including coffee, tea, and alcohol (14).

Q: Is the betel nut related to the betel leaf?
A: No. Almost all betel nut users wrap their betel nuts in betel leaf (*Piper betle*), also called betel vine or pan, which is not related to betel nut but is of the same genus as kava (*Piper methysticum*). *Piper betle* flower or leaf contains aromatic phenolic compounds that stimulate catecholamine release *in vitro* (3). Betel leaves contain oxalic acid, tannin, other phenols (especially chavicol), and terpenes (1). Betel vine is a slender, perennial vine indigenous to Malaysia but cultivated in other parts of Asia for at least 2,000 years. Epidemiologic studies done in the 1940s in India indicate that chewing tobacco with lime results in greater carcinogenic effect than chewing tobacco with betel quid. Betel leaf extract is antimutagenic against DMBA, benzo[a]pyrene, and several tobacco-specific *N*-nitrosamines *in vitro*, and reduced the incidence of benzo[a]pyrene-induced forestomach tumors in Swiss mice (18). Betel vine is susceptible to insects, bacteria, and fungi; if the plant is treated, its leaves may contain heavy pesticide (and fungicide) residues (1).
Steamed leaves of betel vine have been used topically for facial bleaching. Its use has resulted in contact leukomelanosis; after initial hypopigmentation, hyperpigmentation with confetti-like hypopigmentation developed in 15 Taiwanese women (19).

Q: What else is in a betel quid?
A: Ingredients of quids vary but always include betel nut and betel leaf and usually lime (calcium hydroxide), which is often obtained by burning coral or shells. Tobacco is a common additive to betel quids and has been shown to increase the carcinogenicity of the quid. The carcinogenicity of betel quids could be reduced significantly by increasing the ratio of betel leaf to betel nut and leaving out tobacco (1). In Taiwan, *Piper betle* flowers may be added (13). Astringent substances may also be added to betel quids. Cutch (black or dark catechu) is extracted from the heartwood of the cutch or khair tree, *Acacia catechu*. Katha or catha (not to be confused with *Catha edulis*, or khat) is a more purified form of cutch. Gambier (gambir or pale catechu) comes from the tropical Asian shrub *Uncaria gambir* (1).
Other flavorings may include turmeric, cardamon, fennel, nutmeg, coconut, licorice, or tamarind. A clove may be used to fasten the quid, providing additional flavoring.

Bilberry

 10 Second Take

Bilberry fruits are delicious and harmless; the dried fruit may help diarrhea. There are few data to support the use of bilberry leaf, which may be toxic.

 Basics

LATIN NAME

Vaccinium myrtillus, Vaccinium corymbosum

FAMILY

Ericaceae

OTHER COMMON NAMES

Blueberry, European blueberry (*V. myrtillus*), huckleberry, whortleberry, hurtleberry

DESCRIPTION

Bilberry is a dwarf shrub that grows in sandy areas and woods in the northern United States and in Europe, especially northern and central Europe.

PART USED

Fruit, leaf

KNOWN ACTIVE CONSTITUENTS

- *Fruit:* Tannins and anthocyanosides are the active ingredients in bilberry fruit. Dried bilberries contain 5% to 10% catechins; about 30% invertose; and small amounts of flavonone glycosides and anthocyanosides, especially glycosides of malvidin, cyanidin, and delphinidin (1).
- *Leaf:* The leaf contains 0.8% to 6.7% catechol tannins. It also contains leucoanthocyans, flavonoids, phenolic carboxylic acids, iridoids, small amounts of quinolizidine alkaloids, and trace amounts of arbutin and hydroquinone. The chromium content of the leaves, at 9.0 ppm, is extremely high, and the manganese content is also said to be high (2).

MECHANISM/PHARMACOKINETICS

- *Fruit:* Tannins precipitate proteins. This protein deposition on the surface of mucosal membranes is thought to create a protective film that may decrease the absorption of toxins and blunt the effect of irritants. The predominant tannins in bilberries are catechins, which are water-soluble pentahydroxyflavanol tannins resistant to acid hydrolysis (1).
- *Leaf:* An active glycoside hypoglycemic principle called neomyrtillin was extracted in the 1920s (3). The high percentage of chromium in the leaf may also contribute to this herb's antidiabetic effects (2) (see chromium).

 Evidence

CLINICAL TRIALS

- Bilberry fruit for night vision

—A double-blind placebo-controlled trial in 14 patients with hypertensive or diabetic retinopathy reportedly improved angiographic patterns on ophthalmoscopy after 1 month of ingesting bilberry extract (about 115 mg anthocyanins per day) (4).
—The most recent trial, a double-blind, placebo-controlled, crossover study of young males with good vision tested placebo against bilberry extract (160 mg, containing 25% anthocyanosides, t.i.d.), each given for 3 weeks with a 1-month washout period (5). Outcome measures were changes in night visual acuity and night contrast: There were no differences between the active and placebo treatments.

- Bilberry fruit for dysmenorrhea

—A randomized, double-blind, placebo-controlled trial in 30 women with dys-menorrhea tested a bilberry extract (160 mg containing 25% anthocyanosides b.i.d.) starting 3 days before menses was expected to start (6). The study found significant differences between groups for pelvic and lumbosacral pain, breast tenderness, nausea and vomiting, and a feeling of abdominal heaviness; there was no difference in headache.

- Bilberry leaf for diabetes

—No recent trials were identified. However, bilberry leaf extracts were widely used as hypoglycemic agents before the availability of insulin and were later used to reduce insulin requirements (3). A study published in 1927 found that bilberry leaf extracts reduced glycosuria and postprandial hyperglycemia in adult-onset diabetics but rarely had an effect on juvenile-onset diabetes (7). Apparently, the effects of a single dose of myrtillin, the active principle, could be seen for several weeks. No obvious adverse effects were noted on chronic administration.

ANIMAL/IN VITRO

- An aqueous extract of bilberries significantly reduced copper-mediated oxidation of low density lipoprotein (LDL) particles (8).
- A dried hydroalcoholic extract of bilberry leaf significantly decreased plasma glucose levels and triglycerides in streptozotocin-diabetic rats; subsequent experiments suggest that bilberry may be useful specifically in dyslipidemia associated with impaired clearance of triglyceride-rich lipoproteins (9).
- Pharmacologic tests done in the 1920s showed that myrtillin reduced postprandial hyperglycemia and glucosuria in normal dogs and reduced glucosuria in pancreatectomized dogs (10). *Vaccinium* anthocyanosides also may reduce diabetes-induced capillary damage (10).

OTHER CLAIMED BENEFITS/ACTIONS

- *Fruit:* diarrhea, dysentery (dried fruit).
- *Leaf:* vision improvement, retinal disease, other microvascular disease, strengthens capillaries, venous insufficiency, prevention of postoperative bleeding, diabetes, rheumatism, gastrointestinal problems, kidney problems, hemorrhoids, circulatory disorders, heart conditions, skin astringent (topical).

 Risks

ADVERSE REACTIONS

- *Fruit:* none
- *Leaf:* no adverse events have been reported. However, large or long-term doses of leaf extracts should be avoided, given the data on animal toxicity.

PREGNANCY/LACTATION

- *Fruit:* safe to use during pregnancy or lactation
- *Leaf:* should be avoided during pregnancy and lactation

ANIMAL TOXICITY

- *Fruit:* no studies identified
- *Leaf:* High doses or prolonged use of bilberry leaf in animals caused cachexia, anemia, icterus, and excitation. Death can occur at doses of 1.5 g/kg/day (2).

 Dose

COMMON DOSAGE FORMS

- *Dried fruit:* 4 to 8 g taken with fluid t.i.d. or 5 to 20 g crushed berry as decoction or cold macerate.
- *Bilberry leaf* is usually taken in tea (it should not be taken for prolonged periods).

 Common Questions and Answers

Q: Why are dried rather than fresh berries used for diarrhea?
A: Drying concentrates and increases the tannin content. Apparently tannin precursors convert to tannins during the drying process (2).

Q: What are other tannin-containing herbs?
A: Plants containing tannins are commonly used to treat diarrhea. Guava, for example, is used for this purpose in Mexico and Thailand. The BRAT diet (bananas, rice, applesauce, and tea), recommended by North American physicians for childhood diarrhea, makes use of the tannins in tea. The acronym enables physicians to enjoy the moment between informing parents that their child should be put on the BRAT diet and explaining what the acronym means.

Biotin

 10 Second Take

Biotin is a benign B vitamin. Deficiency, uncommon in the general population, causes alopecia. Patients on long-term anticonvulsants should be supplemented.

 Basics

DESCRIPTION

- Biotin is a water-soluble B vitamin necessary for energy metabolism.
- It is an essential cofactor for four CO_2-fixing carboxylase enzymes, including acetyl-CoA carboxylase, pyruvate carboxylase, propionyl-CoA carboxylase, and β-methylcrotonyl CoA carboxylase. Each of these catalyzes a critical step in intermediary metabolism. The U.S. population consumes about 28 to 42 μg/day of biotin, and the Western European population consumes 50 to 100 μg/day.
- It is not stored in the body.

FOOD SOURCES

- Biotin is widely distributed in foods.
- Good food sources include liver (about 100 μg/100 g), egg yolk (about 50 μg/ 100 g), yeast (about 100 μg/100 g), soybeans (about 60 μg/100 g), cereals, legumes (especially sprouted legumes), and nuts.
- The only vegetables that are significant sources of biotin are mushrooms, cauliflower, and sea vegetables (1).
- Intestinal bacteria produce a significant amount of biotin (2).

MAIN FUNCTIONS/PHARMACOKINETICS

- Biotin acts as a coenzyme in four carboxylases that are involved in "fixation" of CO_2 in animal cells, gluconeogenesis and reversal of glycolysis, fatty acid synthesis, and leucine degradation.
- Oral doses of biotin are 100% bioavailable, even in large doses, but administration of a single large dose may increase renal losses (3).

 Evidence

CLINICAL TRIALS

- Brittle nails

—A trial of biotin (2.5 mg p.o. q.d.) in women with brittle nails found improved morphology and a 25% increase in nail thickness, assessed by electron microscopy (4).

OTHER CLAIMED BENEFITS/ACTIONS

Increases hair growth

 Clinical Considerations

DEFICIENCY SIGNS AND SYMPTOMS

- Scaly dermatitis (especially around the eyes, nose, and mouth).
- Alopecia, often with loss of hair color.
- Depression.
- Lassitude, lethargy.
- Hallucinations.
- Paresthesias.
- *In infants:* periorificial dermatitis, conjunctivitis, alopecia (including eyebrows and eyelashes), hypotonia, withdrawn affect, developmental delay.
- Biotin deficiency is uncommon in normal populations; it can be induced by biotinidase deficiency, excessive intake of raw egg white, malabsorption syndromes, or prolonged use of total parenteral nutrition (TPN) without biotin supplementation. Biotinidase deficiency, an inborn error of metabolism, results in an inability to release biotin from degraded carboxylases. This recycling mechanism is important for biotin conservation, so biotin deficiency can result (5).
- "Egg white injury" disease is biotin deficiency induced by consumption of raw egg white, which contains the glycoprotein avidin (which binds biotin at four sites and prevents its absorption) (6).
- Marginal biotin deficiency is not uncommon during pregnancy. In several animals, biotin deficiency is teratogenic at levels that do not obviously affect the pregnant animal (7).

FACTORS DECREASING AVAILABILITY/ABSORPTION

- Holoenzyme synthetase deficiency
- Biotinidase deficiency
- Propionicacidemia
- β-methylcrotonyl glycinuria
- Alcoholism
- Inflammatory bowel disease
- Malabsorption syndromes
- Excessive intake of raw egg white
- Anticonvulsants
- Antibiotics

LABORATORY TESTS

- Blood biotin levels are not an early or sensitive indicator of impaired biotin status. Biotin deficiency results in increased 3-hydroxy-isovaleric acid excretion, decreased bisnorbiotin excretion, and accumulation of odd-chain fatty acids in plasma. Biotin deficiency is best established retrospectively based on whether symptoms improve with biotin administration (8).
- Whole blood biotin (normal values) 200 to 500 pg/mL.
- Urinary biotin (normal values) 6 to 100 μg/24 hours.

Risks

ADVERSE REACTIONS

• Toxicity has not been seen in patients receiving up to 200 mg orally and 20 mg intravenously for treatment.

DRUG INTERACTIONS

• Antibiotics

—Large or long-term doses of antibiotics can decrease biotin levels in humans, probably because the gut bacterial source of biotin is eliminated. Commonly used doses for a week or less are thought to have little effect.

• Anticonvulsants

—Long-term anticonvulsant therapy can lead to biotin depletion severe enough to interfere with amino acid metabolism. Phenobarbital, phenytoin, carbamazepine, and primidone have all been implicated (see questions and answers).

• Lipoic acid

—Biotin and lipoic acid are structurally similar, and potentially the two could compete for uptake (5).

 Dose

ADEQUATE INTAKE

Infants and Children
0 to 6 months	5 μg/day
7 to 11 months	6 μg/day
1 to 3 years	8 μg/day
4 to 8 years	12 μg/day

Males
9 to 13 years	20 μg/day
14 to 18 years	25 μg/day
19 to 50 years	30 μg/day
51 + years	30 μg/day

Females
9 to 13 years	20 μg/day
14 to 18 years	25 μg/day
19 to 50 years	30 μg/day
51 + years	30 μg/day
Pregnant	30 μg/day
Lactating	35 μg/day

CORRECTING DEFICIENCY

1 to 10 mg p.o. q.d.
100 μg. q.d. i.v.

• Oral doses are well absorbed; divided doses are recommended because a single large dose may increase renal losses (3).

 Common Questions and Answers

Q: Are the symptoms of biotin deficiency and biotinidase deficiency the same?
A: Not quite. Although both result in periorificial dermatitis, alopecia, conjunctivitis, ataxia, and developmental delay, biotinidase deficiency can also cause seizures, irreversible neurosensory hearing loss, and optic atrophy, which are not seen in biotin deficiency (there is one case of cerebral atrophy and an apparent stretching of the optic nerve in a patient with biotin deficiency) (8). Biotinidase deficiency may cause additional problems because of the breakdown of biotin-dependent enzymes, thus causing accumulation of metabolites.

Q: Why do anticonvulsants induce biotin deficiency?
A: There are several mechanisms that may account for this; the process may be multifactorial. Primidone and carbamazepine inhibit biotin uptake from the intestine. Phenobarbital, phenytoin, and carbamazepine displace biotin from biotinidase, which may affect transport, cellular uptake, or availability of biotin. Increased excretion of metabolites suggest that anticonvulsants may also accelerate biotin catabolism (8).

Q: Is there a connection between biotin deficiency and sudden infant death syndrome (SIDS)?
A: Two researchers have hypothesized that biotin deficiency could be related to SIDS via a pathogenic mechanism similar to that which causes a fatal hypoglycemic disease in chicks. Apparently hepatic levels of biotin are lower in the livers of babies who died of SIDS when compared with those who died from other causes. This is only a hypothesis; much more work would be needed to establish whether or not there is a connection (8).

Black Cohosh

 10 Second Take

Black cohosh may be helpful for menopausal symptoms but should not be used for longer than 6 months. Long-term effects on breast and endometrium have not been established.

 Basics

LATIN NAME

Cimicifuga racemosa (L.) Nutt. or *Actaea racemosa* L.

FAMILY

Ranunculaceae

OTHER COMMON NAMES

Black snakeroot, bugbane, bugwort, rattleroot, rattletop, rattleweed, macrotys

DESCRIPTION

• Black cohosh is a perennial woodland plant with small white flowers arranged in spikes.
• Native to North America, it also grows in Europe and north Asia.
• It was used in North American Indian medicine. Insects avoid it, which accounts for some of its common names.

PART USED

Root, rhizome

KNOWN ACTIVE CONSTITUENTS

• Formononetin, a phytoestrogen, was reported in a methanol extract of the dried rhizome of *C. racemosa* (1); more recent analyses have not identified formononetin (2).
• A recently identified compound, fukinolic acid (2-*E*-caffeoylfukiic acid) is estrogenic (see animal/*in vitro* toxicity) (3). Other apparent active compounds are triterpene glycosides (including actein and cimicifugoside), resins (15% to 20%, including cimicifugin), caffeic, and isoferulic acids (4).

MECHANISM/PHARMACOKINETICS

• It is unclear whether black cohosh is estrogenic (see animal/*in vitro* estrogenicity studies). In humans, a resinous component, acteina, reportedly causes peripheral vasodilation and increased peripheral blood flow in patients with peripheral arterial disease (5).

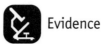 Evidence

CLINICAL TRIALS

• Hot flashes, menopausal symptoms

—A recent randomized, double-blind, placebo-controlled trial in 85 breast cancer survivors (69 completed) found that black cohosh reduced excessive sweating but not hot flashes. Subjects (59 on tamoxifen) took one tablet twice daily of placebo or black cohosh (Remifemin, not identified as such in the article) for 2 months. (6). Hot flash frequency and intensity decreased in both groups with no significant difference between groups. Excessive sweating decreased significantly more in the treatment group than in the placebo group. Other symptoms (palpitations, headaches, poor sleep, depression, irritability) improved equally in both groups; health and well-being scores did not change in either group. Two months is relatively short for this kind of trial.
—A 6-month treatment-controlled study in 60 women who had undergone hysterectomy but maintained at least one ovary compared Remifemin to three estrogen regimens: estriol (1 mg/day), conjugated estrogens (1.25 mg/day), or estrogen-progestin therapy (estradiol 2 mg and norethisterone acetate 1 mg) (7). Black cohosh was equivalent to the other treatments at 4, 8, 12, and 24 weeks, as measured by a modified Kupperman index.
—Another randomized, placebo-controlled trial in 80 menopausal women compared Remifemin (4 tablets/day) to placebo or conjugated estrogens 0.625 mg/day (8). At 12 weeks, Kupperman index and Hamilton anxiety scores were significantly lower in the treated groups compared with the placebo group; black cohosh was somewhat better than estrogen treatment. This is one of the few studies that asked women about hot flashes separately from other symptoms. Daily hot flashes decreased from 4.9 to 0.7 in the Remifemin group, from 5.2 to 3.2 in the estrogen group, and from 5.1 to 3.1 in the placebo group.
—An open, randomized, 12-week study of 60 women compared Remifemin liquid (40 drops b.i.d.) to conjugated estrogens 0.625 mg/day or diazepam 2 mg/day. All treatments improved the Kupperman index, a depression scale, and an anxiety scale (9).
—A 6-month study testing two different doses of black cohosh extract (40 mg or 127 mg/day) found no advantage to the higher dose (10).

• Hormone levels

—Three of four studies show that black cohosh does not affect luteinizing hormone (LH) or follicle-stimulating hormone (FSH). A 6-month study of 152 women using different doses of Remifemin tablets (40 mg or 127 mg/day) found no changes in LH, FSH, prolactin, estradiol, or sex hormone binding globulin (11). The Jacobson trial found no change in LH or FSH levels in 51 participants who underwent blood tests (6). Remifemin 4 tablets/day did not affect LH or FSH levels in the Lehmann-Willenbrock study (7).
—Only one trial, in 110 women with menopausal symptoms, found that those treated with Remifemin (8 mg extract/day 8 weeks) had significantly lower mean LH levels than a control group; FSH levels were unchanged (12). However, the report of this study does not include levels of hormones drawn before the study began, so the two groups may have had different baseline LH levels.

• Vaginal effects

—One placebo-controlled, double-blind trial of black cohosh in 80 women showed estrogenic changes in vaginal cells at 12 weeks (8), but another study of different doses of black cohosh (40 mg or 127 mg/day) in 152 women found no changes in vaginal cells at 6 months (10).

OTHER CLAIMED BENEFITS/ACTIONS

• Labor preparation, induction, and facilitation (specifically strengthening or restarting contractions)
• Cough
• Induction of menses
• Dysmenorrhea
• Premenstrual syndrome
• Rheumatoid arthritis
• Sciatica
• Tinnitus
• Sedative

Risks

ADVERSE REACTIONS

• Adverse birth outcome

—Neurologic complications were reported in a post-dates baby after labor induction with a mixture of black cohosh and blue cohosh given during a home birth (13). After a normal labor, a 3,840 g female was born with no spontaneous breathing. Mechanical ventilation was necessary, and hypoxic injury of the basal ganglia and parasagittal area was demonstrated by computed tomography (CT) scan; at 3 months of age, the baby had lower limb spasticity and required nasogastric feeds. Blue cohosh, which contains the vasoconstrictive and oxytocic glycoside caulosaponin, is more likely to be associated with this adverse event than black cohosh.

• Endometrial hyperplasia

—The Jacobson study notes one case each of endometrial hyperplasia, vaginal bleeding, hysterectomy, and dilation and curettage (D&C) among black cohosh-treated women (all were also taking tamoxifen) (6). Although vaginal bleeding and endometrial hyperplasia have been associated with tamoxifen, no information is provided that would reassure the reader that black cohosh did not contribute to the adverse event (see questions and answers).

• Other

—One case of arrhythmia (not otherwise defined, but classed as a "minor" adverse event) was reported in a trial of black cohosh in a black cohosh-treated patient who was not taking tamoxifen (6).
—Black cohosh can cause stomach discomfort or frontal headaches (4).

• Estrogenicity studies (Animal/*In vitro*)

—Increased uterine weight was seen in two studies of ovariectomized mice given black cohosh (14,15); two other studies showed no estrogenic effects in either mice given oral doses (16,17) or rats given injected doses (16).
—*In vitro* studies are mixed, but most show no estrogenicity. Recent tests of black cohosh in *in vitro* assays showed no estrogenic activity (17,18,19). Six *in vitro* cell culture studies (two reported only as abstracts) found that extracts of black cohosh did not stimulate the growth of breast cancer cells (17,19–23); four found inhibition of growth at some doses (19,21–23). Two other studies found that black cohosh significantly increased the growth of breast cancer cells compared with untreated control cells. One found that the effect was similar to 17 beta-estradiol (14). Another study (reported as an abstract), found that ethanolic extracts of black cohosh (0.1 to 10 μg/mL) significantly increased the number of MCF-7 cells; a higher 100 μg dose had no effect (24). Adding an estrogen antagonist (ICI 182,780) abolished the proliferative effect of black cohosh. A constituent of black cohosh, fukinolic acid, increased growth of MCF-7 breast cancer cells; again, the effect was similar to estradiol (3).
—The only *in vivo* study identified (reported as an abstract) tested Remifemin in five groups of rats with DMBA-induced mammary tumors (25). Rats were ovariectomized after 5 to 9 weeks of neoplastic growth, and then were given no treatment, oral mestranol (450 μg/kg), or Remifemin in doses equivalent to 1×, 10×, or 100× human dosage. Ovariectomy caused tumor regression in all animals; mestranol but not black cohosh increased tumor growth after ovariectomy. No estrogenic effects were noted on histologic examination of uterine tissue; prolactin, FSH, and LH were unaffected. Conclusions cannot be drawn from this abstract without seeing a more complete presentation of data.

PREGNANCY/LACTATION

• May precipitate labor
• See also adverse effects

Dose

COMMON DOSAGE FORMS

• *Dried root or rhizome:* 40 to 200 mg/day.
• *Liquid extract:* (1:2) 1.5 to 3.0 mL/day.
• *Tincture:* (1:10, 60% ethyl alcohol) 0.4 to 2 mL/day (or equivalent to 40 mg root or rhizome/day) (4).
• *Ointments* or *salves* containing black cohosh have also been used.
• Commercial black cohosh preparations are usually standardized to triterpene saponins that include actein and cimicifugoside.
• Remifemin contains 20 mg of black cohosh extract per tablet and is standardized to 1 mg triterpenes, calculated as 26-deoxyactein (erroneously reported in many sources as 27-deoxyactein) per tablet. The current recommended dose is 20 mg twice daily. *Note: Both the formulation and dosage of Remifemin have changed over time. First a liquid, now tablets, the dosage of extract in each tablet has increased from 2 mg to 20 mg. Studies done with earlier versions may not be applicable to the current version.*

Common Questions and Answers

Q: Is it safe to use black cohosh indefinitely?
A: Black cohosh traditionally has not been used long term, and all published studies have only followed women for 6 months or less. There are no adequate published human data regarding long-term safety. Two studies, published only as abstracts, note no change in endometrial thickness, but longer, adequately reported studies must be done. One study administered Remifemin, approximately 136 mg/day for a mean of 98 days, to 28 postmenopausal women (26); the second administered *Cimicifuga* extracts (otherwise unidentified) to 50 postmenopausal women for 6 months (27). Neither noted a change in endometrial thickness. *In vitro* and in *in vivo* estrogenicity tests are mixed. Although no cases of endometrial carcinoma have been reported, I am concerned about unopposed stimulation of the endometrium with long-term use. Phytoestrogens in black cohosh are not the same as phytoestrogens present in beans and grains and may not be as benign.

Black Haw and Cramp Bark

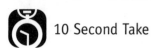 10 Second Take

 Basics

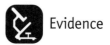 Evidence

Black haw and cramp bark are benign plants used primarily to treat dysmenorrhea.

Basics

LATIN NAME

Viburnum prunifolium L. and *Viburnum opulus* L. Aiton

FAMILY

Caprifoliaceae

OTHER COMMON NAMES

Black haw: Sweet viburnum, American sloe, stagbush, sheep-berry, nanny-berry bush, beach haw, sweet haw
Cramp bark: guelder rose, snowball tree, red elder, rose elder, high bush cranberry

DESCRIPTION

• Tall shrubs, native to North America, black haw and cramp bark are both related to the elder. Both have large, nearly flat-topped heads of white flowers.
• Black haw has blue-black fruit; it grows in woodland and thickets, as well as being planted as an ornamental.
• Cramp bark grows 5 to 10 feet high and has deep red edible but bitter berry clusters.

PART USED

Dried bark from branch, trunk, or root

KNOWN ACTIVE CONSTITUENTS

• *Black haw:* Contains the biflavone amentoflavone (4,5,7-trihydroxyflavone), four iridoid glucosides, triterpenes (α- and β-amyrin, oleanolic acid, ursolic acid), coumarins (scopoletin, scopolin, aesculetin), organic acids, and hydroxycinnamic acid derivatives and small amounts of alkaloids, arbutin, β-sitosterin, and tannins (1,2). Black haw contains about 0.2% salicin (3).
• *Cramp bark:* Contains a sesquiterpene dialdehyde fraction called viopudial. Also DL-catechin, epicatechin, and other phenolics; triterpenes (α- and β-amyrin, oleanolic acid, ursolic acid); D-glucosides; volatile oil; fatty acids; hydroxycinnamic acid derivatives; arbutin; esculetin; iridoid glycoside esters; scopolin; and scopoletin.

MECHANISM/PHARMACOKINETICS

• Scopoletin and aesculetin in black haw are spasmolytics, but these occur in such small amounts that they are unlikely to be important (1,2). The methanolic extract contains compounds that act on uterine musculature but are apparently not sympathomimetics (4).

Evidence

CLINICAL TRIALS

• No clinical trials identified.

ANIMAL/IN VITRO

• Black haw extracts have yielded conflicting results in isolated uterine muscle tests; most show a spasmolytic effect of black haw extract (1,2). Most of these reports predate 1970; some date to 1916. The picture is even more confusing because black haw was commonly adulterated with *Acer spicatum,* which may have confounded published reports (1,2). Intravenous administration of black haw extract (500 μg/kg to 10 mg/kg) or fractions increased blood pressure in normotensive rats (1,2).
• A sesquiterpene dialdehyde fraction called viopudial from cramp bark has uterine antispasmodic activity in isolated smooth muscle preparations; viopudial also lowers heart rate and blood pressure in rats, dogs, and cats. Aqueous extracts of bark from several *Viburnum* species, including *V. opulus,* had a cardiotonic effect on isolated frog and dog hearts (1,2).

OTHER CLAIMED BENEFITS/ACTIONS

Black haw

• Dysmenorrhea
• Amenorrhea
• Menorrhagia
• Preventing miscarriage
• Morning sickness
• Menopausal complaints

Cramp bark

• Dysmenorrhea
• Amenorrhea
• Easing labor
• Muscle spasms
• Asthma
• Hypertension
• Fibromyalgia
• Pelvic pain
• Preterm labor
• Bedwetting
• Topical oil preparations may be used for leg cramps, muscle soreness, and migraines

Risks

- No risks identified.
- There is a theoretical concern that oxalates in black haw (not cramp bark) could increase the risk of calcium oxalate kidney stones (5) (see questions and answers).

 Dose

COMMON DOSAGE FORMS

Cramp bark

- *Fluid extract:* (1:1, 45% to 55% ethanol) 10 to 30 drops daily (adolescents); up to 1/2 tsp several times daily (adult)
- *Powder:* 1 to 4 g
- *Infusion* or *decoction:* 1 g herb/cup, b.i.d. or t.i.d.
- *Tincture:* 2 to 4 mL t.i.d.
- For dysmenorrhea, treatment is usually begun 2 to 3 days before expected menses

Black haw

- *Infusion:* 1 g b.i.d. to t.i.d.
- *Tincture* (1:5) 5 to 10 mL t.i.d.
- *Fluid extract* (1:1) 1 to 4 mL several times daily

 Common Questions and Answers

Q: What is the connection between black haw and kidney stones?
A: Black haw contains oxalates, and it is thought that dietary intake of oxalates can increase the risk of calcium oxalate kidney stones. I'm not particularly worried about black haw predisposing patients to nephrolithiasis for two reasons. The first is that black haw is used mainly to treat dysmenorrhea and so is not commonly taken for long periods. The second reason is that black haw is not extremely high in oxalates anyway. Oxalates are a common dietary component of beans, berries, greens, peanuts, wheat germ, many vegetables, and chocolate. In someone who is taking black haw regularly, it may make sense to take each dose with a calcium supplement. Intake of calcium with oxalate-containing meals may be protective; calcium binds to oxalates in the gastrointestinal tract, thus reducing absorption.

Q: What is the difference between the two species of *Viburnum*?
A: They are generally used for the same purposes; herbalists generally consider cramp bark (*V. opulus*) to be a weaker and safer herb.

Bloodroot

 10 Second Take

Bloodroot has antibacterial properties and may be helpful in mild periodontal disease, but studies are mixed. Some constituents may have caustic effects. Anticancer effects have not been proven.

 Basics

LATIN NAME

Sanguinaria canadensis L.

FAMILY

Papaveraceae

OTHER COMMON NAMES

Red root, tetterwort, Indian red paint, red puccoon

DESCRIPTION

- Bloodroot is a perennial herb that grows in rich woods.
- It is commonly distributed in North America.
- In spring, a distinctive, lobed, single leaf and white flower arise from each bud of the root stalk.
- The entire plant (but especially the root and rhizome), when broken, releases an orange-red fluid.

PART USED

Dried rhizome, root

KNOWN ACTIVE CONSTITUENTS

- Bloodroot contains benzophenanthridine alkaloids; the highest concentrations occur in the rhizome.
- Sanguinarine and its derivatives are the most common alkaloids (50%); other alkaloids include chelerythrine (25%), sanguilutine, sanguirubine, chelirubine, and chelilutine (1).

MECHANISM/PHARMACOKINETICS

- Sanguinarine is an aromatized, heterocyclic, iminium ion; its biologic activity is based on nucleophilic substitution; quaternary nitrogen compounds bind readily to proteins and lipids, rendering this compound active across a broad range of organisms (2).
- Sanguinarine has antiinflammatory activity and inhibits neutral protease enzyme activity.

 Evidence

CLINICAL TRIALS

- Periodontal disease

—There are a number of trials of Sanguinaria oral rinses and toothpaste for periodontal disease, and Sanguinaria-containing products are commonly sold. Most earlier trials were methodologically flawed and have been omitted here; even the more recent trials are rarely double-blind. Results from trials are mixed. There is little to indicate that Sanguinaria-containing products are effective in severe disease; it is possible that these products are beneficial in milder cases or as an adjunctive treatment.
—In a randomized double-blind trial in 34 patients with periodontal disease, those receiving Sanguinaria-containing toothpaste and oral rinse as an adjunct to scaling, root planing, and oral hygiene instruction showed no additional improvement over standard therapy alone (3).
—In a 6-month double-blind placebo-controlled parallel-design trial in 120 participants found that Sanguinaria/zinc oral rinses (with or without Sanguinaria toothpaste) were more effective than placebo for plaque and gingival inflammation (4).
—In a recent 14-week controlled trial, 60 patients with periodontitis received scaling and root planing and were followed by a 2-week oral care regimen that included 0.2% chlorhexidine gluconate oral rinse. After that, patients were randomized to toothpaste and oral rinses with or without sanguinarine. At 14 weeks, patients in the Sanguinaria group had 32% fewer bleeding sites than the control group (5).
—A randomized 9-month trial in 180 patients with moderate to severe periodontitis found that subgingival administration of doxycycline hyclate was more effective than 5% sanguinarine chloride at all time points (6). Two multicenter trials failed to show a consistent benefit of 5% sanguinarine (in a biodegradable delivery system) over control (7).
—Combined use of Sanguinaria-containing oral rinse and toothpaste was tested against placebo in a 60 participants with moderate levels of plaque and gingivitis. At 28 weeks, scores in the Sanguinaria group were 21% lower for plaque, 25% lower for gingivitis, and 43% lower for bleeding on probing (8).
—A 3-week crossover trial of dental students compared two oral rinses, one containing Sanguinaria and zinc and one containing chlorhexidine gluconate (tap water was used as a control) found an antiplaque effect only for chlorhexidine (9).

ANIMAL/IN VITRO

- Sanguinarine differentially reduces viability of human epidermoid carcinoma A431 cells compared to its effects on normal human epidermal keratinocytes (NHEKs) (10).
- In isolated guinea pig atria, sanguinarine has a concentration-dependent positive inotropic effect (11). It prolongs ventricular refractory period (2).
- In vitro, Sanguinaria inhibits neutrophil chemotaxis, oxidative metabolism, and degranulation (12). In vitro, sanguinarine has antibacterial activity against both gram-positive and gram-negative bacteria, antifungal activity, and activity against trichomonas (13).

OTHER CLAIMED BENEFITS/ACTIONS

- Sore throats
- Fevers
- Burns
- Skin cancers
- Warts
- Condyloma acuminata
- Nasal polyps
- Breast cancer
- Expectorant
- Bronchitis, asthma, emphysema, croup
- Emetic

Risks

ADVERSE REACTIONS

In trials of oral rinses, occasional soft tissue irritation has been noted.

ANIMAL TOXICITY

• Reproductive and toxicologic studies in rats and rabbits found that maternal oral toxicity levels were 60 mg/kg/day in rats and 25 mg/kg/day in rabbits (14). Subchronic effects of sanguinarine include anorexia and diarrhea (2). No developmental toxicity was observed, although increased postimplantation loss and reduced body weight in offspring were noted at doses that caused maternal toxicity (14). *Sanguinaria* extract administered orally to rats was not carcinogenic (13).

• The acute LD_{50} of sanguinarine in rats is 1,658 mg/kg; intravenously the acute LD_{50} is 29 mg/kg. The acute oral LD_{50} of two alkaloid extracts was 1,440 mg/kg for one and 1,250 mg/kg for the other (15). No toxic effects were noted in rats fed 150 ppm sanguinarine in the diet or treated with sanguinarine by gavage (up to 0.6 mg/kg body weight) for 30 days. The acute dermal LD_{50} in rabbits is >200 mg/kg (15).

 Dose

COMMON DOSAGE FORMS

• *Tincture:* 1 to 2 mL t.i.d.
• *Decoction:* (1 tsp rhizome in 1 cup water, brought to a boil and then allowed to steep 10 minutes)
• *Poultice* or *paste*

 Common Questions and Answers

Q: How is bloodroot used to treat cancers?
A: It is applied topically as a salve or paste. "Fell's treatment," popular in the 19th century, was a mixture of bloodroot, flour, water, and zinc chloride (16). If the tumor had broken through skin, the paste was applied topically. If not, nitric acid was used to erode the skin and expose the tumor, after which the paste was applied. Because this process was slow, Fell also made incisions through eschar 1/2 in. apart and inserted strips of cotton coated with paste into the incisions daily. *Sanguinaria* ointment was also applied to affected lymph glands, and Fell also gave small amounts internally, sometimes combined with arsenic, water hemlock extract, or dandelion extract. It is claimed that masses often were destroyed within 10 to 14 days. Fell published a treatise in 1857 claiming that remissions or cures were seen in 25 cases (mainly breast cancer) (17). *Sanguinaria* was part of a fixative paste used in Moh's chemosurgery technique for excising basal-cell and squamous-cell carcinomas on the nose; this paste was in use until at least 1962 (18).

Q: What is the connection between sanguinarine and epidemic dropsy?
A: Tropical dropsy or epidemic dropsy was common in India from the 1880s to the 1930s. It was characterized by gastrointestinal disturbances, lower extremity edema, cardiac hypertrophy, and anemia and a distinctive form of glaucoma in about 25% of those affected. The disease was linked to the consumption of Mexican prickly-poppy (*Argemone mexicana* L.) seed oil, which contains small amounts of sanguinarine (berberine, allocryptopine, and protopine are the predominant alkaloids). Although initial experiments showed increased ocular pressure with sanguinarine, later research demonstrated only transient changes in intraocular pressure with no effect on steady-state fluid dynamics (2).

Blue Cohosh

 10 Second Take

Blue cohosh contains alkaloids that are cardiotoxic and irritating to mucous membranes. Adverse birth outcomes have been associated with its use as a labor promoter.

 Basics

LATIN NAME

Caulophyllum thalictroides (L.) Michx.

FAMILY

Berberidaceae

OTHER COMMON NAMES

Papoose root

DESCRIPTION

• A perennial plant with greenish yellow flowers and blue berries, the leaves and stems of blue cohosh appear to be coated with a bluish film.
• Common in eastern North America, it favors moist, rich woodlands.

PART USED

Root, rhizome

KNOWN ACTIVE CONSTITUENTS

• The leaves and seeds contain glycosides and alkaloids, including anagyrine, baptifoline, magniflorine, and *N*-methylcytisine (caulophylline).
• Also contains caulosaponin, citrullol, leontin, gum, resin, and phytosterol (1).
• Blue cohosh rhizomes may contain up to 290 ppm anagyrine, and dietary supplements may contain 5 to 850 ppm *N*-methylcytisine (2).

MECHANISM/PHARMACOKINETICS

• *N*-Methylcytisine appears to have nicotinic effects, elevating blood pressure and stimulating both respiration and intestinal motility, although it is far less toxic than nicotine (3).
• No information on human pharmacokinetics is available.

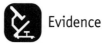 Evidence

CLINICAL TRIALS

No clinical trials identified.

ANIMAL/IN VITRO

• Caulosaponin has been shown to constrict coronary vessels in rats and carotid arteries in cattle and hogs; it causes contractions in isolated rat intestine. Blue cohosh extract causes tonic contraction in isolated rat or guinea pig uteri. The aglycone of caulosaponin also has oxytocic effects.
• In rabbits, methylcytisine demonstrates hyperglycemic action when given intravenously (4).

OTHER CLAIMED BENEFITS/ACTIONS

• Amenorrhea
• Abortifacient
• Menses induction
• Threatened abortion
• Dysmenorrhea
• Uterine atony
• Rheumatic pain
• Arthritis
• Labor pain

Risks

ADVERSE REACTIONS

• Nicotinic toxicity

A case of nicotinic toxicity was reported in a 21-year-old female, 6 weeks pregnant, attempting to achieve abortion by taking 10–20 doses of blue cohosh tincture (along with 15 cups/day of slippery elm tea and vaginally inserted parsley dipped in slippery elm tea) (4a). She presented with abdominal pain, bilious vomiting, tachycardia, hyperthermia, abdominal muscle fasciculations, and diffuse muscular weakness. Symptoms resolved with intravenous hydration. Ultrasound revealed a viable pregnancy.

• Adverse birth outcomes (see also pregnancy/lactation and questions and answers)

—Myocardial infarction and severe congestive heart failure in an infant was associated with maternal ingestion of three times the recommended dose of blue cohosh for about a month before parturition (5). The infant had symptoms consistent with cardiogenic shock and was on a respirator for 3 weeks. At 2 years of age the child still had cardiomegaly and reduced left ventricular function. No analysis of the preparation was performed, so botanical identity remains unconfirmed.
—A case report notes neurologic complications in a post-term baby after labor induction with a mixture of black cohosh and blue cohosh (6). The pregnancy had been uneventful and labor apparently normal. Caulosaponin and caulophyllosaponin are known to have vasoconstrictive and cardiotoxic effects.
—The Food and Drug Administration (FDA) Special Nutritionals Adverse Event Monitoring System database contains two additional cases, including stroke in an infant and aplastic anemia in another after maternal ingestion of blue cohosh.

• Children have been poisoned by eating the seeds (7).
• Black cohosh is a mucous membrane irritant. Severe gastrointestinal pain may be caused by ingesting leaves and seeds, presumably because of glycoside content (4).
• Dermatitis has been reported from handling the rootstock (4).

ANIMAL TOXICITY

• For methylcytisine, the LD_{50} in mice is 21 mg/kg intravenously, 51 mg/kg intraperitoneally, and >500 mg/kg orally. Intravenous LD_{50} for caulosaponin is 11.8 mg/kg in mice and 20.3 mg/kg in rats. Large doses result in increased activity, ataxia, and terminal clonic convulsions. When 5 mg/kg/day was administered subcutaneously to rats, neither gross toxicity nor gross pathologic changes in internal organs were noted. Histologic examination revealed slight edema in renal tubules, thickened arterial walls of the spleen, and a toxic effect on cardiac muscle. Oral doses of caulosaponin and caulophyllosaponin (0.1 g) in small cats showed no adverse effect other than a mild purgative effect (4).
• A 0.5% solution of caulosaponin in propylene glycol resulted in marked inflammation in the rabbit eye, when compared with propylene glycol alone (4).
• The alkaloid anagyrine, which occurs in blue cohosh root, also occurs in lupine, and overconsumption of lupine by cows has been linked to a congenital deformity called "crooked calf disease." A dose-related effect can be experimentally produced in cattle; no effect was seen in sheep or hamsters.

PREGNANCY/LACTATION (SEE ALSO RISKS)

• A survey of 172 certified nurse-midwives (CNMs) found that almost two-thirds of the 90 CNMs who used labor-stimulating herbs used blue cohosh and almost half used black cohosh (8). Twenty-one percent of the CNMs who used these herbs reported complications, including nausea, meconium, and transient fetal tachycardia. (The use of blue cohosh during pregnancy may cause abortion or premature labor.)

 Dose

COMMON DOSAGE FORMS

• *Dried rhizome/root:* 0.3 to 1.0 g in capsules or infusion t.i.d.
• *Liquid extract:* [1:1 in 70% ethanol (EtOH)] 0.5 to 1.0 mL t.i.d.

 Common Questions and Answers

Q: What is the relationship between black cohosh and blue cohosh?
A: The two are not related botanically (cohosh means rough root, which describes both) but are often used together for menstrual disorders and childbirth.

Q: Are there any reports of birth defects associated with blue cohosh?
A: No. However, there is a case report of congenital malformation (vascular anomalies, skeletal dysplasia, and anemia) in an infant that may have been due to maternal ingestion of goat milk contaminated with lupine (which also contains anagyrine) (9). The skeletal deformities were similar to those found in crooked calf disease (bowed or twisted limbs, permanently rigid joints, spinal curvature).

Q: Do roasted seeds have a different effect from raw seeds?
A: The roasted seeds have reportedly been used as a coffee substitute. De Smet notes that one source states that roasted, but not raw, seeds are harmless, but does not reference this claim. It probably is true, though; if roasting did not get rid of the severe gastrointestinal cramps associated with the raw seeds, the herb presumably would not have lasted long as a coffee substitute.

Blue-Green Algae

 10 Second Take

The *Aphanizomenon* and *Anabaena* species of blue-green algae have the potential to produce hepatotoxins and neurotoxins; their use should be avoided.

 Basics

LATIN NAME

Aphanizomenon flos-aquae, Anabaena flos-aquae, and other genera

FAMILY

Oscillatoriaceae

OTHER COMMON NAMES

Super blue green algae

DESCRIPTION

• *Aphanizomenon* and *Anabaena* are cyanobacteria (called blue-green algae, although they are not true algae) that are in the same family as Spirulina.
• Unlike Spirulina, however, *Aphanizomenon* and *Anabaena* have no history of use as a food for humans and can produce potent toxins.

KNOWN ACTIVE CONSTITUENTS

• No information is available on beneficial components. Some strains of *Aphanizomenon* and *Anabaena flos-aquae* have been found to produce microcystins (which are hepatotoxic) and neurotoxins. Two of these neurotoxins, anatoxin-a and anatoxin-a(s), appear to be unique to cyanobacteria. Anatoxin-a has been found in both *Anabaena* and *Aphanizomenon*. *Anabaena* is the only cyanobacterium that contains anatoxin-a(s) (1).
• Other neurotoxins identified in some strains of *Aphanizomenon* and *Anabaena* include the carbamate alkaloids saxitoxin and neosaxitoxin. Saxitoxins, also produced by dinoflagellates associated with "red tides," can kill shellfish and cause paralytic shellfish poisoning in humans who ingest contaminated shellfish. Hepatotoxic cyclic peptides found in cyanobacteria include microcystins (consisting of seven amino acids) and nodularins (consisting of five amino acids).

MECHANISM/PHARMACOKINETICS

• The neurotoxins found in cyanobacteria affect acetylcholine in different ways. Anatoxin-a, found in both *Aphanizomenon* and *Anabaena,* mimics acetylcholine but cannot be broken down by acetylcholinesterase. Anatoxin-a is an extremely potent nicotinic agonist; (+)—anatoxin-a is between 3 and 50 times more potent than (−)-nicotine and 20 times more potent than acetylcholine (2). In addition, anatoxin-a evokes dopamine release from rat striatal synaptosomes (3).
• Anatoxin-a(s) (found in *Anabaena*) is a naturally occurring organophosphate that irreversibly inhibits acetylcholinesterase and, thus, functions much like the synthetic organophosphates, including the pesticides parathion and malathion (1). Saxitoxin and neosaxitoxin (found in *Anabaena* and *Aphanizomenon*) inhibit acetylcholine release.
• Microcystins (found in *Anabaena* and in *Aphanizomenon flos-aquae* and many other blue-green algae) are liver toxins that inhibit protein phosphatases; this distorts the cytoskeleton of hepatocytes, causing them to shrink and separate. This affects the integrity of the cells in the sinusoidal capillaries, thus causing bleeding into the liver (1). The World Health Organization has set the acceptable standard for microcystins at one part per million (see questions and answers).

 Evidence

CLINICAL TRIALS

• No clinical trials identified.

ANIMAL/IN VITRO

• No animal trials (of therapeutic effects) were identified.
• An *in vitro* study showed that methanol extracts of *Aphanizomenon,* along with four other cyanobacteria, showed antibacterial effects against *Aeromonas hydrophila, Bacillus cereus,* and *Bacillus subtilis* (4).

Risks

ADVERSE REACTIONS

• An *Anabaena* and *Microcystis* bloom in Brazil was associated with 2,000 cases of gastroenteritis and 88 deaths (mostly in children). An epidemic of neurologic symptoms and hepatic injury in a hemodialysis unit was traced to microcystin-contaminated water used in dialysis; about 60 patients died (5).
• Ingestion of microcystin-contaminated pond and ditch water (in concentrations as high as 160 pg/mL) has been associated with higher rates of liver cancer in China (5).
• Ingestion of saxitoxins can cause paralytic shellfish poisoning.
• Direct contact with water containing cyanobacterial blooms (usually through recreational activities) has been associated with cases of skin reactions, conjunctivitis, rhinitis, vomiting, diarrhea, and atypical pneumonia (6). The author notes that only circumstantial evidence linked all of the previously mentioned illnesses to cyanobacteria, and that other causes (including bacterial contamination) were often not excluded.

ANIMAL TOXICITY

• The LD_{50} of anatoxin-a is 200 to 250 μg/kg (5). In mice, the LD_{50} of anatoxin-a(s) is 20 μg/kg (intraperitoneally). As noted previously, microcystins are hepatotoxic and anatoxins are neurotoxic. Toxin-producing algal blooms (often with mixed genera of cyanobacteria) are a serious problem because they can pollute water supplies with toxins. Fatal poisonings of dogs, sheep, and other livestock have been reported; dogs have been noted to eat toxic cyanobacteria, which may contain compounds that both attract and kill (7). Toxic algal blooms have also caused massive fish and shellfish kills.
• A novel C-18 lipid named mueggelone, isolated from *Aphanizomenon flos-aquae*, has a significant inhibitory effect on fish larval development (8).

 Dose

COMMON DOSAGE FORMS

• Oral, usually in capsule form, typically 2 g or more daily

 Common Questions and Answers

Q: Why is blue-green algae sold if it is so toxic?
A: Not all blue-green algae are toxic. Spirulina, for example, is safe to ingest and never produces microcystins or anatoxins. *Aphanizomenon* and *Anabaena* are two of only 12 genera of cyanobacteria (out of 500 to 1,500) that have been implicated in animal deaths (1). Both of these genera, however, are available in the United States; *Aphanizomenon* is much more commonly sold as a dietary supplement than *Anabaena*. Within toxic genera, not all strains produce toxins; even within a single strain, toxin production can vary (the reasons for this variability are unclear, but several factors that affect toxin production include light, phosphorus, and nitrogen) (9).
Although no cases of acute human toxicity from commercially sold blue-green algae have been reported, I would not assume these products are safe. These cyanobacteria are harvested from lakes rather than being cultivated and could be contaminated with microcystin-producing strains (techniques exist for removing most microcystins from algae but it is not clear that these techniques are used by all manufacturers). Although large amounts of anatoxin would cause obvious illness, it is not clear whether commercially sold *Aphanizomenon* contains small amounts of anatoxin and what the long-term implications of ingestion are.

Q: Why would people consume something with no proven benefits and potential toxicity?
A: Blue-green algae have been touted as a panacea, which may be why people start taking it, but they may continue because they find it "energizing." This may be a placebo effect, but there is a much more worrisome possibility. There are no harmless ingredients in *Aphanizomenon* or *Anabaena* that have stimulating effects, and, if the effect is real, it may be a subtle sign of toxicity. Anatoxin is a potent stimulator of nicotinic receptors and can cause dopamine release from cells in the corpus striatum. The "buzzed" feeling some patients report may be due to doses of anatoxin too small to cause acute toxicity but large enough to cause psychoactive effects.

Boldo

 10 Second Take

Boldo leaf preparations are used in South America and Europe for digestive problems and are safe for short-term use. The essential oil is toxic.

 Basics

LATIN NAME

Peumus boldus Molina

FAMILY

Monimiaceae

DESCRIPTION

• Boldo is a leathery-leafed tree native to central and southern Chile, which is still the only country where it grows in abundance.
• Its average height is 6 to 12 m (8 to 36 ft) high. If its trunk is severed, it regrows as a bush, with several main stems.

PART USED

Leaf

KNOWN ACTIVE CONSTITUENTS

• Boldo contains isoquinoline alkaloids (up to 0.5%), primarily boldine (2% to 19% of alkaloids).
• Boldo leaves contain 1.2% tannins and 2% to 3% essential oil (containing up to 45% of the toxic terpene ascaridole and 30% cineole) (1).
• Boldo also contains monoterpenic hydrocarbons (primarily p-cymene and α-pinene) and flavonoids, especially glycosides of rhamnetin, isorhamnetin, and kaempferol (2).

MECHANISM/PHARMACOKINETICS

• No human pharmacokinetic data are available. Boldine is excreted renally in rats (2).
• Boldine has antioxidant effects in vitro, preventing chemically induced peroxidation of red blood cell membranes and spontaneous peroxidation of membranes in brain homogenates.
• It is an efficient scavenger of hydroxyl radicals (1).

 Evidence

CLINICAL TRIALS

• No clinical trials identified.

ANIMAL/IN VITRO

• A hydroethanolic extract of boldo and pure boldine each showed significant protection against hepatotoxicity in isolated rat hepatocytes. In vivo, a dried hydroethanolic extract of boldo (containing 0.06% to 0.115% of boldine) at 500 mg/kg reduced carbon tetrachloride-induced hepatotoxicity in mice by 70%; boldine (10 mg/kg) reduced hepatotoxicity by 49% (2).
• A laxative effect was produced in rats after oral administration of 400 or 800 mg/kg hydroethanolic extract q.d. × 8 weeks (2).
• Antiinflammatory effects were noted in the carrageenan-induced rat paw edema test; the effect was dose dependent (2).
• Boldine inhibits peristalsis of the small intestine in anesthetized cats and relaxes smooth muscle in a dose-dependent manner in isolated rat ileum (apparently through anticholinergic effects) (1).

OTHER CLAIMED BENEFITS/ACTIONS

• Hepatobiliary disorders
• Increased bile flow
• Antihelminthic
• Constipation
• Rheumatism
• Headache
• Earache
• Dyspepsia
• Dysmenorrhea
• Sedative
• Syphilis, gonorrhea

Risks

ADVERSE REACTIONS

• None known. However, the essential oil contains ascaridole, a toxic terpene, so boldo is not recommended for long-term use. Boldo should not be used in biliary obstruction.

PREGNANCY/LACTATION

• No data available. However, it should not be used during pregnancy.

ANIMAL TOXICITY

• Doses as high as 3 g/kg resulted in no acute toxicity in rats. Subcutaneous injection of 5 mg/kg of total alkaloids into dogs produced vomiting, diarrhea, and seizures; the dogs recovered within an hour. LD_{50} of a hydroethanolic extract of boldo administered intraperitoneally was 6 g/kg; for pure boldine the LD_{50} was 250 mg/kg and for total alkaloids 420 mg/kg (2). Essential oil of boldo is quite toxic. Oral doses of 0.07 g/kg cause seizures in rats; the LD_{50} is 0.13 g/kg (3).

 Dose

COMMON DOSAGE FORMS

• *Dried leaves:* 3 g cut drug or 3 to 5 g total daily dose as infusion or decoction.
• *Tincture:* (1:5, 80% ethanol) 1 to 3 mL q.d.
• *Fluid extract* (80% ethanol): 0.5 to 1 mL q.d.
• Boldo should not be used longer than 4 weeks; use of the essential oil is not recommended.

 Common Questions and Answers

Q: Has boldo ever been used in conventional medicine?
A: The essential oil of boldo has a history of use in conventional medicine as an antihelminthic. The essential oil contains up to 45% ascaridole, the specific antihelminthic principle (1).

Borage

10 Second Take

Borage leaves and flowers are edible but should not be consumed regularly or used medicinally because of the presence of hepatotoxic compounds. Borage seed oil, however, is safe.

Basics

LATIN NAME

Borago officinalis L.

FAMILY

Boraginaceae

OTHER COMMON NAMES

Burrage, bee bread, ox's tongue, cool tankard, bugloss

DESCRIPTION

• Borage is a large annual (up to 60 cm high) that is indigenous to Europe and north Africa and naturalized to North America.
• It has bristly leaves and stems and blue, star-shaped flowers with a central, prominent black cone of anthers.

PART USED

Aerial parts (leaf and flower), seed oil

KNOWN ACTIVE CONSTITUENTS

• Borage leaf contains 11% mucilage, up to 3% tannins, allantoin, silicic acid, organic acids, and potassium nitrate. Borage herb also contains seven pyrrolizidine alkaloids (PAs) in levels up to 8 mg/kg (see questions and answers) (1).
• Borage seeds contain up to 33% oil, including linoleic acid (37% to 39%), γ-linolenic acid (20% to 22%), and oleic acid (17% to 19%). Although PAs can be isolated from the seeds, borage seed oil has been found to be devoid of PAs (1).

MECHANISM/PHARMACOKINETICS

• No information is available on mechanism or pharmacokinetics of borage herb.
• Gamma-linolenic acid (GLA) is metabolized to dihomo-γ-linolenic acid (DGLA), the fatty acid precursor to the antiinflammatory prostaglandin E_1. DGLA also may competitively inhibit 2 series prostaglandins and 4 series leukotrienes (2).
• There is quite a bit of information available on the dangers of PAs (see questions and answers).

Evidence

Borage seed oil or black currant (Ribes nigrum) seed oil are often used as a substitute for evening primrose oil, because all are high in gamma-linolenic acid. Borage oil contains the highest amount of GLA, followed by black currant and evening primrose oil. Most trials have been done with evening primrose oil (see entry).

CLINICAL TRIALS

• Eczema

—A double-blind, placebo-controlled study of 160 patients with stable, moderately severe eczema randomized to borage oil 500 mg or placebo for 24 weeks as an adjunct to the use of a steroid cream (diflucortolone-21-valerate) (3). There were no significant differences in medication use or clinical improvement between the two groups.

• Rheumatoid arthritis

—A randomized, double-blind, placebo-controlled trial in 37 patients with rheumatoid arthritis and active synovitis tested the effect of 12 capsules of borage oil (0.6 mL borage oil per capsule) for a daily dose of 7.2 mL borage oil containing 1.4 g/day gamma-linolenic acid (4). Twenty-seven patients completed the study. The placebo group, which received an equivalent amount of cottonseed oil, did not show significant improvement in any measure. In contrast, patients receiving borage seed oil experienced a 36% reduction in tender joints, a 45% reduction in tender joint score, a 28% reduction in swollen joint count, and a 41% decrease in swollen joint score. Overall clinical response was significantly better in the treated group. Adverse effects were mild gastrointestinal symptoms with a similar incidence in both groups; no patients treated with borage oil dropped out because of adverse effects (one placebo-treated patient dropped out because of a rash).

• Platelet aggregation
A double-blind, placebo-controlled study of borage seed oil (3 g/day × 6 weeks) in 30 healthy males found no effect of the treatment on spontaneous or induced platelet aggregation (5).

ANIMAL/IN VITRO

- An ethanolic extract of borage was tested against herpes virus and poliovirus *in vitro;* no antiviral effect was demonstrated (1).

OTHER CLAIMED BENEFITS/ACTIONS

- Diuretic
- Fever reduction
- Increase milk flow
- "Blood purifier"
- Pulmonary problems
- Pharyngitis
- Wounds (topical)
- Dermatitis (topical)
- Eye problems (topical, as eyewash)

 Risks

ADVERSE REACTIONS

- None reported. However, there is a theoretical risk of hepatotoxicity with long-term consumption of borage leaves.

DRUG INTERACTIONS

- None known. However, this herb should be avoided in patients who are taking hepatotoxic drugs.

PREGNANCY/LACTATION

- No data available. Caution dictates that unsaturated PAs be avoided during pregnancy and lactation.

ANIMAL TOXICITY

- Guinea pigs fed dried borage, a 15% decoction, or borage tincture for 5 weeks showed no acute adverse effects; however, some animals developed fatty liver.
- In mice, 0.1 mL borage seed oil daily by gavage showed no adverse effects other than a weak laxative effect (1).

 Dose

COMMON DOSAGE FORMS

- *Leaf infusion:* 2 to 4 cups/day
- *Borage seed oil capsules:* 2 to 9 capsules a day

 Common Questions and Answers

Q: Aren't PAs quite toxic?
A: About half of them are. Saturated PAs are nontoxic. Unsaturated PAs are converted to pyrroles by mixed-function oxidases in the liver. Pyrroles are potent alkylating agents that can cause cellular destruction or abnormal growth patterns; this is thought to be the mechanism by which PAs cause hepatotoxicity (6). Toxic PA-containing herbs such as comfrey (*Symphytum* species), *Heliotropium, Senecio,* and *Crotalaria* species should be avoided, and the regular use of borage leaves or flowers should be avoided as well. Borage leaves contain small amounts of the PAs lycopsamine and amabiline (the latter is an unsaturated PA) (7). A rare (but, because it is saturated, nontoxic) PA thesinine is found in the flowers and seeds; mature seed also contains a small amount of amabiline.
However, the primary current medicinal use of borage is in the form of borage seed oil. Although unsaturated PAs have been isolated from borage seed, borage seed oil has been found to be devoid of PAs, at least down to 5 μg/g (1). The German standard is that the daily dose of botanical drugs should not provide more than 10 μg of unsaturated Pas.

Q: Is borage seed oil safe to consume over the long term?
A: Probably, but it is hard to say. The longest trial for borage oil was 6 months, and no significant adverse effects occurred during that time. Significant levels of toxic PAs have not been demonstrated in borage oil. However, prolonged administration of gamma-linolenic acid could theoretically increase the conversion of dihomo-gamma-linolenic acid to arachidonate, causing a slow accumulation of arachidonate, an inflammatory mediator that could counteract antiinflammatory effects of borage oil (or any other treatment containing gamma-linolenic acid) (8). If arachidonate accumulates in tissues (an effect that has not been demonstrated in humans), arthritis symptoms may be exacerbated after discontinuation of treatment.

Q: Is it ok to use borage as a vegetable or tea?
A: An occasional salad with borage leaves is fine. Borage leaves have a cooling cucumber flavor; the leaves and flowers are said to be components of Pimm's #1 cup. It should not be eaten regularly as a vegetable, and borage teas, or other preparations containing borage leaf, should not be regularly consumed.

Boron

10 Second Take

Boron (boric acid, borax, borate) is a low-toxicity nutrient apparently involved in bone health. Topical boric acid may be effective for candidal vaginitis.

Basics

DESCRIPTION

• Boron is a nonmetallic element ubiquitous in rocks, soil, and water. Known to be necessary to vascular plants, boron is abundant in human diets but is not yet considered an essential nutrient (1).
• Boron is distributed throughout tissues, but bone, teeth, and fingernails contain the highest concentrations (2).

FOOD SOURCES

• Legumes, fruits, and nuts are high in boron; the boron content of other food crops varies with soil content (3).
• Boron tends to concentrate in leaves and fruit.
• Wine, cider, and beer are high in boron.
• Mean adult male intake is 112 μmol (1.21 mg) to 141 μmol (1.52 mg) daily (1).

MAIN FUNCTIONS/PHARMACOKINETICS

• The function of boron is not clear; the only consistent finding in animals deprived of boron is growth retardation. However, it may be a factor in bone mineralization. Boron may act as a metabolic regulator by complexing with a variety of substrates (including sugars, polysaccharides, pyridoxine, riboflavin, and pyridine nucleotides). It also may play a role in cell membrane function or stability.
• Ninety percent of ingested boron is absorbed. It is excreted mainly in urine within 3 to 7 days.
• Absorption of vaginally administered boric acid was evaluated in a single subject; about 6% was absorbed, and the blood half-life was about 10.5 hours (4).

Evidence

CLINICAL TRIALS

• Effects on calcium metabolism and bone density

—Boron is probably a factor in bone metabolism, but the exact effect is unclear and mediated by various factors. In a study of 12 postmenopausal women, boron supplementation after boron depletion decreased urinary excretion of calcium and magnesium (5). A placebo-controlled study of boron supplementation (3 mg daily for 10 months) in 11 sedentary and 17 active women found that boron decreased serum phosphorus concentrations (this effect was lower in active women) but did not affect serum calcium (6). In what appears to be the same study group, bone mineral density increased over time in the athletic group and decreased in the sedentary group; however, boron did not appear to influence this (7).
—In 11 postmenopausal women, supplemental boron decreased urinary calcium and urinary oxalate in participants fed a low-magnesium diet but increased urinary calcium in magnesium-supplemented participants (8).

• Effect on hormones

—Boron supplementation after boron deprivation resulted in lower serum calcitonin in a study of 15 men and women (5). In this study, the only significant effect on 17β-estradiol levels was found in postmenopausal women on estrogen, in whom 17β-estradiol increased significantly (5). An earlier study by the same investigator found that boron supplementation after boron deprivation significantly increased both 17β-estradiol and testosterone (9). Another study in six postmenopausal women, however, did not confirm these results (3).
—In 18 men supplemented with 10 mg boron daily for 4 weeks, plasma estradiol concentrations increased significantly; there was not a significant difference in testosterone, plasma lipids, or the oxidizability of low-density lipoprotein (10).

• Osteoarthritis

—It is claimed that arthritis is less common in regions where boron intake is high (11). A small, placebo-controlled trial of 20 patients with osteoarthritis compared placebo to boron 6 mg/day for 8 weeks (12). Only 15 patients completed the trial. It is claimed that the average condition of all patients' joints was significantly better in the boron group and that there was less pain on passive movement in patients on boron. However, there appear to have been marked differences between the two groups to begin with, with those in the placebo group appearing to be more severely affected and consuming twice the amount of analgesics at baseline than the treatment group.

• Brain function

—Boron may play a role in brain function. Several studies of dietary boron and cognitive performance involving a total of 23 women and 5 men found that when compared with a period of high boron intake, low dietary boron resulted in significantly poorer performance on tasks emphasizing attention and short-term memory (13).

• Ergogenics

—A controlled study in 19 male bodybuilders compared the effect of placebo versus 2.5 mg boron for 7 weeks on testosterone, lean body mass, and strength measurements (14). Both groups demonstrated significant increases in total testosterone, lean body mass, and strength measurements, but boron supplementation did not affect any of these variables.

• Candidal vaginitis

—A double-blind trial of intravaginal capsules of boric acid (600 mg) or nystatin (100,000 units) each inserted q.h.s. × 14 days found a cure rate (defined as absence of symptoms, with negative microscopy and culture) of 92% for boric acid after 7 to 10 days and 64% for nystatin (4). At 30 days, the cure rate for boric acid was 72% and for nystatin was 50%. Symptom relief was equivalent for the two drugs. Occasional slight watery discharge was noted.
—A case series of 92 women with chronic candidal vaginitis unresponsive to conventional therapy (topical miconazole, topical clotrimazole, gentian violet tampons, and oral nystatin were tried sequentially) tested boric acid vaginal suppositories (600 mg b.i.d. × 2 weeks) (15). The treatment was repeated once if necessary. After the second treatment, 38 women who still did not have completely normal microscopy were told to insert one capsule daily during menstruation for 4 months. At 6-month follow-up, 78 women (85%) were cured (by microscopy); another 12 (13%) could control infections with periodic treatment.

ANIMAL/IN VITRO

• In marginally vitamin D deficient chicks, boron stimulates growth and partially prevents leg abnormalities (1). Numerous influences, including nutritional variables, affect the responsiveness of bone to dietary boron. Different effects are found in different animal models, and, even in the same animals, different effects were sometimes seen in femurs and vertebrae of the same animals (16).
• Boric acid has a fungistatic effect on treatment isolates of *Candida albicans* (4).

OTHER CLAIMED BENEFITS/ACTIONS

• Osteoporosis
• Arthritis
• Menopausal symptoms

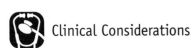 Clinical Considerations

DEFICIENCY SIGNS AND SYMPTOMS

• In stressed animals, boron deprivation impairs calcium metabolism, brain function, and energy metabolism, and may impair immune function.

LABORATORY TESTS

• Boron levels may be measured in serum, plasma, urine, or tissues.

 Risks

ADVERSE REACTIONS

• Acute toxicity may cause nausea, vomiting, diarrhea, dermatitis, and lethargy.
• Chronic toxicity can cause poor appetite, nausea, weight loss, decreased sexual activity, and decreased sperm count and mobility.
• Two infants exposed to borax for several weeks developed anemia, patchy dry erythema, scanty hair, and seizures (1).

DRUG INTERACTIONS

• It is possible that boron increases 17β-estradiol levels in women on estrogen replacement therapy; the clinical implications of this are unclear.

ANIMAL TOXICITY

• Boron has low toxicity when administered orally. In animals, toxicity signs begin to occur after dietary doses exceed 9.25 μmol (100 μg)/g.
• Rats receiving 150 mg/L drinking water exhibited depressed growth, aspermia, impaired ovarian development, and lack of incisor pigmentation. At 300 mg/L rats exhibited decreased plasma triacylglycerols, protein, and alkaline phosphatase and lower amounts of bone fat and calcium. Pigs fed 8 mg boron/kg body weight developed osteoporosis associated with reduced parathyroid activity (2).

 Dose

RECOMMENDED DAILY ALLOWANCE

• No recommended daily allowance (RDA) has been established for boron.
• An acceptable safe intake of boron may be up to 13 mg/day (1).
• Daily adult intakes of boron are in the range of 1.7 to 4.3 mg/day (3).

UPPER LIMITS

Infants and Children
0 to 6 months	Not determinable
7 to 12 months	Not determinable
1 to 3 years	3 mg/day
4 to 8 years	6 mg/day

Males
9 to 13 years	11 mg/day
14 to 18 years	17 mg/day
19 to 50 years	20 mg/day
51+ years	20 mg/day

Females
9 to 13 years	11 mg/day
14 to 18 years	17 mg/day
19 to 50 years	20 mg/day
51+ years	20 mg/day

Pregnant
≤ 18 years	17 mg/day
19 to 50 years	20 mg/day

Lactating
≤ 18 years	17 mg/day
19 to 50 years	20 mg/day

Conversion
1 μmol = 10.8 μg

 Common Questions and Answers

Q: Wasn't boron used as a food preservative?
A: Borax (sodium borate) and boric acid were commonly used as food preservatives from the 1870s to about the 1930s. In 1904 it was reported that humans consuming more than 500 mg/day for 50 days demonstrated disturbed appetite, digestion, and health. Boron began to be viewed as a health hazard and by the 1950s was banned throughout the world as a food preservative.

Burdock

 10 Second Take

Burdock root is edible and safe; no information is available on long-term intake of leaves or fruit. Therapeutic efficacy of burdock has not been demonstrated in clinical trials.

 Basics

LATIN NAME

Arctium lappa L.

FAMILY

Asteraceae/Compositae

OTHER COMMON NAMES

Lappa root, Bardane root

DESCRIPTION

• Burdock is a large, biennial, common bur-bearing plant native to Europe, northern Asia, and North America.

PART USED

Root, and occasionally leaves or fruit

KNOWN ACTIVE CONSTITUENTS

• Burdock root contains up to 45% inulin. It also contains volatile oil, tannin, sitosterol, stigmasterol, resin, mucilage, fatty oil, sugar, acids, γ-guanidino- n-butyric acid, and sulfur-containing acetylenic compounds (arctinones, arctinols, arctinal, and arctic acids). The essential oil contains phenylacetaldehyde, benzaldehyde, methoxypyrazines, costic acid, lactones, and numerous polyacetylenes (1).
• Burdock leaves contain inulin, tannin, mucilage, triterpene alcohols, lupeol, phytol, taraxasterol, stigmasterol, and sitosterol, as well as traces of essential oil (1).
• Burdock fruit contains fatty oil, lappaurin, arctiin, arctin, arctigenin, matairesinol, sesquilignan derivatives, lappanaesthin, resin, and wax. Arctium species seeds contain about 22% fatty oil, about two thirds of which is linoleic acid. Other fatty acids include oleic acid, palmitic acid, and linolenic acid.

 Evidence

CLINICAL TRIALS

No clinical trials identified.

ANIMAL/IN VITRO

• Anticancer effects

—In rats, arctiin was tested against 2-amino-1-methyl-6-phenylimidazo[4,5-b]pyridine (PhIP)-induced mammary carcinogenesis (0.2% or 0.02% arctiin after PhIP initiation) and on 2-amino-3, 8-dimethylimidazo [4,5-f]quinoxaline (MeIQx)-associated hepatocarcinogenesis. Control rats were fed 0.2% or 0.02% arctiin or basal diet alone during the experimental period. Animals were killed at the end of week 48. There was no difference in incidence of mammary carcinomas among the PhIP-treated groups, but multiplicity of tumors and number of colon aberrant crypt foci were significantly decreased in arctiin-treated rats (0.7 $\pm$ 0.7, $p < 0.05$ at the 0.2% dose; 1.0 $\pm$ 1.1, $p < 0.05$ at the 0.02% dose) compared with the PhIP-treated controls (2.1 $\pm$ 2.5) (2). However, arctiin exhibited a weak cocarcinogenic influence on MeIQx-induced hepatocarcinogenesis.
—An animal study from 1966 demonstrated inhibition of the growth of Ehrlich ascites carcinoma in mice (3).
—Benzaldehyde, isolated from burdock, has shown antitumor activity in some animal models. Burdock root has shown mixed results in animal tumor systems (4). A desmutagenic factor has been isolated from burdock and shown to reduce the mutagenicity of DAB (2-nitro-1,4-diaminobenzene) (5). Lignan derivatives from A. lappa induced differentiation of mouse myeloid leukemia cells in vitro. Aliphatic esters were more effective than aromatic esters, and the most active derivative was n-decanoate, which induced differentiation of more than half of the cells at a concentration of 2 μmol.

• Hypoglycemic effects

—A burdock root tincture, administered subcutaneously, resulted in a relatively weak hypoglycemic effect in rats made diabetic by alloxan (1). A more recent study of burdock leaves administered orally to mice as 6.25% of their diet for 43 days found no effect on glucose homeostasis in normal mice. In mice made diabetic by streptozotocin on day 28, an aggravation of hyperglycemia and diabetes symptoms was noted: Basal glucose concentrations rose by 41% (6). Fluid intake and rate of weight loss also increased in burdock-treated mice. Pancreatic insulin concentration, glycated hemoglobin, and insulin-induced hypoglycemia were not affected.
—Rat studies from the 1930s indicate a significant hypoglycemic effect and negligible toxicity of Arctium majus roots (7).

• Antiinflammatory

—Subcutaneous administration of A. lappa root extract decreased carrageenan-induced rat paw edema and demonstrated free radical scavenging activity in vitro (8).

• Antimicrobial effect

—Two components of fresh burdock root have demonstrated bacteriostatic and fungistatic properties; only traces of these compounds were found in dried, commercial root (9,10).

• Prevention of hepatotoxicity

—Administration of A. lappa root extract in mice reduced carbon tetrachloride-induced or acetaminophen-induced acute liver damage (11).

OTHER CLAIMED BENEFITS/ACTIONS

• Anti-cancer agent
• "Blood cleanser"
• Psoriasis (topical)
• Acne (topical)
• Antiinflammatory (topical)
• Diuretic
• Hypoglycemic

Risks

 Dose

 Common Questions and Answers

ADVERSE REACTIONS

• There are no adverse effects reported from consuming burdock root (a common vegetable in Japan and increasingly in North America).
• Young burdock leaves may also be consumed as a vegetable; there is no information available on long-term ingestion of burdock leaves or seeds.
• Contaminated burdock tea

—There are two reports of anticholinergic poisoning from consumption of burdock tea (12,13), but the atropine-like alkaloid isolated from the tea does not occur in burdock. These cases were clearly due to contamination of the tea with a poisonous plant (most likely the root of the deadly nightshade *Atropa bella-donna*), which looks similar to burdock root (9).

• Dermatitis

—Contact dermatitis has been reported in three cases in which people used burdock root plasters as antiinflammatory agents (14).

• Burdock ophthalmia (see questions and answers)

ANIMAL TOXICITY

• Oil from the seeds of *Arctium* species caused no toxic effects in mice when administered in oral or subcutaneous doses up to 0.7 mL (*A. minus*) or 0.1 to 0.2 mL (*A. tomentosum*) (1).

COMMON DOSAGE FORMS

• *Dried root:* 2 to 6 g t.i.d., usually in decoction or infusion
• *Liquid extract:* (1:1 in 25% alcohol) 2 to 8 mL t.i.d.
• *Tincture:* (1:10 in 45% alcohol) 8 to 12 mL t.i.d.

Q: Isn't burdock part of Essiac?
A: Yes, burdock is part of the Essiac herbal mixture used to treat cancer. There are no prospective trials on Essiac, although there have been some negative animal studies and a retrospective case series showing no benefit (see Essiac). Prospective trials of Essiac are being planned in Canada.

Q: What is burdock ophthalmia?
A: Burdock ophthalmia can result from contact with the fruits, or burs (not an issue for those consuming burdock for culinary or medicinal reasons, this is an issue for hikers or those gathering burdock). The barbs on burdock burs can cause serious ocular reactions if they imbed in the conjunctiva or cornea. The barbs are tiny and may be missed on examination. The presence of linear scratch marks in random directions on the cornea is a characteristic sign; conjunctival injection, lid edema, and eventually corneal edema with decreased visual acuity may also occur (1).

Q: What is the connection between burdock and Velcro?
A: It is said that the inventor of Velcro was inspired by how well the hooked shape of the burdock burs adhered to clothing.

Calcium

 10 Second Take

Calcium intake decreases rates of osteoporosis, colorectal neoplasia, nephrolithiasis, and possibly pregnancy-induced hypertension (PIH).

 Basics

DESCRIPTION

Calcium, an essential mineral, is important in neuronal excitability, muscle contraction, and blood coagulation.

FOOD SOURCES

• Dairy products, beans, tofu, corn tortillas processed with lime, *Brassica* species (broccoli, kale, bok choy, mustard, turnip, and collard greens)

MAIN FUNCTIONS/PHARMACOKINETICS

• Calcium comprises 39.9% of bone mineral; 99% of total body calcium is in bone. Ionized calcium reversibly binds proteins and is the most common signal transduction element in cells. It is, thus, crucial to nerve and muscle function.
• A major cofactor for extracellular enzymes and proteins, calcium is involved in cell proliferation, differentiation, neuronal adaptation, and movement (1).

 Evidence

CLINICAL TRIALS

• Osteoporosis and fracture prevention

—In older people, bone loss can be reduced by calcium. Five randomized controlled trials (RCTs) of calcium supplementation (two included vitamin D) demonstrated decreased bone loss in the hip (2). A recent RCT in 176 men and 213 women older than 65 years found that 500 mg calcium plus 700 IU vitamin D$_3$ daily for 3 years reduced bone loss and nonvertebral fractures (11 occurred), compared with placebo (26 nonvertebral fractures occurred, $p = 0.02$) (3). Total body bone mineral was significantly higher in the treatment group at 1, 2, and 3 years; bone mineral density changes were similar between groups at year 3.
—In a placebo-controlled trial of 3,270 older French women (mean age 84 years), hip and other fractures were reduced 26% in a group supplemented with 1,200 mg (30 mmol) calcium and 20 μg (800 IU) vitamin D (4). Several smaller studies also demonstrated decreased fracture rates (2).
—Calcium intake in adolescents is crucial for maximizing peak bone mass. An RCT in 70 prepubertal, nondeficient twin pairs found

that calcium citrate malate (1,000 mg/day for 3 years) enhanced the rate of increase in bone density (5).

• Colorectal lesions

—A randomized, double-blind, 4-year trial of calcium carbonate (3 g daily, containing 1,200 mg elemental calcium) in 930 subjects found that the adjusted risk ratio for any recurrence of colorectal adenomas was 0.85 (6).
—A single-blind, year-long diet study randomized 70 subjects with a history of colonic adenomatous polyps to control diet or 1,200 mg/day calcium via low-fat dairy products (7). Increased calcium intake reduced colonic epithelial cell proliferation and restored markers of normal cellular differentiation.
—A case-control study of 448 patients with colorectal neoplasia (cancer, adenomas, or dysplasia) found a protective effect for calcium supplementation (odds ratio 0.51) (8).

• Hypertension

—Results are mixed in trials of calcium and blood pressure. One review found that 24 trials of calcium supplementation reported a significant reduction in blood pressure in at least a subset; 13 reported no difference (9). An earlier review identified 19 RCTs of calcium supplementation (excluding trials of pregnant women); only 2 showed a significant reduction in systolic and diastolic blood pressure; 11 showed no effect and six were equivocal (10). Another review noted a variable response to calcium supplementation (including increased blood pressure in some hypertensive patients) (11).
—A recent trial of calcium supplementation (1.5 g daily × 8 weeks) in 116 African-American adolescents found a small but significant reduction in diastolic, but not systolic, blood pressure among those with low dietary calcium intake (12).

• Pregnancy-induced hypertension

—A Cochrane systematic review of calcium and PIH identified nine placebo-controlled RCTs; calcium significantly decreased hypertension relative risk [(RR) 0.80, 95% confidence interval (CI) 0.73 to 0.88], especially in women at high risk of hypertension (RR 0.35, 95% CI 0.21 to 0.57) and with low dietary calcium (RR 0.49, 95% CI 0.38 to 0.62) (13). An analysis of 22 trials since 1983 concluded that calcium supplementation lowers the risk of PIH, especially where calcium intake is low (14). Another meta-analysis found net blood pressure reductions in 10 of 12 trials (15).
—The largest RCT compared calcium carbonate (2 g daily) to placebo in 4,589 women (16). Calcium significantly, but slightly, reduced the incidence of hypertension; blood pressure did not decrease significantly. These results, at odds with all previous RCTs, may be because the study was done in a country where calcium intake is high (14).

—A randomized, double-blind trial compared calcium (600 mg) and linoleic acid (450 mg) to placebo in 86 primigravidas at high risk for pre-eclampsia (17). Significantly fewer treated women (9.3%) developed pre-eclampsia compared with controls (37.2%).

• Premenstrual syndrome

—A randomized, double-blind trial of 497 healthy women with premenstrual syndrome found that calcium carbonate (1,000 mg elemental calcium daily) for 3 months reduced symptoms significantly more (48% reduction) than placebo (30%) (18).

• Caries

—A calcium-fortified chewing gum, compared with conventional gum, ameliorated the cariogenic effects of sucrose (19).

 Clinical Considerations

DEFICIENCY SIGNS AND SYMPTOMS

• Paresthesias in distal extremities and perioral area, then muscle cramping, hyperreflexia, carpopedal spasm, laryngospasm, tetany, and seizures. Signs and symptoms are most common when calcium falls abruptly, usually appearing when calcium is less than 2.5 mg/dL.

FACTORS DECREASING AVAILABILITY/ABSORPTION

• Hypoparathyroidism, hyperphosphatemia, achlorhydria, malabsorption syndromes, pancreatitis, vitamin D deficiency, renal failure, magnesium deficiency, aging, oxalic acid (in rhubarb, spinach, etc.), phytic acid (in bran, outer husks of grain), fiber, excessive dietary phosphate, excessive protein intake, hyperalimentation, medications (including furosemide, anticonvulsants, aluminum-containing antacids, glucocorticoids, and parenteral magnesium), and EDTA.

FACTORS INCREASING AVAILABILITY/ABSORPTION

• Hyperparathyroidism, hyperthyroidism, granulomatous disease, renal failure, malignancies, excessive ingestion, hypervitaminosis A and D, thiazide diuretics, lithium, milk-alkali syndrome.

LABORATORY TESTS

• Normal serum calcium levels are 80 to 105 mg/L (conventional units) or 2.0 to 2.6 mmol/L (SI units).
• Low serum calcium usually indicates a parathyroid problem (dietary deficiency rarely lowers serum calcium because of skeletal reserves).

Risks

ADVERSE REACTIONS

• Extremely high supplemental, but not dietary, calcium intake (greater than 2,500 mg/day), can cause hypercalcemia or nephrolithiasis (see questions and answers). Constipation, bloating, and excess gas may occur with supplementation.

DRUG INTERACTIONS

• In 20 patients on long-term levothyroxine, concurrent administration of calcium carbonate (1,200 mg elemental calcium) reduced thyroxine (T_4) levels and increased serum thyrotropin (20).
• Calcium may impede absorption of atenolol, salicylates, bisphosphonates, fluoride, iron, and tetracyclines.

Dose

COMMON DOSAGE FORMS

Calcium carbonate, calcium citrate, tricalcium phosphate, dicalcium phosphate, bone meal, dolomite, oyster shell

ADEQUATE INTAKES

Infants and Children
0 to 6 months	210 mg/day
7 to 12 months	270 mg/day
1 to 3 years	500 mg/day
4 to 8 years	800 mg/day

Males
9 to 13 years	1,300 mg/day
14 to 18 years	1,300 mg/day
19 to 50 years	1,000 mg/day
51+ years	1,200 mg/day

Females
9 to 13 years	1,300 mg/day
14 to 18 years	1,300 mg/day
19 to 50 years	1,000 mg/day
51+ years	1,200 mg/day

Pregnant
≤18 years	1,300 mg/day
19 to 50 years	1,000 mg/day

Lactating
≤18 years	1,300 mg/day
19 to 50 years	1,000 mg/day

UPPER LIMITS

Infants and Children
0 to 6 months	Not determinable
7 to 12 months	Not determinable
1 to 3 years	2,500 mg/day
4 to 8 years	2,500 mg/day

Males
9 to 13 years	2,500 mg/day
14 to 18 years	2,500 mg/day
19 to 50 years	2,500 mg/day
51+ years	2,500 mg/day

Females
9 to 13 years	2,500 mg/day
14 to 18 years	2,500 mg/day
19 to 50 years	2,500 mg/day
51+ years	2,500 mg/day

Pregnant	2,500 mg/day
Lactating	2,500 mg/day

• Treatment of deficiency

—Asymptomatic deficiency: oral calcium. Symptomatic patients: parenteral calcium (10 mL of 10% calcium gluconate or 5 mL of calcium chloride)

Common Questions and Answers

Q: What is the best supplemental calcium?
A: Calcium carbonate is inexpensive and as bioavailable as citrate malate if taken with meals; calcium lactate and phosphate are also well absorbed. When taken fasting, calcium citrate malate is best absorbed.

Q: Do calcium supplements contain lead?
A: Yes, if derived from bone or dolomite. Chelates and refined preparations contain the least lead; dolomite, "natural source," and bone meal contained the most (21). Because there are lead-free choices, why add avoidable dietary lead?

Q: Why should calcium be taken with meals?
A: Amino acids chelate calcium and increases calcium absorption. Also, taking calcium with meals reduces the risk of nephrolithiasis.

Q: Doesn't calcium cause nephrolithiasis?
A: No. Although many of us learned that stone-formers should avoid dietary calcium, the opposite is true. Calcium binds oxalate in the gastrointestinal tract, thus preventing absorption.
High dietary calcium is safe. The Masai ingest more than 5,000 mg calcium daily and do not have higher rates of renal stones or hypercalcemia (22). In the Nurse's Health Study I (91,731 women), women with the highest dietary calcium intake had a relative risk of kidney stone formation of 0.65, compared with those with the lowest calcium intake (23). In the Health Professionals Follow-Up Study (45,619 men); the relative risk for men with the highest dietary intake was 0.56 compared with those with the lowest intake (24). In 1,309 women, those with renal stones consumed almost 250 mg/day less calcium than did women without stones (25).
Supplemental calcium, however, was associated with increased incidence of renal stones (RR 1.20) in the Nurse's Health Study (23). Two thirds took supplements between meals or with low-oxalate meals. Advise patients to take calcium supplements with the largest meal of the day.

Q: Why should stone formers drink mineral water?
A: Mineral water provides both calcium and hydration. A study of 40 calcium oxalate-forming stone patients and 40 healthy volunteers compared French mineral water (containing 202 ppm calcium and 36 ppm magnesium) to tap water (containing 13 ppm calcium and 1 ppm magnesium) (26). Both regimens favorably altered risk factors (oxalate excretion, relative supersaturation of calcium oxalate, brushite, and uric acid), but mineral water was superior. A single dose of mineral water (containing 172 mg calcium) inhibited intact parathyroid hormone and decreased markers of bone resorption (27).

Q: What is the home test for calcium tablet solubility?
A: Place a calcium tablet in 6 oz. of white vinegar at room temperature and stir occasionally. The tablet should dissolve within 30 minutes (28). This tests only solubility not bioavailability.

Q: How does sodium intake affect calcium?
A: Sodium and calcium share some transport systems in the proximal tubule, and each 100 mg increase in sodium intake increases calcium excretion 0.5 to 1 mg. (29). In 381 healthy white pubertal females, urinary sodium was one of the most important determinants of calcium excretion (30).

Calendula

 10 Second Take

Calendula is a safe herb. Clinical trial data is lacking but the herb may have promise as an antiinfective.

 Basics

LATIN NAME

Calendula officinalis L.

FAMILY

Compositae/Asteraceae

OTHER COMMON NAMES

Marigold, pot marigold, marybud, gold-bloom

DESCRIPTION

- Calendula is an aromatic, annual or biennial plant with orange-yellow flowers.
- It is native to central, eastern, and southern Europe.

PART USED

Flower

KNOWN ACTIVE CONSTITUENTS

- Triterpenoids (oleanolic acid glycosides, triterpene alcohols), sesquiterpenoids, carotenoids, flavonoids, polysaccharides, and sterols, predominately faradiol monoester (1).

 Evidence

CLINICAL TRIALS

No clinical trials identified.

ANIMAL/IN VITRO

- Antimicrobial and molluscicidal effects

—Hydroalcoholic extracts have shown antibacterial, antifungal, and antiviral effects *in vitro* (1). An organic extract of calendula demonstrated anti-HIV activity in an *in vitro* MTT/tetrazolium-based assay (2). At 500 μg/mL, the organic extract protected Molt-4 human lymphocytic cells from fusion and cell death for up to 24 hours when cultivated with infected U-937/HIV-1 cells.
—A 70% hydroalcoholic flower tincture exhibited marked virucidal activity against influenza virus and suppressed the growth of herpes simplex virus *in vitro* (1).
—Two experiments done before 1979 demonstrate activity against trichomonas (1); the effect is due to oxygen-containing terpene alcohols and lactones in the essential oil (3).
—Leaves and flowers of calendula exhibited marked potency in killing snail vectors of schistosomiasis; offspring of snails previously exposed to low doses were more sensitive to tested extracts (4).

- Wound healing activity

—Calendula promotes reepithelialization, formation of granulation tissue, and regeneration of dermal collagen in skin wounds. A freeze-dried aqueous extract of calendula demonstrated angiogenic activity in the chick chorioallantoic membrane assay; the authors suggest that water-soluble flavonoids induce hyaluron deposition and increase the rate of neovascularization (5). Strong bioadhesive qualities of polysaccharides from calendula have been demonstrated on porcine buccal mucous membranes (6).

- Antiinflammatory effects

—Very mild inhibition of inflammation was seen in the carrageenan-induced rat paw edema test; indomethacin (5 mg/kg) inhibited edema by 45%, whereas an oral dose of 100 mg/kg calendula flower extract inhibited edema 11% (7). A mild dose-dependent antiinflammatory effect of topical calendula extracts was seen in a croton oil ear test in mice. Both a hydroalcoholic 70% extract and a CO_2 extract (containing only lipophilic constituents) were tested. The CO_2 extract was far superior, but the effect was quite mild; a dose of 120 μg/ear (corresponding to about 2.9 mg crude drug) demonstrated only 10% of the effect of indomethacin (8). Triterpenoids have been shown to be the most active antiinflammatory principles. Faradiol, derived from calendula, was equal in potency to indomethacin (9,10).
—The most abundant and the most active triterpenoid compound is the faradiol monoester; it has been suggested that this compound be used for standardizing calendula extracts. Free faradiol (which does not occur in the crude extract but is derived by hydrolysis) is more than twice as active as the faradiol ester.

- Cancer

—A triterpene-containing fraction given orally to mice inoculated with Ehrlich mouse carcinoma prevented the development of ascites and increased survival time compared with controls (1).

OTHER CLAIMED BENEFITS/ACTIONS

Oral preparations

- Fevers
- Cancer
- Menses induction
- Muscle spasms

Topical preparations

- Wound healing
- Leg ulcers
- Bruises
- Burns
- Oropharyngeal inflammation

 Risks

- None known. However, caution should be used in those with known sensitivity to members of the Compositae family.

PREGNANCY/LACTATION

- No data available. However, *in vitro* uterotonic effects have been reported (11) and caution dictates that oral calendula should be avoided during pregnancy and lactation. There is probably no harm in topical applications.

ANIMAL TOXICITY

- For mice, the LD_{50} of aqueous extract was 375 mg/kg intravenously and 580 mg/kg intraperitoneally; subcutaneous administration of a hydroalcoholic extract showed an LD_{50} of 45 mg/mouse. Intravenous administration in rats showed an LD_{50} of 526 mg/100 g (1).
- Chronic toxicity studies have shown no toxicity of aqueous extracts in rats, mice, and hamsters (1).

 Dose

MODE OF ADMINISTRATION

Usually topical, occasionally oral

COMMON DOSAGE FORMS

- *Dried florets:* 1 to 4 g, usually as tea or infusion t.i.d.
- *Liquid extract:* (1:1 in 40% alcohol) 0.5 to 1 mL t.i.d.
- *Tincture:* (1:5 in 90% alcohol) 0.3 to 1.2 mL t.i.d.
- *Topical ointment:* 2% to 5%, equivalent of 2 to 5 g in 100-g ointment.
- *Infusion, liquid extract,* or *diluted tincture* (one part tincture to three parts hot water) may be used topically on compresses.

Capsicum, Chili Pepper, or Cayenne

 10 Second Take

Evidence supports topical application of chili peppers for several painful cutaneous disorders and neural dysfunction.

 Basics

LATIN NAME

Capsicum annuum L., *C. frutescens* L.

FAMILY

Solanaceae

OTHER COMMON NAMES

Paprika, red pepper, hot pepper, Tabasco pepper

DESCRIPTION

• *Capsicum annuum,* an annual herb up to 1 m in height, grows in mild temperate to semitropical areas of Europe, Mexico, and the United States (among others).
• Cayenne is a blend of capsicums. *Capsicum frutescens* (hot pepper, bird pepper, Tabasco pepper), a small spreading shrub native to tropical America, is cultivated in Africa and Asia.
• *Capsicum chinense* (Scotch bonnet pepper, habanero pepper), perhaps the hottest pepper, probably originated in the Amazon basin and is now widely cultivated.

PART USED

Dry, ripe fruit

KNOWN ACTIVE CONSTITUENTS

• Capsaicin (*trans*-8-methyl-*N*-vanillyl-6-nonenamide) and dihydrocapsaicin are the main pungent principles; (−)-capsaiciniol is a nonpungent analog of capsaicin isolated from *C. frutescens* (1).
• It is a good source of Vitamin B_1, vitamin C, and especially vitamin A (2).

MECHANISM/PHARMACOKINETICS

• Capsaicin depletes tissues of substance P; chronic administration desensitizes sensory neurons through a calcium-channel blocking effect.
• Axoplasmic transport and synthesis of neuropeptides are also affected (3). Capsaicin also inhibits the isoenzymes CYP1A2 and CYP2E1 (1).

 Evidence

CLINICAL TRIALS

Musculoskeletal

• Arthritis

—A double-blind, placebo-controlled multicenter study in 113 arthritic subjects tested capsaicin cream against vehicle q.i.d. for 12 weeks. Capsaicin-treated patients reported greater reduction of pain on visual analog scale at the end of the first and third month and also experienced less joint tenderness and pain on passive range of motion. Forty-six percent of patients experienced burning or stinging that resolved over time; at week 12 only 7% of patients experienced burning (4). Seventeen patients withdrew (11 capsaicin-treated, two of whom withdrew because of adverse effects attributed to capsaicin: moderate burning and knee pain).
—One double-blind controlled study of 21 patients found that topical capsaicin cream reduced tenderness and pain 40% in osteoarthritis patients; there was no effect on patients with rheumatoid arthritis (5).

• Fibromyalgia

—A 4-week, placebo-controlled study of 45 fibromyalgia patients found that topical capsaicin (0.025%) resulted in less tenderness at trigger points compared with the placebo-treated group; there was no significant difference in visual analog pain scores (6). Grip strength increased significantly only in the capsaicin group.

Dermatology

• Pruritis

—Three of five double-blind placebo-controlled studies showed a significantly better response of capsaicin over placebo (3).

• Psoriasis

—Three placebo-controlled studies indicate a benefit of capsaicin treatment for psoriasis (3). Itching, scaling, and erythema were significantly lower with capsaicin in two controlled trials. In the third trial, the combined psoriasis score was reduced significantly more with capsaicin than vehicle.

Gynecology

• Vulvar vestibulitis

—Topical capsaicin (0.025%) was compared with vehicle in 14 women with vulvar vestibulitis; the nine subjects who had completed the study at the time of its presentation experienced a mean reduction of pain of 77% (7).

Neurology

• Headache

—Two controlled studies of capsaicin cream applied topically to the ipsilateral nostril to treat cluster headache found a beneficial effect. One study used a burning placebo; 57% of those treated with capsaicin and 17% of those treated with camphor had a positive response.

• Diabetic neuropathy

—Topical capsaicin may be useful for diabetic neuropathy; one placebo-controlled study of 252 patients found that 69.5% of patients treated with 0.075% capsaicin cream improved (by physician's global index) compared with 53.4% of those on placebo; a significant difference. Intensity of pain (measured by visual analog scale and calculated as percent improvement from baseline) was also significantly less in the capsaicin group (8).

• Postherpetic neuralgia

—An uncontrolled trial of topical 0.025% capsaicin cream in 33 older patients with postherpetic neuralgia found that almost 80% of the capsaicin-treated patients experienced some relief from their pain after 6 weeks (9).

• Polyneuropathy

—A randomized double-blind placebo-controlled study tested capsaicin cream (0.075% applied q.i.d.) against placebo for chronic distal painful polyneuropathy in 40 patients (39 completed). Outcome measures included a visual analog scale of pain severity, pain relief, and activities of daily living, and patient and investigator assessment. Capsaicin cream was no more effective than placebo for any indices; in the first month, several indices favored the placebo (10).

• Postmastectomy pain syndrome

—A small, controlled study of 23 patients found capsaicin cream helpful in postmastectomy pain syndrome. Five of 13 patients receiving the capsaicin cream reported good to excellent results compared with 1 out of 10 placebo-treated patients. There was no significant difference between groups on visual analog scale for pain (11); however, pain severity and overall pain relief were significantly better in the capsaicin-treated group (11).

• Swallowing reflex

—A controlled study of capsaicin in 20 older patients with cerebral thrombosis or dementia resulting from cerebral arterial sclerosis found a dose-dependent beneficial effect of capsaicin on latent time of swallowing (12).

Urology

• Overactive bladder

—Intravesical capsaicin may be effective in patients with urge incontinence resulting from neurologic impairment. The only prospective double-blind placebo-controlled trial to date in 12 paraplegic patients found that instillation of 100 mL 1 mM capsaicin in 30% alcohol for 30 minutes, compared with alcohol alone, resulted in significant regression of urine leakage episodes and sensory urgency in all capsaicin-treated patients; only one placebo-treated subject subjectively improved (13). Adverse effects in both groups were suprapubic pain, increased incontinence, or macroscopic hematuria during the first week and one urinary infection in each group. One capsaicin-treated patient experienced autonomic dysreflexia.

Miscellaneous

• Carbohydrate oxidation

—Capsicum ingestion may stimulate carbohydrate oxidation. In a crossover study, 8 male long-distance runners exercised for an hour after a breakfast with or without 10 g of hot red pepper. Red pepper significantly elevated respiratory quotient and blood lactate levels at rest and during exercise; plasma triacylglycerol concentrations during exercise were significantly higher after the red pepper meal (14). There was no significant difference in oxygen consumption.

• Gastroenterologic effects

—A prospective crossover study in 12 healthy adults infected with *Helicobacter pylori* compared the effect of jalapeno peppers (6 subjects), fresh garlic (10 subjects), and bismuth subsalicylate (11 subjects) on *H. pylori*, as assessed by median urease activity. Bismuth had a marked inhibitory effect; neither garlic nor capsaicin had any effect (15).
—A controlled study in 18 volunteers given water with or without 20 g chili pepper, followed half an hour later by 600 mg aspirin, found that gastroduodenal mucosal damage (assessed by endoscopy) was reduced significantly after treatment (16).

ANIMAL/IN VITRO

• Capsaicin inhibits the effect of several carcinogens, including benzo[α]pyrene and the tobacco-specific nitrosamine, 4-(methylnitrosamino)-1-(3 pyridyl)-1-butanone (NNK).
• Capsaicin inhibits growth of HeLa, ovarian carcinoma, mammary adenocarcinoma, and human promyelocytic leukemia cells in culture.
• In animals, capsaicin stimulates lipid mobilization from adipose tissue (17) and reduces inflammation (18).

 Risks

ADVERSE REACTIONS

• Burning, stinging, itching, and erythema are commonly reported with initial use of capsaicin cream; in one psoriasis trial, 18% discontinued use of the cream because of burning (3).
• Local burning or stinging usually disappears after a few doses. Patients should be counseled to wash their hands after applying the cream and to avoid touching their eyes.

DRUG INTERACTIONS

• In rats, concomitant administration of capsicum increased theophylline peak plasma levels and area under the curve (19).
• Also in rats, chronic administration of capsicum extract reduced the oral bioavailability of aspirin, possibly through gastrointestinal effects. A single administration of 300 mg/kg capsicum extract reduced aspirin in blood to undetectable levels and reduced salicylic acid bioavailability by 59%. Chronic administration of 300 mg/kg capsicum extract q.d. × 4 weeks reduced salicylic acid bioavailability by 76%, compared with controls (20).

 Dose

COMMON DOSAGE FORMS

• *Capsules:* 400 to 500 mg up to t.i.d.
• *Tincture:* 1:10 (g/L), 90% ethanol: 5 to 10 drops in water.
• Also used in topical preparations, including oils, creams, ointments, and poultices. Commercial capsaicin preparations, commonly available over-the-counter (OTC), usually contain 0.025 or 0.075% capsaicin and are applied up to q.i.d.

 Common Questions and Answers

Q: Do chili peppers increase the risk of stomach cancer?
A: It is extremely unlikely, but studies are mixed. Although a case-control study in Mexico found that consumers of chili peppers were at greater risk of stomach cancer (age and sex-adjusted odds ratio 5.49), compared with nonconsumers, an Italian case control study found that chili consumption was protective against stomach cancer. Chili pepper consumption is quite high in Mexico (about 20 g/day), and the overall rate of gastric cancer is low (1). Capsaicin appears to be gastroprotective and to inhibit carcinogenesis in several models (1); however, other studies have found capsaicin to be mutagenic (21). I am with the folks who think chili peppers are good for you.

Q: What is the connection between gophers and chili peppers?
A: Given a choice, pocket gophers will avoid capsicum-spiked soil. An experiment found that gophers preferred soil without capsicum; mean soil contact time was decreased by 46% when they were exposed to soil enriched with 1.5% capsicum-oleoresin. Soil-digging behavior, unfortunately, was minimally affected.

Caraway

 10 Second Take

Caraway seed is a safe herb in normally used quantities, whether used in cooking or medicinally for gastrointestinal spasm.

 Basics

LATIN NAME

Carum carvi L.

FAMILY

Umbelliferae/Apiaceae

DESCRIPTION

• A biennial plant up to 3 ft high with white to faint pink blossoms.
• Native to Europe, caraway often grows along roadsides or in meadows. It also grows in Egypt, Morocco, Australia, and China.

PART USED

Fruit (seed)

KNOWN ACTIVE CONSTITUENTS

• Caraway contains 3% to 7% essential oil, which contains up to 65% (*S*)-(+)-carvone, up to 40% (*R*)-(+)-limonene, and less than 1.5% carveol and dihydrocarveol.
• The herb also contains up to 20% petroselinic acid and oleic acid, protein, carbohydrates, phenolic acids, and flavonoids (1).

MECHANISM/PHARMACOKINETICS

• Components of caraway increase gastric tone and appear to have relaxant effects on smooth muscle (see *in vitro* studies). Human pharmacokinetic data are not available for caraway or its constituents. In mice, (*S*)-(+)-carvone is absorbed within 35 minutes after application to shaved abdominal skin. In rabbits (*S*)-(+)-carvone is oxidized to hydroxycarvone and conjugated with glucoronic acid (1). Gastroduodenal motility was tested by stationary manometry after administration of a fixed preparation of peppermint oil 90 mg and caraway oil 50 mg. In six volunteers, both enteric and nonenteric-coated preparations decreased the frequency and amplitude of contractions during the migrating motor complex, indicating a local effect on smooth muscle relaxation (2).

 Evidence

CLINICAL TRIALS

Dyspepsia

• No clinical trials were identified for caraway alone. Three controlled trials of a fixed combination of peppermint oil 90 mg and caraway oil 50 mg were identified. A randomized, double-blind, placebo-controlled trial tested a combination product (2 capsules daily) against cisapride (10 mg t.i.d.) in 118 patients with functional dyspepsia for 4 weeks (3). Pain scores by visual analog scale were reduced by 4.65 points with the essential oil product and by 4.16 points with cisapride. Comparable results in the dyspeptic discomfort score and in the Clinical Global Impression (CGI) were also seen. Adverse events (primarily gastrointestinal) were mild and similar between the two groups.
• Another double-blind, placebo-controlled trial in 45 dyspepsia patients (39 completed) tested three capsules daily of a combination product (90 mg peppermint oil with 50 mg caraway oil in each enteric-coated capsule) (4). After 4 weeks of treatment, 63.2% of the treatment group was free of pain compared with 25% of patients in the control group. Pain intensity improved in 89.9% of those treated compared with 45% in the placebo group. The condition of 52.6% of patients receiving the herb product was judged "very much better" by the CGI scale compared with 25% of those receiving placebo. Side effects were mild; three patients dropped out from the placebo group and four from the treatment group (one treated patient reported substernal burning, nausea, and severe eructation).
• In another study, 96 subjects with dysfunctional dyspepsia were assigned to placebo or the peppermint/caraway combination (1 capsule b.i.d.) for 4 weeks. Compared with baseline, the average intensity of pain, sensations of pressure or heaviness, and CGI improved significantly more in the treated group than in the placebo group (5).
• A commercial combination product containing hydroethanolic extracts of four herbs (100 mL contained 3.7 g caraway, 8.13 g fennel, 9.26 g peppermint, and 1.92 g wormwood) was compared with metoclopramide in 60 subjects for the treatment of upper abdominal complaints (including pain, nausea, heartburn, retching, and gastric cramping) (6). Patients took 25 drops t.i.d. (20 minutes before meals) of the herbal product or metoclopramide (total daily dose about 24 mg). After 2 weeks, significant differences favoring the herb treatment were seen in epigastric pain, nausea, heartburn, and gastric spasm.

ANIMAL/IN VITRO

• Antispasmodic effects

—An alcohol extract of caraway reduced chemically induced spasm in guinea pig ileum in a dose-dependent manner. In another experiment, caraway oil (27 mg/L) decreased phasic contractions by 50% in guinea pig tracheal smooth muscle, but no effect was seen in electrically stimulated guinea pig ileum (1). Available data are not entirely consistent on this point; alcohol extracts may have different effects on smooth muscle than essential oils; there is some evidence that essential oils of caraway and other antispasmodic herbs actually increase smooth muscle tone and stimulate bowel motility (7).

• Respiratory effects

—(*S*)-(+)-carvone, administered by steam inhalation, increased the volume and decreased the specific gravity of respiratory tract fluid in rabbits (1).

• Anticancer effects

—Topical or dietary caraway oil reduced 9,10 dimethyl-1,2-benzanthracene (DMBA) and croton oil-induced skin tumors in mice (8). Administered orally as 3% of the diet or applied topically (0.2 mL twice weekly), caraway oil significantly reduced the number of mice bearing tumors, number of papillomas, and volume of papillomas, compared with controls. Caraway oil also inhibited the development of carcinomas, which occurred in 4/24 control animals and none of the treated animals. In addition, some papillomas actually regressed in treated animals. Caraway oil also inhibited *N*-nitrosodiethylamine-induced lung and forestomach tumors in mice (9). Anticancer effects are thought to be due to the high concentration of limonene.

• Antimicrobial effects

—Alcohol extracts of caraway have shown antibacterial and antifungal effects in many test organisms, including *Escherichia coli*, *Staphylococcus aureus*, *Candida albicans*, *Streptomyces venezuelae*, and species of *Aspergillus*, *Epidermophyton*, and *Trichophyton* (1).

OTHER CLAIMED BENEFITS/ACTIONS

• Gastrointestinal spasm
• Flatulence
• Colic
• Increase milk production

Risks

ADVERSE REACTIONS

- Nausea
- Eructation

PREGNANCY/LACTATION

- Pregnant or lactating women should avoid ingestion of caraway oil (see questions and answers). Caraway oil is purported to have abortifacient effects.
- Caraway seed in amounts used in foods is probably safe.

ANIMAL TOXICITY

- Acute LD_{50} of caraway oil in rats is 3.5 mL/kg and 6.68 g/kg. In rabbits, the LD_{50} of dermally administered caraway oil is 1.78 mL/kg.
- In chronic toxicity studies, 1% dietary (S)-$(+)$-carvone fed to rats for 16 weeks caused growth retardation and testicular atrophy. In another study, 0.1% (S)-$(+)$-carvone fed to rats for 28 weeks and 0.25% for 1 year had no effect (1). A 12-week toxicity study in rats determined that the maximal acceptable daily intake was 1.0 mg (S)-$(+)$-carvone/kg body weight (1).

 ## Dose

COMMON DOSAGE FORMS

- Adult: 1 to 5 g crushed fruit daily as infusion, in divided doses (usually q.i.d., taken between meals).

Children:

—0–1 years of age: 1 g daily or 1 teaspoon of infusion in their bottle.
—1–4 years of age: 1 to 2 g daily or 1 teaspoon of infusion in their bottle.
—4–10 years of age: 1 to 4 g daily.
—10 years and older: adult dose.

- Essential oils should be avoided in infants, children, pregnant and lactating women and used only with great caution in other cases.

 ## Common Questions and Answers

Q: Does caraway seed in foods have any medicinal effect?
A: Maybe. In fact it is interesting that caraway seed is often added to cabbage and rye bread, foods with a reputation for causing flatulence! It is also used in as one of the herbs in "digestive" liqueurs.

Q: Can caraway be used in lactating women?
A: Caraway is reputed to increase milk production. Small amounts of seed in foods or teas or infusions made from seed are not a problem. However, essential oil of caraway (a much stronger form of the herb) should not be used in lactating women.

Carnitine

10 Second Take

Carnitine (L-carnitine, "vitamin Bt") is benign; evidence supports its use for intermittent claudication.

Basics

DESCRIPTION

• Carnitine is formed in the liver and kidney from lysine and methionine. L-propionyl-carnitine is a naturally occurring derivative.

FOOD SOURCES

• Muscle meats, liver, milk, and yeast. Dietary intake is not necessary when lysine and methionine ingestion is adequate (1).
• Human milk contains 28 to 95 nmol carnitine/mL. Milk-based formulas contain similar amounts; soy or casein-based formulas contain little carnitine (2).

MAIN FUNCTIONS/PHARMACOKINETICS

• Carnitine, a carrier molecule, is vital to lipid metabolism; it transports acyl acids across cell membranes and is required for carrying long-chain fatty acids into mitochondria for β-oxidation. Carnitine is also necessary for ketogenesis in liver and kidney (1).
• Absorbed rapidly from the intestine, carnitine is cleared renally; more than 90% is usually reabsorbed. Skeletal muscle contains 97% of total carnitine (3). Carnitine concentrations are very high in the epididymis (4).

Evidence

CLINICAL TRIALS

• Peripheral vascular disease

—Carnitine benefits intermittent claudication. A double-blind randomized controlled trial (RCT) in 155 subjects with severe claudication found that L-carnitine (1 g b.i.d. × 6 months) significantly increased peak walking time (54% vs. 25% improvement in the placebo group, $p < 0.001$); walking distance, speed, and claudication onset time also improved significantly (5). Some improvements were apparent at 3 months.
—Another randomized double-blind study in 22 patients (Fontaine class II) found that carnitine (1 g t.i.d. × 90 days) significantly improved claudication distance, blood flow velocity, plasminogen inhibitor-1 activity, and erythrocyte deformity (6).
—A double-blind RCT in 485 subjects found that propionyl-L-carnitine (1 g b.i.d. × 12 months); improved maximal walking distance (but not initial claudication distance) significantly only in those with baseline

walking distances less than 250 m (7). A double-blind trial of 245 patients found that propionyl-L-carnitine (500 mg b.i.d. escalated to up to 1,500 mg b.i.d. × 24 weeks) improved maximal walking capacity but not time to claudication (8). In another report on the same trial, carnitine improved emotional, but not physical, function (9).
—A double-blind crossover RCT of 20 patients with intermittent claudication found that carnitine significantly improved walking distance (10).
—In 20 type II diabetics with peripheral vascular disease, propionylcarnitine 1,500 mg/day × 6 months significantly improved ankle/arm pressure index, Windsor index, walking distance, and variation in walking distance over placebo (11).

• Angina

—Several trials support using carnitine for angina. A double-blind, placebo-controlled RCT tested L-propionylcarnitine (500 mg t.i.d. × 6 weeks) in 74 patients with more than two anginal attacks a week despite treatment. Compared with placebo, carnitine increased the time to 0.1 mV ST-segment depression and increased exercise duration slightly. Heart rate, blood pressure, maximal exercise, and number of anginal attacks were not affected (12).
—A crossover RCT compared diltiazem (180 mg q.d. × 3 weeks, then 360 mg × 3 weeks) to L-propionylcarnitine (1,500 mg q.d. × 6 weeks) in 46 patients with stable, exercise-induced angina; both treatments significantly improved exercise duration, time to ST depression, ST segment depression at maximal exercise, and number of anginal attacks (13). Only diltiazem improved resting and maximal heart rate, diastolic blood pressure, and rate-pressure product.
—A double-blind crossover RCT of 44 men with stable chronic angina found that carnitine (1 g b.i.d. × 4 weeks), compared with placebo, significantly increased maximal exercise load and caused less ST segment depression; there was no difference in blood pressure, heart rate, or time to ST segment depression (14).

• Myocardial infarction

—A controlled trial of 22 patients with acute myocardial infarction found that L-carnitine (40 mg/kg/day × 5 days) did not significantly reduce necrotic area, measured by MB-CPK release (15).

• Heart failure

—A double-blind multicenter RCT of 537 patients with mild to moderate heart failure found no benefit of propionyl-L-carnitine (1 g b.i.d. × 6 months) over placebo on exercise capacity (16).
—A placebo-controlled trial in 50 patients with left ventricular dysfunction [NYHA class II, ejection fraction (EF) less than 45%] found that l-propionylcarnitine (500 mg t.i.d. × 6 months), but not placebo, improved left ventricular shortening fraction, left ventricular EF, stroke volume, cardiac index, and systemic vascular resistance (17). The

treated group also improved significantly more in exercise time (1.4 minutes) than the placebo group (0.36 minutes).

• Alzheimer's and age-related cognitive impairment

—A double-blind, placebo-controlled RCT of 30 patients with mild to moderate dementia found that patients given acetyl levocarnitine hydrochloride (2.5 g/day × 3 months, then 3 g/day × 3 months) demonstrated less deterioration in timed cancellation tests and the digit span test than those assigned to placebo (18). There were no differences in other neuropsychologic test results.
—A double-blind, placebo-controlled RCT of acetyl-carnitine (2 g/day × 1 year) in 130 Alzheimer's patients found that acetyl-carnitine decreased rate of progression, measured by the Blessed Dementia scale (19).
—A double-blind RCT of acetyl-L-carnitine (1 g t.i.d. × 1 year) in 229 patients with early-onset dementia found no differences between groups in decline (20).
—In a single-blind study in which 481 subjects in geriatric and neurologic units received placebo for the first and fifth months, and 1,500 mg L-acetylcarnitine for the second through fourth months, subjects given L-acetylcarnitine significantly improved in affect, the mini mental status examination, and the Randt memory test (21).

• Ergogenics/weight loss

—Studies of carnitine on exercise performance have been inconsistent (22). A review of 20 published studies of carnitine and exercise performance found that most studies ≤1 month showed no benefit (23). Several studies by one group found that supplementing for 1 to 6 months prevented training-associated decrease in muscle carnitine and increased activity of pyruvate dehydrogenase and electron transport chain enzymes.
—A double-blind, placebo-controlled study in 36 moderately overweight women (28 completed) tested l-carnitine (2 g b.i.d. × 8 weeks) as an adjunct to walking 30 minutes four times weekly (24). There were no differences between groups in total body mass, fat mass, or other variables; five treated subjects dropped out of the study because of nausea or diarrhea.

• Hemodialysis

—In eight older trials that tested the effect of carnitine on lipids in hemodialysis patients, results were mixed (25). A more recent double-blind placebo-controlled trial of 38 patients found that up to 6 months of L-carnitine infusions (20 mg/kg) caused no significant changes in lipids (25).
—An RCT in 24 patients found that L-carnitine (1 g intravenously after dialysis treatments for 6 months), compared with placebo, reduced erythropoietin use (26). It is theorized that L-carnitine deficiency may promote erythropoietin resistance in dialyzed patients.

• Chronic fatigue syndrome

—A crossover study in 30 CFS patients compared amantadine with L-carnitine, each given for two months (27). Amantadine was poorly tolerated (15 patients were unable to complete 8 weeks) and did not improve clinical parameters. L-carnitine significantly improved 12 of 18 parameters (one patient discontinued because of diarrhea).

• Peyronie's disease

—A randomized 3-month trial of 48 patients with Peyronie's disease (15 acute, 33 chronic) compared acetyl-L-carnitine (1 g b.i.d.) to tamoxifen (20 mg b.i.d.) and found acetyl-L-carnitine significantly more effective in reducing pain and inhibiting disease progression (28).

• Leg ulcers

—A double-blind pilot RCT in 15 sickle cell patients with chronic leg ulceration found no advantage of adjunctive propionyl-L-carnitine (2 g b.i.d. × 12 weeks) over placebo in ulcer healing rates (29).

• Hyperthyroidism

—A randomized, placebo-controlled, complex crossover trial of L-carnitine (2 or 4 g/day × 2 to 4 months) in 50 women concluded that both doses of carnitine reduced symptoms of hyperthyroidism (30).

• Pediatrics

—A placebo-controlled crossover RCT in 47 children with seizures found no significant effect of adjunctive carnitine (100 mg/kg/day × 4 weeks) on well-being scores (31).
—An uncontrolled trial in 14 pediatric patients with valproic acid-induced hyperammonemia found that L-carnitine (1 g/m^2/day in two doses) normalized ammonia levels (32).

OTHER CLAIMED BENEFITS/ACTIONS

• Arrhythmias
• Cardiac myopathy
• Mitral valve prolapse
• Hyperlipidemia
• Alzheimer's disease, other memory disorders
• Renal disease
• Hepatic disease
• Chronic obstructive pulmonary disease
• AIDS
• Muscular dystrophies
• Diabetes

 Clinical Considerations

DEFICIENCY SIGNS AND SYMPTOMS

• In myopathic carnitine deficiency, muscle weakness is paramount; excessive lipids may be found in muscle tissue (2). Primary systemic carnitine deficiency may resemble Reye's syndrome, causing episodes of hyperammonemia, hypoglycemia, hypoprothrombinemia, and possibly metabolic encephalopathy.

FACTORS DECREASING AVAILABILITY/ABSORPTION

• Lipid storage diseases, organic aciduria, diabetes, muscular dystrophy, hyperthyroidism, congenital carnitine deficiency, protein malnutrition, choline deficiency (see questions and answers), renal disease, hemodialysis, enteral feeding with protein hydrolysate formulas

LABORATORY TESTS

• Carnitine levels are determined spectrophotometrically or through radioisotope assay (which is 10 times more sensitive). Both depend on the carnitine acetyltransferase reaction (3).

 Risks

ADVERSE REACTIONS

• L-carnitine may cause diarrhea or agitation.
• D-carnitine has been associated with muscle pain (33) and should not be used.

 Dose

Doses of up to 3 g/day appear to be benign.

 Common Questions and Answers

Q: Do vegetarians risk carnitine deficiency?
A: Probably not. Carnitine, as its name suggests, is found mainly in meat, but lysine and methionine can be converted into carnitine (although vegetarian diets are often low in methionine). One study found that vegetarians (including lactovegetarians), especially children, had significantly lower plasma and urinary carnitine levels than nonvegetarians (34). However, it is unknown how risk of deficiency correlates with carnitine levels. Only two cases of diet-induced carnitine deficiency have been reported; one in a 12-year-old strict vegetarian, and another in a child switched from a milk-based to a soy-based formula. Both children most likely had carnitine biosynthesis defects (2).

Q: Is carnitine essential?
A: Only for mealworm larvae, although some evidence suggests that premature infants may need it as well (1). Some consider carnitine "conditionally essential" because there are many opportunities for impairment of carnitine function (3).

Carotenoids

10 Second Take

Dietary carotenoids are associated with decreased risk of cardiovascular disease and cancer; however, β-carotene supplementation does not decrease the risk of any disease.

Basics

DESCRIPTION

• Carotenoids are orange, yellow, and red pigments present in many vegetables and fruits.
• There are more than 600 carotenoids, all of which are polyisoprenoids that possess numerous conjugated double bonds.
• About 50 carotenoids serve as vitamin A precursors, including the most common carotenoids in human serum: lutein, lycopene, zeaxanthin, β-cryptoxanthin, β-carotene, and α-carotene.

FOOD SOURCES

• Carotenoids are found in many vegetables and fruits, as well as in red palm oil. β-Carotene is found in orange, red, and dark green vegetables and fruits (carrots and pumpkins are especially high in β-carotene).
• Lycopene is found in tomato products, watermelon, guava, and in smaller amounts in pink grapefruit.

MAIN FUNCTIONS/PHARMACOKINETICS

• Carotenoids enhance cell-to-cell communication, enhance differentiation of cells, modulate the immune response, and may affect reproductive performance (1).
• Besides being important precursors of vitamin A, carotenoids quench singlet oxygen and have both antioxidant and prooxidant properties, depending on the environment. Carotenoids can form radical cations or anions (highly reactive molecules that can react with other free radicals to create nonradical products) or can interact with other molecules, restoring the carotenoid to the ground state while producing a new free radical. Antioxidant properties usually predominate in physiologic conditions.

Evidence

Epidemiologic studies have linked intake of foods high in β-carotene with decreased risk of cancer of the lung, head and neck, gastrointestinal tract, breast, and prostate, as well as ischemic heart disease, stroke, and age-related macular degeneration (2). However, β-carotene supplementation trials in those at high risk of lung cancer or cardiovascular disease have found either no benefit or increased risk.

CLINICAL TRIALS

• Cancer prevention

—Two of three randomized controlled trials of the effect of β-carotene on lung cancer risk found an adverse effect of supplementation; the third found no effect. In the Alpha-Tocopherol Beta-Carotene Cancer Prevention (ATBC) Study, 29,133 Finnish smokers 50 to 69 years old were treated with β-carotene 20 mg for 5 to 8 years. There was a higher rate of lung cancer [relative risk (RR) 1.18] and total mortality (RR 1.08) in the group treated with β-carotene than in those treated with placebo (3).
—The Carotene and Retinol Efficacy Trial (CARET) tested β-carotene (30 mg/day) and retinyl ester (25,000 IU) against placebo in smokers and asbestos workers; the trial was prematurely terminated after 4 years because of increased lung cancer (RR = 1.28) and increased total mortality (RR = 1.17) in the supplemented group (4).
—In the Physicians Health Study, there were no differences between those supplemented with β-carotene capsules (50 mg every other day) and the unsupplemented group in lung cancer incidence, cancer deaths, or deaths from any cause (5).

• Pancreatic cancer

—In the ATBC trial, β-carotene had no effect on the incidence of pancreatic cancer or rate of mortality (6).

• Skin cancer

—In a study of 1,805 participants previously diagnosed with nonmelanoma skin cancer, there was no difference in recurrence of basal-cell or squamous-cell skin cancers by β-carotene supplementation (50 mg/day over 5 years) compared with placebo (7).

• Precancerous conditions

—Although dietary intake of carotenoids is linked with a lower rate of cervical cancer, two randomized, placebo-controlled trials of β-carotene supplementation (10 mg/day × 3 months in 333 women or 30 mg/day × 9 months in 98 women) found no difference between treatment and placebo in regression of cervical dysplasia (8). A recent, longer randomized placebo-controlled trial of 141 women with minor squamous atypia or cervical intraepithelial neoplasia (CIN)-1 tested 30 mg β-carotene, 500 mg vitamin C, or both for 2 years and found no effect of either supplement (9).
—In clinical trials, β-carotene supplements reduced oral leukoplakia but had no effect on colorectal adenomas or sputum atypia (1).

• Cardiovascular disease prevention

—The incidence of cardiovascular disease deaths in the ATBC study was increased 11% in the β-carotene-supplemented group (3); among the 1,862 participants who had had a previous myocardial infarction, there were significantly more deaths from fatal coronary heart disease in the β-carotene group (10). The incidence of cardiovascular disease deaths was increased 26% in the CARET study (4); there was no difference in cardiovascular disease rates in the total population of the Physician's Health Study (those with prior angina or coronary revascularizations, however, did seem to benefit) (5). In the ATBC study, β-carotene had no effect on fatal coronary heart disease (11).

• Diabetes prevention

—In the Physicians Health Study, β-carotene supplementation for an average of 12 years had no effect on the risk of type II diabetes (12).

• Photosensitivity

—Carotenoids can lessen photosensitivity caused by porphyrins by quenching excited species formed by the interaction of porphyrins with light. Both β-carotene and canthaxanthin have been used to treat erythropoietic porphyria and other photosensitivity diseases; β-carotene is preferable because canthaxanthin can cause a reversible retinopathy (13).
—A recent study found that 25 mg mixed carotenoids (primarily β-carotene) with or without vitamin E (500 IU RRR-α-tocopherol) daily for 3 months reduced ultraviolet-light-induced erythema (14).

Carotenoids

 Risks

ADVERSE REACTIONS

• Dietary and supplemental carotenoids are generally safe because they are stored in fat cells and tissues. Most are nontoxic even at high doses. Combining β-carotene and alcohol, however, can cause hepatotoxicity.
• Hypercarotenosis, a yellowish discoloration of the skin (including palms and soles, which differentiates it from jaundice) is a benign effect of high doses of carotenoids.
• Canthaxanthin can cause a reversible retinopathy.
• Anovulation and amenorrhea have been associated with carotenemia, but there is no evidence that carotenoids affect reproductive function (see questions and answers).

DRUG INTERACTIONS

• β-Carotene supplementation may reduce plasma levels of other carotenoids, but these interactions have not been well-delineated (15).
• In humans, studies have been mixed on whether carotenoids interfere with the metabolism of α-tocopherol (15).
• Alcohol interacts with β-carotene, resulting in hepatotoxicity (alcohol also appears to enhance the toxicity of vitamin A, while promoting vitamin A deficiency) (16). In baboons, ethanol delays blood clearance of β-carotene (17).

ANIMAL TOXICITY

• β-Carotene does not interfere with reproductive function in rats given up to 1,000 mg/kg orally per day. Two-year chronic toxicity studies have found no increased tumors in rats or mice; vacuolated cells with eccentric nuclei were noted in the livers of dogs and mice but not rats (18).

 Clinical Considerations

DEFICIENCY SIGNS AND SYMPTOMS

• Carotenoids are not necessary if preformed vitamin A is present in the diet (see vitamin A).

FACTORS DECREASING AVAILABILITY/ABSORPTION

• Inadequate bile flow, lipid malabsorption, reduced gastric acidity, increased dietary intake (absorption efficiency decreases as intake increases), vitamin E supplementation, fiber (especially pectins), lack of fat in diet, olestra, incomplete release of carotenoids from food matrix. Studies are mixed on whether supplementation with β-carotene decreases serum levels of other carotenoids (19).

FACTORS INCREASING AVAILABILITY/ABSORPTION

Dietary intake

LABORATORY TESTS

Plasma concentrations, measured by high-pressure liquid chromatography (HPLC)

 Dose

There is no standard dose of carotenoids; doses used in clinical trials are described previously.

 Common Questions and Answers

Q: What is the connection between carotenemia and amenorrhea?
A: Since 1971, sporadic reports of diet-induced carotenemia have been associated with menstrual dysfunction (20,21). This effect has not been noted in women receiving β-carotene supplements for photosensitivity, even when hypercarotenemia is present (22). Almost all of these women with carotenemia and menstrual dysfunction were vegetarian; hypercarotenemia may be simply a marker for a vegetarian diet, which in turn is associated with increased fecal excretion and, thus, decreased blood levels of estradiol. The effect may be due to other compounds in carrots; rabbits that have been fed large amounts of carrots show diminished ovarian secretion of progesterone (23).

Q: Isn't it impossible to overdose on β-carotene?
A: Excess β-carotene is deposited in fat and skin, causing harmless hypercarotenosis. Until recently, it was thought that even very high doses of β-carotene were nontoxic. However, a primate study found hepatotoxicity when high doses of β-carotene were combined with ethanol. One could say that high-dose β-carotene supplements should not be used in alcoholics; I would go further and say that no one should use high-dose supplements. Given the amount of data on lack of benefit and possible risk, only those with photosensitivity diseases should consider β-carotene supplementation.

Q: Why has β-carotene been so unsuccessful in clinical trials?
A: The association of serum β-carotene levels with decreased risk of cancer and heart disease may have been merely a marker for intake of carotenoids (or other protective factors in fruits and vegetables). One reason that supplementing with β-carotene may have an adverse effect is that it may displace other dietary carotenoids. Maria Linder, PhD, author of *Nutritional Biochemistry,* has suggested that use of isolated β-carotene may increase formation of oxidation products (24).

Cartilage (Shark and Bovine)

10 Second Take

Shark and calf cartilage have been promoted as cancer treatments. These are benign therapies with interesting *in vitro* properties, but there is no credible human evidence supporting efficacy as a cancer treatment.

Basics

DESCRIPTION

• Cartilage is usually obtained from sharks (which have no bones, only cartilage) or cattle (typically from calf trachea).

KNOWN ACTIVE CONSTITUENTS

• Shark cartilage contains about 40% proteins, 5% to 20% glycosaminoglycans (the most plentiful of which is chondroitin sulfate), and calcium salts (1).
• Several fractions inhibit angiogenesis *in vitro*; exact molecular identification has not been achieved (2).

MECHANISM/PHARMACOKINETICS

• Proposed mechanisms for the anticancer effect of cartilage include antiangiogenesis effects, inhibition of metalloproteinases (enzymes used by tumors to invade tissue), and stimulation of macrophages and other cytotoxic cells.
• Mucopolysaccharides in bovine cartilage also may inhibit tumor cell division. None of these proposed mechanisms has been proven.

Evidence

CLINICAL TRIALS

• Cancer

—A trial of shark cartilage in 60 patients with advanced cancer found no anticancer activity or improvements in quality of life (3). Twenty-four men and 36 women (97% with stage 4 cancer) with cancer of the breast (18), colon (16), lung (14), prostate (8), lymphatic system (3), or brain (1) received 1 g/kg of shark cartilage orally each day (in three divided doses) for at least 12 weeks. After 6 weeks, if no response was seen, the dose was increased to 1.3 g/kg. No complete or partial responses were seen; 10 of 50 assessable patients had stable disease for 12 weeks or more (range 12 to 45.7 weeks). Five patients died, and five withdrew because of gastrointestinal toxicity. Twenty-two patients (36.7%) had progressive disease by the 6-week evaluation point; five more developed progressive disease by 12 weeks. There were no significant changes in quality of life scores. Twenty-one adverse events were noted, 14 of which were gastrointestinal (nausea, vomiting, constipation).
—A case series, published as an opinion piece, claimed a partial or complete response in 31 patients with assorted advanced malignancies who were treated with oral or subcutaneous bovine cartilage (Catrix, which is powdered beef trachea) (4). Several of these cases appear quite interesting; however, heterogeneity in prognoses, prior treatment, concurrent treatment, doses, duration, and mode of administration render interpretation of this case series problematic.
—Another case series of nine patients treated with bovine cartilage (Catrix-S 5% solution, the injection form of Catrix) administered the therapy subcutaneously (100 mL × 3 weeks, then 150 mL for an additional 1 to 38 weeks) (5). This series found progressive disease in eight patients but a complete response in one patient with metastatic renal cell carcinoma. Bilateral lung metastases and a flank mass resolved during therapy (5).
—Another study of oral shark cartilage powder, presented only in abstract form at an American Society of Clinical Oncology meeting, tested oral (Catrix 3 g daily) and subcutaneous bovine cartilage (from 50 mL biweekly up to 150 mL/day) in four different schedules of administration to treat patients with metastatic renal cell carcinoma. Of 22 evaluable patients, 3 had durable partial responses and one had stable disease (6).

• Antiangiogenic effects

—The effect of orally administered liquid shark cartilage extract (not otherwise defined) on wound granulation tissue formation was tested in a randomized, double-blind controlled trial of 29 men who received placebo or one of two doses of shark cartilage extract (7 or 21 mL daily) (2). Participants took the extracts for 23 days; on day 12, an inert polyvinyl alcohol sponge (within perforated silicone tubing) was inserted subcutaneously in the arm; it was removed and examined on Day 23 for indirect measures of angiogenesis (endothelial cell density and factor VIII immunostaining). Mean endothelial cell density was significantly lower in those who ingested shark cartilage (no dose-response effect was seen), compared with placebo. Hydroxyproline content of sponges did not differ. No adverse effects or toxicity was noted; there were no changes in blood chemistry, urinalysis, or bleeding times.
—An antiangiogenic fraction of shark cartilage was found to have antiinflammatory effects on cutaneous irritation in humans (7). The authors suggest that these effects could be beneficial in psoriasis.

• Wound healing

—Topically applied sterile, powdered bovine cartilage was tested in humans in a controlled study using paired, experimentally inflicted wounds. Paired incisions were made, then "a light frosting" of cartilage applied to treated wounds, and then wounds were sutured closed. After 7 to 14 days, wounds were excised and tensile strength measured. In 12 of 15 wound pairs, the wound treated with cartilage was stronger. Overall, increased tensile strength in treated wounds was 42% (8).

• Osteoarthritis

—Chondroitin sulfate, the most prevalent glycosaminoglycan in cartilage, has a beneficial effect on arthritis (see chondroitin sulfate).

ANIMAL/IN VITRO

- Animal and *in vivo* studies have shown some antineoplastic effects against lung cancer and leukemia in rodents (1). A recent study of two commercial shark cartilage extracts found that oral administration in doses from 5 to 100 mg for up to 25 days after implantation of SCCVII carcinoma in mice had no effect on growth of the primary tumor or development of metastases (9). Another study of a fraction found that intraperitoneal injection in mice suppressed sarcoma-180 cell growth and B-16-F10 mouse melanoma cell metastasis (10).
- Powdered shark cartilage has limited activity in colon, breast, ovarian, and astrocytoma cell lines, with more pronounced growth suppression in myeloma cells (exposed to continuous high doses) and Lewis lung carcinoma cell lines (1).
- Antiangiogenic properties

—Several fractions of shark cartilage extracts have shown antiangiogenic effects (2,7,10). Inhibition of endothelial cell proliferation (a marker for antiangiogenesis) was noted in the human umbilical vein endothelial cell proliferation assay; a concentration-dependent reduction in 3H-thymidine uptake was noted (IC50 366.4 $\pm$ 4.63 μg/mL). Combining tumor necrosis factor-alpha and shark cartilage was more effective at reducing endothelial cell proliferation then either alone (11). Specificity for vascular endothelium was demonstrated; there was no effect on human astrocytoma cells or fibroblasts.

- Antiinflammatory, analgesic, and wound healing effects

—Cartilage powder or extract decreased time to healing in experimentally inflicted wounds in both diabetic (12) and nondiabetic rats (13,14); another rat experiment found that bovine cartilage reduced the adverse effects of cortisone on wound healing (15).

OTHER CLAIMED BENEFITS/ACTIONS

- Arthritis
- Wound healing

 Risk

ADVERSE REACTIONS

- No serious risks have been noted. Cartilage is usually well tolerated.
- In the Miller study of 60 patients, 14 of 20 adverse effects were gastrointestinal (nausea, vomiting, and constipation). Dysgeusia (bad taste in the mouth) and dyspepsia are not uncommon common complaints in those receiving shark cartilage. Although unusual, fatigue, nausea, fever, dizziness, and hypercalcemia have been reported. Discomfort at the injection site has also been noted in studies that used injections.

 Dose

COMMON DOSAGE FORMS

- No standard dosage has been identified; for treatment of cancer, doses as high as 110 g daily are used.
- *Powdered shark cartilage* (Catrix and others) may be administered orally in capsules, pills, in slurries, or as a liquid extract.
- *Powdered cartilage* is also used topically.
- *Powdered cartilage* has been administered as an enema.
- *Subcutaneous injection* of a sterile, pH-balanced, volume-and solids-adjusted form of powdered cartilage (Catrix-S) has also been used.

 Common Questions and Answers

Q: What is the Cuban study?
A: A 16-week study of Catrix was conducted in Cuba by William Lane (author of *Sharks Don't Get Cancer*). Never published, this study received wide publicity because it was covered on the TV show *60 Minutes* (CBS Feb 28, 1993) in which it was claimed that of 29 participants, 15 were evaluable and 3 of these showed a response to the treatment (16). Questions have been raised about whether cancer diagnoses were biopsy-confirmed, how responses were determined, and so forth. Because details have never been published, this study cannot be evaluated.

Q: Is it true that cancer is unknown in sharks?
A: No. In fact the prevalence of cancer among sharks is unknown. It is true that most cancers found in cartilaginous fish (including skates and rays, as well as sharks) are melanomas and soft tissue sarcomas.

Cascara

 10 Second Take

Cascara is an anthranoid-containing herb with laxative effects. Its effects are milder than other anthranoid-containing plants, but it can still cause significant potassium loss.

 Basics

LATIN NAME

Rhamnus purshiana DC

FAMILY

Rhamnaceae

OTHER COMMON NAMES

Cascara sagrada, buckthorn, chittem bark, sacred bark

DESCRIPTION

• A deciduous tree, 18 to 54 feet high, cascara has reddish-brown bark; thin, acutely pointed leaves; greenish flowers; and purplish fruit. Native to the Pacific coast of North America, cascara grows as far east as Montana and as far north as southeast British Columbia.

PART USED

Dried bark (see questions and answers)

KNOWN ACTIVE CONSTITUENTS

• A mixture of hydroxyanthracene derivatives
• Cascarosides A, B, C, D, E, and F (*O*- and *C*-glycosides) comprise up to 70% of the total complex; aloins and chrysaloins comprise up to 30%; and a mixture of hydroxyanthracene *O*-glycosides comprise up to 20%.

MECHANISM/PHARMACOKINETICS

• Anthranoids are compounds based on anthraquinone, dianthrone, or anthrone structures. Most anthranoids in plants are found in the glycoside form; these hydrophilic molecules pass unabsorbed through the stomach and large intestine, requiring the intervention of intestinal bacteria to split off the sugar and release the active aglycone anthrone. Aglycone anthrones include rhein, aloe-emodin, emodin, alizarin, chrysophanol, and lucidin. Anthrones are highly reactive (anthrones are 100-fold more cytotoxic than anthraquinones) and are primarily responsible for the laxative effect of anthranoid-containing plants (1).
• Cascarosides are *O*- and *C*-glycosides that are hydrolyzed by bacteria to aloins and chrysaloins, which then are respectively cleaved to aloe-emodin anthrone or chrysophanol anthrone. Aloe-emodin can in turn be oxidized to rhein. The main active metabolite is aloe-emodin-9-anthrone.
• In humans, an unestimated but probably small amount of aglycone anthrones is absorbed; after absorption, anthranoids are converted primarily to corresponding glucuronide and sulfate derivatives and excreted mainly in urine and bile (the kidneys retain some anthranoid derivatives) (2). In animal experiments, more than 20% of aloe-emodin is absorbed (bioavailability is lower, however, because aloe-emodin oxidizes quickly to rhein and an unknown metabolite) (3).
• Anthraquinones affect secretory and absorption mechanisms; mechanisms are thought to include inhibition of the sodium-potassium pump, increased mucosal permeability of the colonic mucosa, and possible effects on Meissner's plexus or prostaglandin-mediated effects (2). Anthraquinones are thought not to increase peristalsis; only the anthrones appear to have this effect.
• Pharmacokinetics studies have not been done on cascara specifically, but a human pharmacokinetics study of a preparation containing a mixture of aloins and their 3-rhamnosides found that 16.4 mg hydroxyanthracene derivatives/day for a week resulted in only tiny amounts of the metabolite aloe-emodin in plasma (less than 2 ng/mL), and this was achieved only sporadically (3).

 Evidence

CLINICAL TRIALS

No clinical trials identified.

ANIMAL/IN VITRO

• Cascarosides do not induce diarrhea in mice, rabbits, guinea pigs, rhesus monkeys, and most Wistar rats, apparently because of differences in intestinal bacterial flora.
• Mice and cats become more susceptible to cascarosides after being fed a high-protein diet, which apparently alters gut flora (2).

OTHER CLAIMED BENEFITS/ACTIONS

• Psoriasis
• Weight loss

 Risks

ADVERSE REACTIONS

• Fluid and electrolyte loss (potassium loss may be clinically significant)
• Abdominal spasms and pain
• Diarrhea
• Decreased peristalsis (chronic use can cause damage to the smooth muscles and myenteric plexi)
• Finger clubbing (chronic use of anthranoid laxatives) (4,5)
• Cholestatic hepatitis: One case of intrahepatic cholestasis and portal hypertension has been associated with cascara use (6)
• Laxatives should not be used in those with intestinal obstruction or ileus.
• Other effects

—Pseudomelanosis coli
—Discolored urine or feces (yellowish-brown or red discoloration—the color is pH-dependent) (see questions and answers).

DRUG INTERACTIONS

• Cardiac glycosides—potassium loss from anthranoid-containing laxatives may predispose those on cardiac glycosides to cardiac arrhythmias.
• Any laxative has the potential to interfere with concomitantly administered oral drugs by decreasing intestinal transit time.

ANIMAL TOXICITY

• Little data available. Aloin has low toxicity in rats and mice.
• In rats, senna and cascara glycosides may be weak promoters of colon carcinogenesis (7) (see questions and answers).

Dose

COMMON DOSAGE FORMS

• *Dried bark, cut or powdered:* 0.3 to 1 g q.d.; infusion made with 1.5 to 2 g (daily dose, single or split dose).
• *Other preparations:* equivalent to 20 to 30 mg hydroxyanthracene derivatives (calculated as cascaroside A) total daily dose.
• The proper dose of laxative is always the smallest effective dose. Not recommended for children younger than 10 years.
• Not recommended for periods of longer than 1 to 2 weeks without medical advice. Defecation occurs about 6 to 12 hours after oral administration.
• Cascara is not usually found in laxative teas because of its unpleasant taste (some preparations are treated with alkali, alkaline earths, or magnesium oxide to reduce bitterness) (7a).

 Common Questions and Answers

Q: Is it really acceptable to use cascara in lactating women?
A: Yes. Although anthraquinones are partially excreted into milk, the risk of the infant developing diarrhea is apparently minimal (5). Cascara and senna are two of only seven drugs that the American Academy of Pediatrics considers compatible with breast feeding (the other five are cimetidine, atropine, cascara, cisapride, loperamide, and magnesium sulfate) (8). Some anthraquinones, however, including aloe-emodin and emodin, are genotoxic, so some question the use of anthraquinone in breast-feeding mothers (5). Apart from effects on the infants, anthraquinone laxatives are not completely benign and should be reserved for cases in which bulk-forming agents with adequate hydration have failed.

Q: Why is fresh bark never used?
A: Fresh bark contains large amounts of anthrones. The bark is normally stored for a year or heated under aerobic conditions to decrease the anthrone level. The emetic principle (apparently resulting from monoanthrones and their *O*-glycosides) in fresh bark is destroyed on prolonged storage or by heating (9).

Q: What is pseudomelanosis coli?
A: Pseudomelanosis coli is a harmless, abnormal discoloration of the colonic mucosa (typically a reticular pattern of dark lines resembling alligator skin; histologically, dark granules are noted in the macrophages of the lamina propia). Seventy-three percent of chronic anthraquinone users manifest it, rendering it a reliable marker for chronic laxative abuse (10). Melanosis has also been reported in the gastric mucosa, but this is unusual. Pigmentation is reversible within 4 to 12 months after cessation of laxative use (10).

Q: Are all anthranoid-containing herbs fairly interchangeable?
A: No. Cascara is safer than other anthranoid-containing herbs, because cascarosides are not as easily metabolized to anthrones as are sennosides. Anthraquinone *O*-glycosides occur in substantial amounts in Chinese rhubarb (*Rheum officinale*) and are probably more highly absorbed gastrointestinally than other compounds. Anthrone *C*-glycosides and dianthrone *O*-glycosides are preferred to anthraquinones, because intestinal absorption of the aglycones in the former is much lower than with the anthraquinones (2).

Q: Isn't there a link between colon cancer and anthranoid laxatives?
A: It is not clear whether or not anthranoid laxatives increase the risk of colorectal cancer in humans. One prospective study of 1,095 patients found that the incidence of pseudomelanosis coli (a marker of chronic anthranoid laxative use) was 6.9% for patients with normal colons, 9.8% for patients with adenomas, and 18.6% for patients with colorectal carcinomas (11). A retrospective study of 3,049 patients who underwent colorectal endoscopy, however, found that the incidence of pseudomelanosis coli was 3.13% in patients without pathologic changes, 8.64% in those with colorectal adenomas, and 3.29% in those with colorectal carcinomas. Because pseudomelanosis coli resolves within 4 to 12 months, these studies can only pick up relatively recent chronic use. Two case-control studies published in German found no link between anthranoid laxative use and colorectal cancer (3).
In rats, senna and cascara glycosides may be weak promoters of colon carcinogenesis (7). On their own, these glycosides did not increase preneoplastic lesions called aberrant crypt foci (ACF). However, rats treated with a carcinogen and the highest dose of glycosides had more ACF than those treated only with the carcinogen.

Cat's Claw

10 Second Take

Cat's claw has some interesting immunostimulatory qualities *in vitro,* but there is no clinical evidence of benefit.

Basics

LATIN NAME

Uncaria tomentosa (Wildd.) DC.

FAMILY

Rubiaceae

OTHER COMMON NAMES

Uña de gato, garabato, samento, kug kukjaquil (Peru), rangaya (Panama)

DESCRIPTION

- *Uncaria tomentosa* is a woody climbing vine (a liana) that can grow to 20 m in height and bears distinctive claw-like structures on its stem.
- It grows in South and Central America. More than 20 plants in 12 different families have the common name *uña de gato* (Spanish for cat's claw).

PART USED

Inner bark

KNOWN ACTIVE CONSTITUENTS

- There are two chemotypes of *U. tomentosa,* one containing pentacyclic and one containing tetracyclic indole and oxindole alkaloids. Pentacyclic oxindole alkaloids include isopteropodine, pteropodine, isomitraphylline, uncarine F, mitraphylline, speciophylline, akuammigine, tetrahydroalstonine, and isoajmalicine. Tetracyclic alkaloids include rhynchophylline, isorhynchophylline, corynoxeine and isocorynoxeine, hirsutine, dihydrocoryneantheine, hirsuteine, and corynantheine (1).
- Eight quinovic acid glycosides, four polyhydroxylated triterpenes, and the precursor alkaloid 5α-carboxystrictosidine, oleanolic acid, and ursolic acid have been isolated (2,3). β-Sitosterol, stigmasterol, and campesterol have been isolated in a steroid fraction of bark (1).

MECHANISM/PHARMACOKINETICS

- Mechanism of action has not been well established. Water decoctions of *U. tomentosa* and *U. guianensis* had antioxidant effects and suppressed tumor necrosis factor (TNF)-α (4,5). Basal prostaglandin (PG) E_2 production was not affected, although LPS-induced PGE_2 release was significantly reduced at high doses (5). Pentacyclic oxindole alkaloids increase phagocytosis by granulocytes (6).

Evidence

CLINICAL TRIALS

- Osteoarthritis

—A placebo-controlled trial of freeze-dried *U. guianensis* in 45 patients with osteoarthritis of the knee assigned 30 subjects to treatment and 15 to placebo for 4 weeks (5). Activity-associated pain, patient assessment, and medical assessment significantly favored the cat's claw preparation over placebo; however, knee pain at rest, pain at night and knee circumference were unaffected.

- Immune stimulation

—13 HIV-positive participants (11 male, 2 female) took 20 mg/day *U. tomentosa* root in a hydrochloric acid extract containing 12 mg total pentacyclic oxindole alkaloids per gram for 2.2 to 5 months (1). There were no significant changes in T4:T8 cell ratios. Relative and absolute lymphocyte counts increased significantly (from a mean of 24.0% ± 78 to 33.7 ± 8.1); mean leukocyte numbers were unchanged.

ANIMAL/IN VITRO

- Immunostimulation/anticancer effects

—Extracts of *U. tomentosa* (0.025 to 0.1 mg/mL) stimulated interleukin (IL)-1 and IL-6 production by rat alveolar macrophages in a dose-dependent manner; IL-1 and IL-6 production was also enhanced in lipopolysaccharide-stimulated macrophages (7). Several experiments have demonstrated enhancement of phagocytosis by several alkaloids (1).
—Five of six oxindole alkaloids tested from *U. tomentosa* (isopteropodine, pteropodine, isomitraphylline, uncarine F, and speciophylline but not mitraphylline) inhibited the growth of leukemia call lines HL60 and U-937 in a dose-dependent manner. Uncarine F was most potent against leukemia cells (IC_{50} of 21.7 μmol/L in HL60 cells and 29.0 μmol/L in U-937 cells), and these doses did not inhibit human bone marrow progenitor cells (8). The methods used in this experiment have been questioned, and unpublished attempts by others to reproduce this experiment were unsuccessful (9).
—An aqueous extract of *U. tomentosa* appeared to act as a selective estrogen receptor modulator, reducing estradiol binding to poorly differentiated infiltrating ductal carcinoma cells (10).

- Mutagenesis

—*U. tomentosa* extracts demonstrate a protective effect against photomutagenesis in *Salmonella typhimurium* exposed to 8-methoxypsoralen (8-MOP) plus ultraviolet-A (UVA) (11). Urine from smokers increases mutagenicity in *S. typhimurium;* after one subject ingested an aqueous extract of *U. tomentosa* daily for 15 days, mutagenicity of urine was reduced (11).

- Antiviral effects

—At high concentrations, antiviral effects of quinovic acid glycosides against vesicular stomatitis virus were noted. There was no effect against rhinovirus (2).

- Antiinflammatory effects

—Fractionated extracts of *U. tomentosa* have shown antiinflammatory effects in the rat paw edema test (3).

- Leukopenia

—An aqueous extract of *U. tomentosa* depleted of indole alkaloids (C-Med-200) was evaluated in a doxorubicin-induced leukopenia rat model (12). Untreated rats were compared with rats that received daily gavage with C-Med-100 × 16 days; a third group received a granulocyte colony stimulator (Neupogen, injected subcutaneously × 10 days) as a positive control. Both treated groups recovered significantly faster than the control group.

OTHER CLAIMED BENEFITS/ACTIONS

- Cancer treatment or prevention
- Contraception
- Arthritis
- AIDS
- Inflammatory bowel disease
- Diverticulitis
- Gastritis
- Ulcers
- Asthma
- Diabetes
- Viral infections
- Genitourinary tract inflammation/gonorrhea
- Cirrhosis
- Menstrual disorders

Risks

ADVERSE REACTIONS

• Allergic interstitial nephritis

—There is one case report of a 35-year-old woman with systemic lupus erythematosus (SLE) and renal insufficiency who was treated intermittently with immunosuppressive therapy (13). One month after a creatinine level of 2.0 mg/dL (the patient's baseline) was recorded, the patient's level rose to 2.9 mg/dL and subsequently to 3.6 mg/dL, without manifestations of acute SLE. Her only new medicine was cat's claw 1 capsule q.i.d. (regular medications included prednisone, atenolol, metolazone, furosemide, and nifedipine). She was diagnosed with acute allergic interstitial nephritis and told to discontinue the herb. One month later her serum creatinine was 2.7 mg/dL.

ANIMAL TOXICITY

• In a 4-week oral toxicity study in rats, an aqueous extract of *U. tomentosa* in a dose of 1,000 mg/kg/day caused a significant increase in lymphocytes and decrease in neutrophils and increased kidney weight (kidney histology was normal). In an acute oral toxicity study in mice, acute LD_{50} was >16 g/kg (1).
• An *in vitro* test of aqueous extracts of *U. tomentosa* on Chinese hamster ovary cells and bacteria (*Photobacterium phosphoreum*) found no toxicity (14).

 Dose

COMMON DOSAGE FORMS

• *Teas*
• *Capsules*
• *Tablets*
• *Extracts* (aqueous or dry)
• *Traditional preparation* (boiling about 20 g sliced root bark in 1 L of water for 45 minutes, decanting, and adding water to achieve original volume) for a 10-day supply would provide about 4 mg of oxindole alkaloids a day.

 Common Questions and Answers

Q: Isn't cat's claw used for contraception?
A: Peruvian Indians have used an infusion of the root bark to prevent conception. It is said that drinking the tea 3 months in a row during menses helps prevent pregnancy for up to 4 years. I could not find any evidence supporting this claim.

Catnip

 10 Second Take

Catnip is a benign herb (although an overdose effect has been reported in a toddler). Recreational drug effects are probably exaggerated.

 Basics

LATIN NAME

Nepeta cataria

FAMILY

Labiatae

OTHER COMMON NAMES

Catmint

DESCRIPTION

• Catnip is a perennial herb in the mint family.
• Indigenous to Europe and cultivated in the United States, catnip has been used medicinally in humans and recreationally in both cats and humans.

PART USED

Leaf

KNOWN ACTIVE CONSTITUENTS

• Catnip contains 7-methylcyclo-pentapyranones (also called methylcyclopentanoid monoterpenes or simple iridoids).
• The *cis-trans* isomer nepetalactone comprises 70% to 99.9% of the essential oil and the *trans-cis* isomer *iso* nepetalactone or epinepetalactone comprises 0.1% to 30% of the oil (1).
• Other iridoids include dihydronepetalactone, isodihydronepetalactone, neonepetalactone, and 5,9,-dehydronepetalactone. It has also been reported to contain a sesquiterpene (1).

MECHANISM/PHARMACOKINETICS

• No information is available on mechanism of action or pharmacokinetics. Nepetalactone, however, is chemically similar to the valepotriates, sedating compounds found in valerian (2).

 Evidence

CLINICAL TRIALS

No clinical trials identified.

ANIMAL/IN VITRO

• Cats experience a well-documented response to the smell of catnip that usually involves a sequence of sniffing, licking and chewing with head shaking, chin and cheek rubbing, and rolling and body rubbing (1). The response lasts about 15 minutes, and there is a refractory period of about an hour. The response is inherited as an autosomal dominant gene. Catnip has no effect on cats when it is administered orally.
• Mice fed catnip as 10% of a meal experienced amphetamine-like effects including increased locomotion, rearing behavior, and seizures, as well as decreased sodium pentobarbital-induced sleeping time (3). Tolerance appeared to develop to these effects over time.

OTHER CLAIMED BENEFITS/ACTIONS

• Insomnia
• Anxiety
• Colic
• Dyspepsia
• Tonic
• Intoxicant
• Colds
• Respiratory problems (smoked)

Risks

ADVERSE REACTIONS

• A 19-month-old toddler who consumed raisins soaked in catnip tea (and who had the tea bag in his mouth) became first listless and then obtunded and hypotonic (4). Sixty hours after admission, the patient had a bowel movement and rapidly recovered; he was discharged the next day.

PREGNANCY/LACTATION

Catnip is reputed to be a uterine stimulant and so should not be used during pregnancy.

 ## Dose

COMMON DOSAGE FORMS

Usually taken as tea.

 ## Common Questions and Answers

Q: Can catnip be used as a recreational drug?
A: People have smoked catnip recreationally, but it is not clear whether it has psychoactive effects in humans. One report describes four cases of short-lived euphoria in catnip smokers (5). The plant pictures accompanying the report identified marijuana as catnip and vice versa. The picture mix-up does not disqualify the written report (in all likelihood the author had nothing to do with the pictures), but it is certainly possible that any psychoactive effects of catnip are merely placebo effects.

Q: Do other animals exhibit the catnip response?
A: This has been well studied. No, at least for dogs, rabbits, mice, rats, guinea pigs, and fowl. Even among felines (*Felis* species), there are species differences. One researcher found that lions and jaguars are extremely sensitive, whereas tigers, pumas, leopards, and bobcats have little to no response. Another researcher tested at least one animal in the following species and found at least one responder among lions, tigers, leopards, jaguars, snow leopards, clouded leopards, bobcats, lynx, pumas, Asiatic golden cats, ocelots, and margay cats. No response was found in cheetahs, servals, a swamp cat, a Pallas' cat, a leopard cat, an African golden cat, fishing cats, jaguarundis, and a pampas cat (1).

Q: Do other substances affect cats the same way?
A: Yes. Valerian (*Valeriana officinalis*) attracts cats (it is also said to attract rats). *Teucrium marum* (cat thyme), *Viburnum opulus* (cramp bark), and a variety of other plants have been reported also to attract cats; in addition, several species of ants and beetles secrete substances that attract cats. All of these compounds are methylcyclopentapyranones.

Chamomile

 10 Second Take

Chamomile is a benign, pleasant-tasting herb used for stomach complaints and as a mild sedative. Occasional allergic reactions have been reported.

 Basics

LATIN NAME

Matricaria recutita L., also *Chamomilla recutita* (L.) Rauschert or *Matricaria chamomilla* sensu L.

FAMILY

Asteraceae/Compositae

OTHER COMMON NAMES

German chamomile, Hungarian chamomile, Sweet false chamomile, blue chamomile, wild chamomile, scented mayweed

DESCRIPTION

• A small, branched annual up to 18 in. high, with small white daisy-like flowers.
• It is widely distributed in waste places and extensively cultivated.
• It is distinguished from other chamomiles by the hollow, rather than solid, conical receptacle on which its yellow tubular florets are arranged.

PART USED

Flowers

KNOWN ACTIVE CONSTITUENTS

• The volatile oil contains $(-)\alpha$-bisabolol; bisabolol oxides A, B, and C; bisabolone oxide; chamazulene; chamaviolin; and spathulenol. Flavonoids include flavones, flavonols, apigenin, luteolin, quercitrin, and others. Sesquiterpene lactones include matricin, matricarin, and desacetylmatricarin.
• Coumarins include umbelliferone and herniarin (1).
• Oleanolic acid and β-sitosterol were recently identified in the essential oil (2).

MECHANISM/PHARMACOKINETICS

• Apigenin has antispasmodic effects on isolated guinea pig ileum; chamazulene, α-bisabolol, apigenin, and other flavonoids have antiinflammatory effects (3). Apigenin is a ligand for the central benzodiazepine receptor (4).
• A human dermal penetration study of the chamomile flavonoids apigenin, luteolin, and apigenin 7-O-β-glucoside demonstrated that these flavonoids are not merely adsorbed at the skin surface but penetrate into deeper skin layers (5).

 Evidence

CLINICAL TRIALS

• Eczema

—A proprietary chamomile topical cream (Kamillosan, containing 2% ethanolic extract of chamomile flowers) was compared either to placebo or to 0.5% hydrocortisone in a trial of 69 participants with atopic eczema; one treatment was applied to the left arm, the other to the right (6). The chamomile cream was clearly distinguishable in color and odor from the other two creams. At 2 weeks, all groups improved similarly in pruritus, erythema, and desquamation. A benefit for Kamillosan is claimed, but no statistical analysis is given, and data presented do not appear to support conclusions.

• Oral mucositis

—Although an uncontrolled trial in 98 cancer patients indicated that chamomile mouthwash might be effective in preventing or treating oral mucositis (7), a double-blind, placebo-controlled trial did not support this hypothesis. One hundred sixty-four patients entering their first cycle of 5-fluorouracil (5-FU)-based, five consecutive day chemotherapy were randomized to either chamomile or placebo mouthwash three times daily for 2 weeks; all patients also received oral cryotherapy for 30 minutes with each dose of 5-FU (8). Physicians scored stomatitis severity on a scale from 1 to 4; patients also completed self-assessment scores using the same scale. Daily mean mucositis scores did not differ between the chamomile group and the placebo group. No toxicity was noted.

• Common cold

—Inhaled chamomile vapors may help the common cold. Sixty patients with colds were randomly allocated to four groups; all treated themselves with steam inhalation. Three groups received different doses of a chamomile extract (13, 26, or 39 mL of an alcohol extract), which were mixed into a liter of water that had been boiled and then cooled to 50°C. The control group received only the 35% alcohol solution to administer in the same manner (9). After a single treatment, patients estimated symptoms on a visual analog scale. The sum of the total analog scores (STAS) was statistically different between control and the highest dose of chamomile, and the sum of differences of discomfort intensity (SDDI) was statistically different between control and the 26 and 39 mL doses of chamomile.

• Colic

—In a randomized, double-blind, placebo-controlled trial, a mixed herb tea containing chamomile was tested in 72 colicky 2- to 8-week-old infants (10). Sixty-eight infants completed the study. Tea was offered at every episode of colic, up to 150 mL/dose up to three times daily, for 7 days. Besides chamomile, the herb tea also contained vervain (*Verbena officinalis*), licorice (*Glycyrrhiza glabra*), fennel (*Foeniculum vulgare*), and balm (*Melissa officinalis*), natural flavors, and glucose; the placebo tea contained only glucose and natural flavorings. The herb tea eliminated colic in 57% of 33 infants, whereas placebo eliminated colic in 26% of 35 infants. The mean colic score was also significantly improved in tea-treated infants. Number of night wakings was not different between the two groups.

• Radiation dermatitis

—Topical chamomile ointment was tested against almond ointment in the prevention of acute radiation skin reaction in a placebo-controlled trial of 50 breast cancer patients receiving radiation treatment (11). Each patient served as her own control by applying one cream above the mastectomy scar and one cream below the scar. Acute skin reaction was assessed by physicians on a 4-point scale; patients also evaluated symptoms of pain and itching. No statistically significant difference was found between the areas treated with chamomile or almond ointment.

—A comparison of hydrocortisone 1% cream, chamomile cream (Kamillosan), and a witch hazel (*Hamamelis virginiana*) preparation found that only the hydrocortisone cream reduced ultraviolet (UV)-radiation induced erythema (12).

ANIMAL/IN VITRO

• Apigenin has anxiolytic effects in mice without causing sedation or muscle relaxation (4).
In an *in vitro* study of isolated rat mast cells, chamazulene and α-bisabolol did not affect degranulation of rat mast cells; the *trans* en-yne dicycloether partly inhibited degranulation in concentrations above 10^{-4}M (13).

OTHER CLAIMED BENEFITS/ACTIONS

• Tonic
• Dyspepsia
• Colic
• Insomnia
• Fevers
• Sedative
• Antiinflammatory (topical)
• Wounds and sores (topical)
• Colds (inhaled)
• Antibacterial, antifungal

Risks

ADVERSE REACTIONS

- Allergy to members of the Compositae family are not uncommon, especially among those allergic to ragweed. Chamomile allergy is less common than is thought (see questions and answers).
- An enema made from chamomile (Kamillosan) given during labor to a 35-year-old woman with no history of atopy resulted in anaphylaxis and fatal asphyxia of the newborn (14); skin prick test with the chamomile preparation was strongly positive. Two reports of anaphylaxis from chamomile tea have been reported (15,16), but in neither of these cases was a definitive identification of the plant made (see questions and answers).
- A case of severe asthma occurred after a 58-year-old tea trader inhaled a chamomile aerosol to treat influenza, and chronic respiratory symptoms are reported to be higher in workers processing teas containing chamomile (17).
- In a study of chamomile extract administered by steam inhalation, up to 40% of those receiving the highest dose reported transient, mild dizziness (9).

PREGNANCY/LACTATION

- Chamomile is reputed to be a safe herb for pregnant or lactating women; however, a chamomile enema during labor resulted in anaphylaxis (see adverse effects).

ANIMAL TOXICITY

- Acute toxicity is low.
- In rabbits, acute oral and acute dermal LD_{50} values of essential oil of chamomile was greater than 5 g/kg (3).

 Dose

COMMON DOSAGE FORMS

- *Dried flowerheads:* 2 to 5 g (usually as tea or infusion) t.i.d. to q.i.d., between meals. Infusion may be used as a gargle or externally as a rinse or poultice.
- *Liquid extract:* (1:1 in 45% alcohol) 1 to 4 mL t.i.d.

 Common Questions and Answers

Q: Are the dangers of chamomile as an allergen exaggerated?
A: Yes. It is likely that neither of the cases of anaphylaxis resulting from tea were actually caused by true chamomile. Neither report identified the herb by genus and species, and neither analyzed the preparation for a positive identification. The herb is identified only as "chamomile," a term that can cover not only true German chamomile but also Roman or English chamomile [*Chamaemelum nobile* (L.) All., formerly *Anthemis nobilis* L.] or *Anthemis cotula* L. "dog's chamomile" or "stinking dog fennel" (this plant smells like chamomile with undertones of garbage). Even the potential of chamomile to cause contact dermatitis is probably exaggerated. A critical review of 50 reports of allergic contact dermatitis attributed to chamomile found that most of the articles referred to *Anthemis cotula* or its relatives. *Anthemis cotula* is extremely high in the sesquiterpene lactone anthecotulide, whereas true chamomile generally contains only traces (in species cultivated for drug use, anthecotulide is generally not detectable) (17).
However, people sensitized to specific sesquiterpene lactones may cross-react to others, and chamomile is not an uncommon sensitizer among florists and gardeners; occasional patients are sensitized through the use of Compositae-containing cosmetics or massage oils. In individuals receiving patch tests for contact dermatitis, 118 of 3,851 (3.1%) reacted to a Compositae mix; of these, 56.5% reacted to (correctly identified) chamomile (18).

Chamomile, Roman

 10 Second Take

Roman chamomile is a benign herb used for similar indications as German chamomile.

 Basics

LATIN NAME

Chamaemelum nobile, formerly *Anthemis nobilis*

FAMILY

Compositae/Asteraeeae

OTHER COMMON NAMES

English chamomile, garden chamomile, lawn chamomile, sweet chamomile, true chamomile, or double chamomile

DESCRIPTION

A fragrant, white-flowered, branched, creeping perennial, up to a foot high, native to southern and western Europe.

PART USED

Flowers

KNOWN ACTIVE CONSTITUENTS

• Volatile oil has aliphatic esters, especially n-butyl angelate and isoamyl angelate.
• Chamazulene renders the essential oil blue. Sesquiterpene lactones, including the germacranolides nobilin, 3-epinobilin, 1,10-epoxynobilin, and 3-dehydronobilin.
• Also other hydroxyperoxides, flavonoids (including apigenin and luteolin), phenols, and small amounts of coumarins and thiophene derivatives (1).

MECHANISM/PHARMACOKINETICS

• Apigenin has antispasmodic effects on isolated guinea pig ileum; chamazulene, α-bisabolol, and apigenin have antiinflammatory effects (2). Apigenin is a ligand for the central benzodiazepine receptor (3).
• A human dermal penetration study of the chamomile flavonoids apigenin, luteolin, and apigenin 7-O-β-glucoside demonstrated that these flavonoids are not merely adsorbed at the skin surface but penetrate into deeper skin layers (4).

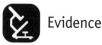 Evidence

CLINICAL TRIALS

No clinical trials identified.

ANIMAL/IN VITRO

• There are few studies of Roman chamomile, but several compounds that occur in this and other chamomiles have been tested. In rats, the antiinflammatory activity of sesquiterpene lactones with α-methylene-γ-lactone ring (as present in nobilin) has been demonstrated (1).
• Some hydroperoxides have been shown to have moderate antibacterial activity (5).

OTHER CLAIMED BENEFITS/ACTIONS

• Sedative
• Mild analgesic
• Increases appetite
• Antiemetic
• Antispasmodic
• Irritable bowel
• Dysmenorrhea
• Flatulence
• Antiinflammatory (topical)

Risks

ADVERSE REACTIONS

Contact dermatitis

PREGNANCY/LACTATION

• This herb is reputed to have abortifacient effects and should not be consumed during pregnancy.

ANIMAL TOXICITY

Acute toxicity is relatively low; acute LD_{50} values in rats exceed 5 g/kg (6).

 Dose

COMMON DOSAGE FORMS

• *Dried flowerheads:* 1 to 4 g usually as infusion t.i.d. to q.i.d. between meals.
• *Liquid extract:* (1:1 in 70% alcohol) 1 to 4 mL t.i.d.
• Infusion may be applied topically.

 Common Questions and Answers

Q: Does this herb cause emesis or treat emesis?
A: Roman chamomile does not cause emesis. Several sources note that high doses of Roman chamomile can cause emesis; all of these references can be tracked back to the 1982 edition of *Martindale: The Extra Pharmacopeia.* More recent editions have dropped this adverse effect. Roman chamomile is used to treat nausea and vomiting; although there is a theoretical concern that high doses of anthemic acid could cause vomiting, it is of little clinical relevance.

Q: Are Roman chamomile and German chamomile interchangeable?
A: Both of these chamomiles are used for many similar purposes, serving as digestives, antispasmodics, and sedatives. Although they differ in essential oil and chemical composition, many compounds (including sesquiterpene lactones and flavonoids) are common to both. German chamomile (*Matricaria recutita* L.) is more commonly used medicinally.

Chaparral

10 Second Take

Although a constituent of chaparral has some anticancer qualities *in vitro,* there is no reliable clinical evidence of benefit. Chaparral is hepatotoxic and should not be used internally.

Basics

LATIN NAME

Larrea tridentata (Sessé & Moc. ex DC.) Coville

FAMILY

Zygophyllaceae

OTHER COMMON NAMES

Greasewood, creosote bush, *hediondilla, gobernadora*

DESCRIPTION

- A small woody, evergreen desert shrub with thorny stems and fleshy leaves that thrives in poor, sandy soil.
- It is common in the southwestern United States and Mexico.
- The plant has a pungent, acrid odor.

PART USED

Leaf

KNOWN ACTIVE CONSTITUENTS

- The lignan nordihydroguaiaretic acid (NDGA) constitutes 5% to 10% of the dry weight of leaves.
- Major secondary components are waxes, volatile compounds, saponins, and phenolics (the latter account for up to 91% of extractable dry weight). Phenolic compounds include flavonoid aglycones and glycosides, NDGA, and related lignans (including secoisolariciresinol, enterolactone, enterodiol, matairesinol, guaiaretic acid, dihydroguaiaretic acid, guaiaretic acid diquinone, and didehydrolarreatricin) (1).

MECHANISM/PHARMACOKINETICS

- NDGA has antioxidant effects and inhibits cyclooxygenase and lipoxygenase pathways of arachidonic acid metabolism (2).
- Some components of chaparral have estrogenic and antiimplantation effects (1).
- NDGA competes with estradiol for binding to α-fetoprotein and demonstrates estrogenic effects in an assay using pS2 expression (an estrogen-responsive protein in ER + MCF breast cancer cells) (3).

Evidence

CLINICAL TRIALS

- Psoriasis

—In a trial of four patients with stable plaque psoriasis, NDGA was tested in concentrations of 0.5%, 1.0%, 2.0%, and 3.0% w/v. All concentrations were tested in all patients, using a grid system on selected plaque. Betamethasone 17-valerate 0.025% ointment was used as an active control. Each treatment was applied daily for 14 days (with occlusion); patients were examined and the area photographed each day. Only the steroid cream-treated squares appeared normal after 10 days; other treated areas showed no change other than reduction in scaling, attributable to occlusion (4).

- Cancer

—There is a case report of regression of rapidly growing recurrent malignant melanoma (previously excised three times) of the cheek in an 85-year-old man who, after refusing further medical treatment, began drinking 2 to 3 cups daily of chaparral tea; 10 months later the lesion had shrunk from 3 to 4 cm to 2 to 3 mm, satellite lesions had disappeared, a previous large, tender mass in the right inframandibular area had disappeared, and the patient had gained 25 pounds (5).
—On the basis of the previous case and some experimental data, the National Cancer Institute (NCI) sponsored a yearlong clinical trial of NDGA in patients with advanced malignancy; some patients drank chaparral tea and others received pure NDGA (250 to 3,000 mg/day) (6). Of 45 evaluable outcomes, four remissions were reported (apparently including the malignant melanoma patient mentioned previously). The other remissions were another patient with melanoma (3-month remission), a patient with testicular choriocarcinoma metastasized to the lung (remission of 2 months), and a patient with lymphosarcoma (regression lasted 10 days). None of these "remissions" was lasting. Apparently this report, published in the *Rocky Mountain Medical Journal* (7), lacks relevant clinical detail (6).

ANIMAL/IN VITRO

- Cancer

—NDGA and chaparral extracts have had mixed (predominately negative) effects in various animal tumor models (6).

- Renal effects

—NDGA has been used to induce renal cystic disease in rats (2). In mice, NDGA markedly reduces both toxic and carcinogenic effects of the renal carcinogen ferric-nitrilotriacetate (8).

- Immunosuppression

—In an *in vivo* model of allograft rejection in mice, NDGA had a beneficial effect (compared with a vehicle control) in preventing infiltration and subsequent cytotoxicity of sensitized effector cells without compromising basic cell functions (9).

OTHER CLAIMED BENEFITS/ACTIONS

- Kidney problems
- Colds
- Arthritis
- Tuberculosis
- Chickenpox
- Gastrointestinal complaints
- Rheumatism (topical)
- Cuts, sores, bruises, burns (topical)
- Contraception
- Weight loss
- Liver tonic

Risks

ADVERSE REACTIONS

• Hepatotoxicity

—Numerous cases of hepatotoxicity associated with chaparral ingestion have been reported. A review of 18 adverse effects associated with chaparral (11 associated with chaparral capsules or tablets and four associated with mixed products containing chaparral; for two patients no information on product was available) reported to the Food and Drug Administration (FDA) between 1992 and 1994 found that there was evidence of hepatotoxicity in 13 cases. The pattern was consistent and included jaundice; marked increases in liver function tests; and histopathologic features of hepatocellular necrosis, cholestasis, cholangitis, and cirrhosis (the predominant pattern of injury was drug-induced or toxic cholestatic hepatitis) (10). In 10 of these cases there was sufficient documentation to show that ingestion of chaparral and hepatotoxicity were related. Another report of two cases describes a 42-year-old woman who developed hepatitis 2 months after starting chaparral and a 71-year-old man who developed hepatitis 3 months after ingesting chaparral leaf daily; in the latter case the illness resolved with discontinuation and recurred with rechallenge (11). In another case, a severe cholangiolitic hepatitis was demonstrated in a patient who had taken chaparral tablets (160 mg/day) for 2 months (12).

• Autoimmune syndrome

—A 40-year-old man developed a positive Coombs test after beginning a regimen of four chaparral tablets daily (13). After discontinuing the herb both direct and indirect antiglobulin tests decreased and became negative. Rechallenge with chaparral after 8 weeks resulted in a positive direct antiglobulin test after 5 weeks and a positive indirect antiglobulin test after 16 weeks (there was no evidence of decreased red cell survival).

DRUG INTERACTIONS

• None reported. However, it would be expected that combination with other hepatotoxic drugs or herbs could increase the risk of hepatic injury.

ANIMAL TOXICITY

• NDGA is a known nephrotoxin and is used to induce renal cysts in rats (14).
• LD_{50} in rats is 100 mg/kg in propylene glycol-water and 5,500 mg/kg orally. LD_{50} is 800 mg/kg intraperitoneally with peanut oil. NDGA administered at 0.2% level chronically in drinking water of hamsters was without ill effect.

Dose

COMMON DOSAGE FORMS

• The oral ingestion of chaparral is not recommended. It is often taken as tea, usually ½ cup up to q.i.d. Externally it is used as a poultice or as a salve.

Common Questions and Answers

Q: Wasn't NDGA used in foods?
A: Yes. Up until 1967 (when more effective antioxidants were introduced), NDGA was used in the United States as a food preservative in lard, oils, candies, baking mixes, frozen foods, and so forth at levels up to 0.02% (5).

Q: Why aren't there more cases of liver injury reported?
A: As with other herb or drug hepatotoxins, there is varying susceptibility to hepatotoxic effects.

Q: Where does the Spanish name for this plant (*gobernadora* means governess) come from?
A: The plant crowds out other plants. Apparently the plant concentrates salts from the soil and falling leaves deposit these salts on the surface of the soil, creating an inhospitable environment for other plants.

Q: Are some preparations of chaparral more toxic than others?
A: Teas may be much safer than tablets, capsules, or alcohol extracts. Most (although not all) cases of chaparral toxicity have been linked to capsules or tablets, which may be much more toxic than teas simply because eating the leaves provides a larger dose of NDGA and other compounds; a hot water infusion is not very efficient at extracting these compounds. High-pressure liquid chromatography (HPLC) chromatograms of a methanolic extract of chaparral compared with chaparral tea found that the methanolic extract extracted much more NDGA (and other lignans) than the aqueous extract (1). Alcohol extracts of chaparral, tablets, and capsules are currently available; their use should be strongly discouraged. Chaparral tea is most likely less toxic but may not be completely benign. Given the lack of evidence of any benefit, all internal uses of chaparral should be discouraged. There is no evidence that external application is harmful (or, for that matter, beneficial).

Charcoal, Activated

10 Second Take

Besides gastric decontamination, activated charcoal (activated carbon, active carbon, medical coal) is a safe treatment for uremic pruritus, flatulence, diarrhea, and possibly as adjunctive treatment for neonatal hyperbilirubinemia.

Basics

DESCRIPTION

• Activated charcoal is adsorbent carbon made by heating wood or other organic matter to 800°C to 900°C in the presence of steam and the absence of air; this produces a very porous material that adsorbs odors, toxins, and dissolved organic matter (1).

KNOWN ACTIVE CONSTITUENTS

Carbon

MECHANISM/PHARMACOKINETICS

• Activated charcoal binds small molecular weight compounds by adsorption. It acts within the gastrointestinal tract and is not systemically absorbed. Its effect in hyperbilirubinemia is probably due to binding bilirubin in the gastrointestinal tract and interrupting its enterohepatic circulation.

Evidence

Activated charcoal is commonly used in emergency departments for absorbing drugs in the gastrointestinal tract. Gut decontamination trials are not covered.

CLINICAL TRIALS

• Flatulence/Gas

—A placebo-controlled study of 99 adults (69 in India and 30 in the United States) tested activated charcoal on breath hydrogen concentration (which correlates with hydrogen production in the colon). Charcoal (four capsules, each containing 260 mg) or placebo was given to each participant, with the same dose repeated 1 hour later. Lactulose was given between charcoal doses to create intestinal gas. Symptoms of bloating, abdominal cramps, and loose stools were recorded. Activated charcoal reduced breath hydrogen levels and symptoms significantly compared with placebo (2). Activated charcoal was not effective if given with or after lactulose.
—A small placebo-controlled crossover trial by the same investigator compared activated charcoal (260 mg/capsule), simethicone (20 mg/capsule), and placebo in 10 volunteers who ate beans (3). After taking fasting breath samples, four coded capsules were given to each subject, with the dose repeated at 1 hour. Baked beans were consumed 30 minutes after the first dose. One volunteer did not produce H_2; in the nine others charcoal significantly reduced peak breath H_2 levels and symptoms compared with placebo. Simethicone had no benefit over placebo.

• Uremic pruritus

—A double-blind crossover study found that activated charcoal (6 g q.d. × 8 weeks) relieved pruritus in 10 of 11 hemodialysis patients (4).
—An uncontrolled trial in 23 hemodialysis patients with severe pruritus (10 underwent a 1-week placebo run-in, during which symptoms remained stable) tested activated charcoal (6 g q.d. × 6 weeks) (5). Pruritus disappeared in 10 patients and improved in 10 other patients; effects lasted several weeks.

• Cholestasis of pregnancy

—An open study randomized 19 women (during 20 pregnancies) with cholestasis of pregnancy to activated charcoal (50 g in a water suspension t.i.d. × 8 days) and found no effect on pruritus but significantly decreased serum bile acids (6). Compared with baseline, mean bile acids decreased by about 50% in the charcoal group and increased in controls. The difference between groups was statistically significant at 8 days.

• Neonatal hyperbilirubinemia

—A controlled study of 30 neonates with hyperbilirubinemia compared phototherapy and charcoal (7.5 mL to 10 mL of slurry, containing 0.98–1.3g activated charcoal in 10% dextrose, before every meal) with phototherapy alone (7). Significantly faster and greater declines in blood bilirubin levels were noted in the charcoal-treated group. Treatment was discontinued in one baby due to vomiting; no other adverse effects were noted.

• Diarrhea

—A German study compared tannalbuminate (TA)/ethacridinlactate (EL) to charcoal for travelers diarrhea in 186 German tourists in Turkey. TA/EL was more effective in normalizing stool frequency and decreasing pain; complaints of moderate to severe abdominal pain were 50% in the TA/EL group and 82.2% in the charcoal group (8).
—A randomized controlled (unclear whether blinded) study of 39 Indonesian children with acute gastroenteritis and severe dehydration tested orally administered activated charcoal as an adjunct to intravenous and oral rehydration (9). The charcoal was given until 1 day after cessation of diarrhea. Endpoints were number of days in the hospital with diarrhea, total amount of oral rehydration solution used, and total amount of lactated Ringer's solution used. The group that received charcoal used significantly less oral rehydration therapy (ORT) and lactated Ringer's solution and averaged significantly fewer days of diarrhea 2.125 days (± 0.80), compared with 3.0 days (± 1.17) for controls.

- Hypercholesterolemia

—The only published double-blind trial found no effect of activated charcoal. Twelve hypercholesterolemic patients were randomized to activated charcoal (5 g t.i.d.) or control (unactivated charcoal 5 g t.i.d.) for 12 weeks (10). Twelve patients (largely overlapping the first group) took part in an increased-dose study, receiving 10 g t.i.d. for 12 weeks. Significantly decreased cholesterol was noted in only two patients (one received 15 g/day and another received 30 g/day). Hematologic and biochemical parameters did not change.

One patient in the 30-g charcoal group died, apparently from recurrent myocardial infarction. Several participants noted loose stools; mean stool weights increased in all groups. Fat excretion did not increase; however, two patients treated with anticoagulants required an increased dose, but there was no change in prothrombin time overall.

—A crossover study in seven patients with hypercholesterolemia found more positive results; this study compared four doses of charcoal (4, 8, 16, and 32 g/day) with bran (8 g/day); each phase lasted 3 weeks. Charcoal decreased total and low density lipoprotein (LDL)-cholesterol and increased the ratio of high density lipoprotein (HDL)-cholesterol to LDL-cholesterol in a dose-dependent manner. The 32-g dose reduced total cholesterol by 29% and LDL by 41%; HDL increased in 6 of 7 patients (11). In a second crossover study published in the same report, 10 patients with severe hypercholesterolemia received activated charcoal (16 g daily in divided doses), cholestyramine 16 g, cholestyramine 8 g plus activated charcoal 8 g, or bran (control). In the charcoal-only group, total cholesterol was reduced 23%, LDL-cholesterol decreased 29%; in the cholestyramine group, total cholesterol decreased 31% and LDL 39%; and the combination lowered total cholesterol 30% and LDL 38%. All active regimens improved HDL/LDL ratios. Triglycerides increased with cholestyramine but not with charcoal. Some improvement in lipid parameters persisted during the bran phase.

—A small uncontrolled trial in seven patients with hypercholesterolemia treated with 24 g/day charcoal in divided doses for 4 weeks found that the treatment decreased total cholesterol 25% and LDL-cholesterol 41% and increased HDL-cholesterol 8% (there was no effect on triglycerides) (12).

ANIMAL/IN VITRO

- Activated charcoal lowers bilirubin levels in hyperbilirubinemic rats. *In vitro*, activated charcoal binds bile acids (6).

 Risks

ADVERSE REACTIONS

- Activated charcoal in the doses discussed here is quite safe; the main concern is its propensity to adsorb concurrently administered medications. Charcoal blackens stools because it is not absorbed; this is completely benign. Occasional constipation and loose stools have been reported in clinical trials.
- Even in the large repeated doses used in treating acute ingestions, charcoal is still safe (more than 100,000 patients were treated with activated charcoal, in cases reported to the American Association of Poison Control Centers, and yet reported adverse events are rare) (13). These unusual events include aspiration pneumonitis, empyema, bronchiolitis obliterans, and several cases of intestinal obstruction resulting from charcoal bezoars (13). Most of these cases involved multiple doses in the treatment of ingestions of drugs with antiperistaltic activity, but in one case small-bowel obstruction developed after administration of 350-g charcoal for treatment of theophylline toxicity (adhesions were present at the ileocecal valve) (14). The risk of aspiration pneumonia is low even in intubated patients; a retrospective review of 50 overdose patients who required intubation and then were treated with activated charcoal found that only two patients (4%) developed new infiltrates (15).

DRUG INTERACTIONS

- Activated charcoal is used in overdoses because it adsorbs many substances. It has the potential to adsorb many orally administered drugs (or dietary supplements) and should be administered between meals and as far away from medication as practicable.
- *Coumarins:* In one trial, two patients on coumarin anticoagulants required an increase in dosage while taking charcoal (10).
- *Vitamins:* Up to 30-g charcoal daily apparently does not affect vitamin absorption (see questions and answers).
- *Oral contraceptives*: Activated charcoal (5 g q.i.d.) taken at least 3 hours after an oral contraceptive did not increase the risk of breakthrough ovulation (16).

 Dose

COMMON DOSAGE FORMS

- Doses have ranged from 2 g to 150 g depending on study and indication
- Hypercholesterolemia: 24 to 32 g
- Uremic pruritus: 6 g q.d.
- Cholestasis of pregnancy: 50 mL activated charcoal in slurry t.i.d.
- Gas: 1 g b.i.d. to q.i.d.

 Common Questions and Answers

Q: Does activated charcoal benefit hypercholesterolemia in some patients?
A: It may benefit a subset of patients, but it is not clear what this subset is. The effect is not consistent enough to be clinically useful. The therapy has other limitations; the large doses required, as well as its propensity to adsorb many medications, makes it an inconvenient long-term therapy.

Q: Because charcoal blackens stools, won't patients know whether they are receiving charcoal in a controlled trial?
A: One of the trials mentioned previously used inactivated charcoal, which also blackens stools, as a control.
Other trials have addressed this point by supplementing all participants with iron, which also blackens stools. The downside to adding iron is that it adds an additional variable; iron can cause gastrointestinal symptoms including nausea and constipation.

Q: Does activated charcoal lower serum vitamin levels?
A: Apparently not, even in doses of 30 g daily. Two trials looked at vitamin levels; Neuvonen found that serum vitamin A, D, and E levels were unaffected, and Hoekstra found no changes in levels of vitamin A, B$_{12}$, E, carotene, or folic acid (10). Both trials lasted at least 3 months, long enough to note decreases if charcoal interfered with vitamin absorption.

Chocolate/Cocoa/Cacao

10 Second Take

Chocolate is rich in antioxidants, magnesium, and compounds that are similar to cannabinoids. Humans often overdose on this herb without ill effects.

Basics

LATIN NAME

Theobroma cacao L. ssp. Cacao

FAMILY

Sterculiaceae or Byttneriaceae

DESCRIPTION

• Chocolate comes from the beans of the cacao tree, a 20-ft. tall evergreen that originated in South America and was brought into Mexico by the Mayas before the seventh century AD. Its species name, Theobroma, is Greek for "food of the gods."
• The words chocolate and cocoa are derived from the Aztec; chocolate means "bitter water" and cocoa is an 18th century corruption of the tree's name "cacao."
• Originally an unsweetened beverage flavored with chili peppers, Europeans invented the sweet form of hot chocolate. The use of chocolate in confectionary dates only from 1828, when the use of a screw press to separate cocoa butter from chocolate became popular. Defatted cocoa powder was one result of this innovation, and the other was cocoa butter, which could now be added to chocolate to create the smooth candies that are so popular today (1).

PART USED

Fruit (bean)

KNOWN ACTIVE CONSTITUENTS

• Chocolate contains the methylxanthines theobromine, theophylline, and caffeine.
• The caffeine content of chocolate is much lower than that of tea or coffee; by weight, the caffeine content of cocoa is 0.009%, coffee 0.04%, black tea 0.06%, and green tea 0.01% (2).
• Chocolate contains significant amounts of flavonoid polyphenols. Cocoa powder has more phenols by weight than bakers (unsweetened) chocolate, which has more phenols than milk chocolate.
• A study comparing the catechin content of chocolate and tea found that dark chocolate contained the most catechins (53.5 mg/100 g), milk chocolate contained 15.9 mg/100 g, and an infusion of black tea (1 g per 100 mL water) contained only 13.9 mg/100 mL (3). The type of catechins differed; chocolate contained only (+)-catechin and (−)-epicatechin, whereas tea contained only low concentrations of those catechins. However, tea contained more types of catechins, including high concentrations of (−) epigallocatechin gallate (EGCG) and (−)-epicatechin gallate, as well as low concentrations of (−) epigallocatechin and (+)-gallocatechin.
• Chocolate contains 0.4 to 6.6 μg/g phenylethylamine (similar in structure to amphetamine) (4). Chocolate also contains phenylalanine and tyrosine, both precursors to norepinephrine and dopamine (5). In addition, chocolate contains three unsaturated N-acylethanolamines (NAEs) that may act as cannabinoid mimics (see animal/in vitro and questions and answers). It is unclear whether these substances directly activate cannabinoid receptors or increase levels of anandamide, a brain lipid that mimics the effect of marijuana (6).
• Chocolate and cocoa powder are very rich sources of magnesium; chocolate contains 100 mg/100 g, and cocoa powder contains 520 mg/100 g (4).

MECHANISM/PHARMACOKINETICS

• Although the pharmacokinetics of purified methylxanthines are well established, little is known about the pharmacokinetics of chocolate.
• Platelet activation may be decreased by altered eicosanoid synthesis (see antioxidant effects).

Evidence

CLINICAL TRIALS

• Chocolate "addiction"

—A placebo-controlled, double-blind crossover study tested the effects of progesterone or alprazolam in perimenstrual craving for chocolate or sweets (7). Forty-four women fulfilled criteria for cyclic chocolate craving and 44 for cyclic sweet cravings (34 fulfilled criteria for both). After a 2-month baseline assessment and a 1-month placebo run-in, treatments (placebo, alprazolam, or oral micronized progesterone) were administered from the beginning of the third week to the second day of menses. None of the treatments decreased craving for chocolate or sweets.

—An experimental study aimed at separating physiologic from sensory factors found no evidence for a physiologic basis for chocolate craving (8). This crossover study compared the effect of chocolate bars, cocoa capsules, white "chocolate," white chocolate plus cocoa capsules, placebo, or nothing on satiation of chocolate craving in 72 students who served as their own controls. (White chocolate is made from a cocoa butter base and does not contain the pharmacologic components of chocolate or cocoa.)

Only 34 students turned in at least one observation for each treatment (this study is notable for having more dropouts than completers). Milk chocolate was the standard for craving relief. White chocolate produced intermediate scores; cocoa capsules, however, did not reduce craving any more than placebo.

—A case series noted a high rate of chocolate craving among MDMA (Ecstasy) abusers. MDMA causes long-term serotonin (5-HT) depletion, and the authors of this case series postulate that eating chocolate may have been an unconscious effort to raise 5-HT levels.

• Epidemiology

—Total intake of catechins from chocolate and tea was estimated in a representative sample of the Dutch population. Tea was the most important source of catechins, supplying 55% of the total daily intake, but chocolate was an important source as well, contributing 20% of total intake (3).

- Cardiovascular risk factors

—Low density lipoprotein (LDL) oxidation lag time was measured in 12 male volunteers, who then consumed 35 g of cocoa (2). Before cocoa ingestion, LDL oxidation lag time was 61.2 minutes. Two hours after cocoa intake, oxidation lag time was prolonged to 70.3 minutes; 4 hours after ingestion oxidation lag time had returned to 64.4 minutes.

—A study of 13 volunteers (including 6 women) gave 10 participants an 80-g semisweet chocolate bolus (9). Two hours later, epicatechin levels increased 12-fold (compared with baseline), plasma total antioxidant capacity increased 31%, and plasma 2-thiobarbituric acid reactive substances decreased 40%; in three controls who consumed low-procyanidin vanilla chips, no significant changes from baseline were seen.

—A randomized, double-blind crossover study found that compared with low-procyanidin chocolate, high-procyanidin chocolate increased plasma prostacyclin (32%) and decreased plasma leukotrienes (29%) (10). The authors suggest that altered eicosanoid synthesis may be the mechanism by which platelet activation is decreased (10).

ANIMAL/IN VITRO

- Cardiovascular risk factors

—Compared with water or a caffeine-containing beverage, cocoa consumption significantly suppressed *ex vivo* adenosine diphosphate (ADP) or epinephrine-induced human platelet activation and platelet microparticle formation (11). Delayed platelet-related primary hemostasis was demonstrated by prolonged collagen-epinephrine-induced closure time.

—*In vitro*, cocoa phenols inhibited human LDL oxidation by 75% (12). A 41-g (1.5 oz.) piece of milk chocolate contains 205 mg phenol, equivalent to the 210 mg phenol found in a 140 mL (5 oz.) serving of red wine. The authors suggest that the pairing of red wine and chocolate may have cardiovascular, as well as gustatory, benefits.

- Immunoregulatory effects

—Cacao liquor polyphenols inhibited reactive oxygen species (hydrogen peroxide and superoxide anion) in activated granulocytes and human peripheral blood lymphocytes (13).

OTHER CLAIMED BENEFITS/ACTIONS

- Mood elevation, anxiolytic, aphrodisiac, diuretic, alopecia, malaria, fever

 Risks

ADVERSE REACTIONS

- Nephrolithiasis

—It is possible that chocolate could contribute to renal stone formation in susceptible individuals. One study found that a single chocolate bar caused less pancreatic stimulation than sucrose (as determined by glucose, insulin, and C-peptide levels) but caused a significant increase in triglyceridemia, calciuria, and oxaluria (14).

- Migraine

—Chocolate has been implicated as a migraine trigger, but this has been called into question (see questions and answers).

 Dose

MODE OF ADMINISTRATION

p.o. p.r.n.

 Common Questions and Answers

Q: Why should one take calcium supplements with chocolate?
A: Combining calcium and chocolate reduces fat absorption. A randomized, double-blind, crossover trial in 10 men tested the effects of chocolate 98 to 101 g/day with or without added calcium (0.9 g calcium/day) for 2 weeks (15). Calcium supplementation reduced absorption of cocoa butter by 13% (it was calculated that the absorbable energy value of the chocolate was reduced by 9%). LDL-cholesterol was reduced by 15%; there was no effect on high density lipoprotein (HDL)-cholesterol. The addition of calcium did not change the taste of the chocolate, according to several confectionary experts who acted as tasters.

Q: Just how similar are compounds in chocolate to marijuana?
A: The substances are structurally related, although clearly marijuana is stronger. Passions run high on this point. A recent publication sought to reassure those worried that chocolate might lead to the hard stuff by reporting that NAEs in chocolate were no higher than in soybeans, hazelnuts, oatmeal, and millet (16). Researchers also tested anandamide and the endocannabinoid 2-arachidonoylglycerol (found in milk and cocoa) in an *in vivo* test used to assess cannabimimetics. Although the compounds were active in four of five behavioral tests, they were only active at much higher concentrations than delta[9]-tetrahydrocannabinol (THC). Another experiment found that most of these compounds were hydrolyzed in the gastrointestinal tract and that less than 5% of orally administered compounds entered the bloodstream. Critics of this study charge that it definitively answered a question that no one had asked (17). One response points out that the finding that NAEs do not cause overt cannabis-like effects was hardly a surprise because no one had claimed that marijuana and chocolate have comparable psychoactive effects. The two most prevalent NAEs in chocolate (N-oleylethanolamine and N-linoleylethanolamine) were not tested at all. NAEs may act synergistically and may prevent anandamide degradation rather than acting as anandamide agonists.

Q: So can chocolate cause a false-positive urine test for drugs?
A: No, but an intrepid lawyer tried that defense, arguing that his client's positive urine immunoassay for cannabinoids was due to ingestion of a large amount of chocolate (18). However, testing revealed no cross-reactivity of the NAEs, N-oleoylethanolamine or N-linoleoylethanolamine, with marijuana cannabinoids. The accused was convicted.

Q: Doesn't chocolate cause migraines?
A: Although chocolate is thought to trigger headaches, especially migraines, a double-blind study has cast doubt on that theory. Sixty-three women with chronic headache (50% migraine, 37.5% tension-type, and 12.5% mixed) followed a diet restricted in vasoactive amine-rich foods for 2 weeks before undergoing provocative trials with two samples of chocolate and two samples of carob presented in random order (19). Participants maintained diaries throughout the study, recording diet and headache. Chocolate was no more likely to provoke headache than was carob in any of the headache groups. Participants' belief in whether chocolate ingestion was related to headache did not correlate with the results.

Q: Why isn't chocolate perishable?
A: Although chocolate is a very fatty food, it does not become rancid because it is so rich in antioxidants. This quality was exploited during World War II, when there were times during combat when U.S. troops were rationed three chocolate bars a day as their only meals (12).

Chondroitin

 10 Second Take

Chondroitin is a harmless treatment for osteoarthritis; clinical trial evidence supports its efficacy.

 Basics

DESCRIPTION

• Chondroitin sulfate is a glycosaminoglycan found in the proteoglycans of articular cartilage, as well as other connective tissues (1).
• It is made of alternating sequences of sulfated residues of uronic acid (β-D-glucoronic) and α-D-N-acetyl-galactosamine linked by β bonds (2).
• Most chondroitin used in dietary supplements comes from cow trachea, but it is also taken from shark cartilage and other types of cartilage.

MECHANISM/PHARMACOKINETICS

• Mechanism is not known. Chondroitin has antiinflammatory activity and benefits cartilage metabolism *in vitro* (1). Chondroitin-sulfate is apparently absorbed as high-molecular-mass polysaccharide and partially depolymerized or desulfated low-molecular-mass polysaccharide chains. It has been suggested that high-molecular-mass chondroitin sulfate reaches the blood circulation through the lymphatic system. After ingestion, chondroitin sulfate and its depolymerized derivatives can be detected in synovial fluid and cartilage (3).
• The half-life of chondroitin sulfate in humans is 8.6 hours ($\pm$ 0.7), C_{max} is 6.6 μg/mL ($\pm$ 0.7), and T_{max} 1.0 hours ($\pm$ 0.3) (3). After intravenous administration, 53% is excreted by the kidneys; after oral administration, 19% is excreted by the kidneys (3). After absorption in the stomach and intestine, it is distributed to the liver, kidneys, synovial fluid, and cartilage.

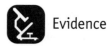 Evidence

CLINICAL TRIALS

• A meta-analysis of 15 double-blind, placebo-controlled (DBPC) trials of glucosamine or chondroitin for osteoarthritis identified nine chondroitin trials that fulfilled criteria; the pooled effect size was large for small trials (1.7) and for large trials (0.8) (using the Cohen scale, an effect over 0.8 is a large effect) (4). Although these trials showed a beneficial effect, most trials were of poor methodologic quality (including particular deficiencies associated with inflation of treatment effects), so the authors of this meta-analysis note that the actual treatment effects may be lower. However, a commentary on this study notes that the quality of the trials was comparable to studies of nonsteroidal antiinflammatory drugs (NSAIDs) in osteoarthritis (1).

Chondroitin

• An oddly designed treatment-controlled double-blind trial randomized 146 volunteers (126 completed) with unilateral or bilateral knee osteoarthritis, who had stopped other treatments for at least 15 days, either to chondroitin (400 mg t.i.d.) or diclofenac (50 mg t.i.d.); each dose in both groups was given with a placebo (5). The trial lasted 6 months. Apparently the chondroitin group received chondroitin for 3 months and then placebo only for 3 months, whereas the diclofenac group received diclofenac for 1 month and placebo for 5 months. Groups were assessed on spontaneous pain, pain on load, average consumption of acetaminophen (paracetamol), and the Lequesne Index (a scored functionality test). All measures improved in both groups; on day 45, Lequesne scores were equivalent between groups. The chondroitin group, still receiving chondroitin, continued to improve during months 2 and 3 compared with the second group (now being treated with placebo alone). Gastrointestinal symptoms were reported by three people in each group. At the 6-month mark, there were significant differences between groups favoring chondroitin on the Lequesne index, spontaneous pain, pain on load, and mean number of analgesics consumed. The unusual design of this trial, however, makes comparisons between groups difficult to make.

• A study in 24 patients compared orally administered chondroitin sulfate (0.8 g q.d. × 10 days) with placebo on biochemical parameters of synovial fluid in osteoarthritis patients scheduled for joint aspiration (3). Compared with baseline, treated patients had significant changes, with increased hyaluronate, decreased collagenolytic activity, decreased phospholipase A_2 PLA_2, and decreased N-acetylglucosaminidase (NAG); there were no significant changes in proteins or leukocytes. The placebo-treated group had no changes over baseline.

• Keratoconjunctivitis sicca

—Because chondroitin absorbs water, it has been used in conjunction with hyaluronic acid as a topical hydrating agent in the treatment of dry keratoconjunctivitis sicca. A study of 20 patients compared eyedrops containing chondroitin, hyaluronic acid, or both with an artificial tear solution (6). There was no consistent preference among patients; however, the five patients with severe dry eyes preferred solutions containing chondroitin.

• Snoring

—On the theory that reducing turbulent flow by coating nasal mucosa with a friction-reducing agent would reduce snoring, nasal administration of topical chondroitin sulfate (3 g/100 mL solution, 8 mg/instillation) was tested in a double-blind, placebo-controlled crossover study in seven non-apneic patients (including four women). No significant difference in total sleep time or sleep characteristics was found; however, time spent snoring, as a percentage of total sleep time, decreased significantly from 46.5% to 31.3% (7). There were interindividual differences; the treatment did not affect two of seven patients but dramatically affected others (in one case reducing time spent snoring from 61.6% to 8%). Equivalent noise levels did not change. The treatment was well tolerated.

ANIMAL/IN VITRO

• In rats implanted with sponges, the antiinflammatory effect of orally administered chondroitin is comparable to that of ibuprofen and indomethacin in measures of polymorphonuclear cell infiltration and macrophage infiltration; however, indomethacin and ibuprofen were more effective than chondroitin sulfate in edema (3).

 Risks

ADVERSE REACTIONS

Mild gastrointestinal symptoms have been reported.

 Dose

The usual dose is 400 mg t.i.d.

Chromium

10 Second Take

Trivalent chromium is a trace mineral important in glucose tolerance; supplementation may be helpful in diabetics.

Basics

DESCRIPTION

• Trivalent chromium is a transition element that is an essential trace mineral.
• Hexavalent chromium is a strong oxidizing agent and a pulmonary carcinogen.

FOOD SOURCES

• Whole grains, nuts, seeds, raisins, prunes, brewer's yeast, mushrooms, asparagus, beer, wine (1), and dark chocolate (2) are good sources.
• Meat (especially processed meat) and dairy products also contain chromium; acidic foods can take up chromium from stainless steel containers or cookware (which contain 11% to 30% chromium).
• Average intake is 10 to 60 μg/day (1). Chromium content in drinking water may range from 0.4 to 8.0 μg chromium/L, the mean is 1.8 μg chromium/L (3).

MAIN FUNCTIONS/PHARMACOKINETICS

• Chromium potentiates insulin action and is involved in normal metabolism of cholesterol, fat, and glucose. Absorption of chromium compounds from the gut is only about 0.5% to 2%; most ingested chromium is excreted unchanged in feces (2).
• Although small amounts of hexavalent chromium are in the diet, stomach acidity reduces hexavalent to trivalent chromium. After absorption, chromium binds to transferrin and distributes widely in the body. The kidney excretes most of absorbed chromium; about 10% is excreted in bile and small amounts in hair, nails, sweat, and milk.

Evidence

CLINICAL TRIALS

• Diabetes

—A review of 16 trials of chromium in subjects with insulin-dependent diabetes mellitus (IDDM) found that 3 trials showed no effects, whereas 13 showed improvements on at least some measures (glucose levels, insulin levels, or lipids) (4). The reviewer points out that 200 μg or less is clearly ineffective; almost all of the positive studies involved doses of 400 μg a day or more. Chromium picolinate is more bioavailable than chromium chloride. All five studies that used chromium picolinate had positive results, and 1,000 μg a day was more effective than 200 μg a day. In one of the larger, more recent, double-blind placebo-controlled studies, 180 Chinese adults with noninsulin dependent diabetes mellitus (NIDDM) were given chromium picolinate (1.92 μmol or 9.6 μmol b.i.d.) for 16 weeks. Fasting blood glucose was lower in the high-dose group at 2 and 4 months; there was no significant difference between the low-dose group and placebo. Both chromium-treated groups, compared with placebo, had lower fasting insulin concentrations and 2-hour insulin concentrations at 2 and 4 months; glycosylated hemoglobin (HbA$_{1c}$) levels decreased significantly in both treated groups at 4 months, with a significant dose-related effect (5).

• Impaired glucose tolerance

—A review of 15 controlled studies of identifiable chromium compounds in impaired glucose tolerance found that 3 reported negative findings and 12 reported positive findings (6). A placebo-controlled study of 17 volunteers fed a low-chromium diet for 14 weeks, after which they received chromium (4 μmol or 200 μg) or placebo for 5 weeks and then were crossed over to the other treatment, found no change in nine subjects with normal glucose tolerance. However, eight subjects with impaired glucose tolerance tests deteriorated further during the placebo period and improved significantly during chromium supplementation (7).
—Chromium appears to normalize both high and low blood sugar levels; one study found that the blood glucose of nondiabetic persons with good glucose tolerance was unchanged by supplemental chromium, whereas the blood glucose of persons with 90-minute glucose levels greater than 5.56 mmol/L (after glucose challenge of 1 g/kg body weight) decreased. Those who tended towards low blood sugar levels (90-minute glucose levels less than fasting) had increased blood glucose after supplementation (4).

• Lipids

—Of eight controlled trials with identified chromium compounds, four found positive results and four found negative results; doses were equivalent to 4 μmol (200 mg)/day (6). Two studies of the relationship of serum chromium levels to coronary artery disease (CAD) in a total of 122 participants (including 82 with CAD) found that mean chromium levels were significantly lower in the 82 participants with CAD than in controls (6).

• Ergogenics

—Chromium is popular as a bodybuilding aid. Studies, however, have been mixed, with better studies showing that supplementation makes no difference in lean body mass, percentage of body fat, or strength (8,9).

Risks

ADVERSE REACTIONS

• Trivalent chromium generally has low toxicity; ingestion of up to 1 mg/day has resulted in no signs of toxicity. The reference dose established by the Environmental Protection Agency (EPA) is 350 times the upper limit of estimated safe and adequate daily dietary intake (ESADDI) (200 μg). An exception is chromium sulfate, a corrosive trivalent compound that was fatal in a 48-year-old woman, who developed hemorrhagic gastroenteritis, pancreatitis, and cardiogenic shock after ingesting 48 g of chromium sulfate (3).
• Tannery workers are exposed to high levels of trivalent chromium; stainless steel welding generates hexavalent chromium (10).
• Hexavalent chromium, including chromic acid and dichromate, is quite toxic, and doses of as little as 0.5 to 0.8 g have been lethal.
• Acute chromic acid exposure causes acute gastroenteritis, gastrointestinal hemorrhage, yellow-green vomitus, hematemesis, and acute tubular necrosis with kidney failure. Treatment of poisoning with hexavalent compounds is symptomatic; the efficacy of hemodialysis, dimercaprol (BAL), and exchange transfusion has not been established (3).
• Hexavalent chromium is a known human lung carcinogen (causing squamous and small-cell carcinomas). Chromate dusts cause conjunctivitis, lacrimation, nose and throat irritation, rhinitis, epistaxis, and ulceration or perforation of the nasal septum (3).
• Topical exposure to hexavalent chromium can cause irritant or allergic contact dermatitis.
• A case report in which a 35-year-old man experienced ill-defined cognitive symptoms on three separate occasions after taking 200 to 400 μg chromium picolinate has been published (11). The description of symptoms ("feeling funny" "a disruption or short-circuiting of his thinking," and "thought processes slowed") are extremely vague and not consistent with what is known about chromium.

Clinical Considerations

DEFICIENCY SIGNS AND SYMPTOMS

- In humans given total parenteral nutrition (TPN) containing little or no chromium, deficiency can cause glucose intolerance, weight loss, and, in one case, peripheral neuropathy that reversed with chromium chloride supplementation (2).
- In animals, deficiency causes:

—Increased circulating insulin
—Hyperglycemia
—Hypercholesterolemia
—Increased fat deposition
—Decreased sperm count
—Shortened life span

Factors Decreasing Availability/Absorption

- Calcium or magnesium-containing antacids decrease absorption.
- Physical trauma or intense exercise increases urinary excretion.
- In animals, zinc, iron, and chromium appear to compete for absorption; deficiency of one of these minerals increases absorption of the others.
- High sugar diets enhance chromium loss in urine (2,9).

FACTORS INCREASING AVAILABILITY/ABSORPTION

- Vitamin C (enhances chromium absorption), aspirin, indomethacin

LABORATORY TESTS

- Laboratory indicators of chromium status are limited in usefulness; there are no chromium-specific enzymes, and levels are so low that they are difficult to measure (9).
- Plasma concentrations reflect recent exposure to both hexavalent and trivalent chromium; in the general population these concentrations are usually between 1 to 3 nmol (0.052 to 0.156 μg/L). Intracellular chromium reflects hexavalent chromium levels because only the hexavalent form penetrates erythrocytes. Chromium in erythrocytes is four to six times that in plasma, so whole blood chromium would be expected to be two to three times higher than serum levels (3).
- Urine reflects absorption over the past 1 to 2 days; concentrations should be less than 10 μg chromium/L in the general population (3).
- Levels of chromium in hair cannot distinguish external from internal sources; concentrations in hair may be up to 1,000 times higher than in serum (3).

 ## Dose

COMMON DOSAGE FORMS

Adequate Intakes

Infants and Children
0 to 6 months	0.2 μg/day
7 to 12 months	5.5 μg/day
1 to 3 years	11 μg/day
4 to 8 years	15 μg/day

Males
9 to 13 years	25 μg/day
14 to 18 years	35 μg/day
19 to 50 years	35 μg/day
51+ years	30 μg/day

Females
9 to 13 years	21 μg/day
14 to 18 years	24 μg/day
19 to 50 years	25 μg/day
51+ years	20 μg/day

Pregnant
≤18 years	29 μg/day
19 to 50 years	30 μg/day

Lactating
≤18 years	44 μg/day
19 to 50 years	45 μg/day

Conversion
1 μmol = 50 μg

 ## Common Questions and Answers

Q: What is GTF?
A: GTF is glucose tolerance factor, a water-soluble complex in brewer's yeast and other biologic extracts of which chromium is thought to be an important part. A few small studies have shown that high-chromium brewer's yeast is superior to chromium salts in ameliorating glucose tolerance (1). Brewer's yeast is certainly an inexpensive way to get chromium; 1 g of brewer's yeast provides about 45 μg chromium. Several months may be required to see an effect (1).

Q: Isn't there concern about mutagenic effects of other types of chromium (besides hexavalent chromium)?
A: High concentrations of chromium picolinate and picolinic acid (but not chromium chloride or nicotinate) appeared to be mutagenic in an assay of Chinese hamster ovary cells (2). Supplementation trials in humans, with doses up to 200 μg (3.8 μmol) have not shown toxicity, but these are short-term trials. There are no long-term human toxicity data available.

Q: Are any herbs high in chromium?
A: Yes. Black pepper is quite high in chromium (although for most people this is not a significant dietary source). Interestingly, several herbs traditionally used to treat diabetes, including blueberry leaves, artichokes, sage, and shepherds purse, are high in chromium, containing 3 to 9 μg/g (1).

Cinnamon

10 Second Take

Cinnamon has antifungal and smooth-muscle-relaxing effects (although clinical trials are lacking); the oil can be a dermal and mucosal irritant.

Basics

LATIN NAME

Cinnamomum cassia auct. or *Cinnamomum aromaticum* Nees

FAMILY

Lauraceae

OTHER COMMON NAMES

- *Cinnamomum cassia:* Cassia, Saigon cinnamon, Chinese cinnamon, rou gui (Mandarin), Nikkei (Japanese), Yukkye (Korean)
- *Cinnamomum verum* or *Cinnamomum zeylanicum:* Ceylon cinnamon, Seychelles cinnamon

DESCRIPTION

- Cinnamon bark, besides being a common dessert spice, is a common ingredient in Chinese herbal mixtures. It is also a common ingredient in toothpaste and mouthwashes.
- Evergreen trees up to 10 m high. The leathery leaves, highest in eugenol, smell of cloves.
- Probably native to Sri Lanka, the primary importer of cinnamon; Malaysia, Madagascar, and the Seychelles also import cinnamon.

PART USED

Inner bark, twigs (in Chinese medicine), occasionally flowers

KNOWN ACTIVE CONSTITUENTS

- The essential oil is the most important constituent (usually 0.5% to 2.5% of the bark); Saigon cinnamon contains up to 6% essential oil.
- Cinnamon oil contains 65% to 80% cinnamaldehyde, *trans*-cinnamic acid (5% to 10%), eugenol, other phenylpropanoids, tannins, mucilage, oligomeric procyanidins, and traces of coumarins (1).

MECHANISM/PHARMACOKINETICS

- It is unclear whether cinnamon oil constituents are absorbed through skin.
- Metabolites in urine include hippuric acid, benzoic acid, and cinnamic acid.

Evidence

CLINICAL TRIALS

- An uncontrolled trial of three HIV positive participants with oral candidiasis found that three of five improved after receiving an oral cinnamon preparation for a week (2).

ANIMAL/IN VITRO

- Antifungal effects

—Cinnamic aldehyde is the active fungitoxic agent; it is active against a number of pathogens causing respiratory tract mycoses, including *Aspergillus niger, Aspergillus fumigatus, Aspergillus nidulans, Aspergillus flavus, Candida albicans, Candida tropicalis, Candida pseudotropicalis,* and *Histoplasma capsulatum* (3). Cinnamic aldehyde is in the vapors of the essential oil and has been suggested as an inhaled therapy for respiratory tract mycoses.
—Essential oil of *C. zeylanicum* inhibited 80% of the dermatophyte strains tested in one study, producing inhibition zones greater than 10 mm in diameter (4). An *in vitro* study found that *C. zeylanicum* and commercial cinnamon powder were active against *Candida* species, including fluconazole-resistant species (2). Preparations of cinnamon candies and gums had a weaker effect.

- Other antimicrobial effects

—*In vitro*, cinnamon inhibits the growth of various bacteria; cassia flower oil and cinnamaldehyde were reported to be active against herpes virus and adenovirus (5).

- Cardiovascular effects

—Cinnamophilin, a lignan isolated from *Cinnamomum philippinense,* appears to be a novel thromboxane A_2 receptor antagonist. Cinnamophilin appears to inhibit platelet aggregation and counteract chemically induced contraction in rat aortic and guinea pig tracheal preparations (6). It also appeared to have calcium-channel blocking activity in rat thoracic aorta (7). In a rat heart preparation, cinnamophilin in a concentration of 10 mmol converted six of nine episodes of ischemia-reperfusion arrhythmia to normal sinus rhythm. Cinnamophilin prolonged action potential duration and suppressed maximal rate of rise of the action potential upstroke (8).
—Cinnamaldehyde demonstrated a hypotensive effect in dogs and guinea pigs and cinnamaldehyde caused positive inotropic and chronotropic effects in isolated guinea pig heart preparations (5).

- Cancer/immune stimulation

—*In vitro*, 2'-hydroxycinnamaldehyde and 2'-benzoxycinnamaldehyde inhibited the growth of 29 kinds of human cancer cells and the *in vivo* growth of SW-620 human tumor xenografts in nude mice (9). The key functional group in the antitumor effect of cinnamaldehyde analogs appears to be the propenal group (10).
—*In vitro,* an extract of *C. cassia* stimulated proliferation of human lymphocytes, enhancing cytotoxic T lymphocyte but not natural killer cell activity (11). This activity appeared to be associated with glycoproteins of about 100 kDa. Another study found that 2'-hydroxycinnamaldehyde and 2'-benzoxycinnamaldehyde accelerated T-cell differentiation and inhibited lymphocyte proliferation induced by two of three compounds (12).

- Gastrointestinal/smooth muscle effects

—Cinnamophilin counteracted chemically induced contraction in rat aortic and guinea pig tracheal preparations (6).
—Cinnamon oil and cinnamaldehyde inhibited gastric motion in rats and dogs, inhibited intestinal propulsion in mice, and reduced gastric erosions in stressed mice. An aqueous extract of Chinese cinnamon reduced serotonin-induced ulcers in mice (5). Although the ulcer experiments used reasonable therapeutic doses, most of the experiments described previously used high doses (often 5 to 10 mg/kg i.v. or 250 to 500 mg/kg i.p.) (5).

- Antioxidant effects

—Etheric, methanolic, and aqueous extracts of cinnamon exhibited antioxidant effects *in vitro* and have been proposed as possible food preservatives (13).

OTHER CLAIMED BENEFITS/ACTIONS

- Dysmenorrhea
- Styptic
- Bloating
- Flatulence
- Gastrointestinal cramps
- Colic
- Diarrhea
- Dyspepsia
- Colds and flu

Risks

ADVERSE REACTIONS

• Squamous cell carcinoma

—A case report attributed squamous cell carcinoma of the tongue in a 24-year-old woman to repeated and prolonged exposure to cinnamon-flavored gum (14).

• Dermal and mucosal irritation

—Cinnamaldehyde is a dermal irritant. A 10×12cm second-degree burn (surrounded by a 3- to 4-cm first-degree burn) was reported in an 11-year-old student who broke a vial of cinnamon oil in his rear pants pocket and left the area unwashed for 48 hours (15).
—Although almost any substance that comes into contact with skin or mucosa can cause irritation in sensitive individuals, cinnamaldehyde may be the leading substance responsible for allergic reactions caused by perfumes or cosmetics (5). In patch tests, cinnamon oil in concentrations as low as 0.01% has caused reactions (5). Cross-reactions may occur in those allergic to Peru balsam (*Myroxylon balsamum*) or cloves (*Syzygium aromaticum*).
—Chronic exposure to oral hygiene products has caused urticaria, stomatitis with vesiculation of oral mucosa, cheilitis, and eczema (16), and oral blistering and orofacial granulomatosis have been reported.
—Cinnamon oil has been abused among schoolchildren. Thirty-two cases of cinnamon oil abuse (all among adolescent boys) were reported to the Pittsburgh Poison Center within a 5-month period in 1988 to 1989. Ingestion of cinnamon oil on toothpicks, hard candy, or fingers dipped in cinnamon oil resulted in reported feelings of warmth and facial flushing. Oral burning, nausea, or abdominal pain was reported by some of those exposed orally; several boys had facial erythema. All responded to dilution with oral fluids or, in the case of dermal exposure, soap and water decontamination. Two had splashed cinnamon oil into their eyes and were treated with irrigation; one was treated for conjunctivitis (16).

DRUG INTERACTIONS

• Cinnamon interferes with tetracycline and methacycline dissolution *in vitro;* in the presence of cassia (2 g in 100 mL), about 20% of tetracycline hydrochloride dissolved within 30 minutes (compared with 97% dissolution in plain water) (5).

PREGNANCY/LACTATION

• Some advise that the herb not be used in the presence of gastric ulcers or during pregnancy (1); others note that only prolonged use of the essential oil need be restricted in pregnancy (see questions and answers).

ANIMAL TOXICITY

• Acute (up to 3 g/kg $\times$ 24 hours) and chronic (100 mg/kg/day $\times$ 90 days) oral toxicity studies of ethanolic extract of *C. zeylanicum* in mice found no acute or chronic mortality (17). Compared with controls, chronic dosing resulted in a reduction in weight gain, a reduction in liver weight, decreased hemoglobin, and increased reproductive organ weights and sperm counts (18).
• In mice, the LD_{50} for cinnamaldehyde has been reported to be 132 mg/kg i.v., 610 mg/kg i.p., and 2,225 mg/kg p.o. (5). The LD_{50} in rats for volatile oil of Ceylon cinnamon is 4,160 mg/kg p.o. and for cassia oil 5,200 mg/kg p.o. An aqueous extract of cinnamon was nontoxic (LD_{50} 4,980 mg/kg i.p.). A dose of 70 mg cinnamaldehyde administered orally to rats for 8 weeks resulted in no toxicity.
• Dietary levels up to 2,500 ppm resulted in no macroscopic effects. A dose of 10,000 ppm cinnamaldehyde added to the diet of rats over a 16-week period resulted in slight swelling of hepatic cells and hyperkeratosis of the squamous portion of the stomach; another researcher reported nephritis (5).
• Dermal LD_{50} of cinnamaldehyde is 0.59 mg/kg, 0.69 mg/kg for Ceylon cinnamon, and 0.32 mg/kg for cassia oil, although other researchers have found low dermal absorption (5).
• In mice, 125 to 500 mg/kg i.p. and 250 to 1,000 mg/kg p.o. decreased spontaneous motor activity. A dose of 500 mg/kg p.o. of Ceylon cinnamon oil depressed operant conditioning behavior in rats. No effect was seen in doses $\leq$150 mg/kg (5).

 ## Dose

COMMON DOSAGE FORMS

• *Dried bark:* 2 to 4 g in divided doses
• *Infusion:* made from 0.5 to 1 g bark b.i.d. to t.i.d., usually with meals
• *Liquid extract:* (1:1 in 70% alcohol) 0.5 to 1 mL t.i.d.

 ## Common Questions and Answers

Q: Isn't cinnamon used as an abortifacient?
A: There is no evidence that *Cinnamomum* species have abortifacient effects. In the Middle Ages, cinnamon did have that reputation; however, cinnamon was often confused with *Cassia fistulosa,* a different species that contains anthraquinones, the cathartic substances found in laxative herbs such as senna and cascara sagrada. It is believed that stimulation of intestinal motility may increase uterine muscle activity, so this may be where the reputation came from. Cinnamon does have teratogenic effects in chick embryos (5).

Coenzyme Q$_{10}$

 10 Second Take

Coenzyme Q$_{10}$ is a safe supplement that may be beneficial in congestive heart failure (CHF) and before cardiac surgery. There is no reliable evidence for its effect as treatment for cancer, Parkinson's disease, periodontal disease, or aerobic capacity, but it may reduce cardiac toxicity from anthracyclines.

 Basics

DESCRIPTION

• Coenzyme Q$_{10}$ (CoQ10, ubiquinone, 2-3-dimethoxy 5-methyl-6-decaphenyl benzoquinone) is a naturally occurring fat-soluble quinone found in high concentrations in mitochondria, particularly in the myocardium.
• Its structure is similar to vitamin K. Although it serves vital functions, coenzyme Q$_{10}$ is nonessential because the quinone moiety is synthesized from tyrosine and the polyprenyl side chain is synthesized from acetyl-CoA (1).

FOOD SOURCES

• Dietary sources, including meat and poultry, may contribute up to a quarter of coenzyme Q$_{10}$ in the human body (1).

MAIN FUNCTIONS/PHARMACOKINETICS

• Involved in adenosine triphosphate (ATP) production, coenzyme Q$_{10}$ also transports electrons during cellular respiration and oxidative phosphorylation and regulates the reduced form of nicotinamide adenine dinucleotide (NADH) and succinate dehydrogenase in the respiratory transport chain. Its reduced form, ubiquinol, functions as an antioxidant (2).
• Oral administration of 30 mg causes a peak level of 1 μg/mL within 6 hours; a second peak occurs after 24 hours (this suggests enterohepatic recycling). Administration of 100 mg t.i.d. resulted in steady-state levels of 5.4 μg/mL. The plasma half-life is about 34 hours (2).

 Evidence

CLINICAL TRIALS

• Myocardial infarction

—A placebo-controlled study in 144 patients after acute myocardial infarction tested the effect of 120 mg/day of coenzyme Q$_{10}$ for 4 weeks (3). The incidence of angina was significantly less in the treated group compared with the placebo group (9.5% vs. 28.1%). Total arrhythmias (9.5% vs. 25.3%) and total cardiac events, including nonfatal infarction and cardiac deaths, were also significantly reduced in the treated group (15% vs. 30.9%).

• Angina

—The effects of coenzyme Q$_{10}$ in angina are unclear. A double-blind placebo-controlled crossover trial of 12 patients with stable angina found that coenzyme Q$_{10}$ (50 mg t.i.d. × 4 weeks) increased exercise time (406 ±114 seconds) significantly compared with placebo (345 ± 102 seconds) but did not reduce frequency of angina (4).
—A crossover study in 20 patients found that 60 mg/day coenzyme Q$_{10}$ for 4 weeks found that, compared with baseline, coenzyme Q$_{10}$ treatment significantly decreased angina attacks (by 1.9 episodes/week), decreased nitroglycerine consumption, and increased exercise duration (5).

• CHF

—A Danish meta-analysis identified 14 controlled trials of patients with CHF receiving adjuvant coenzyme Q$_{10}$ (60 to 200 mg/day); 8 met criteria for meta-analysis. Seven of eight studies demonstrated significant improvement in measures of heart function, including ejection fraction, stroke volume, cardiac output, cardiac index, and end diastolic volume index (6).
—Two more recent studies, however, not included in the previously mentioned meta-analysis, found no benefit for coenzyme Q$_{10}$. A double-blind crossover trial in which 30 patients (27 completed) with ischemic or idiopathic dilated cardiomyopathy and chronic left ventricular dysfunction (ejection fraction 26% ± 6%) were treated with placebo or coenzyme Q$_{10}$ (33 mg t.i.d.) for 3 months, coenzyme Q$_{10}$ did not significantly improve resting left ventricular ejection fraction, cardiac volumes, or quality of life indices (7).
—A randomized, double-blind, placebo-controlled trial of 55 patients (46 completed) with CHF (NYHA III and IV, with ejection fraction less than 40%) receiving standard therapy tested the adjunctive effect of coenzyme Q$_{10}$ (200 mg/day) against placebo for 6 months (8). There were no significant differences from baseline in either groups in ejection fraction and peak oxygen consumption, and exercise duration remained unchanged in both the coenzyme Q$_{10}$ and placebo groups.

• Hypertension

—A placebo-controlled study in 59 patients tested coenzyme Q$_{10}$ (60 mg b.i.d.) in 30 patients against a B-complex vitamin (placebo) in 29 hypertensive subjects for 8 weeks and found that, compared with placebo, coenzyme Q$_{10}$ significantly decreased systolic and diastolic blood pressure (9).

• Tissue reperfusion injury

—In one study, 30 patients undergoing elective vascular surgery requiring aortic cross-clamping were randomized to coenzyme Q$_{10}$1 (50 mg/day) or placebo for 7 days preoperatively. Concentrations of malondialdehyde, conjugated dienes, creatine kinase, and lactate dehydrogenase (LDH) were significantly lower in treated group (10). An unblinded trial of coenzyme Q$_{10}$ (150 mg × 7 days) versus no treatment in 40 patients undergoing elective coronary artery bypass graft (CABG) found that concentrations of malondialdehyde, conjugated dienes, and creatine kinase were lower than in the treated group, which also had a significantly lower incidence of ventricular arrhythmias during recovery period. The number of patients requiring inotropic agents did not differ between groups but dosage of dopamine required to maintain stable hemodynamics was lower in the treated group (11).
—Acute supplementation, however, does not appear to help postoperative outcomes. A randomized double-blind trial compared placebo to 600 mg coenzyme Q$_{10}$ (in divided doses 12 hours before surgery) in 20 patients with good left ventricular function undergoing elective coronary revascularization. There was no difference between the two groups in postoperative levels of myoglobin, creatine kinase MB fraction, or cardiac troponin T (12).

• Exercise capacity

—A double-blind placebo-controlled trial of coenzyme Q$_{10}$ (120 mg/day × 6 weeks) on aerobic capacity and lipid peroxidation was conducted during exercise in 19 adults (8 of whom were older than 60). Coenzyme Q$_{10}$ did not affect time to exhaustion, maximal oxygen uptake, or serum malondialdehyde concentration in either younger or older adults (13). Two other controlled studies, each of 18 adults, showed a similar lack of effect of coenzyme Q$_{10}$ (14,15).

• Parkinson's disease

—An uncontrolled pilot study of three doses of coenzyme Q$_{10}$ (400, 600, or 800 mg daily in divided doses for 1 month) in 15 participants with Parkinson's disease found no change in the mean score on the motor section of the Unified Parkinson's Disease Rating Scale (16). Substantial increases in plasma coenzyme Q$_{10}$ levels were noted, and it was well tolerated. There were no changes in electrocardiogram (EKG), complete blood count (CBC), or blood chemistries; however, two of five patients who took 800 mg/day were noted to have three to five hyaline casts (one also had three to five granular casts) in urinalyses taken at the end of the study.

- Cancer

—Lower levels of coenzyme Q$_{10}$ have been noted in cancer patients, and several small uncontrolled studies claim a beneficial effect in women with breast cancer. However, no appropriately controlled clinical trials were identified (17). A small study in 20 children with acute lymphoblastic leukemia and non-Hodgkin's lymphoma who were being treated with anthracyclines added coenzyme Q$_{10}$ (100 mg b.i.d.) as an adjunctive treatment in 10 patients (18). Both groups experienced significantly decreased percentage left ventricular fractional shortening. Interventricular septum wall thickening decreased only in the unsupplemented group; two patients in the unsupplemented group had septum wall motion abnormalities compared with none in the supplemented group.

- Diabetes

—A randomized double-blind placebo-controlled trial in 34 patients with Type 1 diabetes tested coenzyme Q$_{10}$ (100 mg) versus placebo for 3 months; there were no differences between groups in HbA$_{1c}$, mean daily glucose, mean insulin dose, hypoglycemic episodes, cholesterol, or well-being on a visual analog scale.
—Diabetes mellitus with mitochondrial DNA (ntDNA) 3243 (A-G) is an X-linked mutation that results in progressive insulin secretory effect and neurosensory deafness; it is also called maternally inherited diabetes mellitus and deafness (MIDD) (19). In a study that compared 28 MIDD patients with 16 controls, coenzyme Q$_{10}$ (150 mg/day × 3 years) prevented progressive hearing loss and improved blood lactate after exercise; it had no effect, however, on the diabetic complications or other clinical symptoms. Coenzyme Q$_{10}$ had no effect on the insulin secretory capacity in participants with the mutation who had either impaired or normal glucose tolerance and who were studied in parallel (19).

- Periodontal disease

—A beneficial effect of coenzyme Q$_{10}$ on periodontal disease has been claimed. According to a review and critique of the dental literature, both controlled studies were methodologically flawed (20). According to this reviewer, a study of 18 patients (21) provided only vague assessments of clinical improvement rather than reproducible measurements. A larger double-blind study of 56 patients compared placebo with coenzyme Q$_{10}$ (60 mg × 12 weeks); no difference was seen in gingival redness, bleeding, or pus discharge, but a significant difference in tooth mobility was noted at 4 and 12 weeks (22). Although probing depth scores improved in both groups at 12 weeks, apparently there was not a significant difference between the two groups.

- Low density lipoprotein (LDL) oxidation

—A double-blind placebo-controlled crossover trial in 19 men with CHD and hypercholesterolemia tested lovastatin (60 mg/day) with or with coenzyme Q$_{10}$ (180 mg per day) for 6 weeks each (23). Although blood LDL ubiquinol concentrations increased, the lag time in copper-mediated oxidation increased only by 5%. This was statistically significant but probably not clinically significant.

- Lipid peroxidation

—In an uncontrolled study, malonyldialdehyde and 4-hydroxynonenal concentrations decreased significantly in paint and lacquer workers (who are exposed to organic solvents that can cause lipid peroxidation) after 4 weeks of treatment with coenzyme Q$_{10}$ (24).

- Oxidative DNA damage

—Coenzyme Q$_{10}$ in oil ($n = 20$) or as granulate ($n = 20$), each in a dose of 30 mg t.i.d., had no effect on oxidative DNA damage (assessed by urinary excretion of 8-oxo-7,8-dihydro-2′-deoxyguanosine, a repair product of oxidative DNA damage) in smokers (25).

 Clinical Considerations

FACTORS DECREASING AVAILABILITY/ABSORPTION

- *Statins:* In 17 men treated with simvastatin (20 to 40 mg/day for a mean of 4.7 years), discontinuing simvastatin for 4 weeks increased coenzyme Q$_{10}$ levels 32%; resumption of treatment caused coenzyme Q$_{10}$ levels to decrease 25% (26).
- Advanced cardiac failure is associated with lower levels of tissue coenzyme Q$_{10}$ (27). Plasma coenzyme Q$_{10}$ levels are decreased in subjects with hyperlipidemia and in smokers (28). Cancer, mitochondrial disease, and mevalonate kinase deficiency are also associated with low coenzyme Q$_{10}$ levels.
- Phenylketonuria (PKU) is associated with reduced serum coenzyme Q$_{10}$, most likely because dietary restrictions reduce intake; also, tyrosine availability may be diminished in PKU (1).

LABORATORY TESTS

- Coenzyme Q$_{10}$ serum levels can be measured by high-pressure liquid chromatography (HPLC); however, appropriate reference levels are not well established.
- Studies in normal participants have found normal values to range from 0.3 to 3.84 μg/mL, with most readings clustering between 0.6 to 1.0 μg/mL.

 Risks

ADVERSE REACTIONS

- Coenzyme Q$_{10}$ is very safe. Adverse events have been limited to occasional reports of gastrointestinal upset.
- A 35-year-old woman with mitochondrial encephalopathy developed urticaria after treatment with coenzyme Q$_{10}$ and bromazepam; skin tests for both were negative, but an oral provocation test with ubiquinone (not bromazepam) was positive (29). As coenzyme Q$_{10}$ was considered a necessary treatment for this patient, rush desensitization was done and effectively desensitized the patient.

DRUG INTERACTIONS

- Warfarin

—A 72-year-old woman on warfarin developed less responsiveness to the drug after starting to take coenzyme Q$_{10}$ regularly. After discontinuing coenzyme Q$_{10}$, warfarin responsiveness returned (30).

 Dose

Usual doses are 90 to 390 mg/day.

Coltsfoot

10 Second Take

Coltsfoot contains hepatotoxic unsaturated pyrrolizidine alkaloids (PAs) and should not be consumed internally.

Basics

LATIN NAME

Tussilago farfara L.

FAMILY

Compositae

OTHER COMMON NAMES

Coughwort, horsehoof, foal's foot, and bull's foot

DESCRIPTION

• An early flowering perennial up to 30 cm high, with large, horseshoe-shaped leaves, which are white-felted on the underside.
• Common in Eastern Europe, Italy, and the Balkans, coltsfoot has yellow flowers and seeds in a dandelion-like ball.

PART USED

Flower, leaf

KNOWN ACTIVE CONSTITUENTS

• Mucilage (6% to 10%), inulin, tannins (5%), small amounts of flavonoids, plant acids, triterpenes, and sterols (1). Sesquiterpene lactones (tussilagone and petasitolid) and unsaturated PAs senkirkine and senecionine. North American coltsfoot contains up to 140 mg/kg senkirkine in flower buds and up to 49 mg/kg in mature whole plants. Senecionine is present in amounts up to 7 mg/kg in flower buds and up to 1 mg/kg in mature whole plants (2). Coltsfoot also contains the saturated (nontoxic) PAs tussilagine and isotussilagine.
• Chinese coltsfoot contains smaller amounts of PAs than European (or North American) coltsfoot. In one study senkirkine content was as much as 47 ppm in plants of Chinese origin and less than 0.03 ppm in plants of Swiss origin (3).

MECHANISM/PHARMACOKINETICS

• Tussilagone administered intravenously produces a rapid pressor effect in dogs (0.02 to 0.3 mg/kg), cats (0.02 to 0.5 mg/kg), and rats (0.4 to 4.0 mg/kg); in addition, it stimulates respiration (4).
• A methylene chloride extract of T. farfara buds inhibited platelet activating factor and appeared to have calcium channel blocking effects (5).

Evidence

CLINICAL TRIALS

No clinical trials identified.

OTHER CLAIMED BENEFITS/ACTIONS

• Cough
• Bronchitis
• Sore throat
• Asthma (in smoking mixture)

Risks

ADVERSE REACTIONS

• Maternal use of a mixed-herb tea containing 9% coltsfoot tea throughout a pregnancy resulted in hepatic venoocclusive disease in an infant, who lived only 38 days after birth. It is likely that this tea did not actually contain coltsfoot (6) (see questions and answers).
• The presence of unsaturated PAs in this plant makes it inadvisable to consume it (see questions and answers).

PREGNANCY/LACTATION

• See adverse reactions.
• All products containing unsaturated PAs should be avoided during pregnancy or lactation (PAs are excreted into milk in rats and mice) (7).

ANIMAL TOXICITY

• In a carcinogenicity study that lasted 600 days, 12 rats were fed Chinese coltsfoot buds as 16% of the diet. Eight of 12 rats in this high-dose group developed hemangioendothelial sarcoma of the liver; one developed hepatocellular adenoma, one developed hepatocellular carcinoma, and one developed bladder papilloma. One hemangioendothelial sarcoma of the liver occurred in a group of 10 rats fed 8% coltsfoot (7).
• In mice, the acute LD_{50} of tussilagone is 28.9 mg/kg (4).

Dose

COMMON DOSAGE FORMS

- Oral ingestion of coltsfoot is not recommended.
- *Tea, infusion, or decoction:* 0.6 to 2 g dried herb t.i.d.
- *Liquid extract:* (1:1 in 25% alcohol) 0.6 to 2 mL t.i.d.
- *Tincture:* (1:5 in 45% alcohol) 2 to 8 mL t.i.d.
- *Syrup:* (liquid extract 1:4 in syrup) 2 to 8 mL t.i.d.

 Common Questions and Answers

Q: Why is there a question about whether coltsfoot actually caused hepatoocclusive disease in the infant of the woman who drank coltsfoot tea throughout her pregnancy?
A: Analysis of the tea showed that it contained no senkirkine but did contain 0.6 mg/kg senecionine. This raises the suspicion that the plant in this tea was not coltsfoot at all. In coltsfoot, the senkirkine to senecionine ratio is usually 10:1. The fact that only senkirkine was present suggests that the tea actually contained butterbur (*Petasites hybridus*). Later analysis showed that the tea contained both *Petasites hybridus* and *Tussilago farfara* (2). Unfortunately, both plants are referred to as coltsfoot (8). However, no preparation containing unsaturated PAs can be recommended during pregnancy or, to my mind, any other time either.

Q: Are even small amounts of PAs dangerous?
A: Not all PAs are dangerous; it is the unsaturated ones we need to worry about (saturated PAs are nontoxic). There is great individual variability in susceptibility. According to Commission E, the daily dose of coltsfoot teas should not contain more than 10 μg PAs and daily dose of extracts or fresh juice no more than 1 μg. However, establishing a safe dose of such a toxic class of compounds is tricky, and I do not believe that there is a safe chronic dose of unsaturated PAs (PA toxicity is cumulative).

Q: Is there such a thing as PA-free coltsfoot?
A: Not yet, but a research program is underway to cultivate PA-free coltsfoot by plant selection and *in vitro* culturing methods (9). It is possible to remove PAs through processing.

Q: What are PAs?
A: PAs comprise about 200 compounds present in more than 350 plant species, including several medicinal plants. *Tussilago farfara, Cynoglossum officinale, Echium plantagineum,* and *Alkanna tinctoria* contain toxic PAs, as well as species of *Petasites, Senecio, Eupatorium, Symphytum, Heliotropium,* and *Crotalaria.* PAs contain a necine base composed of two five-membered rings. Toxic PAs contain unsaturated necine rings; PAs with saturated necine rings are nontoxic (e.g., *Echinacea* species and *Arnica montana* contain only saturated PAs). PAs are absorbed intestinally and reach the liver through the portal vein. Oxidation of unsaturated PAs by mixed-function oxidases and cytochromes lead to toxic pyrrole derivatives, which are highly reactive electrophiles that can alkylate DNA. Many of these can bind to liver macromolecules and are hepatotoxic in humans (7).

PAs have been associated with many cases of acute and chronic venoocclusive disease. Most cases have been associated with grain contamination by *Heliotropium* or *Senecio* species. Medicinal teas made from herbal material contaminated with *Senecio* and *Crotalaria* are used in Jamaica and have been associated with hepatic damage, especially in children.

An unusual epidemic of central nervous system toxicity in 200 patients associated with contamination of food grains occurred in Uzbekistan, USSR in 1942 to 1951. *Trichodesma incanum,* which contains 1.5% to 3.1% PAs (mainly trichodesmine and incanine), caused Ozhalanger encephalitis in the USSR. Ten days after exposure those affected developed headaches, nausea, and vomiting, followed by delirium and coma. Forty-four persons died, primarily of respiratory depression.

Pulmonary toxicity has also been reported, often associated with severe pulmonary hypertension. In fatal cases of PA ingestion, estimated daily intake has ranged from 0.5 mg/kg to 3.3 mg/kg (7).

Comfrey

10 Second Take

Comfrey contains hepatotoxic alkaloids and should not be ingested internally; topical use on unbroken skin is probably safe.

Basics

LATIN NAME

Symphytum officinale L.

FAMILY

Boraginaceae

OTHER COMMON NAMES

Boneset, knit bone, common comfrey (*S. officinale*); prickly comfrey (*Symphytum asperum* Lepechin); Russian comfrey (*Symphytum* x *uplandicum* Nyman).

DESCRIPTION

• A bristly perennial herb with hairy, lanceolate, alternate leaves and small purple flowers, 5 to 150 cm in height, native throughout all of Europe and naturalized in North America.

PART USED

Root, leaf

KNOWN ACTIVE CONSTITUENTS

• Allantoin 0.6% to 0.8%, pyrrolizidine alkaloids (PAs) 0.02% to 0.07%, intermedine, acetylintermedine, lycopsamine, acetyllycopsamine, symphytine, symlandine, and echimidine (in some sources) (see questions and answers) (1,2). Mucilage may be present in comfrey root up to 29%, and tannins may compose 2.4% of dried leaves (3).

• The PA content of comfrey varies. Not only does species matter (see questions and answers), but roots contain significantly higher concentrations of PAs than leaves (4), and younger, smaller leaves have a higher alkaloid content than older leaves (5). There is extreme variability in the PA content of commercially available comfrey products; for example, levels of the PA lycopsamine ranged from undetectable to 5.3 ppm in various comfrey products (6). An analysis of two brands of comfrey-pepsin preparations found total pyrrolizidine content to be 2,900 mg/kg in the brand containing roots and 270 mg/kg in the brand containing leaves (7).

MECHANISM/PHARMACOKINETICS

• Allantoin is claimed to be a cell proliferant, promoting granulation and tissue regeneration. The mucilage would be expected to have an emollient action.
• PAs are absorbed from the intestine and reach the liver via the portal vein. After hydrolytic cleavage, cytochromes and mixed function oxidases oxidize PAs to pyrrole derivatives, highly reactive electrophilic alkylating compounds that covalently bind to protein, RNA, and DNA (8). Because these reactions take place in the liver, it is the organ most affected.
• In animals, metabolism of PAs varies considerably with species; humans are much more susceptible than rodents. Rats and mice are the most susceptible lab animals; rabbits and guinea pigs are quite resistant. Although chickens and turkeys are susceptible, Japanese quail are highly resistant (9).

Evidence

CLINICAL TRIALS

• No clinical trials identified.

ANIMAL/IN VITRO

Symphytum leaf extracts have demonstrated mild analgesic activity, and wound-healing effects have been demonstrated in rats (2).

OTHER CLAIMED BENEFITS/ACTIONS

• Broken bones
• Wound healing
• Contusions, sprains, dislocations (topical)
• Antiinflammatory
• Arthritis
• Bronchitis
• Cholecystitis
• Gallstones
• Gastritis
• Diarrhea

Risks

ADVERSE REACTIONS

• Hepatic venoocclusive disease

—Comfrey has been implicated in several cases of hepatic venoocclusive disease, including two fatal cases. In the first of these, a 23-year-old man presented with hepatic venoocclusive disease and severe portal hypertension; light microscopy and hepatic angiography demonstrated occlusion of sublobular veins and widespread hemorrhagic necrosis of hepatocytes (10).
—An unpublished case was reported to the USP Practitioners Reporting Network of a man who drank comfrey tea and subsequently died of liver damage (details are unavailable) (11).
—At least two cases of hepatic venoocclusive disease have involved comfrey-pepsin capsules. One was in an older woman admitted with hepatic venoocclusive disease, portal hypertension, and cirrhosis who had taken six comfrey-pepsin capsules per day for the 6 months before admission, and another was in a 49-year-old woman who had been taking six comfrey-pepsin pills for 4 months before admission.
—Other cases of hepatic venoocclusive disease occurred in a 47-year-old woman who was drinking 10 cups of comfrey tea daily, as well as ingesting comfrey pills, for more than a year, and in a 13-year-old boy given a comfrey root preparation to treat Crohn's disease (11).
—In fatal cases, total comfrey ingestion has been estimated to be 6 to 167 mg/kg. In nonfatal cases of hepatic venoocclusive disease, total ingestion has been estimated at 2 to 27 mg/kg.

ANIMAL TOXICITY

• In rats, a diet containing 33% comfrey leaf was tolerated, but a diet containing 4% comfrey root was poorly tolerated. Hepatocellular adenomas occurred in all groups fed comfrey; none of the control animals developed hepatocellular adenomas. Other tumors included hemangioendothelial sarcomas, urinary tract papillomas and carcinomas, pituitary and adrenal cortical adenomas, colonic adenomas, retroperitoneal teratoma, and lymphatic leukemia (5).
• In a study designed to test low-dose toxicity of comfrey, eight young adult rats received 50 mg/kg of comfrey-derived alkaloids weekly for 6 weeks. Pathologic changes in the liver included vascular congestion, mild necrosis, loss of definition of hepatocyte cellular membranes, endothelial sloughing, loss of hepatocyte microvilli, and bleb formation on the sinusoidal borders of hepatocytes (12).

 Dose

COMMON DOSAGE FORMS

• Internal ingestion of comfrey is not recommended.
• *Dried root or rhizome:* 2 to 4 g t.i.d.
• *Infusion or decoction:* 5 to 10 g chopped or powdered dried root b.i.d. or t.i.d.
• *Liquid extract:* (1:1 in 25% alcohol) 2 to 4 mL t.i.d.
• Topical preparations include poultices, ointments, mucilaginous decoctions (containing 10% to 15% root), and so forth.
• The German Commission E recommends that topical preparations not contain more than 100 μg unsaturated PAs (daily dose) and should not be used longer than 4 to 6 weeks in a year.

 Common Questions and Answers

Q: Are some species of comfrey safer to consume than other species?
A: Probably, but why take a chance? Most genotypes of common comfrey (*S. officinale*) do not contain echimidine, which is likely the most toxic of the PAs found in comfrey (1,13). Prickly comfrey (*Symphytum asperum* Lepechin) does contain echimidine, as does *Symphytum x uplandicum* (Russian comfrey, a hybrid of common comfrey and prickly comfrey). Also, products are not necessarily accurately labeled regarding species. Even if a product contains only common comfrey, this species is not devoid of hepatotoxic compounds. Common comfrey contains symphytine and other unsaturated PAs and cannot be considered safe.

Q: Aren't comfrey leaves eaten as a vegetable?
A: Yes, comfrey leaves may be used as a salad green, cooked greens, or used in soups and various other dishes. Blanched stalks may be used like asparagus, and peeled roots are sometimes used in soups. In addition, roasted roots may be combined with other plants and used as a coffee substitute. Even Russian comfrey has been used as food; leaves may be boiled, steamed, or used in soups and other dishes; they have also been ground into a flour apparently used for thickening gravies and soups (14). Because 90% of total plant alkaloids may be in the form of *N*-oxides, which are highly water-soluble, cooked greens would probably have a lower toxic potential if the cooking water is thrown away (13).

Q: Is the use of topical comfrey preparations dangerous?
A: Probably not, if they are not used on broken skin; PAs are poorly absorbed through the skin. In rats, percutaneous absorption of alkaloids was 20 to 50 times lower than absorption following oral administration in rats (15).

Q: What are PAs?
A: See "Coltsfoot" questions and answers.

Copper

10 Second Take

Copper is essential, but high doses are toxic.

Basics

DESCRIPTION

• Copper, a transition metal, is an essential trace mineral (the third most abundant, after zinc and iron, in the human body).
• An adult contains about 50 to 120 mg (0.79 to 1.9 mmol) copper.

FOOD SOURCES

• Shellfish, nuts, seeds, legumes, whole grains, bran, liver, and other organ meats contain 0.3 to 2 mg copper/100 g. Mushrooms, tomatoes, potatoes, bananas, grapes, and chocolate contain 0.1 to 0.3 mg/100 g (1).
• Water can also be a significant dietary source (see questions and answers).
• Average intake is about 1.0 mg/day (2).

MAIN FUNCTIONS/PHARMACOKINETICS

• Copper is essential for the formation and maintenance of connective tissue, myelin, and melanin. An important catalyst for iron absorption and flux in and out of cells, copper is also vital to the function of many enzymes, including amine oxidases, ferroxidases (including ceruloplasmin, an antioxidant), cytochrome c oxidase (which functions in cellular respiration), dopamine-β-hydroxylase, lysyl oxidase (which helps cross-link elastin and collagen), superoxide dismutase (an antioxidant), and tyrosinase (involved in melanin formation) (2). Copper-binding proteins include metallothionein, albumin, transcuprein, and blood-clotting factor V (1).
• Absorbed intestinally, copper is transported to the liver through the portal vein and incorporated into ceruloplasmin (the most common transport form). The primary route of elimination is biliary; urinary excretion accounts for about 3%. Biologic half-life is 13 to 33 days.

Evidence

CLINICAL TRIALS

• Bone turnover

—A double-blind crossover study in 24 adults (12 women) found no effect of 3 mg $CuSO_4$, 3 mg Cu-glycine chelate, or 6 mg Cu-glycine chelate (each given for 6 weeks, alternating with 6-week periods of placebo administration) on biochemical markers of bone turnover (3).

• Arthritis

—A crossover study compared copper bracelets to placebo (aluminum) bracelets, each worn for 1 month (4). Of 77 subjects with evaluable data, 37 preferred the copper bracelet, 10 preferred the aluminum bracelet, and 30 found the treatments equivalent. Although a benefit is claimed, copper was superior only if those who rated the treatments equivalent were excluded.

OTHER CLAIMED BENEFITS/ACTIONS

• Antiinflammatory, arthritis, lowers cholesterol

Risks

ADVERSE REACTIONS

• Acute toxic exposure

—The estimated lethal dose in an untreated adult is 10 to 20 g copper. Gastrointestinal symptoms occur at whole blood concentrations >2.87 mg copper/L, and hepatorenal dysfunction and/or shock appear at whole blood levels >7.98 mg copper/L. Ingesting 0.25 to 0.5 g copper sulfate (about 40 copper by weight) or liquid containing >30 ppm copper causes nausea, vomiting, and abdominal pain (5).
—Cupric or copper sulfate causes a metallic taste; vomiting (usually greenish blue); and sometimes diarrhea, hematemesis, or melena. Acute copper poisoning can cause lethargy, rhabdomyolysis, renal dysfunction, hemolysis refractory hypotension, and coma.
—Inhaled copper may cause mucosal irritation or metal fume fever (symptoms include fever, chills, myalgias, headache, malaise, and dry throat). Metal fume fever is now rare because of industrial changes (5).

• Chronic copper exposure

—Chronic copper exposure can cause greenish hair; cuticles may be lost. Chronic copper poisoning causes hepatic toxicity.

• Gastrointestinal effects

—A trial in 60 women tested graded levels of copper (0, 1, 3, and 5 mg copper sulfate/L in tap water, administered for 2 weeks, followed by 1 week of tap water) (6). Copper did not cause diarrhea, but nausea, abdominal pain, and vomiting were significantly related to copper levels $\geq$3 mg copper/L. Most symptoms disappeared quickly.

• Treatment of toxicity

—Persistent vomiting usually renders the use of emetics or gastric lavage redundant. Activated charcoal is used but there are no data on efficacy. Chelation is recommended in severe poisoning [usually intravenous $CaNa_2$ ethylenediaminetetraaceetic acid (EDTA) or intramuscular dimercaprol (BAL); D-penicillamine may be used in nonallergic patients], but effectiveness is not well documented. (5).

• Treatment of Wilson's disease

—D-penicillamine 0.5 to 1.0 g p.o. b.i.d.
—Trientine 0.25 to 0.5 g p.o. t.i.d.
—Zinc acetate 50 mg t.i.d.

ANIMAL TOXICITY

• Maximal tolerated dose is about 250 mg copper/kg/day; above that, hepatic centrilobular necrosis occurs.
• There is a large interspecies variation; sheep are the most sensitive species; dogs are more sensitive than humans; mice are more resistant than rats.

Clinical Considerations

DEFICIENCY SIGNS AND SYMPTOMS

• Although dietary intake of copper in the United States is often below the recommended intake, frank deficiency is rare.
• Copper toxicity is also rare.
• Anemia
• Leukopenia
• Neutropenia
• Osteoporosis (in growing bones; possibly accompanied by metaphyseal flaring and fractures at metaphyseal margins)
• Hypercholesterolemia
• In animals, copper deficiency causes cardiac hypertrophy, altered lipid and glucose metabolism, hypercholesterolemia, decreased fertility, and decreased immune response (2).

Copper

FACTORS DECREASING AVAILABILITY/ABSORPTION

• Zinc (high intake enhances intestinal metallothionein, which complexes with copper in intestinal cells, rendering it unabsorbable).
• Iron (excessive intake of inorganic iron salts causes competition for intestinal transporters).
• Although high dietary intake of vitamin C reduces ceruloplasmin activity, body copper levels are not reduced (2, personal communication).
• Antacids, diarrhea, celiac disease, and sprue.

FACTORS INCREASING AVAILABILITY/ABSORPTION

• Impaired biliary excretion (can cause hepatic copper accumulation), pregnancy, inflammatory conditions, hematologic disease, infectious diseases, cardiovascular disease, uremia, diabetes, cancer, postsurgery.
• Copper-associated diseases

—An autosomal recessive metabolic disease, Wilson's disease causes a defect in an adenosine triphosphate (ATP)-dependent copper transporter; impaired ability to excrete copper causes accumulation. Neurologic symptoms, renal tubular dysfunction, hepatic disease, and Kayser-Fleischer rings (corneal copper deposits) may occur. Treatment is lifelong.
—A fatal X-linked disorder occurring in 1 in 50,000 to 100,000 live births, Menkes' disease is characterized by symptoms of copper deficiency (except for anemia and neutropenia). Copper, even if injected, is poorly absorbed and accumulates in intestinal mucosa, kidney, and fibroblasts (2). Symptoms include mental retardation and poorly pigmented hair and skin.
—Three copper-associated childhood diseases may be identical. Indian childhood cirrhosis (ICC), common until the 1970s, has been attributed to copper leaching into milk boiled in brass or copper storage vessels (5).
—Endemic Tyrolean infantile cirrhosis (138 cases of infantile liver cirrhosis in rural Western Austria over 75 years) was also linked to milk stored in untinned copper or brass vessels and may be identical to ICC (7). Susceptibility appeared to be an autosomal recessive trait. The disease disappeared after 1974, apparently because of a change in storage and cooking vessels. Endemic Tyrolean infantile cirrhosis is not a variant of Wilson's disease (8).
—"Non-Indian childhood cirrhosis" or "idiopathic copper toxicosis," attributed to copper in drinking water, was identified in Australia, German, Kuwait, Singapore, and the United States. It involves hepatic insufficiency manifesting early in life, with hepatic copper concentration 400 to 4,000 μg copper/g dry weight (neonatal normal 295 μg copper/g) and cirrhosis.

LABORATORY TESTS

• Normal ranges (labs vary)

—serum copper 10 to 24.6 μmol/L (64 to 156 μg/dL)
—ceruloplasmin 180 to 400 mg/L (18 to 40 mg/dL)
—erythrocyte superoxide dismutase (SOD) 0.47 ± 0.067 mg/g (1).
—urine copper levels up to 50 μg copper/L (In symptomatic Wilson's disease, 24-hour urine level usually greater than 100 μg copper.)

• Tests for copper status are not ideal and are not sensitive to marginal deficiency. Serum ceruloplasmin, considered the most reliable indicator of copper status, is an acute phase reactant, so levels can rise in many conditions. Red cell superoxide dismutase activity may be as sensitive as ceruloplasmin. Urinary copper varies greatly. Hair, nails, and saliva are not reliable for assessing copper status (1).

Dose

RECOMMENDED DIETARY ALLOWANCE

Infants and Children
0 to 6 months	200 μg/day (adequate intake)
7 to 12 months	220 μg/day (adequate intake)
1 to 3 years	340 μg/day
4 to 8 years	440 μg/day

Males
9 to 13 years	700 μg/day
14 to 18 years	890 μg/day
19 to 50 years	900 μg/day
51+ years	900 μg/day

Females
9 to 13 years	700 μg/day
14 to 18 years	890 μg/day
19 to 50 years	900 μg/day
51+ years	900 μg/day
Pregnant	1,000 μg/day
Lactating	1,300 μg/day

UPPER LIMITS

Infants and Children
0 to 6 months	Not determinable
7 to 12 months	Not determinable
1 to 3 years	1,000 μg/day
4 to 8 years	3,000 μg/day

Males
9 to 13 years	5,000 μg/day
14 to 18 years	8,000 μg/day
19 to 50 years	10,000 μg/day
51+ years	10,000 μg/day

Females
9 to 13 years	5,000 μg/day
14 to 18 years	8,000 μg/day
19 to 50 years	10,000 μg/day
51+ years	10,000 μg/day

Pregnant
≤18 years	8,000 μg/day
19 to 50 years	10,000 μg/day

Lactating
≤18 years	8,000 μg/day
19 to 50 years	10,000 μg/day

• World Health Organization (WHO) recommends that women ingest no more than 10 mg copper/day and that men ingest no more than 12 mg/day (1).

Conversion
1 mmol = 63.54 mg
1 mg = 16 μmol

Common Questions and Answers

Q: Do copper levels in water affect health?
A: It is unclear, but water is a major source of dietary copper. The median concentration of copper in water is 4 to 10 μg copper/L (most not bioavailable).
The U.S. Environmental Protection Agency (EPA) Maximum Contaminant Level (MCL) is 1.3 mg copper/L, but this is based on taste, not toxicity data, which is scant. The WHO has proposed a limit of 31.48 μmol (2 mg)/L, a level at which even babies show no toxic effects (9).
In adults, the Lowest Observable Adverse Event Level (LOAEL) is 5.3 mg. Massachusetts residents who drank water with up to 8.8 mg copper/L over 22 years had no excess deaths from liver disease. Another study in Massachusetts residents who drank water containing 8.5 to 8.8 mg copper/L found no increase in deaths from cirrhosis or other liver diseases in children younger than 6 years (5). Death, however, is a fairly high standard for toxicity.

Q: Is copper related to cardiovascular disease?
A: It's unclear. Copper deficiency can cause hypercholesterolemia (2). A Finnish study in 1,666 men found that serum copper concentrations in the two highest quartiles (1.02 to 1.16 mg/L and ≥1.17 mg/L) were associated with increased risk of myocardial infarction (relative risk of 3.5 and 4.0, respectively) (10). However, serum copper levels are not a good measure of body copper. Because ceruloplasmin is an acute phase reactant, increases in serum copper and ceruloplasmin may be due to inflammation (2).

Cranberry

10 Second Take

Cranberry products are harmless and have antibacterial and antiadherence qualities that may be useful in preventing bacteriuria and urinary tract infections (UTIs).

Basics

LATIN NAME

Vaccinium macrocarpon Aiton

FAMILY

Ericaceae

OTHER COMMON NAMES

None identified

PART USED

Fruit

KNOWN ACTIVE CONSTITUENTS

- Flavonoids, anthocyanins (odain), catechin, triterpenoids, β-hydroxybutyric acid, citric, malic, glucoronic, quinic and benzoic acid, ellagic acid, and vitamin C (1).
- Vitamin C is 13.5 mg/100 g raw cranberries, quinic acid 1.05%, malic acid 0.78%, citric acid 1.06%, dextrose 2.81%, and fructose 0.82% (2).

MECHANISM/PHARMACOKINETICS

- Cranberries (and blueberries, which are in the same *Vaccinium* genus), prevent bacteria from adhering to uroepithelial cells (3,4). Both cranberries and blueberries contain polymeric compounds that appear to be responsible for this effect (5).
- A recent article identified these inhibitors as proanthocyanidins (a form of condensed tannins); purified versions of these exhibited antiadherence effects at concentrations of 10 to 50 μg/mL (6).

Evidence

CLINICAL TRIALS

- UTI treatment

—A Cochrane review identified no controlled trials (there were two uncontrolled trials) of cranberry products for treating UTIs that fulfilled inclusion criteria (7).

- UTI prevention

—A Cochrane review (8) of cranberry products in preventing UTIs identified four trials. Three of four trials indicated that cranberries were effective for at least one outcome; however, the methodologic quality of the four included trials was poor, and two of four trials used a bacteriologic rather than a clinical endpoint.
—A parallel group study of 192 elderly women (9) randomized the women to 300 mL of cranberry juice or placebo juice daily; 153 were included in the final analysis. Only 4% (20 out of 473) of the urine samples from the cranberry group had bacteriuria and pyuria associated with urinary tract symptoms, compared with 7% (37 out of 498) in the placebo group; however, the reviewers note that it is unclear whether the samples included the baseline urine samples in the denominator. In addition, it is not clear whether the groups were comparable at baseline; the placebo group had a higher rate of UTIs in the months preceding the study.
—An unblinded and problematic crossover study in The Netherlands randomized 38 men and women, to either 30 mL cranberry juice or water (10). The dropout rate was 55%. Of 17 people who completed the trial, 3 had a UTI for the whole study period, 7 had no UTI during the study period and 7 had one or more episodes. Apparently only the latter group was included in the final analysis; among these seven there were fewer occurrences of UTI when cranberry juice was being taken.
—One small crossover trial of 19 women with recurrent UTIs randomized participants to either cranberry capsules or placebo (11). The dropout rate was high; only 10 participants completed the trial. Six of 21 UTIs during the study occurred while participants were taking the cranberry capsules. Compared with the placebo phase, 7 of 10 participants exhibited fewer UTIs during the cranberry phase (two participants had the same number of UTIs, and one participant experienced one more UTI).

—A Canadian crossover trial randomized 40 children with neuropathic bladder managed by clean intermittent catheterization to either cranberry juice or water. Only 21 completed the study (12). The percentage of months with a positive culture and UTI symptoms was 17% (19/112) in the cranberry group, compared with 17.1% (10/117) in the water group. The percentage of months with a positive culture and no UTI symptoms was 24.1% (27/112) in the cranberry group and 17.1% (20/117) in the water group. There were 19 withdrawals/dropouts from the study. Seventeen withdrawals were from the cranberry group; of these, 12 gave reasons related to taste (9), caloric load (2), and cost (1).

- Reduction of bacteriuria

—Cranberry juice acidifies the urine but also decreases bacterial adherence (3). In one study, 153 elderly women drank 300 mL a day of cranberry juice or a placebo juice matched for taste, appearance, and vitamin C content. Those who drank the placebo drink had more than twice the incidence of bacteriuria and pyuria as those who drank the cranberry juice.
—A double-blind placebo-controlled 6-month crossover study of cranberry concentrate on rates of bacteriuria and symptomatic UTI in 15 children with neurogenic bladder receiving intermittent catheterization found that bacteriuria remained high; there were no significant differences in symptomatic infections, positive urine cultures, or acidification of urine (13).

- Peristomal skin integrity

—A small study of 13 urostomy patients found that daily ingestion of 160 to 320 g of cranberry juice resulted in improvement in five of the six patients who started the study with peristomal skin conditions, even though urine did not become more acidic (14).

ANIMAL/IN VITRO

• Anticarcinogenic effects

—The polymeric proanthocyanidin fraction of four members of the *Vaccinium* genus (lowbush cranberry, bilberry, cranberry, and lingonberry) exhibited potential anticarcinogenic activity in an *in vitro* system that tested the ability to induce Phase II xenobiotic detoxification enzyme quinone reductase and to inhibit induction of ornithine decarboxylase by a tumor promoter (15). Components of the hexane/chloroform fraction of bilberry and of the proanthocyanidin fraction of lowbush cranberry, cranberry, and lingonberry exhibited anticarcinogenic effects.

• Antibacterial/Antiadherence effects

—The effect of a number of fruit juices on the adhesive ability of *Escherichia coli* has been tested; only *Vaccinium* species (which includes both cranberry and blueberry) were beneficial (5). A proanthocyanidin extract from cranberries decreased adherence of P-fimbriated *E. coli* to uroepithelial cell surfaces (16). Cranberry concentrate (pH adjusted) has been tested against a variety of pathogens; after 24 hour incubation in broth, bactericidal activity was demonstrated against *E. coli, Staphylococcus aureus, Pseudomonas aeruginosa, Klebsiella pneumoniae,* and *Proteus mirabilis* (17). Compared with broth, the concentrate reduced colony counts of *Enterococcus faecalis* from 4.1×10^8 to 7.5×10^2 and *Salmonella enteritidis* from 2×10^8 to 3×10.
—Urine obtained after cranberry or ascorbic acid supplementation reduced initial deposition rates and numbers of adherent *E. coli* and *E. faecalis,* but not *P. aeruginosa, Staphylococcus epidermidis,* or *Candida albicans* (18). Cranberry juice inhibited adherence by 75% or more of 77 clinical isolates of *E. coli;* urine taken from 15/22 participants 1 to 3 hours after drinking 15 oz. cranberry cocktail was also noted to have significant antiadherence effects (3).

• Low-density lipoprotein (LDL) oxidation

—A cranberry extract containing 1,548 mg gallic acid equivalents/L inhibited the oxidative modification of LDL particles, measured by a reduction in thiobarbituric acid reactive substances and reduced electrophoretic mobility of LDL (19).

OTHER CLAIMED BENEFITS/ACTIONS

• Blood disorders
• Stomach ailments
• Liver problems
• Wound dressings

 Risks

ADVERSE REACTIONS

None reported. However, cranberry tablets significantly increased urinary oxalate levels in five volunteers (by an average of 43.4%), which could theoretically increase the risk of nephrolithiasis (20).

DRUG INTERACTIONS

None reported

ANIMAL TOXICITY

No information available

 Dose

• No reliable information on dosing is available.
• Cranberry juice cocktail contains 25% juice, whereas cranberry juice drinks contain only about 10% juice.
• Compared with cranberry juice cocktail, fresh or frozen cranberries are four times as potent; cranberry juice concentrate is 27 times as potent; and juice concentrate powder (usually what is in capsules) is 32 times as potent.
• Cranberry sauce is about half the strength of cranberry juice cocktail (1).

 Common Questions and Answers

Q: Doesn't the effect of cranberry juice on hippuric acid explain the action of cranberry?
A: Until recently, it was suggested that the quinic acid caused large amounts of hippuric acid to be excreted in the urine that then acted as an antibacterial agent. Several studies, however, have shown no difference in the levels, or only a transient effect, thus casting some doubt on this theory (7).

Creategin

 10 Second Take

Creatine is popular as an ergogenic aid; limited evidence supports benefits only in high-intensity, short-term exercise. Potential renal effects with long-term use are of concern.

 Basics

DESCRIPTION

• Creatine is a nitrogenous amine found in animal products. Omnivores ingest about 1 g daily; creatine can also be formed in the liver, kidney, and pancreas from glycine, arginine, and methionine (1).
• Creatine comprises 0.3% to 0.5% of muscle weight (about 1.2 kg in a 70-kg male) (2). Most creatine in muscle (60%) is in the form of phosphocreatine and about 40% is in the form of free creatine.

FOOD SOURCES

Meat, fish, and other animal products

MAIN FUNCTIONS/PHARMACOKINETICS

• Creatine is an important source of energy for muscle contraction because it can undergo both rapid and reversible phosphorylation. Phosphorylation of creatine, catalyzed by creatine kinase, forms phosphocreatine; during dephosphorylation a phosphate group is donated to adenosine triphosphate (ADP) forming adenosine triphosphate (ATP).
• This phosphorylation-dephosphorylation reaction provides phosphate for performing high-intensity, short-duration physical activity (1). Three days of creatine ingestion (0.35 g/kg free-fat mass/day) increased total body water and intracellular fluid volumes without affecting extracellular fluid volumes (3).

 Evidence

CLINICAL TRIALS

• Ergogenics

—Creatine research is characterized by many small laboratory studies and very few field studies. Evidence is mixed on the effect of creatine in short-term, high-intensity exercise, and negative trials predominate for other ergogenic effects. A review of creatine supplementation in exercise identified 31 trials of creatine monohydrate supplements on short-term ($\leq$30 seconds) high-intensity performance, thought to be dependent on endogenous levels of ATP and phosphocreatine (1). Twenty-two of these trials were randomized, double-blind, and placebo-controlled, but all were very small (the largest enrolled 36 participants; two thirds enrolled fewer than 20 participants). Most trials used doses of 20 to 25 g/day. Most (23/31) of these trials indicated a positive ergogenic effect; however, only 9 of 22 randomized double-blind placebo-controlled trials showed a benefit.
—Fourteen trials of creatine monophosphate in high-intensity, more prolonged, predominantly anaerobic exercise tests (>30 to $\leq$150 seconds) were identified (1). Nine were randomized, double-blind, placebo-controlled trials. The largest trial enrolled only 32 participants, and only three trials enrolled more than 20 people. Most used doses of creatine $\geq$20 g/day. Five of fourteen trials showed a positive ergogenic effect; only two of nine randomized double-blind placebo-controlled trials showed a benefit. Six of these studies (four in swimmers and two in runners) were field studies. None of the studies that examined creatine supplementation in swim performance found any benefit. In 12 female runners, creatine supplementation (20 g/day × 5 days) did not improve 700-m run time. A single-blind study of creatine supplementation in 10 trained middle distance runners reported a significant benefit.
—Studies in aerobic exercise performance tests (>150 seconds, testing primarily aerobic glycolysis) are even less impressive. Only two of eight studies of creatine monohydrate supplementation (most used 20 g/day) in aerobic exercise performance tests found a benefit of creatine (1). Of the five randomized, double-blind, placebo-controlled trials, only one found a benefit. Only one of five of the field trials found a benefit; one of the field reports found that creatine impaired performance in a forest terrain run.

• Effects on body mass

—Of 19 publications (including 21 groups) that recorded effects on body mass, increased body mass was noted in 13/21 groups (1). Short-term supplementation may increase both total body mass and lean body mass (at least in males); however, most of the increased body mass may be due to water retention (1).

• Chronic heart failure

—A double-blind, placebo-controlled trial in 17 males with congestive heart failure tested the effects of creatine 20 g/day × 10 days. There was no effect on ejection fraction; however, compared with the placebo group, creatine increased performance in knee extensor exercise, cycle ergometry, and peak torque (4).
—Another study found that creatine supplementation (5 g q.i.d. × 5 days) in 20 male congestive heart failure patients increased skeletal muscle endurance and decreased abnormal skeletal muscle metabolic response to exercise in a forearm model of muscle metabolism (5).

• Neuromuscular diseases

—A double-blind, placebo-controlled crossover trial of creatine monohydrate (20 g/day × 4 weeks) in 16 patients with chronic progressive external ophthalmoplegia or mitochondrial myopathy found no significant effects of creatine on exercise performance, eye movement, or activities of daily life (6).
—A double-blind, placebo-controlled crossover clinical study of creatine (20 g/day) in 36 patients with muscular dystrophies tested the effects of creatine monohydrate (20 g/day × 8 weeks) and found a small but significant improvement in muscle strength and daily life activities (7).
—A single-blind study in 21 patients with a variety of neuromuscular diseases gave participants placebo for 11 days, then creatine monohydrate (10 g q.d. × 5 days, then 5 g q.d. × 5 to 7 days). Compared with baseline, creatine but not placebo improved isometric and isokinetic knee strength, handgrip strength, and dorsiflexion ankle strength over baseline (8).

Risks

ADVERSE REACTIONS

• Renal impairment

—Creatine breaks down to creatinine, and those with impaired renal function should not supplement with creatine. In addition, long-term studies on the renal effects of creatinine have not been performed. A 25-year-old man with focal segmental glomerulosclerosis (with frequently relapsing nephrotic syndrome) had maintained normal renal function for years on cyclosporine; renal function deteriorated after starting creatine supplementation (9). One month after discontinuing creatine, his renal function tests normalized.

—In clinical trials, no adverse effects have been associated with creatine supplementation of up to 30 g/day for 1 week or up to 3 g/day for 6 weeks (1). A double-blind, placebo-controlled, 12-week study that included 34 participants (including 14 females) tested the effects of creatine monohydrate (20 g/day × 5 days, then 10 g/day for 51 days). Pooled data showed no significant changes in total protein, serum creatinine, bilirubin, blood urea nitrogen (BUN), or liver enzymes. However, when results were broken down by sex, there was a significant increase in serum creatine phosphokinase (CPK) in men and a significant increase in serum BUN in women at the end of the study. Both abnormalities returned to normal at a follow-up visit 1 month after the study ended (10,11).

DRUG INTERACTIONS

• Caffeine appears to eliminate any ergogenic effect of creatine (1).
• Concurrent use with potentially nephrotoxic drugs should be avoided.

 ## Clinical Considerations

LABORATORY TESTS

Skeletal muscle creatine: normal intracellular concentration 90 to 150 mmol/kg (saturation limit 150 to 160 mmol/kg) (9).

 ## Dose

COMMON DOSAGE FORMS

• 20 to 25 g (0.3 g/kg/day) × 5 days, then maintenance dose of 2 to 5 g/day, is the most commonly tested regimen in clinical trials. However, 3 g/day × 28 days achieves similar intracellular creatine levels, and maintenance doses above 2 g/day (0.03 g/kg/day) appear to have no additional benefit (12).

 ## Common Questions and Answers

Q: Is it legal to use creatine supplementation in athletic competition?
A: Yes, it is an allowable substance.

Cysteine/Cystine

 10 Second Take

Cysteine is a benign amino acid.

 Basics

DESCRIPTION

• Cyst(e)ine (a notation that includes both cysteine and cysteine) is a sulfur-containing amino acid.
• The difference between cysteine and cystine is oxidation state.

FOOD SOURCES

Most protein-containing foods

MAIN FUNCTIONS/PHARMACOKINETICS

• Cysteine may be ingested preformed or formed from methionine and serine via transsulfuration. Cysteine spares methionine by reducing methionine catabolism. Cysteine, a reducing agent, has free SH-groups. Two cysteines can form a disulfide bond, which is how they link strands of proteins. Cysteine is essential for protein synthesis, growth, and nitrogen balance; it is also a precursor of glutathione, co-enzyme A, taurine, and inorganic sulfate (1). Cysteine can enhance iron absorption (2). The half-life of cysteine is 2.5 days (3).

 Evidence

CLINICAL TRIALS

• No clinical trials of cysteine alone were identified.
• A topical cream containing L-cysteine, glycine, and DL-threonine was tested on stasis ulcers of the leg in a randomized, double-blind, placebo-controlled trial (4). Leg ulcers were dressed and treated three times weekly; after 12 weeks healing was significantly better and pain significantly decreased in patients treated with the amino acid combination. The extent to which cysteine contributed to this benefit is unknown.

Risks

ADVERSE REACTIONS

None reported in humans (see animal toxicity)

ANIMAL TOXICITY

• In large amounts, cysteine is neurotoxic in several species, causing retinal damage and damage to cortical neurons. Cats fed a 5% cystine diet seemed well acutely but had acute neurotoxicity after several months. In rodents, 2% to 5% L-cystine diet by weight increases plasma cholesterol concentration (1).

 Clinical Considerations

DEFICIENCY SIGNS AND SYMPTOMS

Measures of nitrogen balance or growth have been used to assess sulfur amino acid adequacy. Most sulfur from sulfur amino acids is excreted in the urine as inorganic sulfate, so urinary sulfur or urinary sulfate levels can indicate sulfur amino acid intake and metabolism. Urinary taurine level also can be used to determine whether there is an adequate supply of sulfur amino acids.

FACTORS DECREASING AVAILABILITY/ABSORPTION

• Infants, especially preterm infants, appear to have a limited capacity for transsulfuration and, thus, a limited capacity to convert methionine to cysteine and taurine. Vegans have reduced urinary taurine excretion compared with omnivores; however, even vegans and their children consuming little taurine are healthy (1).
• Hepatic dysfunction, inborn errors of methionine metabolism, or prematurity can all limit the ability to convert methionine to cysteine (1).

LABORATORY TESTS

• Venous blood 70 to 108 μmol/L (5)
• Urinary output ½ cystine 120 μmol/ 24 hours

 Dose

• Estimated upper-end requirements for sulfur amino acids (methionine plus cysteine)

—Infants 58 mg/kg/day
—Children 27 mg/kg/day
—Older children (age 10 to 12 years) 22 mg/kg/day
—Adults 13 mg/kg/day

Dandelion

 10 Second Take

Dandelion leaf is a benign vegetable and medicinal herb with poorly documented but easily demonstrable diuretic effects.

 Basics

LATIN NAME

Taraxacum officinale Weber ex F.H. Wigg, syn. *Taraxacum vulgare* Schrank

FAMILY

Asteraceae

OTHER COMMON NAMES

Dent de lion, piss-en-lit, lion's tooth, fairy clock, priest's crown, blowball, wild endive, cankerwort, and Irish daisy

DESCRIPTION

- Considered a weed by gardeners, dandelion is an important medicinal herb and nutritious foodstuff.
- Found mainly in temperate zones of the northern hemisphere, dandelion's bright yellow blossoms are a common sight for most of the year.

PART USED

- Root, leaves, or the whole plant may be used medicinally.
- Leaves are used as a vegetable, a coffee substitute is made from the roots, and wine may be made from the flowers.

KNOWN ACTIVE CONSTITUENTS

- Dandelion root contains sesquiterpene lactones, the γ-butyrolactone glucoside taraxacoside, triterpenes (including taraxasterol, taraxerol, and taraxol), and sterols (including stigmasterol and β-sitosterol). The leaves contain sesquiterpene lactones, p-hydroxyphenylacetic acid, amino acids, furan fatty acids, and vitamin A. The flowers contain triterpenes, β-sitosterol, and carotenoids (1).
- Dandelion is very high in potassium; mean leaf potassium content is 4.51% wet weight (w/w) and for roots 2.45% wet weight (2). Mean sodium content for leaves was 0.49% w/w and root 0.33% w/w; calcium was 0.88% w/w for leaves and 0.33% w/w for roots.

 Evidence

CLINICAL TRIALS

No clinical trials identified.

ANIMAL/IN VITRO

- Diuretic effects

—Results on diuretic effects are mixed. One study in mice found that a 4% aqueous extract of dandelion herb (apparently leaves), administered daily for 30 days, was equivalent to furosemide in its diuretic effect (3). Diuresis was measured 5 hours after dosing. Extract of the herb was superior to extract of the root, and a 4% extract of herb was superior to other doses. Urinary sodium and potassium increased; researchers noted that dandelion is an excellent source of potassium (4.25% of dry weight, apparently of leaves) and a poor source of sodium, so that potassium levels should not be depleted.
—Two more recent experiments did not show significant diuresis of root extracts in rodents. One experiment using fractionated extracts of oven-dried dandelion root found no significant diuretic effect of dandelion at 5 hours in saline-loaded mice (2). An ethanol root extract failed to show diuretic or natriuretic activity following oral or intraperitoneal administration in an unspecified number of rodents; potassium excretion doubled (4).

- Analgesic and antiinflammatory activity

—100 mg/kg ethanol root extract intraperitoneally reduced writhing response to phenylquinone in mice and briefly enhanced reaction time (+38% at 180 degrees Fahrenheit) in the hot plate test (4). Carrageenan-induced rat paw edema was partially inhibited (−42% at 3 hours) following intraperitoneal administration of 100 mg/kg ethanol root extract (4).

- Increasing bile flow

—In three studies done between 1931 and 1959, extracts of dandelion increased bile flow in rats and dogs (5).

- Hypoglycemic effects

—Animal studies are mixed but none show an effect in diabetic animals. In rabbits, 1 to 2 g/kg of dandelion given orally produced a hypoglycemic response in normal rabbits at 8 and 12 hours (the 2 g/kg dose reduced glucose levels at 4 hours as well). All levels returned to baseline by 24 hours. There was no effect, however, on rabbits with alloxan-induced diabetes (6). In a study of mice, replacement of part of the diet with dried herb did not affect glucose levels in either diabetic or streptozotocin-diabetic animals (7).

- Antitumor effect

—An aqueous extract, administered intraperitoneally, was reported to have an antitumor effect in mice (1).

—Acute toxicity is very low. In mice, intraperitoneal LD_{50} values were 36.6 g/kg for dandelion root and 28.8 g/kg for whole herb (in this experiment fluid extract of grass was equally toxic) (3). No toxicity was noted in rabbits dosed orally with up to 6 g/kg for up to 7 days (6).

Risks

ADVERSE REACTIONS

• None reported for root, leaves, or flowers. However, a German text from 1974 states that children who consume the milky sap from the flower stem can suffer nausea, vomiting, diarrhea, and cardiac arrhythmia (1).
• Those with occlusion of the bile ducts, cholecystitis, or small bowel obstruction should not use dandelion (8).

DRUG INTERACTIONS

• None known for *Taraxacum officinale.*
• However, *Taraxacum mongolicum* Hand-Mazz., a Chinese herb (*Pu gong ying*), used for its antibacterial and hepatoprotective effects, interacts with a fluoroquinolone. *T. mongolicum* decreased maximum plasma concentrations (C_{max}) of ciprofloxacin by 73% in rats given oral doses (20 mg/kg ciprofloxacin and an aqueous extract of 2 g whole herb/kg) of the two drugs concurrently (9).

 ## Dose

COMMON DOSAGE FORMS

• Dandelion leaf

—Adults: 4 to 10 g of dried herb in capsules or by infusion t.i.d.
—2 to 5 mL tincture (1:5, ethanol 25% V/V) t.i.d.
—5 to 10 mL juice from fresh leaf b.i.d.

• Dandelion root

—Adults: 3 to 5 g of dried herb in capsules or by infusion t.i.d.
—5 to 10 mL tincture (1:5, ethanol 25% V/V) t.i.d.

 ## Common Questions and Answers

Q: Are dandelion leaves an effective diuretic in humans?
A: Probably, although clinical trials have not been done. It has a long folk history in several different cultures for this effect, and some of its common names (the French name *piss-en-lit* means piss in the bed) attest to its effects. Anyone who doubts this need only consume some dandelion greens for dinner to be convinced.
Its extremely high potassium content should prevent potassium depletion. A clinical trial that compares dandelion to loop diuretics for diuresis and effect on serum potassium levels is needed.

Q: Is the effect of dandelion on weight loss merely a diuretic effect?
A: Probably. In one experiment in rats and mice, weight loss occurred in a dose-dependent manner, with whole herb extract being superior to root extract; the results were consistent with the herb's diuretic effect.
A huge daily dose of 8 mL/kg aqueous extract of whole herb for 30 days resulted in a 31.3% weight loss in mice and a 28.2% weight loss in rats (3).

Q: Can I eat dandelion greens out of my yard?
A: Well, you could, but do not serve them to guests. Most yard dandelions are very bitter, especially if you gather them later than early spring. Commercially grown varieties are less bitter; and mildest of all are blanched winter-grown leaves. The bitterness is due to sesquiterpene lactones, and their formation is known to be light-dependent (2).

Danshen

10 Second Take

Danshen, a Chinese herb used to treat cardiovascular disease, can potentiate the effects of warfarin and should not be combined with anticoagulants.

Basics

LATIN NAME

Salvia miltiorrhiza Bunge.

FAMILY

Lamiaceae

OTHER COMMON NAMES

Tan seng, red-rooted sage, salvia root

PART USED

Root, rhizome

KNOWN ACTIVE CONSTITUENTS

Ketone and alcohol derivatives, including tanshinone (I, IIA, IIB), cryptotanshinone, isocryptotanshinone, miltirone, tanshinol (I and II), and salviol (1)

MECHANISM/PHARMACOKINETICS

Tanshinone IIA appears to have calcium channel blocking ability. In rats, 70% of intravenously administered tanshinone IIA was excreted in feces via bile; the rest was excreted in urine (1).

Evidence

CLINICAL TRIALS

No clinical trials identified.

ANIMAL/IN VITRO

- Cardiovascular effects

—Danshen inhibits platelet aggregation *in vitro* and *in vivo*, and demonstrates hypotensive, positive inotropic, and negative chronotropic effects, as well as vasodilatory effects on coronary arteries. Danshen extracts reduce ischemic symptoms in animals with induced myocardial ischemia (1).

- Alcohol intake

—Intragastric administration of 200 mg/kg *Salvia miltiorrhiza* extract significantly reduced ethanol intake by 40% in ethanol-preferring rats, and when given with 2 g/kg ethanol intragastrically, reduced blood ethanol levels up to 60% compared with controls (2). Total fluid intake was unchanged. Reduction in ethanol intake was rapid, and there was no residual effect; ethanol intake returned to pretreatment levels the day after treatment was stopped. When ethanol was administered intraperitoneally, danshen had no effect on blood alcohol levels.

OTHER CLAIMED BENEFITS/ACTIONS

- Angina
- Stroke
- Thrombophlebitis
- Hepatitis
- Other infectious diseases
- Psoriasis and other skin diseases

Risks

ADVERSE REACTIONS

Pruritus, stomach ache, or decreased appetite has been reported with tinctures of this herb (3).

DRUG INTERACTIONS

- Warfarin

—Danshen appears to potentiate warfarin. Two case reports of clotting abnormalities including prolonged prothrombin time (PT) and activated partial thromboplastin time (APTT) in patients mixing danshen and warfarin have been reported. Elevated international normalized ratio (INR) was reported in a 48-year-old woman hospitalized for a chest infection; she had been maintained on a varying dose of warfarin for 15 months and was taking furosemide and digoxin, as well as danshen (4).
—Elevated INR was also reported in a 66-year-old man on warfarin (5) and danshen admitted for melena (subsequently diagnosed with gastric adenocarcinoma). The patient had also been using a topical Chinese medicated oil containing 15% methyl salicylate (Kwan Loong Medicated Oil).
—In rats, danshen appears to decrease the elimination of warfarin (6). It would be prudent to avoid the combined use of danshen with any anticoagulant.

ANIMAL TOXICITY

- No acute toxicity was noted in rabbits administered 2 to 3 g/kg/day aqueous extract for 14 days. LD_{50} in mice was 80.5 ± 3.1 g/kg i.p. (1).
- No chronic toxicity studies were identified.

 Dose

COMMON DOSAGE FORMS

Danshen is usually used as part of a mixture of Chinese herbs.

Devil's Claw

10 Second Take

A nontoxic herb popular for arthritis, devil's claw has not been impressive in clinical trials.

Basics

LATIN NAME

Harpagophytum procumbens DC

FAMILY

Pedaliaceae

OTHER COMMON NAMES

Grapple plant, wool-spider

DESCRIPTION

• A perennial herbaceous plant with branches lying flat on the ground, devil's claw is common in southern Africa.
• The woody, branched fruit is tipped with barbs.

PART USED

Secondary roots (tubers of the lateral roots)

KNOWN ACTIVE CONSTITUENTS

• Harpagoside (an iridoid glycoside), harpagide, and procumbide
• Also contains free cinnamic acid and phenolic glycosides (1)

Evidence

CLINICAL TRIALS

• Back pain

—Two trials of devil's claw indicate that the herb has only mild, if any, beneficial effect in low back pain. A randomized, double-blind, placebo-controlled trial tested the effect of devil's claw on acute exacerbation of low back pain in 197 patients, age 18 to 75 years, with chronic susceptibility to back pain (2). *Harpagophytum* extract WS 1531 in two different doses: 600 mg (51 mg harpagoside) or 1,200 mg (102 mg harpagoside) was tested versus placebo for 4 weeks. The main outcome measure was the proportion of patients free of pain without other analgesics for a minimum of 5 days in the last week of the trial. Secondary outcome measures included change in the Arhus Low Back Pain Index and levels of consumption of tramadol, the only analgesic allowed in the trial.
Out of 183 patients who completed the study, only 19 (3 in the placebo group, 6 in the 600 mg devil's claw group, and 10 in the 1,200 mg group) were pain-free without tramadol for at least 5 days in the fourth week of treatment (13 of these had had pain for less than 6 weeks before the trial). The difference was statistically significant. There was no consistently better effect with a larger dose. The median change in the overall Arhus index decreased about 20% in all three groups; there was no significant difference among groups. Analgesic intake appeared to be related more to pain than to group assignment. Adverse reactions were mild and included nine cases of gastrointestinal upset (four in each devil's claw group and one in the placebo group).
—The same investigator conducted a previous randomized placebo-controlled 4-week trial that tested devil's claw (two tablets t.i.d., equivalent to 6 g of herb containing 50 mg harpagoside) in 118 patients with acute exacerbation of chronic back pain (109 patients completed the trial). Devil's claw did not significantly reduce analgesic intake; the Arhus index improved significantly in both groups, but there was not a significant difference between groups. A post-hoc analysis found that 9 of 51 patients who received devil's claw were pain-free at the end of treatment compared with 1 of 54 patients receiving placebo (3).

• Arthritis

—A randomized, double-blind, 4-month study in 122 subjects with osteoarthritis of the knee and/or hip compared devil's claw (six capsules/day; each containing 435 mg powdered herb) against diacerhein 100 mg/day (an anthraquinone derivative, approved as an osteoarthritis treatment in France and Italy). The study was apparently reported twice (4,5). Both treatments improved pain by Lequesne's index, with no difference between the two treatments. Participants using devil's claw used significantly fewer analgesics than the diacerhein group; adverse events were minor and less common in the devil's claw group.
—In an uncontrolled trial, 13 participants with arthritis (9 had seropositive arthritis, 2 had seronegative rheumatoid arthritis and 2 had psoriatic arthritis) received one tablet containing 410 mg of aqueous extract of *Harpagophytum* t.i.d. before meals for 6 weeks. Participants were allowed to continue their usual medications. Outcome measures included pain, early morning stiffness, Ritchie articular index, grip strength, patient impression, and functional class; subjects were assessed at baseline, after 6 weeks of therapy, and 6 weeks later. There were no significant changes from baseline in any of the parameters measured at any time point; there were no significant changes in blood counts or blood chemistry. The mean erythrocyte sedimentation rate (ESR) rose from 48 mm to 56 mm. One patient dropped out after 4 days because of headache, tinnitus, and anorexia (6).

ANIMAL/IN VITRO

- Inflammation and analgesia

—One study found that pretreatment with intraperitoneal (400 or 800 mg/kg aqueous extract) or intraduodenal (200, 400, or 1,600 mg/kg) administration of *Harpagophytum* significantly reduced carrageenan-induced edema; however, orally administered extracts did not work (see questions and answers) (7).

—One study found a dose-dependent effect of intraperitoneal *Harpagophytum* in reducing carrageenan-induced edema in rats and dose-dependent analgesic effects in the writing test in mice (8). In the same report, harpagoside (also administered intraperitoneally) was ineffective in reducing carrageenan-induced edema.

—Administration by mouth or by gastric gavage appears to be ineffective. A controlled study that compared indomethacin to devil's claw (1 g dried aqueous extract per kilogram p.o.) found the herb ineffective against carrageenan-induced foot swelling (9). Two doses (0.1 g and 1.0 g/kg p.o.) were tested against tap water and indomethacin in adjuvant-induced arthritis and found to be largely ineffective (the larger dose appeared to worsen swelling compared with placebo; this effect was significant only on the seventh day) (9).

—A controlled study that compared aspirin to devil's claw found that doses of devil's claw up to 6,000 mg/kg administered by gastric gavage did not significantly inhibit carrageenan-induced rat paw edema (10). In the same report, a comparison of placebo, indomethacin, and devil's claw (2 g/kg q.d. × 7 days) in adjuvant-induced arthritis found no significant effect of devils claw. *In vitro,* in concentrations up to 10^5 μg/mL, devil's claw did not alter synthetase activity (10).

- Cardiovascular effects

—At high doses (400 mg/kg dried crude methanolic extract), devil's claw administered by gavage decreased blood pressure and heart rate in rats. Harpagoside had the same effect at a lower dose. An antiarrhythmic effect was also demonstrated in intact rats; in isolated rabbit heart *Harpagophytum* and harpagoside, at high doses, demonstrated marked negative inotropic effects (11). A crude methanolic extract of *Harpagophytum* has also shown a protective effect against reperfusion-induced hyperkinetic ventricular arrhythmias in isolated rat heart.

OTHER CLAIMED BENEFITS/ACTIONS

- Antidiabetic
- Arthritis
- Indigestion
- Loss of appetite
- Dyspepsia
- Headache
- Fevers
- Hypercholesterolemia
- Pain associated with pregnancy
- Ulcers, boils, and skin lesions (topical)

 Risks

ADVERSE REACTIONS

- Gastrointestinal upset
- No other side effects were noted in a case series of 630 patients with arthrosis treated with devil's claw aqueous dry extract standardized to 2.5% iridoid glycosides in doses up to 9 g/day for 6 months (12).

ANIMAL TOXICITY

- Devil's claw appears to have minimal toxicity in short-term studies; no chronic toxicity studies have been performed.
- The average lethal dose in mice (of what appears to be a 10% aqueous solution of extract) has been reported as 220 mL/kg; another report found the oral LD_{50} in mice to be greater than 13.5 g/kg.
- In rats given 7.5 g/kg p.o. × 21 days, clinical, hematologic, and gross pathologic findings were unremarkable. In rats, 2.0 g/kg devil's claw administered for 7 days resulted in no adverse hepatic effects (10).

PREGNANCY/LACTATION

In Africa the herb is used to treat pain during pregnancy (it may also be applied as an ointment to the abdomen of a pregnant woman anticipating a difficult delivery).

 Dose

COMMON DOSAGE FORMS

- *Dried tuber:* 1.5 to 3 g as decoction t.i.d.
- *Liquid extract:* (1:1 in 25% alcohol) 0.1 to 2 mL t.i.d.
- *Tincture:* (1:5 in 25% alcohol) 0.5 to 1 mL t.i.d.
- Commercial sources usually contain 1.4% to 2% harpagoside.

 Common Questions and Answers

Q: Is devil's claw more effective when administered by non-oral routes?
A: It is very possible that routes of administration that bypass the stomach are more effective. Animal studies using intraduodenal or intraperitoneal administration of devil's claw have achieved better results. Passage through the stomach appears to inactivate *Harpagophytum*. An acid treatment (0.1 N HCl), meant to replicate gastric acidity, abolished antiinflammatory and analgesic effects of *Harpagophytum* (8). It would be interesting to see how an enteric-coated preparation would fare in a clinical trial.

Q: Why isn't the whole root used?
A: The roots contain the most harpagoside (there are traces in the leaves and none in the flowers, stems, or ripe fruits). Apparently the secondary tubers contain twice as much glucoside as the primary roots.

DHEA

 10 Second Take

DHEA may be useful in lupus, depression, and erectile dysfunction; no reliable evidence supports claims that DHEA prevents cardiovascular disease, cancer, or aging.

 Basics

DESCRIPTION

- DHEA (dehydroepiandrosterone), a C-19 steroid hormone (5-androsten-3β-ol-17-one), produced by adrenal cortex and testes, is a precursor, via pregnenolone, of testosterone and estrogens.
- Hydrosteroid sulfatases convert DHEA to DHEA-sulfate (DHEA-S), the most abundant circulating steroid hormone in humans (concentrations may be 500 times higher than DHEA) (1).

MECHANISM/PHARMACOKINETICS

- Half-life of DHEA is 1 to 3 hours, DHEA-S 10 to 20 hours. DHEA binds weakly and DHEA-S strongly to albumin. Peripheral and adrenal tissues can convert DHEA-S back to DHEA. DHEA enhances neuronal response to N-methyl-D-aspartate (NMDA) and may be a γ-aminobutyric acid (GABA) antagonist, but findings are inconsistent (1).
- DHEA concentrations, high at birth, decrease until 5 years of age and then rise. In men, concentrations peak between 20 and 30 years of age; in women, two peaks occur, at about ages 20 and 40. By age 70 to 80, DHEA and DHEA-S concentrations are only 20% (in men) and 30% (in women) of peak levels (1).

 Evidence

CLINICAL TRIALS

- Erectile dysfunction

—A double-blind randomized controlled trial (RCT) in 40 men (30 completed) with erectile dysfunction and DHEA-S levels less than 1.5 μmol/L tested placebo against DHEA 50 mg q.d. $\times$ 6 months (2). DHEA treatment, compared with placebo, resulted in higher mean scores on the International Index of Erectile Function. DHEA did not affect serum prostate-specific antigen (PSA), prolactin, or testosterone; mean prostate size; or mean post-void residual urine volume.

- Depression

—A double-blind, 6-week RCT compared placebo to DHEA (up to 90 mg/day) in 22 patients with major depression (15 on antidepressants); DHEA decreased Hamilton depression scores significantly more than placebo. Five of 11 DHEA-treated and 1/11 placebo-treated patients experienced a 50% decrease in symptoms (3).
—A double-blind, randomized crossover trial in 17 men and women with midlife-onset dysthymia (15 completed) compared placebo with DHEA (90 mg $\times$ 3 weeks, then 450 mg $\times$ 3 weeks) (4). Significantly more (60%) of the DHEA group than the placebo group (20%) responded (defined as 50% reduction in the Hamilton Depression Scale or Beck Depression Inventory). Significant benefit was noted in the treated group before dose escalation.
—A double-blind RCT compared placebo to DHEA 50 mg/day $\times$ 3 months in 60 perimenopausal women with altered mood and well-being and found no benefit for DHEA (5).

- Cognition

—A double-blind crossover study in 40 healthy older men and women found that 50 mg DHEA for 2 weeks had no effect on psychologic or cognitive parameters (6). DHEA, androstenedione, and testosterone increased in both men and women. Another placebo-controlled trial by the same investigator in 36 younger men found that a single dose of DHEA 300 mg did not affect memory performance (7).

- Endocrine effects

—A trial in 22 postmenopausal women compared DHEA-S 50 mg/day to transdermal estradiol (50 μg/day) or the combination for 3 months (8); improvements in the Kupperman index (a suboptimal measure of menopausal symptoms) and increases in serum estradiol, estrone, and plasma β-endorphin were similar among groups. DHEA-S increased androgen levels but not 17-hydroxyprogesterone, sex hormone binding globulin (SHBG), cortisol, follicle stimulating hormone (FSH), or luteinizing hormone (LH).
—An open, 1-year trial of topical DHEA (10% cream) in 14 postmenopausal women reported estrogenic changes in vaginal epithelium in most participants, endometrial biopsy showed no endometrial changes, and SHBG levels decreased (9).
—In women, DHEA administration can double testosterone and androstenedione levels. DHEA does not appear to influence triiodothyronine (T3), or thyroxine (T4) levels (1).

- Bone

—In a lupus trial, vertebral bone mineral density (BMD) was significantly reduced in the placebo group but maintained in the DHEA group (10).
—The Labrie trial of topical DHEA cream reported significantly increased BMD at the hip (from 0.744 to 0.759 g/cm^2) (9).

- Anorexia

—A randomized (not placebo-controlled) trial in 15 anorexic females tested DHEA (50, 100, 200 mg) for 3 months and found improvements in markers of bone turnover; 53% had at least one menstrual cycle while on therapy (11).

- Body composition

—A crossover RCT in 39 men compared placebo to 100 mg DHEA daily for 3 months and found no changes in body composition, urologic parameters, or sex drive (12). The DHEA-treated group, compared with placebo, had elevated estradiol, free testosterone, mean corpuscular hemoglobin concentration, and serum potassium; significant decreases were noted in blood urea nitrogen (BUN)/creatinine ratio, uric acid, alanine aminotransferase, total cholesterol, and high density lipoprotein (HDL)-cholesterol (however, no results were outside of normal range). Total testosterone, PSA, fasting blood insulin, and T4 did not change.
—In a double-blind crossover trial, DHEA 50 mg $\times$ 3 months administered to 30 participants (17 women) ages 40 to 70 years caused no change in percent body fat or body mass index (13).
—A double-blind RCT in morbidly obese adolescents tested sublingual DHEA 40 mg b.i.d. $\times$ 8 weeks (14). Body weight, body composition, serum lipids, and insulin sensitivity were unaffected; testosterone levels in females significantly increased.
—A placebo-controlled trial of a high dose of DHEA (1,600 mg daily) against placebo in 10 healthy men for 1 month found that DHEA, but not placebo, significantly reduced body fat (31%) and decreased total and low density lipoprotein (LDL)-cholesterol; body weight and serum insulin sensitivity did not change (15).
—In an uncontrolled study of 15 healthy postmenopausal women, topical 10% DHEA cream (3 to 5 g) was applied daily for 12 months (16). Subcutaneous skinfold thickness significantly decreased, (9.8%) mid-thigh muscular area significantly increased (3.5%), and femoral fat significantly decreased (3.8%). There was no effect on weight, body mass index, or waist to hip ratio. HDL, SHBG, glucose, insulin, and insulin growth factor binding protein decreased significantly. Other lipid parameters, insulin growth factor, LH, FSH, and growth hormone (GH) were not affected. The index of sebum secretion increased 73%. Measurements returned to baseline 3 months after active treatment.

- Vaccine adjuvant

—There was no benefit of DHEA over placebo as a vaccine adjuvant in four trials (three using influenza vaccine and one using tetanus toxoid) (1).

- Lupus

—A double-blind RCT in 28 women with mild to moderate systemic lupus erythematosus (SLE) compared placebo to DHEA 200 mg/day for 3 months (17). Compared with placebo, treatment resulted in fewer flares and significant subjective improvement in disease activity; there were no differences between groups in SLE disease activity index scores or prednisone dosages.
—No benefit of DHEA used adjunctively to conventional medications was noted in a double-blind RCT of 21 women (19 completed) with severe active SLE given placebo or DHEA 200 mg for 6 months (10).

- Prevention of chronic disease

—Although observational studies show a possible link between DHEA levels and disease risk, relationships differ and implications are far from clear (see questions and answers). One review found that 8/11 studies of DHEA and/or DHEA-S in men reported an inverse relationship between DHEA-S and DHEA concentrations and risk of cardiovascular disease; three showed no relationship and one showed a positive relationship (18). However, a study of 289 postmenopausal women found that high concentrations of DHEA-S were associated with a higher rate of cardiovascular disease in women (19). Premenopausal breast cancer patients seem to have lower levels of DHEA-S than normal subjects (20,21), but postmenopausal breast cancer patients have higher levels (22,23). A case-control study comparing serum levels of hormones in stored blood from 31 patients later diagnosed with ovarian cancer with 62 controls found that the risk of ovarian cancer increased with higher levels of DHEA and androstenedione (24).

OTHER CLAIMED BENEFITS/ACTIONS

- Antiaging
- Cancer prevention
- Aphrodisiac
- Cardiovascular disease prevention
- Diabetes
- Weight loss

 ## Clinical Considerations

FACTORS DECREASING AVAILABILITY/ABSORPTION

- Critical illness
- SLE
- Noninsulin dependent diabetes mellitus (NIDDM)
- Rheumatoid arthritis (RA) (DHEA-S)
- Depression may be associated with blunted circadian variation of DHEA concentrations
- Dexamethasone (DHEA, DHEA-S)
- Carbamazepine (DHEA-S)
- Aminoglutethamide (DHEA-S)
- Insulin (DHEA, DHEA-S) (1)

FACTORS INCREASING AVAILABILITY/ABSORPTION

- Exercise
- Smoking (DHEA-S)
- *Calcium-channel blockers:* Diltiazem raised both DHEA and DHEA-S in obese hypertensive men but not women; amlodipine and nitrendipine increased DHEA-S in men (1).
- Metformin increased serum DHEA-S concentrations and decreased insulin levels in men. Benfluorex (an insulin-sensitizing agent) increased DHEA and DHEA-S concentrations and reduced glucose-stimulated insulin response in insulin-resistant men.
- Alprazolam (DHEA)
- Retinol (DHEA-S)

 ## Risks

ADVERSE REACTIONS

- Insomnia
- Acne (women)
- Increased facial or body hair (women)
- Nasal congestion
- Headache
- Fatigue
- In one of eight subjects, serum lactate dehydrogenase (LDH) tripled and aspartate aminotransferase increased 1.5 fold after DHEA 1,600 mg daily; levels returned to normal within 1 month of discontinuation (1).
- A 51-year-old man (without prior psychiatric history) was hospitalized for mania 4 months after beginning DHEA (25 to 50 mg/day) (25). Manic symptoms were noted within 2 weeks of DHEA initiation.

 ## Dose

COMMON DOSAGE FORMS

- Oral dosages range from 50 to 1,600 mg/day.
- Oral, transdermal, intravenous, subcutaneous, and vaginal routes have been used.
- Micronization enhances absorption.
- *Quality note:* Products may not contain labeled amounts; one study found that only 7/16 products contained DHEA 90% to 110% of labeled claim (26).

 ## Common Questions and Answers

Q: Why is DHEA considered a panacea?
A: Because DHEA levels decrease with age, proponents believe that DHEA supplementation prevents aging. Although most observational studies have shown an association of low endogenous DHEA levels and higher rates of cardiovascular disease in men (not women), the association is unclear and there is no evidence that DHEA supplementation reduces risk.
Although animal studies have shown some remarkable effects of DHEA against cancer, other diseases, and obesity, most animal models have little to no circulating DHEA to start with and, thus, experience dramatic drug effects with supplementation. Rodents have almost undetectable levels of DHEA, and other primates have much lower amounts than do humans. Against endogenous background levels present in humans, DHEA is not impressive and may even have adverse effects in women.

Echinacea

10 Second Take

Echinacea, an immune stimulant, may be helpful in treating but not preventing colds.

Basics

LATIN NAME

Echinacea pallida (Nutt.) Nutt, *Echinacea purpurea* (L.) Moench., *Echinacea angustifolia* DC.

FAMILY

Compositae/Asteraceae

OTHER COMMON NAMES

Purple coneflower, purple Kansas coneflower, red sunflower, and comb flower

DESCRIPTION

• Echinacea, a decorative plant, has daisy-like flowers (purple, dark pink, sometimes white, yellow, or red) and a prominent central cone; its petals (actually ray flowers) often point earthward.

PART USED

Aerial parts or root

KNOWN ACTIVE CONSTITUENTS

• Caffeic acid derivatives, alkamides, poly-acetylenes (ketoalkenes/ketoalkynes), glyco-proteins, and polysaccharides. Alkylamides are thought to be the most active constituents; it is unclear which alkylamides are most active (also, alkylamides from *E. purpurea* differ from those of *E. angustifolia*)(1).
• Cichoric acid, a caffeic acid derivative, may be the most active constituent of fresh squeezed juice preparations, but only traces are present in *E. angustifolia* roots. Echinacoside, another caffeic acid derivative, is present in the roots of *E. angustifolia* and *E. pallida* but is almost absent from *E. purpurea* roots (1).
• Ketodialkenes and ketodialkynes, present in *E. pallida* roots, are absent from the roots of *E. angustifolia* and *E. purpurea*. Hydrophilic polysaccharides and glycoproteins, prominent in expressed juice and in extracts of aerial parts, are found in lesser concentrations in roots. High molecular weight hydrophilic polysaccharides and glycoproteins may only be bioavailable in parenterally administered preparations (1).

MECHANISM/PHARMACOKINETICS

• Mechanisms of action include stimulation of phagocytosis, activation of macrophage cytotoxicity, and stimulation of tumor necrosis factor-alpha, interleukin-1, and interferon-B2.

Evidence

CLINICAL TRIALS

• Prevention of upper respiratory infections (URIs)

—None of the placebo-controlled randomized controlled trials (RCTs) of echinacea-only products for the prevention of URIs found a benefit. A three-armed trial in 302 subjects (289 were analyzed) compared *E. angustifolia* root extract to *E. purpurea* root extract and placebo (2 × 50 drops daily 5 times/week × 12 weeks); there was no difference among groups in the time to occurrence of the first URI or in the proportion of groups that developed URIs (2). Another trial, published twice, tested pressed juice of *E. purpurea* herb extract (4 mL twice daily for 8 weeks) in 109 subjects and found no benefit on the incidence, duration, or severity of colds or URIs (3,4). The only trial using a rhinovirus challenge found no effect of echinacea (an uncharacterized extract containing 0.16% cichoric acid) on the incidence of experimentally induced infection or colds (5).

• Treatment of URIs

—Seven randomized, placebo-controlled trials, with a total of 1,354 subjects, found echinacea beneficial for URI treatment in at least one treated group. Tested extracts included: *E. pallida* root (6,7); pressed juice (8,9); *E. purpurea* root (10,11); two doses of Echinaforce (containing *E. purpurea* root 5%, herb 95%) (11); and Echinacea Plus tea, containing *E. purpurea* herb, *E. angustifolia* herb, and a dry extract of *E. purpurea* root in a 6:1 ratio (12). Most formulations (all but two extracts of *E. purpurea* root) were significantly better than placebo in the primary outcome measures. Most trials examined duration of symptoms; the Hoheisel study (sometimes classified as a prevention trial) administered echinacea at first onset of symptoms and found a significant reduction in proportion of participants who developed a "real cold," as well as shorter duration of symptoms.

• Immune stimulation

—A systematic review of controlled clinical trials of echinacea products for immune modulation identified 26 controlled clinical trials (18 randomized, 11 double-blind) (13). Nineteen trials examined infection prevention or treatment; four examined side effects of cancer therapies and three trials tested modulation of immune parameters. A beneficial effect was claimed for 30/34 trials; however, studies were methodologically flawed.
—Echinacea (greater than 0.1 μg/kg) or ginseng extract (10 μg/kg) significantly enhanced natural killer cell function in normal individuals, chronic fatigue syndrome patients, and AIDS patients (14). Both herbs also increased antibody-dependent cellular cytotoxicity of peripheral blood mononuclear cells (from all patient groups) against human herpes virus-6 infected H9 cells.
—A double-blind study in 24 healthy men found that an ethanolic *E. purpurea* root extract (30 drops t.i.d. × 5 days) increased phagocytosis by 120%, a significant difference from placebo (which increased phagocytosis by 20%). Phagocytotic activity normalized within 6 days (15).

ANIMAL/IN VITRO

• Immune stimulation

—Expressed juice of *E. purpurea* herb (5.0 mg/mL) stimulated phagocytosis in several *in vitro* assays (a high dose of 12.5 mg, however, reduced phagocytosis) (15). An ethanolic extract of *E. purpurea* root (5 mg extract t.i.d. × 2 days) tripled phagocytosis in the carbon clearance test in mice (14).
—In another study, 100 μg of *E. purpurea* polysaccharides equaled 10 units macrophage-activating factor in stimulating peritoneal and bone marrow macrophages to cytotoxicity against P-815 cells (15).
—Oral *E. purpurea* extract for 14 days increased natural killer cell numbers in aging mice (16).

—Acidic arabinogalactan polysaccharides from *E. purpurea* activated macrophage cytotoxicity against tumor cells and *Leishmania enriettii* and stimulated production of tumor necrosis factor-alpha, interleukin-1, and interferon-B2 (17).

—Another experiment found similar results with concentrations greater than 1 μg; purified polysaccharides had no effect on T lymphocytes but modestly increased proliferation of B lymphocytes (18). The authors mention but do not detail a mouse experiment in which intraperitoneal injection of purified polysaccharides did not affect survival (18).

—Echinacea-treated rats showed significant augmentation of primary and secondary IgG response to key hole limpet hemocyanin (19).

—Polysaccharides from *E. purpurea* cell cultures restored resistance against lethal infections of *Listeria monocytogenes* and *Candida albicans* in experimentally immunosuppressed mice (20).

—Phototoxic effects of *E. purpurea* root extracts against fungi (including *C. albicans* and other species of *Candida*) have been attributed to ketoalkenes and ketoalkynes (21).

—A polysaccharide and glycoprotein-containing fraction of *E. purpurea* root showed effects against herpes simplex and influenza viruses; polyacetylenic compounds from *E purpurea* root have antibacterial activity against *Escherichia coli* and *Pseudomonas aeruginosa* (15).

• Antioxidant effects

—Several polyphenols isolated from echinacea reduced oxygen radical-induced collagen degradation, suggesting that topical echinacea extracts may be useful for preventing ultraviolet radiation-induced photodamage of the skin (22).

—Methanol extracts of freeze-dried roots of *E. angustifolia, E. pallida,* and *E. purpurea* had free radical scavenging effects and suppressed low density lipoprotein (LDL) oxidation (23).

• Wound healing

—Guinea pig wounds treated with a topical ointment containing 0.15 mL *E. purpurea* juice were significantly smaller compared with untreated controls (15).

OTHER CLAIMED BENEFITS/ACTIONS

• Urinary tract infections
• Vaginal candidiasis
• Wounds (topical)
• Skin conditions (topical)
• Cancer

 Risks

ADVERSE REACTIONS

• Four cases of anaphylaxis, 12 cases of acute asthma, and 10 cases of urticaria/angioedema attributed to echinacea were reported to the Australian Adverse Drug Reactions Advisory Committee; 3 of 5 cases evaluated by the reviewers had positive skin prick tests (24).
• With oral products, unpleasant taste is the most common side effect, allergic skin reactions may also occur. Parenteral administration of *E. purpurea* squeezed sap [Echinacin (R)] may cause shivering, fever, and muscle weakness (25).
• Acute disseminated encephalomyelitis

—A 49-year-old woman treated with intramuscular injections of a homeopathic product [containing *E. angustifolia* D2 1.1 mL, lachesis D8 (snake venom) 0.3 mL, and "echinacea comp Hevert inject" 0.3 mL], administered with her own blood, developed numbness and weakness in her arm and was diagnosed with acute disseminated encephalomyelitis (26). Given confounding factors, it is difficult to attribute these effects to echinacea.

PREGNANCY/LACTATION

• A controlled study compared 206 women who reported gestational use of echinacea to the Motherisk program (112 reported first trimester use) with 206 controls; there were no significant differences between groups for major or minor malformations (27).

ANIMAL TOXICITY

• In rats, oral doses of expressed juice of *E. purpurea* herb (up to 8,000 mg/kg × 4 weeks) caused no pathologic changes on necropsy. LD_{50} acute dose in rats is >15,000 mg/kg orally and greater than 5,000 mg/kg intravenously; in mice oral LD_{50} is >30,000 mg/kg and > 10,000 mg/kg intravenously (15).

 Dose

COMMON DOSAGE FORMS

• *Echinacea angustifolia* root

—*Dried root:* 1 g
—*Liquid extract:* (1:5 in 45% ethanol) 0.5 to 1 mL t.i.d.
—*Tincture:* (1:5 in 45% ethanol) 2 to 5 mL t.i.d.

• *Echinacea purpurea* herb

—*Juice:* 6 to 9 mL expressed juice, or equivalent preparations (daily dose)
—*External:* Semisolid preparations containing at least 15% pressed juice
—*Children:* Proportion of adult dose by age or body weight

• *Echinacea purpurea* root

—300 mg crude drug t.i.d.
—*Tincture:* (1:5, ethanol 55%) 60 drops t.i.d.

• Usually, echinacea is not administered for longer than 8 weeks. For chronic administration, breaks are advised (schedules vary by source and include alternating weeks; 3 out of 4 weeks; 1 month on, 2 weeks off, etc.). No data support one regimen over another.
• *Quality note:* Extracts of *E. purpurea* root may be inferior to *E. pallida* root or *E. purpurea* herb. Standardized extracts of echinacea are available, but it is unclear to which compound echinacea should be standardized.

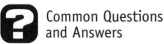 Common Questions and Answers

Q: Should patients with HIV or autoimmune disease avoid echinacea?
A: Theoretically, stimulation of T cells could encourage viral replication. However, a phase I study, published in a nutraceutical journal, in 14 men with HIV (9 on antiretrovirals) found that *E. angustifolia* (1,000 mg t.i.d. × 12 weeks) significantly reduced viral load (28). A double-blind placebo-controlled crossover study in HIV-positive patients compared placebo to *E. angustifolia* (1 g t.i.d. × 16 weeks); preliminary results in 12/61 patients, reported in 1998 as an abstract, revealed marked increase in natural killer (NK)-mediated lysis of HIV-transfected cells only during the treatment period (29). Even if echinacea is beneficial temporarily, the effects of echinacea are thought to diminish with time. Longer, better studies are needed. I no longer discourage HIV-positive patients from using echinacea, but I do not recommend it either. Concerns that echinacea worsens autoimmune disease are also theoretical; no cases have been reported. Echinacea can cause allergic reactions; I advise atopic and asthmatic patients against taking echinacea.

Elderberry, Elder flower

 10 Second Take

Dried or cooked elder flowers or berries are benign. There is limited preliminary evidence for an antiviral activity of elder fruit extract.

 Basics

LATIN NAME

Sambucus nigra L., *Sambucus canadensis* L.

FAMILY

Caprifoliaceae

OTHER COMMON NAMES

Sambucus, black elder flower, European elder flower (*Sambucus nigra*), American elder, Canadian elder, and common Eastern elderberry (*Sambucus canadensis*)

DESCRIPTION

• Elderberry is a tall shrub with white flowers and black fruits that is native throughout Europe, west and central Asia, and north Africa; it is now naturalized in the United States.
• The herb is primarily collected in Eastern Europe.

PART USED

• Flowers, dried
• Fruit, cooked or dried

KNOWN ACTIVE CONSTITUENTS

• Up to 3% flavonoids (primarily flavonol glycosides and free aglycones); up to 9% minerals, primarily potassium; phenolic compounds; triterpenes, triterpene acids; 0.03% to 0.3% volatile oil containing 66% free fatty acids (linoleic, linolenic, and palmitic acids) and approximately 7% alkanes.
• Pharmacopeial grade dried elder flower must contain no less than 0.8% total flavonoids.

 Evidence

CLINICAL TRIALS

• A problematic double-blind study of individuals with less than 24 hours of flu symptoms (at least three of four of the following: fever, myalgia, nasal discharge, and cough) treated 40 patients either with placebo or with a standardized elderberry syrup (2 tablespoons per day for children and 4 tablespoons per day for adults) (1). Serologic tests were done for influenza A and B. Symptom severity and persistence and "complete cure" were recorded over 6 days. Thirteen patients (including eight in the control group) apparently were excluded after the study began because of negative virologic tests, missed treatments, or missed physician visits. Of the 27 patients who completed the trial, antibody titers were not significantly different between the two groups. Significantly more patients in the treated group than in the placebo group were asymptomatic by the fifth day. Problems with this study include incomplete reporting and statistical reporting, a high rate of post-enrollment exclusion of patients, and different viral infections between the two groups (two in the treated group did not have influenza).

ANIMAL/IN VITRO

• A standardized elderberry extract reduced hemagglutination and inhibited replication of 70 human influenza viruses *in vitro* (1).
• Elderberry bark contains lectins (proteins or glycoproteins that agglutinate cells by binding carbohydrates in a specific and reversible manner). Lectins are used in the laboratory for various biologic applications, including blood group determination, and as probes for analyzing cell surface carbohydrates by cell agglutination. Elderberry bark provides sialic acid-specific lectins that can be used to study sialic acids on the surfaces of cancer cells (2). A lectin-related protein, SNLRP, derived from elderberry bark is a novel ribosome inactivating protein with an inactive B chain (devoid of carbohydrate binding activity) (3).

OTHER CLAIMED BENEFITS/ACTIONS

• *Flower:* colds, flu, fever, sore throat, blood purifier, eczema, and dermatitis (topically applied)
• *Fruit:* laxative, diuretic, fevers, sciatica, and neuralgia

Risks

ADVERSE REACTIONS

• Raw or undercooked fruit should not be consumed because it can cause nausea and vomiting (4). Several picnickers who drank fresh elderberry juice developed symptoms including nausea, vomiting, weakness, dizziness, numbness, and stupor (5). Red-fruit elders (*Sambucus racemosa*) should be avoided. Leaves, stems, bark, and roots can cause severe diarrhea.

 Dose

COMMON DOSAGE FORMS

• *Tea or infusion:* 2 to 5 g dried flower drunk as hot as possible t.i.d.
• *Liquid extract:* (1:1 in 25% alcohol) 2 to 5 mL t.i.d.
• *Tincture:* (1:5 in 25% ethanol) 10 to 25 mL t.i.d.

 Common Questions and Answers

Q: What are other uses of elder?
A: Elderberries are used to make wine, jams, pies, syrups, or juices; flowers are sometimes used for flavoring salads (one source says they should not be washed or the fragrance will be lost); flowers are also sometimes made into fritters (6).
Elder flower water used to be a popular cosmetic. Made of boiling water poured over elder blossoms steeped for several hours, mixed with alcohol and strained, elder flower water is an old home remedy for clearing the complexion of freckles or blemishes and for softening the skin.
The stems have a large porous pith and have been hollowed out for use as whistles.

Eleuthero

 10 Second Take

Eleuthero is a relatively safe adaptogenic herb; most clinical studies have not supported an ergogenic effect.

 Basics

LATIN NAME

Eleutherococcus senticosus (Rupr. & Maxim.) Maxim., formerly *Acanthopanax senticosus* (Rupr. & Maxim.) Harms

FAMILY

Araliaceae

OTHER COMMON NAMES

Siberian ginseng, eleuthero ginseng, eleutherococc, thorny ginseng, touch-me-not, devils shrub, Taiga root, and thorny Ussurian pepperbush

DESCRIPTION

• A slender, thorny shrub, eleuthero grows in northern China, Korea, Japan, and the southeastern part of the former USSR.
• Eleuthero is not ginseng and contains no ginsenosides (the two belong to different genera, but both are in the family Araliaceae).

PART USED

• Roots and rhizomes
• Russian material may contain mainly rhizomes; Korean material contains mainly roots; Chinese material contains both (1).

KNOWN ACTIVE CONSTITUENTS

• Eleuthero contains triterpene saponins, lignans, coumarins, phenylpropanoids, steroids, carbohydrates, xanthones, and flavones (1). The term eleutherosides includes compounds in different chemical classes. There may be as many as 14 eleutherosides; eleutherosides A to G are present in concentrations of 0.6% to 0.9% in roots and 0.6% to 1.5% in stems (2). Eleutheroside B is syringin. Eleutheroside D or E (different optical isomers) is syringaresinol di-*O*-β-D-glucoside, also known as liriodendrin; this is thought to be the most pharmacologically active eleutheroside.
• Together, eleutherosides B and E constitute about 80% of glycosides in eleuthero (2). Triterpenoidal saponins are found only in very small quantities in eleuthero rhizomes but occur in significant amounts in the leaves (1).

MECHANISM/PHARMACOKINETICS

• *In vitro,* extracts of eleuthero bind to progestin, mineralocorticoid, glucocorticoid, and estrogen receptors (3).

 Evidence

CLINICAL TRIALS

• Ergogenics

—Most of the better studies of eleuthero have shown no effect on ergogenics. A randomized, double-blind, crossover study in 10 endurance cyclists tested the effects of eleuthero (Endurox 1,200 mg/day) or placebo, each given for 7 days before cycling for 120 minutes at 60% maximal oxygen consumption (VO₂ max) followed by a simulated 10-km time trial (4). Participants were asked to try to keep their diet consistent before each phase. There was no difference between groups at any steady-state time interval or during the cycling time trial.
—In a double-blind study, 20 distance runners were randomized to an eleuthero extract, 60 drops (3.4 mL, containing eleutherosides B and E and alcohol 30% to 34%) or placebo daily for 6 weeks (5). At baseline, then every 2 weeks for 8 weeks, participants completed a 15-minute submaximal treadmill run and a maximal treadmill run to volitional exhaustion (one test was done 2 weeks after treatment ended). No significant difference was observed for any measure, including heart rate, ventilatory equivalent for oxygen ($\dot{V}_E/\dot{V}O_2$) expired minute volume/oxygen consumption, respiratory exchange ratio, rating of perceived exertion, maximal time to exhaustion, serum lactate, or psychologic measures.
—A placebo-controlled crossover trial comparing Asian ginseng (*Panax ginseng*) to eleuthero on cycle ergometry found no difference between eleuthero and placebo on VO₂ max; ginseng, however, did have a beneficial effect (6).
—A small, single-blind, placebo-controlled trial in six young male athletes (21 to 22 years old) tested the effects of 8 days of eleuthero extract 2 mL b.i.d. (each milliliter contained 0.53 mg eleutheroside B and 0.12 mg eleutheroside D) on maximal working capacity by bicycle ergometry. Participants were tested three times over 3 days to establish a baseline and then were tested after being given first placebo and then eleuthero (7). Total work and time to exhaustion were significantly greater after eleuthero, compared with both the placebo phase and baseline; maximal oxygen uptake and oxygen pulse were significantly higher in the eleuthero phase compared with baseline but not significantly different from the placebo phase.
—A study on physical fitness and lipid metabolism randomized 35 participants to an eleuthero preparation (Taiga Wurzel, 25 drops t.i.d.) and 15 participants to echinacea (40 drops t.i.d.) for 1 month (8). Compared with baseline, total cholesterol, low density lipoprotein (LDL), triglycerides, and free fatty acids decreased significantly in the eleuthero group; there were no changes in the echinacea group. Liver function tests and

other blood chemistries did not change significantly in either group. At 30 days, a significant increase in maximal oxygen uptake was seen in the eleuthero-treated group but not the echinacea-treated group (apparently this study was done on a subset of 10 from each group).

• Immune markers

—A placebo-controlled study in 36 healthy volunteers compared an ethanolic eleuthero preparation (10 mL, containing 1.96 g 1:1 ethanolic root extract, t.i.d. daily × 4 weeks) to observe effects on cellular immune status (9). The eleuthero-treated group experienced an increase in the absolute numbers of lymphocytes, particularly helper T cells; suppressor T cells and B lymphocytes also increased significantly. There was no increase in total white blood cells (WBCs), and no side effects were observed.

ANIMAL/IN VITRO

• A review of adaptogens notes that eleuthero protected rats from prolonged irradiation and mitigated weight loss in diabetic rats (10). Intraperitoneal injection of an aqueous root extract reduced blood sugar levels in mice (1).
• In mice, eleuthero decreased spontaneous mammary gland tumors, decreased spontaneous leukemia, inhibited urethane-induced lung adenomas, and inhibited indole-induced myeloid leukemia. Eleuthero also inhibited 6-methylthiouracil-induced thyroid tumors in rats. Cytoprotective effects have been shown *in vitro* (1).
• Hexobarbital-induced sleeping time was increased in mice given eleuthero extract intraperitoneally acutely (40 to 320 mg/kg) or chronically (80 to 320 mg/kg × 4 to 5 days) (11). *In vitro,* eleuthero inhibited hexobarbital metabolism by 66%, compared with controls (11).

OTHER CLAIMED BENEFITS/ACTIONS

• Bronchitis
• Heart ailments
• Hypertension
• Insomnia
• Rheumatism
• Hypercholesterolemia
• Impotence
• Cancer
• Arthritis
• Chronic lung ailments
• Stress

Risks

ADVERSE REACTIONS

• See pregnancy/lactation.
• Russian clinical trials identified no serious toxicity, although two trials noted that eleuthero should not be given to those with high blood pressure (12). Cases of tachycardia and insomnia have also been reported in Russian clinical studies.

DRUG INTERACTIONS

• Digoxin

—A 74-year-old man whose digoxin levels had been maintained in a consistent range for many years experienced a sudden rise in digoxin levels to 5.2 nmol/L after taking capsules purportedly containing Siberian ginseng (13) (concurrent medications included acetaminophen, cimetidine, oxazepam, aspirin, and magaldrate). Although the therapeutic range for digoxin is 0.6 to 2.6 nmol/L, this patient was completely asymptomatic with digoxin levels of 5.2 nmol/L (EKG was unchanged, and there were no other signs or symptoms of digoxin poisoning). This suggested that the herb interfered with the assay for digoxin rather than actually increasing serum digoxin levels. Although the implicated capsules tested negative for digoxin and digitoxin, the capsules were not tested to confirm that they contained eleutherosides. The question has been raised whether this is a case of substitution of *Periploca sepium* for *Eleutherococcus*, especially because *Periploca* does contain cardiac glycosides (14). However, the patient had no symptoms of cardiac glycoside overdose, so interference with the digoxin assay by whatever was in the preparation seems the most likely explanation.

PREGNANCY/LACTATION

• A case of neonatal hirsutism was reported in a baby whose mother took purported Siberian ginseng (615 mg b.i.d., Jamieson Natural Sources, Toronto) throughout her pregnancy and while breastfeeding (15). The mother had noticed increased hair growth during her pregnancy. The baby, examined at 2 weeks of age, had thick black pubic hair; hair over the entire forehead; swollen, red nipples; and enlarged testes. 17-hydroxyprogesterone, testosterone, and cortisol levels were normal. The preparation was not analyzed by the authors of the case report, but bulk lots of purported Siberian ginseng powder from the Canadian manufacturer of the product revealed no trace of eleutherosides. Mass spectrometry led to the identification of the powder as root bark of Chinese silk vine (*Periploca sepium,* Asclepiadaceae) (16). Confusion may have arisen because the Chinese term *wu-jia-pi* refers to eleuthero, whereas the term *jia-pi* usually applies to *Periploca*. In immature male rats given *Periploca,* no signs of androgenicity were seen (17).
• In Wistar rats given 10 mg/day total eleutherosides per kilogram body weight for 16 days, no teratogenic effects were seen. Eleuthero in the diet of pregnant sheep or minks caused no adverse effects on offspring. In rats, 13.5 mL fluid extract per kilogram body weight during pregnancy (6th to 15th day) did not cause adverse effects on fetuses (1).

ANIMAL TOXICITY

• Toxicity is very low. LD_{50} for powdered root is about 30 g/kg body weight in mice. Oral LD_{50} of 33% ethanolic extract in mice was 14.5 g/kg; a single dose of 3 g freeze-dried root extract was not fatal to mice.
• At very high doses, sedation, ataxia, tremor, and vomiting occur in animals (however, this effect may be due to alcohol in the preparation rather than eleuthero). In rats, daily feeding of 33% ethanolic extract (equivalent to 10 mg/kg total eleutherosides) by gastric tube for 2 months caused no significant changes in body weight or other toxic effects. A dose of 5 mg/kg of 33% ethanolic extract in drinking water given to rats for 320 days did not cause toxic effects or mortality.

 Dose

COMMON DOSAGE FORMS

• *Dried root/rhizome:* 0.6 to 3 g total daily dose
• *Teas:* 2 to 3 g powdered or cut root
• *Infusion:* 2 to 3 g in 150 mL water
• *Fluid extract:* 1:1 (g/mL) 2 to 3 mL
• *Tincture:* 1:5 (g/mL) 10 to 15 mL
• Eleuthero is usually used for a month at a time. When used for a longer time, it is common to take a break for 2 to 3 weeks.
• *Quality note:* Eleuthero has been substituted for *Panax ginseng* (1). Chinese silk vine (*Periploca sepium*) has been misidentified as eleuthero.

 Common Questions and Answers

Q: What is an adaptogen?
A: Adaptogens are gentle normalizing agents that have a variety of nonspecific effects that help to bring an organism back to homeostasis. The classic definition, by Brekhman, is "a) an adaptogen should be innocuous and cause minimal disorders in the physiological functions of an organism; b) the action of an adaptogen should be non-specific, i.e., it should increase resistance to adverse influences of a wide range of factors of physical, chemical and biological nature; c) an adaptogen may possess normalizing activity irrespective of the direction of the foregoing pathologic changes" (10).

Ephedra

10 Second Take

Although traditional use of ephedra for respiratory problems does not appear to be unsafe, its use in weight loss, bodybuilding, or energizing products (or as a recreational drug) is dangerous and has resulted in strokes, myocardial infarction, and death.

Basics

LATIN NAME

Ephedra sinica Stapf, *E. equisetina* Bunge, *E. gerardiana* Wall ex Stapf, *E. intermedia* Schenk & C.A. Mey, *E. distachya* L.

FAMILY

Ephedraceae

OTHER COMMON NAMES

Chinese ephedra, ma huang, cao ma huang, horsetail

DESCRIPTION

• A perennial evergreen, small shrub (20 to 90 cm high) with short, slender green branches and tiny, scale-like leaves; the plant appears leafless.

PART USED

Dried stem, aerial parts

KNOWN ACTIVE CONSTITUENTS

• The active alkaloids are ephedrine, pseudoephedrine, norephedrine, and norpseudoephedrine; ephedra also contains small amounts of $(-)N$-methyl ephedrine and $(+)N$-methyl pseudoephedrine. Amounts vary by species but may range from 0.5% to 2.0% alkaloids; the combination of $(-)$ephedrine and $(+)$pseudoephedrine account for approximately 90% of total alkaloids. *E. intermedia* is unusual in that it has a higher proportion of pseudoephedrine than ephedrine.

MECHANISM/PHARMACOKINETICS

• Ephedrine is an orally active sympathomimetic amine with a longer duration of action than epinephrine. Pseudoephedrine is weaker than ephedrine but has similar actions. Both ephedrine and pseudoephedrine stimulate alpha$_1$, beta$_1$, and beta$_2$ adrenoceptors (1).

• Systemic effects of ephedrine include bronchodilation, increased peripheral resistance, increased heart rate, increased blood pressure, urinary retention, increased respiratory rate, increased body temperature, and pupillary dilation (2). C_{max} occurs approximately 2 hours after ingestion, although one study found a C_{max} of 3.9 hours (3).

• In a randomized crossover pharmacokinetics study, three commercial ma huang products were compared with a 25 mg ephedrine capsule in 10 participants. Pharmacokinetic parameters were similar for synthetic and botanical ephedrine (4).

Evidence

CLINICAL TRIALS

• Weight loss

—Nine placebo-controlled trials of ephedrine/caffeine (usually 20 mg ephedrine/ 200 mg caffeine t.i.d.) for weight loss, with a total of about 400 subjects, are split between positive (5–9) and negative (10–13) trials. One treatment-controlled 15-week trial in 103 subjects (81 completed) found ephedra 20 mg/caffeine 200 mg equivalent to 15 mg dexfenfluramine b.i.d. (14). In clinical trials, adverse events, including hypertension, palpitations, insomnia, and headache, were more common in ephedra-treated subjects.

• Ergogenics

—Two double-blind, placebo-controlled trials by the same investigator found a benefit of ephedrine/caffeine on, respectively, high-intensity aerobic performance in 12 untrained males (15) and on run times in nine recreational runners (16); however, in the more recent trial, 25% experienced nausea and vomiting after exercise.

• Sexual arousal in women

—In a double-blind, placebo-controlled crossover trial in 20 sexually functional women, ephedrine sulfate (50 mg) significantly facilitated the initial stages of physiologic sexual arousal, measured by vaginal pulse amplitude responses to erotic films; however, it had no significant effect on subjective ratings of sexual arousal (17). Physiologic sexual responses were not increased during presentation of a nonerotic travel film. Significant increases in heart rate were seen approximately 42 minutes after ingestion.

• Heart rate and blood pressure

—Twelve normotensive adults (including six women) age 23 to 40 were given four capsules of a ma huang product (375 mg each). Heart rate and blood pressure were measured at baseline and 8 hours and 17 hours after ingestion. Half the participants experienced a statistically significant increase in 12-hour heart rate (from approximately 72 beats per minute to 81 beats per minute) (3). Between

hours 8 and 11, four participants had statistically significant increases in systolic blood pressure, whereas two had a significant decrease in diastolic blood pressure.

ANIMAL/IN VITRO

• An extracted fraction of ephedra inhibits complement *in vitro,* causing a dose-dependent loss of C2 hemolytic activity (18).

OTHER CLAIMED BENEFITS/ACTIONS

• Weight loss
• Stimulant
• Nasal congestion
• Allergic rhinitis
• Colds
• Sinusitis
• Asthma
• Urticaria
• Enuresis
• Narcolepsy

Risks

ADVERSE REACTIONS

• Hundreds of adverse events have been associated with ephedra, including reports of stroke, myocardial infarction, chest pain, seizures, insomnia, nausea and vomiting, fatigue, and dizziness (19). A review of 140 adverse events associated with ephedra-containing products reported to the Food and Drug Administration (FDA) between June 1997 and March 1999 found that 31% of cases were considered definitely or probably related and 31% possibly related (20). Among these three categories, 10 deaths and 13 cases of permanent disability resulted. Also in the definitely, probably, or possibly related categories, 47% of adverse events involved cardiovascular symptoms (most commonly hypertension, followed by palpitations or tachycardia) and 18% involved the central nervous system (stroke and seizures). Between 1993 and 1997, the FDA received reports of 34 deaths and about 800 medical and psychiatric complications linked to ephedra (2). Many deaths occurred among young healthy adults, many of whom used an over-the-counter (OTC) product called "Herbal Ecstasy."

• Suicide

—An ephedra-containing product was used to commit suicide (21).

• Stroke

—As with cocaine, fatalities are often associated with cerebral vascular abnormalities (22).

• Hypersensitivity myocarditis

—A 39-year-old African-American hypertensive man taking two to six capsules daily of ma huang for 3 months (the patient was also taking vitamins, pravastatin, and furosemide) developed hypersensitivity myocarditis attributed to ephedra (23).

• Nephrolithiasis

—A 27-year-old man who was taking 4 to 12 tablets daily of an energy supplement called Pro-Lift (ProPerformance, Pittsburgh, Pennsylvania) containing 170-mg ma huang extract per tablet experienced six episodes of renal colic and four hospitalizations in a 7-month period (21). Gas chromatography and mass spectrometry identified the substrate of the stones as combinations of ephedrine, norephedrine, and pseudoephedrine.
—The Louis C. Herring and Co. kidney stone database revealed over 200 stones with a similar profile; the incidence was approximately 0.064% (21).

• Psychiatric complications

—Ephedrine-induced psychosis was first described in 1968; psychotic and affective changes may occur (2). As with amphetamine, ephedrine produces paranoia with a clear sensorium. A review of 20 cases of ephedrine-induced psychoses found delusions in all cases, auditory hallucinations in 90%, visual hallucinations in 45%, affective disturbance in 30%, and agitation with insomnia in 55% (24). Delusions and audio or visual hallucinations may occur, as well as mania. Ephedrine psychosis may last days or weeks and resolves without treatment (2).
—A 45-year-old man with no history of psychiatric illness or substance abuse, not taking any concurrent medications, developed symptoms of mania 1 month after initiating a regimen of ma huang capsules (25).
—Another 39-year-old man with no history of psychiatric disorder or substance abuse who had been consuming an ephedra compound in both pill and powder concentrate form to lose weight developed typical symptoms of mania that resolved completely on discontinuation of ephedra (26).

• Hepatitis

—There is one unconvincing case report of hepatitis diagnosed in a 33-year-old woman about 3 weeks after she began to take "a Chinese medicine product containing ma huang" (27). Symptoms began several days after ingestion. There are no other reports of hepatotoxicity associated with ephedra. No other ingredients in the product are revealed nor was any analysis done of the product. Hepatotoxicity is not uncommon with several other herbs nor with drugs that may be mixed with herbs in Chinese patent medicines, so this case cannot be reasonably attributed to ephedra.

DRUG INTERACTIONS

• Intracerebral hemorrhage

—The combination of ephedra with phenylpropanolamine or with caffeine increases the risk of all major adverse effects, including stroke, intracranial hemorrhage, seizures, mania, and psychosis. The combination of ephedra and caffeine has substantially higher side effects than the consumption of either alone.
—A 68-year-old man with chronic obstructive pulmonary disease (COPD) suffered an intracerebral hemorrhage and necrotizing angiitis of the small vessels attributed to the use of an OTC combination product antiasthma pill that contained theophylline 0.025 g, ephedrine 0.01 g, caffeine 0.015 g, and theobromine 0.025 g (28). The patient had taken four to six tablets a day for 10 years and had used the medication 2 hours before the onset of the stroke. It is unclear to what extent, if any, ephedra contributed to this outcome.

 Dose

COMMON DOSAGE FORMS

• The use of ephedra products other than for respiratory conditions, and under the supervision of a knowledgeable health care practitioner, is not recommended. Doses are provided for information only.
• Adult

—Herb preparations corresponding to 15 to 30 mg total alkaloid/dose, calculated as ephedrine. Maximum daily dosage is 300 mg total alkaloid, calculated as ephedrine, according to Commission E.

• Children

—Herb preparations corresponding to 0.5 mg total alkaloid per kilogram of body weight per dose. Maximum daily dosage is 2 mg total alkaloid per kg of body weight, according to Commission E.

 Common Questions and Answers

Q: Are OTC ephedra products safe?
A: Ephedra is a common and dangerous component of OTC weight loss or bodybuilding supplements. In 1996, sales of drugs containing ephedra totaled $6.5 billion. Amounts of ephedra alkaloids may vary widely; nine commercial supplements had a range of ephedrine-type alkaloids contents of 1.08 to 13.54 mg (4).
Ephedra has been traditionally used (primarily for asthma and other respiratory conditions) in both Western and Eastern herbalism (various forms including toasted with honey are used in traditional Chinese medicine). Adverse effects have not been linked with this traditional use. The use of this herb for weight loss, bodybuilding, energy-boosting, or recreational use has no traditional precedent and is clearly dangerous. Derivatives of ephedra are also present in OTC drugs. Ephedrine, in doses up to 25 mg/tablet, is common in OTC oral asthma medications. Pseudoephedrine is commonly used as a decongestant and in cough and cold products (1). These products have better warning labels than dietary supplements but can still result in adverse effects.

Q: Is Mormon tea ephedra?
A: Yes, but Mormon tea (*Ephedra nevadensis*) does not contain ephedrine. There are 40 different species of ephedra, and none of the species that grow in North and Central America contain alkaloids (29).

Q: Can't ephedra be used to manufacture speed (methamphetamine)?
A: Ephedra can provide starting material for synthesizing methamphetamine and the sale has been regulated in several states because of this. However, ephedra is no longer the primary commercial source for ephedrine because it is much easier to synthesize ephedrine than it is to extract ephedrine from ephedra (29). In addition, ephedrine drug products (including OTC bronchodilators for asthma) can also be used to manufacture speed (19).

Essiac

10 Second Take

Essiac, a commonly used herbal cancer therapy, is benign. There is no reliable evidence of increased survival or beneficial effects on disease progression.

Basics

DESCRIPTION

• Essiac is a Canadian herbal cancer treatment. The primary ingredients are burdock root (*Arctium lappa* L.), turkey rhubarb (*Rheum palmatum* L.), slippery elm (*Ulmus rubra* Muhl or *Ulmus fulva* Michx), and sheep sorrel (*Rumex acetosella* L.).
• Other ingredients may include watercress, (*Nasturtium officinale* R. Br.), blessed thistle (*Cnicus benedictus* L.), red clover (*Trifolium pratense* L.), and kelp (*Laminaria digitata* Lmx.).
• Derived from a traditional First Nations Ojibwa cancer treatment, Essiac was popularized by Rene Caisse, a Canadian nurse who was given the recipe in 1922 by a patient reportedly cured of breast cancer. Caisse named the mixture (Essiac is Caisse spelled backwards) and modified the formula, administering it to hundreds of cancer patients over 40 years (one herb was administered by injection and the others in a tea). The formula was further modified between the 1950s and 1970s by Caisse and an American physician, Dr. Charles Brusch. Watercress, blessed thistle, red clover, and kelp were added to the formula, and the entire mixture was administered orally. Before her death in 1978, Caisse gave the formula to the Resperin Corporation in Ontario. It is now manufactured as Essiac (Essiac Products, New Brunswick, Canada). Flor-Essence (Flora, British Columbia), another Canadian product, is thought to be the eight-herb formula developed by Caisse and Brusch (1). At least 40 different "Essiac" products are available in North America, Australia, and the United Kingdom; its use is very popular. In Canada, Essiac is available through Health Canada Emergency Drug Release program to patients who have exhausted conventional treatments.

Evidence

CLINICAL TRIALS

• No prospective clinical trials have been completed. A retrospective review done by the Canadian government in the early 1980s on voluntarily submitted physician reports of 86 cancer patients found no evidence that progression of cancer was altered by Essiac. Forty-seven patients received "no benefit," 17 patients died, 8 patient reports could not be evaluated, 5 required fewer analgesics, 1 had "subjective improvement," 4 were "stable," and 4 had an "objective response." On follow-up of the 8 patients in the "stable" or "objective response" categories, 2 had died, 3 had disease progression, and 3 were in stable condition. It was the opinion of the Bureau of Human Prescription Drugs that prior conventional treatment could have accounted for lack of disease progression in these patients (2).
• In 1978, the Health Protection Branch of Health Canada began a clinical trial of Essiac in 58 terminal cancer patients, but the trial was discontinued in 1983 because of a lack of physician participation. The researchers concluded that the product appeared to be nontoxic but that the limited data from the trial were inadequate to confirm any survival; quality of life and pain control were not evaluated (3).

ANIMAL/IN VITRO

• Essiac

—Several flavones, polysaccharides, and polyphenols common to the four main herbs in Essiac have shown some antitumor or immunomodulatory effects in preliminary studies in cell culture or mice (3). Emodin, for instance, found in turkey rhubarb and sheep sorrel, reduces the activation of cooked-food mutagens (4).
—According to the Office of Technology Assessment (OTA) report, Memorial Sloane-Kettering tested Essiac in the S-180 mouse sarcoma model and a variety of animal leukemia and solid tumor models; no antitumor effect was seen (2). These experiments have been criticized because of problems with the test systems and possibly inappropriate preparation and storage of the herbs; the results of testing were apparently never published (1). In 1983 the U.S. National Cancer Institute (NCI) found no antitumor effect of Essiac in the mouse lymphocytic leukemia P388 tumor system (2). The Sloane-Kettering studies found no evidence of acute toxicity; NCI found lethal toxicity at the highest doses given to mice (2).

• Burdock

—Benzaldehyde, isolated from burdock, has shown antitumor activity in some animal models. Burdock root has shown mixed results in animal tumor systems (2). A desmutagenic factor has been isolated from burdock and shown to reduce the mutagenicity of 2-nitro-1, 4-diaminobenzene (DAB) (5).

• Turkey rhubarb

—Turkey rhubarb contains anthraquinones, including aloe emodin, which inhibit tumor initiation and growth (1). Most tests of turkey rhubarb in animal tumor models have been negative; a positive effect was found at one dose (but not at a higher dose) in the sarcoma 37 animal system (2).

• Sheep sorrel

—No activity was found in the mouse leukemia system. Aloe emodin and emodin have been isolated from sorrel (see previous discussion) (2).

• Slippery elm

—No antitumor effect was found in the mouse leukemia model. Beta-sitosterol and a polysaccharide isolated from slippery elm have been reported to have antitumor activity in animal tumor models (2).

OTHER CLAIMED BENEFITS/ACTIONS

• Cancers
• Strengthens the immune system
• Improves appetite
• Pain relief
• Improves quality of life

Risks

ADVERSE REACTIONS

- No serious adverse effects reported
- Essiac may cause nausea, vomiting, or diarrhea if taken with or close to meals.

DRUG INTERACTIONS

- None reported

 Dose

COMMON DOSAGE FORMS

- Essiac is usually taken as a tea one to three times a day, at least 1 hour before or 2 hours after meals. In its bottled form, recommended doses are 2 oz. diluted in an equal amount of warm water once a day for 10 days, then half the dose per day for 1 or 2 years. Amounts are then gradually reduced to two or three times weekly.
- Different methods of preparation are recommended by different sources. Spring or unfluoridated water is often recommended for brewing, and most sources call for refrigeration after preparation.

 Common Questions and Answers

Q: Isn't burdock toxic?
A: Not at all. Burdock root is a commonly eaten vegetable in Japan and is becoming increasingly available in North America as well. It is completely harmless. The myth of its toxicity comes from two reports of anticholinergic toxicity from consumption of burdock tea (6,7), but the atropine-like alkaloid isolated from the tea does not occur in burdock. These cases were clearly due to contamination of the tea with a poisonous plant, most likely the deadly nightshade root (*Atropa bella-donna*), which closely resembles burdock root (8). Deadly nightshade is a common herb contaminant that has been found in lots of comfrey, nettle, mate, and other herbs.

Eucalyptus

 10 Second Take

Topical eucalyptus oil preparations may help headache and tinea and repel mosquitoes. Eucalyptus oil should not be used internally by anyone or externally by children.

 Basics

LATIN NAME

Eucalyptus globulus Labill.

FAMILY

Myrtaceae

OTHER COMMON NAMES

Australian fever tree leaf, blue gum tree leaf, fever tree leaf, malee, and Tasmanian blue gum leaf

DESCRIPTION

• *Eucalyptus globulus* vs is a fast-growing tree up to 60 m tall.
• It has oval leaves when young; mature leaves are gray-green and scimitar-shaped.

PART USED

Essential oil, leaf

KNOWN ACTIVE CONSTITUENTS

• Eucalyptus oil contains 1,8-cineole (70% to 85%) and other monoterpenes, including α-pinene, β-pinene, limonene, and *p*-cymene, and a few sesquiterpenes (1). Medicinal oils (usually distilled from *Eucalyptus globules*) contain primarily 1, 8-cineole (eucalyptol).
• Eucalyptus citriodorae is an aromatic oil that contains predominately citronellol (2). Leaf and bark may contain significant amounts of tannins. Kino is dried exudate from the bark (eucalyptus kino or red gum comes from *Eucalyptus rostrata*; botany bay kino, containing 28% kino tannin and 48% catechin, comes from *Eucalyptus globulus* or *Eucalyptus resinifera* (2).

MECHANISM/PHARMACOKINETICS

• Cineole dose-dependently inhibits the production of tumor necrosis factor-α, interleukin-1β, leukotriene B$_4$, and thromboxane B$_2$ in human blood monocytes *in vitro* (3).
• Inhaled cineole (eucalyptol) in humans has a plasma half-life of 35.8 minutes (1).

 Evidence

CLINICAL TRIALS

• Antifungal effects

—Eucalyptus oil in ointment (1% v/v) was tested in 50 patients with tinea pedis, tinea corporis, or tinea cruris. After 2 weeks of treatment all patients had negative potassium hydroxide (KOH) tests. All patients improved; 60% were cured (4).

• Nasal congestion

—A single-blind parallel study in 234 participants with respiratory tract infections compared vaporized eucalyptus oil, camphor, menthol, and steam. Eucalyptus oil was significantly better than other treatments in reducing nasal congestion (1).
—Several studies in patients with colds have found no benefit of eucalyptus oil over placebo for nasal congestion (1).
—Camphor, eucalyptus, and menthol vapor stimulated cold receptors in the nose but had no effect on nasal resistance to airflow (5).

• Cough

—In 20 participants who inhaled air, placebo (pine oil), or menthol dissolved in eucalyptus oil (3:1 ratio), treatment reduced citric acid-induced cough (6). It is unclear what eucalyptus contributed to this effect.

• Headache

—A double-blind placebo-controlled crossover study in 32 healthy men examined the effects of topical applications of ethanol and peppermint oil, eucalyptus oil, both oils, and placebo (7). Both peppermint preparations significantly reduced electromyographic (EMG) activity of the temporalis muscle; eucalyptus or ethanol caused no change. Induced pain was similar among groups. Performance-related activity (a measure of mood state) increased significantly only in the combination group; irritability significantly decreased in both groups receiving peppermint.

• Plaque

—A 4-day trial compared chewing gums containing eucalyptus extract, funoran, or neither (control) on plaque formation (8). Gum was chewed after meals; no other oral hygiene measures were used. Compared with controls, both treatment gums significantly reduced plaque.

• Insect repellent (topical)

—Both a eucalyptus-based insect repellent (PMD) and diethyltoluamide (deet) provided 98% protection from *Cilicoides inpuntatus* biting for 8 hours after application (9). A eucalyptus-based preparation was equivalent to deet against *Anopheles gambiae* and *Anopheles funestus* mosquitoes in Tanzania (10).

—Smoke from eucalyptus leaves was 72.2% efficacious for repelling mosquitoes (11). A mosquito repellent based on *Eucalyptus maculata* oil actually attracted the biting midge *Cilicoides imicola* (12).

ANIMAL/IN VITRO

• Respiratory tract effects

—Eucalyptus oil (7.5 g/m^3); pine needle oil (9.4 g/m^3); and a combination of menthol, eucalyptus oil, and pine needle oil caused dose-dependent decreased ciliary beat frequency in nasal respiratory cells from humans (13).
—In guinea pigs, eucalyptus oil 5% (inhaled or i.p. 50 mg/kg) had an antitussive effect; codeine was stronger (1).
—Eucalyptus oil (50 mg/kg), administered by gavage, increased respiratory tract fluid in guinea pigs by 172%; smaller increases were seen in rats, rabbits, cats, and dogs. No changes were seen in specific gravity or chloride content of respiratory tract fluid. Eucalyptus oil given by steam inhalation to urethane-treated rabbits did not affect respiratory tract fluid output; deaths occurred at 20 g/kg.

• Antimicrobial effects

—Eucalyptus oil has antibacterial properties against *Streptococcus,* pathogenic strains of *Proteus, Klebsiella, Escherichia coli, Salmonella typhi, Pseudomonas, Staphylococcus aureus, Bacillus anthracis, Bacillus subtilis,* and *Micrococcus glutamicus* (1). Essential oil of *Eucalyptus pauciflora* showed strong antifungal activity at 1.0 μL/mL against human pathogenic fungi (including *Epidermophyton floccosum, Microsporum andouinii, Microsporum canis, Microsporum gypseum, Microsporum nanum, Trichophyton mentagrophytes, Trichophyton rubrum, Trichophyton tonsurans,* and *Trichophyton violaceum*); no adverse effect was noted on mammalian cells in concentrations up to 5% (4).

OTHER CLAIMED BENEFITS/ACTIONS

• Eucalyptus leaf: bronchial disease, nasal congestion, bronchitis, throat inflammation.
• Kino: throat irritation, diarrhea, and dysentery (2).

Risks

ADVERSE REACTIONS

- Eucalyptus oil-containing preparations should not be ingested internally and should not be topically applied to babies or young children.
- Eucalyptus leaf preparations can cause nausea, vomiting, or diarrhea.
- They should not be used in gastrointestinal tract inflammation, bile duct inflammation, or liver disease.
- Poisoning

—Eucalyptus oil ingestion can be toxic but effects are variable. As little as 4 mL of oil has resulted in adult fatalities. Overdose symptoms include epigastric burning, abdominal pain, vomiting, pinpoint pupils, bronchospasm, and tachypnea, followed by respiratory depression, coma, and convulsions. The odor of eucalyptus may be detected on the breath (1).
—A thorough review noted an 1893 report documenting the death of a child who ingested approximately 15 mL eucalyptus oil; a 1925 article noted eight deaths among adults who ingested 4 to 560 mL eucalyptus oil (however, some patients have survived after ingesting 60 mL) (14). An adult who ingested 120 to 220 mL survived with dialysis and mannitol administration.
—Eucalyptus oil was commonly associated with hospitalization in Victoria, Australia. A survey of ingestions in 109 children younger than 5 years found that 90 incidents involved vaporizer solutions (15).
—An analysis of 41 cases of eucalyptus oil poisoning in children younger than 14 years in southeast Queensland over 7 years found that 33 children (80%) remained entirely asymptomatic (including all children reported to have ingested greater than 30 mL eucalyptus oil) (16). There was no relationship between the amount of oil ingested and presence or severity of symptoms. Half of the symptomatic children received no treatment. Twenty-two children (four symptomatic) underwent gastrointestinal contamination (primarily with activated charcoal). Fourteen children (five symptomatic) were hospitalized overnight; 27 were discharged home from the emergency department. Symptomatic children had good outcomes whether or not gastrointestinal decontamination was performed.
—The sickest child, a 4-month-old boy who ingested up to 30 mL eucalyptus oil, developed drowsiness, hypertonia, hyperreflexia, bilaterally upgoing planter reflexes, and cyanosis on passage of a nasogastric tube. Three hours after treatment with activated charcoal, fluids, and oxygen, planter reflexes normalized; generalized hyperreflexia (with normal tone) persisted. At 3 years of follow-up, development was normal.
—A retrospective analysis of 109 children hospitalized in Melbourne for eucalyptus oil poisoning found that 41% were asymptomatic, 30% had minor poisoning (ataxia, vomiting, abdominal pain, or miosis), 25% moderate poisoning (drowsiness, obtundation, or a score of 8 to 14 on the Glasgow coma scale), 3% had major poisoning (unconsciousness unresponsive to verbal command, Glasgow coma scale score of 3 to 7 for any duration without hypoventilation), and 1% had life-threatening poisoning (unconsciousness with hypoventilation) (14).
—Even topical application can cause systemic toxicity; a 6-year-old girl presented with slurred speech, ataxia, and muscle weakness progressing to unconsciousness following widespread application of a eucalyptus oil preparation for urticaria. Symptoms resolved within 6 hours of scrubbing the skin (16).

- Management of eucalyptus oil poisoning

—Minor depression of consciousness is expected after ingestion of 2 to 3 mL 100% oil; significant depression after more than 5 mL.
—Children who ingest any amount of eucalyptus oil should receive medical attention; nasogastric administration of activated charcoal is difficult to justify in asymptomatic patients and gastric lavage is also questionable (especially in young children because lavage can cause complications) (14).
—*Asymptomatic patients if presentation is more than 1 hour after ingestion:* No treatment.
—*Recent large ingestion:* Gastric lavage under endotracheal anesthesia.
—*Obtunded patients:* Should be frequently monitored.
—*Unconscious patients:* Endotracheal intubation, gastric lavage, whole bowel irrigation, and activated charcoal.
—*Hypoventilation or severe pneumonitis:* Mechanical ventilation (14).

DRUG INTERACTIONS

- Although there are no reports of drug interactions, eucalyptus oil induces hepatic microsomal enzyme activity.
- In rats, eucalyptol reduces the effect of pentobarbitone (2). Aerosolized eucalyptol given to rats for 4 days decreased amphetamine, pentobarbital, aminopyrene, and zoxazolamine given 24 hours after the last aerosol (phenylbutazone was not affected) (17).

PREGNANCY/LACTATION

Eucalyptus oil or leaf preparations are not advisable during pregnancy and lactation.

ANIMAL TOXICITY

- In rats, the oral LD_{50} of eucalyptus oil is 4.44 g/kg; in mice the oral LD_{50} is 3.32 g/kg. The oral LD_{50} in rats of 1,8-cineole was 2.40 g/kg.
- The dermal LD_{50} of 1,8-cineole in rabbits was more than 5 g/kg (1). Deaths occurred in rabbits given 20 g/kg eucalyptus oil by steam inhalation.

 Dose

COMMON DOSAGE FORMS

Leaf

- *Dried leaf:* 1.5 to 3 g as infusion b.i.d.
- *Fluid extract:* 1:1 (g/mL): 2 to 3 mL b.i.d.
- *Tincture:* 1:5 (g/mL): 10 to 15 mL b.i.d.
- Steam vapors of aqueous infusion may be inhaled.

Oil

- Internal use: Not recommended; doses provided for information only

—*Oil:* 0.05 to 0.2 mL per dose; daily dose, 0.3 to 0.6 mL
—*Capsules:* 100 to 200 mg b.i.d. for 5 doses

- *By inhalation:* 12 drops per 150 mL of boiling water or a 1.5% V/V solution up to t.i.d.
- External use

—*Liniment:* 25% V/V of oil
—*Ointment:* 1.3% V/m applied up to t.i.d.
—*Tincture (hydroethanolic):* (containing 5% to 10% essential oil) may be applied locally

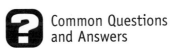 Common Questions and Answers

Q: What is the connection between cryptococcosis and eucalyptus?
A: Although *Cryptococcus neoformans* var. *neoformans,* an opportunistic fungal pathogen, is found worldwide, *Cryptococcus neoformans* var. *gatti,* which can also cause cryptococcosis, occurs primarily in association with *Eucalyptus camaldulensis* and *E. tereticornis* (18). There also may be an alternative environmental niche for *C. neoformans* var. *gatti,* which can occur in areas without these two species (19).

Evening Primrose, Evening Primrose Oil (EPO)

10 Second Take

Evening primrose oil (EPO) is benign. Evidence supports its use for diabetic neuropathy and rheumatoid arthritis; no benefit for psoriasis, hot flashes or premenstrual syndrome has been shown. Trials on eczema are mixed.

Basics

LATIN NAME

Oenothera biennis L.

FAMILY

Onagraceae

DESCRIPTION

• A biennial herb native to North America, evening primrose grows to 60 cm.
• Its yellow, four-petaled flowers open in the evening.

PART USED

Seed oil

KNOWN ACTIVE CONSTITUENTS

Seeds contain 24% fixed oil containing 65% to 80% linoleic acid and 7% to 14% gamma-linolenic, also called gamolenic acid (GLA) (1).

MECHANISM/PHARMACOKINETICS

• GLA is metabolized to dihomo-γ-linolenic acid (DGLA), which produces the antiinflammatory prostaglandin E_1.
• DGLA also may competitively inhibit 2 series prostaglandins and 4 series leukotrienes (2).

Evidence

CLINICAL TRIALS

• Labor induction

—Midwives sometimes recommend oral or topical EPO to speed cervical ripening. A survey of the American College of Nurse-Midwives found that 90/172 certified nurse-midwives (CNMs) used herbal preparations to stimulate labor; of these, 60% used EPO (3). A retrospective study compared the medical records of 54 women prescribed EPO during pregnancy (500 mg p.o. t.i.d. × 1 week starting at week 37, then 500 mg p.o. q.d. until labor) with the records of 54 women not prescribed EPO (4). The two groups fared similarly on most outcome measures, but labor lasted an average of 3 hours longer in the EPO group. This study has several problems: there were significant differences between groups (infants in the EPO group were significantly larger; compliance was not assessed, etc.).

• Diabetic neuropathy

—Two trials found a benefit of EPO in diabetic neuropathy. A randomized, double-blind, placebo-controlled 1-year study in 111 patients with mild diabetic neuropathy tested EF4 (12 capsules, each containing 40 mg of GLA) (5). EPO was significantly superior to placebo in 8/10 neurophysiologic parameters and 5 of 6 neurologic assessments. No adverse events were noted. Hemoglobin A_{1c} levels deteriorated in both groups during the trial.
—Another double-blind placebo-controlled trial of 22 patients with distal diabetic polyneuropathy tested 360 mg GLA for 6 months on neuropathy symptoms and signs, nerve conduction studies, and thermal threshold measurements (6). Compared with placebo, the treated group had significantly improved neuropathy symptoms, motor nerve conduction velocity (MNCV), compound muscle action potential (CMAP), median and sensory nerve action potential (SNAP) amplitude, and heat and cold threshold.

• Rheumatoid arthritis

—A study of 49 patients with rheumatoid arthritis compared placebo with EPO (540 mg GLA) or an EPO/fish oil product (450 mg GLA and 240 mg eicosapentaenoic acid) (2). Compared with placebo, significantly more patients in both treated groups reduced analgesic intake (2). A study of 37 patients with rheumatoid arthritis compared GLA with cottonseed oil; 24 weeks of treatment with GLA improved pain, ability to perform tasks, and physician global assessment (7).
—Another double-blind placebo-controlled study of 40 patients with rheumatoid arthritis and nonsteroidal anti-inflammatory drug (NSAID)-induced gastrointestinal lesions compared 6 g daily of EPO (540 mg GLA) to olive oil for 6 months (8). Neither group improved much; morning stiffness was significantly less at 3 months in the GLA group; olive oil was significantly better than GLA in reducing pain and articular index at 6 months.

• Premenstrual syndrome

—A systematic review of seven placebo-controlled trials of EPO for premenstrual syndrome identified seven trials; only two were properly randomized and controlled (9). Both enrolled 38 women and tested EPO (Efamol) capsules (8 or 12 capsules daily). Neither found a benefit for EPO.

• Mastalgia

—EPO is approved for the treatment of mastalgia in the United Kingdom, but no randomized controlled trials were identified. Several case series claim a benefit for EPO (10–13).

• Breast cysts

—A trial of 200 women (185 completed) with at least one aspirated breast cyst compared EPO (6 capsules daily) to placebo (paraffin) for 1 year (14). There was no difference in overall recurrence rate between the treated and placebo group.

• Hot flashes

—In a randomized double-blind controlled trial, 56 menopausal women (35 completed) with at least three hot flashes daily received EPO (2,000 mg with 40 mg vitamin E b.i.d. × 6 months) or control (paraffin) (15). EPO was not superior to placebo in any measure. Both groups experienced decreased nighttime hot flashes; only the placebo group improved in daytime hot flashes.

• Hepatitis B

—A randomized controlled trial (no mention is made of blinding) of 24 patients (20 completed) with hepatitis B showed no benefit for EPO (4 g daily × 12 months) against placebo (16). There was no evidence of histologic benefit, and no patient's blood became negative for surface antigen. At 12 months, mean serum alanine transaminase (ALT) level was similar between the two groups; at 6 months ALT levels were statistically higher in the EPO group than in the placebo group.

- Psoriasis

—A double-blind, placebo-controlled, 28-week trial tested 12 capsules daily of a mixed product (each capsule contained EPO 430 mg, fish oil 107 mg, and vitamin E 10 mg) for psoriasis. No benefit of treatment was seen in psoriasis severity or transepidermal water loss (17). A 9-month trial tested a similar product (Efamol Marine), providing a total daily dose of 480 mg GLA, 240 mg eicosapentaenoic acid (EPA), and 132 mg docosahexaenoic acid (DHA) in 38 patients with psoriatic arthritis. During the third month of the study, patients attempted to reduce their intake of NSAIDs (18). Severity, percentage of body affected, and itch were unchanged; NSAID requirements remained the same and there was no change in arthritis activity. Serum thromboxane B_2 rose and leukotriene B_4 fell in the treated group, indicating a possible effect on prostaglandin metabolism.

- Atopic dermatitis

—A 16-week, double-blind, placebo-controlled trial of 60 children with atopic dermatitis found no benefit for EPO (Epogam, with 40 mg GLA and 10 mg vitamin E per capsule, 8 to 12 capsules daily) (19). Over 16 weeks, both groups improved significantly; there was no significant difference between the two groups.
—Another double-blind placebo-controlled trial in patients with atopic eczema tested EPO (eight capsules daily of Efamol—each capsule contained 360 mg linoleic acid, 50 mg oleic acid, and 45 mg GLA) in 25 patients (20). Inflammation decreased in both groups; EPO-treated patients had significantly less inflammation than those receiving placebo.
—In 17 children and 15 adults, a randomized double-blind crossover trial found that 3 weeks of treatment with Efamol (four capsules b.i.d. for adults, two capsules b.i.d. for children) resulted in modest but significant improvement on both physician and patient assessments (21).
—A double-blind controlled crossover study in 99 adults and children with atopic eczema compared three doses of Efamol; only the highest dose (six capsules b.i.d.) showed a significant clinical improvement (22).
—A meta-analysis of nine controlled trials (four parallel, five crossover) of Epogam (not including trials mentioned previously) found that parallel trials favored EPO over placebo; there was no significant difference between EPO and placebo in the crossover trials (23).
—A double-blind placebo-controlled trial in 39 patients with stable hand dermatitis tested Epogam (600 mg GLA daily × 16 weeks; patients were observed for another 8 weeks) (24). Clinical parameters improved in both groups, with no significant difference between groups. No changes in lipid composition of plasma red cells or epidermis were noted, and no changes were seen in biopsied skin.
—EPO is approved to treat atopic dermatitis in the United Kingdom.

- Pruritis in dialysis patients

—A study of 16 dialysis patients compared EPO to linoleic acid (2 g/day × 6 weeks) (25). The EPO-treated group experienced significantly increased DGLA (a precursor of antiinflammatory prostaglandin E_1) with no concomitant change in arachidonic acid (a proinflammatory precursor of prostaglandin E_2). Although the EPO-treated group improved significantly in three uremic skin symptoms, pruritus was not significantly affected.

OTHER CLAIMED BENEFITS/ACTIONS

- Cancer
- Attention deficit/Hyperactivity disorder

 Risks

ADVERSE REACTIONS

- No serious adverse events have been reported.
- Side effects reported in trials include nausea, indigestion, softening of stools, and headache.

 Dose

- Adults: 3 to 8 g
- Children: 2 to 4 g

 Common Questions and Answers

Q: Doesn't EPO cause seizures?
A: Although the assertion that EPO causes seizures or decreases seizure threshold in phenothiazine-treated patients has been repeated in many publications, there have been no reliable published reports of such an effect. EPO was briefly used to differentiate temporal lobe epilepsy from schizophrenia. A report of new-onset nocturnal seizures has been reported in a 45-year-old woman, beginning about a month after consuming capsules containing EPO, black cohosh, and vitex (26). Products were not analyzed, and the case is sketchily presented. The only reference for an EPO-phenothiazine interaction is an anonymous entry in the Data Sheet Compendium 1994–1995 (27), for which details are unavailable. Phenothiazines decrease seizure threshold on their own, so an interaction report would have to be well-documented to be credible.

Eyebright

 10 Second Take

There is no evidence of efficacy of this herb for eye irritations or other indications.

 Basics

LATIN NAME

Euphrasia officinalis L., *Euphrasia rostkoviana* Hayne, and other *Euphrasia* species

FAMILY

Scrophulariaceae

OTHER COMMON NAMES

Euphrasy

DESCRIPTION

• An annual herb indigenous to Europe and North America, eyebright is 10 to 30 cm high, with toothed leaves and white or lilac, violet-veined flowers, with a yellow spot on the flower's lower lip.
• It prefers dry grasslands. It is hemiparasitic and must grow among other plants; nodules on its roots attach to roots of other nearby plants (1).

PART USED

Aerial parts

KNOWN ACTIVE CONSTITUENTS

• None of the components of eyebright are known to be active for what it is used for. It contains iridoid glycosides, lignans, phenylpropane glycosides, flavonoids, tannins, and phenol-carboxylic acids (2).
• Phenol-carboxylic acids may have some antibacterial properties (1).

 Evidence

CLINICAL TRIALS

• No clinical trials identified.

OTHER CLAIMED BENEFITS/ACTIONS

• Conjunctivitis
• Blepharitis
• Styes
• Eye injuries
• Eyestrain
• Coughs, colds
• Skin conditions
• Earache
• Headache
• Rhinitis
• Sore throat

Risks

ADVERSE REACTIONS

The use of nonsterile preparations in the eye should not be encouraged.

 Dose

COMMON DOSAGE FORMS

- *Tea, infusion, or decoction:* 2 to 4 g dried herb
- *Liquid extract:* (1:1 in 25% alcohol) 2 to 4 mL t.i.d.
- *Tincture:* (1:5 in 45% alcohol) 2 to 6 mL t.i.d.
- *Eye bath or compress:* 2% decoction used externally t.i.d. to q.i.d.

 Common Questions and Answers

Q: What is the history behind this herb?
A: The word Euphrasia comes from the Greek name of one of the three graces, Euphrosyne (gladness), the grace known for joy and mirth (the connection apparently comes from the herb's reputation for preserving eyesight, said to bring gladness). It has been used at least since the 14th century. The use of this herb is apparently an example of the Doctrine of Signatures; the purple-veined white flower resembles a bloodshot eye (3).

Fennel

10 Second Take

Fennel is a delicious vegetable, and medicinal use of the seeds is safe. However, the essential oil should be avoided.

Basics

LATIN NAME

Foeniculum vulgare Mill.

FAMILY

Apiaceae/Umbelliferae

OTHER COMMON NAMES

Wild fennel (F. vulgare); sweet fennel, Florence fennel, finocchio (F. vulgare var. dulce), and vegetable sweet anise

DESCRIPTION

• Foeniculum comes from the Latin and means "fragrant hay."
• A perennial, licorice-scented herb up to 5 feet high with lacy leaves and bright yellow flowers in umbels.
• The wild form of fennel is native to the Mediterranean. Sweet fennel (finocchio) is a cultivar that is used as a vegetable.

PART USED

• Dried ripe fruit (commonly called seed).
• The "bulbs" (actually the enlarged bases of stalks) are eaten as a vegetable.

KNOWN ACTIVE CONSTITUENTS

• Fennel has 2% to 6% essential oil that contains trans-anethole (60% to 95%), fenchone (1% to 30%), and estragole (3% to 8%; however, one anethole-free variety contains 80%) (1). Also contains α-pinene, β-pinene, β-myrcene, and p-cymene.
• Oil of bitter fennel contains more than 60% anethole and more than 15% fenchone; oil of sweet fennel contains more than 80% anethole (2).

Evidence

CLINICAL TRIALS

• Gastrointestinal complaints

—A commercial combination product containing hydroethanolic extracts of caraway, fennel, peppermint, and wormwood (100 mL contained 3.7 g caraway, 8.13 g fennel, 9.26 g peppermint, and 1.92 g wormwood) was compared with metoclopramide (about 24 mg daily) in 60 participants for the treatment of upper abdominal complaints (including pain, nausea, heartburn, retching, and gastric cramping) (3). Patients took 25 drops 20 minutes before meals three times daily of the herbal product or metoclopramide. After 2 weeks, significant differences favoring the herb treatment were seen in epigastric pain, nausea, heartburn, and gastric cramping.

ANIMAL/IN VITRO

• Anethole and fenchone administered by inhalation to rabbits in doses up to 243 mg/kg produced a dose-dependent decrease in the specific gravity of respiratory tract fluid; fenchone but not anethole increased the volume of respiratory fluid (2).
• An alcohol extract of bitter fennel induced spasms in guinea pig ileum. A dose of 2 to 3 g/kg body weight decreased induced ileal spasms in cats. In rabbits, a dose of 24 mg/kg of a fennel preparation (not otherwise identified) increased gastric motility in vivo.
• An alcohol extract 100 mg/kg decreased carrageenan-induced rat paw edema.
• Estrogenic effects were demonstrated in oophorectomized rats fed acetone extract of sweet fennel (0.5 to 2-5 mg/kg) for 10 days; estrogenic effects were also demonstrated in male rats after 15 days (2).
• An ethanol extract of F. vulgare had a diuretic effect in rats, analgesic and antipyretic effect in mice, and (at a dose of 500 mg/kg) increased bile flow by 33% in rats (4).
• The growth of Staphylococcus aureus and Bacillus subtilis was inhibited by an ethanol extract (4); fennel oil has been reported to be active against Escherichia coli, Streptococcus pyogenes, and S. aureus (2).

OTHER CLAIMED BENEFITS/ACTIONS

• Stimulates lactation
• Stimulates menstruation
• Eye disorders
• Dyspepsia
• Bloating, flatulence
• Antimicrobial
• Colds
• Diarrhea, indigestion
• Weight loss, appetite suppression

Risks

ADVERSE REACTIONS

- There is a case report of fennel-associated asthma in a 9-year-old atopic child, but in general, allergic potential is low (1).
- Ingestion of the distilled oil of fennel has been associated with hallucinations, and quantities as small as 1 to 5 mL can cause pulmonary edema, respiratory problems, and seizures (5).
- In humans, dermal application of fennel infusion increases inflammation caused by ultraviolet light and other stimuli (1).

ANIMAL TOXICITY

- In chronic feeding studies, oral doses of anethole up to 1,000 to 2,500 ppm caused no effects; some hepatocellular toxicity has been noted at levels greater than 3,000 ppm; deaths occurred above 10,000 ppm (1).
- The LD_{50} of bitter fennel oil is 4.5 mL/kg in rats (1). In rabbits, 21 g fennel oil p.o. is lethal. The acute dermal LD_{50} in rabbits is greater than 5 mL/kg (1).
- An ethanol plant extract administered orally did not cause any deaths in doses up to 3 g/kg. At the 3g/kg dose, the only negative effects noted were piloerection and reduced locomotor activity (4).

 Dose

COMMON DOSAGE FORMS

- *Tea or infusion:* (made from freshly crushed dried fruit) 2 to 5 g b.i.d. to q.i.d. between meals
- *Syrup or honey:* 10 to 20 g total daily dose
- *Compound fennel tincture:* 5 to 7.5 g total daily dose
- *Oil:* 0.1 to 0.6 mL, equivalent to 0.1 to 0.6 g of herb (total daily dose)

- Children

Fruit (total daily dose)
0 to 1 year:	2 to 4 g as infusion
1 to 4 years:	3 to 5 g
4 to 10 years:	4 to 6 g
10 and above:	adult dose

Syrup or honey (total daily dose)
1 to 4 years:	3 to 6 g
4 to 10 years:	6 to 10 g
10 and above:	adult dose

- Some caution that doses above 7 g should not be used for more than 2 weeks.

 Common Questions and Answers

Q: Which variety of fennel is better for cooking?
A: Sweet fennel is cultivated as a vegetable; it has a larger bulb (actually the enlarged base of the stem) than wild fennel and is preferred for culinary purposes. Although the bulb of the plant is what is normally eaten, the stalks have also been used as a vegetable, and all parts of the plant have been used as flavoring.

Q: Does fennel have the same potential as licorice to cause hypertension or hypokalemia?
A: No. Fennel and anise share the distinctive flavor of licorice, but not the same physiologic effects. The licorice flavor comes from anethole, which is present in all three plants. Anise and fennel are in the same family (Apiaceae), whereas licorice is in a different family altogether (Fabaceae).

Q: Why haven't you mentioned that this plant resembles hemlock?
A: It is traditional when talking about fennel to warn foragers that wild fennel resembles hemlock. I have not mentioned it because it is difficult for me to believe that anyone paying the slightest bit of attention could confuse the two plants. Although the leaves are somewhat similar (as are many members of the parsley family, Apiaceae), hemlock smells rank; fennel smells like licorice.

Fenugreek

10 Second Take

Fenugreek is a benign herb used in both food and medicine. It may have lipid-lowering effects, especially in diabetics (but there is no convincing evidence that it lowers blood sugar levels).

Basics

LATIN NAME

Trigonella foenum-graecum L

FAMILY

Leguminosae/Fabaceae

OTHER COMMON NAMES

Methi (India); chilbe (Israel)

DESCRIPTION

• An annual plant up to 0.6 m high, fenugreek has clover-like leaves and white pea-like flowers.
• It is native to Asia and southeastern Europe and is used as a spice, as well as medicinally, in traditional Arabian, Greek, Indian, and Chinese medicine.

PART USED

Seed

KNOWN ACTIVE CONSTITUENTS

• Fenugreek contains steroidal saponins, primarily diosgenin. In diabetic dogs, about 57% of a saponin-rich fraction was hydrolyzed to sapogenins (diosgenin, smilagenin, gitogenin) in the gastrointestinal tract (1).
• Fenugreek also contains 20% to 30% protein (especially the amino acids lysine and tryptophan) (2), 32.4% gel fiber (3), and 0.13% trigonelline.

MECHANISM/PHARMACOKINETICS

• No information is available on mechanism or pharmacokinetics.
• Diosgenin is thought to be the component responsible for lowering cholesterol, but nonsteroidal saponins may also contribute to this effect (1).

Evidence

CLINICAL TRIALS

• Diabetes and hyperlipidemia

—In one trial, 60 patients (15 female) with non-insulin dependent diabetes mellitus (NIDDM) were treated with 25 g powdered fenugreek seed divided into two doses, consumed 15 minutes before meals (3). Forty patients were concurrently receiving oral hypoglycemics. Blood samples were collected at the end of a week (prior to treatment administration) and at 4, 8, 12, and 24 weeks. Mean serum cholesterol decreased significantly from 241 $\pm$ 6.2 mg/dL to 207 $\pm$ 6.7 mg/dL, a 14% decrease, primarily resulting from reduced low density lipoprotein (LDL) and very low density lipoprotein (VLDL). Other significant changes included decreased triglycerides and increased high density lipoprotein (HDL).
—Trigonelline (500 mg) had a transient hypoglycemic effect (lasting 2 hours) in 5/10 diabetic patients (4). Increasing doses up to 3,000 mg/day had no effect on diurnal blood glucose.
—A dose of 2.5 g b.i.d. $\times$ 3 months did not affect blood lipids or blood sugar in healthy individuals (5). However, in diabetic patients with cardiovascular disease, the same dose significantly lowered total cholesterol and triglycerides without affecting HDL-cholesterol.
—Germinated fenugreek seed powder (12.5 or 18 g/day in a single dose) was tested in 20 hypocholesterolemic adults for 1 month; the higher dose caused significant reduction in total cholesterol and LDL levels (6). HDL, VLDL, and triglycerides did not change in either group.

ANIMAL/IN VITRO

• A defatted, saponin-rich fraction of fenugreek (containing 53.9% fiber and 4.8% steroid saponins), in a dose of 1.86 g/kg significantly lowered cholesterol, blood glucose, and glucagon (there was no effect on insulin) in normal dogs, and significantly decreased cholesterol and blood glucose in alloxan-diabetic dogs. The lipid extract had no effect (7).
• 4-hydroxyisoleucine, an amino acid extracted from fenugreek seeds, potentiates insulin secretion. Intravenous glucose tolerance tests in normal rats or oral glucose tolerance tests in normal dogs improved after administration of 4-hydroxyisoleucine (18 mg/kg) (8). In diabetic rats, one intravenous dose (50 mg/kg) partially restored glucose-induced insulin response but did not affect glucose tolerance. The same dose administered for 6 days decreased basal hyperglycemia, basal insulinemia, and improved glucose tolerance. In vitro, glucose-induced insulin release from islets of NIDDM rats was potentiated, indicating that direct pancreatic B cell stimulation occurs (9).
• A dose of 50 mg/kg had significant hypoglycemic effects in rats, lasting 24 hours; in rabbits, a dose of 250 mg/kg of trigonelline inhibited the hypercholesterolemic effect of cortisone (0.5 mg/kg) when administered with or before cortisone, but had no effect when administered 2 hours after cortisone (4).
• In mice, administration of fenugreek seed extract (0.11 g/kg body weight) for 15 days decreased triiodothyronine (T3), increased T4 and increased body weight (10). Decreased superoxide dismutase activity was noted, but there were no changes in hepatic lipid peroxidation or catalase.

OTHER CLAIMED BENEFITS/ACTIONS

• Breast enlargement
• Dyspepsia
• Anorexia
• Gastritis
• Externally for gout, wounds, eczema, leg ulcers, and boils

Risks

ADVERSE REACTIONS

• Fenugreek may give an odor to the urine that can result in a false diagnosis of maple syrup urine disease (see questions and answers).

PREGNANCY/LACTATION

• No information available. However, fenugreek is a widely consumed culinary herb and would be expected to be safe.

ANIMAL TOXICITY

• In an acute toxicity study in mice, debitterized fenugreek powder administered intragastrically produced no toxicity in doses up to 5 g/kg; no change was seen in organ weight or histology (11).
• In a 90-day subchronic toxicity study, fenugreek in doses up to 10% of the diet in weanling rats had no effect on daily food intake or growth. No changes in organ weight, histology, hematology, liver enzymes, cholesterol, urea, or creatinine were noted (11).

 Dose

COMMON DOSAGE FORMS

• *Seeds:* 1 to 6 g t.i.d.
• *Preparations:* cold macerate 0.5 g t.i.d.
• *External use:* The powdered herb may be made into a paste for use as a warm poultice.

 Common Questions and Answers

Q: How is fenugreek used in foods?
A: Fenugreek is amazingly versatile. Besides being used to flavor curries and salads, fenugreek has another life as a flavor enhancer in processed foods; it is the main flavoring in imitation maple flavor. The maple-like aroma scents the urine, and several individuals underwent workups for maple syrup urine disease after ingesting fenugreek tea (12,13). Its complex taste is used to maximize flavor in coffee extract and vanilla extract; it is also used to flavor butterscotch, rum, licorice, pickles, and cheese. The roasted seeds can be used as a coffee substitute (14). Fenugreek was also one of the ingredients in Lydia Pinkham's Vegetable Compound, a 19th century patent medicine for women's conditions.

Feverfew

10 Second Take

Evidence supports the use of dried feverfew leaf for migraine prophylaxis. It is benign, although some users experience mouth ulcers or gastrointestinal symptoms.

Basics

LATIN NAME

Tanacetum parthenium (L.) Schulz Bip/ formerly *Chrysanthemum parthenium* (L.) Bernh.

FAMILY

Asteraceae/Compositae

OTHER COMMON NAMES

Altamisa, Santa Maria

DESCRIPTION

• A perennial herb, feverfew is a member of the chrysanthemum family and has small, daisy-like flowers.

PART USED

Leaf, aerial parts

KNOWN ACTIVE CONSTITUENTS

• Sesquiterpene lactones, especially germacranolides (including parthenolide and 3-beta hydroxyparthenolide), sesquiterpenes, monoterpenes, polyacetylene compounds, and flavonoids (1). Melatonin is also present (2.45 μg/g in fresh green leaf; 2.19 μg/g in freeze-dried green leaf) (2).
• Flowerheads contain as much as four times the parthenolide of leaves (3). Parthenolide levels in the leaf also increase up to fourfold after the plant flowers (1). Parthenolide in dried leaves may exceed 1% or may be entirely absent (4).
• Although parthenolide is commonly thought to be the most active compound, there is no evidence that parthenolide is active in preventing or treating migraine; other constituents are likely to be responsible for antimigraine activity (2).

MECHANISM/PHARMACOKINETICS

• The mechanism of action is unknown, and no information on pharmacokinetics is available.
• Aqueous feverfew extracts inhibit platelet aggregation induced by adenosine diphosphate (ADP), collagen, or thrombin but not arachidonic acid. In platelets, phospholipase A_2 is inhibited, but thromboxane B_2 production is not affected. Most studies show no effect of feverfew extracts on cyclooxygenase production; effects on the arachidonic acid pathway are more likely (3).

Evidence

CLINICAL TRIALS

• Migraine prophylaxis

—A systematic review of six randomized, double-blind, placebo-controlled trials (four crossover) of feverfew for migraine prophylaxis found that four of six trials showed a positive effect (5). These trials are summarized briefly.
—In a randomized, double-blind crossover trial, 72 migraine patients (59 completed) were given placebo or dried whole feverfew leaf (82 mg, containing 0.62% parthenolide) for 4 months and then were crossed over to the other group (6). While receiving feverfew, patients had fewer and less severe migraines, with less vomiting; the duration of individual attacks remained the same.
—In a crossover trial, 57 participants took feverfew (100 mg powdered leaf, containing 0.2% parthenolide) daily for 2 months, and then the participants were randomized to continued feverfew or placebo for 1 month, after which they were crossed over to the other group for one month (7). During the initial phase, feverfew decreased pain intensity compared with baseline. During the placebo-controlled crossover, pain intensity, severity of nausea and vomiting, and sensitivity to noise and light were significantly less during the feverfew phase compared with the placebo phase.
—A trial in 147 subjects, published only in abstract form, tested placebo against three daily doses of feverfew (6.25 mg, 18.75 mg, and 56.25 mg/day of a super-critical carbon dioxide feverfew leaf extract ×3 months) on frequency of migraine and found a significant reduction in attacks; the 18.75-mg dose appeared superior to the other two doses (8).
—Another trial tested the effects of feverfew withdrawal in regular users. In this study, 17 participants with migraine who had been using feverfew leaf daily for 2 to 4 years were randomized to capsules containing 50 mg of dried feverfew per day or placebo for 6 months (9). Patients receiving feverfew showed no change in migraine incidence; those receiving placebo had a significant increase in frequency and severity of migraines, nausea, and vomiting. Two patients whose migraines had been in complete remission while self-treated with feverfew suffered severe migraines while on placebo and withdrew from the study to resume feverfew treatment. "Post-feverfew syndrome" (rebound of migraine symptoms, anxiety, sleep difficulties, and muscle and joint stiffness) occurred in 10% of regular feverfew users who were switched to placebo.

—A crossover trial in 50 patients (44 completed) tested the effect of feverfew capsules (143 mg/day containing 0.35% parthenolide, in a 90% ethanol extract) for 4 months on severity of migraines and number of work days lost; no change was seen in either measure (10). (An alcohol extract may be less effective than dried leaves.)
—A crossover study tested the effect of 100 mg feverfew/day for 2 months in 20 participants on serotonin uptake and platelet activity, as well as migraines, and found no effect (11). This study is reported only as an abstract of a poster presentation, with no information as to the nature of the feverfew preparation or details about outcome measures (12).

• Rheumatoid arthritis

—In a double-blind placebo-controlled trial, 41 female patients with rheumatoid arthritis inadequately controlled with nonsteroidal antiinflammatory drugs (NSAIDs) were given either one capsule of feverfew (70 to 86 g) or placebo for 6 weeks (13). The addition of feverfew to NSAID treatment did not make a significant difference in functional capacity, stiffness, pain, grip strength, sedimentation rate, rheumatoid factor, or immunoglobulins.

• Platelet aggregation

—Platelets from 10 participants who had taken feverfew for 3.5 to 8 years were subjected to platelet aggregation studies and found to be normal (14). ADP and thrombin-induced aggregation was similar to four controls (former feverfew users who had discontinued the herb at least 6 months before the test); a few feverfew users (number not given) had attenuated response to serotonin and a prostaglandin (PG) endoperoxide.

ANIMAL/IN VITRO

• Feverfew extract and parthenolide inhibit mitogen-induced proliferation of human peripheral blood mononuclear cells *in vitro*; however, cytotoxicity occurs after incubation for 48 to 72 hours (3). Feverfew extract, administered intraperitoneally, inhibits collagen-induced bronchoconstriction in guinea pigs (possibly because of phospholipase A_2 inhibition) (3).
• Antifungal and antimicrobial effects of parthenolide, essential oil, and eudesmanolides isolated from feverfew have been demonstrated *in vitro* (3).

OTHER CLAIMED BENEFITS/ACTIONS

• Tinnitus
• Vertigo
• Arthritis
• Fever
• Menstrual disorders
• Labor difficulties
• Stomachache
• Toothache
• Insect bites

Risks

ADVERSE REACTIONS

- Aphthous ulcers
- Oral pain, lip swelling, dry tongue
- Loss of taste
- Indigestion
- Diarrhea
- Flatulence
- Nausea and vomiting
- Post-feverfew syndrome (rebound of migraine symptoms, anxiety, sleep difficulties, and muscle and joint stiffness) (9)
- Feverfew should not be used by patients with known sensitivities to ragweed or other members of the Asteraceae family such as chamomile or yarrow.

ANIMAL TOXICITY

- No toxic effects were seen in short-term feeding studies in rats given the equivalent of more than 100 times the human daily dose daily for 5 weeks or in guinea pigs given the equivalent of 150 times the human daily dose daily for 7 weeks (3).

 ## Dose

COMMON DOSAGE FORMS

- *Leaf, fresh:* two to three medium-sized leaves/day
- *Leaf, freeze-dried:* 50 mg daily
- *Aerial parts, dried:* 50 to 200 mg/day
- Standardized extracts of feverfew, containing at least 0.2% of parthenolide, are available. However, parthenolide is probably only a marker compound (15).
- Alcohol extracts are available but may be ineffective; a single trial on an alcohol extract found no effect (10).

 ## Common Questions and Answers

Q: Does feverfew work for treatment of acute migraine?
A: No studies have been done on this, but some migraine patients report that taking a dose of extract or eating a few leaves of feverfew during the prodromal phase of a migraine can avert a headache. Some migraineurs grow the plant on a windowsill to have ready access to the fresh leaves.

Q: How common are aphthous ulcers, and do they still occur if the herb is taken in capsules?
A: Even capsules of dried feverfew can cause aphthous ulcers, apparently through a systemic effect (2). In a survey of 300 feverfew users, aphthous ulcers from chewing fresh leaves were reported by 11.3% of users, and 6.5% reported digestive disturbances (9).

Q: Does it matter what kind of feverfew is used?
A: There are several controversies about feverfew quality. Sesquiterpene lactones are regarded as the active constituents in feverfew, and parthenolide is the main sesquiterpene lactone in European feverfew. North American feverfew (and feverfew grown in some parts of Europe) may not contain any parthenolide, although other sesquiterpene lactones are present (15). Even if parthenolide is only a marker compound, preparations standardized for parthenolide are available and I think preferable, if only because all successful studies on the herb so far have used parthenolide-containing European feverfew. Even if parthenolide is only a marker compound, its presence provides some assurance of similarity. Another controversy centers around whether only strains of feverfew that have a single row of florets are effective; there is no evidence to support this claim (2). Some think fresh leaves are most effective; given the variation of (unknown active) compounds in variants, however, dried preparations are a reasonable choice. Another quality claim is that freeze-dried leaves are more effective than air-dried leaves, but there is no evidence for that. Prolonged storage of dried feverfew does decrease parthenolide content; at room temperature, parthenolide decreases 20% in 1 year and 50% in 2 years (2).

Fish oil

10 Second Take

Fish oil is benign and may reduce cardiovascular risk; it has promise for other conditions.

Basics

DESCRIPTION

• Fish oil contains the omega-3 (n-3) polyunsaturated fatty acids (PUFAs) eicosapentaenoic acid (EPA, 20:5–3) and docosahexaenoic acid (DHA 22:6–3), which can also be formed from EPA.

FOOD SOURCES

• The fattiest fish (herring, menhaden, sardines, and anchovies) contain more than 8% fat and are the best sources of n-3 PUFAs (1). Salmon, mackerel, bluefish, and swordfish are very good sources; tuna and cod liver oil are good sources. The fat of seals, polar bears, and other marine mammals that eat fish are high in n-3 PUFAs.
• Supplements are usually made from menhaden, sardines, and anchovies (1). The name "menhaden" comes from a Narragansett Indian word that means "they manure," probably reflecting their use as fertilizer.

MAIN FUNCTIONS/PHARMACOKINETICS

• EPA and DHA are precursors to eicosanoids [including prostaglandins (PG), leukotrienes, and thromboxanes] and are important membrane constituents (1). Marine oils decrease prostaglandin E_2 metabolites; decrease thromboxane A_2 (a potent vasoconstrictor and platelet aggregator); increase thromboxane A_3 (a weak vasoconstrictor); decrease leukotriene B_4 (which induces inflammation); increase leukotriene B_5 (a weak inflammation inducer); and increase prostacyclin PGI3 (a vasodilator that inhibits platelet aggregation) (2). N-3 long-chain PUFAs also lower interleukin (IL)-1 and increase IL-2 production (1). EPA reduces the synthesis of very low density lipoprotein (VLDL) (3).

Evidence

CLINICAL TRIALS

• Cardiovascular disease/risk factors

—Most prospective cohort studies report an inverse relationship between fish consumption and cardiovascular mortality (3).
—In one study, 11,324 patients with recent myocardial infarctions (MI) were randomized to n-3 PUFAs (1 g/day), vitamin E (300 mg/day), both, or placebo for up to 2 years (4). Fish oil, but not vitamin E, decreased the relative risk of coronary heart disease (death, nonfatal MI, or stroke) by 15%.
—In another study, 2,033 men were randomized to reduced fat, increased fiber, or eating fatty fish two to three times/week (or supplementing with 500 mg n-3 PUFAs/day) (5). After 2 years, the fish and fish oil group had a 29% reduction in total mortality. A randomized controlled trial (RCT) in 232 patients with coronary artery disease found no difference between placebo and fish oil (6 g/day × 3 months, then 3 g/day × 21 months) in reducing cardiovascular events or in minimal lumen diameter (6).
—A 1-year RCT compared placebo with fish oil (EPA 1.08 g/day) or mustard oil (alpha-linolenic acid, 2.9 g/day) in 360 patients with suspected MI (7). Both treatments decreased total cardiac event incidence (fish oil 24.5%; mustard oil 28%) compared with placebo (34.7%).
—A review of 56 studies (36 crossover, 20 parallel) concluded that fish oils significantly lower triglycerides, decrease VLDL, and slightly increase low-density lipoprotein (LDL) (8); high-density lipoprotein (HDL) and total cholesterol were unaffected.
—A meta-analysis of 31 placebo-controlled trials ($n = 1,356$) found that fish oil (< 3 to 15 g/day) significantly reduced systolic (mean 3.0 mm Hg) and diastolic blood pressure (mean 1.5 mm Hg) (9). A dose-response relationship was seen in hypertensive patients; there was no effect in normotensive participants.
—A meta-analysis of seven trials concluded that fish oil reduced restenosis rates after coronary angioplasty (10), but recent studies found no benefit. One placebo-controlled RCT of 59 patients with coronary heart disease and normal lipids found that fish oil (6 g daily for an average of 28 months) lowered triglycerides 30% but did not affect cholesterol, minimal lumen diameter, or stenosis (11).
—In a 2 × 2 factorial study, 814 patients were randomized to fish oils (5.4 g n-3 PUFAs) or placebo for 19 weeks, beginning 6 days before percutaneous transluminal angioplasty (12). Later, 653 patients were randomized to low molecular weight heparin or control. Quantitative coronary angiography at about 18 weeks showed no significant differences between groups in restenosis rates, minimal lumen diameter, or ischemic events.

—A double-blind placebo-controlled RCT in 500 patients tested n-3 PUFAs (5.1 g/day) starting at least 2 weeks before angioplasty (13). Restenosis rates were similar between groups at 6 months. Fish oil 4 g/day, compared with no treatment in 610 patients after coronary artery bypass graft, reduced vein-graft occlusions at 1 year (14).
—In 60 healthy volunteers, fish oil benefited heart rate variability in men but not women (15).
—A placebo-controlled 12-week RCT in 55 patients (49 completed) found that 5.2 g n-3 PUFAs significantly benefited heart rate variability over placebo (16).
—A double-blind placebo-controlled trial of 79 patients with ventricular arrhythmias found that significantly more (44%) of the fish oil group than the placebo group (15%) experienced 70% reduction of ventricular premature complexes (17).

• Cancer

—In 60 cancer patients, 18 g n-3 PUFAs daily, compared with placebo, significantly prolonged survival (18). In 28 pancreatic cancer patients, EPA (titrated to 6 g/day × 12 weeks) stabilized weight (19).
—In 22 cachectic cancer patients, maximum tolerated dose of fish oil was 0.3 g/kg/day (about 21 g, or 13 g PUFAs) (20).

• Inflammatory bowel disease

—A review concluded that n-3 PUFAs are potentially effective for Crohn's disease and ulcerative colitis (21).
—A small crossover study in 10 patients with active ulcerative colitis found sulfasalazine superior to PUFAs (5.4 g/day) (22).

• Diabetes

—A meta-analysis of 26 trials that included diabetics found that fish oil (typically ≈ 3 g PUFAs) did not affect HbA_{1c}, lowered triglycerides almost 30%, and slightly increased LDL (23).

• Rheumatoid arthritis

—A meta-analysis of 10 papers ($n = 395$) found that fish oil for 3 months significantly reduced tender joints score and morning stiffness (24).

• Systemic lupus erythematosus (SLE)

—In 11 adolescents with pediatric SLE, fish oil significantly decreased triglycerides, but 5/11 remained dyslipoproteinemic (25).
—A double-blind crossover study in 26 patients with lupus nephritis found no effect of fish oil on proteinuria, glomerular dilatation rate, a disease activity index, or steroid consumption; lipids improved (26).

• Dermatologic conditions

—Three studies found a benefit for fish oil (1.8 to 12 g PUFAs) on psoriasis (27–29), but one double-blind study in 145 participants (5 g PUFAs × 4 months) found no difference compared with placebo (30).
—Two studies found a benefit for fish oil on eczema (31,32).

- Asthma

—A Cochrane review of RCTs on asthma found eight trials (6 parallel, 2 crossover, 7 placebo-controlled, one dose-ranging) (33). There was no consistent effect on FEV_1, peak flow rate, symptoms, medication use, or bronchial hyperreactivity; a pediatric study found that fish oil with dietary manipulation improved peak flow and reduced medication use.

- Cystic fibrosis

—A placebo-controlled trial in 16 cystic fibrosis patients colonized with *Pseudomonas aeruginosa* found that EPA (2.7 g daily × 6 weeks) significantly improved sputum volume and pulmonary function tests (34).

- Renal conditions

—Two RCTs on IgA nephropathy found a benefit for fish oil; two found none (35).
—Sixty-six renal transplant patients received 6 g fish oil or placebo for a year. Treated patients had higher median glomerular filtration rate and effective renal plasma flow, lower mean arterial pressure, and fewer rejections (8 vs. 20); there was no difference in kidney survival (36).
—However, another study of 50 patients treated with adjunctive fish oil (6 g/day) or placebo for 3 months found no significant difference between groups in renal function, rejection episodes, and so forth (37).
—A double-blind RCT in 24 participants receiving hemodialysis grafts compared 400 mg/day fish oil to placebo, starting 2 weeks after graft placement (38). At 1 year, primary patency rates were significantly higher in the treated group (75.6%) than controls (14.9%).

- Psychiatric conditions

—A 4-month, double-blind, placebo-controlled study in 30 patients with bipolar disorder found longer remissions and fewer relapses in those given adjunctive fish oil (15 g, containing 9.6 g/day n-3 PUFAs) compared with placebo (39).
—A Cochrane review of four schizophrenia trials ($n = 204$) concluded that limited data suggest a benefit of EPA (40).

- Dysmenorrhea

—In a placebo-controlled crossover RCT in 42 adolescents with dysmenorrhea, fish oil (EPA 1.8 g, DHA 720 mg × 2 months), but not placebo, significantly reduced symptom scores from baseline (41).

- Pregnancy

—Fish oil may prevent preterm birth, but few data support benefit on other pregnancy outcomes. An RCT in 533 women compared fish oil (4 g/day, 2.7 g n-3 PUFAs), placebo, or no supplementation from week 30 of pregnancy (42). Length of gestation was significantly longer (by 4 days) and birthweight higher in the treated group.
—The Fish Oil Trials in Pregnancy (FOTIP) studies included six simultaneously conducted multicenter trials. Pregnant women with previous preterm birth ($n = 232$), intrauterine growth retardation (IUGR, $n = 280$), pregnancy-induced hypertension (PIH, $n = 386$), or who were carrying twins ($n = 579$) were randomized to placebo or fish oil (2.7 g n-3 PUFAs/day) from about 20 weeks gestation (43). Two therapeutic trials enrolled 79 women with pre-eclampsia and 63 with suspected IUGR to 6.1 g n-3 PUFAs/day from about 33 weeks. In women with previous preterm birth, fish oil reduced the risk of preterm delivery from 33.3% to 21.3% (OR 0.54, 95% CI 0.30 to 0.98); there was no difference in twin pregnancies or rates of recurrence for other outcomes.
—Another double-blind RCT of 223 pregnant women at high risk of PIH or IUGR also found no effect of fish oil (2.7 g PUFAs/day, with 1.62 g EPA and 1.08 g DHA) on either outcome (44).

ANIMAL/IN VITRO

Not covered

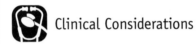 Clinical Considerations

DEFICIENCY SIGNS AND SYMPTOMS

Not well established

FACTORS DECREASING AVAILABILITY/ABSORPTION

Pregnancy

FACTORS INCREASING AVAILABILITY/ABSORPTION

None identified

LABORATORY TESTS

Fatty acid analysis is usually carried out in platelets.

 Risks

ADVERSE REACTIONS

- Nausea, loose stools, and "fishy" breath
- Doses >4 g/day increase bleeding time and decrease platelet count (2).
- An autopsy study noted increased risk of hemorrhagic stroke associated with high levels of n-3 PUFAS in perirenal fat (45).
- Lipoid pneumonia was associated with ingestion of cod liver oil capsules in a 63-year-old woman smoker with probable esophageal reflux (46).
- Theoretically, chronic intake of peroxidation products in improperly stored PUFAs could be harmful (47).

DRUG INTERACTIONS

None reported

 Dose

COMMON DOSAGE FORMS

- Fish oil supplements may contain from 30% to 66% n-3 PUFAs. An upper limit of 10% daily dietary intake of PUFAs is suggested (45).
- Doses are daily total of n-3 PUFAs (usually EPA plus DHA).
- Asthma: 1 to 3 g
- Atherosclerosis/prevention of restenosis after grafting: 3 to 6.5 g
- Bipolar disorder: 9.6 g
- Cancer: cachexia 6 g; treatment 18 g
- Cardiovascular risk factors: 1 to 4 g
- Cystic fibrosis: 2.7 g
- Diabetes: 3 to 9 g
- Heart rate variability: 2 to 6.6 g
- Hypertension: 3 to 15 g
- IgA nephropathy: 2.7 to 3 g PUFAs
- Inflammatory bowel disease: 2.7 to 5.4 g
- Prevention of preterm birth: 2.7 g PUFAs
- Rheumatoid arthritis: 2.7 to 18 g (usually 3 to 6 g)

Flaxseed or Linseed

 10 Second Take

Whole flaxseed is benign when used as a bulk-forming agent. The safety of long-term use of large amounts of ground flaxseed has not been established.

 Basics

LATIN NAME

Linum usitatissimum L.

FAMILY

Linaceae

DESCRIPTION

• An annual herb with blue flowers, flax is one of the oldest and most commonly cultivated plants.
• Its fiber is used to make linen, and flaxseed oil is used on wood and, increasingly, as a dietary supplement.
• Seeds are used in breads or cereals or are sometimes sprouted. In Ethiopia, seeds are combined with water and honey as a drink and roasted seed paste is eaten on bread. Roasted seeds may be used as a coffee substitute, and in Transylvania the leaves are used as a vegetable (1).

PART USED

Dried, ripe seeds

KNOWN ACTIVE CONSTITUENTS

• The seed contains 3% to 6% mucilage (found in the epidermis of the seed husk), which can be hydrolyzed to galactose, arabinose, rhamnose, xylose, galacturonic acid, and mannuronic acid.
• Flaxseed contains fixed oil (30% to 45%), primarily triglycerides of linolenic, linoleic, and oleic acids; 25% protein; the lignan precursor secoisolariciresinol glycoside; and 0.1% to 1.5% cyanogenic glycosides (2). Seventy percent of the oil in flaxseed is polyunsaturated; alpha-linolenic acid comprises most of the fatty acids (3). One gram of seeds has 4.7 kcal.

MECHANISM/PHARMACOKINETICS

• Linseed contains soluble fiber that forms a gel in the intestinal tract, thus softening stools.
• Linseed delays gastric emptying in healthy volunteers (2).
• Supplementation with flaxseed powder 10 g/day for three menstrual cycles resulted in increased urinary excretion of the lignans enterodiol and enterolactone (threefold to 285-fold increase); there were no differences in excretion of isoflavonoids or the lignan matairesinol (4).

 Evidence

CLINICAL TRIALS

• Constipation

—Two studies in patients with constipation have demonstrated decreased transit time and increased stool weight (2). Another study found that 50 g milled flaxseed daily for 4 weeks increased the number of weekly bowel movements by 30% (5).

• Hot flashes

—A 12-week trial in 145 postmenopausal women tested the effects of a phytoestrogen-rich diet versus usual diet on menopausal symptoms (6). Women in the treated group ate 2 teaspoons of ground flaxseed along with 80 g tofu, two glasses of soy milk, and 1 teaspoon of miso daily. This phytoestrogen-rich diet resulted in significantly increased sex hormone binding globulin (SHBG); menopausal symptoms decreased significantly from baseline in both groups with no significant difference between groups.

• Lipids

—A randomized crossover study in 29 participants (including seven women) with hyperlipidemia tested the effects of muffins containing partially defatted flaxseed (about 50 g/day) or wheat bran on lipids. Each intervention contained 20 g fiber/day and was administered for 3 weeks with a 2-week washout period (7). Consumption of wheat bran did not affect lipids. Compared with baseline, flaxseed muffin consumption significantly reduced total cholesterol (5.5 μmol/L $\pm$ 1.2%), low density lipoprotein (LDL)-cholesterol (9.7 μmol/L $\pm$ 1.8%), and apolipoprotein B (5.9 μmol/L $\pm$ 1.5%). Ratios of LDL to high-density lipoprotein (HDL) and of apolipoprotein B to apolipoprotein A-1 were not affected, and triglyceride levels were significantly increased (10.2 μmol/L $\pm$ 4.8%). Serum thiol concentrations were significantly decreased after flaxseed compared with controls.
—A controlled study in 10 adults tested the effects of 50 g flaxseed/day in muffins against unsupplemented muffins for 4 weeks (5). Compared with baseline, total cholesterol was significantly reduced by 6% and plasma LDL was reduced by 8% in the flax group; at 4 weeks, however, there was no difference between groups in total or LDL-cholesterol. Levels of the antioxidants retinol and alpha-tocopherol were unchanged, and there were no differences between groups in products of lipid peroxidation.

• Other cardiovascular risk factors

—Eleven healthy male volunteers were randomized to consume 40 g of flaxseed oil or sunflower seed oil for 23 days. Eicosapentaenoic acid in platelets did not change in the sunflower seed group but more than doubled in the group treated with flaxseed oil (8). Collagen-induced but not adenosine diphosphate-induced platelet aggregation response was reduced.
—The effect of four diets was tested in 15 obese people (9). During the first and fourth month, participants ate a saturated/high-fat diet. During the second month the participants ate a low-fat diet high in alpha-linolenic acid and during the third month a low-fat diet high in oleic acid. Systemic arterial compliance rose significantly during the alpha-linolenic acid period. Systemic arterial compliance was also higher during the oleic acid period but significantly lower then during the alpha-linolenic acid period. Total cholesterol levels, mean arterial pressures, and glucose tolerance did not change during any intervention.

• Rheumatoid arthritis

—A double-blind, placebo-controlled study randomized 22 patients with rheumatoid arthritis either to flaxseed oil or safflower seed oil for 3 months. The group receiving flaxseed showed increased bleeding time but no significant changes in clinical, subjective, or laboratory parameters (10).

• Lupus nephritis

—A study of nine patients with lupus nephritis (eight completed) tested the effects of flaxseed in three doses (15, 30, and 45 g/day) each for 4 weeks (11). There were no differences in systemic lupus erythematosus disease activity index among groups. Compared with baseline, total cholesterol was significantly reduced in the 30- and 45-g groups. Blood viscosity was significantly reduced only at the 30-g dose (this effect was maintained after the 5-week washout period). All three doses inhibited platelet activating factor-induced platelet aggregation and significantly elevated complement. Serum creatinine was significantly reduced from baseline in the 30- and 45-g doses; levels returned to baseline after the 5-week washout period.

• Menstrual cycle/reproductive hormone effects

—A study in 18 women compared supplementation with flaxseed powder (10 g/day) for three cycles to unsupplemented cycles (12). Luteal phases were significantly longer during ovulatory cycles during flax consumption compared with ovulatory control cycles (12.6 ± 0.4 days vs. 11.4 ± 0.4 days). There were no differences in estradiol, estrone, progesterone, dehydroepiandrosterone (DHEA), prolactin, or SHBG concentrations. During the flax cycles, luteal phase progesterone/estradiol ratios were significantly higher, and midfollicular phase testosterone levels were significantly higher than during unsupplemented cycles.

—A randomized crossover study in 28 post-menopausal women compared two doses of ground flaxseed (5 or 10 g/day) against an unsupplemented diet during three 7-week feeding periods. There was a significant increase in urinary 2-hydroxyestrogen (2-OHE) excretion during the flaxseed period, and the urinary 2-OHE_1 : $16\alpha\text{-OHE}_1$ ratio increased in a dose-related fashion (13). Total urinary levels of $16\alpha\text{-OHE}_1$, however, were not affected (see questions and answers).

• Effects on glucose

—Flaxseed decreased postprandial hyperglycemia in eight noninsulin-dependent diabetics (2,14) (see questions and answers).

ANIMAL/IN VITRO

• Chemoprotective effects against mammary and colon cancer have been demonstrated in animals (13) (see questions and answers).

OTHER CLAIMED BENEFITS/ACTIONS

• Cancer prevention, irritable bowel syndrome, gastrointestinal complaints, gastritis, diverticulitis, coughs, sore throat, rheumatoid arthritis, abscesses, ulcers, and inflamed skin (topical)

 Risks

ADVERSE REACTIONS

• Anaphylaxis

—One case of IgE-mediated anaphylaxis has been linked to flaxseed hypersensitivity. Hypersensitivity to linseed is considered rare (14).

• Potential cyanide exposure (see questions and answers).

DRUG INTERACTIONS

Soluble fibers may decrease absorption of drugs absorbed in the intestinal tract.

 Dose

COMMON DOSAGE FORMS

• *Seeds:* 5 to 10 g whole, bruised, cracked, or crushed seeds, soaked in water and taken with plenty of fluids b.i.d. to t.i.d.
• *External:* 30 to 50 g crushed or powdered seed may be used as a warm, moist poultice or compress.
• Children

—0 to 6 years: Only under medical supervision.
—6 to 12 years: Half the adult dosage.

 Common Questions and Answers

Q: What is the danger of cyanide poisoning with ingestion of linseed?
A: Although no cases of cyanide poisoning associated with flaxseed ingestion have been reported, this is a theoretically plausible risk with ground flaxseed (there is no danger from whole flaxseed used as a bulk-forming laxative, because the seeds are not absorbed from the gastrointestinal tract). Linseed contains linamaron, a cyanogenic glycoside, and the potential cyanide yield of different batches of flaxseed ranges from 4 to 12 mmol/kg (15).

Hydrogen cyanide is converted into thiocyanate by the mitochondrial enzyme rhodanase; however, ingestion of large amounts of cyanide overwhelms this detoxification system (16). Flaxseed clearly increases levels of the cyanide metabolite thiocyanate. Two males were given 60 g ground linseed daily for 10 days; thiocyanate levels in 24-hour urinary excretion increased sevenfold, from 32 μmol (range 26 to 40 μmol/L) to 247 μmol (191 to 330 μmol/L); equivalent to cyanide exposure of more than 0.25 mmol/day (15). The authors note that grinding seeds may increase hydrolysis of glucosides to cyanohydrins or increase access of glucosides to intestinal glucosidase, either of which might increase cyanide in the gut. Low levels of hydrogen cyanide were noted in a person after ingestion of 100 g linseed. Hydrogen cyanide blood levels did not increase significantly in 20 participants who ingested 30 or 100 g of cracked linseed initially followed by 45 g daily for 5 weeks (16). Thiocyanate levels, however, increased in both serum and urine (urinary excretion increased 75%, a level similar to that of heavy smokers) (16).

Flaxseed is traditionally used whole or cracked as a laxative or as a crunchy additive to breads and cereals; it is not traditionally eaten in large quantities. Only recently has the consumption of large amounts of flaxseed been promoted, and the effects of long-term consumption of large amounts of ground flaxseed has not been established.

Q: Does flaxseed oil have the same effects of fish oil?
A: Probably not. Ingestion of dietary flaxseed does not increase docosahexaenoic acid (DHA). In fact, one study found that dietary intake of alpha-linolenic acid was inversely related to tissue concentrations of docosahexaenoic acid, raising the possibility that linoleic acid consumption may displace DHA (17).

Q: Why is flaxseed thought to prevent cancer?
A: In animals, flaxseed has chemoprotective effects, inhibiting mammary tumor growth and decreasing some markers of colon cancer risk. One trial found a significant increase in urinary 2-OHE excretion during flaxseed supplementation, and an increase in the ratio of 2-OHE$_1$ to 16α-OHE$_1$ in urine (13). Both 2-OHE$_1$ and 16α-OHE$_1$ are metabolites of endogenous estrogens; the 16α-OHE$_1$ metabolite is associated with increased risk of breast cancer, whereas 2-OHE metabolites appear to be protective.
Although the effects of flaxseed on estrogen metabolism may be promising, there have been no clinical trials to date of flaxseed for chemoprevention.

Q: Does it make sense to take flaxseed oil for hot flashes?
A: No. The lignan phytoestrogens in flaxseed will not be found in flaxseed oil. Even flaxseed has not been shown effective against hot flashes (6).

Folic Acid (Folate)

 10 Second Take

Folate, a benign B vitamin, prevents neural tube defects, lowers homocysteine levels, and reduces side effects of methotrexate.

 Basics

DESCRIPTION

• Folate, a B vitamin, comprises the pteroylglutamates (which vary in level of reduction of the pteridine ring, one-carbon substitutions, and number of glutamate residues). Endogenous folates exist in various labile forms, often peptide-linked.
• Folic acid (pteroylglutamic acid) is the stable pharmaceutical form (1). Folinic acid (N 5-formyl tetrahydrofolate) is an active metabolic derivative.

FOOD SOURCES

• Folates are in most natural foods. Rich sources include yeast, liver, other organ meats, vegetables, fruits, whole grains, nuts, and seeds.
• Cooking or processing destroys folate.
• Since 1998, the FDA has required fortification of enriched grains with folic acid.

MAIN FUNCTIONS/PHARMACOKINETICS

• Folate coenzymes are important to metabolic reactions involving transfer of one-carbon units. Folate (and vitamin B_{12}) is necessary for the methylation of homocysteine to methionine and for the synthesis of S-adenosylmethionine. Folate is also required for the synthesis of purines and the regulation of DNA synthesis.
• Folate, absorbed in the small bowel, is excreted in both urine and bile (1). The body contains 5 to 10 mg (11.3 to 22.6 μmol) folate, half in the liver.

 Evidence

CLINICAL TRIALS

• Neural tube defects

—A Cochrane review of four trials including 6,425 women found that periconceptional use of folate significantly reduced the incidence of neural tube defects [odds ratio (OR) 0.28, 95% confidence interval (CI) 0.15 to 0.53] (2).

• Other pregnancy effects

—A Cochrane review of 21 studies of folate supplementation in pregnancy found improved hemoglobin levels and folate status and possibly reduced incidence of low birthweight (3).

• Side effects of methotrexate

—A Cochrane review of folic acid, folinic acid or folate in patients with rheumatoid arthritis identified seven trials including 307 patients (4). Folic acid, but not the more costly folinic acid, significantly decreased (79%) mucosal and other side effects. Disease activity parameters were not affected.

• Cognition and mood

—In one study, 15% to 38% of depressed adults had deficient or borderline levels of folate (5). Depressed patients with low serum folate are less likely to respond to fluoxetine (6). A double-blind trial of adjunctive methylfolate (15 mg/day ×6 months) in 41 depressed ($n = 24$) or schizophrenic ($n = 17$) participants with deficient or borderline folate levels found that folate, compared with placebo, significantly improved the mean clinical outcome score at 3 and 6 months (7). Another double-blind, placebo-controlled 10-week RCT found that folate (500 μg) added to fluoxetine (20 mg/day) significantly improved outcomes over placebo in women, but not men (8).
—Among 30 nuns in a longitudinal study of aging and Alzheimer's disease, serum folate and neocortical atrophy were highly correlated (9).
—Seventy-two treated patients with epilepsy received placebo, folate (5 mg/day), thiamin (50 mg/day), or folate and thiamin for 6 months (10). Thiamin, but not folate levels, improved several neuropsychologic functions.

• Cancer prevention

—Folate with vitamin B_{12} may reduce squamous metaplasia with cellular atypia in heavy smokers (11).
—Folate deficiency may be a factor in cervical dysplasia, but two placebo-controlled 6-month supplementation trials of folate (5 to 10 mg/day) in women with mild to severe cervical intraepithelial neoplasia (CIN) (most subjects had CIN 1) found no differences between groups (12,13).
—Alcohol-associated increased risk of breast cancer may be reduced by adequate folate intake (14).

• Cardiovascular disease/ hyperhomocysteinemia

—Folic acid is the most effective single therapy for hyperhomocysteinemia; however, vitamins B_6 and B_{12} are also important, and combined therapy is best. A dose of 400 μg daily is effective; higher daily doses are needed only in renal failure (15). Two reviews found that most cross-sectional and case-control studies support an association between hyperhomocysteinemia and cardiovascular risk; prospective studies are more mixed (15,16).
—One study found that combining folic acid (2.5 mg), vitamin B_6 (25 mg), and vitamin B_{12} (250 μg) reduced atherosclerosis progression (17).
—An RCT of 158 healthy siblings of patients with premature atherothrombotic disease (134 completed) tested placebo versus folic acid (5 mg) and vitamin B_6 (250 mg/day) for 2 years (18). Vitamin treatment significantly decreased homocysteine levels and decreased abnormal exercise electrocardiograms but did not affect ankle-brachial pressure indices or carotid or peripheral arterial outcome variables.

• Diarrhea

—A RCT of 106 boys (6 to 23 months) with diarrhea of less than 3 days duration found no benefit of folic acid (5 mg q8 × 5 days) over placebo in stool output or oral rehydration solution intake (19).

• Gingival hyperplasia

—Two controlled trials found no benefit of folic acid (3 mg × 4 months and 5 mg × 1 year) on phenytoin-induced gingival hyperplasia (20,21). A small study of eight institutionalized disabled residents found a small benefit of 5 mg folic acid for 6 months following gingivectomy (22).

 Clinical Considerations

DEFICIENCY SIGNS AND SYMPTOMS

• Symptoms of megaloblastic anemia may include weakness, tiredness, dyspnea, diarrhea, anorexia, syncope, headache, palpitations, and sore tongue. Folate deficiency may also cause irritability, forgetfulness, hostility, and paranoia (1).

FACTORS DECREASING AVAILABILITY/ABSORPTION

• Alcohol (decreases intrahepatic circulation of folate); poor diet; malabsorption syndromes; methotrexate; triamterene; pentamidine; trimethoprim; pyrimethamine; colchicine; other folic acid antagonists (see questions and answers); anticonvulsants (phenytoin, diphenylhydantoin, primidone); barbiturates; cycloserine; metformin; excessive lysine or methionine; congenital deficiency of dihydrofolate reductase; methyltetrahydrofolate transmethylase or formiminotransferase; nonconjugase defects or conjugase inhibitors; liver disease; pregnancy; lactation; kidney dialysis; increased hematopoiesis; and chronic exfoliative dermatitis (1).

FACTORS INCREASING AVAILABILITY/ABSORPTION

Good diet

LABORATORY TESTS

• Serum folate > 13.5 nmol/L is normal, 6.7 to 13.2 nmol/L is low, and < 6.7 nmol/L is deficient.
• Red blood cell folate > 360 nmol/L is normal, 315 to 358 nmol/L is low, and < 315 nmol/L is deficient (23).
• A microbiologic assay using *Lactobacillus casei* (which requires folate for growth) is used to measure serum and red blood cell folate (1).
• In folate malabsorption, administration of 100 μg (226.67 nmol) folic acid daily will produce a hematologic response in patients with folic acid deficiency but not B_{12} deficiency (1).

 Risks

ADVERSE REACTIONS

• Daily doses of up to 10 mg folic acid are nontoxic in healthy nonpregnant persons.
• Folic acid may mask pernicious anemia (because of vitamin B_{12} deficiency) by preventing identification of megaloblasts; however, serum B_{12} levels can be used to exclude pernicious anemia in patients receiving folic acid supplements (24).

DRUG INTERACTIONS

• Methotrexate, triamterene, pentamidine, other folic acid antagonists; anticonvulsants (phenytoin, diphenylhydantoin, primidone); barbiturates; cycloserine; metformin; zinc (see questions and answers)

ANIMAL TOXICITY

• Massive doses of folic acid in rats cause renal toxicity by precipitating crystalline folic acid. Intravenous folic acid (45 to 125 mg or 102 to 283.3 μmol) caused seizures in normal rats; lower doses caused seizures in rats with induced cortical lesions (1).

 Dose

RECOMMENDED DIETARY ALLOWANCE (25)

Infants and children

0 to 6 months	65 μg/day (adequate intake)
7 to 12 months	80 μg/day (adequate intake)
1 to 3 years	150 μg/day
4 to 8 years	200 μg/day

Males

9 to 13 years	300 μg/day
14 to 50 years	400 μg/day
51+ years	400 μg/day

Females

9 to 13 years	300 μg/day
14 to 50 years	400 μg/day
51+ years	400 μg/day
Pregnant	600 μg/day
Lactating	500 μg/day

UPPER LIMITS

Infants and Children

0 to 6 months	Not determinable
7 to 12 months	Not determinable
1 to 3 years	300 μg/day
4 to 8 years	400 μg/day

Males

9 to 13 years	600 μg/day
14 to 18 years	800 μg/day
19 to 50 years	1,000 μg/day
51+ years	1,000 μg/day

Females

9 to 13 years	600 μg/day
14 to 18 years	800 μg/day
19 to 50 years	1,000 μg/day
51+ years	1,000 μg/day

Pregnant

± 18 years	800 μg/day
19 to 50 years	1,000 μg/day

Lactating

± 18 years	800 μg/day
19 to 50 years	1,000 μg/day

Conversion: 1 mg = 2.26 μmol

• In folate malabsorption, therapeutic doses may be up to 1 mg/day; higher doses are not more effective. The maintenance dose is usually 0.1 mg/day (1).

 Common Questions and Answers

Q: Should epileptic patients be supplemented with folic acid?
A: Yes, especially if they are taking phenytoin. Very high intravenous doses of folic acid may reverse the effect of anticonvulsants, but this is not relevant to normal oral doses. Even high intravenous doses do not affect most epileptics: Six subjects given 75 mg folic acid over 30 minutes had no electroencephalographic (EEG) changes; one had transient EEG abnormalities after receiving 150 mg i.v. over 30 minutes; and one had a seizure after 14.4 mg (EEG abnormalities were noted after 7.2 mg i.v. over 3 minutes) (24). Phenytoin competes with folate and can halve serum folate levels in epileptic patients (26). Folic acid may be a cofactor in converting phenytoin to inactive metabolites, thus preventing accumulation of reactive intermediate epoxides (26). Phenytoin and folic acid should be initiated concurrently; folic acid initiated after deficiency occurs may decrease phenytoin levels, causing a "pseudo-steady-state" in which phenytoin appears to be at steady-state concentration but is not (26).

Q: Does folic acid help vitiligo or infertility?
A: An uncontrolled study in 15 patients with vitiligo found a benefit for a combination of folic acid (2 mg b.i.d.), vitamin B_{12} (100 mg intramuscularly every 2 weeks), and vitamin C (500 mg b.i.d.) for 1 to 2 years (numbers are averages; patients received different dosages) (28). Repigmentation (beginning after 3 months) was complete in six patients and 80% for two patients.
An uncontrolled study in 65 infertile males with idiopathic round cell syndrome found that folinic acid (15 mg/day ×3 months) significantly increased the number and motility of spermatozoa and decreased round cells (29). Twenty-four pregnancies resulted within 6 months after therapy ended.

Q: Will folic acid interfere with folate antagonists?
A: This is controversial. Folate antagonists include methotrexate, aminopterin, trimethoprim, trimetrexate, and triamterene. In patients with rheumatoid arthritis, folic acid supplementation reduces side effects without compromising drug efficacy, although clearly a balance must be sought (30).

Q: Does folic acid intake decrease zinc levels?
A: Daily doses of 10 to 15 mg over 6 months to 4 years do not appear to interfere with zinc status (24).

Foxglove

10 Second Take

Foxglove is a toxic herb that should not be used medicinally.

Basics

LATIN NAME

Digitalis purpurea L., *D. lanata* Ehrh. (Grecian foxglove)

FAMILY

Scrophuliaraceae

DESCRIPTION

• *D. purpurea* is a biennial herb that grows up to 6 ft tall with purple to white flowers (spotted inside the lower part) on a long raceme.
• *D. lanata* has long narrow leaves and smaller yellow-brown flowers.
• Foxgloves are native to Europe but are cultivated as ornamentals in North America.

PART USED

Leaf

KNOWN ACTIVE CONSTITUENTS

• Digitalis glycosides. Besides digitoxin, gitaloxin, and gitoxin (which together compose about 0.16% of foxglove leaves) (1), about 30 other glycosides (including purpurea glycosides A and B and glucogitaloxin) have been identified in *D. purpurea* (2). Glycoside concentrations vary with the plant source and conditions of growth, and, because many of these are secondary glycosides derived by hydrolysis of sugars from the primary glycosides, postharvest treatment of the plant also affects glycoside content (2).
• Digitoxin can be obtained from either *D. purpurea* or *D. lanata*; digoxin is present only in the leaves of *D. lanata* (3). Nearly 70 glycosides have been detected in the leaves of *D. lanata*. All are derived from five different aglycones, designated lanatosides A to E. The three that are common to *D. purpurea* and *D. lanata* are digitoxigenin, gitoxigenin, and gitaloxigenin (3).

MECHANISM/PHARMACOKINETICS

• Glycosides derived from digitalis inhibit sodium-potassium adenosine triphosphatase (ATPase), increasing intracellular sodium and stimulating sodium calcium exchange; these compounds act on the cardiovascular system.
• Digoxin has a positive inotropic and vagomimetic effect and also decreases activation of the sympathetic nervous system (3a). Digoxin has become a more popular drug than digitoxin because it acts more rapidly and is more rapidly eliminated than digitoxin. Digoxin is more hydrophilic, binds less to plasma proteins, and is mainly eliminated by the kidneys. Digitoxin is metabolized more slowly through the liver (4).

Evidence

CLINICAL TRIALS

No clinical trials of foxglove identified.

Risks

ADVERSE REACTIONS

• Foxglove is poisonous, and antidigoxin Fab fragments are not particularly effective in foxglove poisoning. Most cases of toxicity have resulted from mistaking the plant for comfrey. In one case, a 46-year-old Asian woman presented to the emergency room with nausea, lethargy, dizziness, and weakness after ingesting four large foxglove leaves 4 hours previously (5). Her electrocardiogram (EKG) showed sinus and junctional brady-cardia with intermittent second-degree atrioventricular (AV) block; her digoxin level was 0.8 ng/mL and remained at that level despite a total of four vials of Digibind given over 24 hours (beginning 24 hours after exposure). She was discharged 2 days later with transient AV block but asymptomatic.

• Three men who shared a "comfrey" salad were admitted to the hospital with nausea, vomiting, and irregular heart rates. One had a high-grade AV block, runs of idionodal tachycardia, and an accelerated idionodal rhythm. The second had first-degree and second-degree sinoatrial block with occasional atriventricular nodal escape beats, and the third had a normal EKG with sinus bradycardia (rate 46 beats/minute). All had serum digoxin concentrations in the low therapeutic range. The two patients with arrhythmia were treated with diuresis, potassium, and eventually peritoneal dialysis (6).

• In another case, a 70-year-old man was admitted, with vomiting, diarrhea, confusion, and visual disturbances; EKG monitoring revealed complete heart block with a ventricular rate of 40 beats/minute, requiring a temporary pacemaker (7). In all of these cases, people mistook foxglove for comfrey.

• An apparently accidentally adulterated mixture of herbs meant for "internal cleansing" resulted in two cases of digoxin poisoning. In the first case a 23-year-old woman presented with complete heart block; serum digoxin was 3.66 ng/mL. She was treated with 10 vials of digoxin-specific Fab (Digibind) without clinical response. The next day, when the serum digoxin level was 2.29 ng/mL, she was treated with choles-tyramine and improved clinically. She was discharged the next day, with a serum digoxin level of 1.91 ng/mL. In the other case, a 46-year-old woman was hospitalized for evaluation of visual disturbances, nausea, vomiting, shortness of breath, palpitations, and a feeling of chest pressure. She had been using the same internal cleansing program as the patient described previously. Her serum digoxin level was 0.9 ng/mL and creatine kinase levels were elevated, with a normal MB fraction. The dietary supplement mixture tested positive for the presence of cardiac glycosides. The problem was eventually traced to a supply of plantain contaminated with *D. lanata* (8).

• A 22-year-old man took an intentional overdose of a homemade foxglove extract (made from three wheelbarrows of foxglove leaves mixed with vodka and filtered to yield 8 oz of extract) (9). After experiencing nausea 90 minutes after ingestion, the man ingested potassium chloride, purportedly an antidote, and then presented to the hospital about 4 hours after ingestion. EKG showed Mobitz Type I second-degree heart block and repolarization changes consistent with cardiac glycoside poisoning. Activated charcoal (50 g q4 × 24 hours) and i.v. meto-clopramide were given; an hour later symptomatic bradycardia was observed, at which time digoxin-specific Fab fragments were administered. A total of 37 vials (4,000 mg) was administered over 24 hours, causing only transient clinical and EKG improvement after each administration. Cholestyramine was added every 6 hours to interrupt enterohepatic recirculation of glycoside. Nausea and bradycardia improved with declining digitoxin fluorescence-polarization immunoassay (FPIA) levels over 11 days. Serum digitoxin levels showed no evidence of increased elimination or altered distribution with Fab therapy. Analysis of the extract revealed 465 mg/g cardioactive glycosides.

Dose

COMMON DOSAGE FORMS

Foxglove is a poisonous herb and should not be used medicinally.

Common Questions and Answers

Q: Is the administration of antidigoxin Fab fragments effective in plants containing cardiac glycosides?
A: Depends on the plant. This treatment is quite effective for oleander poisoning but is not very effective in foxglove poisoning. With foxglove Fab fragments cannot be dosed based on digitoxin or digoxin immunoassay levels, probably because of nonassayable cross-reacting glycosides. After 37 vials of Fab fragments at a cost of $11,000 were given to a patient who attempted suicide by foxglove, the authors retrospectively calculated that 100 vials (4,000 mg, an impracticable amount) would have been necessary to have an effect (9).
In contrast, antidigoxin Fab is effective in reversing oleander-induced arrhythmias. Accidental poisoning by oleander is common in the tropics and subtropics; fatal poisonings have been reported from many parts of the world. Suicide attempts using yellow oleander seeds have become such a common problem in Sri Lanka that a randomized controlled trial could be done with antidigoxin Fab. Sixty-six patients who presented with a serious cardiac arrhythmia were randomized to either 1,200 mg of antidigoxin Fab or saline placebo. The presenting arrhythmia had resolved completely after 2 hours in 15 treated patients and 2 controls; after 8 hours, 24 treated patients and 5 controls were in sinus rhythm (10).

Q: Is there any truth to the argument that foxglove is safer than digoxin?
A: No. Some think that foxglove is safer than digoxin because, purportedly, chronic users of foxglove experience nausea before development of dangerous arrhythmias, whereas toxic levels of digoxin can be attained without nausea. This is a specious and dangerous argument. I do not know whether it is true that foxglove is more likely to cause nausea than digoxin, but the varying levels of glycosides in foxglove and the narrow therapeutic window render dosing a game of Russian roulette. Nausea is hardly a specific enough symptom to substitute for digoxin levels. With foxglove, neither the laboratory tests nor the antidotes available for digoxin are reliable. Drugs are far safer.

Garlic

10 Second Take

Garlic is benign and can lower cholesterol and decrease platelet aggregation. Avoid use before surgery.

Basics

LATIN NAME

Allium sativum L.

FAMILY

Liliaceae (Alliaceae)

DESCRIPTION

Garlic, widely used in great culinary traditions, also has a long history of medicinal use.

PART USED

Bulb

KNOWN ACTIVE CONSTITUENTS

• Alliin ((+)-*S*-allyl-L-cysteine sulfoxide) is the main sulfur-containing amino acid. Garlic also contains (+)-*S*-methyl-L-cysteine sulfoxide, gamma-L-glutamyl peptides, *S*-allyl cysteine, other amino acids, steroids, and adenosine. When cell membranes are breached, as in crushing or chopping, alliin (*S*-allyl-L-cysteine sulfoxide) contacts the enzyme alliinase and converts to allicin (diallyl thiosulfinate), a thermally unstable compound that has the characteristic garlic smell (1). Allicin is metabolized very quickly, primarily to allyl mercaptan; no allicin is found in the blood after eating garlic.

MECHANISM/PHARMACOKINETICS

• Cardiovascular

—Garlic has antioxidant effects, inhibits cholesterol synthesis, and inhibits platelet aggregation. Allicin inhibits lipid peroxidation at a concentration of 0.18 mM. Allicin and ajoene (another organosulfur compound) inhibit cholesterol biosynthesis in rat hepatocyte cell lines (1). Garlic powder extract reduced cholesterol esters and free cholesterol in smooth muscle cells cultured from human aortic atherosclerotic plaques (2). Allicin, ajoene, and other sulfur-containing compounds in garlic inhibit platelet aggregation (3).

• Cancer prevention

—Possible mechanisms of action affecting carcinogenesis include induction of hepatic enzymes, enhancement of glutathione peroxidase activity, and enhancement of glutathione S-transferase activity (3). Garlic also reduces ornithine decarboxylase and lipoxygenase activity.

Evidence

CLINICAL TRIALS

• Hypercholesterolemia

—A review of garlic for hypercholesterolemia identified 45 randomized controlled trials (RCTs) (40 placebo-controlled, 34 double-blind) (4). Twenty-two trials tested a commercial dehydrated garlic preparation standardized to 1.3% alliin. Pooled data from placebo-controlled trials found that, compared with placebo, total cholesterol (TC) levels in treated groups were reduced 0.19 mmol/L (7.2 mg/dL) after 4 to 6 weeks of therapy (14 trials) and 0.44 mmol/L (17.1 mg/dL) after 8 to 12 weeks (24 trials); there was no difference at 20 to 24 weeks (6 trials). An analysis limited to standardized garlic preparations found that TC was reduced by 0.26 mmol/L (10.2 mg/dL) after 4 to 6 weeks (8 trials) and by 0.5 mmol/L (19.2 mg/dL) after 8 to 12 weeks (12 trials). In 17 trials that examined triglycerides (13 used a standardized preparation), triglyceride levels at 8 to 12 weeks were reduced 0.21 mmol/L (19.1 mg/dL). Garlic reduced both low density lipoprotein (LDL) and high density lipoprotein (HDL); in 13 trials, at 8 to 12 weeks, garlic preparations reduced LDL by 0.16 mmol/L [6.2 mg/dL, 95% confidence interval (CI) 0.02 to 0.3 mmol/L]. In 14 trials that examined HDL, the average reduction was 0.02 mmol/L (0.9 mg/dL, 95% CI −0.03 to 0.07 mmol/L).
—Another meta-analysis of 13 double-blind, placebo-controlled RCTs of garlic preparations in those with TC ≥200 mg/dL (5.17 mmol/L) found that garlic reduced TC levels from baseline significantly more than placebo (weighted mean difference in the garlic group was 0.41 mmol/L) (95% CI −0.66 to −0.15 mmol/L) and in the placebo group was 15.7 mg/dL (95% CI −25.6 to −5.7 mg/dL) (5). In six diet-controlled studies with high methodologic scores there was no difference between garlic and placebo groups. An analysis of five trials that provided information on LDL and HDL levels found no difference between garlic and placebo.
—A recent double-blind, placebo-controlled trial of a commercial garlic preparation (not included in the meta-analyses mentioned previously) tested two doses of garlic (500 or 1,000 mg dehydrated powder/day) in 51 moderately hypercholesterolemic adults for 12 weeks (6). No significant differences between groups were seen for TC, HDL, LDL, or triglyceride levels.

• Blood pressure

—Only 3 of 30 trials (23 placebo-controlled) on blood pressure noted that garlic significantly decreased diastolic blood pressure (2% to 7%), and only one noted decreased systolic blood pressure (approximately 3%) in the treated group, compared to the control group (4).

• Glucose

—Only 1 of 12 trials that assessed effects of garlic on glucose, a 4-week trial of a standardized preparation in nondiabetics, found a significant reduction. None found an effect on glycosylated hemoglobin, serum insulin, or C-peptide levels (4). Five of six trials that examined spontaneous platelet aggregation reported results. Four found significantly decreased platelet aggregation; one found significantly decreased epinephrine-induced but not adenosine diphosphate (ADP)-induced platelet aggregation (4).

• Atherosclerotic plaque

—A double-blind, placebo-controlled RCT tested the effect of garlic powder (900 mg/day) in 280 patients (152 completed) with advanced atherosclerotic disease on plaque volume by B-mode ultrasound (7). Over 4 years, the placebo group increased plaque volume 15.6%, whereas the garlic group decreased 2.6%. This trial had a very high dropout rate.

• Antifungal effects

—A study of 34 Venezuelan soldiers with culture-positive tinea pedis were treated with 0.4% (w/w) topical ajoene cream b.i.d. for 7 days (8). Treatment completely cured 79% of patients; an additional 7-day course cured remaining patients. All patients were culture-negative immediately after and 90 days after cessation of treatment.

• Tick bites

—A double-blind, placebo-controlled crossover RCT tested garlic (1,200 mg/day p.o.) against tick bites in 100 Swedish Marines (80 completed). The first phase lasted 8 weeks with a 2-week washout period; the second phase lasted 10 weeks (9). Among 80 completers, tick bites were significantly reduced during the garlic phase. Relative risk (RR) by intention to treat analysis was 0.79 (95% CI 0.65 to 0.96); RR of completers was 0.70 (95% CI 0.54 to 0.90).

• Peripheral vascular disease

—A placebo-controlled, double-blind RCT of 80 patients (64 completed) with Stage II peripheral artery disease compared standardized garlic tablets (400 mg b.i.d.) with placebo and found a significant increase in pain-free walking distance during the last 6 weeks of the 12 week trial (10). Both groups received physical therapy twice weekly. Compared with baseline, the treated group walked 46 m further (28.5% increase) at the end of the trial, whereas the control group walked 31 m further (18.1%). It is not clear from the report whether this difference was significant; a Cochrane review (of only this single study) concluded that there was no difference between groups (11).

- Plasma viscosity/platelet aggregation

—In 10 volunteers, 900-mg standardized garlic powder reduced plasma viscosity, increased fibrinolytic activity, and increased capillary blood flow (1). A double-blind, placebo-controlled RCT of 120 patients with cerebrovascular risk factors found that 800 mg garlic q.d. × 4 weeks decreased platelet aggregation 56.3% (12). Allicin also decreases platelet aggregation (13).

- Cancer prevention

—A meta-analysis of 18 studies on garlic and cancer risk found that garlic reduced colorectal cancer risk; the random-effects RR estimates for consumption of garlic (eight studies) was 0.66 (95% CI 0.48 to 0.91) (14). Most studies examined dietary garlic; if a study of garlic supplements and one that included garlic, onions, and pepper as a single exposure category are excluded, differences were no longer significant. For stomach cancer (five studies) the random-effects RR was 0.61 (95% CI 0.37 to 1.03); without the garlic supplement study, the difference was still significant, RR 0.53 (95% CI 0.3 to 0.92). The authors note that effect estimates were heterogeneous; there may have been publication bias and total vegetable consumption may have confounded results.
—A review of epidemiologic studies (mostly case-control studies, two prospective) found that 19/20 studies showed that regular consumption of garlic and onions reduced the risk of cancer (particularly gastrointestinal tract cancers) (15). In the parts of Georgia known for Vidalia onions, the stomach cancer mortality rate (among whites) is only a third the national level and half the state level (16).

OTHER CLAIMED BENEFITS/ACTIONS

- Upper respiratory infections
- Influenza
- Parasites
- Diabetes
- Hepatic disease
- Gallbladder disease
- Lead poisoning
- Leprosy
- AIDS

 Risks

ADVERSE REACTIONS

- Gastrointestinal upset, abdominal pain, fullness, anorexia, flatulence, and body odor.
- Dermatitis, pemphigus, and occupational asthma (see questions and answers).
- Burns from topically applied garlic, especially in children, have been reported (17,18).
- Garlic should be avoided before surgery (see questions and answers).

DRUG INTERACTIONS

- Anticoagulants

—Anticoagulation effect may be additive with other anticoagulant drugs (19) (see questions and answers)

PREGNANCY/LACTATION

- No adverse effects have been reported.
- Garlic flavors breast milk, an effect that may actually improve milk intake of babies (20).

 Dose

COMMON DOSAGE FORMS

- *Dried powdered bulb:* 600 mg q.d. to 4 g t.i.d. (usually 600 to 1,000 mg q.d.)
- *Tincture:* [1:5 in 45% ethanol (EtOH)]: 2 to 4 mL t.i.d.
- *Oil:* 0.03 to 0.12 mL t.i.d.
- *Juice:* 2 to 4 mL
- Chewing raw garlic converts alliin to allicin within seconds. Enteric-coated dried garlic tablets reduce deactivation of alliinase by stomach acid.
- Alliin/allicin equivalents: One clove of garlic or 1.0 gm garlic powder usually contains the equivalent of 6 to 10 mg of alliin, which is equivalent to approximately 3 to 5 mg allicin; 1 mg alliin is equivalent to 0.45 mg allicin (1).

 Common Questions and Answers

Q: What dermatologic reactions are associated with garlic?
A: Contact hypersensitivity to garlic is an occupational hazard of food handlers. After a positive patch test, a placebo-controlled rechallenge confirmed the diagnosis of garlic-induced systemic contact dermatitis in a patient who experienced prolonged hand dermatitis while taking commercial garlic tablets (21).
Garlic poultices may cause lesions typical of a chemical burn (17).
One case of diet-related superficial pemphigus has been reported (22). Garlic provoked acantholysis in human skin cells from four of seven donors (23).

Q: Can garlic affect bleeding time?
A: Yes. Garlic should be avoided for at least 1 week preoperatively. Excessive bleeding during a transurethral prostatic resection (TURP) in a 72-year-old man taking garlic tablets was reported (24).
A 32-year-old woman with a heavy dietary garlic intake had a prolonged clotting time ($12\frac{1}{2}$ minutes) before mammoplasty, significant oozing during surgery, and a 200-cc hematoma that was removed 1 week postoperatively. Clotting time dropped to 6 minutes 1 week after discontinuing garlic (25).
Spontaneous spinal epidural hematoma resulting in paraplegia in an 87-year-old patient was attributed to chronic heavy use of garlic (26).

Q: How is garlic linked to asthma?
A: Occupational asthma and/or rhinitis have occurred in workers regularly exposed to garlic dust. Seven of 12 garlic workers in Spain with respiratory symptoms responded positively to inhalation challenge with garlic dust; serum IgE and skin tests supported the findings. Many workers were also sensitized to related *Allium* species such as leek and onion (27).

Germander

10 Second Take

Germander is a hepatotoxic herb that should not be used medicinally.

Basics

LATIN NAME

Teucrium chamaedrys L.

FAMILY

Labiatae/Lamiaceae

OTHER COMMON NAMES

Common germander, wall germander

DESCRIPTION

• Germander is a variable perennial herb, a member of the mint family, that grows in woods and thickets.
• It is native to Europe and found also in the Mideast.

PART USED

Flowering herb

KNOWN ACTIVE CONSTITUENTS

• Neo-clerodane diterpenoids, especially teucrin A. Flavonoids (diosmine, isoquercitin, cirsiliol, cirsimaritin), choline, tannins, and sterols including β-sitosterol, a phenyl-propanoid glycoside named teucrioside.
• Essential oil contains 31 compounds, predominately caryophyllene and humulene.

MECHANISM/PHARMACOKINETICS

• Mouse experiments show that constituents of *T. chamaedrys* are transformed by cytochrome P450 3A into hepatotoxic metabolites (probably epoxides) (1). These damaging metabolites were partially inactivated by glutathione and possibly epoxide hydrolase. Studies in isolated rat hepatocytes confirmed that the furano-neo-clerodane diterpenoid fraction (also purified teucrin A or teuchamaedryn A) were hepatotoxic (2). Glutathione levels decreased, as did protein thiols (which affects cytoskeleton-associated proteins, leading to formation of plasma membrane blebs, the rupture of which lyses the cell). Germander diterpenoids (100 μg/mL) increase cytosolic Ca 2^+, activate calcium-dependent tissue transaminase, fragment internucleosomal DNA, decrease cell ATP, and cause overexpression of proapoptosis gene products, causing apoptosis within 2 hours (3).

Evidence

CLINICAL TRIALS

No clinical trials identified.

ANIMAL/IN VITRO

• Extracts of *Teucrium* reportedly inhibit the growth of HeLa cells.
• Two diterpenoids, teucvin and teucvidin, showed no antitumor effect against P388 lymphocytic leukemia in mice. Teucvin reportedly is a potent amebicidal agent (4).

OTHER CLAIMED BENEFITS/ACTIONS

• Diuretic
• Weight loss aid
• Diarrhea
• Hemorrhoids
• Wounds
• Increased bile flow
• Mouthwash
• Expectorant
• Tonic

Risks

ADVERSE REACTIONS

• Hepatitis

—Twenty-six cases of hepatitis were reported in France after the use of Belgian weight-loss capsules or teas containing *T. chamaedrys* (5). Seven of these cases were detailed in the *Annals of Internal Medicine* in 1992 (6). In the review of 26 cases, doses taken ranged between 450 and 1,600 mg per day (these are normal daily doses); no relationship with dose or duration could be established. After a mean of 9 weeks (range 2 to 18 weeks) patients developed acute symptomatic hepatitis with minimal cholestasis, jaundice, and elevated levels of alanine transaminase (ALT) and aspartate transaminase (AST). Liver biopsy showed centrilobular or panlobular hepatocyte necrosis. Two patients had transient portal hypertension without encephalopathy. Patients recovered in 1.5 to 6 months, but hepatitis swiftly recurred in 12 patients who were accidentally rechallenged. Most of these cases did not result in serious long-term outcomes; however, one patient still had inflammatory lesions on liver biopsy 2 years after the acute hepatitis, and another (who had been reexposed to germander) showed signs suggestive of chronic active hepatitis (5). Antinuclear and antismooth muscle antibodies were demonstrated in two patients with germander-induced hepatitis (4).

—Since that 1992 report, several other cases have been reported, including a fatal case of massive hepatic necrosis in a 68-year-old woman after accidental readministration of germander (7).

—One case of cirrhosis was reported in a 54-year-old woman who had taken germander for 11 months (4).

—Recently, two cases of germander-associated hepatitis were reported in Canada (8).

 ## Dose

COMMON DOSAGE FORMS

• Use of this herb is not recommended; dosages provided for information only
• Dried herb in capsules or tea (daily doses range from 600 to 1,600 mg)
• Herbal liqueur

 ## Common Questions and Answers

Q: Can the use of germander ever be clinically justified?
A: No. Although the frequency of germander-associated hepatitis is low, germander lacks unique actions that would justify its clinical use. Its popularity undoubtedly stemmed from its reputation as a weight-loss product. Although there are no clinical trials of this use, the nausea and anorexia associated with liver dysfunction certainly could lead to weight loss. As with drugs, there are no safe herbal weight-loss products (excepting those that are merely ineffective).

Q: Does American germander have the same toxicity as common germander?
A: American germander, *Teucrium canadense,* contains several of the same constituents as *T. chamaedrys,* including the neo-clerodane diterpenoids, which are the suspected cause of hepatotoxicity. Although there have been no published cases of *T. canadense*-associated hepatotoxicity, there has been a suspicion raised that at least some of the hepato-toxicity linked with purported skullcap (*Scutellaria lateriflora*) preparations is actually attributable to American germander, which is widely used as a substitute for or in combination with skullcap. Given the severity and unpredictability of hepatotoxicity, caution dictates that all *Teucrium* species and products be avoided.

Q: How common is germander-associated hepatitis?
A: The frequency of germander-associated hepatitis is low (it has been estimated at one case per 4,000 months of treatment) (4). Although there is no single variable that links the patients who developed hepatitis, many were also taking nonsteroidal antiinflam-matory drugs (NSAIDs), some of which have hepatotoxic effects; it is possible that an herb-drug interaction increases susceptibility to hepatitis.

Germanium (Ge)

 10 Second Take

Germanium compounds are toxic (primarily to the kidney) and should not be used. Some compounds may have anti-cancer potential and should be researched further.

 Basics

DESCRIPTION

• Germanium (atomic number 32, atomic weight 72.6) is a naturally occurring trace element in argyrodite and germanite and cadmium-containing zinc ores (1).
• It is used in the electronics industry as a semiconductor.
• Germanium dietary supplements have been popular as tonics and anticancer agents in Japan since the 1970s; use has spread since then. Dietary supplements may contain inorganic germanium, usually germanium dioxide (GeO_2), or organic germanium, carboxyethyl germanium sesquioxide (Ge132). Germanium-lactate-citrate (Ge-lac-cit), a preparation marketed as organic germanium, actually contained inorganic germanium. Germanium sesquioxide (Ge132) is synthetic but can be easily contaminated with germanium dioxide (GeO_2), which is commonly used as starting material (2).

FOOD SOURCES

• Tiny amounts of germanium are found in many foods; only four of 125 foods analyzed contained average germanium levels greater than 2 ppm (2).
• Canned tuna may contain 3 ppm, and tomato juice and baked beans may contain 5 ppm (1).
• Most plants contain less than 1 ppm, but shiitake mushrooms, garlic, and pearl barley contain higher quantities (1).
• Typical daily intake is 0.4 to 1.5 mg (5.5 to 20.7 μmol) (3). In the United Kingdom daily intake is about 367 μg (2).

MAIN FUNCTIONS/PHARMACOKINETICS

• Germanium deficiency has not been established. No germanium-specific essential function has been demonstrated in humans, other animals, or plants (2).
• Dietary germanium appears to be well absorbed from the intestine; excretion is primarily renal. After a single oral dose of Ge132 (100 mg) in 11 healthy volunteers (including one woman) given 100 mg Ge132, urinary excretion of germanium peaked at about 3 hours and returned to a predosing level at 24 hours. In humans given Ge132, the absorption rate was 30% and urinary excretion was quite rapid (2). In animals, the biologic half-life of germanium was 1 to 2 days in rats (liver and whole body) and only about 2 hours in mouse lung, liver, and kidneys (2).

 Evidence

CLINICAL TRIALS

• Several trials of spirogermanium, an azaspiran organogermanium compound, in patients with advanced cancers were not impressive (2). The treatment caused pulmonary toxicity in two cases and neurotoxicity in 40% of those with advanced disease (1).
• Other evidence

—An interesting case report notes complete remission of pulmonary spindle cell carcinoma in a 47-year-old women with an unresectable 3.4 × 4.5 cm tumor that encircled the pulmonary artery and had invaded the esophagus and pericardium (4). After unsuccessful chemotherapy and radiation treatment (the patient had worsening symptoms and radiographic evidence of tumor progression), the patient discontinued conventional treatment and began self-treatment with bis-betacarboxyethygermanium sesquioxide, starting at 7.2 g/day, then tapered. Three months later, chest radiographs showed 60% clearing of the left lung; at 5 and 7 months, thoracic computed tomography (CT) scans showed that the mass had almost completely disappeared. The patient continued on low-dose germanium sesquioxide and showed no evidence of recurrent disease more than 4 years later.

ANIMAL/IN VITRO

• Organic germanium compounds (including germanium sesquioxide) have shown antitumor, anticancer, antimicrobial, analgesic, and immunomodulating effects in animals (2). In rats, a low intake of germanium affects the mineral composition in bone and liver (3,5).

 Clinical Considerations

LABORATORY TESTS

• *Urine:* mean levels range from 0.078 to 1.26 mg/L
• *Serum:* About 0.29 mg/L
• *Plasma:* About 0.154 ± 0.02 mg/L (2)
• Germanium dioxide accumulates in kidneys, liver, spleen, hair, and nails. Germanium sesquioxide accumulates to a lesser degree primarily in kidneys, liver, and spleen (2). In normal human tissues, germanium ranges from 0.0009 ppm in lymph nodes to 9.00 ppm in the kidney (2). The average content of germanium in the body is 20 mg (6).

Germanium (Ge)

Risks

ADVERSE REACTIONS

• At least 32 cases of germanium poisoning have been reported. A 1997 review identified 31 reported cases of poisoning resulting from germanium products, including nine (29%) that were fatal (2). Anemia and renal dysfunction were noted in all cases. Anorexia, weight loss, fatigue, muscle weakness, nausea, and vomiting were also common. Hyperplastic bone marrow, hepatosteatosis, myopathy, or neuropathies (including sensory impairment, truncal ataxia, and cerebellar ataxia) may be seen. Duration of use ranged from 2 to 36 months, and total germanium intake ranged from 15 to 324 g (2).

• Since the previously mentioned review, a case of sensory ataxia and renal failure was reported in a 63-year-old woman who had taken inorganic germanium (36 mg/day × 6 years) (7).

• Glomeruli are evidently spared damage. Urinalysis is characteristically normal; renal biopsy characteristically shows vacuolar degeneration of tubular epithelial cells. Swollen mitochondria with electron-dense inclusions may be seen in renal or muscle biopsy (2). Renal failure has persisted for 2 years after discontinuation of germanium, and other symptoms may persist many months after germanium use is discontinued. In nails, hair, and kidneys, germanium levels may be high 10 months after cessation of use (2).

• In clinical trials with germanium sesquioxide, adverse gastrointestinal and cardiac effects were noted; 62.9% of older adults who took 10 mg germanium sesquioxide for 12 weeks had abnormal electrocardiograms (2). Spirogermanium caused pulmonary toxicity in two cases and neurotoxicity in 40% of those with advanced disease (1).

• Calculated lowest effect levels by adverse events in humans (2)

Inorganic	0.9 to 6.7 mg/kg/d
GeO_2	0.7 to 23 mg/kg/d
Ge132	1.7 to 5.6 mg/kg/d
Ge-lac-cit	0.8 to 8.0 mg/kg/d

DRUG INTERACTIONS

• Diuretics

—A case of diuretic resistance was reported in a 63-year-old man with membranous glomerulonephritis, taking furosemide and cyclosporine (8). Ten days after initiating several dietary supplements, including 10 to 12 tablets daily of a germanium-ginseng preparation called Uncle Hsu's Korean ginseng, he developed edema and hypertension requiring hospitalization. After discharge, the patient rechallenged himself with the supplements and required readmission 2 weeks later. The authors noted that diuresis became effective 48 hours after the supplements were withheld, and that germanium toxicity may cause lipofuscin granule accumulation in the ascending limb of the loop of Henle, where loop diuretics act.

ANIMAL TOXICITY

• Acute oral toxicity is low. LD_{50} for GeO_2 was 3.7 g/kg for rats and 6.3 g/kg for male mice. LD_{50} for Ge132 was 11.0 to 11.7 g/kg in rats, and 6.3 to 12.5 g/kg in mice (2). In a 40-week pair-feeding study, the lowest observed adverse effect dose (LOAEL) of germanium for decreased growth, anemia, and renal dysfunction was 26 mg/kg body weight/day; for GeO_2 the LOAEL was 37.5 mg/kg body weight/day. Rats fed GeO_2 0.15% for 23 weeks have developed myopathy; the same dose can cause neuropathy after 8 months (2).

• Characteristic renal dysfunction can be observed in rats given GeO_2 in drinking water (500 ppm × 6 months) (2); the effect of Ge132 is not as clear. In rats, tumorigenicity and teratogenicity studies with germanium have been negative (2).

Common Questions and Answers

Q: Don't some herbs contain significant levels of germanium?
A: Ginseng, aloe, and garlic were reported to contain germanium in parts per million levels in the late 1980s, but this determination turned out to be erroneous. More sensitive analytical techniques determined that the levels of germanium in these herbs are in parts per billion (2).

Ginger

 10 Second Take

Ginger is a commonly used culinary and medicinal herb that is benign and may be helpful for nausea and vomiting.

 Basics

LATIN NAME

Zingiber officinale Roscoe

FAMILY

Zingiberaceae

OTHER COMMON NAMES

Common ginger, zingiber

DESCRIPTION

• Ginger is a tropical plant used as a spice, as well as medicinally.
• It is a common ingredient in almost half of Chinese and Japanese herbal medicines.

PART USED

Rhizome

KNOWN ACTIVE CONSTITUENTS

• Monoterpenes including geranial (α-citral) and neral (β-citral) and sesquiterpenes, including β-sesquiphellandrene, β-bisabolene, α-curcumene, and α-zingiberene.
• Drying decreases monoterpenes and increases sesquiterpenes.
• Ginger also contains phenolic ketones, mainly gingerols and their derivative shogaols (1).

MECHANISM/PHARMACOKINETICS

• In rats, 3 mg of 6-gingerol/kg was cleared within minutes from plasma; serum protein binding was 92.4% and total body clearance was 16.8 mL/minute/kg (2).
• Because pharmacologic effects have been demonstrated 3 hours after intravenous administration, gingerol may be sequestered in tissues or may be effective in extremely low concentrations (1).
• Gingerols inhibit lipoxygenase and affect prostaglandin synthetase activity *in vitro*. Ginger also appears to inhibit thromboxane synthetase and raise prostacyclin levels without increasing prostaglandin levels (1).
• One report examined the effect of 5 g of ginger daily for 7 days in seven women and found that mean thromboxane levels decreased by almost 37% (1).

 Evidence

CLINICAL TRIALS

• Morning sickness

—A randomized, double-blind placebo-controlled trial in 70 women with nausea and vomiting of pregnancy compared ginger (1 g daily) to placebo for 4 days (3). Nausea severity was rated by a visual analog scale and number of vomiting episodes in the 24 hours before treatment compared with episodes during treatment. Visual analog scores and number of vomiting episodes decreased significantly in the ginger group, compared with the placebo group.
—In a double-blind crossover trial of 30 women with morning sickness (27 completed), each woman received ginger capsules (250 mg q.i.d.) or placebo for 4 days. After a 2-day washout period, each woman was crossed over to the other group for 4 days; 70.4% of the women preferred the ginger, which reduced both emesis and the degree of nausea (4).

• Postoperative nausea and vomiting

—Two of three studies showed a benefit of ginger. A double-blind, randomized study in 60 women undergoing major gynecologic surgery compared placebo with ginger (1 g p.o. 1.5 hours before surgery) or metoclopramide 10 mg (i.v. at induction of anesthesia); placebo pills and injections were used to preserve blinding (5). The incidence of nausea was significantly lower in the ginger-treated group than in the placebo group; the effect of metoclopramide was similar to ginger. The placebo group used significantly more antiemetic postoperatively than the treated groups.
—In a double-blind study that compared ginger (2g) and metoclopramide (10 mg) with placebo in 120 women undergoing laparoscopic gynecologic surgery, ginger equaled metoclopramide in preventing postoperative nausea and vomiting (6).
—Another placebo-controlled trial of 108 women undergoing gynecologic laparoscopic surgery (under general anesthesia, with preoperative diazepam) tested 500 mg and 1,000 mg of ginger given 1 hour before surgery. This dose was ineffective in reducing the incidence of postoperative nausea and vomiting (7).

• Chemotherapy-induced nausea and vomiting

—A small trial of 11 patients who regularly experienced nausea after taking 8-MOP before photophoresis found that ginger (1590 mg 30 minutes before 8-MOP) reduced nausea scores by two thirds (8).

• Motion sickness

—A placebo-controlled trial of eighty naval cadets unaccustomed to heavy seas found that ginger (1 g every hour for 4 hours) reduced the number of vomiting episodes and cold sweats but did not significantly reduce nausea or vertigo (9).
—Seven seasickness treatments, including ginger, were compared in 1,741 volunteers embarking on a whale safari in Norway (10). Medications were cinnarizine 25 mg; cinnarizine 20 mg with domperidone 15 mg; cyclizine 50 mg; dimenhydrate 50 mg with caffeine 50 mg; ginger 250 mg (Zintona); meclizine 12.5 mg with caffeine 50 mg; and scopolamine 0.5 mg. Vomiting and retching were endpoints. At least some seasickness was reported by 18.2% to 26.8% of the participants. Questionnaires were returned by 1,489 volunteers (85.5%); there was no significant difference among treatments. The lack of a placebo control makes this trial difficult to interpret.
—Studies in preventing laboratory-induced motion sickness have been mixed. In one study, 36 undergraduates ingested capsules of dimenhydrinate, powdered ginger, or a placebo herb and then were blindfolded and placed in a tilted rotating chair for whichever of the following came first: 6 minutes, emesis, three triplings in the magnitude of nausea, or pleas for freedom (11). None of the participants in the placebo and dimenhydrinate groups could stay in the chair for 6 minutes, but half of those in the ginger group did.
—Another laboratory study of eight volunteers found ginger more effective than placebo in controlling induced dizziness (12).
—However, another study of induced motion sickness in 28 volunteers compared three preparations of ginger (500 mg or 1,000 mg dried root or 1,000 mg fresh root) to scopolamine (0.6 mg p.o.) or placebo (13). Neither powdered nor fresh ginger prevented motion sickness. Disordered gastric motility and decreased gastric emptying (associated with motion sickness) were not significantly affected by ginger.

• Gastroduodenal motility

—The effect of ginger extract (2×100 mg) on gastroduodenal motility was assessed by stationary manometry in 12 healthy volunteers (14). Oral ginger improved gastroduodenal motility in the fasting state and after a standard test meal.

• Osteoarthritis

—A double-blind, controlled crossover study in patients with osteoarthritis of the hip or knee tested ginger extract against ibuprofen or placebo (each given for 3 weeks with a 1-week washout period between treatments) (15). Acetaminophen use was allowed if needed. There was no difference between ginger and placebo; ibuprofen improved a visual analogue scale of pain and the Lequesne index. No serious adverse events occurred.

ANIMAL/IN VITRO

- Ginger prevents emesis in several species of animals (2).
- Cholesterol-lowering effects, cholagogic effects, hepatoprotective effects, decreased gastric secretion, and inhibition of gastric lesions have been demonstrated in animal studies (1).
- Shogaol has antitussive effects in animals.
- *In vitro,* ginger extracts demonstrate potent antioxidant effects; inhibit DNA damage induced by lipid peroxidation; and demonstrate modest antibacterial, antifungal, molluscicidal, ascaricidal, and antirhinoviral activity (1).

OTHER CLAIMED BENEFITS/ACTIONS

- Arthritis
- Coughing
- Congestion
- Headaches
- Low back pain (injected)
- Diarrhea
- Suppressed menses
- Indigestion
- Burns, aches, pains, bruises, and cysts (topical)

 Risks

ADVERSE REACTIONS

- Dyspepsia
- Bezoar

—A few cases of bezoar have been reported; most cases involved the consumption of preserved ginger by children or the elderly (1).

DRUG INTERACTIONS

- *Sulfaguanidine:* In rats, ginger enhances absorption of sulfaguanidine up to 150% (1).

PREGNANCY/LACTATION

See questions and answers

 Dose

MODE OF ADMINISTRATION

p.o., topical (in baths)

COMMON DOSAGE FORMS

- *Powdered root:* 0.5 to 2.0 g daily in single or divided doses
- For motion sickness, usually 500 to 1,000 mg taken 30 minutes before travel, repeated as needed
- *Candied root* or *ginger candy*

 Common Questions and Answers

Q: Is it safe to use ginger during pregnancy?
A: Some herbalists warn against using ginger during pregnancy. Although useful for morning sickness, ginger has traditionally been used for "suppressed menses" and may have abortifacient properties. This effect has not been shown in humans. Thromboxane synthetase inhibition has been demonstrated *in vitro,* but clinical trials show no effect (see next question).

In a double-blind, placebo-controlled crossover trial of ginger for nausea and vomiting of pregnancy in 30 women, one patient experienced a spontaneous abortion; another underwent induced abortion for non-medical reasons. Three patients were excluded from analysis. Twenty-five patients went to term, and all infants born were normal in terms of appearance, birthweight, and Apgar scores (4).

Although the cautious may choose to avoid large doses (greater than 1,000 mg/day) in pregnancy, there appears to be no harm in using smaller doses. Ginger is such a common ingredient in Asian cooking that it is unlikely to cause harm. Doses used medicinally are not much higher than doses received through food.

Q: Does ginger increase bleeding time?
A: No, at least not in usual doses. No cases of ginger-related bleeding have been reported, and this is one of the very few herbs for which platelet function tests have been done. Although ginger is a potent thromboxane synthetase inhibitor *in vitro,* clinical studies are reassuring. The first of these, a placebo-controlled crossover trial, administered 2 g of dried ginger to eight male volunteers; platelet function and bleeding time was assessed immediately before, 3 hours after, and 24 hours after ingestion. Ginger did not affect bleeding time, platelet count, or platelet function (16). Very high doses of dried ginger, however, may affect platelets. A controlled trial tested a single dose of placebo against 10 g powdered ginger in 20 patients with coronary artery disease; ginger significantly reduced adenosine diphosphate (ADP)- and epinephrine-induced platelet aggregation (17). Another study in the same publication tested 4 g powdered ginger daily for 3 months in 10 to 30 patients with coronary artery disease (the number is not clear from the report); this dose of ginger had no effect on ADP- and epinephrine-induced platelet aggregation; lipids and glucose were also unaffected (17).

Another crossover trial in 18 healthy volunteers (including 9 women) compared the effect of placebo, 15 g raw ginger root, or 40 g cooked stem ginger, each given for 2 weeks (18). There was no significant effect of either dose on platelet cyclooxygenase activity, assessed by *ex vivo* maximally stimulated thromboxane B_2 production. In summary, although very high doses of dried ginger may reduce platelet aggregation, culinary use and ordinary medicinal use do not appear to affect bleeding.

Q: What is "ginger paralysis"?
A: Ginger preparations contaminated with tri-*O*-tolyl phosphate were responsible for a significant number of fatalities and cases of paralysis in the United States in 1930. There is nothing in ginger that causes this effect.

Ginkgo

10 Second Take

Ginkgo is useful in treating dementia, age-related memory problems, and intermittent claudication, but it can increase the risk of bleeding.

Basics

LATIN NAME

Ginkgo biloba L.

FAMILY

Ginkgoaceae

OTHER COMMON NAMES

Maidenhair tree

DESCRIPTION

• *Ginkgo biloba*, an ancient tree, existed 100 million years ago. A common urban planting, it has distinctive fan-shaped leaves.

PART USED

• Leaf
• Seed (Chinese medicine)

KNOWN ACTIVE CONSTITUENTS

• Leaf

—Ginkgolides are diterpene terpenoids with a unique cage-like structure, bearing tertiary butyl substituents that are rare in nature. Divided into types A, B, C, and J, ginkgolides differ only in the position and number of hydroxyl groups. Another terpenoid, bilobalide, and ginkgo flavonol glycosides are also thought to be active. Proanthocyanadins and amino acids are also present.

MECHANISMS/PHARMACOKINETICS

• Ginkgo leaf extracts inhibit phospholipase A, lipid peroxidase, and protein kinase C; increase blood flow through small vessels; have neuroprotective effects; scavenge free radicals; and reduce platelet aggregation (1).
• Ginkgolide B appears to be the most active platelet activating factor antagonist (2). Ginkgo appears to increase the density of muscarinic receptors, beta-adrenoreceptors, and thyrotropin-releasing hormone receptors and to increase acetylcholine receptors. It may also influence dopaminergic neurons (3).
• Although ginkgo extracts reversibly inhibit monoamine oxidase $(MAO)_A$ and MAO_B in rat brain *in vitro*, a functional test in mice showed no MAO inhibition (4), and positron emission tomography in 10 participants treated with 120 mg/day of the standardized extract Egb 761 showed no changes in labelled MAO_A or MAO_B (5).

Evidence

CLINICAL TRIALS

• Dementia

—A meta-analysis (6) identified more than 50 studies on ginkgo leaf extracts and dementia, including Alzheimer's; however, only four double-blind, placebo-controlled randomized controlled trials (RCTs), with a total of 424 participants, met all inclusion criteria. Overall, there was a significant 3% difference favoring ginkgo in the ADAS-Cog (Alzheimer's Disease Assessment Scale-Cognition) ($p < 0.0001$). The authors concluded that there is a small but significant effect of 3- to 6-months treatment with 120- to 240-mg ginkgo extract on cognition in Alzheimer's disease.
—A systematic review of nine randomized, double-blind, and placebo-controlled studies also concluded that ginkgo is more effective than placebo for dementia (7).
—A recent trial (not included in the previously mentioned studies) tested Egb 761 (Schwabe's standardized extract) 160 or 240 mg/day in 214 patients with Alzheimer's or vascular dementia for 24 weeks (after 12 weeks ginkgo users were re-randomized to ginkgo or placebo; initial placebo users remained on placebo throughout) (8). An intention-to-treat analysis showed no effect of ginkgo on neuropsychologic tests, clinical assessment, behavorial assessment, or self-perceived health and memory status.

• Memory

—A double-blind study of 31 outpatients older than 50 years with mild to moderate memory impairment found a benefit of 120 mg/day on some but not other tests of cognitive function at 12 and 24 weeks (9).
—A double-blind placebo-controlled trial in 40 cognitively intact participants 55 to 86 years old given Egb 761 180 mg/day or placebo for 6 weeks found no significant difference between groups in the trail-making test or the Wechsler Memory Scale-Revised; compared with baseline, there was a significant difference between groups favoring ginkgo in the Stroop Color and Words Test (10).

• Seasonal affective disorder (SAD)

—A double-blind placebo-controlled RCT found no benefit for ginkgo (PN246, Bio-Biloba) for 10 weeks or until symptoms occurred in 27 patients with SAD (11).

• Cerebral insufficiency

—A meta-analysis found that 26/40 controlled trials showed that ginkgo benefited cerebral insufficiency (a syndrome, not accepted in the United States, encompassing difficulties with memory and concentration, confusion, fatigue, depression, tinnitus, and headache). Most studies were metho-dologically poor; eight well-performed trials showed a significant benefit for ginkgo (12).

• Schizophrenia

—A study of ginkgo extract as an adjunct to haloperidol in 82 treatment-resistant chronic schizophrenics found that the ginkgo group improved significantly on the Scale for the Assessment of Positive Symptoms and the Scale for the Assessment of Negative Symptoms (SANS); the haloperidol-only group improved significantly only on SANS (13). Superoxide dismutase (SOD) levels decreased significantly only in the ginkgo group.

• Intermittent claudication

—A meta-analysis of eight placebo-controlled, double-blind RCTs found that ginkgo significantly increased pain-free walking distance (weighted mean difference: 34 m, 95% CI 26 to 43 m) (14).
—A review of 15 controlled trials of ginkgo for intermittent claudication found a benefit in all trials; however, only two trials were of acceptable methodologic quality (15).
—A 24-week study (not included in the previously mentioned reviews) compared Egb 761 120 or 240 mg/day in 74 patients with peripheral arterial occlusive disease (Fontaine's stage II); pain-free walking distance increased in both groups (60.6 m in the 120-mg group and 107.0 m in the 240-mg group) (16).

• Tinnitus

—A review of five RCTs (four placebo-controlled, one treatment-controlled) found ginkgo 120 to 160 mg/day superior to placebo for tinnitus in four studies; the only study that found no benefit tested a suboptimal dose of 29.2 mg extract/day (17). Endpoints were heterogenous and included patient preference, loudness of tinnitus by audiometer, and specialist evaluation.
—The largest trial to date (not in the previously mentioned review), a double-blind, placebo-controlled trial of 1,121 healthy people with tinnitus, tested a standardized extract (LI 1370, Lichter Pharma) t.i.d. × 12 weeks. In this study, 478 pairs, in which all completed at least one questionnaire, were analyzed (18). This trial, performed entirely by phone and mail, found no difference between groups in tinnitus at weeks 4, 12, or 14.
—Two trials of ginkgo combined with laser treatment found no benefit of adjunctive ginkgo for tinnitus (19,20).

• Stroke

—A double-blind placebo-controlled trial of 55 patients with ischemic stroke found no benefit for ginkgo extract (40 mg q6 × 4 weeks) (21).

- Sexual dysfunction

—No RCTs were identified. An open trial of standardized ginkgo extract (60 mg q.d. to 240 mg b.i.d. × 4 weeks) in 30 males and 33 females with antidepressant-induced sexual dysfunction [most on selective serotonin reuptake inhibitors (SSRIs)] found a benefit (22); another open trial of ginkgo (300 mg t.i.d. × 1 month) in 9 men and 13 women with SSRI-induced sexual dysfunction did not (three women and no men reported partial improvement) (23). Neither report identifies the ginkgo formulation. In an open trial reported only in abstract form, ginkgo extract (60 mg q.d. × 12 to 18 months) improved blood supply by duplex ultrasonography in 60 patients with arterial erectile dysfunction unresponsive to papaverine (24).

- Premenstrual syndrome (PMS)
A double-blind, placebo-controlled study in 143 women with PMS found that ginkgo extract (80 to 160 mg b.i.d. × 2 cycles) significantly improved breast tenderness and emotional symptoms (25).

- Multiple sclerosis

—A double-blind, placebo-controlled RCT of 104 patients with an acute exacerbation of remitting-relapsing multiple sclerosis found no effect of ginkgolide B (120 mg or 180 mg intravenously b.i.d. × 7 days) on functional status or disability scales on day 15, 30, or 60 (26).

- Ocular blood flow

—A crossover trial in 11 healthy volunteers compared placebo and ginkgo extract (40 mg t.i.d. × 2 days) (27). Compared with baseline, ginkgo, but not placebo, significantly increased end-diastolic velocity in the ophthalmic artery.

- Clastogenic factors

—In 30 Chernobyl cleanup workers with clastogenic factors (persistent markers of oxidative stress caused by radiation), standardized ginkgo extract (40 mg t.i.d. for 2 months) reduced clastogenic activity of plasma to control levels; the effect persisted for at least 7 months (28).

ANIMAL/IN VITRO

Not covered

OTHER CLAIMED BENEFITS/ACTIONS

- Leaf: heart tonic, lung tonic, asthma, chilblains
- Seed: cough

 Risks

Adverse Reactions

- Leaf extract: bleeding

—Ginkgo has been implicated in cases of subarachnoid hemorrhage (29), subdural hematoma (30,31), and postoperative bleeding (32). (Also see drug interactions.)

- Leaf extract: seizures

—Two cases of seizures within 2 weeks of initiating ginkgo (unidentified, unanalyzed preparations) in well-controlled epileptics were reported (33).

- Leaf extract: other adverse events

—In trials, gastrointestinal complaints and headaches, but no serious adverse reactions, have been reported.
—Coma, reversed by flumazenil, was reported in an 80-year-old Alzheimer's patient 2 days after initiating both trazodone and ginkgo (34). Trazodone is the likely culprit.

- Fruit: contact dermatitis

—Contact with ginkgo fruit (which contains ginkgolic acid, similar to poison ivy allergens) has caused contact dermatitis. A patient who ingested ginkgo fruit (not considered edible) developed stomatitis and proctitis (35).

- Seed: seizures, other neurological effects

—Ginkgo seeds contain an antipyridoxine neurotoxin, ginkgotoxin (4'-O-methylpyridoxine), 99% of which is inactivated by boiling (36). Seed poisoning causes vomiting, irritability, and seizures within 1 to 12 hours. Poisoning should be treated with pyridoxal phosphate 2 mg/kg and anticonvulsants (37). 4'-O-methylpyridoxine is recirculated via enterohepatic circulation, so levels may stay high for hours. Recently, a 2-year-old girl developed vomiting and diarrhea 7 hours after ingesting 50 to 60 roasted ginkgo seeds and seized 2 hours later; 4-methoxypyridoxine levels were as high as 360 ng/mL (37). She was treated with pyridoxal phosphate and diazepam and was asymptomatic the next day.
Fatalities have occurred from consumption of 15 to 574 pieces (37). During food shortages in China and Japan, overconsumption of ginkgo seeds caused a syndrome called Gin-nan sitotoxism with a 27% mortality rate (36).

DRUG INTERACTIONS

- Anticoagulants

—Increases bleeding risk. A 78-year-old woman, stable on warfarin, had an intracerebral hemorrhage 2 months after initiating ginkgo (38).
—A 70-year-old man on daily aspirin for 3 years experienced spontaneous hyphema a week after starting ginkgo (39).

 Dose

- Standardized leaf extract (Egb 761 and others) contains 22% to 27% flavonol glycosides (including quercetin, kaempferol, and their glycosides) and 5% to 7% terpene lactones (consisting of 2.8% to 3.4% ginkgolides A, B, and C and 2.6% to 3.3% bilobalide). Usual dose 40 mg b.i.d. to t.i.d.

? Common Questions and Answers

Q: Is ginkgotoxin present in leaf extracts?
A: A recent analysis shows that it is present in tiny quantities (36). Although leaf extract has not shown toxic effects in animal or human studies, long-term, high-dose safety studies are lacking. As a precaution, long-term ginkgo users should take 50 mg of vitamin B_6 daily.
Ginkgolic acids can cause rash; Germany, but not the United States, limits ginkgolic acids to 5 ppm.

Q: Why would anyone eat those foul-smelling seeds?
A: Americans often recoil at the thought of eating ginkgo seeds because they have smelled rotten fruit, which smells remarkably similar to dog feces because of short-chain carboxylic acids that are products of hydrolysis. Fresh seeds, however, shorn of their pungent pericarps, are odorless. Boiled before eating, ginkgo seeds are delicious and highly prized in Asia.

Ginseng

10 Second Take

Ginseng, a tonic herb, has corticosteroid and hypoglycemic effects.

Basics

LATIN NAME

Panax ginseng C.A. Meyer, other *Panax* species

FAMILY

Araliaceae

DESCRIPTION

- *Panax ginseng,* native to eastern Asia, is widely used in China, Japan, and Korea. *P. notoginseng* (1) F.H. Chen is from southwest China and *P. quinquefolius* L. (American ginseng) is cultivated in North America.
- Red ginseng is steam-treated; white ginseng is bleached with SO_2 before drying.

PART USED

Roots (main or lateral); root hairs are considered inferior

KNOWN ACTIVE CONSTITUENTS

- There are 2% to 3% ginsenosides (dammarane saponins) in the protopanaxatriol class (Rg_1, Rg_2, Rf, Re) and the protopanaxadiol class (Rc, Rd, Rb_1, and Rb_2). Also, an oleanolic saponin, polysaccharides, polyacetylenes, peptides, and lipids (1). Total ginsenosides are higher in than *P. ginseng*; Rb_1 is dominant in both, but the Rb_1:Rg_1 ratio is much higher in American ginseng. *P. quinquefolius* contains no Rf or Rg_2(2).

MECHANISM/PHARMACOKINETICS

- Ginseng has corticosteroid-like actions, hypoglycemic activity and affects neurotransmitter activity. A ginsenoside extract from *P. ginseng* demonstrated affinity for progestin, mineralocorticoid, and glucocorticoid receptors *in vitro* (3). In rats, ginseng saponins increase adrenocorticotropic hormone (ACTH) and corticosterone secretion (4). Ginseng inhibits platelet aggregation; a lipophilic fraction potently inhibits thromboxane A_2 production (5).
- In animals, Rg_1 is rapidly absorbed, metabolized, and distributed throughout many tissues; however, neither the saponin nor metabolites cross the blood-brain barrier (6). Urine and feces are the main routes of excretion. In rats, gastrointestinal absorption of Rg_1 is 1.9%, Rb_1 0.1%, and Rb_2 3.7%. Ginsenosides have low bioavailability; decomposition products may be more active (3). Absorption may require metabolism by intestinal bacteria. Rb_1 is associated with sedation, Rg_1 with mild stimulation.

Evidence

CLINICAL TRIALS

- Diabetes/glycemic effects

—A double-blind, placebo-controlled trial of two doses of (apparently Asian) ginseng extract (100 mg or 200 mg q.d. × 8 weeks) in 36 noninsulin-dependent diabetes mellitus (NIDDM) patients found that ginseng improved mood, vigor, well-being, and psychomotor performance (7). A dose of 200 mg significantly reduced HbA_{1c} and increased physical activity (but baseline values are not given).

—Three randomized controlled trials (RCTs) by the same investigator tested American ginseng. A placebo-controlled crossover study in 12 healthy participants found that 1, 2, or 3 g of ginseng reduced postprandial glycemia in a time-dependent but not dose-dependent manner (8). In 10 healthy participants and 9 participants with Type II diabetes given 3 g American ginseng 40 minutes before glucose challenge (9), ginseng reduced postprandial glycemia in both groups; concurrent administration reduced glycemia only in diabetics. Ten Type II diabetics were randomized to placebo, 3, 6, or 9 g of ginseng 120, 80, 40, or 0 minutes before glucose challenge. All doses reduced area under the curve (AUC) and incremental glycemia at 30, 45, and 120 minutes (10).

- Menopausal symptoms

—A double-blind RCT of 384 menopausal women found no difference between placebo and a standardized ginseng extract (100 mg G115, Pharmaton, × 16 weeks) on hot flashes, follicle stimulating hormone (FSH), estradiol levels, endometrial thickness, vaginal maturity index, vaginal pH, or scales assessing psychologic well-being index or menopausal symptoms (11).

- Impotence

—In 90 men with erectile dysfunction, Korean red ginseng (1,800 mg. q.d. × 3 months), compared with trazodone (25 mg q.h.s.) or placebo, significantly improved patient satisfaction, libido, rigidity, and tumescence and reduced early detumescence (12). Frequency of intercourse, premature ejaculation, morning erections, testosterone levels, and other measures were unchanged from baseline in all groups.

- Fertility

—In 66 men, ginseng extract (4 g/day) increased sperm counts from 15 million/mL to 29 million/mL in men with idiopathic oligospermia and from 5 million/mL to 25 million/mL in men with varicocele; normal controls increased from 85 million/mL to 93 million/mL (13). Motility also increased more in treated participants than controls. Testosterone levels increased in all groups.

- Ergogenics

—A review identified 11 controlled trials (10 described as double-blind, 7 reported only as abstracts) of ginseng and ergogenic performance. Seven found no effect; four found a positive effect. Six of seven trials since 1996 found no effect (14).

- Stress/adaptogenic properties

—A double-blind RCT of ginseng extract (G115, 200 or 400 mg/day × 8 weeks) found no effect on mood disturbance in 83 healthy participants (15). A double-blind placebo-controlled study in 112 healthy participants found no benefit of an Asian ginseng extract (400 mg q.d. × 8 to 9 weeks) in concentration, memory, or subjective experience (16). A placebo-controlled study of a commercial ginseng-multivitamin/multimineral preparation among 60 geriatric inpatients found no differences between groups in length of stay, activities of daily living, cognitive function, or somatic symptoms (17).

—A double-blind study of a multivitamin with or without ginseng in 625 patients with stress or fatigue found that ginseng significantly improved quality of life at 4 months (18).

- Cancer prevention

—Three epidemiologic studies (two case-control, one prospective cohort) in Korea, by the same investigator, linked ginseng intake with reduced cancer risk (19–21). (Ginseng intake could be a marker for other health-promoting behaviors.)

- Immunomodulation

—A double-blind RCT in 227 participants found that standardized ginseng extract (100 mg/day × 4 weeks before polyvalent influenza vaccination) used as a vaccine adjuvant reduced incidence of colds or flu (inexplicably combined), compared with placebo (22). Natural killer cell (NK) activity and antibody titers were higher in the ginseng-treated group at weeks 8 and 12.

—Ginseng (at 10 μg/kg concentration) enhanced NK activity in peripheral blood mononuclear cells from healthy participants and those with AIDS or chronic fatigue syndrome (23).

- Bronchitis

—A randomized, non-blinded trial tested ginseng extract (G115, 100 mg b.i.d. × 9 days) as an adjunct to antibiotics in 75 patients with acute exacerbation of chronic bronchitis. Bacterial clearance was faster in the ginseng-treated group than in controls (24). Only 44 cases were evaluated.

- Alcohol clearance

—In a crossover study, 14 participants consumed 72 g/kg 25% ethanol over 45 minutes; blood alcohol levels were 35.2% lower when subjects consumed 3 g ginseng extract with alcohol (25).

OTHER CLAIMED BENEFITS/ACTIONS

- Aphrodisiac
- Memory or performance enhancer
- Increased resistance to stress or disease

 Risks

ADVERSE REACTIONS

- Cerebral arteritis

—A 28-year-old woman who ingested about 200 mL of an extract made of 25 g ginseng stewed with rice wine developed severe headache, nausea, vomiting, and chest tightness within 8 hours; cerebral angiogram 6 days later revealed cerebral arteritis (26). Symptoms resolved over the next 10 days.

- Hypertension

—There are two case reports of hypertension reported in ginseng users (27).

- Estrogenic effects

—A 72-year-old woman experienced vaginal bleeding after taking a Swiss-Austrian ginseng formula (28).
—Another 44-year-old menopausal woman experienced episodes of uterine bleeding related to seasonal use of a ginseng-containing Chinese face cream (29). Rechallenge caused uterine bleeding 4 weeks later. Endometrial biopsy showed a disordered proliferative pattern.
—A 62-year-old oophorectomized woman had an estrogenized vaginal smear while taking ginseng; the effect disappeared 5 weeks after discontinuation and reappeared 2 weeks after rechallenge (30). Estrogen levels were not affected. No estrogens were identified in the ginseng tablet; however, saponins in a methanolic ginseng extract competed strongly for estrogen and progesterone receptors in human myometrial cytosol.
—Mastalgia with diffuse nodularity was reported in a 70-year-old woman taking powdered ginseng (31). Prolactin levels were normal. Cessation of use resolved symptoms, and rechallenge reproduced symptoms.
—Only one of these products was analyzed to exclude steroid adulteration.

- Mania

—A 35-year-old depressed woman interrupted her lithium and amitriptyline and began taking ginseng daily (32). Ten days later she was hospitalized for an acute manic episode.

- Stevens-Johnson syndrome

—A case of Stevens-Johnson syndrome was reported as possibly associated with ginseng (33); however, the patient used ginseng regularly and had recently taken antibiotics and a nonsteroidal antiinflammatory drug (NSAID), rendering this association improbable.
—Insomnia, anxiety, diarrhea, and skin eruptions may occur with ginseng use (8).
—Hypertension related to chronic ginseng ingestion has been reported (34) (see questions and answers).
—Traditional contraindications include acute illness, fever, menstrual irregularity, cardiac disorders, and bleeding disorders (27).

DRUG INTERACTIONS

- Phenelzine

—Combined use caused headache, insomnia, and tremulousness in a 64-year-old woman (35) and may have precipitated manic symptoms in a 42-year-old depressed patient (36) (manic symptoms were atypical, and the patient was also taking bee pollen, lorazepam, and triazolam).

- Warfarin

—A 47-year-old man stable on warfarin [international normalized ratio (INR) 2 to 3], (who was also taking diltiazem, nitroglycerine, and salsalate) ingested ginseng for 2 weeks, after which INR decreased to 1.5 (37). A subsequent rat study showed no effect of a single oral dose (2 mg/kg) or steady-state ginseng (0.2 mg/kg daily × 6 days) on the pharmacokinetics or pharmacodynamics of warfarin (38). Also, vitamin K was not detectable in ginseng.

- Caffeine

—Combined use with caffeine or other stimulants may increase side effects.

- Alcohol

—Enhanced alcohol clearance (see clinical trials)

PREGNANCY/LACTATION

- Ginseng is traditionally contraindicated in pregnant and lactating women and in children (except for specific conditions).

ANIMAL TOXICITY

- In mice, up to 6 g/kg intraperitoneally and a single 30 g/kg dose of a 5:1 extract was safe. Subacute toxicity studies at 1.5 to 15 mg/kg/day caused no adverse effects. Oral doses up to 15 mg/kg in male or female rats caused no adverse effects in two generations of offspring (3).

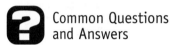 Dose

COMMON DOSAGE FORMS

- *Dried roots:* 0.5 to 3.0 g/day (chewed, in capsules, or as tea). Chronic daily doses are usually 0.4 to 0.8 g/day.
- *Liquid extract:* (1:2): 1 to 6 mL/day
- *Decoction:* made from 1 to 10 g dried root/day
- Courses of treatment may last 2 weeks to 3 months; (root-free periods of 2 weeks to 2 months are recommended). Ginseng is taken more than 2 hours away from food.

 Common Questions and Answers

Q: What is "ginseng abuse syndrome?"
A: This is a term coined in an uncontrolled study of 144 ginseng users (39). Fourteen participants reported nervousness, irritability, insomnia, and morning diarrhea. All were heavy caffeine users, so reported symptoms may be due to an interaction. Still, long-term, high-dose use (some used up to 15 g/day) is not recommended.

Q: What is the quality of commercial preparations?
A: Variable. Of 50 commercial ginseng products sold in 11 countries, 6 (including 2 sold in the United States) contained no detectable ginseng (40). Ginsenosides ranged from 1.9% to 9.0% by weight in the products that contained ginseng. One U.S. product contained ephedra.

Glucosamine

 10 Second Take

Glucosamine is a low-toxicity compound used to treat arthritis; efficacy has been demonstrated in clinical trials.

 Basics

DESCRIPTION

• Glucosamine is a small molecule, molecular weight 179.17, with a pKa of 6.91 (1); it is important in the formation of glycoproteins and connective tissue polysaccharides/ glycosaminoglycans, including those in cartilage.

FOOD SOURCES

• Glucosamine is found in low concentrations in meat (skin contains significant amounts).
• Commercially, it is derived from chitin, found in the shells of arthropods, including shrimp, lobster, and crab.

MAIN FUNCTIONS/PHARMACOKINETICS

• Glucosamine is a major substituent of glycosaminoglycan chains, including those in aggrecan, a proteoglycan that helps to provide hydrophilic properties, an important part of cartilage resilience (2). Cultured chondrocytes produce more aggrecan when media contains glucosamine.
• Glucosamine and N-acetyl-D-glucosamine (NAG) are constituents of connective tissue glycosaminoglycans (GAGs) and substrates for their biosynthesis; in addition, glucosamine and NAG inhibit their degradation (3). After an oral dose, glucosamine is incorporated into plasma glycoproteins; bioavailability is about 26% (4).

 Evidence

CLINICAL TRIALS

• A meta-analysis of glucosamine and chondroitin identified six studies of glucosamine for arthritis of the knee (5). Although these trials showed a beneficial effect, most trials were of poor methodologic quality (including particular deficiencies associated with inflation of treatment effects), so the authors of this meta-analysis note that the actual treatment effects may be lower. However, a commentary on this study notes that the quality of the trials was comparable to studies of nonsteroidal antiinflammatory drugs (NSAIDs) in osteoarthritis (6).
• A recent double-blind randomized controlled trial (RCT), not included in the previously mentioned meta-analysis, compared placebo with glucosamine (500 mg t.i.d.) for 2 months in 98 patients with osteoarthritis of the knee (7). Glucosamine was not better than placebo for reducing pain.
• Four trials have compared glucosamine to ibuprofen and found glucosamine to be as least as effective as ibuprofen (1200 mg daily dose). A double-blind RCT in 45 participants with temporomandibular joint osteoarthritis compared glucosamine sulfate (500 mg t.i.d.) with ibuprofen (400 mg t.i.d.) for 90 days (8). Participants were allowed to use acetaminophen. Both groups improved; in the third month those taking glucosamine had a significantly greater decrease in functional pain improvement and acetaminophen used than participants taking ibuprofen. A double-blind 1-month treatment-controlled trial of 200 patients with arthritis of the knee found glucosamine sulfate 500 mg t.i.d. as effective as ibuprofen in relieving symptoms (9). A double-blind 8-week study in 40 patients with osteoarthritis found that glucosamine sulfate 500 mg t.i.d. was more effective than ibuprofen (400 mg t.i.d.) in relieving pain (10). A double-blind study of 178 Chinese patients with osteoarthritis of the knee randomized half to receive glucosamine (500 mg t.i.d.) and half to receive ibuprofen (400 mg t.i.d.) (11). Both treatments improved pain and swelling to a similar extent; glucosamine was better tolerated than ibuprofen.
• A double-blind placebo-controlled RCT of 212 patients with knee osteoarthritis compared oral glucosamine (1,500 mg/day) with placebo for 3 years (12). Controls had a mean joint-space loss after 3 years of −0.31 mm (95% CI −0.48 to −0.13). Glucosamine-treated patients had no significant joint-space loss (−0.06 mm, 95% CI −0.22 to 0.09). Symptoms improved only in the glucosamine group.

ANIMAL/IN VITRO

• Antiarthritic effects have been demonstrated in animal models (6), including a recent placebo-controlled, blinded study in dogs that demonstrated that prior treatment with glucosamine hydrochloride and chondroitin sulfate protected against chemically-induced synovitis, associated bone remodeling, and lameness (13).

OTHER CLAIMED BENEFITS/ACTIONS

• Tendonitis
• Prevention of muscle injuries
• Repairs damaged cartilage

Clinical Considerations

LABORATORY TESTS

None identified

 Risks

ADVERSE EVENTS

• In clinical trials, glucosamine appears to be safe; some people have reported gastrointestinal discomfort.
• Insulin resistance

—Although not reported in humans, there is reason to be concerned about potential insulin resistance in adults with noninsulin-dependent diabetes mellitus (NIDDM). Although fasting glucose levels were not affected in either a 4-week or a 3-year study (14), insulin levels have not been studied in diabetics taking glucosamine (see questions and answers).

• An immediate hypersensitivity reaction to glucosamine sulfate in an elderly female patient has been reported (15).

ANIMAL TOXICITY

Insulin resistance (see questions and answers)

 Dose

• The usual dose is 500 mg t.i.d.; occasionally 1,500 mg q.d. is used.
• It may take several weeks to notice an effect.

 Common Questions and Answers

Q: Why is there reason to think that glucosamine may be a problem in diabetics?
A: Although one study has looked at fasting glucose levels in those treated with glucosamine and found no effect (14), insulin levels have not been studied in diabetics taking glucosamine. Two studies tested short-term glucosamine infusion in nondiabetics. One, in 18 participants, found no effect on insulin sensitivity (16); the other, in 10 participants, found no effect on glucose-stimulated insulin secretion but did find an increase in fasting glucose levels and the glucose threshold of glucose-stimulated insulin secretion (17).
Glucosamine increases insulin resistance in both normal and diabetic animals, through mechanisms that are not clear (2). Intravenous doses as low as 0.1 mg/kg significantly reduce glucose uptake in skeletal muscle (18). In rats, glucosamine induced significant insulin resistance both at the level of the whole body and in rectus abdominis muscle and blunted the increase in muscle glycogen normally induced by insulin (19). Time-dependent inhibition in postreceptor insulin signaling (necessary for glucose transport and glycogen storage) was also seen. In rats, severe impairment in insulin secretion induced by glucose or arginine were seen after intravenous infusion of 3.5 mg/kg/minute, which may indicate an adverse effect on beta cells (20). There is enough disturbing animal evidence to make it imperative to study the effect of glucosamine on insulin levels in diabetics.

Glutamine (Gln, Q)

 10 Second Take

Glutamine is harmless; parenteral supplementation may benefit critically ill or injured patients. Little evidence supports supplementation in gastrointestinal conditions, cancer, or chemotherapy-associated complications.

 Basics

DESCRIPTION

• Glutamine is a conditionally essential amino acid (it may become essential under highly abnormal conditions, especially in catabolic states such as severe injury, cancer, or infection).
• Glutamine is important as a nitrogen shuttle, cellular energy source, and component of proteins.
• It is the most abundant amino acid in the blood (1).

FOOD SOURCES

Most protein-containing foods

MAIN FUNCTIONS/PHARMACOKINETICS

• Glutamine is the most important nitrogen transporter, particularly for transporting ammonia from peripheral tissues to the kidney (which excretes it as ammonia) or to the liver (which converts it to urea).
• Glutamine also supplies cellular fuel and supplies carbon and nitrogen for metabolic intermediates.
• It is needed for the synthesis of purine and pyrimidine nucleotides and the formation of glucosamine. Hydrolysis of the amide group forms ammonia and glutamate (2). In catabolic states, nutritional support that includes glutamine spares muscle mass.

 Evidence

CLINICAL TRIALS

• Gastrointestinal disorders

—Glutamine is very important to gut structure and function, apparently stimulating mucosal growth and supporting intestinal immune surveillance (2). Large doses (more than 20 g/daily) of parenterally administered glutamine inhibit gut mucosal atrophy (3).
—Effects of oral or enteral supplementation, however, have not been impressive. A double-blind controlled trial of orally administered glutamine (4 g or 8 g/day × 28 days) in patients with AIDS who had abnormal intestinal permeability found no benefit in the glutamine-treated group (4). A study in children with active Crohn's disease found no benefit of a glutamine-enriched diet (5).

• Complications of cancer treatment

—A review of glutamine for the treatment of gastrointestinal disorders concluded that there is little evidence of benefit for chemotherapy-associated mucositis (6). More recent studies, not included in the previous review, have also been unimpressive; effects on mucosal protection are mixed, and improvement in pain was seen only in a subset of one study. In 24 patients with metastatic colorectal cancer, glutamine significantly reduced chemotherapy-induced mucositis and gastrointestinal ulcerations; however, there was no effect on chemotherapy-associated clinical side effects (7).
—A randomized, double-blind, controlled study randomized 66 patients scheduled for 5-fluorouracil chemotherapy to glutamine (4 g b.i.d. × 14 days) and 68 to placebo; all participants received oral cryotherapy (30 minutes of sucking on ice chips) before chemotherapy. There were no significant differences in mucositis scores between the two groups (8).
—In 193 bone marrow transplant patients, a swish-and-swallow formulation of glutamine (1g/m² /dose q.i.d.) was compared with placebo (glycine). Glutamine-treated autologous bone marrow transplant patients experienced less mouth pain and consumed fewer opiates, but there was no effect in allogeneic bone marrow transplant patients (9). Another study by the same author in 24 patients found that glutamine (2 g amino acid/m² b.i.d.), compared with glycine placebo, significantly improved chemotherapy-associated stomatitis (10).
—A study of glutamine (10 g t.i.d.) in 65 patients with advanced breast cancer receiving doxifluridine found no effect on diarrhea, response rates, median time to response, or median duration of response (11).

• Hospital course

—Small studies suggest that glutamine may reduce the length of hospital stays after resection for colorectal cancer or after bone marrow transplantation (3).
—A trial that randomized 84 intensive care patients to parenteral feeding with or without glutamine 25 g (glutamine replaced other amino acids isonitrogenously) found that supplemented feeds appeared to reduce mortality. Survival between groups was similar for the first 20 days but a later benefit was seen; significantly more patients receiving glutamate than those receiving unsupplemented parenteral nutrition (24 vs. 14) were alive at 6 months (3).
—In 72 patients with multiple trauma, those treated with glutamine-supplemented enteral nutrition had significantly less pneumonia, bacteremia, or sepsis than those receiving enteral nutrition without additional glutamine (12).

• Ergogenic effects

—Acute ingestion of L-glutamine (0.03 g/kg) in 10 trained males resulted in no effect on high-intensity exercise performance or buffering potential (13).

ANIMAL/IN VITRO

• Cancer

—Tumor cells use glutamine for growth; however, rodent studies appear to show that glutamine benefits animals without causing cancer to grow. In a rat sarcoma model, oral glutamine does not stimulate tumor growth but actually increases intracellular methotrexate and the effectiveness of methotrexate treatment. Glutamine also protects rats from acute and chronic radiation injury (1). A glutamine-supplemented diet reduced enterocolitis and mortality in rats treated with methotrexate and accelerated healing in rats given 5-fluorouracil (2).

OTHER CLAIMED BENEFITS/ACTIONS

• Cancer
• Gastrointestinal disorders

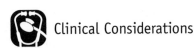 Clinical Considerations

 Risks

 Dose

LABORATORY TESTS

The free amino acid concentration in venous blood is 51 to 181 μmol/L.

No risks identified.

COMMON DOSAGE FORMS

Not established; most oral supplementation trials have used doses of 4 to 8 g/day.

RECOMMENDED DIETARY ALLOWANCE

Normally glutamine is not needed because it is produced endogenously.

Glycine (Gly, G)

 10 Second Take

Glycine is a safe amino acid that may be beneficial in reducing negative symptoms in schizophrenia.

 Basics

DESCRIPTION

• Glycine is the smallest amino acid in the body.
• It is a nonessential amino acid consisting of a single carbon molecule attached to an amino and carboxylic group.

FOOD SOURCES

• Most protein-containing foods.
• Endogenously, serine and glycine are readily interconverted by the addition or removal of a hydroxymethyl group (1).

MAIN FUNCTIONS/PHARMACOKINETICS

• Glycine is a major constituent of collagen. Glycine conjugation is important for detoxifying drugs. Glycine may also regulate glutamine metabolism within hepatocytes (1). In the central nervous system, glycine functions as an inhibitory neurotransmitter; also, a glycine site within the *N*-methyl-D-aspartate (NMDA) receptor complex must be activated in order for the receptor complex to function properly.
• A precursor for glutathione, creatine, and purine biosynthesis, glycine is also incorporated into porphyrins (hemoglobin and cytochromes) and may have a role in protecting tissues from ischemia, hypoxia, and reperfusion injury (2).

 Evidence

CLINICAL TRIALS

• Schizophrenia

—No trials have shown a beneficial effect of glycine on positive symptoms (hallucinations, disorganized thought); studies are mixed on negative symptoms (alogia, flat affect, anhedonia, apathy, motor retardation).
—A double-blind, placebo-controlled, crossover trial was performed in 22 treatment-resistant schizophrenic patients to assess the effect of a glycine solution (0.8 g/kg/day, a mean dose of approximately 60 g/day) or a taste-matched placebo solution as adjunctive treatment to antipsychotic medication (3). In this 6-week trial, glycine treatment resulted in a 30% ($\pm$16%) decline in negative symptoms [measured by the Positive and Negative Symptom Scale (PANSS); no significant changes in negative symptoms were observed during placebo treatment. Cognitive symptoms improved by 16% and depression improved by 17% during glycine treatment; no improvements were seen with placebo treatment. Changes in positive symptoms were not significantly different between treatment and placebo. Both glycine and serine serum levels increased.
—Another placebo-controlled 8-week study of 14 male schizophrenic patients found that 0.4 g/kg body weight (about 30 g/day) of glycine dissolved in juice as adjunctive treatment to neuroleptic and anticholinergic medications improved negative symptoms in all seven patients; only two of seven placebo-treated patients improved in negative symptoms (4). Neither group improved on positive symptoms, general psychopathology, or extrapyramidal side effects. After this study, all patients received glycine for an additional 8 weeks, in an open-label phase; those previously treated with glycine showed no further improvement, but those previously treated with placebo showed significant improvement in negative symptoms.
—A double-blind, placebo-controlled 12-week study of 19 patients with chronic, treatment-resistant schizophrenia tested the effect of glycine (30 g/day) as adjunctive treatment to optimal doses of clozapine (400 to 1,200 mg/day) (4a). Evaluations were done biweekly using the Brief Psychiatric Rating Scale, the Scale for the Assessment of Negative Symptoms, and the Simpson-Angus movement scale. Glycine was ineffective for decreasing positive or negative symptoms. In addition, it appeared to interfere with clozapine; patients treated with clozapine alone experienced a 35% reduction in positive symptoms.
—Earlier clinical trials using lower doses of glycine (5 to 15 g/day) either found no effect of glycine on schizophrenia or found some effect only on negative symptoms (5). Cycloserine, a partial glycine agonist, is currently undergoing study and appears promising.

ANIMAL/IN VITRO

• In animal models, glycine has cytoprotective effects in the stomach, kidney, liver and cardiovascular system against a variety of chemical insults (1). Representative studies follow. A study in rats given the liver carcinogen W Y-14,643 found that glycine (as 5% of the diet) did not inhibit early foci formation but significantly decreased their ability to progress to tumors (6).
• Intravenous glycine improved survival after hemorrhagic shock in rats in a dose-dependent manner. Although 20% of saline-treated rats survived 72 hours after shock, glycine administered in a dose of 45 mg/kg increased survival to 78% (7).
• Two studies have found that dietary glycine prevents cyclosporine A-induced nephrotoxicity in rats. Rats fed a diet containing glycine (5%) for 3 days before cyclosporine treatment were compared with rats maintained on a control diet. Dietary glycine prevented or significantly reduced kidney damage resulting from cyclosporine in all parameters studied (8). Another study found similar results and noted that glycine minimized hypoxia and blocked free radical reduction without altering cyclosporine A blood levels (9).
• Alcohol-induced liver injury

—In rats exposed to ethanol continuously to cause alcoholic liver injury, administration of glycine after cessation of alcohol resulted in about a 30% more rapid recovery of liver enzyme level levels (serum aspartate aminotransferase and alanine aminotransferase), lower hepatic pathology scores and lower rates of steatosis than rats fed a controlled diet (10).

Clinical Considerations

FACTORS DECREASING AVAILABILITY/ABSORPTION

• Several hereditary collagen diseases (osteogenesis imperfecta, Ehlers-Danlos syndrome type IV, and epidermolysis bullosa pruriginosa) are due to the substitution of other residues for glycine in collagen; mutations in glycine receptors can also cause hereditary motor disorders (1).
• Glycine synthesis is marginal in early life; it may be conditionally essential in the neonate (1).

LABORATORY TESTS

• Free amino acid concentration in blood plasma is 179 to 587 μmol/L in venous blood and 226 μmol/L in arterial blood. Urinary output of glycine is 1,380 μmol/24 hours. Its half-life in plasma is 12 hours (11).

 ## Risks

ADVERSE REACTIONS

• None identified. There have been several clinical trials using glycine orally or parenterally; no safety concerns have been identified.

 ## Dose

COMMON DOSAGE FORMS

• Clinical trials have used doses of 5 to 30 g/day.

 ## Common Questions and Answers

Q: Why haven't there been more clinical trials of glycine?
A: Probably because it is widely viewed as having no pharmacologic effect. Glycine is often used as a placebo in amino acid studies, especially as a nitrogen source in control solutions. The possible activity of glycine makes it an inappropriate control. Some researchers have recommended that it be replaced by a mixture of nonessential amino acids (1).

Goldenseal

 10 Second Take

There are no clinical trials of goldenseal, an endangered plant, although trials exist for berberine (available in other, nonendangered plants).

 Basics

LATIN NAME

Hydrastis canadensis L.

FAMILY

Ranunculaceae (Hydrastidaceae)

OTHER COMMON NAMES

Yellow root, orange root, Indian turmeric, eye root, jaundice root, Indian dye, ground raspberry, and yellow puccoon

DESCRIPTION

• Goldenseal, a perennial, grows up to 30 cm high, with a hairy stem and lobed, sharply toothed, hairy leaves with small greenish white flowers and a compound berry.
• Goldenseal grows in rich shady woods in the eastern United States.

PART USED

Root, rhizome

KNOWN ACTIVE CONSTITUENTS

• Isoquinoline alkaloids, especially hydrastine (1.5% to 4%), berberine (benzyltetrahydroxyquinoline) (about 2.5%), and canadine (about 0.5%).
• Minor alkaloids include canadaline, hydrastadine, and isohydrastadine (1). Activity is attributed to hydrastine and berberine.

MECHANISM/PHARMACOKINETICS

• Berberine is not well absorbed orally; in rats, doses as high as 1 g/kg resulted in only traces of berberine in a few tissues. In rats, less than 1% of parenterally administered berberine is excreted unchanged in urine; the remainder undergoes hepatic biotransformation. The elimination half-life of berberine chloride following intraperitoneal or oral administration is 5 to 6 hours. No human pharmacokinetic data are available, but it is known that a significant quantity of berberine is excreted unchanged in urine (2).

 Evidence

CLINICAL TRIALS

• All clinical trials identified used berberine sulfate, not goldenseal (the amount of goldenseal that would have to be consumed to achieve these levels of berberine is unrealistically high).
• Giardiasis

—A clinical trial of berberine from *Berberis aristata* for giardiasis in more than 300 pediatric patients (5 months to 14 years) compared several doses of berberine (5 to 10 mg/kg/day × 5 or 10 days) with metronidazole 20 mg, quinacrine hydrochloride 5 mg, and furazolidine 5 mg. Ten days of berberine 10 mg/kg/day was effective and comparable to the pharmaceutical drugs (3).

• Trachoma

—A study of 190 children with trachoma compared drops and ointment containing placebo, 0.2% berberine, 0.2% berberine with 0.5% neomycin, or sodium sulfacetamide (20% drops, 6% ointment). Each was used t.i.d. × 3 months (4). The treatments were roughly equivalent in relieving signs and symptoms; 83.33% in the berberine group, 87.5% in the berberine/neomycin combination group, 72.72% in the sulfacetamide group, and none in the placebo group achieved clinical cure. However, only the combination treatment was significantly better than placebo in achieving microbiologic cure.

• Diarrhea

—Two of three trials of berberine and diarrhea found negative results. A randomized, placebo-controlled double-blind trial in Burma tested berberine with or without tetracycline on acute watery diarrhea (5). Patients were randomized to placebo q.i.d., berberine 100 mg q.i.d., tetracycline 500 mg q.i.d., or both berberine and tetracycline q.i.d. (placebos were used to equalize the number of pills and capsules).
—In 215 patients with non-cholera diarrhea, none of the treatments were more effective than placebo. In 185 patients with cholera, tetracycline was effective, significantly reducing the number of motions, duration of diarrhea, and volume of required intravenous and oral fluid. Berberine, however, was not significantly different than placebo. Berberine reduced cyclic adenosine monophosphate concentration 77%, possibly indicating a small, clinically insignificant antisecretory effect.
—A higher dose of berberine (200 mg every 6 hours) given with tetracycline (500 mg every 6 hours) was compared to tetracycline alone in a double-blind trial of 74 adult patients with cholera. There were no differences between groups in volume of stools, number of motions, or duration of diarrhea (5a).

—A randomized, controlled, non-blinded trial in Bangladesh of 165 adults with acute diarrhea caused by enterotoxigenic *Escherichia coli* (ETEC) and *Vibrio cholerae* examined the effect of a single dose of berberine sulfate (400 mg orally). Thirty-three patients with ETEC diarrhea were compared with 30 controls who received 100 mL water by mouth (a suboptimal placebo; berberine is bitter and stains stools yellow). Sixty-one patients with cholera were randomized to 400 mg berberine or no treatment; 41 patients were randomized to tetracycline or combined treatment (400 mg berberine q8 × 3 hours plus 1 g tetracycline). In patients with ETEC, berberine significantly reduced stool volume at 8, 16, and 24 hours. At 24 hours the mean stool volume in the treated group was reduced 48% compared with controls. Significantly more in the berberine group (42%) stopped having diarrheal stools within 24 hours, compared with 20% of controls (6).
—In patients with cholera, a single 400-mg dose of berberine reduced stool volume at 16 hours and 24 hours after treatment; there was no difference between groups at 8 hours. Those who received 1,200 mg berberine with tetracycline fared no better than those who received tetracycline alone. Few side effects were noted (transient nausea, abdominal discomfort and complaints about the bitter taste) (6).

• Congestive heart failure

—Twelve patients with congestive heart failure were given berberine 0.02 or 0.2 mg/kg/minute intravenously × 30 minutes (7). The higher dose significantly decreased systemic vascular resistance (48%), pulmonary vascular resistance (41%), right atrial (28%) and left ventricular end-diastolic pressures (32%), and increased cardiac index (45%), stroke index (45%), and left ventricular ejection fraction (56%) (all *p* <0.01). Four patients developed repeated runs of ventricular tachycardia with *torsades des pointes* 1 to 20 hours after the infusion.

CASE REPORT

• Gastric secretion

—A 1956 study on a fistulous subject tested the effect of several bitters and found increased gastric secretion after the administration of *Hydrastis* fluid extract (8).

ANIMAL/IN VITRO

• Cardiovascular effects

—Injected berberine lowers blood pressure, is vasoconstrictive, and stimulates bile secretion. Berberine or goldenseal root extract opposes the action of epinephrine (9). In dogs, berberine lowers peripheral vascular resistance and increases inotropic activity.

• Skin cancer

—In mice, berberine suppressed skin tumors induced by DMBA and telocidin (10).

• Uterine contractility

—Hydrastine and berberine affect uterine contractility and have central nervous system effects in very large doses when injected. However, these alkaloids are not absorbed following oral administration (9). Goldenseal causes strong uterine contractions in isolated mouse uterus, especially pregnant mouse uterus (2).

• Effects on bilirubin

—Berberine-containing plants have been associated with neonatal jaundice (11). Berberine appears to displace bilirubin *in vitro* and *in vivo*. *In vitro,* berberine was about 10 times as effective as phenylbutazone in displacing bilirubin. Intraperitoneal administration of berberine (10 and 20 μg/kg daily × 1 week) to rats significantly decreased mean bilirubin serum protein binding and persistently elevated steady-state serum concentrations of total bilirubin (12).

• Antimicrobial effects

—Goldenseal extract and several major alkaloids (berberine, canadine, canadaline, β-hydrastine) were active against *Staphylococcus aureus, Staphylococcus sanguis, Escherichia coli, Pseudomonas aeruginosa,* and *Candida albicans;* different alkaloids contributed markedly different effects (13).

• Immunomodulatory effects

—Rats treated with goldenseal root extract over 6 weeks showed increased primary IgM response during the first 2 weeks (14).
—Berberine was immunosuppressive in a mouse model of autoimmune tubulo-interstitial nephritis (15).

• Anticancer effects

—*In vitro,* berberine inhibits COX-2 transcriptional activity in colon cancer cells at concentrations higher than 0.3 mM; the effect is dose dependent (16).
—Berberine inhibits *N*-acetyltransferase activity in human bladder tumor cells (17), and induces apoptosis in human leukemia HL-60 cells, associated with downregulation of nucleophosmin/B23 and telomerase activity (18). Berberine had an antitumor effect on six types of esophageal cancer cells *in vitro* (19).

OTHER CLAIMED BENEFITS/ACTIONS

• Mouth sores (topical)
• Eye irritation (topical)
• Menorrhagia
• Liver ailments
• Gastritis and other stomach ailments
• Rattlesnake bites

 ## Risks

ADVERSE REACTIONS

• Berberine is well tolerated in doses up to 0.5 g.
• Nausea, emesis, and gastrointestinal discomfort have been reported.
• Possible mucosal ulceration.
• Ventricular tachycardia with *torsades des pointes* (berberine).

DRUG INTERACTIONS

May interfere with tetracycline (5)

PREGNANCY/LACTATION

• No information available. However, its use is not recommended during pregnancy.

ANIMAL TOXICITY

• The oral LD_{50} in mice of berberine is 3.29 mg/10 g (orally administered berberine sulfate). In cats, 25 mg/kg induces sedation and 100 mg/kg is lethal. In rats, oral doses of 100 mg/kg berberine sulfate are well tolerated. A dose of 25 mg/kg berberine sulfate administered orally for 10 days to cats was not associated with any gross microscopic changes; however, doses of 50 or 100 mg/kg induced hemorrhagic inflammation of the intestines. In dogs, 2.75 g of berberine administered produced gastrointestinal irritation and inflammation and paralysis.

 ## Dose

COMMON DOSAGE FORMS

• *Decoction, capsules, other preparations:* 0.5 to 1 g t.i.d.
• *Tincture:* (1:10 in 60% alcohol) 2 to 4 mL t.i.d.
• *Liquid extract:* (1:1 in 60% alcohol) 0.3 to 1 mL t.i.d.

 ## Common Questions and Answers

Q: Can goldenseal cause false-negative drug testing?
A: No. The rumor that goldenseal will prevent standard testing procedures from detecting opiates in the urine has a long history, but a study found no effect. Codeine (120 mg) was given to several subjects and then goldenseal (15.6 g) given over the next 2½ days. Goldenseal did not mask the detection of opiates in urine. Apparently, administration of goldenseal to horses increases urine volume, specific gravity, and acidity, causing a significant decrease in total morphine excreted 5 to 6 hours after dosing. However, this is unlikely to interfere with the urine test used in humans. The myth that goldenseal compromises urine opiate testing apparently comes from a turn-of-the-century novel by John Uri Lloyd called *Stringtown on the Pike* (20). Some myths never die.

Q: Where does the name come from?
A: The cup-like scars of previous annual stems on the rhizome look like the wax seals formerly used to seal envelopes (21).

Q: Why shouldn't goldenseal be used?
A: Goldenseal is endangered, has no unique medicinal uses that have been validated, and should not be used medicinally. Substitutes include goldthread [*Coptis trifolia* (L.) Salisb.], which contains berberine coptine; *Coptis chinensis* Franch. (a Chinese cultivated variety with large roots); Oregon grape [*Mahonia aquafolium* (Pursh) Nutt.] or barberry (*Berberis vulgaris* L.), all of which contain berberine.

Gotu Kola

10 Second Take

Gotu kola is a benign Ayurvedic tonic herb; recent controlled trials indicate a benefit of a fraction of the herb for chronic venous insufficiency.

Basics

LATIN NAME

Centella asiatica (L.) Urban., *Hydrocotyle asiatica* L.

FAMILY

Apiaceae

OTHER COMMON NAMES

Pennywort, Asiatic pennywort, *Mandukaparni*, *Brahma-manduki* (Hindi), *Tsubo-kusa* (Japanese), *Luei Gong Gen* or *Tungchian* (Chinese), and *idrocotile* (Italian)

DESCRIPTION

• A slender trailing perennial herb with long, prostrate stems.
• It is indigenous to the tropics of both hemispheres, including Africa, Australia, Asia, Central America, South America, and the southern United States. It is particularly common in swampy areas of India, Sri Lanka, Pakistan, and the Islamic Republic of Iran.
• The leaves are eaten raw, cooked or in teas; in Thailand the juice of the leaves is mixed with water and sweetened.

PART USED

Aerial parts, entire plant

KNOWN ACTIVE CONSTITUENTS

• The triterpenes asiatic acid and madecassic acid (approximately 2%) and their triterpene ester glycosides asiaticoside and madecassoside.
• One study found the following amounts of these terpenoid compounds: asiatic acid 7.02 mg/g, asiaticoside 9.21 mg/g, madecassic acid 7.89 mg/g, and madecassoside 0.051 mg/g (1).
• The essential oil contains large amounts of an unidentified terpene acetate, as well as *trans*-β farnesene, germacrene D, and β-caryophyllene (1).

MECHANISM/PHARMACOKINETICS

• Asiaticoside is converted to asiatic acid, and equimolar doses of asiatic acid 12 mg or asiatoside 24 mg showed comparable bioavailability in 12 volunteers tested; steady-state area under the curve (AUC) 0 to 12 hours was 614 ± 250 ng.h/mL after asiatic acid and 606 ± 316 ng.h/mL after asiaticoside (2).
• Peak plasma concentrations of total triterpenic fraction (TTFCA) found that single 30 or 60 mg doses did not affect peak plasma concentrations but that chronic dosing (30 or 60 mg daily) increased peak plasma concentrations, AUC 0 to 24 hours, and half-life (3).

Evidence

CLINICAL TRIALS

• Venous insufficiency

—A placebo-controlled study compared two doses of TTFCA from *Centella asiatica* in patients with venous hypertension (ambulatory venous pressure > 42 mm Hg) for 4 weeks (4). Twenty patients received TTFCA 60 mg t.i.d., 20 patients received 30 mg t.i.d., and 12 patients received placebo. Ten normal participants received TTFCA 60 mg t.i.d. After 4 weeks of treatment there was a significant, dose-dependent decrease of capillary filtration rate (assessed by venous occlusion plethysmography), ankle edema and ankle circumference, and symptoms in the venous hypertension patients. Patients also improved in a novel test, the ankle edema coin tester (time to disappearance of marks made by "coins" placed under a sphygmomanometer cuff inflated for 10 minutes at 70 mm Hg). There were no significant changes in the placebo group or in normal participants treated with TTFCA.
—In another randomized double-blind placebo-controlled study of 94 patients (86 women) aged 20 to 80 years with venous insufficiency of the lower limbs, a reconstituted mixture of asiatic acid, madecassic acid, and asiaticoside (TECA) was tested in two doses (30 or 60 mg b.i.d.) (5). A significant improvement in the TECA group was seen for edema, symptoms of fullness in the lower limbs, and overall patient evaluation. Venous distensibility measured by mercury strain gauge plethysmography (limb volume increase under cuff pressure). Compared with placebo, the 120-mg TECA group experienced significant improvement in lower limb heaviness, standing lower limb pain, and global evaluation of efficacy; the 60-mg dose was not significantly better than placebo for these parameters. For edema, both doses of TECA were significantly better than placebo. Although venous distensibility improved in both treated groups and worsened in the placebo group, these differences were not statistically significant. The incidence of side effects did not differ among groups; two patients in the TECA group discontinued because of gastric pain.
—In a double-blind, placebo-controlled trial of TTFCA (30 mg b.i.d. or 60 mg b.i.d.) in 87 patients with chronic venous hypertensive microangiopathy, a dose-related improvement in microcirculatory parameters was found (6).

- Anxiety

—A double-blind, placebo-controlled trial of gotu kola (12 g crude powder, in a single dose mixed with grape juice) in 40 participants found that gotu kola significantly reduced the acoustic startle response (ASR) (reflex blinking in response to loud noise; a response aggravated by fear, anxiety, stress-related disorders, and anxiogenic substances) (7). There was no effect on mood, heart rate, or blood pressure.

—A review of gotu kola found numerous reports of benefit of extracts for dermatologic conditions, including wound healing, burns, scleroderma, prevention of keloid formation, skin ulcers, cellulites, and leprosy; most of these reports are more than 30 years old (1).

ANIMAL/IN VITRO

- Antimicrobial effects

—Although a publication in 1950 noted that asiaticoside treatment resulted in faster recovery of guinea pigs from tuberculosis, another publication from 1951 noted that asiatic acid was not therapeutic and actually hastened development of the disease (1).

—A dry powder of gotu kola had no direct action on the viability or acid-fastness of *Mycobacterium tuberculosis* H37rv *in vitro* (8). Isolated constituents may do better; another study found that liposomal asiaticoside showed better activity against *Mycobacterium leprae* and *M. tuberculosis* than free asiatocoside both in *in vitro* and *in vivo* studies in mice (9).

—A water extract of gotu kola was active against herpes simplex virus 1 and 2 in a plaque inhibition assay (10).

- Wound healing/radiation dermatitis

—Topical application of asiaticoside has significant wound healing activity in both normal wound healing in guinea pigs (0.2% solution) and delayed-type wound healing in diabetic rats (0.4% solution). In addition, asiaticoside was active orally at 1 mg/kg in the guinea pig punch wound model (11). In experimental wounds in rats titrated extract of *Centella asiatica* (TECA) stimulated extracellular matrix accumulation; asiatic acid and asiaticoside were the most active triterpenes (12). Another study of an aqueous extract of *Centella asiatica* on induced wounds in rats found increased collagen content, increased tensile strength, faster epithelialization, and faster wound contraction, compared with control wounds (13). Both collagen and glycosaminoglycan synthesis were stimulated. Asiaticoside (0.2%) topically applied twice daily for 7 days in two experimental wounds increased levels of several antioxidants in newly formed tissues (14).

—In rats, an extract of *Centella asiatica* caused an earlier but significantly less severe, skin reaction in acute radiation dermatitis but was not as effective as tetrandrine (15).

- Ulcers

—An extract of gotu kola significantly inhibited stress-induced gastric ulcers (16); another study found hastened scar formation in duodenal tissue after chemically induced ulceration in Wistar rats (1).

- Stress reduction

—An ethanol extract of *Centella asiatica* demonstrated significant antistress activity similar to diazepam in rats (17). Mild sedative and anxiolytic effects have been demonstrated in mice (18).

- Cancer

—Oral administration of *Centella asiatica* extract, as well as a partially purified fraction, retarded the development of solid and ascites tumors and increased the lifespan of tumor-bearing mice (19).

OTHER CLAIMED BENEFITS/ACTIONS

- Leprosy
- Liver problems
- Fevers
- Analgesic
- Antiinflammatory
- Aphrodisiac
- Psychiatric problems
- Contraceptive
- Lupus
- Eczema
- Psoriasis

 Risks

ADVERSE REACTIONS

- *Centella asiatica* is a weak sensitizer; although occasional cases of contact dermatitis are reported, the risk of acquiring contact sensitivity to this plant or its constituents is low (20).
- Clinical studies have demonstrated good tolerance to *Centella* extracts and to asiaticoside (1).

ANIMAL TOXICITY

- In mice and rabbits, the toxic dose of asiaticoside is 40 to 50 mg/kg body weight.
- In mice and rabbits, subcutaneous administration of 0.04 to 0.05 g asiaticoside/kg body weight was toxic; doses of 0.2 to 0.25 g/kg body weight increased blood coagulation time (1).
- Orally, 1 g asiaticoside/kg body weight is not toxic; oral toxicity of standardized extract and asiaticoside is reported to be low.
- Topical asiaticoside produced papillomas and one dermal sarcoma in hairless mice (1).

 Dose

COMMON DOSAGE FORMS

- *Standardized extracts* (of a triterpenic extract, standardized to contain 40% asiaticoside, 29% to 30% asiatic acid, 29% to 30% madecassic acid, and 1% to 2% madecassoside) 20 to 40 mg t.i.d.
- Standardized preparations available in Europe include Centelase, Madecassol, and TECA
- *Dried leaf:* 0.6 g b.i.d. to t.i.d.
- *Infusion:* made from 0.6 g herb t.i.d. (up to a total daily dose of 2 to 4 g).
- *Tincture (1:5):* 10 to 20 mL per day
- *Fluid extract (1:1):* 2 to 4 mL per day
- Topical: Infusions may be used to soak compresses
- Children

—Should not be used for children younger than 2 years.
—In older children, low-strength preparations should be used.

- Older adults

—Low-strength preparations should be used.

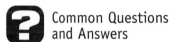 Common Questions and Answers

Q: Where does the name gotu kola come from?
A: In Sinhalese, gotu kola means cup-shaped leaf.

Hawthorn

 10 Second Take

Hawthorn is a benign herb that may be very useful for patients with congestive heart failure (CHF) or arrhythmias.

 Basics

LATIN NAME

Crataegus laevigata (Poir) DC, syn. *Crataegus oxyacantha* L., *C. monogyna* Jacq., and other species

FAMILY

Rosaceae

OTHER COMMON NAMES

Haw, may, may-bush, whitethorn, maythorn, hogapple

DESCRIPTION

• A shrub or tree, usually with long thorns on its branches, hawthorn has white flowers in late spring and red fruit in the fall.
• There are approximately 280 species.
• Hawthorn fruits have been eaten fresh, dried, or preserved by many groups and are currently used in jams in Europe and fruit candies and wine in China (1).

PART USED

Flower, leaf, fruit

KNOWN ACTIVE CONSTITUENTS

• Fruit

—Procyanidins (0.1% to 6.9%) are the primary active constituent in fruit; these are mostly (−) epicatechin subunits, with a small amount of diastereoisomeric (+) catechin. The fruit contains 0.3% to 0.5% triterpene acids including ursolic acid, crataegolic acid, flavonglycosides, and flavone-*C*-glycosides (hyperoside, vitexin-2″-*O*-rhamnoside, vitexin, and isovitexin) (2). Other components include quercetin derivatives, rutin, sugar (35%), and vitamin C.

• Leaf and flower

—Flavonoids (0.5% to 1.5%) including hyperoside, vitexin-2″-*O*-rhamnoside, and acetylvitexin-2″-*O*-rhamnoside are the main active constituents in leaves and flowers. Other compounds include flavans and procyanidins (1.9% to 3.8%), pentacyclic triterpenoid acids (0.6%) (including ursolic acid, crataegolic acid, and oleanolic acid), flavanol aglycones and flavonol-*O*-glycosides (including quercetin, kaempferol, hyperoside), the flavone-*C*-glycosides (primarily vitexin 0.02%), and flavone-*C*-*O*-glycosides (including vitexin-2″-*O*-rhamnoside) (3).

MECHANISM/PHARMACOKINETICS

• Pharmacokinetic data on the oligomer procyanidins show that these compounds are readily absorbed after oral administration and easily taken up by tissues. After oral administration of ^{14}C-labeled flavans/procyanidins in mice, 65% of trimer procyanidins were detected in the blood 1 hour after administration; 81% was detectable in organs at 7 hours (2). No pharmacokinetics data on specific procyanidins in hawthorn are available.
• The mechanism of action of hawthorn is unknown. Hawthorn extracts have antioxidant and vasodilatory effects; it is thought that the mechanism of action for a positive inotropic effect is phosphodiesterase inhibition.

 Evidence

CLINICAL TRIALS

• CHF

—A randomized, placebo-controlled trial of 209 patients (197 completed) with NYHA Class III heart failure tested two doses of a commercial preparation of hawthorn leaves and flowers (Schwabe's WS 1442, 450 mg or 900 mg twice daily) as an adjunctive treatment for 16 weeks (4). Maximal tolerated workload was significantly increased in the 1,800 mg group, compared to placebo; there was no difference between the 900 mg dose and placebo. Both hawthorn doses decreased typical symptoms of heart failure, compared to placebo. Hawthorn was well tolerated.
—A randomized placebo-controlled trial of 78 patients with NYHA Class II heart failure found that a commercial preparation of hawthorn leaves and flowers resulted in increased working capacity and decreased symptoms at 1 and 2 months (5). In the group receiving hawthorn (200 mg t.i.d.), working capacity by bicycle ergometry increased significantly from 79 watts at baseline to 107 watts 2 months later (benefits were apparent at 1 month). The placebo group increased from 71 watts at baseline to 76 watts at 2 months. Systolic blood pressure (at maximal exercise load) decreased from 171 to 164 mm Hg in the *Crataegus* group; there was no significant difference in diastolic pressure.
—Several studies published in German have found improvement in cardiac function parameters (cardiac output, exercise tolerance, blood pressure, heart rate) with *Crataegus* preparations (6). One of these trials compared hawthorn (LI132 Faros 300 mg t.i.d.) to captopril (12.5 mg t.i.d.) in 132 patients with Class II cardiac insufficiency. Improvement was measured by bicycle ergometry at 8 weeks. The hawthorn group increased from 83 watts to 97 watts, whereas the group receiving captopril improved from 83 watts to 99 watts. Hawthorn was associated with fewer side effects than captopril.

• Hypercholesterolemia

—An uncontrolled study of a hawthorn drink fortified with vitamin C and zinc (250 mL b.i.d. × 1 month) was carried out on 30 hyperlipidemic volunteers (7). Compared with baseline, the drink significantly reduced serum cholesterol, triglycerides, low density lipoprotein (LDL), apolipoprotein-B, and serum malondialdehyde; there was no effect on high density lipoprotein (HDL) or apolipoprotein-A1. Total cholesterol was reduced from 7.31 ± 1.04 μmol/L to 6.19 ± 1.56 μmol/L, triglycerides from 1.93 ± 0.92 μmol/L to 1.75 ± 0.96 μmol/L, and LDL from 3.95 ± 1.14 μmol/L to 3.54 ± 0.96 μmol/L.

ANIMAL/IN VITRO

• In a rat model, hawthorn reduced reperfusion-induced ventricular fibrillation. In rats subjected to left coronary artery ischemia for 7 minutes, followed by reperfusion for 15 minutes, ventricular fibrillation occurred in less than 20% of animals receiving hawthorn extract (0.5 mg/kg or 5 mg/kg), compared with 88% of the animals in the control group (8). In isolated rat myocardial cells, hawthorn extract increased both the amplitude and duration of cell contractions in a dose-dependent manner (30 μg/mL to 120 μg/mL); at higher doses (90 μg/mL to 180 μg/mL), the extract lengthened the refractory period from 144 minutes to 420 minutes (8).

• Hawthorn was tested in isolated normal and atherosclerotic segments taken from human coronary arteries from heart transplant patients. Administration of hawthorn resulted in vascular relaxation (14% of resting tonus) in normal arterial segments and 8% vascular relaxation in atherosclerotic segments.

• In dogs and cats, *Crataegus* and several of its fractions increased coronary heart flow when injected into the coronary artery. Intravenous injection decreased blood pressure in rats, cats, and dogs (3).

• *In vitro* studies of guinea pig hearts showed that *Crataegus* increased coronary blood flow, had positive inotropic and chronotropic effects, and potentiated the effect of cardiac glycosides.

• An alcohol extract of *Crataegus* appeared to inhibit the effect of a hyperlipidemic diet in rats; an aqueous extract was reported to decrease lipid levels in rats fed a normal diet (2). Antioxidant effects have been demonstrated *in vivo* (3).

• Mild central nervous system (CNS) depression, including an increase in barbiturate-induced sleeping time and reduced motility, has been noted in mice given hawthorn extracts (9).

OTHER CLAIMED BENEFITS/ACTIONS

• Sedative/hypnotic
• Hypercholesterolemia
• Hypertension
• Dyspepsia

 Risks

ADVERSE REACTIONS

• Hawthorn is remarkably safe. No serious adverse effects have been reported.
• Minor symptoms reported by patients receiving hawthorn are unusual but include nausea, gastrointestinal upset, palpitations, headache, and dizziness.

DRUG INTERACTIONS

• May potentiate the effect of cardiac glycosides; digitalis dosages may need to be adjusted in patients taking *Crataegus*.

ANIMAL TOXICITY

• An acute oral toxicity study of a standardized hawthorn extract (WS 1442, standardized to 18.75% oligomeric procyanidins) in rats and mice found no deaths or clinical signs at doses as high as 3,000 mg/kg (10). Intraperitoneal administration caused sedation, piloerection, dyspnea, and tremor. LD_{50} was 1,170 mg/kg in mice and 750 mg/kg in the rat

• A 26-week chronic oral toxicity study using the same extract in rats and dogs found a no-effect level of 300 mg/kg/day in both species. In dogs given 30, 90, or 300 mg/kg, spleen weights were reduced compared with controls; no morphologic changes were seen (10).

 Dose

COMMON DOSAGE FORMS

• *Dried fruits:* 0.3 to 1 g t.i.d.
• *Tincture (fruit):* 20 to 40 drops (1 to 2 mL) t.i.d.
• *Tincture (herb and flower):* 20 drops b.i.d. to t.i.d.
• *Fluid extract (fruit):* 10 to 20 drops (0.5 to 1 mL) t.i.d.
• *Infusion:* 1 cup t.i.d.
• Also may be taken in jams, candies, or wine
• Germany's Commission E suggests a minimum daily dosage of 5 mg flavonoids calculated as hyperoside, 10 mg total flavonoids or 5 mg oligomeric procyanidins.
• Hawthorn extracts have also been used intravenously.

Common Questions and Answers

Q: Is hawthorn safe for long-term use?
A: Yes, hawthorn is remarkably safe and may be used indefinitely. It may take several months to see an effect.

Histidine (His, H)

 10 Second Take

Histidine is a benign amino acid that has been tested unsuccessfully for narcolepsy, weight loss, and anemia; it does appear to inhibit platelet aggregation.

 Basics

DESCRIPTION

Histidine is an essential aromatic amino acid that is part of most proteins.

FOOD SOURCES

Most protein-containing foods

MAIN FUNCTIONS/PHARMACOKINETICS

• Histidine is in most proteins.
• An important contributor to intracellular metabolism, it is needed for the formation of purines and pyrimidines. It is a substituent of carnosine and is the precursor of histamine. Plasma half-life is 6 hours (1).

 Evidence

CLINICAL TRIALS

• Anemia

—A randomized double-blind study of 16 uremic patients and 26 dialysis patients tested the effects of L-histidine 4 g/day versus placebo for a mean of 17.5 weeks. Hemoglobin and packed red cell volume increased slightly in both groups, but there was no statistical difference between the two groups (in fact, only the placebo group improved significantly over baseline) (2).

• Narcolepsy

—In an effort to determine whether histidine is a waking factor, L-histidine was administered to three patients with narcolepsy (20 g/day × 14 days), four normal volunteers (32.4 g/day × 5 days), and one patient with progressive systemic sclerosis (48.6 g/day × 16 days). No effect was seen on nocturnal electroencephalogram (EEG) sleep patterns nor in narcolepsy symptoms (3).

• Platelet effects

—Eighteen healthy subjects were given placebo or L-histidine 3 g/day for 7 days. L-histidine reduced spontaneous platelet aggregation significantly and inhibited the generation of platelet thromboxane B_2 but did not affect platelet prostaglandin E_2 synthesis (4).

- Weight loss

—L-histidine has been tested as an anorectic agent in eight normal volunteers who received 4 g/day of L-histidine in a double-blind crossover study. L-histidine therapy did not significantly change appetite, taste, or smell perception; food intake or body weight; serum zinc levels; or urinary histidine excretion (5).

- Rheumatoid arthritis

—Although several studies indicate that patients with rheumatoid arthritis (RA) have lower levels of histidine compared with family members without RA (6), a randomized, placebo-controlled, double-blind 30-week long trial of oral histidine (4.5 g daily) or placebo for the treatment of RA in 60 patients found no advantage in clinical measurements for histidine over placebo (7). Outcomes included grip strength, walking time, tender or swollen joints, morning stiffness, hematocrit, and sedimentation rate. No adverse effects were noted; a small decrease in rheumatoid factor titer and a small increase in hematocrit, relative to baseline, were noted in the histidine group. Salicylate levels were significantly different between the two groups, indicating that the placebo group may have increased their aspirin intake.

ANIMAL/IN VITRO

- Histidine and carnosine are both singlet oxygen scavengers; both improve functional recovery of isolated perfused rat hearts. Carnosine was more potent and more effective (8).
- In mice, both low and high levels of dietary L-histidine increased urocanic acid, a histidine derivative, in the skin and appeared to increase sensitivity to ultraviolet B immune suppression (9). A histidine supplement increased growth rate in mice; it appeared to stimulate increased absorption of zinc and also to affect the thickness of the growth plate in bone (10).

 Risks

ANIMAL TOXICITY

- In rats fed L-histidine in doses up to 2.5% of their diet for 104 weeks, increases in red blood cell count, hemoglobin, and hematocrit were seen at the highest dietary levels.
- Tumor incidence was not significantly different between the control group, the group receiving 1.25% histidine, and the group receiving 2.5% histidine (11).

CLINICAL CONSIDERATIONS

- Requirements

—It is not entirely clear that histidine is essential to adult humans; it is clearly essential to infants, who need 28 mg/kg/day. It is thought that adults need 8 to 12 mg/kg/day, but the actual requirement may be less than 2 mg/kg/day.

LABORATORY TESTS (1)

- 32 to 97 μmol/L in venous blood
- Urinary output 900 μmol/24 hours

Hops

10 Second Take

In addition to imparting a bitter depth of flavor to beer, hops contain a novel phytoestrogen and several potentially anticarcinogenic compounds that deserve further research. No clinical trials have been done on hops for sedation.

Basics

LATIN NAME

Humulus lupulus L.

FAMILY

Cannabinaceae

OTHER COMMON NAMES

Common hops, European hops

DESCRIPTION

• Hop is a prickly, twining perennial climber, with lobed, toothed leaves.
• Male and female flowers grow on separate plants; although the male flowers are small and grow in loose bunches, the female flowers are yellowish-green and cone-like, about 4 cm long.

PART USED

Dried female flowers (strobiles)

KNOWN ACTIVE CONSTITUENTS

• Hops contain a bitter resin that contains 2% to 10% alpha acids (phloroglucinol derivatives including humulone, cohumulone, and adhumolone) and 2% to 6% beta acids (primarily lupulone, colupulone, and adlupulone). Both are denatured during storage. Volatile oils (up to 1%) include myrcene; monocyclic terpenes including limonene and phellandrene; pinenes; sesquiterpenes; monoterpene alcohols; and an aliphatic alcohol, 2-methyl-3-butene-2-ol, which increases on storage and is thought to be a breakdown product of lupulon and humulon (1).
• 8-prenylnaringenin, a potent phytoestrogen, has been identified in hops (2). Several unique prenylated flavonoids have been isolated from hops.

MECHANISM/PHARMACOKINETICS

• No information on pharmacokinetics is available. Humulones and lupulones have antioxidant effects, including radical scavenging activities and lipid peroxidation inhibiting activity (3).

Evidence

CLINICAL TRIALS

A randomized double-blind trial, published in German, compared a hops-valerian preparation to a benzodiazepine and apparently found the treatments equivalent (4).

ANIMAL/IN VITRO

• Anticancer effects

—Three of six flavonoids derived from hops showed dose-dependent decrease in growth of MCF breast cancer, HT-29 colon cancer, and A-2780 ovarian cancer cells in vitro (5). Humulone, in a dose of 1 mg, inhibited the tumor-promoting effect of TPA-induced skin tumor formation after 9,10 dimethyl-1, 2-benzanthracene (DMBA) initiation in mice (and also reduced inflammation in two experiments) (6).
—Hops contain several unique prenylated flavonoids, some of which may have anticarcinogenic effects by inhibiting cytochrome P450 enzymes that convert procarcinogens to carcinogens. Two hops flavonoids, isoxanthohumol and 8-prenylnaringenin, were potent and selective inhibitors of cDNA-expressed human CYP1A2 (metabolism was almost eliminated with 25 μM 8PN and 100 μM isoxanthohumol), and another flavonoid, xanthohumol, inhibited cDNA CYP1A1 and CYP1B1 (7) (see questions and answers).

• Antidiabetes effects

—Colupulone lowered serum glucose levels after glucose injection in nondiabetic Swiss Webster mice (8).

• Sedation

—An alcoholic extract of hop flowers was shown to have a tranquilizing effect. 2 methyl-3-butene-2-ol is sedative in mice (1).

• Antimicrobial effects

—Several flavones have potent antifungal effects in vitro. The essential oil and solvent extracts of hops were active against gram-positive bacteria and Trichophyton mentagrophytes but had no effect on gram-negative bacteria or yeast (1).

OTHER CLAIMED BENEFITS/ACTIONS

• Appetite stimulant
• Premature ejaculation
• Irritable bowel syndrome
• Gastrointestinal cramps
• Gynecologic disorders
• Sedative
• Analgesic
• Kidney problems
• Insomnia

Risks

ADVERSE REACTIONS

- Amenorrhea or irregular menses have been reported in female hops pickers and have been attributed to phytoestrogens absorbed transdermally (see questions and answers).

ANIMAL TOXICITY

- The oral LD_{50} of lupulone is 525 mg/kg in mice and 100 mg/kg in rats.
- The powdered flowers have very low toxicity; in rats the acute toxicity level is 3 g/kg, and the subacute toxicity is 300 mg/kg/day (1).

 ## Dose

COMMON DOSAGE FORMS

- *Tea:* 10-g dried strobiles in 200 to 300 mL water/day.
- *Capsules, other preparations:* 0.5 to 1 g q.d. to q.i.d.
- *Infusions, decoctions:* 0.5 to 1 g up to q.i.d.
- *Liquid extract:* (1:1, 45% ethanol) 0.5 to 1 mL up to q.i.d.
- *Tincture:* (1:5, 60% ethanol) 1 to 2 mL q.d. to q.i.d.
- Hops are also used in baths or topical creams and lotions and are said to soften skin. They are also slept on, as hops pillows (volatile oils released while sleeping are said to have a sedative effect).

 ## Common Questions and Answers

Q: Which phytoestrogens are in hops?
A: Hops do appear to have estrogenic effects, and menstrual irregularities in female hops pickers have been attributed to phytoestrogens. However, hops appear to contain unusual phytoestrogens, not the ones common in other plants (coumestrol, genistein, and daidzein). This phytoestrogen in hops was previously thought to be xanthohumol, but a recent study using sensitive bioassays found that xanthohumol showed no activity. 8-prenylnaringenin, a potent phytoestrogen, was recently isolated from hops. 8-prenylnaringenin was more potent than coumestrol, genistein, or daidzein in several assays, including stimulation of alkaline phosphatase in Ishikawa Var I cells and competitive displacement from rat uterine cytosol by [2,4,6,7-3H]17B-estradiol) (2).

Q: Can hops interact with drugs?
A: Possibly. *In vitro,* prenylated flavonoids from hops inhibited cDNA-expressed human CYP1A2 (7), so, theoretically, serum levels of theophylline and other drugs that are metabolized by this enzyme could increase. It is not clear whether compounds from hops affect CYP 3A4, which metabolizes about a quarter of all drugs. CYP3A4 was not inhibited in Henderson's *in vitro* study. Two earlier mouse studies, however, found inhibition of CYP3A isoenzymes from dietary brewers yeast; subsequently colupulone from hops adsorbed onto yeast during the brewing process was identified as the inducing agent (9,10).

Q: So does drinking beer prevent cancer?
A: I would not go that far. Only a few grams of hops are used in brewing a liter of beer. Still, compared to other alcoholic beverages, beer may be a better choice than some. Of course alcohol intake is associated with gastrointestinal, breast, and other cancers, but beer may indeed contain some healthful compounds. Not only does it contain chromium and B vitamins but several flavonoids from hops have anticancer effects *in vitro*. 8-prenylnaringenin is found in levels up to 300 nM (100 μg/L) (2). One of the most potent hops flavonoids that inhibits the transformation of procarcinogens to carcinogens, isoxanthohumol, is the most prevalent flavonoid in beer, although it is not the most prevalent flavonoid in hops. Isoxanthohumol inhibits carcinogen-induced mutagenesis and formation of DNA adducts. (7).
It would be interesting if beer turns out to have health benefits, especially because beer was once thought quite unhealthful. The planting of hops was forbidden by Henry VI; Henry VIII forbade the addition of hops and sulfur in the brewing of ale. It had been said of hops that it was "a wicked weed that would spoil the taste of the drink and endanger the people" (11).

Q: Where does the name come from?
A: *Humulus* may come from humus, as the plant prefers moist rich soil. The Latin name *lupulus* means small wolf and was given to the plant by Pliny the Elder because of its tendency to wind around trees. Hops can strangle small willows with light climbing embraces, the way a wolf strangles a sheep (12). The word hops appears to be derived from the Anglo-Saxon *hoppan,* which means to climb.

Horse Chestnut

10 Second Take

Horse chestnut seed extracts (HCSEs) are benign, even in pregnancy. They can decrease symptoms resulting from venous insufficiency and may lessen leg edema from other causes.

Basics

LATIN NAME

Aesculus hippocastanum L.

FAMILY

Hippocastanaceae

OTHER COMMON NAMES

Buckeye, Spanish chestnut

DESCRIPTION

• A deciduous tree up to 30 m high with white flowers and prickly globular fruits, horse chestnut is native to Asia Minor.

PART USED

Seed

KNOWN ACTIVE CONSTITUENTS

• There are 3% to 10% mixed triterpene glycosides (saponins), collectively called escin or aescin. More than 30 different saponins have been identified. Aescin can be fractionated into β-aescin, which contains 22-O-acetyl compounds; cryptoaescin with 28-O-acetyl compounds; and α-aescin (a mixture of β-aescin and cryptoaescin).
• Horse-chestnut seed also contains flavonoids, sterols, essential oil, and 30% to 60% starch (1). The seed pericarp contains saponins and proanthocyanidins.

MECHANISM/PHARMACOKINETICS

• Aescin inhibits hyaluronidase at a very high dose (inhibitory concentration $[IC]_{50} = 149.9\ \mu M$) (hyaluronidase breaks down hyaluronic acid, the primary constituent of extravascular matrix around capillary walls) (1). HCSE (900 mg, standardized to 150 mg aescin) reduced the activity of enzymes that catalyze the breakdown of proteoglycans (a major component of capillary walls); this could reduce vascular leakage (1). Aescin enhances prostaglandin $(PG)F_{2\alpha}$ generation in veins (1) and also increases leukocytes in limbs affected by chronic venous insufficiency (2). Aescin reduces lower leg plasma extravasation (capillary filtration) by venous occlusion plethysmography (3).
• Both immediate-release and slow-release preparations resulted in maximum plasma concentrations between 1.9 and 3.3 hours. Terminal half-lives ranged between 17.8 to 21.2 hours for rapid-release forms and 18.5 to 24 hours for slow-release oral forms (1). The oral bioavailability of an aescin solution is only 1.5%. There is a pronounced first-pass effect. Only 0.1% of the dose is detected in urine (1). Plasma protein binding is 84%. Aescin from HCSE and aescin solution are equally bioavailable. In subjects who took 50 mg aescin in capsules (Venostatin retard), maximum plasma levels were 20 to 30 ng/mL 2 to 3 hours after ingestion (4).

Evidence

CLINICAL TRIALS

• A systematic review of double-blind randomized controlled trials of oral HCSE for patients with chronic venous insufficiency identified 16 trials that fit criteria; two were excluded because they were duplicate publications and one because a combination product was used (2). Trials ranged from 2 weeks to 12 weeks, and total daily doses of aescin were 100 to 150 mg/day. Of the eight placebo-controlled trials (four parallel groups, four crossover), all showed a benefit for HCSE including decreased lower-leg volume, decreased calf and ankle circumference, protective effects against edema, and a 22% decrease in capillary filtration rate. Leg pain, pruritus, and fatigue also decreased. Five treatment-controlled randomized controlled trials (RCTs) demonstrated efficacy of HCSE; three trials found HCSE equivalent to rutosides and one found it superior. One trial tested HCSE against compression therapy or placebo; both treatments were better than placebo and HCSE was superior to compression.
• In a randomized controlled crossover trial of HCSE in 50 pregnant women with lower extremity edema, participants received placebo or 600 mg HCSE, standardized to 100 mg aescin, for 20 days. There were significant reductions in foot circumference and pain, fatigue, swelling, and itching after HCSE treatment compared with placebo (5).
• A placebo-controlled study in 70 participants found that 2% aescin gel significantly reduced tenderness to pressure in experimentally-induced hematoma (6).
• Two placebo-controlled studies found that HCSE 80 mg or 360 mg (standardized to 90 mg aescin) increased venous tone and decreased venous capacity; intravenous administration of 20 mg had no effect on venous tone (1).

ANIMAL/IN VITRO

- Vascular leakage decreased after treatment with HCSE (2). In anesthetized dogs, local application of HCSE antagonized clamping-induced venous distension; intravenous administration (2.5 to 5 mg/kg i.v.) increased femoral venous pressure and flow without affecting arterial parameters. HCSE 50 to 400 mg/kg p.o. reduced chemically-induced cutaneous capillary hyperpermeability in rats and rabbits and increased skin capillary resistance in guinea pigs fed a scurvy-promoting diet (7). HCSE (200 mg/kg p.o.) reduced induced lymphatic edema in rats. HCSE has antioxidant effects *in vitro* and *in vivo* (7).
- Aescin inhibits hypoxia-induced activation of endothelial cells and the neutrophil adherence. Aescin (Reparil) (250 ng/mL or 0.22 μM) inhibited the adherence of HL60 (neutrophil-like cells) to hypoxic endothelium in perfused human umbilical vein exposed to hypoxic conditions (8). Aescin also decreased the subsequent production of superoxide anion and of leukotriene B_4. Alterations of the venous wall that occur in varicose veins may be prevented by maintenance of an intact endothelium during blood stasis in the lower limbs and prevention of neutrophil adherence and activation.
- Aescin enhanced venous tone in isolated rabbit, canine, and human veins (1) and, in venous endothelial cells subjected to hypoxia, attenuated the drop in adenosine triphosphate (9).
- *In vitro,* aescin delayed uric acid crystallization at very high concentrations (greater than 10 mg/L) (10). This level would be extremely difficult to reach clinically.

OTHER CLAIMED BENEFITS/ACTIONS

- Varicose veins
- Hemorrhoids
- Asthma
- Bronchitis
- Expectorant
- Hematoma
- Sprains, strains

 Risks

ADVERSE REACTIONS

- Gastrointestinal symptoms, dizziness, nausea, headache, and pruritus (2).
- An observational study in more than 5,000 patients found that mild adverse reactions occurred in 0.6%. Gastrointestinal symptoms and calf spasm were most common. Immediate-release preparations are associated with more stomach upset than slow-release preparations (11).

CONTRAINDICATIONS

Hypersensitivity

PREGNANCY/LACTATION

Horse chestnut extract is well tolerated in pregnant women (12).

ANIMAL TOXICITY

- In acute toxicity studies, the oral LD_{50} of HCSE is 990 mg/kg body weight in mice, 2,150 mg/kg in rats, 1,530 mg/kg body weight in rabbits, 130 mg/kg body weight in dogs (13), and 1,120 mg/kg in guinea pigs (1). LD_{50} by intraperitoneal administration was 342 mg in mice; by intravenous administration it was 138 mg/kg in mice, 165 mg/kg in rats, 465 mg/kg in guinea pigs, and 180 mg/kg in rabbits (1).
- Oral chronic dosing studies of HCSE in rats showed no evidence of toxicity up to 400 mg/kg for 34 weeks; in dogs, doses above 80 mg/kg over 34 weeks caused gastric irritation (13).

 Dose

COMMON DOSAGE FORMS

- Horse chestnut seed extract (HCSE)

—Dry extract 5.0 to 8.0:1 (w/w) (standardized to 16% to 20% triterpene glycosides calculated as anhydrous aescin): 250 to 313 mg extract b.i.d. corresponding to daily dose of 100 mg aescin. The slow-release form is preferred.

- Less common dosage forms

—*Bark:* 1 g as decoction b.i.d. to t.i.d for diarrhea. Bark infusion is also used in baths or in topical dressings.
—*Leaf:* 1 g as tea: two or three cupfuls of the infusion a day as a cough remedy.

Hydrazine Sulfate, Hydrazine Sulphate

 10 Second Take

Three of four U.S. randomized controlled trials showed no benefit of hydrazine sulfate for cancer. Hydrazine sulphate may improve nutritional status. Significant toxicity is associated with high doses.

 Basics

OTHER COMMON NAMES

Sehydrin

DESCRIPTION

• Hydrazine sulfate is an industrial chemical used in rocket fuel, insecticides, and rust-prevention agents, as well as in the refinement of metals, and as an alternative cancer therapy.
• History

—The main promoter of the drug is Dr. Joseph Gold, a research oncologist with the Syracuse Cancer Research Institute, who has based his work on the research of Dr. Otto Warburg, a 1931 Nobel Prize winner. Dr. Warburg theorized that although normal cells metabolize glucose aerobically, cancer cells metabolize glucose largely anaerobically, an inefficient process that requires the body to increase gluconeogenesis, an energy-intensive process. Because phosphoenol pyruvate carboxykinase (PEP-CK) is vital to gluconeogenesis, Dr. Gold theorized that blocking this enzyme would block the energy-wasting process of gluconeogenesis, thus reducing cachexia. Hydrazine sulfate was the most effective of a number of chemicals tested. (Most researchers believe that cachexia results from complex metabolic changes, including lipolysis caused by substances released by the tumor.) Dr. Gold subsequently noted some antitumor effect in animals (1).

MECHANISM/PHARMACOKINETICS

• Hydrazine sulfate inhibits PEP-CK and monoamine oxidase (MAO).
• Availability

—Hydrazine sulfate has Investigational New Drug status in the United States. It may be obtained legally in Canada with a medical prescription from distributors approved by the Health Protection branch of Health Canada. Its costs are not covered either by private or public insurance in North America.

 Evidence

CLINICAL TRIALS

• Lung cancer

—There are one positive and two negative controlled trials of lung cancer. Sixty-five patients with stage IIIb or IV non-small-cell lung cancer received either hydrazine sulphate or placebo in conjunction with conventional chemotherapy (2). Median survival for patients with an initial performance status of 0 or 1 (lower scores indicate higher performance) was significantly higher in the hydrazine sulfate treated group but not in those with an initial performance status greater than 2 nor in the group overall. Subjects on hydrazine sulfate ate more and albumin status improved.
—In 243 patients with unresectable non-small-cell lung cancer randomized to hydrazine sulfate or placebo in combination with cisplatin and etopiside, disease progression was worse in the hydrazine sulfate group (3). There was no significant difference in the groups in terms of median survival time, quality of life assessment, weight change, albumin levels, or toxicity.
—In another study, 291 patients with stage IIIb or IV non-small-cell lung cancer were randomized to either hydrazine sulfate or placebo for one month in conjunction with conventional chemotherapy (4). There were no differences in survival, tumor regression, weight gain, or nutritional status between evaluable members of the two groups (drop-out rates were greater than 80% in each group).

• Colorectal cancer

—In a placebo-controlled trial of 128 patients with metastatic colorectal cancer resistant to 5-fluorouracil (5-FU), no statistically significant benefit was seen in the hydrazine sulfate group in survival, tumor regression, or quality of life. The trial was prematurely halted when interim analysis showed decreased survival in the hydrazine sulfate treated group (5).

• Cachexia

—A placebo-controlled trial of 38 cachectic cancer patients found that hydrazine sulfate improved glucose tolerance in cancer patients (6). Several problematic studies showed beneficial effects on weight gain or maintenance in cancer patients (7,8).

ANIMAL/IN VITRO

• In mice, hydrazine sulfate has been shown to inhibit the growth of Walker 256 intramuscular carcinoma, B-16 mouse melanoma, and Murphy-Sturm lymphosarcoma but not L-1210 solid leukemia (9). Another experiment shows enhancement of chemotherapeutic effect by hydrazine sulfate in intramuscular carcinoma (10).
• In two human prostate cancer cell lines, hydrazine sulfate had no effect. *In vivo,* hydrazine sulfate had no effect on implanted Dunning rat prostate MAT-LyLu cells (11).
• In mice, hydrazine sulfate reduced endotoxin-induced mortality (12). This effect was lost at high doses.

OTHER CLAIMED BENEFITS/ACTIONS

• Breast cancer
• Colorectal cancer
• Lymphoma (Hodgkin's and non-Hodgkin's)
• Lung cancer
• Thyroid cancer
• Melanoma
• Neuroblastoma

Hydrazine Sulfate, Hydrazine Sulphate

 Risks

ADVERSE REACTIONS

- Anorexia
- Dizziness
- Drowsiness
- Excitation
- Impaired motor function
- Liver damage at high doses
- Nausea and vomiting
- Numbness of the extremities
- Peripheral neuritis
- Pruritus
- Seizures
- Hepatorenal failure

—A 55-year-old man with squamous cell carcinoma of the maxillary sinus presented with a 2-week history of rash, pruritus, malaise, and jaundice (13). The patient had refused conventional therapy and had been using hydrazine sulfate (180 mg/day) for 4 months, discontinuing the regimen when symptoms appeared. The patient developed fulminant hepatorenal failure and died. Autopsy of the liver and kidneys showed autolysis of the kidneys and submassive bridging necrosis of the centrilobular and midzonal areas of the liver; there was no evidence of preexisting liver disease.

DRUG INTERACTIONS

- Monoamine oxidase inhibitor (MAOI) dietary precautions should be observed in patients using hydrazine sulfate.
- Alcohol must be avoided while using hydrazine sulfate.
- Sedative-hypnotics.

—Concurrent use of tranquilizers, barbiturates, benzodiazepines, other sedative-hypnotics, or alcohol can decrease effectiveness and increase toxicity of hydrazine sulphate. Also, the effect of sedative drugs may be prolonged.

PREGNANCY/LACTATION

Pregnant women should not use hydrazine sulfate.

ANIMAL TOXICITY

Hydrazine sulfate appears to act as a carcinogen or cocarcinogen in several animal species (1).

 Dose

COMMON DOSAGE FORMS

- *Oral (60 mg capsules):* 60 mg q.i.d. × 4 days, then 60 mg b.i.d. × 3 days, then 60 mg t.i.d. × 30 to 45 days. After 2 to 6 weeks, the cycle repeats. Doses should be taken with meals.
- *Injection:* 60 mg (15 mL) as previously discussed in the oral form but no need to administer near mealtime.

 Common Questions and Answers

Q: Is hydrazine sulfate the same as hydrazine?
A: Hydrazine sulfate is one type of hydrazine; different members of this class of compounds can have quite different effects.

Q: Are any currently used drugs related to hydrazine?
A: Yes. Many hydrazine analogues were screened for anticancer activity; only one is used today for that purpose. Procarbazine, an *N*-methyl-hydrazine, is used with other drugs to treat a variety of tumors (14); it is approved for treating Hodgkin's disease and is part of the mechlorethamine, vincristine (Oncovin), procarbazine, and prednisone (MOPP) regimen. Isoniazid, used to treat tuberculosis, is also a hydrazine compound.

Hypericum or St. John's Wort

10 Second Take

St. John's wort (SJW), an effective antidepressant, can cause phototoxicity and interact with many drugs.

Basics

LATIN NAME

Hypericum perforatum L.

FAMILY

Hypericaceae/Guttiferae

OTHER COMMON NAMES

Klamath weed, goatweed

DESCRIPTION

• A common roadside weed with yellow flowers; the petals and leaves of St. John's wort (SJW) have numerous, punctate glands.

PART USED

Flowering tops (leaves, unopened buds, and flowers)

KNOWN ACTIVE CONSTITUENTS

• Hyperforin and hypericins (the napthodianthrones hypericin and pseudohypericin). Also many flavonoids, including rutin (especially in leaves), quercetin (especially in flowers), and kaempferol; luteolin; myricetin; quercitrin; isoquercitrin; gentisic acid; and leucocyanidin.

MECHANISM/PHARMACOKINETICS

• Mechanism of action has not been clearly defined. *In vitro* (at very high concentrations unlikely to be attained clinically), SJW inhibits serotonin, norepinephrine, and dopamine; the most potent effect appears to be on gamma-aminobutyric acid$_A$ (GABA$_A$) and GABA$_B$ receptors. SJW has weak monoamine oxidase (MAO) inhibiting effects *in vitro,* but not *in vivo* (1) (see questions and answers). SJW inhibits the binding of naloxone to μ-, δ-, and κ-opioid receptors (2).

• Phototoxic photosensitivity from SJW is due to hypericins, photoactive quinones that produce singlet oxygen and free radicals when exposed to light. In the dark, hypericin can reduce oxygen to superoxide radicals, forming semiquinone radicals.
• After one 1,800-mg dose of SJW extract LI 160 in 12 participants, the mean serum level of total hypericins by high-pressure liquid chromatography (HPLC) was 43 ng/mL, far below levels estimated to be phototoxic ($>$ 100 ng/mL) (3).
• Drug interactions appear to be due to induction of CYP3A4 and effects on the adenosine triphosphate (ATP) transporter P-glycoprotein. SJW does not appear to affect CYP1A2 (4).
• Clinical pharmacokinetics studies of a 0.1% hypericin preparation resulted in t_{max} 2.5 hours, c_{max} 4.3 ng/mL, and half-life 6 hours; 0.3% preparation resulted in t_{max} 4 to 6 hours, c_{max} 1.5 to 14.2 ng/mL, and half-life 24.8 to 26.5 hours; pseudohypericin t_{max} was 2 to 4 hours, c_{max} 2.7 to 30.6 ng/mL, and half-life 16.3 to 36 hours (5). Steady-state concentrations are reached after 4 to 7 days. After steady-state administration (3 $\times$ 300 mg/day for 7 days), the mean serum level of hypericins was 12.5 ng/mL (3).

Evidence

CLINICAL TRIALS

• Depression

—Most trials have found SJW effective in treating mild to moderate depression. A meta-analysis of 23 controlled trials (20 double-blind) with 1,757 patients found SJW superior to placebo in 15 placebo-controlled trials [odds ratio (OR) 2.67, 95% confidence interval (CI) 1.78 to 4.01] and as effective as standard antidepressants in 8 trials (6). Most trials were 4 to 8 weeks in duration. Single-herb preparations were tested in 14/15 placebo-controlled trials and 6/8 treatment-controlled trials (the rest tested combinations). Of 13 single-herb placebo-controlled trials that provided data on treatment responders, 55.1% of treated participants improved compared with 22.3% receiving placebo. Single-herb preparations were equivalent to low-dose tricyclic antidepressants (OR 1.10, CI 0.93 to 1.31). Fewer on SJW (19.8%) reported symptoms, compared with 52.8% on standard antidepressants. The trials in this meta-analysis were heterogeneous and used varying diagnostic criteria and dosages of herb.

—Recent trials, not including those mentioned previously, include a double-blind, placebo-controlled, multicenter randomized controlled trial (RCT) of 200 adult outpatients (67.0% female; 85.9% white) with major depression and Hamilton depression (HAM-D) 17-item scale scores of $\geq$20 who received placebo or a standardized extract of SJW 300 mg (Lichtwer Pharma GmbH) t.i.d. $\times$ 8 weeks; after 4 weeks, if needed, the dose was increased to 1,200 mg daily (7). There were no differences between groups in linear rate of change of HAM-D scores, Beck Depression Inventory, Hamilton rating scale for anxiety (HAM-A), or three other scales. The number of remissions was significantly higher in the treated group 14/98 (14.3%) than in the placebo group [5/102 (4.9%)]. Significantly more of those treated with SJW than with placebo (41% vs. 25%) experienced headache.

—Two recent double-blind placebo-controlled RCTs compared SJW to fluoxetine. One tested Ze 117(250 mg b.i.d.) against fluoxetine (20 mg q.d.) for 6 weeks in 240 patients with mild to moderate depression (8); the other tested a dry extract (LoHyp 57, 400 mg b.i.d.) against sertraline (10 mg b.i.d.) $\times$ 6 weeks in 149 participants (129 female) (9). Both trials found the treatments equivalent.

—Two recent trials found SJW equivalent to imipramine. One compared SJW extract (350 mg t.i.d.) to imipramine (100 mg/day in divided doses) for 8 weeks in 263 patients (197 women) with moderate depression (10); the other tested ZE 117 (250 mg b.i.d. $\times$ 6 weeks) against imipramine (75 mg b.i.d.) in 324 patients with mild to moderate depression (11). In both trials, treatments were equivalent.

• HIV infection

—Hypericin has marked antiviral activity *in vitro,* but a Phase I study of oral or i.v. hypericin in 30 HIV-infected adults found unacceptable phototoxicity and no benefit on viral load. All patients receiving multiple i.v. doses of 0.5 mg/kg and most receiving 0.25 mg/kg experienced moderate to severe phototoxicity (12).

• Neuropathic pain

—A double-blind, placebo-controlled crossover RCT in 54 participants with painful polyneuropathy found no benefit for SJW (Calmigen, Sanopharm A/S, Denmark) 3 tablets daily, containing 900 μg hypericins for 5 weeks (13).

OTHER CLAIMED BENEFITS

• Anthelminthic, antiinflammatory, anxiety, insomnia, diuretic, dyspepsia, insomnia, menopausal symptoms, migraines, nocturnal enuresis, premenstrual syndrome, sciatica, trigeminal neuralgia, wounds, ulcers, bites, urticaria, sunburn, myalgia (oil macerate, topical), sunburn prevention/treatment (oil macerate, topical), and oral cavity pain (infusion, gargled)

Risks

ADVERSE REACTIONS

• Photosensitivity

—A 61-year-old woman using SJW for 3 years developed elevated itchy erythematous lesions in light-exposed areas that resolved after discontinuation of SJW (14). A 35-year-old woman who took SJW (ground whole herb, 500 mg/day × 1 month) developed subacute polyneuropathy after sun exposure (15). Symptoms improved in 2 weeks and disappeared over 2 months.
—Photosensitivity, especially in fair-skinned individuals, appears to be dose-related. LI 160 caused increased erythema in light-sensitive volunteers exposed to ultraviolet A (UVA) after receiving 600 mg SJW t.i.d. × 15 days (1). However, another study of LI 160 tested single dose (6 or 12 tablets, containing 5,400 or 10,800 μg hypericin) and multiple doses of SJW (6 tablets with 1,800 μg hypericin × 1 day, then 3 tablets with 2,700 μg hypericin daily × 1 week) (16). Erythema threshold after UVB, UVA or solar-simulated radiation did not change. SJW did not influence erythema index or melanin index (the single dose apparently affected UVB-induced pigmentation).
—Hypericum gel applied to a sprained ankle, followed by ultrasound treatment and sunlight exposure, resulted in second-degree burns (17). Two women developed bullae after topical SJW and sun exposure (18). Phototherapy in a 63-year-old man taking SJW (six pills/day) resulted in follicular edema, urticarial edema, and burning pain (18).
—Topical SJW is less photosensitizing than oral or i.v. administration. Topical hypericum oil (hypericin 110 μg/mL) and hypericum ointment (hypericin 30 μg/mL) combined with solar simulated radiation in 16 volunteers did not change visual erythema scores, but the more sensitive photometric measurement detected increased erythema index after hypericum oil treatment (19).

• Mania (20,21)
• Gastrointestinal symptoms, including nausea
• Anxiety (22)
• Fatigue
• Erectile dysfunction
• Headache
• Adynamic ileus was reported in a 67-year-old woman with diabetes 2 weeks after starting SJW.

DRUG INTERACTIONS

• SJW induces cytochrome P450 isoenzyme CYP3A4 and P-glycoprotein 4.
• SJW lowers serum levels of the following drugs (in clinical studies or multiple well-documented case reports)

—Digoxin (23)
—Anticoagulants (warfarin and phenprocoumon) (24)
—Indinavir (25)
—Amitriptyline (26)
—Cyclosporine
—Oral contraceptives (27)
—Irinotecan

• SJW may lower levels of the following drugs (single case reports or inadequately documented case series)

—Theophylline (28)

• Other drug interactions

—Carbamazepine pharmacokinetics are not affected by SJW (300 mg standardized to 0.3% hypericin t.i.d. × 14 days) (29).
—Serotonin reuptake inhibitors (SRIs) (paroxetine, sertraline) or atypical antidepressants (nefazodone, venlafaxine): Mild serotonin syndrome (nausea, vomiting, anxiety, restlessness, diaphoresis) has been reported when SRIs or atypical antidepressants are combined with SJW, especially in older adults. Paroxetine was associated with excessive sedation in one case report (30).
—Sertraline and SJW added to testosterone resulted in mania in one case report (31).
—General anesthesia: Hypotension unresponsive to vasopressors during general anesthesia was reported in a 23-year-old woman who had been taking SJW for 6 months preoperatively (32). The patient was taking no other preoperative medications and had previously undergone anesthesia with a similar type and dose of anesthetic without problems.

PREGNANCY/LACTATION

• Two women who took SJW during pregnancy experienced no untoward events (33). (See animal toxicity.)

ANIMAL TOXICITY

• Rats fed SJW as 5% of their diet for 119 days experienced no adverse effects on the liver or any significant tissue lesions. Hepatic enzymes were induced. In chronic toxicity studies in rats and in dogs, only nonspecific symptoms of toxicity were seen (reduced body weight and slight pathologic changes in liver and kidneys, probably resulting from increased metabolic load) and some histopathologic changes in the adrenals. No effects were seen on fertility or reproduction (1).
• Forty-eight CD-1 mice were randomized to 180 mg/kg/day hypericum or placebo for 2 weeks before conception and throughout gestation (34). There were no differences between groups in physical milestones, reproductive capability, perinatal outcomes, or growth and development of first- or second-generation offspring.

Dose

COMMON DOSAGE FORMS

• Oral

—Standardized extracts (0.3% hypericin or 3% to 5% hyperforin) 300 mg t.i.d.
—Powder: 2 to 4 g t.i.d.
—Infusion: 2 to 4 g infused in water t.i.d.
—Tincture: (1:10) 2 to 4 mL t.i.d.
—Fluid extract: Equivalent to 0.4 mg to 1.0 mg total hypericin a day, in divided doses
—Powdered extract: Equivalent of 0.4 mg to 1.0 mg total hypericin a day, in divided doses
—300 to 900 mg extract a day, in divided doses (total hypericin 0.4 mg to 2.7 mg a day)
—Dosages are usually halved for children.

• Topical

—Oil macerate of flowers
—Leaf infusion
—Leaf fomentation
—Gels and salves

Common Questions and Answers

Q: Should patients taking SJW observe monoamine oxidase inhibitor (MAOI) dietary restrictions?
A: No. MAO inhibition effects have not been reported in humans. An older *in vitro* study of hypericin indicated MAO inhibition (35); however, more recent studies of hypericin affinity for three neurotransmitter reuptake sites found MAOI activity insignificant (36), and *in vivo* studies show no MAOI effects (37).

Q: Does SJW cause cataracts?
A: Reports associating SJW with cataracts stem from an *in vitro* study in which light-activated hypericin (at about 1,000 times therapeutic plasma concentrations) induced photopolymerization of alpha-crystallins from calf lenses (38). This test, in which a concentration of hypericin inconsistent with achievable serum levels was applied directly on an avascular lens preparation in the absence of antioxidants normally present in sera, is of questionable clinical significance. No eye problems have been reported in any of the many SJW trials.

Inositol

 10 Second Take

Inositol is a benign nutrient; evidence supports its use in respiratory distress syndrome in preterm infants, depression, panic disorder, and obsessive-compulsive disorder.

 Basics

DESCRIPTION

• Inositol is a nonessential nutrient that is part of the vitamin B complex.
• The stereoisomer myoinositol is made from glucose-6-phosphate by cyclization. A component of membrane phospholipids, it is a precursor for the phosphatidyl-inositol cycle, an intracellular second-messenger system for several neurotransmitters. It is usually present as part of phosphatidylinositol (which is abundant in plasma membranes of all cells).
• Plasma and several tissues (including the lens and epididymis) contain free inositol (1).

FOOD SOURCES

• Inositol is ubiquitous both in animal products (which contain free inositol and inositol phospholipid) and plants (which often contain inositol hexaphosphate or phytic acid) (2).
• Humans consume about 1 g/day of inositol. A normal adult synthesizes about 4 g (22 nmol/day) of inositol in the kidneys; other organs that can synthesize inositol from D-glucose include the testes, brain, liver, and mammary glands.
• Breast milk is very high in inositol (both free inositol and the derivative 6-β-galactinol); colostrum is even higher (2).

MAIN FUNCTIONS/PHARMACOKINETICS

• Inositol is rapidly metabolized and has about one third of the calories of glucose. Humans given 3 g of inositol experienced a tripling of blood inositol levels (3); 12 g/day orally increased inositol levels in cerebro-spinal fluid by 70% in eight patients (4).
• Inositides are abundant in the brain and may be involved in neurotransmission. Inositol is one of several substances that regulates phospholipase C (an enzyme that breaks down phosphatidylinositol).

 Evidence

CLINICAL TRIALS

• Respiratory distress syndrome (RDS) in preterm infants

—A Cochrane systematic review of inositol as a treatment for RDS in preterm infants identified three randomized controlled trials (5). The risk of death, bronchopulmonary dysplasia, retinopathy of prematurity, and intraventricular hemorrhage was significantly reduced. The risk of necrotizing enterocolitis and sepsis was not affected.

• Panic disorder

—A double-blind, placebo-controlled, crossover trial in 25 patients with panic disorder (21 completed) tested the effects of inositol 6 g b.i.d. dissolved in juice; both treatment and placebo phases lasted 4 weeks (6). The frequency and severity of panic attacks decreased significantly more after treatment than placebo. Among the 11 patients who used lorazepam, medication use did not differ between the phases. Two patients on inositol complained of sleepiness.
—A double-blind, placebo-controlled crossover trial of seven patients with panic disorder found that a single dose of 20 g inositol had no effect on pharmaceutically induced panic attacks (7).

• Bulimia

—A double-blind crossover trial in 12 patients with bulimia nervosa compared 18 g/day inositol with placebo; each phase lasted 6 weeks (8). Inositol treatment resulted in significantly improved scores, compared with placebo, on the Global Clinical Impression, the Visual Analogue Scale, and the Eating Disorders Inventory.

• Obsessive-compulsive disorder (OCD)

—A placebo-controlled study of 15 patients (including eight women) with OCD previously treated with clomipramine or selective serotonin reuptake inhibitors (SSRIs) (either without response or with unacceptable side effects) tested placebo against inositol (18 g/day, given as 2 teaspoons in juice t.i.d.) (9). Each phase lasted 6 weeks. Inositol was significantly more effective than placebo in 6 weeks. Differences between the two groups were not statistically significant at 3 weeks. There were no reported side effects.

• Depression

—A double-blind, controlled trial of inositol in 39 depressed subjects (22 with major depression and 6 with bipolar disorder) tested the effects of inositol (12 g/day) or placebo for 4 weeks (10). There was a high dropout rate; 11 patients dropped out in the first week. Although both groups improved, Hamilton depression scores in the treated group decreased significantly more than the placebo group at 4 weeks (there was no difference at 2 weeks). Four of the seven treated patients who dropped out in the first week reported symptoms; two had mild psychotic symptoms, one reported weakness and tremor, and one a cutaneous burning sensation. Other side effects included nausea and flatulence. There were no abnormalities in blood chemistry or liver function tests; two patients experienced "mild increase in fasting blood sugar."
—A double-blind placebo-controlled study in 27 depressed patients tested inositol against placebo as an adjunct to SSRIs for 4 weeks (11). Inositol added no benefits to SSRI treatment.

• Cognitive impairment

—A double-blind crossover trial compared placebo to 6 g inositol daily for 1 month in 11 Alzheimer's patients (12). CAMCOG scores were not significantly different between groups; orientation and language improved significantly more in the inositol group than the placebo group.
—A double-blind crossover trial of 6 g inositol daily for 5 days during a series of electroconvulsive treatments (ECTs) in 12 patients showed no effect on ECT-induced memory impairment (13).

• Other psychiatric/behavioral

—A double-blind crossover trial in 12 schizophrenic patients found no benefit of 12 g inositol daily for 1 month (14). A double-blind crossover trial of inositol 200 mg/kg/day in nine autistic children showed no benefit (15).
—A review of inositol notes that inositol appears to benefit conditions responsive to SSRIs (depression, panic disorder, and OCD) but does not appear to benefit schizophrenia, Alzheimer's disease, or attention deficit hyperactivity disorder (16).

ANIMAL/IN VITRO

• A review of inositol treatment in animals notes that in rats, inositol treatment improved behavior in depression and anxiety models; in monkeys, there was no effect on amphetamine-induced hyperactivity, apomorphine-induced stereotypy, or memory tasks (17).
• Orally administered inositol hexaphosphate (phytic acid) decreased the number and size of carcinogen-induced colonic tumors in rats and mice; in treatment models, phytic acid inhibited tumor size and improved survival in mouse and rat fibrosarcoma models (18).

Inositol

 Clinical Considerations

 Risks

 Common Questions and Answers

DEFICIENCY SIGNS AND SYMPTOMS

• In rats, gerbils, and other animals fed an inositol-deficient diet, accumulation of hepatic or intestinal fat as triglycerides occurs. Female gerbils developed severe intestinal lipodystrophy and in later stages developed weight loss, alopecia, exudative dermatitis, and death (2).

FACTORS DECREASING AVAILABILITY/ABSORPTION

• Lithium (see questions and answers)
• Depression

FACTORS INCREASING AVAILABILITY/ABSORPTION

• Breast milk, but not formula, increases serum inositol levels in infants (2).

LABORATORY TESTS

• One study found serum free inositol concentration averaged 33 μmol/L in normal participants and 240 μmol l/L in dialysis patients. Serum inositol concentrations are very high in term neonates, decreasing to adult concentrations by 6 months of age (2).

ADVERSE REACTIONS

• Only minor side effects, including sleepiness, nausea, and flatulence, have been reported with inositol use. Inositol administered to bipolar patients and normal controls did not affect thyroxine (T_4) or thyroid-stimulating hormone (TSH) in either group (19).

DRUG INTERACTIONS

• Lithium, possibly (see questions and answers)
• Inositol hexaphosphate forms complexes with copper, zinc, manganese, iron, and calcium (in descending order) and may reduce the bioavailability of these minerals (18,20).

Q: What is the relationship between inositol and lithium?
A: In animals, inositol reverses lithium effects, and inositol has been proposed as a treatment for lithium-induced side effects. Two studies, however, found opposite results. An open trial of 12 lithium-treated patients experiencing lithium side effects (polyuria, tremor, or skin lesions) reported improved or resolved side effects in 12 patients (3). However, another study of dietary inositol in euthymic bipolar patients showed no effect of inositol on tremor, thirst, or other lithium-induced side effects (19).
Lithium does not appear to affect inositol levels: A double-blind study of chronic lithium on myo-inositol concentrations in 11 participants found no effect of lithium ($n = 7$) compared with placebo ($n = 4$) given for 7 days (21).

Iodine (I$_2$)

 10 Second Take

Iodine supplementation can prevent mental retardation and physical pathologic conditions in those who are deficient, but there is little evidence supporting the supplementation of those who are replete.

 Basics

DESCRIPTION

• Iodine is a nonmetallic element.
• Elemental iodine comes from iodide that is oxidized by sunlight to elemental iodine, a volatile compound; iodine from the atmosphere is eventually returned to the soil by rain.

FOOD SOURCES

• The iodine content of both animal and vegetable foods is dependent on the iodine content of soil on which produce is grown or animals raised.
• Organic iodine is found in many seaweeds, marine fish, and shellfish.

MAIN FUNCTIONS/PHARMACOKINETICS

• Iodine is an essential part of the thyroid hormones thyroxine (T$_4$), 3,5,3′,5′ tetraiodo-thyronine, and 3,5,3′-triiodothyronine (T$_3$). There are 15–20 mg of iodine in an adult human; 70% to 80% is in the thyroid gland, the only storage site of iodide in the body. Iodine is incorporated into the iodine-containing amino acid monoiodothyronine (MIT), diiodothyronine (DIT), T$_3$, T$_4$, and thyroglobulin.
• Inorganic iodide is rapidly absorbed in the stomach and small intestine. Usually less than 10% of iodine absorbed by the gut appears in the thyroid; however, in deficiency states, 80% or more may be absorbed (1).

 Evidence

CLINICAL TRIALS

• Iodine deficiency disorders

—Iodine supplementation is a proven public health measure. In Papua New Guinea, a controlled trial of iodized oil injection in women before pregnancy proved that iodine reduces cretinism in newborns (2). The addition of iodine to irrigation water in an iodine-deficient area of China decreased neonatal and infant mortality; it also increased sheep production and annual yearly income (3)!

• Fibrocystic breasts

—A small, double-blind, controlled, idiosyncratic study tested the effects of orally administered molecular iodine (0.07 to 0.09 mg/kg body weight) in 23 participants; 33 received a control mixture of coloring and quinine (4). Participants were assessed every 2 months and were followed for a mean of 191 days. Asked to evaluate improvements in lumps and pain, 33% of controls (11 women) improved compared with 65% (15 women) in the treated group; it is not clear whether this was statistically significant. Evaluation by a physician found a significant improvement in the treated group versus the control group.
—A previous uncontrolled study in the same report showed that aqueous molecular iodine therapy resulted in side effects in 10.9% of subjects. Side effects included acne, nausea, diarrhea, hair thinning, increased pain, hyperthyroidism, hypothyroidism, skin rash, and headaches. There was no change on mammograms. This was an unclear report of a poorly designed study, and the incidence of side effects is impressive.

 Clinical Considerations

DEFICIENCY SIGNS AND SYMPTOMS

• People who live far from the sea (the main source of iodine) are susceptible to iodine deficiency. Other geographic risk factors include mountainous areas, because glaciation and higher rainfall (which causes runoff) deplete soil; iodine deficiency is also common in river valleys susceptible to repeated flooding. Seafood is the richest dietary source of iodine, containing 300 to 3,000 ng/g (5).
• Iodine deficiency is the largest single cause of preventable brain damage and mental retardation (6). Cretinism is common in India, Indonesia, and China and also occurs in Africa and the Andean region of South America. The neurologic form predominates in all areas except Zaire where the myxedematous form predominates (2).
• In 1990, almost one third of the world's population was at risk for iodine deficiency. After the World Summit for Children in the same year, iodine supplementation programs were implemented worldwide; the population areas of iodine deficiency disorder (IDD) dropped from 28.9% in 1994 to 13.7% in 1997 (7).
• In the fetus, iodine deficiency can cause congenital anomalies, neurologic cretinism (mental retardation, deaf mutism, spastic diplegia, squint), or the less common myxedematous hypothyroid cretinism (which can cause dwarfism and mental retardation); both are associated with increased perinatal and infant mortality. Physical and mental retardation can occur in children and adolescents. In all age groups from neonate to adults, iodine deficiency can cause impaired mental function, goiter, and increases the susceptibility of the thyroid gland to radiation. The brain is particularly sensitive to hypothyroidism, which can cause subtle effects including slow responses, slow reaction times, and apathy (2).

FACTORS DECREASING AVAILABILITY/ABSORPTION

• Inadequate dietary intake, dietary thiocyanates (see questions and answers)

FACTORS INCREASING AVAILABILITY/ABSORPTION

• Excessive iodization of salt or other food, deficiency

LABORATORY TESTS

• Urinary iodine

100 to 200 μg/L	Satisfactory
50 to 99 μg/L	Mild IDD
20 to 49 μg/L	Moderate IDD
<20 μg/L	Severe IDD (2)

Iodine (I$_2$)

 Risks

ADVERSE REACTIONS

• Thyroid effects

—Asians consume seaweed, which is quite high in iodine. On the Japanese island of Hokkaido, inhabitants consume up to 80,000 μg iodine a day (2). Healthy people can consume large amounts of iodine without apparent ill effect. High dietary intake of iodine decreases the incidence of nontoxic diffuse goiter and toxic nodular goiter without affecting the incidence of Graves' disease or Hashimoto's disease (2). Studies are mixed on whether or not iodine supplementation can aggravate or induce autoimmune thyroiditis. A large-scale study is needed to answer the question (6).

• Iodine-induced hyperthyroidism (IIH)

—In people with chronic iodine deficiency, acute increase in iodine intake can cause hyperthyroidism. IIH is a common complication of new iodine-supplementation programs; it is most common among people older than 40 years with autonomous nodular goiters (6). IIH is really an iodine deficiency disorder. Iodine deficiency increases thyrocyte proliferation and mutation rates; nodules may become autonomous and then can cause hyperthyroidism after iodine supplementation. IIH can occur with intakes above 0.20 mg/day (2). Iodine supplementation can also aggravate or even induce autoimmune thyroiditis.
—An increased incidence of goiter among Peace Corps volunteers in Niger, West Africa, was linked to excess iodine from iodine-based antimicrobial filters used for water purification; the use of two-stage iodine-resin ceramic water filters was associated with a 3.9-fold increased risk of thyroid dysfunction (8).

• Acute poisoning

—Iodine is a respiratory irritant (however, respiratory exposure is limited by its low vapor pressure). Acute iodine intoxication can cause burning pain in the mouth and throat, thirst, nausea, abdominal pain, diarrhea, albuminuria, and shock. Lips may be stained brown and vomitus blue (if stomach contents include starches). A dose of 2 to 4 g can be fatal in humans (9).

ANIMAL TOXICITY

• Iodine deficiency in animals can cause thyroid insufficiency and reproductive failure, retarded fetal development, abortion, stillbirth, or birth of weak hairless offspring, often associated with prolonged gestation and parturition and retention of placental membranes (2).

 Dose

RECOMMENDED DIETARY ALLOWANCE

Infants and children

0 to 6 months	110 μg/day (adequate intake)
7 to 12 months	130 μg/day (adequate intake)
1 to 3 years	90 μg/day
4 to 8 years	90 μg/day

Males

9 to 13 years	120 μg/day
14 to 18 years	150 μg/day
19 to 50 years	150 μg/day
51+ years	150 μg/day

Females

9 to 13 years	120 μg/day
14 to 18 years	150 μg/day
19 to 50 years	150 μg/day
51+ years	150 μg/day
Pregnant	220 μg/day
Lactating	290 μg/day

UPPER LIMITS

Infants and children

0 to 6 months	Not determinable
7 to 12 months	Not determinable
1 to 3 years	200 μg/day
4 to 8 years	300 μg/day

Males

9 to 13 years	600 μg/day
14 to 18 years	900 μg/day
19 to 50 years	1100 μg/day
51+ years	1100 μg/day

Females

9 to 13 years	600 μg/day
14 to 18 years	900 μg/day
19 to 50 years	1100 μg/day
51+ years	1100 μg/day

Pregnant

≤18 years	900 μg/day
19 to 50 years	1100 μg/day

Lactating

≤18 years	900 μg/day
19 to 50 years	1100 μg/day

• Correction of deficiency

—Iodine supplementation has been accomplished with iodized salt, bread, oil, or sugar. Iodized salt (20 to 40 mg/kg) has been most popular and has been used since the 1920s. Iodized oil injected intramuscularly has been used to prevent endemic goiter and cretinism. One injection can last for more than 4 years. Iodized oil can also be given orally but does not last as long. Poppy seed oil contains 480 mg iodine/mL. Iodized peanut, walnut, and soybean oils have also been developed (2). The usual dose is 1 mL p.o. or i.m. (dose is somewhat controversial). The oral dose should be repeated every 6 months, and the intramuscular dose repeated in 3 to 5 years (2).
—Infants of iodine-deficient pregnant women treated up to the end of the second trimester were normal; later treatment or treatment after birth had some beneficial effect on brain growth and developmental achievement but did not change neurologic status (2).

 Common Questions and Answers

Q: Is goiter always caused by iodine deficiency?
A: No. Either iodine deficiency or excess can cause goiter. Iodine deficiency is the most common cause of goiter. A sometimes overlooked cause of (usually myxedematous) goiter is certain foods. Inadequately soaked or undercooked cassava is the primary culinary culprit. Cassava contains the thioglycoside linamarin, which hydrolyzes in the gut to cyanide and is then metabolized to thiocyanate, which inhibits uptake of iodide by the thyroid. In Zaire, goiter and severe hypothyroidism have been associated with undercooked cassava. Millet, sweet potato, various beans, and several industrial pollutants also contain goitrogenic substances (1).

Ipriflavone

10 Second Take

Ipriflavone, a synthetic isoflavone, is promoted for osteoporosis prevention; evidence of efficacy, however, is mixed, and it has been associated with lymphopenia.

Basics

DESCRIPTION

• Ipriflavone (IP) (7-isopropoxyisoflavone) is a synthetic isoflavone, structurally similar to plant-derived isoflavones, that is sold as a dietary supplement.

MECHANISM/PHARMACOKINETICS

• IP appears to inhibit osteoclasts and stimulate osteoblasts; both of these actions may be through modulation of intracellular free calcium.

Evidence

CLINICAL TRIALS

• Bone mineral density (BMD) in menopausal women

—The largest, most recent, and best trial to date found no benefit of IP on bone. The Ipriflavone Multicenter European Fracture Study, conducted in Belgium, Denmark, and Italy, randomized 474 postmenopausal white women with osteoporosis (less than 0.86 g/cm^2) of the lumbar spine to placebo or IP 200 mg t.i.d. for 3 years (1). A total of 292 women completed the trial. Both groups received calcium (500 mg/day). IP caused no difference from baseline or between groups in annual percentage change in BMD at spine, hip, or forearm; new vertebral fractures were similar between groups, and biochemical markers were similar between groups. IP was associated with lymphocytopenia (see adverse effects). Other smaller placebo-controlled trials favor a beneficial effect of IP on BMD of the vertebrae or radius.
—A 2 year, placebo-controlled multicenter Italian RCT of 255 postmenopausal women (all received 1 g calcium daily; 196 completed) with low radial BMD measured by dual photon absorptiometry (DPA) found a significant benefit for IP 200 mg t.i.d. in maintaining radial BMD compared with the control group at 1 and 2 years (2). Another publication reports two multicenter studies (3); one, however, is clearly a republication of the study discussed previously. The other study enrolled 198 women; entry criteria, treatment, duration, and analysis appeared identical to the study just described; however, BMD measurements were taken at the vertebra and dual-energy x-ray absorptiometry (DXA) was used. In the intention to treat analysis, the placebo group lost 1.1% vertebral BMD at year 2; there were no changes from baseline in the IP-treated group.
—Another 2-year study randomized 56 postmenopausal white women (40 completed) with low vertebral bone density (measured by DXA) to IP (200 mg t.i.d.) or placebo; both groups also received calcium 1,000 mg (4). In the intention to treat analysis the placebo group lost more bone (−3.8%) than the IP (−1.2%); the between-group differences were significant only at year 2.
—Fifty-seven postmenopausal women with osteopenia or osteoporosis were randomized to either 600 mg IP or 0.8 g/day calcium lactate for 1 year (5). Decreases in lumbar BMD measured by DXA appeared to be similar between groups.
—A double-blind study of 40 postmenopausal women treated with IP (600 mg/day) or placebo (all received calcium 1,000 mg/day) found that after a year, BMD in the spine and forearm, measured by DXA, was significantly reduced from baseline in the placebo group and remained stable in the IP group (6).

• Vertebral fractures

—Three studies have examined vertebral fracture endpoints. The Alexandersen study discussed previously found no benefit. Two smaller double-blind, placebo-controlled studies of women older than 65 years with vertebral fractures claim a benefit for IP 200 mg t.i.d. (all women received calcium 1 g/day).
—The first study, in the *Italian Journal of Mineral Electrolyte Research,* enrolled 49 women (only 27 completed the 2-year trial) (7). Radial BMD (measured by DPA) increased in the treated group and did not change in the placebo group; the difference between groups was significant at year 1 and 2. Four patients in the IP group had at least one new vertebral fracture by x-ray examination; eight patients in the placebo group had new vertebral fractures. However, these numbers are uninterpretable because the denominators are not given (these numbers include women who were treated for 1 or 2 years and who received x-ray evaluation at year 1, year 2, or both).
—In the second 2-year randomized double-blind study of 100 women (84 completed) older than age 65 years with osteoporosis and at least one previous vertebral fracture, IP 200 mg t.i.d. was compared to placebo (all received calcium 1 g daily) (8). Radial BMD increased in the treated group and decreased in the placebo group. Between-group differences were significant at 6, 12, and 24 months. Two new vertebral fractures occurred in the treated group and 11 new vertebral fractures occurred in the placebo group (it is not stated how many patients this represents or whether this was statistically significant). Analgesic use decreased significantly in the IP group, whereas it increased in the placebo group.

• IP as adjunct to vitamin D or estrogen

—Ninety-eight postmenopausal oophorectomized women 45 to 65 years were randomized to IP 600 mg daily ($n = 28$), vitamin D ($n = 15$) 1 μg, both ($n = 20$), or neither ($n = 35$). Seventy-nine women completed the 18-month study. All groups lost vertebral bone (measured by DXA), but the combined treatment significantly reduced bone loss at all timepoints compared with all other groups. At 18 months the combination group had lost 0.33% of vertebral bone, the IP group 2.37%, vitamin D 1.15%, and controls 3.70%.

- IP and estrogen

—There is some evidence that IP may be helpful as an adjunct to low-dose estrogen, but studies are inconsistent.

—In one study, 116 recently oophorectomized Japanese women were randomized to placebo, conjugated equine estrogens (CEE) (0.625 mg/day), IP 600 mg/day, or CEE and IP (9). At 48 weeks, vertebral BMD (measured by DXA) was reduced significantly by 6.1% in the placebo group, 3.9% in the CEE group, and 5.1% in the IP group; however, there was no significant change in the combined-therapy group (vertebral BMD decreased 1.2%).

—A double-blind, 1-year multicenter study in 83 postmenopausal women assigned participants to a double placebo ($n = 24$), placebo and CEE 0.3 mg/day ($n = 31$), or CEE 0.3 mg/day plus IP 200 mg t.i.d. ($n = 28$) (10). "Valid completers" in the placebo group showed decreased forearm bone density (measured by DPA) at 1 year; the CEE group lost an average of 1.4%, whereas the CEE plus IP group experienced significantly increased BMD ($+5.6\%$, $p < 0.01$). The difference was significant ($p < 0.05$).

—Another 1-year study randomized 105 white early postmenopausal women to control (calcium 500 mg), low-dose hormone replacement therapy (HRT) (25 mg/day transdermal 17 beta-estradiol plus medrogestone 5 mg/day × 12 days/month), high-dose HRT (50 mg/day transdermal 17 beta-estradiol plus medrogestone 5 mg/day × 12 days/month), IP 600 mg/day, or IP combined with low-dose HRT (11). Compared with baseline, vertebral BMD (measured by DPA) significantly changed only in the control group, in which vertebral BMD decreased 3.41%.

—Another study randomized 80 (52 completed) postmenopausal women age 40 to 49 to IP 200 mg t.i.d., CEE 0.3 mg/day, or IP 400 mg plus CEE 0.3 mg/day (all treatment groups also received calcium 500 mg/day). Compared with baseline, vertebral bone density (measured by DXA) decreased significantly in the control and low-dose CEE groups and increased significantly in both IP groups at 1 and 2 years (12). The difference between both IP groups and the other two groups was significant. IP had no effect on vaginal maturation index, which predictably improved in both groups receiving CEE.

- IP versus calcitonin

—Forty postmenopausal women with BMD greater than 2 standard deviations (SD) below the mean for age-matched controls were studied in a controlled but not blinded study comparing salmon calcitonin to IP over a year (13). Both treatments significantly increased BMD (4.3% in the IP group and 1.9% in the calcitonin group); the between-group difference was significant.

- Gonadotropin-releasing hormone (GnRH)-induced bone loss

—A randomized study of IP in preventing GnRH-induced bone loss tested leuprolide alone versus leuprolide with IP in 102 women with uterine fibroids (14). BMD of the lumbar spine, measured by DXA, was reduced in both groups after 6 months but IP significantly mitigated bone loss (which was −5.26% in the leuprolide-only group and −3.70% in the IP-supplemented group ($p < 0.01$ between groups).

- Stroke patients

—BMD decreases in paralyzed limbs. A randomized three-armed study of 103 patients with hemiplegia after stroke compared 600 mg IP, 1 mg vitamin D_3, or no treatment for 12 months (15). BMD on the hemiplegic side decreased 1.4% in the IP group, 3.8% in the vitamin D_3 group, and 5.4% in the control group (IP was significantly better than the other two groups).

Risks

ADVERSE REACTIONS

- In the largest study to date, IP was associated with a significant decrease in lymphocyte concentrations, an effect that started 6 months after treatment began (1). Twenty-nine women developed lympho-cytopenia during the study; two additional women had lymphocytopenia at 36 months. Lymphocytopenia was subclinical, and, after discontinuation, 52% recovered to baseline levels within 1 year and 81% by 2 years.
- Data from 60 studies performed in Europe and Japan, with a total of 2,769 treated patients, showed a similar incidence of adverse reactions for those treated with IP (14.5%) and those treated with placebo (16.1%) (16). Gastrointestinal complaints including heartburn, vomiting, abdominal pain, constipation, and diarrhea accounted for 77.9% of the adverse reactions observed in the treatment. Skin rashes, pruritus, headache, depression, drowsiness, fatigue, and tachycardia have also been reported.
- An article summarizing IP safety data notes transient changes in liver and kidney function tests, as well as hematologic parameters. It is stated that slight elevation of liver enzymes occurred in both the treated and control group; however, the data on the control group are not presented (16). The percentage of patients with out-of-range laboratory values ranged from 0.42% (total proteins) to 3.66% (leucocytes); however, without data on the placebo-treated patients, these numbers are uninterpretable.

DRUG INTERACTIONS

- Acenocoumarol—IP increases anticoagulant effect (16)
- Oral hypoglycemics—no effect (16)
- Estrogen—IP is not estrogenic (17) but appears to potentiate the activity of estrogen (18).
- Theophylline—increased serum levels in one patient (19)

Dose

COMMON DOSAGE FORMS

- 200 mg p.o. t.i.d.
- A dosage reduction is recommended in patients with renal dysfunction (20).

—400 mg/day (creatinine clearance 40 to 80 mL/minute)
—200 mg/d (creatinine clearance less than 40 mL/minute)

Iron (Fe)

 10 Second Take

Iron deficiency is common. Supplementation may help breath-holding spells.

 Basics

DESCRIPTION

• Iron, the most abundant trace element in humans, is required by most organisms. Ferrous iron (Fe^{2+}) oxidizes to ferric iron (Fe^{3+}), which reduces back to ferrous iron, so iron is an important catalyst of redox reactions. Iron is stored in ferritin or hemosiderin.

FOOD SOURCES

• Meat is high in naturally chelated heme iron. Non-heme iron from plants is poorly bioavailable, and oxalates, phytate, tannins, and bioflavonoids in plants further decrease bioavailability (1). Fruit juice contains some iron; some European ciders and wines contain more than 16 mg iron/L. City water usually contains less than 5 mg/L; well water may be higher. The so-called reduced iron used to fortify cereal and flour is finely powdered, insoluble, poorly absorbed metallic iron (such as ferric pyrophosphate), which must be oxidized and then reduced in the duodenum; most passes through the gastrointestinal tract unchanged (2). Although breast milk and cow's milk contain similar amounts of iron, iron is more bioavailable in breast milk (3).

MECHANISM/PHARMACOKINETICS

• Two thirds of iron in the body circulates in erythrocytes as part of hemoglobin; iron is recycled from degraded erythrocytes (1). Each milliliter of blood contains about 0.5 mg iron. Myoglobin contains iron, as do heme-containing cytochromes and iron-sulfur proteins involved in electron transport and oxidative phosphorylation, cytochrome P450 enzymes, ribonucleotide reductase, tyrosine and tryptophan hydroxylases, myeloperoxidase, catalase, and tryptophan oxygenase (1).
• Iron balance is maintained primarily by regulating absorption, which occurs intestinally (especially at the duodenum), rather than by regulating excretion (primarily via bile). Average daily intake in Europe and North America is 10 to 20 mg (about 1 mg/day is absorbed). Men excrete 0.9 to 1.05 mg/day. It is difficult to lose iron except by bleeding.

 Evidence

CLINICAL TRIALS

• Restless legs syndrome (RLS)

—Iron deficiency has been linked with RLS in older adults (4,5). However, a double-blind, placebo-controlled randomized controlled trial (RCT) in 28 participants with RLS found no benefit of ferrous sulfate ($FeSO_4$ 325 mg b.i.d. × 12 weeks) on quality of sleep or nights without symptoms (6).

• Breath-holding spells (BHS)

—Iron deficiency anemia (by hemoglobin levels) is common in children with BHS (7). A double-blind, placebo-controlled trial in 67 children with BHS tested $FeSO_4$ 5 mg/kg/day × 16 weeks (8). In the treated group versus controls, 17 (51.5%) versus 0 had a complete response and 12 (36.4%) versus 2 (5.9%) had a partial response.

• Growth

—An RCT of 407 Ethiopian families found that compared with children whose food was cooked in aluminum pots, children whose families received iron pots had significantly higher hemoglobin concentrations, less anemia, and better growth (9). Meats cooked in iron had twice as much iron and legumes had 1.5 times as much iron as food cooked in aluminum or clay pots.
—An Indonesian placebo-controlled RCT of 47 iron-replete children (12 to 18 months old) found that weight gain was significantly less in the group that received $FeSO_4$ (3 mg/kg/day × 4 months) (10).

• Learning

—An RCT in 81 high school girls with non-anemic iron deficiency (normal hemoglobin with serum ferritin less than 12.0 μg/L) found that $FeSO_4$ (650 mg b.i.d. × 8 weeks), compared with placebo, improved iron status and performance on verbal learning and memory tests (11).

• Exercise

—A placebo-controlled RCT in 42 iron-depleted, nonanemic women found that $FeSO_4$ (100 mg/day × 6 weeks) improved adaptation to aerobic exercise (12).

• Pregnancy

—A Cochrane review of 20 trials found that iron supplementation prevented low hemoglobin at birth or postpartum but did not affect other maternal or fetal outcomes (little data came from communities where iron deficiency is common) (13).

• Cardiovascular disease

—Studies are mixed. Although most found no relationship between iron intake or status and cardiovascular disease risk, most studies examined only serum ferritin (on its own not an adequate measure of iron status).

—A large epidemiologic study found that Finnish men with serum ferritin ≥ 200 μg/L had twice the risk of myocardial infarction (MI) of those with lower serum ferritin [relative risk (RR) 2.2, 95% confidence interval (CI) 1.2 to 4.0] (14). However, three later prospective studies of serum ferritin and coronary heart disease (CHD) and four of five case-control or cross-sectional studies found no association. None of five studies found an association between cardiovascular disease and transferrin saturation (15). A study in 9,920 men and women ages 35 to 79 years (followed for about 16 years) found a significantly higher risk of dying of acute MI in those with very high serum ferritin (>175 μg/L) than those with levels <120 μg/L (RR 2.18, 95% CI 1.01 to 4.74 for men and RR 5.53, 95% CI 1.69 to 18.12 for women) (16).
—A recent prospective study of 7,983 older adults in The Netherlands found that heme iron, but not total dietary iron, was linked to MI [RR for highest vs. lowest tertile was 1.83 (95% CI 1.16 to 291, p for trend 0.008)] (17). Other compounds in meat could have confounded results (fat was controlled for).
—Although hereditary hemochromatosis and other iron overload syndromes have been linked to cardiovascular disease, recent studies question this (18). An autopsy study found a low prevalence of coronary artery disease among patients with iron-overload syndromes (19).
—A recent systematic review of 12 prospective epidemiologic studies (including many discussed previously) with 7,800 CHD cases concluded that there is not strong evidence for an association between iron status [serum ferritin, transferrin saturation, and total iron-binding capacity (TIBC)] and CHD (20).
—NHANES II found no correlation between serum ferritin and total mortality or deaths from cardiovascular disease; however, African-American men with serum ferritin less than 50 μg/L had significantly higher all-cause mortality (21).

 Clinical Considerations

DEFICIENCY SIGNS AND SYMPTOMS

• Iron deficiency anemia

—Iron deficiency, the most common cause of anemia, affects 40% of the world's population (2). African-Americans, Mexican Americans, Native Americans, and Inuits are at very high risk. Estimated deficiency rates in white middle-class Americans are: children 5%, reproductive age women 10% to 20%, pregnant or postpartum women 30% to 60%, postmenopausal women 5% to 10%, men (20 to 44 years) 1% to 5%, men (45 to 70 years) 5% to 10%, and men and women older than 70 years 10% to 30% (2).

TREATMENT OF DEFICIENCY (18)

- Adults: FeSO$_4$ 300 mg (60 mg elemental iron) q.d.
- Infants: 2 to 3 mg/kg elemental iron
- Children and adolescents: 30 mg/day elemental iron

FACTORS DECREASING AVAILABILITY/ABSORPTION

- Lack of dietary iron; dietary tannins; phytates; oxalates; other phenolic compounds (form insoluble precipitates); antacids (renders iron insoluble); tea ($\downarrow$60%); coffee ($\downarrow$40%); rapid transit time, malabsorption syndromes; achlorhydria; infection/inflammation (Linder); menses (women lose about 0.6 mg/iron/day); pregnancy, birth, lactation (during pregnancy and lactation iron requirements increase 1 to 2.5 mg/day; 3 to 4 mg iron/day is transferred to the fetus during the last trimester of pregnancy); blood loss (trauma, blood donation, etc.)

FACTORS INCREASING AVAILABILITY/ABSORPTION

- Dietary factors (Vitamin C, fructose, fumarate, lysine, histidine, cysteine, methionine, citrate increase absorption)
- Excessive supplementation
- Chronic alcoholism (alcoholic cirrhosis may slightly increase hepatic iron)
- Transfusional hemosiderosis
- Porphyria cutanea tarda
- Shunt hemochromatosis (after portal-systemic shunt placement, especially end-to-side anastomoses)
- Exposure to alcoholic beverages brewed in steel or iron barrels
- Iron overload diseases
- Hereditary hemochromatosis: autosomal recessive inborn error of metabolism; homozygosity frequency 0.3% to 0.5%, carrier rate 10% to 15% in northern European Caucasians; causes cirrhosis, diabetes, and hyperpigmentation; can also cause fatigue, arrhythmias, and cardiomyopathy and increases risk of hepatic carcinoma
- Hereditary sideroblastic anemia: rare sex-linked disorder
- Congenital atransferrinemia: extremely rare, probably autosomal recessive; inability to synthesize transferrin
- Congenital ceruloplasminemia: rare autosomal recessive disease; excessive iron in brain, liver, and pancreas
- Congenital cataract with hyperferritinemia (may occur without iron overload)

—Superficial hemosiderosis of the central nervous system (CNS) (very rare: recurrent subarachnoid hemorrhages cause iron deposits in the meninges; may be associated with ataxia) (2)

- Treatment

—Hereditary hemochromatosis: removal of 500 mL blood one to three times per week over 1 to 2 years, until falling venous hemoglobin concentration does not normalize within a week. After that, phlebotomy (500 mL) every 2 to 6 months (goal is ferritin ≤20 μg/L)
—Iron overload associated with porphyria cutanea tarda: phlebotomy
—Secondary hemochromatosis: parenteral administration of iron chelators
—Transfusion hemosiderosis: long-term chelation with desferrioxamine

LABORATORY TESTS (1)

Serum ferritin (ng/mL)

	Median	Range
Adult males	69 to 140	<6 to 400
Adult females	34–39	<3 to 200
At birth	101	
1-month old	356	
6 months to puberty	30	7 to 142
Pregnant women (32 to 40 weeks, without iron supplementation)	12	

 Risks

ADVERSE REACTIONS

- Iron poisoning

—Iron is the most common cause of fatal pediatric poisonings in the United States (21). Thirty mg elemental iron/kg is toxic; ingestion of 60 mg/kg has caused death (typically, a fatal dose is greater than 250 mg/kg) (22).
—Within 2 hours, vomiting, diarrhea, abdominal pain, hematemesis, lethargy, shock, and acidosis may occur. Patients may be asymptomatic 2 to 12 hours after ingestion, but treatment (which may include hemodialysis, peritoneal dialysis, and exchange transfusions) must not be delayed. At 12 to 48 hours, shock, seizures, pulmonary edema, acidosis, anuria, hyperthermia, and death may occur. Survivors may manifest pyloric stenosis, antral stenosis, hepatic cirrhosis, or CNS damage 2 to 6 weeks after ingestion (23).

- Cancer

—Iron workers have an increased risk of respiratory tract neoplasia; inhaled iron may be a carcinogen (or may carry carcinogens) (24).

 Dose

RECOMMENDED DIETARY ALLOWANCE

Infants and children

0 to 6 months	0.27 mg/day (adequate intake)
7 to 12 months	11 mg/day
1 to 3 years	7 mg/day
4 to 8 years	10 mg/day

Males

9 to 13 years	8 mg/day
14 to 18 years	11 mg/day
19 to 50 years	8 mg/day
51+ years	8 mg/day

Females

9 to 13 years	8 mg/day
14 to 18 years	15 mg/day
19 to 50 years	18 mg/day
51+ years	8 mg/day
Pregnant	27 mg/day

Lactating

≤18 years	10 mg/day
19 to 50 years	9 mg/day

UPPER LIMITS

Infants and children

0 to 6 months	40 mg/day
7 to 12 months	40 mg/day
1 to 3 years	40 mg/day
4 to 8 years	40 mg/day

Males

9 to 13 years	40 mg/day
14 to 18 years	45 mg/day
19 to 50 years	45 mg/day
51+ years	45 mg/day

Females

9 to 13 years	40 mg/day
14 to 18 years	45 mg/day
19 to 50 years	45 mg/day
51+ years	45 mg/day
Pregnant	45 mg/day
Lactating	45 mg/day

 Common Questions and Answers

Q: Can vitamin C cause iron overload?
A: No, large chronic doses of vitamin C do not increase serum ferritin. However, those at risk for iron overload syndromes should avoid vitamin C supplements (1).

Isoleucine (Ile, I)

 10 Second Take

Isoleucine is a safe, essential amino acid; there is limited evidence that combined branched amino acids improve appetite, but clinical trials have not supported other claims.

 Basics

DESCRIPTION

• Leucine is one of three branched-chain essential amino acids (BCAAs); the others are isoleucine and valine.

FOOD SOURCES

Most protein-containing foods

MAIN FUNCTIONS/PHARMACOKINETICS

• The hydrophobicity of BCAAs make them important to protein formation; BCAAs also affect response to infection (1). BCAAs make up about a third of muscle protein and are an important constituent of other tissues (2).
• The plasma clearance half-life of isoleucine is 2 days.

 Evidence

CLINICAL TRIALS

• No clinical trials for isoleucine alone were identified.
• BCAA and phenylketonuria

—A mixture of valine, isoleucine, and leucine was administered to 16 adolescents and young adults with phenylketonuria in a double-blind crossover study comprising four 3-month periods (3). Time to completion of the Attention Diagnostic Methods (which requires substantial attention with mental processing) was significantly faster during the period in which the amino acid mixture was administered. There was not a significant change seen on the Continuous Performance Test.

• BCAA in amyotrophic lateral sclerosis (ALS)

—A double-blind, placebo-controlled trial compared BCAAs (L-leucine 12 g, isoleucine 8 g, and L-valine 6.4 g, with pyridoxal phosphate 160 mg daily) to L-threonine (4 g daily) or placebo for 6 months in 95 patients with ALS. Every 2 months, muscle strength, muscle torque, forced vital capacity (FVC), activities of daily living involving upper and lower limbs, and timed tasks were tested. Both the placebo group and the threonine group lost weight, whereas the BCAA-supplemented group gained weight; the difference was significant. Estimated decline in FVC was 2.5 times greater in both groups supplemented with amino acids, compared with placebo. No other significant differences were seen among treatment groups. The amino acids were well tolerated, but the authors point out that adverse effects of these amino acids on pulmonary function could not be ruled out (4). Long-term effects of this mixture also are unknown. Another trial of BCAA for ALS was halted after 126 participants were recruited because of what appeared to be excess mortality among randomized active treatment (24 BCAA, 13 placebo); there was also no evidence of efficacy in disability scales between the two groups (5).

- BCAA and tardive dyskinesia (TD)

—An uncontrolled 2-week trial in nine men with neuroleptic-induced TD tested the administration of a BCAA medical food three times a day for 2 weeks (6). Compared with baseline, frequency of TD movements (collected by videotape and analyzed in blinded random sequence) decreased significantly; movements decreased at least 38% in all subjects.

- BCAA and appetite

—A double-blind study in 28 cancer patients compared BCAA (4.8 g daily) with placebo; improvements in appetite were seen in 55% of the treatment group compared with 16% of those in the placebo group (7).

- BCAA in protein wasting associated with bedrest

—Nineteen healthy subjects were randomized into two groups; one group received 30 μmol/day of BCAAs, whereas the other received the same amount of nonessential amino acids. BCAA supplementation attenuated nitrogen loss during short-term bedrest (8).

OTHER CLAIMED BENEFITS/ACTIONS

- Muscular dystrophy
- Improves healing
- Improves athletic performance

 Clinical Considerations

FACTORS INCREASING AVAILABILITY/ABSORPTION

- Maple syrup urine disease (MSUD) or branched chain α-ketoaciduria is the group of inherited disorders of leucine, isoleucine, and valine metabolism. Infants do not manifest symptoms until they start eating protein-containing food; the most deficient in enzymes may die within 10 days of birth. Progressive neurologic dysfunction and urine and ear wax that smells of caramel or maple syrup characterize this disease. Screening should be done in the first week of life. Long-term management of MSUD involves dietary manipulation designed to maintain plasma concentrations of BCAAs 3 to 4 hours after a meal in a specific range (isoleucine, 40 to 90 μmol; leucine, 80 to 200 μmol; and valine, 200 to 425 μmol).

LABORATORY TESTS

- Isoleucine 110 μmol/24 hours
- 40 to 99 μmol/L venous blood

Dose

RECOMMENDED DIETARY ALLOWANCE (9)

- Infants 3 to 4 months   70 mg/kg/day
- Children 2 to 5 years   31 mg/kg/day
- Children 10 to 12 years   28 mg/kg/day
- Adults   10 to 23 mg/ kg/day

Karela or Bitter Melon

10 Second Take

Bitter melon is a vegetable that is also used medicinally for diabetes. High doses of extract are toxic to animals, especially pregnant ones, and a leaf infusion has caused hypoglycemic coma in children. Cooked fruit appears benign.

Basics

LATIN NAME

Momordica charantia L.

FAMILY

Cucurbitaceae

OTHER COMMON NAMES

Karela (Hindi), karla (Marathi), parakkachedi (Tamil), susharl (Sanskrit) bitter gourd, balsam-pear, cundeamor (Spanish). In Jamaica, a cultivated form is called carilla, or goo-fah; a smaller wild variant is called cerasee in Jamaica and sorossie in the Dominican Republic.

DESCRIPTION

- Bitter melon is an annual, climbing vine with showy flowers, cultivated throughout the tropics but especially in India, China, East Africa, the Caribbean, Central America, and South America.
- Its warty, cucumber-like fruit, unripe, is eaten as a vegetable and used medicinally for diabetes.
- The name may come from "mordere" (to bite) because of its bitten appearance.

PART USED

Unripe fruit, seeds, aerial parts

KNOWN ACTIVE CONSTITUENTS

- The fruit contains the insulinomimetic proteins P-insulin and V-insulin, the steroidal glycoside charantin (a mixture of sitosterol and stigmastadienol glycosides, also called sterolins), saponins, and cucurbitacin steroidal glycosides called momordicosides and momordicines.
- Also contains acylglucosylsterols, linolenoylglucopyranosylclcrosterol, amino acids, and phenolic compounds (1). Momordica antihuman immunodeficiency virus protein, molecular weight 30 kD, is an antiviral protein derived from karela.

MECHANISM/PHARMACOKINETICS

- No human pharmacokinetics data are available.
- Hypoglycemic effects have been demonstrated for charantin, insulinomimetic proteins, and an alkaloid-rich fraction of karela fruit juice.
- Karela appears to inhibit intestinal glucose uptake and may inhibit hepatic gluconeogenesis (2).

Evidence

CLINICAL TRIALS

- No placebo-controlled trials were identified; there are many uncontrolled trials. The most recent trial, in 100 participants with non-insulin dependent diabetes mellitus (NIDDM), found that consumption of an aqueous suspension of bitter melon fruit reduced both fasting and postprandial glucose levels significantly in 86 participants; 5 experienced reduction in fasting but not postprandial glucose (3).
- Different preparations may have different effects. A study of nine Asians with NIDDM found that 50 mL of an aqueous extract of karela given with a 50-g oral glucose load reduced glucose concentrations of patients with NIDDM by more than 20% within 1 hour; insulin levels were not affected (4). In the same report, daily consumption of fried karela for 8 to 11 weeks did not significantly affect glucose tolerance but did reduce glycosylated hemoglobin.
- Another study compared powdered fruit (5 g t.i.d. × 21 days) in five diabetics with aqueous extract (100 g in 100 mL water q.d.) in seven diabetics. The powdered fruit did not significantly decrease blood sugar from baseline; the aqueous fruit extract, however, significantly decreased blood sugar 54% from baseline (compared with 25% in the powder-treated group) at the 3-week timepoint. The difference between groups was significant. Glycosylated hemoglobin decreased significantly from 8.37 ± 0.39 to 6.95 ± 0.46 (5). Participants were followed for an additional 4 weeks; the hypoglycemic effect increased over time.
- Daily consumption of powdered karela fruit for 7 weeks improved both glucose tolerance and fasting blood glucose levels in eight patients with NIDDM (6).
- In another trial, karela juice significantly improved glucose tolerance in 13 of 18 patients tested (7).
- Powdered karela seed administered orally (amount not reported) significantly reduced postprandial blood sugar values from 350–380 mg% to 150–180 mg% in 20 diabetic patients, including 14 with NIDDM and 6 with insulin dependent diabetes mellitus (IDDM). Headache and increased appetite were reported (8).
- A polypeptide derived from karela called P-insulin or V-insulin, administered subcutaneously, has been reported to cause significant hypoglycemic effects in nine diabetics (9); another similar study found an effect in 11 IDDM patients but no effect in 8 NIDDM patients (10).

ANIMAL/IN VITRO

- Diabetes

—Diabetes studies in rabbits, rats, and mice have demonstrated hypoglycemic effects of karela fruit, juice, or extract, but results have not been entirely consistent. One study of rats found that fruit or seed extract improved glucose tolerance in diabetic animals but that chronic administration of fruit extract was lethal (11). Fasting blood sugar was not affected in normal or streptozocin-diabetic rats.

—The development of cataracts was delayed in karela treated streptozotocin-diabetic rats (5).

—*In vitro* studies of fruit extract have found stimulation of insulin release from isolated pancreatic islet cells. Insulin-like activity including increased glucose uptake into muscle, stimulation of lipogenesis, and inhibition of lipolysis on tissue preparations has been demonstrated *in vitro* (1).

- Cancer

—Topical application of karela peel reduced 9,10 dimethyl-1,2-benzanthracene (DMBA)-induced papillomas in mice (seed and whole fruit extract were much less effective) (12). In human breast cancer-bearing SCID mice, MAP30, an antiretroviral protein isolated from karela (10 µg/injection every other day × 10 injections), significantly increased survival (13).

- Other effects

—Karela has been shown to lower cholesterol in normal rats (14). Some analgesic and antiinflammatory effects have been demonstrated in animals (1).

- Antiviral effects

—MAP30 is active against HIV and herpes simplex virus (HSV) (including acyclovir-resistant strains) (15). Sperm are not affected even by very high doses of MAP30 (1,000 times the maximum effective concentration), raising the possibility that this compound could be used in nonspermicidal vaginal microbicides (16).

OTHER CLAIMED BENEFITS/ACTIONS

- Tonic
- Emetic
- Laxative
- Colds, other viral infections
- Fever
- Gastroenteritis
- Tumors
- Abortifacient

 Risks

ADVERSE REACTIONS

- Seizures and hypoglycemic coma have been reported in two children, aged 3 and 4 years, within 2 hours of ingesting a tea of *Momordica charantia* leaves and vine. Both patients recovered uneventfully (17).
- Abdominal pain and diarrhea have been reported in diabetic patients consuming karela juice or dried juice powder equivalent to 250–500 g of fruit (18). Headache and increased appetite were reported in one trial (8).

DRUG INTERACTIONS

- MAP30 potentiates the effect of the weak HIV antagonists dexamethasone and indomethacin in a test measuring reduction of p24 expression in infected MT-4 lymphocytes (19).
- One case reported as an interaction between karela and chlorpropamide is in actuality a sketchy anecdote about a Pakistani woman who reported less glycosuria after consuming curry with multiple ingredients (curry is composed of multiple herbs) including karela.

PREGNANCY/LACTATION

- Bitter melon demonstrates marked toxicity in pregnant animals (see animal toxicity).
- It has a reputation as an abortifacient and should not be used during pregnancy.

ANIMAL TOXICITY

- Antifertility effects have been demonstrated in several species. Male dogs treated for 60 days with 1.75 g/day of karela fruit extract developed testicular lesions; daily oral administration of fresh karela leaf juice in female mice reversibly reduced fertility. Uterine bleeding has been induced in pregnant rats given karela; pregnant rats and rabbits given 6 mL/kg karela juice orally suffered uterine hemorrhage and death within hours (1).
- Although nonpregnant rats and rabbits did not suffer this acute effect, chronic dosing at this level resulted in more than 80% of animals dying within 25 days. Intraperitoneal administration of 15 to 40 mL/kg of karela juice was lethal to rats within 18 hours (1).
- In animals, hepatotoxicity has been demonstrated (elevated hepatic enzymes and congestion of hepatic central veins) (1).

 Dose

MODE OF ADMINISTRATION

Oral, enema (rare)

COMMON DOSAGE FORMS

- Boiled, steamed, fried or sautéed karela is eaten as a vegetable.
- Karela juice (usually made by crushing and straining unripe fruit): about 50 mL is taken once or twice daily.
- Karela infusion or decoction (made from the aerial parts of the plant): taken once or twice a day.

 Common Questions and Answers

Q: The animal toxicity information is not reassuring. Is this herb dangerous?
A: Bitter melon appears to have very toxic effects in pregnant animals. No reports of uterine rupture or hepatotoxicity have been reported in humans, but karela does have a reputation as an abortifacient and it makes sense not to use it during pregnancy.
It is true that most vegetables seem more benign than this herb. Lack of human adverse effects may be due to species differences in susceptibility or perhaps to the inactivation of toxic compounds by heat, because karela is not eaten raw. It may also have to do with dose; bitter melon is not consumed as a staple and is often used as one of several ingredients in a dish. There is no danger in its traditional food uses, but bitter melon clearly has pharmacologic effects, and it is unknown whether long-term daily intake of karela in the form of powder or juice is safe.

Kava

10 Second Take

Clinical trial evidence supports the use of kava for anxiety; however, adverse effects include dystonic reactions, hepatotoxicity, and kava dermopathy.

Basics

LATIN NAME

Piper methysticum G. Forster.

FAMILY

Piperaceae

OTHER COMMON NAMES

Kava-kava, kava pepper

DESCRIPTION

• Widely used in Polynesia, Micronesia, and Melanesia as a ceremonial, tranquilizing beverage, kava (a psychoactive member of the pepper family) is used medicinally for anxiety and insomnia in Europe and the United States.

PART USED

Root, rhizome

KNOWN ACTIVE CONSTITUENTS

• Kavalactones (also called kavapyrones) 3% to 20% (1), including kawain (kavain), dihydrokawain, methysticin, dihydromethysticin, yangonin, and demethoxyyangonin (2).

MECHANISM/PHARMACOKINETICS

• The kavapyrones are centrally acting skeletal muscle relaxants and anticonvulsants. Their effects appear to be due to inhibition of sodium and calcium channels, as well as effects on glutamate systems (3).
• Kava extract has been reported to affect gamma-aminobutyric acid $(GABA)_A$ receptors as shown by enhanced muscimol binding in one study (4). In another study, kava was reported to have no effect on GABA or benzodiazepine binding (5).

Evidence

CLINICAL TRIALS

• Anxiety

—A systematic review of kava for anxiety identified seven double-blind randomized, placebo-controlled trials; six were included in the review, and three with a common endpoint [total Hamilton Anxiety (HAMA) score] were analyzed in a meta-analysis (6). All trials demonstrated a decrease in anxiety, and a meta-analysis of three trials showed a significant difference in reduction of HAMA score compared with placebo. The weighted mean difference was 9.69 [95% confidence interval (CI) 3.54 to 15.83]. Kavapyrone content varied between 60 to 240 mg/day. Adverse events included restlessness, stomach complaints, drowsiness, tremor, headache, and fatigue.
—In the only published treatment-controlled trial identified for kava (equivalent to 210 mg kavapyrones daily) was compared with 15 mg/day oxazepam or 9 mg/day bromazepam for 6 weeks. A total of 164 patients completed the protocol; HAMA ratings did not differ significantly among the three groups (7).
—A placebo-controlled double-blind clinical trial tested a kava constituent, kavain. Thirty-eight outpatients with anxiety associated with neurotic or psychosomatic disturbances were treated with D,L-kavain (Neuronika) or oxazepam (8). Assessed by the Anxiety Status Inventory (ASI) and the Zung Self-Rating Anxiety Scale (SAS), the treatments were equivalent. No adverse drug reactions were reported.

• Performance

—A randomized, double-blind crossover study oxazepam (15 mg the day before testing, 75 mg on the day of testing) to standardized kava extract (200 mg/day × 5 days) in 12 participants. Oxazepam predictably impaired event-related potentials and recognition memory, whereas kava slightly enhanced both (9). (See interactions.)

• Kava and menopausal symptoms

—A study of kava for climacteric symptoms in 40 women using doses of 30 to 60 mg/day for 56 to 84 days found significant improvements in the HAMA scale and Kupperman index (10). Another trial by the same investigator using a higher dose (equivalent to 210 mg kavapyrones/day) in 40 menopausal women also found improvements in symptoms, HAMA, Kupperman index, and Depression Status Inventory (DSI) (11).

ANIMAL/IN VITRO

• A study in mice showed no apparent tolerance development to doses of 100 mg/kg for 7 weeks and only slight tolerance at doses of 150 mg/kg (12). An additive effect was reported in mice using hypnotic doses of kava and alcohol (13).

Risks

ADVERSE REACTIONS

• In short-term studies, side effects (predominately gastrointestinal discomfort, headache, dizziness, and allergic skin reactions) were mild and reversible; the total incidence of reported side effects was only 1.5% to 2.3% (14). However, a study of kava use in aboriginals in Australia found that heavy long-term use of kava was associated with rash; increased gamma-glutamyl transferase; decreased albumin, plasma protein, urea, and bilirubin levels; increased red-cell volume; decreased platelets; decreased lymphocytes; shortness of breath; face puffiness; alkaline urine; hematuria; low specific gravity; decreased BMI; and brisk patellar reflexes. These effects were dose-related (the heaviest users used 440 g dried powder, infused in cold water, per week) (15).
• Vision

—In a single subject who had never used kava before, a heavy dose of traditionally prepared kava administered under experimental conditions resulted in no effect on visual acuity, stereoacuity, or refractive error. However, kava reduced the near point of accommodation, decreased the near point of convergence, disturbed oculomotor balance, and increased pupil diameter (16).

• Kava dermopathy

—Heavy, chronic use of kava results in yellowing of the skin and an ichthyosiform eruption known as kava dermopathy, often accompanied by eye irritation (17). Kava dermopathy is treated by abstention from kava. Although the scaly dermatitis is similar to that seen in pellagra, niacin deficiency has been ruled out as a mechanism: a randomized controlled trial of 100 mg nicotinamide in 29 kava drinkers with kava dermopathy showed no difference between the treatment and placebo groups (18). Stopping kava, however, results in complete resolution of symptoms.

- Sebotropic drug reaction

—Two cases of drug reactions have been reported with kava (19). A 52-year-old woman who had taken kava for 3 weeks developed papules and plaques on her face, thorax, and arms. Biopsy revealed an infiltrate in the reticular dermis. A kava extract patch test was positive (tests in a control group of 20 adults were all negative). A 70-year-old man on multiple drugs (nitrofurantoin, allopurinol, spironolactone, furosemide, mesterolone, and yohimbine) who had been taking kava for 2 to 3 weeks experienced itching after exposure to sunlight, followed by erythematous infiltrated plaques; biopsy revealed lymphocytic infiltrate destroying sebaceous glands. Skin testing and photopatch were negative; lymphocyte proliferation tests revealed significant proliferation only with kava. Biopsies from both patients revealed a lymphocytic attack on sebaceous glands.

- Dyskinesia

—Acute dystonic reactions have been reported in a series of three cases (20). A 28-year-old man (with a history of similar reactions to promethacin and fluspirilene injections) experienced involuntary neck extension and upward deviation of gaze that began 90 minutes after ingesting a single 100-mg dose of kava extract (Laitan) and resolved spontaneously within 40 minutes. A 22-year-old woman presented with tonic rotation of the head, oral and lingual dyskinesia, and painful twisting motions of the trunk within 4 hours of a single 100-mg dose of kava extract (Laitan); biperiden resolved the reaction. In the third case, a 63-year-old woman experienced forceful oral and lingual dyskinesia 4 days after starting kava extract (Kavasporal forte) 150 mg t.i.d.; biperiden resolved the reaction.

- Hepatitis

—A 50-year-old man developed hepatitis after consuming kava (Laitan) (equivalent to 210 to 280 mg kavalactones) daily for 2 months (21). The subject took no other drugs and consumed no alcohol; tests for viral hepatitis, HIV, cytomegalovirus (CMV), and Epstein-Barr virus were negative. The patient required transplant; histology showed hepatocellular necrosis and extensive lymphocytic infiltration. A case of recurring necrotizing hepatitis (22) and fulminant liver failure requiring transplant in a 60-year-old woman were reported; 17 other cases of liver failure associated with kava have been reported to European regulatory authorities (23).

DRUG INTERACTIONS

- Levodopa

—A 76-year-old woman with Parkinson's disease and motor fluctuations noticed increased number and duration of off periods within 10 days of starting kava extract (Kavasporal forte 150 mg b.i.d.); within 2 days of discontinuing drug she returned to baseline (20).

- Benzodiazepines

—A double-blind, randomized crossover trial in 18 participants, presented at a meeting, compared bromazepam (4.5 mg b.i.d.) to kava extract (120 mg kavalactones b.i.d.), and the combination; each treatment was administered for 2 weeks with a 1-week washout between treatments (24). The combination did not appear to affect general well-being or mental performance more than bromazepam alone. Of seven cognitive performance tests, three (vigilance, stress tolerance, and motor coordination) were unchanged with kava but worsened with bromazepam (with or without kava).
—A 54-year-old man on daily doses of alprazolam, cimetidine, and terazosin was hospitalized after experiencing an acute change in mental status 3 days after starting to take kava. He recovered from his lethargy and disorientation within several hours (25). This is a multidrug interaction in which cimetidine is likely to have played an important role. Cimetidine affects microsomal enzymes and reduces the hepatic metabolism of numerous drugs, including diazepam. Cimetidine may have increased alprazolam (and possibly kavalactone) levels, but clearly the addition of kava tipped the balance.

- Alcohol

—Two clinical studies on combining alcohol with kava found different results. A clinical trial in 20 volunteers given 100 mg kava extract t.i.d × 8 days added ethanol (in sufficient doses to achieve blood alcohol levels of 0.05%) on days 1, 4, and 8; no additive effects of kava and alcohol were noted (26).
—Another clinical study in 40 participants (including 20 females) compared the effects of kava, alcohol, or both on performance skills on cognitive and visuomotor tests. Kava alone had little effect on subjective impairment or performance. There was a decrease noted in performance on the Digit Symbol Coding test, but the combination of alcohol and kava produced greater decrements in the divided attention test than alcohol alone (27).

ANIMAL TOXICITY

- Kava extracts have been tested in formal chronic (26 week) toxicity studies in rats (up to 320 mg/kg) and dogs (up to 60 mg/kg). The high dose caused only mild histopathologic changes in liver and kidneys.
- There has been no evidence of mutagenic, teratogenic, or genotoxic potential in standard assays (27).

 Dose

COMMON DOSAGE FORMS

- *Cut rhizome:* 1.7 to 3.4 g/day or other preparations equivalent to 60 to 120 mg kavapyrones/day
- *Fluid extract:* 1:2 (g/mL) 3 to 6 mL/day in divided doses
- *Dry extract with 30% kavapyrones:* 0.2 to 0.4 g
- *Soft extract with 550 mg/g kavapyrones:* 100 to 200 mg/day
- Traditional preparation provides 25 to 300 mg kavapyrones/dose

 Common Questions and Answers

Q: Can one get "drunk" on kava?
A: Apparently. Heavy recreational doses can cause gait disturbance and other signs similar to alcohol intoxication. Interestingly, a 44-year-old motorist arrested in Utah for swerving in and out of traffic lanes appeared to be typically drunk (staggering, slurred speech, and slowed responses) but a breath test showed no evidence of alcohol. The motorist turned out to be suffering the effects of 16 cups of kava. Although the herb is legal, the motorist was convicted of driving under the influence of kava, in the first case of its kind (28). Given the herb's effects on vision (see risks), driving is not a good idea after a heavy dose.

Kelp

10 Second Take

Kelp represents several species of iodine-rich edible seaweed.

Basics

LATIN NAME

Laminaria, Macrocystis, Nereocystis, Fucus species

FAMILY

Phaeophyta

OTHER COMMON NAMES

Kombu

DESCRIPTION

• The term kelp can be applied to a variety of brown seaweeds, primarily in the order Laminariales, which includes *Laminaria, Macrocystis,* and *Nereocystis.*
• Another brown algae, bladderwrack (*Fucus vesiculosis*), in the order Fucales (rockweed), is also called kelp (1).
• Brown algae are annual plants common in temperate and polar climates; they differ from most plants by storing food as laminarin (an unusual polysaccharide) or oil rather than starch.
• Some giant kelps can grow as much as 60 m in one season (2).

PART USED

Whole plant

KNOWN ACTIVE CONSTITUENTS

• Algin, or sodium alginate, a high molecular weight polysaccharide common to all brown algae (amounts vary from 12% to 45%).
• Kelp also contains significant amounts of iodine in highly variable amounts; *Fucus vesiculosis* from the Baltic Sea contains 0.03% iodine, and from the North Sea 0.1%; some species of *Fucus* may contain up to 0.5% iodine (1). Kelp also contains significant amounts of potassium and sodium.

MECHANISM/PHARMACOKINETICS

• Algin is gel-forming and may be responsible for a laxative effect.
• Iodine can stimulate the production of thyroid hormones in those deficient in this mineral.

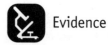

Evidence

CLINICAL TRIALS

• Thermogenic properties

—*Laminaria digitata* and other plants were tested for thermogenic properties in humans. Four subjects were treated with *Laminaria* tincture. Calorimetric and cardiovascular measures were taken at baseline and at five consecutive timepoints 45 minutes apart. A significant rise in heart rate was seen, but no significant change in blood pressure, energy expenditure, or respiratory quotient (3).

• Strontium absorption

—In 14 humans given alginate syrup or bread with stable strontium, absorption of strontium was significantly reduced (4). Radioactive strontium absorption in rats was significantly reduced by sodium alginate from different species of algae, including kelp species, but sodium alginate from *Sargassum siliquastrum* was superior.

ANIMAL/IN VITRO

• Cancer

—Rats fed a diet containing 5% *Laminaria* had a lower risk of developing 9,10 dimethyl-1,2 benzanthracene (DMBA)-induced mammary tumors. Treated rats had a significant delay to the time of tumor ($p = 0.007$) and had fewer adenocarcinomas per rat ($p < 0.05$) (5).
—In rats, intake of two kelp species (as well as several other seaweeds) decreased tumors induced by the carcinogen 1,2-dimethyl-hydrazine (6). *Laminaria* extract also reduced the incidence of sarcoma-180 in mice (7).

OTHER CLAIMED BENEFITS/ACTIONS

• Constipation
• Weight loss
• Bronchitis
• Emphysema
• Asthma
• Indigestion
• Ulcers
• Colitis
• Gallstones
• Genitourinary tract problems
• Arthritis
• Skin problems

Risks

ADVERSE REACTIONS

• Toxic metals

—Fifteen samples of kelp-containing dietary supplements sold in United Kingdom were found to contain low levels of total and inorganic arsenic (not enough to exceed a safe daily dose) (8).
—Relatively high concentrations of cadmium and lead (more than 100 μg/100 g) were found in kelp from the Canadian Arctic (9).

• Iodine

—Iodine concentrations vary widely; a survey of 15 samples of kelp-containing dietary supplements found that in several cases iodine intake could exceed 1,000 μg/day (8).

• Hyperthyroidism

—A 72-year-old woman developed hyperthyroidism while ingesting kelp (Vitalia) tablets. Six months after discontinuing the kelp tablets, her hyperthyroidism had disappeared (10). A similar case was reported in a 50-year-old woman who took six iodine-containing kelp tablets (Kelpasan) containing 200 mg of kelp each; she developed hyperthyroidism within 2 months that resolved spontaneously following discontinuation of tablets (11). A case of iodide-induced goiter in a patient with Hashimoto's thyroiditis has been associated with excessive seaweed consumption (12).
—Seaweed is rich in iodine. Healthy people can consume large amounts of iodine without apparent ill effect; on the Japanese island of Hokkaido, inhabitants consume up to 80,000 μg iodine a day (13). High dietary intake of iodine decreases the incidence of nontoxic diffuse goiter and toxic nodular goiter without affecting the incidence of Graves' disease or Hashimoto's disease (13).

• Carotenodermia

—Carotenodermia from excessive consumption of seaweed to lose weight was reported in a 22-year-old woman (14).

• Rash

—Two cases of acneiform eruption were related to excessive consumption of kelp tablets obtained at the health food store. In both cases the eruptions disappeared when kelp was discontinued (15).

DRUG INTERACTIONS

High dietary iodine levels may interfere with thionamide drugs (13).

 Dose

COMMON DOSAGE FORMS

• *Dried thallus:* 0.8 to 2 g total daily dose
• *Liquid extract:* (1:1, 25% ethanol) 1 to 2 mL total daily dose
• *Tincture:* (1:5, 25% ethanol) 4 to 10 mL daily dose
• Tablets also available

 Common Questions and Answers

Q: Are kelp products used in North America?
A: Yes, in both medicine and food. *Laminaria* "tents", which swell slowly over hours, are used in gynecology as a gentle means of dilating the cervix before induced abortion or other intrauterine procedures.
Algin is used as a thickener in foods and is made into films used as edible sausage casing (16). *Fucus vesiculosis* is used in clambakes to impart a unique flavor to lobsters and clams steamed over it.

Q: Is eating seaweed good for you?
A: Maybe. It certainly is not harmful. Japanese eat large amounts of seaweed that may range from 4.9 to 7.3 g per person per day; in some areas seaweed may compose 25% of the diet. It may be used as a vegetable in soups, sweets, and salads, as well as part of the base of miso soup (7). It has been hypothesized that *Laminaria* may protect against breast cancer in humans; however, there is little epidemiologic evidence to support this.
Some seaweeds may contribute significant amounts of vitamin B_{12} to vegetarian diets. A small study of 21 participants (including one male) who were adherents to a strict uncooked vegan diet called the living food diet found that vegans consuming nori or chlorella (these are not kelp) had serum vitamin B_{12} concentrations twice as high as those not using the seaweed (17).

Khat

 10 Second Take

Khat is a masticatory herb with amphetamine-like sympathomimetic effects. Chronic users often have a staring gaze and brown-stained teeth, but no long-term harmful effects have been clearly shown. Occasional cases of psychosis have been reported.

 Basics

LATIN NAME

Catha edulis (Vahl) Forssk. Ex Endl.

FAMILY

Celastraceae

OTHER COMMON NAMES

Abbyssinian tea, *qat, kaht, kat, gad, tschat, chat, jaad,* and *miraa* (Kenya)

DESCRIPTION

• A small evergreen tree that grows at high altitudes, khat is cultivated in Ethiopia, east and south Africa, and Yemen.
• Khat use is very widespread in Yemen but it is also used commonly in Ethiopia, Kenya, and Djibouti (1).

PART USED

Fresh leaves

KNOWN ACTIVE CONSTITUENTS

• Khat contains sympathomimetic alkaloids including cathine [norpseudoephedrine, or S,S (+)-phenylproponolamine], its diasteromer norephedrine [R,S (−)-phenylpropanola-mine], and cathinone [S(−) alpha-amino prophenone, a keto analog of cathine]. Cathinone is most concentrated in young leaves, where it may compose 70% of the phenylalkylamine fraction (2).
• The alkaloid content of khat varies; 100 g of fresh khat may contain 36 mg cathinone, 120 mg cathine, and 8 mg norephedrine. Young fresh leaves are highest in cathinone.

MECHANISM/PHARMACOKINETICS

• Cathinone is substantially absorbed through the buccal mucosa. After oral administration in capsules, peak serum levels of cathinone are reached within an hour; it is converted to norephedrine and disappears from serum within 6 hours (3).
• Orally administered cathinone is similar to amphetamine but has a more rapid onset of action (3). In six khat-naïve volunteers who received a single oral dose of khat corresponding to 0.8 mg/kg body weight, maximal plasma levels of cathinone were attained within 30 minutes and the elimination half-life was 260 ± 102 minutes (4). An earlier experiment found similar effects of pure cathinone (0.8 mg/kg body weight); the main difference was that, compared with taking pure cathinone, chewing the leaf slowed the absorption of cathinone and caused a later plasma peak. Khat significantly prolonged gastric emptying in a controlled study in 12 healthy volunteers (5).
• Cathinone, although more potent that cathine, is quite unstable, dimerizing spontaneously to an inactive compound (6). Cathine is absorbed slowly from the gastrointestinal tract; little is absorbed through the buccal mucosa.

 Evidence

CLINICAL TRIALS

• No clinical studies of benefit were identified. Clinical studies of adverse effects have been performed (see risks).

ANIMAL/IN VITRO

• In animals, khat alkaloids have sympathomimetic effects, can induce an indirect analgesic effect apparently secondary to its central nervous system stimulating effect, and can cause hyperthermia (3). Anorexic effects are also noted, although this effect is less potent than with amphetamine, and tolerance to the weight-reducing effect disappears more quickly than amphetamine—within a month.
• Cathinone induces locomotor activity, an effect that can be prevented by pretreatment with dopamine antagonists. Cathinone also increases the sensitivity of test animals to external stimulation (3).

OTHER CLAIMED BENEFITS/ACTIONS

• Asthma
• Ulcers
• Reducing fatigue

 Risks

ADVERSE REACTIONS

• Male reproductive tract effects

—Long-term use of khat may cause erectile dysfunction (3). A comparison of 65 khat addicts and 50 non-khat addicts found that semen volume, sperm count, sperm motility, motility index, and percentage of normal spermatozoa were lower among khat addicts (7). Among khat addicts, a mean of 65% of sperm were deformed.

• Memory

—A comparative study among flight attendants presenting for Federal Aviation Administration medical examinations compared 25 daily khat-chewing flight attendants with 39 occasional khat-chewing flight attendants and 24 air crew members who did not chew khat (8). Memory function test scores were significantly lower in khat chewers, and the effect was more pronounced in regular khat chewers than social khat chewers. Regular chewers also experienced a statistically significant shift toward fast frequency bands in electroencephalograms; however, this did not correlate with the memory functions assessed.

• Urodynamics

—A randomized double-blind controlled trial in 11 healthy males tested the results of a khat-chewing session preceded by placebo or indoramin. Khat chewing decreased average and maximum urine flow rates. This effect was inhibited by indoramin, causing the researchers to conclude that urinary side effects may be mediated by stimulation of α_1-adrenergic receptors (9).

• Psychosis

—Khat-related psychosis is well-documented but reports are relatively rare. Khat may cause hypomania or mania, often with grandiose delusions, or a paranoid psychosis often associated with fear, anxiety and possibly auditory hallucinations (10). Phenothiazines have been used to treat khat-induced psychosis (3).

- Immediate and chronic effects of khat use

—Immediate effects of khat use include transient conjunctival and facial congestion, tachycardia, palpitations (sometimes with extrasystole), increased blood pressure, mydriasis, hyperthermia, sweating, increased respiratory rate, and anorexia. Changes in heart rate and blood pressure are more pronounced among naïve users than chronic users.

—Khat users experience moderate euphoria, increased energy, volubility, a labile affect, and other symptoms consistent with mild hypomania. Khat-naïve participants given a single dose of khat (0.8 mg/kg body weight) were evaluated with the Addiction Research Center Inventory Scale. Khat had a significant amphetamine-like effect and caused participants to feel more excited and energetic (4).

—A staring gaze, dilated pupils and brown staining of the teeth are common in heavy khat users. It is unclear whether khat consumption affects periodontal health; however, stomatitis with secondary infections are commonly seen among khat users (3). A survey of 706 Yemenis (638 khat users and 168 non-khat users) that included a history and physical found that the only adverse effects clearly linked to the level of khat consumption were gastrointestinal problems and insomnia (10).

- Dependence/withdrawal

—Although psychic dependence is common, physical dependence does not seem to occur. Tolerance to mood-elevating effects does not appear to occur, although chronic users may cease to experience insomnia, and effects on heart rate and blood pressure are less pronounced in chronic users (3). Discontinuation of khat after heavy use may cause slight trembling, lassitude, mild depression, increased desire for sleep, and nightmares that may have paranoid content (11). Two cases of khat addiction were successfully treated with bromocriptine (12).

DRUG INTERACTIONS

- General anesthesia

—A French report from 1969 noted that khat users are more likely to become psychotic in the postanesthetic phase (1).

- Amoxicillin and ampicillin

—A bioavailability study on 8 healthy males tested the effect of khat chewing on ampicillin and amoxicillin bioavailability. Each antibiotic was tested under fasting conditions, taken right before khat chewing, taken before khat chewing together with food and drinks, taken 2 hours before khat chewing, taken midway through a 4-hour khat-chewing session, and taken 2 hours after that khat-chewing session. Both the extent and the rate of ampicillin bioavailability were substantially reduced by chewing khat at all timepoints tested except when the antibiotic was taken 2 hours after chewing khat. The strongest effect was seen if the drug was administered during a khat-chewing session (13). In contrast, amoxicillin bioavailability was reduced only if the antibiotic was taken during a khat-chewing session.

PREGNANCY/LACTATION

- A study of 1,141 consecutive deliveries in the Yemen Arab Republic found that nonusers of khat (n = 427) had significantly fewer low birth weight babies than khat users (223 occasional users and 391 regular users) (14). There were no differences between groups in rates of stillbirths or congenital malformations.
- Nor-pseudoephedrine has been found to be excreted in breast milk in several lactating, khat-chewing women (15). Nor-pseudoephedrine was also seen in the urine of one infant.

ANIMAL TOXICITY

- Cathinone is less averse than amphetamine in conditioning studies; it causes higher levels of response and tolerance to its anorectic effect is more rapid than amphetamine (1).
- Khat reduces the fertility of female mice and rats and appears to reduce placental blood flow and impair fetal growth in guinea pigs.

Dose

COMMON DOSAGE FORMS

- Fresh, preferably young, leaves are chewed one at a time. The juice is swallowed and the residue expelled.

Common Questions and Answers

Q: Doesn't khat increase the risk of oral cancers?
A: There is no convincing evidence of that. A survey of 706 Yemenis (638 khat users and 168 non-khat users) included oral examinations; no oral cancers were found (10). A 2-year record review of oral, oropharyngeal, and other head and neck malignancies in the Asir region of Saudi Arabia found that 10 of 28 were nonsmoking long-term khat-chewers (16). However, this study is unconvincing, not only because of its small size, but also because it is not at all clear that the prevalence of use was any higher than in the general population.

Q: Is khat used medicinally?
A: Although the use of khat is at least seven centuries old (its use was recommended to combat hunger and fatigue in messengers and soldiers) and it is a home remedy for asthma, khat does not appear to be a traditional remedy of Yemen.

Q: What happens during a khat-chewing session?
A: Khat chewing is often a social event; users usually bring their own leaves, which are chewed one at a time. The juice is swallowed, and the residue stored in the cheek and expelled at the end of the session. A khat-chewing session may last 4 hours, with each consumer consuming 100 to 200 g of leaves. In Yemen, khat chewing is primarily a male habit. In Somalia, women (either in female or mixed groups) regularly consume khat; chewing sessions often include consumption of copious amounts of highly sweetened tea or Coca-Cola.

Q: What is the economic impact of khat?
A: Khat use has a major economic impact. In Yemen, poor families spend up to half of their income on khat. It is estimated that over 40% of irrigated farmland is used for khat cultivation (far more than is used for cereal farming or coffee) (17).

Kombucha

 10 Second Take

There is no scientific basis for claimed benefits of kombucha. Several cases of severe illness have been possibly linked to kombucha.

 Basics

OTHER COMMON NAMES

Kombucha tea, kombucha mushroom, Kargasok tea, Manchurian tea, Dr. Sklenar's kombucha mushroom infusion, and fungus japonicus

DESCRIPTION

• Although often referred to as a "mushroom," kombucha is a fungal infusion composed of a symbiotic mixture of bacteria and yeast (including *Bacterium xylinum, Bacterium gluconicum, Bacterium xylinoides, Acetobacter ketogenum, Pichia fermentans, Saccharomyces apiculatus, Saccharomycodes ludwigii,* and *Schizosaccharomyces pombe*) grown in sweetened tea (1).
• An investigation of two commercially available specimens of kombucha and 32 specimens from private households in Germany revealed yeasts of the genera *Brettanomyces* in 56% of specimens, *Zygosaccharomyces* in 29% of specimens, and *Saccharomyces* in 26% of specimens (2). *Saccharomycodes ludwigii* and *Candida kefyr* were seen only in isolated cases. Three specimens were contaminated, one with *Penicillium* species and two (from the same household) with *Candida albicans.*

PART USED

The fermented tea in which kombucha grows is drunk.

KNOWN ACTIVE CONSTITUENTS

• The fermentation process produces gluconic acid. Alcohol (0.5% to 1%) is also produced, some of which is converted to acetic acid.
• Lactic acid, tartaric acid, malic acid, malonic acid, citric acid, and oxalic acid also are present.
• Caffeine may also be present from the tea in which the kombucha grows.

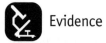 Evidence

OTHER CLAIMED BENEFITS/ACTIONS

• Cancer
• Rheumatism
• Intestinal disorders
• Aging
• HIV infection
• Arthritis
• Insomnia
• Regrowth of hair

 Risks

ADVERSE REACTIONS

• One case of hepatotoxicity has been reported (3). A 53-year-old man with hypothyroidism and fibromyalgia, taking levothyroxine, trazodone, and nabumetone, with infrequent alcohol use, presented with chest tightness, abdominal cramping, dry cough, and a rash. He had been drinking kombucha tea half a cup twice a day for 2 weeks, discontinuing use (9 days before seeking treatment) after noticing abdominal cramping and mild anorexia. Two days after discontinuation he developed an erythematous papular rash on the chest and neck and dark urine. Hepatitis serologies and Monospot test were negative, liver function tests increased, and bilirubin studies were normal. All lab values returned to normal without treatment within a month.
• Two cases of severe illness have been possibly linked to the consumption of kombucha tea. A 59-year-old woman found unconscious in her home developed metabolic acidosis, disseminated intravascular coagulopathy, cardiac arrest, and then died (4). Toxicologic screens were negative. The patient's daughter reported that during the previous 2 months, the patient had drunk 4 oz of kombucha tea daily.
• A previously healthy 48-year-old woman developed pulmonary edema and severe metabolic acidosis; she suffered a cardiac arrest but recovered (4). This patient also reported drinking kombucha tea during the previous 2 months and had obtained the kombucha from the same person as the other patient. Immediately before her illness she had increased her intake of the tea to 12 oz daily and also increased the period of incubation of the mushroom. However, at least 115 other people in town had used kombucha from the same source; no other cases of acute illness were reported. Microbiologic analysis of the tea identified several species of yeast and bacteria, including *Saccharomyces cerevisiae* and *Candida valida.* Analysis did not reveal any known human pathogens or toxin-producing organisms. It is not entirely convincing that either of these cases was due to the consumption of kombucha.

- Four other cases of illness possibly associated with kombucha were reported (5). These included a 55-year-old female diabetic alcoholic who developed jaundice 2 months after beginning daily consumption of kombucha tea. The patient had no signs of chronic liver disease and her aspartate transaminase (AST) was 259 U/L and alanine transaminase (ALT) was 585 U/L. All abnormal laboratory values normalized in 7 weeks.
- A 51-year-old woman taking thyroid hormone and estrogen replacement therapy was admitted after complaining of xerostomia, dizziness, nausea, vomiting, headache, and neck pain. She was released after 2 days and readmitted after reingesting the tea with recurrence of symptoms. On the second admission she also suffered three syncopal episodes. The only laboratory value of note was an elevated caffeine level of 3.8 mg/L 2 days after admission.
- Two other patients presented with apparent allergic reactions an hour after consuming kombucha tea. One patient presented with shaking, shortness of breath, and akathisia; the other presented with shortness of breath and throat tightness. Both patients had hypotension, tachycardia, and tachypnea. Both were released the same day after treatment for allergic reaction.

- Cutaneous anthrax

—An outbreak of skin lesions was reported in 20 patients near Tehran (6). The skin lesions (painless, with a black necrotic center, erythema around margin, and peripheral edema) were diagnosed as cutaneous anthrax. The lesions developed 5 to 7 days after each patient had applied kombucha mushroom topically as a painkiller. The contaminated material had been prepared in a farmyard close to cattle and was contaminated with multiple bacterial organisms. *Bacillus anthracis*, however, was not identifiable in the preparation. Inoculation of an uncontaminated kombucha demonstrated that *B. anthracis* could grow in both the tea and the mushroom.

- Lead poisoning

—Two cases of lead poisoning in a married couple were linked to the consumption of kombucha tea that had been brewed in a ceramic pot. The couple had been drinking the tea for 6 months; apparently lead from the glaze leached into the tea (7).

ANIMAL TOXICITY

- In one study, 48 mice were given Kargasok tea in their drinking water at six concentrations ranging from 0% to 100% for 2 to 8 weeks; 18 rats were given 0%, 15%, or 50% concentrations of the beverage for 12 weeks. Body weight was not affected. Rats treated with both concentrations had nephropathy and nonsuppurative necrosis of the duodenum, pancreas, and intestine. Mice had no lesions even when given 100% concentration of tea (8).
- Another experiment did find an effect of the tea on body weight in mice. Kargasok tea in concentrations of 50% and 100% resulted in significant decreases in food intake and weight in mice fed the tea for 8 weeks (9). Kargasok tea (concentration of 50%) caused weight loss of 16% associated with a 20% to 29% decrease in food intake; decreased food and fluid intake were reversible within 1 week. Concentrations as low as 15% over 2 weeks caused decreased food and fluid intake.

 ## Dose

COMMON DOSAGE FORMS

- The use of kombucha is not recommended.
- Typical daily dose of kombucha "tea": 2 oz at first, increasing to half a cup after 2 weeks.

 ## Common Questions and Answers

Q: Is bacterial contamination of this tea a concern?
A: It is theoretically possible that pathogens could grow in this tea, and it makes sense for immunocompromised patients to avoid it. However, the pH of the tea decreases to 1.8 within 24 hours, which should discourage the growth of most pathogens (4).

Q: Is there any evidence to support an anticancer claim?
A: In the 1960s, Dr. Sklenar developed a cancer therapy centered around kombucha. Dr. Sklenar had his own method for diagnosing cancer that involved iridology (a debunked method of diagnosing disease through examination of the iris) and analysis of the "Sklenar blood picture." An analysis of seven case histories concluded that they were not backed by solid medical data and that there was no reliable evidence that kombucha is an effective treatment for cancer (10).

Lactobacilli

 10 Second Take

Evidence supports using *Lactobacillus* preparations for lactose intolerance. Limited evidence supports the prevention and treatment of pediatric diarrhea and possibly other uses.

 Basics

LATIN NAME

L. acidophilus, L. casei, and other *Lactobacillus* species

OTHER COMMON NAMES

"Yogurt" bacteria

DESCRIPTION

* Lactobacilli are facultatively anaerobic gram-positive rods that inhabit the human oral cavity, gastrointestinal tract, and vagina.
* *Lactobacillus* is considered a "biotherapeutic agent" or "probiotic"; the latter term dates to 1965, when it was used to describe any substance or organism that helps to achieve microbial balance in the intestine (1).

PART USED

Live culture of whole microorganisms, often in fermented milk products

MECHANISM/PHARMACOKINETICS

* Mechanisms of action may include production of antimicrobial substances; competition for nutrients, competition for bacterial adhesion sites; and interference with bacterial attachment; and enzymatic modification of toxin receptors (2).

 Evidence

CLINICAL TRIALS

The use of Lactobacillus preparations as a tolerable dairy source for those who are lactose intolerant and as a means of restoring gut bacteria after antibiotic use is accepted in conventional medicine.

* Prevention of traveler's diarrhea

—*Lactobacillus* preparations do not appear to protect against traveler's diarrhea. A randomized, double-blind, placebo-controlled trial tested the effects of two capsules of *Lactobacillus fermentum* and *L. acidophilus* daily for 3 weeks or until diarrhea occurred in British soldiers in Belize (3). Among the 282 evaluable subjects, there was no difference in the incidence of diarrhea.
—A double-blind placebo-controlled trial tested *Lactobacillus* GG (*Lactobacillus casei* species strain *rhamnosus*) as a prophylactic against traveler's diarrhea in 820 vacationers to southern Turkey. Participants were treated for 7 to 14 days. Among the 756 patients who completed the trial, no significant difference was seen between treated subjects and controls (4).
—A randomized double-blind trial in 50 travelers to Mexico from the United States tested a commercial preparation of lactobacilli administered for 1 week (5). No difference was noted between the placebo group and the treated group either during the week of ingestion or during the next 3 weeks.
—A double-blind, placebo-controlled trial in 48 volunteers tested the effect of Lactinex (a commercial preparation of *L. acidophilus* and *Lactobacillus bulgaricus*) against a challenge with enterotoxigenic *Escherichia coli* (6). No significant differences were noted in attack rate, incubation period, duration of diarrhea, or volume or number of liquid stools.

* Prevention of diarrhea in children

—Most trials show a benefit of *Lactobacillus* preparations in reducing the incidence of diarrhea in children. A double-blind, placebo-controlled trial in 81 hospitalized children (1 to 36 months old) compared orally admin-istered *Lactobacillus* GG to placebo twice daily during hospitalization; *Lactobacillus* significantly reduced the risk of diarrhea (7).
—A placebo-controlled trial in 204 undernourished children (aged 6 to 24 months) in Peru tested the effects of *Lactobacillus* GG in flavored gelatin once daily, 6 days a week, for 15 months (8). Treated children had significantly fewer episodes of diarrhea (5.21 episodes/child/year vs. 6.02 episodes/child/year in the placebo group, *p* = 0.028).

—Even dead lactobacilli appear to have an effect. A placebo-controlled trial in 73 children (40 treated with antibiotics) tested the effects of freeze-dried heat-killed *L. acidophilus* versus placebo as an adjunct to oral rehydration (9). Compared with placebo, the mean duration of diarrhea was significantly decreased in the acidophilus group.
—Not all trials are positive. A crossover study in 287 children in day care tested the effects of standard yogurt, yogurt with *L. casei,* or jellied milk, each given for 1 month with a 1-month washout period between treatments (10). There was no difference in incidence of diarrhea over the 6-month study.

* Treatment of diarrhea

—Most trials show a benefit for *Lactobacillus* to treat pediatric diarrhea. A placebo-controlled trial of *L. casei* GG as an adjunct to oral rehydration in 71 Finnish children (4 to 45 months old) with acute diarrhea (82% with rotavirus) found that *Lactobacillus* significantly reduced days of diarrhea from a mean of 2.4 days in the placebo group (which received pasteurized yogurt) to 1.4 days (11).
—A study of 97 children age 6 to 36 months with acute diarrhea (89% were positive for rotavirus) tested the effects of freeze-dried *Lactobacillus reuteri* against placebo (for up to 5 days) as an adjunct to oral or intravenous rehydration (12). Colonization was demonstrated. The administration of *Lactobacillus* significantly decreased the duration of watery diarrhea with results seen by the second day of treatment; there were no differences in length of hospital stay.
—A study of *Lactobacillus* GG in 287 children (aged 1 month to 3 years) with acute diarrhea tested *Lactobacillus* as an adjunct to oral rehydration solution (13). Duration of diarrhea was significantly less in children receiving *Lactobacillus.*
—A placebo-controlled, double-blind trial in 39 children with acute diarrhea tested the effects of placebo against *Lactobacillus* GG in 39 children mean age 8 months (14). There was not a significant difference in clinical response between the two groups. In premature infants, two studies of *L. casei* GG did not improve intestinal pathogens or provide clinical benefit (2).

* Antibiotic-associated diarrhea

—Trials are mixed on whether or not lactobacilli are helpful. A double-blind, randomized controlled trial of children receiving oral antibiotics tested the effects of *Lactobacillus* GG in 202 children (aged 6 months to 10 years; 188 completed) treated with oral antibiotics as outpatients (15). *Lactobacillus* significantly reduced the incidence of diarrhea and stool frequency.
—In 16 healthy volunteers given erythromycin 400 mg t.i.d. for a week, the effects of yogurt containing *Lactobacillus* GG was compared with pasteurized regular yogurt. *Lactobacillus* treatment resulted in significantly fewer days with diarrhea (2) than did the control yogurt (8).

—A double-blind study in 98 inpatients receiving ampicillin tested Lactinex (a commercial mixture of *L. acidophilus* and *L. bulgaricus*) against placebo q.i.d. for 5 days (16). There was no difference in incidence of diarrhea between the two groups.

—A placebo-controlled pediatric trial of the same preparation administered q.i.d. for 10 days found no benefit in prevention of amoxicillin-induced diarrhea in children (17).

• Pouchitis

—A randomized, placebo-controlled trial of 40 patients with chronic pouchitis (a complication of ileal pouch-anal anastomosis) in remission, tested VSL (containing four strains of lactobacilli, three strains of bifidobacteria, and one strain of *Streptococcus salivarious*) 6 g/day for 9 months (1). Three patients (15%) in the treated group relapsed during the 9-month follow-up compared with zero patients in the placebo group.

• Small bowel bacterial overgrowth

—A study in 19 dialysis patients (including 9 females) tested the effects of two strains of freeze-dried *L. acidophilus* (one capsule containing 10^9 colonies twice daily) (18). Compared with baseline, *Lactobacillus* treatment decreased levels of dimethylamine (DMA) and the carcinogen nitrosodi-methylamine significantly. After an average of 67 days treatment, mean DMA levels dropped 42%; among 10 similar patients receiving placebo, mean serum DMA levels increased 13%. Among six patients who received *Lactobacillus* long-term (107 to 205 days), body weight and caloric intake increased significantly; there was not a significant change in midarm muscle area or serum albumin. Small bowel bacterial overgrowth, common in end-stage kidney disease, increases metabolic activity and methylamine toxins, which are precursors of nitrosamine carcinogens.

• Eczema

—A randomized controlled trial in 27 breast-fed infants with atopic eczema compared hydrolyzed whey formulas containing *Bifidobacterium lactis* or *Lactobacillus* GG to unsupplemented formula (19). After 2 months, severity scores significantly improved in both groups given probiotic-supplemented formulas, compared with the unsupplemented group. The concentration of soluble CD4 in serum and eosinophilic protein X in urine also decreased.

• Asthma

—A double-blind crossover study in 15 adults with moderate asthma tested yogurt with or without live *L. acidophilus,* each provided for 1 month (20). There were no changes in immune parameters, peak flow, spirometry values, or quality of life measures.

• Candidal vaginitis and bacterial vaginosis (BV)

—In an attempted crossover study, 33 women with recurrent candidal vaginitis received 8oz of yogurt with *L. acidophilus* for 6 months compared with 6 months without yogurt (21). Twelve patients violated protocol and eight patients initially assigned to yogurt refused to enter the control phase, apparently because the treatment was so successful. Of the 13 women who completed both arms of the study, the mean number of infections over 6 months with 2.54 ± 1.66 in controls compared with 0.38 ± 0.51 in the treated group, a significant difference.

—A double-blind, placebo-controlled trial tested a vaginal suppository containing freeze-dried *L. acidophilus* (10^8 to 10^9 colony forming units intravaginally b.i.d. × 6 days for 7 to 10 days) in 60 women with BV (22). Immediately after treatment, 16 out of 28 women treated with lactobacilli had normal vaginal wet smears compared with 0 of 29 placebo-treated women; however, there was a high relapse rate after the next menses.

—A poorly designed crossover study of 46 women with recurrent candidal vaginitis or BV compared three 2-month phases; in the first, women consumed yogurt with live *Lactobacillus;* in the second, women consumed pasteurized yogurt; and in the third, patients were to consume no yogurt. They were assessed monthly (23). Only seven participants completed the 6-month trial; only 17 completed both yogurt phases. Among completers there were no differences in positive vaginal cultures for *Candida,* but there were significant differences in number of episodes of BV. The extremely high dropout rate and the inclusion of women with different conditions renders this trial uninterpretable.

• Urinary tract infection (UTI)

—Although no placebo-controlled trials have been performed of urogenital tract colonization with lactobacilli to reduce UTIs, data from uncontrolled trials are interesting. A small pilot study in 10 women with recurrent UTI tested a vaginal suppository containing *L. casei* and *L. fermentum* weekly for 12 to 16 months (24). Eight patients completed the regimen; during the year-long trial there were 11 infections among the eight women, compared with 49 infections in the previous 12 months (a 66.3% reduction). Another uncontrolled trial in 55 premenopausal women (38 completed) compared weekly vaginal suppositories that contained either *Lactobacillus rhamnosus* or lactobacillus growth factor for 1 year. Compared with the previous year, the UTI infection rate decreased 73% for those on lactobacilli and 79% for those receiving lactobacillus growth factor (25).

OTHER CLAIMED BENEFITS/ACTIONS

• Immune stimulation
• Inflammatory bowel disease

 Risks

ADVERSE REACTIONS

• Although lactobacilli are usually benign, they can become pathogenic under some circumstances. Various species of *Lactobacillus* (including *L. acidophilus, L. casei, L. salivarius,* and *L. rhamnosus*) have been isolated in cases of bacterial endocarditis; *L. rhamnosus* and *L. plantarum* have been isolated from bloodstream infections (26). Although lactobacillemia is quite rare, it may be more common in liver transplant patients, among whom eight cases of *Lactobacillus* bacteremia were identified; Roux-en-Y choledochojejunostomy appeared to predispose to this condition (27). A case of oral antibiotic-induced D-lactic acidosis was reported in a patient with enteric overgrowth of *L. acidophilus* (28).

 Dose

COMMON DOSAGE FORMS

• Usually one or two capsules containing 10^9 colony forming units twice daily or 8 oz lactobacilli-containing fermented milk product daily.

 Common Questions and Answers

Q: What other probiotics are promising?
A: Various organisms (including *Enterococcus faecium, Streptococcus thermophilus,* and *Bifidobacterium longum*) have been tested. The most promising is probably the yeast *Saccharomyces boulardii;* three double-blind placebo-controlled trials in a total of 761 patients found a significant reduction in the incidence of antibiotic-associated diarrhea (29). Double-blind, placebo-controlled trials have also demonstrated benefit against *Clostridium difficile* diarrhea, HIV-related diarrhea, and acute diarrhea in infants and adults. *S. boulardii* has been associated with increased thirst and mild constipation, and a 1-year old treated with *S. boulardii* for diarrhea developed fungemia (30).

Lecithin/Phosphatidylcholine

 10 Second Take

Phosphatidylcholine is a benign supplement; clinical trials, however, do not support its use for dementia, tardive dyskinesia, or hypercholesterolemia.

 Basics

DESCRIPTION

• Phosphatidylcholine is a phospholipid that composes more than half of phospholipids in mammalian cells (1).
• Lecithin is the same as phosphatidyl-choline; however, commercial lecithin, which is made from soybeans, may contain only 23% phosphatidylcholine, with the remainder composed of other phospholipids (1).

FOOD SOURCES

• Phosphatidylcholine is abundant in plant and animal foods; rich sources include soybeans, eggs, and muscle and organ meats (2).
• Phosphatidylcholine is the primary source of dietary choline for Americans (who consume between 0.4 to 0.9 g choline/day) (3).

MAIN FUNCTIONS/PHARMACOKINETICS

• Phosphatidylcholine and sphingomyelin are the main choline-containing substances in tissues (phosphatidylcholine constitutes more than 50% of phospholipids in mammalian membranes) (1).
• Phosphatidylcholine is synthesized by phosphorylation of choline to cytidine diphosphocholine, which is then combined with diacylglycerol phosphate, forming phosphatidylcholine and cytidine monophosphate. The other biosynthesis pathway for phosphatidylcholine involves the sequential methylation of phosphatidyl-ethanolamine to phosphatidylcholine by phosphatidylethanolamine-*N*-methyl-transferase, using *S*-adenosylmethionine as the methyl donor (1). Phosphatidylcholine is important in cell signaling and is essential for very low density lipoprotein (VLDL) secretion.

 Evidence

CLINICAL TRIALS

• Dementia

—A Cochrane review of lecithin in the treatment of dementia or cognitive impairment identified 11 randomized trials involving 265 patients with Alzheimer's disease and 21 patients with Parkinson's disease associated dementia. No trials reported clear clinical benefits of lecithin (4).

• Tardive dyskinesia

—A Cochrane collaboration review of cholinergic agents (including choline, lecithin, and other agents) for tardive dyskinesia identified seven studies (another 10 trials were awaiting further data from authors) (5). The studies reviewed to date did not find a significant advantage of lecithin compared with placebo.

• Hypercholesterolemia

—A review of 24 studies on the effect of supplementary lecithin on cholesterol found that most studies were methodologically flawed (lacking appropriate controls, small sample sizes, or inadequate controlling of intake of other foods that could be confounding) (6). In four trials, attempts were made to control for the effect of linoleic acid. The combined results of these four appropriately controlled trials did not find benefits of lecithin on lowering serum cholesterol.

• Fatty liver

—In a double-blind study, 15 patients receiving long-term total parenteral nutrition (TPN) (all of whom had low plasma choline concentrations, and eight of whom had fatty livers at baseline) were given either 20 g lecithin (30% phosphatidylcholine containing about 300 μmol choline moiety/kg/day) or placebo (soy oil) orally b.i.d. × 6 weeks (7). Ten participants completed the study. Lecithin supplementation significantly and progressively increased liver-spleen Houndsfield units by computed tomography (indicating decreased fat) in the lecithin-treated group but not the placebo group. Plasma-free choline increased in the lecithin group and decreased in the placebo group.

• Platelet aggregation

—A study comparing fish oils or soy lecithin on platelet aggregation found that soy lecithin (25 g daily for 15 days) increased platelet adhesion (fish oil decreased platelet aggregation) (8).

ANIMAL/IN VITRO

• Twelve baboons were fed a liquid diet supplemented with polyunsaturated lecithin (4.1 mg/kcal) for up to 8 years. Ethanol or an isocaloric carbohydrate composed 50% of total energy (9). These were compared with 18 baboons fed an equivalent amount of the same diet (again, with or without ethanol) but without lecithin supplementation. Lecithin exerted a significant protective effect against hepatic fibrosis. Septal fibrosis (and cirrhosis in two cases) developed in seven of nine baboons fed the regular diet with ethanol and none of the baboons fed the lecithin-supplemented diet with ethanol.

OTHER CLAIMED BENEFITS/ACTIONS

• Cardiovascular disease

Clinical Considerations

DEFICIENCY SIGNS AND SYMPTOMS

• In humans, choline deficiency can decrease phosphatidylcholine concentrations in erythrocyte membranes (and increase serum alanine transaminase activity). In animals, choline deficiency affects the function of liver, kidneys, and pancreas (1).

FACTORS DECREASING AVAILABILITY/ABSORPTION

• Pregnancy
• Lactation
• Total parenteral nutrition
• Cirrhosis
• Hemodialysis

 ## Risks

ADVERSE REACTIONS

• None identified for phosphatidylcholine. High doses (20 g) of choline can cause dizziness, nausea, diarrhea, and fishy odor resulting from bacterial breakdown to trimethylamines (3).

 ## Dose

RECOMMENDED DIETARY ALLOWANCE (10)

• Intake of phosphatidylcholine is not required because it is synthesized endogenously from choline.
• The following values are for choline:

Adequate intake

Infants and children

0 to 5 months	125 mg
6 to 11 months	150 mg
1 to 3 years	200 mg
4 to 8 years	250mg

Males

9 to 13 years	375 mg
14 to 18 years	550 mg
19 to 50 years	550 mg
51+ years	550 mg

Females

9 to 13 years	375 mg
14 to 18 years	400 mg
19 to 50 years	425 mg
51+ years	425 mg
Pregnant	450 mg
Lactating	550 mg

Lemon Balm

 10 Second Take

Lemon balm is a harmless herb. Two clinical trials of topical preparations for herpes are unimpressive.

 Basics

LATIN NAME

Melissa officinalis L.

FAMILY

Lamiaceae

OTHER COMMON NAMES

Sweet balm, lemon balm, bee balm, and balm mint

DESCRIPTION

• A shade-loving perennial up to a meter in height, Melissa has white flowers in a leafy whorled spike.
• The leaves smell of lemon.
• It is native to the eastern Mediterranean region and western Asia; it is now widely cultivated.

PART USED

Aerial parts (dried or fresh)

KNOWN ACTIVE CONSTITUENTS

• Essential oil containing monoterpinoid aldehydes, primarily geranial, neral, and citronellal; flavonoids, primarily luteolin, quercetin, apigenin, and kaempferol; monoterpene and phenylpropanoid glycosides; rosmarinic acid (up to 4%); caffeic acid; chlorogenic acid; and triterpenes including ursolic acid and oleanolic acid (1).

MECHANISM/PHARMACOKINETIC

• Ethanolic extract of Melissa was able to displace [3H]-(N)-nicotine from nicotinic receptors and [3H]-(N)-scopolamine from muscarinic receptors [inhibitory concentration $(IC)_{50}$ less than 1 mg/mL] (2).
• Rosmarinic acid inhibits several complement-dependent inflammatory processes, particularly C5 convertase in the classical pathway (3).

 Evidence

CLINICAL TRIALS

• Herpes

—It is not clear whether topical application of Melissa is helpful in herpes. A double-blind placebo–controlled trial in 66 patients (52 female) with recurrent oral or genital herpes compared the effect of placebo to a melissa cream containing a dried extract from Melissa leaves (Lo-701, Lomaherpan) on a symptom-rating score that included "complaints," blisters, and affected area (4). Participants were told to apply the cream to the affected area four times daily and to be examined within 24 hours (and again on the second, third, and fifth day). Symptom score on the second day was significantly lower in the treatment group compared with control; however, the total symptom score over 5 days of treatment was not significantly different between groups. Number of blisters did not differ between the groups, nor did physicians judge treatment to be more effective than placebo.
—A controlled trial in 116 patients (70 female) compared the effect of Lomaherpan cream [1% lyophilized Melissa leaf extract (70:1)] with cream base applied two to four times daily over 5 to 10 days in acute herpes infection in those with symptoms lasting less than 72 hours (5). Eighty-five patients had received no prior treatment. The idiosyncratic outcomes included rubor, swelling, vesicles, scabbing, pain, and healing. The only symptoms significantly improved in the Melissa group were rubor and swelling on day 2 (there was no difference on day 5). There was a significant difference favoring Melissa in both physician assessment and patient assessment of healing. Mean area of lesions was significantly less on day 5 (but not on day 2) in the subset of those with herpes labialis.

ANIMAL/IN VITRO

• Sedation

—Sedative and analgesic effects of a freeze-dried hydroalcoholic extract of Melissa have been demonstrated in mice; this extract also potentiated the hypnotic effect of pentobarbital (6). In mice, intraperitoneal administration of the essential oil had no sedative effect, but oral administration in doses over 3.16 mg/kg was sedative (1).

• Thyroid effects

—A freeze-dried aqueous extract of Melissa had a strong dose-related antithyrotropic effect, inhibiting the binding of radiolabeled thyroid-stimulating hormone (TSH) to human thyroid membrane (7). Incubation of freeze-dried aqueous extracts of Melissa and other plants decreased the TSH-binding inhibitory activity of thyroid-stimulating immunoglobulin G found in the blood of patients with Graves' disease (8).

• Antimicrobial effect

—Essential oil of Melissa was more effective than essential oils of either lavender or rosemary on inhibiting growth of bacteria, yeasts, and filamentous fungi (9). Aqueous extracts of Melissa showed potent anti-HIV-1 activity, inhibiting cytopathogenicity in MT-4 cells (10).

• Other effects

—The essential oil of Melissa has a spasmolytic effect in guinea pig ileum, rat duodenum and vas deferens, and rabbit aorta and jejunum. Another study, however, found that an ethanol extract of Melissa did not oppose acetylcholine or histamine-induced spasm in guinea pig ileum (1). In guinea pig tracheal muscle, essential oil had a relaxant effect.

• A methanolic extract of Melissa caused a concentration-dependent inhibition of lipid peroxidation (11).

OTHER CLAIMED BENEFITS/ACTIONS

• Depression
• Liver problems
• Dyspepsia
• Flatulence
• Fevers
• Wound healing
• Memory improvement
• Restlessness, irritability

Risks

ANIMAL TOXICITY

Melissa extract showed only weak sensitizing potential in guinea pigs (12).

 Dose

COMMON DOSAGE FORMS

- *Leaf:* 1.5 to 4.5 g as tea or infusion b.i.d. to t.i.d.
- *Tincture:* (1:5, 45% ethanol) 2 to 6 mL t.i.d.
- *Topical application:* Cream with 1% of a lyophilized aqueous extract (70:1) b.i.d. to q.i.d. (from prodromal signs to several days after lesions heal)

 Common Questions and Answers

Q: Why are beekeepers interested in lemon balm?
A: Honeybees are attracted to the essential oil of *Melissa,* which apparently is chemically similar to a pheromone produced by bees (13).

Leucine (Leu, L)

 10 Second Take

Leucine is a safe, essential amino acid; there is limited evidence that combined branched-chain amino acids (BCAAs) improve appetite, but clinical trials have not supported other claims.

 Basics

DESCRIPTION

Leucine is an essential BCAA.

FOOD SOURCES

Most protein-containing foods

MECHANISM/PHARMACOKINETICS

• The hydrophobicity of BCAAs (leucine, isoleucine, and valine) make them important to protein formation; BCAAs also affect response to infection (1).
• BCAAs make up about a third of muscle protein and are an important constituent of other tissues (2). Leucine stimulates protein synthesis in muscle.
• The plasma half-life of leucine is 5 days.

 Evidence

CLINICAL TRIALS

• Ergogenics

—Exercise significantly decreases leucine levels. A review of leucine supplementation and intensive exercise noted that leucine supplementation (200 mg/kg) 50 minutes before running had no effect on performance (2).
—A randomized double-blind crossover study in 20 male track and field power athletes compared leucine (50.0 ± 3.3 mg/kg body weight daily) with placebo for 10 weeks and found that leucine supplementation prevented decreased serum leucine concentrations, compared with placebo (3).

• Muscular dystrophy

—A double-blind, placebo-controlled trial of 96 patients with Duchenne muscular dystrophy were randomized to placebo or leucine (0.2 g/kg/day) for a year; no benefit for leucine was demonstrated in terms of muscle strength, joint contracture, functional grade and activity, and pulmonary function tests (4).

• BCAA and phenylketonuria

—A mixture of valine, isoleucine, and leucine was administered to 16 adolescents and young adults with phenylketonuria in a double-blind crossover study comprising four 3-month periods (5). Time to completion of the Attention Diagnostic Methods (which requires substantial attention with mental processing) was significantly faster during the period in which the amino acid mixture was administered. There was not a significant change seen on the Continuous Performance Test.

• BCAA in amyotrophic lateral sclerosis (ALS)

—A double-blind, placebo-controlled trial compared BCAAs (L-leucine 12 g, isoleucine 8 g, and L-valine 6.4 g with pyridoxal phosphate, 160 mg daily) to L-threonine (4 g daily) or placebo for 6 months in 95 patients with ALS (6). Every 2 months, muscle strength, muscle torque, forced vital capacity (FVC), activities of daily living involving upper and lower limbs, and timed tasks were tested. Both the placebo group and the threonine group lost weight, whereas the BCAA-supplemented group gained weight; the difference was significant. Estimated decline in FVC was 2.5 times greater in both groups supplemented with amino acids, compared with placebo. No other significant differences were seen among treatment groups. The amino acids were well tolerated, but the authors point out that adverse effects of these amino acids on pulmonary function could not be ruled out. Long-term effects of this mixture also are unknown.
—Another trial of BCAAs for ALS was halted after 126 participants were recruited because of what appeared to be excess mortality among randomized active treatment (24 BCAAs, 13 placebo); there was also no evidence of efficacy in disability scales between the two groups (7).

- BCAA and tardive dyskinesia (TD)

—An uncontrolled 2-week trial in nine men with neuroleptic-induced TD tested administration of a BCAA medical food three times a day for 2 weeks (8). Compared with baseline, frequency of TD movements (collected by videotape and analyzed in blinded random sequence) decreased significantly; movements decreased at least 38% in all participants.

- BCAA and appetite

—A double-blind study in 28 cancer patients compared BCAA (4.8 g daily) with placebo; improvements in appetite were seen in 55% of the treatment group compared with 16% of those in the placebo group (9).

- BCAA in protein wasting associated with bedrest

—Nineteen healthy participants were randomized into two groups; one group received 30 μmol/day of BCAAs, whereas the other received the same amount of nonessential amino acids. BCAA supplementation attenuated nitrogen loss during short-term bedrest (10).

OTHER CLAIMED BENEFITS/ACTIONS

- Improves healing

 Risks

No risks identified.

 Clinical Considerations

FACTORS INCREASING AVAILABILITY/ABSORPTION

- Maple syrup urine disease (MSUD) or branched chain α-ketoaciduria is the group of inherited disorders of leucine, isoleucine, and valine metabolism. Infants do not manifest symptoms until they start eating protein-containing food; the most deficient in enzymes may die within 10 days of birth. Progressive neurologic dysfunction and urine and ear wax that smell of caramel or maple syrup characterize this disease. Screening should be done in the first week of life. Long-term management of MSUD involves dietary manipulation designed to maintain plasma concentrations of BCAAs 3 to 4 hours after a meal in a specific range (isoleucine, 40 to 90 μmol; leucine, 80 to 200 μmol; and valine, 200 to 425 μmol).

LABORATORY TESTS

- 78 to 176 μmol/L venous blood
- Urinary output 809 μmol/24 hours

 Dose

DIETARY REQUIREMENTS

Infants 3 to 4 months	161 mg/kg/day
Children 2 to 5 years	73 mg/kg/day
Children 10 to 12 years	42 mg/kg/day
Adults	14 to 39 mg/kg/day

Licorice

10 Second Take

Real licorice can cause hypertension, hypokalemia, arrhythmias, edema, and preterm birth.

Basics

LATIN NAME

Glycyrrhiza glabra L.

FAMILY

Leguminosae/Fabaceae

OTHER COMMON NAMES

Sweet root

DESCRIPTION

• Licorice, a perennial herb with sweet-tasting roots, is native to the Mediterranean, the Mideast, Russia, and Asia. It is widely used as a flavoring, sweetener, and medicinal herb.

PART USED

Roots, rhizomes

KNOWN ACTIVE CONSTITUENTS

• Triterpenoid saponins, especially glycyrrhizin [also called glycyrrhizic or glycyrrhizinic acid (GL)], which is 50 times sweeter than sugar, and hydroxyglycyrrhizin. Glycyrrhizin concentration varies from 1% to 24% (usually 6% to 14%) (1). Also numerous flavonoids including liquiritin, isoliquiritin, and liquiritoside (2) and coumarin derivatives.

MECHANISM/PHARMACOKINETICS

• GL is hydrolyzed to glycyrrhetinic acid (GA) in the intestine, apparently by intestinal bacteria. Licorice inhibits 11β-hydroxysteroid dehydrogenase, which converts cortisol to cortisone. Cortisol has the same binding affinity as aldosterone (cortisone has a lower binding affinity), so inhibition of 11β-hydroxysteroid dehydrogenase produces high renal levels of cortisol, leading to apparent mineralocorticoid excess (3).
• Peak serum concentration of GL occurs in less than 4 hours, then decreases rapidly. None is detectable at 96 hours. GA peaks at 24 hours, decreases gradually, and is still detectable in most people at 72 hours (1).
• Excretion of metabolites is most likely gastrointestinal; 2% of metabolites appear in urine.

Evidence

CLINICAL TRIALS

• Hepatitis

—A randomized controlled trial (RCT) in 57 patients with chronic hepatitis C found that glycyrrhizin (80, 160, or 240 mg intravenously three times per week), compared with placebo, significantly decreased serum alanine aminotransferase 26% versus 6%, $p < 0.02$. The effect was seen in 2 days, was not dose-related, and disappeared after cessation of therapy (4). There was no effect on viral clearance.

• Ulcers/gastrointestinal bleeding

—A double-blind crossover study of nine volunteers tested 975 mg of aspirin with or without licorice (525 mg t.i.d.); licorice reduced the incidence of human fecal blood loss by 20% (5).
—Once used conventionally to treat peptic ulcer, licorice was abandoned because of side effects (6). Numerous older studies found licorice effective for ulcers; two studies of deglycyrrhizinated licorice (DGL), which contains no GL and reputedly does not cause hypertension, found DGL equivalent to cimetidine (7,8).

• Endocrine effects

—Licorice has glucocorticoid effects, an effect once exploited to treat Addison's disease (9). In 10 volunteers, GA 500 mg/day decreased plasma cortisone (but not cortisol), elevated free cortisol and decreased free cortisone in urine (10). In 11 volunteers, licorice for 10 days increased urinary free cortisol, decreased urinary aldosterone, and decreased plasma renin activity, indicating significant suppression of the renin-angiotensin-aldosterone system (11). This suppression may last for several months (3).
—A small study of seven men found that licorice (7 g, with 500 mg GL daily × 1 week) significantly decreased serum testosterone and 17-hydroxyprogesterone (12). However, a larger study tested 5 to 6 g licorice for 4 days in 20 men and a different brand of licorice in 21 participants (including 10 women) and found no effect of licorice on salivary testosterone (cortisol did increase) (13).
—Licorice increases atrial natriuretic peptide levels (6).
—A case of licorice-related hyper-prolactinemia has been reported (14).

OTHER CLAIMED BENEFITS/ACTIONS

• Chronic fatigue syndrome
• Expectorant
• Antitussive
• Antiinflammatory
• Bronchitis
• Gastrointestinal antispasmodic
• Laxative
• Aphthous ulcers

Risks

ADVERSE REACTIONS

• Licorice toxicity causes pseudoprimary aldosteronism; symptoms may include edema, hypertension, and hypokalemia (15,16).
• Arrhythmias

—Cardiac arrhythmias have been associated with licorice ingestion. A 44-year-old woman who had ingested 40 to 70 g licorice daily for 4 months developed repeated episodes of life-threatening *torsades de pointes* (17). Cardiac arrest, including two deaths, has been associated with licorice use.

• Hypertension (see questions and answers)

—Excessive use of licorice can cause hypertension. Hypertension encephalopathy was reported in a 15-year-old 3 hours after eating 0.5 kg licorice (18); ingestion of 1 kg licorice by a 25-year-old woman with myeloid leukemia caused decerebrate rigidity, tetraparesis, and coma (19).
—Ingestion of 100 g licorice daily × 4 weeks in 30 normotensive participants significantly increased systolic (6.5 mm Hg) but not diastolic blood pressure and decreased serum potassium 0.24 mmol/L. Effects were still apparent 4 weeks after discontinuing licorice (20). Women may be more susceptible; blood pressures were slightly higher for women than men, and 14/19 women gained weight (mean 0.59 kg; one women gained 6.8 kg), although men did not gain weight. In 13 different women given 50 g licorice, systolic blood pressure rose 5.6 mm Hg and diastolic blood pressure rose 3.4 mm Hg.

• Hypokalemia

—Fifty-nine cases of licorice-associated hypokalemic myopathy have been reported; most patients had additional risk factors for hypokalemia, including alcoholism, diarrhea, or diuretic use (21).
—Severe hypokalemia has caused several cases of rhabdomyolysis, including a 62-year-old man on diuretics who developed weakness and pain during Ramadan (during which observers fast during the day and often consume a licorice-containing soft drink during the evening meal). Apparently the fasting, diuretic use, and licorice consumption proved synergistic for hypokalemia (22).
—Rhabdomyolysis and subsequent acute renal failure was reported in a 72-year-old man who had consumed 240 mg GL as an antacid for many years (23). After normalization of serum potassium, rechallenge with 40 mg GL administered intravenously daily caused moderate hypokalemia (2.3 mEq/L).

- Pulmonary edema/congestive heart failure

—Pulmonary edema was reported in a 64-year-old healthy man who ate four packages (1,020 g) of Twizzlers (one of the few American "licorice" brands that contains real licorice) over 3 days; total GL consumed was approximately 3.6 g (9).
—Three previous cases of licorice-associated congestive heart failure were reported (9).

- Preterm birth

—A survey of 1,049 Finnish women who gave birth to singleton infants in 1998 examined the effect of licorice on birth outcome (24). Almost half of mothers surveyed (46%) reported weekly licorice consumption, and only 2.3% of respondents never consumed licorice during pregnancy. Compared with babies exposed to the lowest levels of maternal licorice (less than 250 mg GL/week), babies exposed to the highest levels (≥500 mg GL/week) were significantly more likely to be born before 38 weeks gestation [odds ratio (OR) 2.5, 95% confidence interval (CI) 1.1, 5.5, $p = 0.03$]. Adjustments were made for sex, maternal age, parity, smoking, coffee consumption, and systolic blood pressure. Heavy licorice consumption shortened gestation by a mean of 2.52 days. Possible mechanisms include inhibition of cortisol metabolism (cortisol stimulates corticotropin-releasing hormone from the placenta and is thought to be a parturition trigger) or possibly increased uterine prostaglandin levels through inhibition of 15-β-hydroxyprostaglandin dehydrogenase (a homologue of 11-β-hydroxysteroid dehydrogenase).

DRUG INTERACTIONS

- Corticosteroids

—Licorice potentiates corticosteroids. Oral administration of GL increases the plasma concentration of prednisolone. GA, but not GL, potentiates the effect of hydrocortisone in human lung tissue. Topical GA potentiates the action of hydrocortisone (25).

- Oral contraceptives

—Combined oral contraceptives may increase sensitivity to GL. Hypokalemia and hypertension were reported in two oral contraceptive users who used licorice chewing gum; daily doses of GL were 120 mg and 50 mg (notable because adverse effects usually occur at much higher doses) (26).

- Nitrofurantoin

—DGL may increase nitrofurantoin bioavailability > 50% (1).

- Thiazide diuretics

—Concurrent use increases the risk of hypokalemia.

- Laxatives

—Licorice may potentiate the effect of other laxatives.

- Insulin

—Glycyrrhizin may act synergistically with insulin in suppressing renin and aldosterone (1).

 Dose

COMMON DOSAGE FORMS

- *Powdered dried root:* 1 to 5 g q.d. to t.i.d.
- *Infusion or decoction:* 1 to 5 g t.i.d. Infusion may be made by pouring boiling water over herb and steeping for 30 minutes or by boiling herb for a few minutes and then letting it steep 15 minutes.
- *Liquid extract:* 2 to 5 mL t.i.d.
- *DGL:* 0.4 to 1.6 t.i.d. (for ulcers).

 Common Questions and Answers

Q: What is a safe range of licorice ingestion?
A: Individuals vary in susceptibility to licorice; 100 mg GL daily (about 50 g or 1.75 oz of candy) is enough to produce adverse effects in some people, and most people who consume more than 400 mg GL daily will experience symptoms (3). Some individuals, however, are hypersensitive to glycyrrhizin; doses as low as 20 mg/day GL have produced severe hypokalemia (23).
—A safety study in 39 healthy women tested oral GL (1, 2, and 4 mg/kg body weight) for 8 weeks (27). The authors proposed a no-effect level of 2 mg/kg and extrapolated an acceptable daily intake (ADI) of 0.2 mg/kg body weight. If licorice contains 0.2% of GL, a 60-kg person should ingest no more than 6 g licorice (containing 12 mg GL) a day.

Q: Is licorice toxicity common?
A: Although the prevalence of licorice toxicity is unknown, it is not common; many people consume licorice without ill effects. In Denmark, average licorice consumption is 2 kg per person per year, and no epidemics of licorice toxicity have been reported. One study of Danish schoolchildren (6 to 18 years old) found no linear relationship between licorice consumption and blood pressure (28). No common characteristics of susceptible individuals have been identified (although women seem more susceptible than men).

Q: Is licorice in Chinese medicine dangerous?
A: Almost all reported cases of licorice-induced problems have been from licorice-containing liqueurs, candies, gum, laxatives, or chewing tobacco rather than from the use of licorice as medicine. In Chinese medicine licorice is always used as part of a mixture, and the synergistic effects of mixtures, as well as perhaps dose differences, may prevent problems.

Q: Is licorice a laxative?
A: Yes. Glycyrrhizin is a surfactant, increasing the wettability of bowel contents. It is often combined with anthraquinone-containing herbs (29).

Q: What is licorice used to flavor?
A: Licorice is commonly used to flavor and sweeten herbal teas. It may be added to chewing gum, cigarettes, snuff, chewing tobacco, beer, porter, stout, or root beer. Most "licorice" candies manufactured in the United States are actually flavored with anise; imported candies usually contain real licorice.

Linden

10 Second Take

Linden is a benign herb widely consumed in tea. It is reputed to have an anxiolytic effect, although no clinical trials have been done.

Basics

LATIN NAME

Tilia cordata Miller, *T. platyphyllos* Scopoli

FAMILY

Tiliaceae

OTHER COMMON NAMES

T. platyphyllos Scopoli: lime tree flower, large-leafed linden; *Tilia cordata:* small-leafed linden; *T. x europaea* L.: common European linden, lime leaves, European linden

DESCRIPTION

• *Tilia* is a large deciduous tree that grows up to 130 ft tall, with heart-shaped, toothed leaves (dark green above and pale green below) and greenish-yellow, aromatic flowers.
• The tree is native to Europe and cultivated in North America.

PART USED

Flower

KNOWN ACTIVE CONSTITUENTS

• Mucilaginous polysaccharides (3% to 10%), condensed tannins (2%), flavonoids (1%), kaempferol glycosides, and phenolic acids
• The essential oil contains alkanes C18-31, 2-phenylethyl alcohol and its esters (1.0% to 7.4%), geraniol (0.5% to 5.9%), eugenol (1.0% to 2.5%), and *cis-trans* farnesol (0.3% to 1.6%) (1,2).

MECHANISM/PHARMACOKINETICS

• No information available on pharmacokinetics.
• Components of *Tilia* bind to benzodiazepine receptors (3,4). Sedative qualities have been attributed to farnesol, but farnesol occurs only in small quantities. Flavonol glycosides and phenolic acids have a diaphoretic effect. Emollient properties of the mucilaginous polysaccharides may be responsible for soothing coughs (5).

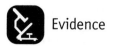

Evidence

CLINICAL TRIALS

No clinical trials identified.

ANIMAL/IN VITRO

• Hypotensive effects

—In rabbits, intravenous administration of an aqueous extract of *Tilia sylvestris* causes decreased diastolic arterial pressure; the dialyzed seed extract was more effective than dialyzed extracts from flowers, bracts, or sapwood (2).
—Earlier animal studies showed that extracts cause hypotensive and vasodilation effects and increased pulse rate (5).

• Sedation/benzodiazepine effects

—A complex fraction with unidentified constituents from an extract of *Tilia tomentosa* flowers was shown to have anxiolytic effects in mice without affecting locomotor activity (4).
—An immunoassay of 12 plants found that fractions of *Tilia* flowers contained low concentrations of benzodiazepine-like agents (3).
—Kaempferol has been identified as a low-affinity ligand in a benzodiazepine receptor binding assay, but kaempferol did not produce sedation or anxiolytic effects in mice (4).

• Iron absorption

—In rats with ligated intestinal segments, *Tilia* increased iron absorption (6).

OTHER CLAIMED BENEFITS/ACTIONS

• Colds
• Cough
• Hypertension
• Restlessness
• Headache
• Skin ailments (topical)

Risks

ADVERSE REACTIONS

• No serious adverse events have been reported; occasional allergic reactions have been reported. It is controversial whether there is cross-reaction between *Tilia* pollen and grass pollen because *Tilia* pollen is usually contaminated with grass pollen (2).

ANIMAL TOXICITY

• The flowers have not been tested for toxicity.
• An aqueous extract from the seeds and sap wood of *Tilia silvestris* was tested for toxicity in white Wistar mice; the lethal dose was 3 to 5 g/kg intraperitoneally (2).

 Dose

COMMON DOSAGE FORMS

• Dried flower

—*2–4 g as tea or decoction* q.d. (in the evening): t.i.d. (both preferably taken hot)
—*Equivalent preparations:* 2 to 4 g daily dose
—*Liquid extract:* (1:1, 25% ethanol) 2 to 4 mL t.i.d.
—*Tincture:* (1:5, 25% ethanol) 4 to 10 mL t.i.d.

 Common Questions and Answers

Q: Aren't large amounts of linden toxic?
A: It is stated in several sources that large amounts of linden are known to be toxic to the heart. All of these references apparently stem from a statement in a German book published in 1979 (7), but there are no published case reports or animal studies that document this effect.
One source (8) also states that tea made from old linden flowers can cause narcotic intoxication, but various experts have disputed this and I think it can be safely ignored.

Lobelia

10 Second Take

Lobeline from lobelia has been studied as an aid in smoking cessation; however, nausea, vomiting, and other side effects should limit its attractiveness.

Basics

LATIN NAME

Lobelia inflata L.

FAMILY

Campanulaceae

OTHER COMMON NAMES

Indian tobacco, puke weed

DESCRIPTION

• An annual or biennial herb, 1 to 2 ft tall with stalked, pale violet-blue flowers. It is common in open woods in meadows of eastern North America.

PART USED

Dried aerial parts

KNOWN ACTIVE CONSTITUENTS

• Piperidine alkaloids (0.2% to 0.6%), primarily lobeline. Minor alkaloids include lobelinine and lobelanidine and carboxylic acids (chelidonic acid and phenyloxypropionic acid) (1). Beta-amyrin palmitate also appears to be active (2); see animal/*in vitro*.

MECHANISM/PHARMACOKINETICS

• Lobeline is a potent ligand at nicotinic cholinergic receptors on neurons (3). Lobeline interacts with the receptor in a novel way (4). Although lobeline has been classified as a nicotinic agonist, it has recently been demonstrated that lobeline inhibits dopamine uptake into synaptic vesicles. The mechanism differs from amphetamine; whereas D-amphetamine inhibits dopamine uptake and promotes release from the synaptic vesicles equally, lobeline is 28 times as potent in inhibiting dopamine uptake as in evoking dopamine release (5). Beta-amyrin palmitate causes release of [3H]norepinephrine in mouse brain synaptosomes (6).

Evidence

CLINICAL TRIALS

• Smoking cessation

—A Cochrane collaboration review found no randomized trials that assessed the long-term effect of lobeline on smoking cessation (7). The effect of lobeline on short-term cessation, however, has been studied. Lobeline has been used for smoking cessation since 1936. In a 1937 study, lobeline (8-mg capsules ad lib up to 18 a day) was tested in 28 smokers and five nonsmokers; four controls were given magnesium capsules (8). Those receiving lobeline experienced gas, heartburn, nausea, vomiting, epigastric pain, faintness, excess salivation, and metallic taste. No participant would take more than three capsules daily for more than 3 days, and some wouldn't take a second dose! A marked rise in blood sugar was noted in two patients. The authors concluded that this dose was not practical.

—There was a spate of trials in the 1950s and 1960s on the use of lobeline-containing products for smoking cessation. Buffering lobeline apparently reduced side effects in some (but not all) studies. A trial in 200 male smokers tested a proprietary formulation called Bantron [2 mg lobeline sulfate and 100 mg of antacids (tricalcium phosphate and magnesium carbonate)] against placebo or lobeline sulfate (2 mg). This was a sophisticated placebo-controlled trial in which some receiving placebo were told they were getting active drug and some receiving active drug were told they were receiving placebo. Bantron significantly reduced the number of cigarettes smoked; at the end of 6 days, more than 80% of those on Bantron stopped smoking, compared with less than 10% of those on placebo or lobeline sulfate (9). This may have been due to differential release of lobeline; a later report found that blood levels of lobeline were higher after use of Bantron than lobeline suspended in cornstarch (10). Physiologic effects of Bantron were also tested; no significant changes were noted in heart rate, blood pressure, respiratory rate, or skin temperature between lobeline and placebo among smokers (nonsmokers experienced a slight rise in pulse, blood pressure, and respiration) (9).

—Other trials of buffered preparations for smoking cessation were not so promising. A placebo-controlled crossover trial in 55 smokers of Lobidan (a buffered preparation containing lobeline sulfate 2 mg, magnesium carbonate 125 mg, and tribasic calcium phosphate 180 mg) found no advantage of Lobidan over placebo (11). Only 29 completed this trial; side effects were similar during the placebo and treatment phases among completers. A French trial of a buffered preparation found a high rate of nausea, vertigo, and tachycardia, also resulting in a high dropout rate (12).

—Before nicotine gum there were lobeline candies. A placebo-controlled double-blind study of 74 participants (63 completed) found that 0.5 mg of lobeline in a cherry-flavored candy (administered every 1 to 2 hours during the first week, every 3 hours during the second week, every 4 hours during the third week, and every 4 to 6 hours during the fourth week) resulted in two thirds of the lobeline group decreasing cigarette consumption by at least half (13.8% stopped completely), compared with the placebo group, in which 14.8% reduced their cigarette intake by at least half and no one stopped entirely (13).

—Another randomized, double-blind placebo-controlled multicenter study of 313 smokers tested the effect of 5 mg of lobeline twice daily, along with 8 mg of D-amphetamine in the morning (apparently to combat fears of weight gain!) (14). Candies containing 0.5 mg lobeline were also supplied with instructions not to exceed 10 doses daily. After 1 week, 66% of treated participants had stopped smoking, and 50% in the placebo group had stopped smoking; the difference was statistically significant. Three patients in the lobeline group reported anorexia. Mild nausea occurred in both groups, but a burning sensation in the mouth or throat was much more common in the lobeline group.

ANIMAL/IN VITRO

- In rats, pretraining lobeline treatment improved performance on learning and memory tasks to an extent similar to nicotine (15). Antidepressant activity in mice has been demonstrated with a crude methanolic extract of *Lobelia inflata* leaves. Beta-amyrin palmitate appears to be one of the active components (2). The mechanism of beta-amyrin palmitate antidepressant activity has been tested in the forced swimming method in mice; the duration of immobility of mice was reduced significantly in a dose-dependent manner (5, 10, 20 mg/kg). The same doses reduced locomotor activity of mice and antagonized methamphetamine-induced locomotor stimulation (16). Noradrenergic activity appears to be activated; in mouse brain synaptosomes, beta-amyrin palmitate caused release of [3H]norepinephrine (6).
- Although lobeline is a potent ligand at nicotinic cholinergic receptors on neurons, chronic administration of lobeline, unlike nicotine, does not upregulate nicotinic receptors. Lobeline is less potent then nicotine in reducing locomotor activity and body temperature in mice but does not produce desensitization; in addition, a nicotinic cholinergic antagonist did not affect lobeline (3). In mice, acute tolerance did not occur but chronic tolerance occurred after 10 days; cross-tolerance between lobeline and nicotine was noted (4).

OTHER CLAIMED BENEFITS/ACTIONS

- Asthma
- Bronchitis
- Spastic colon
- Muscle spasm

 Risks

ADVERSE REACTIONS

- Large doses can cause nausea, vomiting, diaphoresis, tachycardia, hypertension, coma, and death (1).
- Intravenous injections of lobeline HCl in 26 male volunteers caused a sensation of choking, pressure, or fumes in the throat and upper chest at a mean dose of 12 μg per kg; reflex changes in breathing pattern were noted usually immediately before the sensations. A dry cough appeared at a mean dose of 24.3 μg/kg (17).

DRUG INTERACTIONS

- The combination of lobeline and tobacco appears to cause more adverse effects than lobeline alone (13).

PREGNANCY/LACTATION

No information available, but use is not recommended during pregnancy.

 Dose

COMMON DOSAGE FORMS

- The use of lobelia is not recommended.
- *Dried herb:* 0.2 to 0.6 g t.i.d. or 50 to 200 mg as infusion up to t.i.d.
- *Simple tincture of lobelia:* (1:8, 60% ethanol): 0.4 to 1.6 mL up to t.i.d. (1).
- *Lobelia tincture, ethereal:* (approximately 1:5) 0.3 to 1.0 mL up to t.i.d.
- *Liquid extract:* (1:1, 50% ethanol) 0.2 to 0.6 mL t.i.d.
- *Topical application:* Ointment, lotion, plaster, or suppository

Lysine (Lys, K)

10 Second Take

Lysine is a relatively safe amino acid, popular for treating or preventing herpes attacks. However, controlled clinical trials do not support its use for this indication.

Basics

DESCRIPTION

- Lysine is an essential amino acid, molecular weight 146. Lysine monohydrochloride (LMH), once promoted as a protein-enhancing supplement, is sold as a dietary supplement. LMH is mildly salty and can be used as a salt substitute (1).

FOOD SOURCES

- Most protein-containing foods, including all meats and legumes; proteins in grains and nuts are somewhat low in lysine. Average daily consumption of lysine is 8.3 g in nonvegetarians, 5.4 g in lacto-ovo-vegetarians, and 3.7 g in vegans (2).

MECHANISM/PHARMACOKINETICS

- Lysine is used in carnitine synthesis and, thus, is important to the transport of fatty acids. Lysine is very important to protein structure, allowing cross-links in proteins in collagen, elastin, and other tissues.
- Lysine from food is absorbed from the gut and incorporated into proteins all over the body. Excess lysine travels via the portal circulation to the liver where it is catabolized. A strongly conserved amino acid, the half-life of lysine in plasma is 11 days (2). Intravenous administration of 30 g LMH for 30 minutes in adults causes insulin and growth hormone release without elevating blood glucose (arginine and histidine have a similar effect, with arginine producing a greater response than lysine).

Evidence

CLINICAL TRIALS

- Herpes simplex virus (HSV)

—Lysine is popular for treating or preventing HSV infection. Although there is a theoretical basis for effectiveness (HSV has a high requirement for arginine and L-lysine inhibits herpes virus replication *in vitro*), most clinical trials have had negative results. After a brief letter was published observing benefit in oral and genital herpes infections (3), an uncontrolled trial in 45 patients (34 females) with recurrent HSV infections (primarily oral, with a few genital and facial cases) tested the effects of LMH (maintenance dose 312 to 500 mg daily, increasing to 800 to 1,000 mg daily during a recurrence) for varying periods that ranged from 2 months to 3 years (4). The treatment appeared to benefit patients in pain relief and more rapid resolution of episodes.

—Two controlled trials found no benefit in oral herpes. A double-blind, randomized, placebo-controlled trial of 119 patients (including 103 females) with recurrent oral lesions tested L-lysine tablets (500 mg) or placebo; participants were instructed to take two tablets at the first symptom of recurrence and then one tablet b.i.d. for 5 days (5). The trial lasted 48 weeks, during which there were 251 episodes of recurrent herpes labialis. There was no significant difference between groups in rate of healing, appearance of lesion at its worst, or recurrence-free intervals.

—A double-blind, placebo-controlled crossover study tested the effect of 500 mg L-lysine b.i.d. for 12 weeks in 65 participants with recurrent oral herpes (6). There was no washout period. There were no significant differences between groups in number of recurrences, rate of healing, or appearance of lesion at its worst. However, significantly more patients (14) were free of recurrences only during lysine treatment than were recurrence-free only during the placebo period (4).

—Two controlled trials included participants with genital herpes. A double-blind, placebo-controlled trial of oral lysine (400 mg t.i.d. for 4 to 5 months) in 21 patients with severe recurrent genital and/or oral herpes found no difference in frequency or duration of episodes between the two groups (7).

—A double-blind, placebo-controlled trial of lysine (1,000 mg t.i.d. for 6 months) was conducted in 114 participants with oral and/or genital herpes. More than half of the participants (57) dropped out, and seven additional participants in the lysine group were excluded from analysis because of concurrent acyclovir use. The final analysis, of 27 L-lysine-treated and 25 placebo-treated participants, found that the L-lysine group had significantly fewer HSV infections than expected and a faster healing time; the placebo-treated group did not experience these changes (8). The high dropout rate and unclear explanation of how estimates of number and duration of episodes were calculated make this trial difficult to interpret.

—A lysine review notes that although some of the trials described previously asked participants to avoid foods rich in arginine, none used dietary controls or attempted to assess dietary intake of lysine and arginine (1). Animal protein foods have a high lysine/arginine ratio, whereas cereal grains, nuts, and legumes often have a low lysine/arginine ratio. The ratio of lysine to arginine may be more important than absolute lysine intake (1).

- Bone

—A study of supplemental amino acids in 45 postmenopausal women with osteoporosis compared the effects of 800 mg/day of L-lysine, L-valine, or L-tryptophan, each administered for 3 days. Compared with baseline values, lysine significantly increased ^{47}Ca fractional absorption; the other amino acids had no effect (9). The effect lasted at least 24 hours; it was thought that perhaps supplementation stimulated production of a calcium-binding protein by enterocytes.

ANIMAL/IN VITRO

- In rats, supplemental lysine decreases serum cholesterol and significantly reduces stroke risk (1).

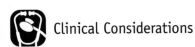 Clinical Considerations

LABORATORY TESTS

- Venous blood 105 to 207 μmol/L
- Urinary output 50 μmol/24 hour (2)

 Risks

ADVERSE REACTIONS

- Lysine is well-tolerated in adults and infants. A daily dose of 40 g caused only mild gastrointestinal complaints (abdominal cramps and transient diarrhea), which disappeared when the dose was reduced (1). Lysine was well-tolerated in infants given up to 6.5 g LMH (containing 5.18 g L-lysine) daily for 3 to 4 days.

ANIMAL TOXICITY

- LD_{50} of LMH in adult male rats was 22 mmol/kg (approximately 4 g/kg) body weight intravenously. No adverse effects of LMH supplementation were seen in rats fed a high-lysine diet for 2 years (1).

 Dose

COMMON DOSAGE FORMS

- Clinical trials have tested doses of 1,000 to 3,000 mg daily. Supplemental divided doses up to 3 g/day L-lysine (3.75 g LMH) appear to be safe in adults and children (1).

RECOMMENDED DIETARY ALLOWANCE (10)

Infants and children

3 to 4 months	103 mg/kg/day
2 to 5 years	64 mg/kg/day
10 to 12 years	44 mg/kg/day
Adults	12–30 mg/kg/day

Magnesium

10 Second Take

Evidence supports magnesium supplementation for ventricular arrhythmias.

Basics

DESCRIPTION

Magnesium, an essential mineral, is the fourth most common mineral in the body.

FOOD SOURCES

Vegetables, fruits, grains, nuts, seeds, animal products, and dairy products

MAIN FUNCTIONS/PHARMACOKINETICS

• Magnesium is essential for all reactions using adenosine triphosphate (ATP) (1). 50% to 60% of body magnesium is in bone. 21% to 27% of dietary magnesium is absorbed intestinally (2). Renal glomeruli filter about 10% of total body magnesium daily; of this, only about 5% is excreted in the urine.

Evidence

CLINICAL TRIALS

• Obstetrics

—Trials of magnesium for preeclampsia and to prevent preterm labor are not covered.

• Asthma

—A Cochrane review of 7 placebo-controlled randomized controlled trials (RCTs) (665 patients) of magnesium in treating acute asthma concluded that intravenous magnesium improved peak flow and reduced hospital admissions only in subjects with severe acute asthma (3).
—A double-blind treatment-controlled RCT of 33 patients found 3 mL nebulized magnesium (3.2% solution, 95 mg) equivalent to salbutamol for acute asthma (4). Another double-blind RCT of 35 patients with acute asthma found a benefit for adjunctive MgSo$_4$ over nebulized salbutamol alone (5).

• Arrhythmias

—Evidence supports using magnesium for ventricular but not atrial arrhythmias (2). In 100 patients undergoing cardiopulmonary bypass, magnesium reduced frequency of postoperative ventricular dysrhythmias more than placebo (6).
—In another trial of 588 patients with complex arrhythmias, intravenous magnesium decreased ventricular ectopic beats, couplets, and non-sustained ventricular tachycardia (7).
—A double-blind trial of 28 children undergoing heart surgery with cardio-pulmonary bypass found that four (27%)

placebo-treated patients developed junctional ectopic tachycardia compared to none in the group receiving magnesium (30 mg/kg i.v. postsurgically) (8).
—In 98 angina patients undergoing coronary artery bypass grafting, MgSo$_4$ during and after surgery (totalling 48 mmol), compared to no treatment, resulted in better myocardial recovery (9).
—After coronary artery bypass surgery in 167 patients, adjunctive MgSo$_4$ did not decrease the incidence of atrial fibrillation more than propranolol alone (10).
—Magnesium alone or adjunctively to sotalol did not benefit patients with persistent atrial fibrillation after elective cardioversion (11).

• Myocardial infarction (MI)

—The Leicester Intravenous Magnesium Intervention Trial (LIMIT 2), a double-blind RCT in 2,316 patients with suspected acute MI, found that magnesium (total of 73 mmol), compared to placebo, significantly reduced all-cause mortality 28 days later by 24% [95% confidence interval (CI) 1-43%] (12). Magnesium reduced left ventricular failure by 25% (95% CI 1-43%). One to 5.5 years later (mean 2.7 years), survivors in the magnesium group had 21% lower mortality from ischemic heart disease (95% CI 5-35%) and 16% lower all-cause mortality than controls (95% CI 2-29%) (13).
—The largest placebo-controlled study, the fourth International Study of Infarct Survival (ISIS-4) randomized 58,050 patients with suspected acute MI to captopril and/or controlled-release mononitrate for one month and/or intravenous MgSo$_4$ (totaling 80 mmol over 24 hours) in a $2 \times 2 \times 2$ factorial design (14). Captopril, but not magnesium, reduced five-week mortality. Magnesium appeared to adversely affect mortality in patients with heart failure or cardiogenic shock (14).
—An RCT in 154 patients with acute MI found no benefit of intravenous magnesium before, during, and after direct coronary angioplasty on infarct size at 30 days (15).
—An RCT found no benefit of intravenous magnesium (10 g over 24 hours) after in-hospital cardiac arrest (16).

• Blood pressure

—Studies of magnesium and blood pressure are mixed (17–20). A recent crossover RCT of 60 hypertensive patients (including 26 women) found that 20 mmol/day (480 mg) magnesium significantly but slightly lowered blood pressure (2.0-3.7 mm Hg) compared to control (21).

• Prevention of hearing loss

—A double-blind, placebo-controlled study in 300 noise-exposed military recruits found that magnesium aspartate (6.7 mmol [167 mg] daily × 2 months) reduced frequency and severity of noise-induced permanent hearing changes (22).

• Leg cramps

—A double-blind crossover RCT of 93 participants (only 42 completed) with nocturnal leg cramps found no benefit of magnesium citrate (900 mg p.o. b.i.d. × 1 month) over placebo (23).
—In 73 women with pregnancy-related leg cramps, magnesium lactate or citrate (15 mmol daily × 3 weeks), compared to placebo, decreased next-day persistence of nocturnal cramps (25% vs 50%) and improved overall ratings; serum magnesium levels did not change (24).

• Detrusor instability

—A double-blind RCT in 40 women with sensory urgency or detrusor instability found that Mg hydroxide (350-700 mg b.i.d. × 4 weeks) improved symptoms in 11/20 subjects (5/20 placebo-treated patients improved). Urodynamic parameters did not change (25).

• Headaches

—Prochlorperazine was superior to intravenous MgSo$_4$ in relieving acute headache pain in 36 patients (26). An RCT in 81 adults found that Mg (24 mmol or 600 mg trimagnesium dicitrate q.d. × 12 weeks) significantly reduced number of days with migraine and attack frequency over placebo (41.6% vs. 15.8% reduction) (27). Duration or intensity of attacks did not change. 18.6% of patients receiving magnesium reported diarrhea and 4.7% gastric irritation. Another placebo-controlled, double-blind 12-week trial of 69 subjects with migraine showed no benefit of magnesium 10 mmol (250 mg) b.i.d. over placebo on number, intensity, or duration of migraines (28).
—Twenty-four women with menstrual migraine received 120 mg. magnesium pyrrolidine carboxylic acid t.i.d. or placebo for the latter half of cycles for 2 months (29). Pain indices decreased in both groups, but magnesium was superior in reducing pain and number of days with headache.

• PMS

—A double-blind RCT of magnesium pyrrolidone carboxylic acid (360 mg t.i.d. during the second half of cycles × 2 months) in 32 women (28 completed) found that magnesium significantly reduced scores on the Menstrual Distress Questionnaire (30).
—A double-blind, placebo-controlled crossover RCT found no benefit of magnesium oxide (200 mg/day × 2 cycles) over placebo in 38 women at one month; magnesium improved only fluid retention in the second month (31).

ANIMAL/IN VITRO EVIDENCE

Not covered

OTHER CLAIMED BENEFITS/ACTIONS

No others identified

Clinical Considerations

To minimize diarrhea, magnesium should be taken in divided doses (3-6 times daily), each with a full glass of water. Inorganic forms (magnesium oxide, magnesium chloride) may be more likely to cause diarrhea than organic forms (magnesium citrate, magnesium aspartate).

- Hypomagnesemia

—Electrolyte and acid-base imbalances should be corrected. Intravenous administration is preferred (intramuscular injection is painful and can lead to fibrosis).
—Adolescents and adults: 1-2 g $MgSO_4$ 7H2O (8.2 to 16.4 mEq magnesium) infused over 5 to 10 minutes, then 6 g infused over 24 hours or until the condition resolves.
—Asymptomatic adolescents and adults with serum levels < 0.5 mmol/L (1.0 mEq/L): oral supplements in divided doses if effective; otherwise intramuscular injection or intravenous infusion (2).
—Symptomatic infants and children (with normal renal function): 3.6 to 6.0 mg (0.15 to 0.25 mmol) or 0.3 to 0.5 mEq/kg body weight as 50% $MgSO_4$ over the first few hours, with an equal dose administered parenterally over the remainder of the day. (Calcium should also be administered initially, with potassium and other electrolytes as needed).
—Chronic malabsorption in children: 12 to 18 mg/kg (0.5 to 0.75 mmol) in multiple divided oral doses. (2).

DEFICIENCY SIGNS AND SYMPTOMS

- Inadequate magnesium intake is common; NHANES III (1988 to 1991) found that magnesium intake was lower than the recommended dietary allowance (RDA) in males and females ages 12 to 60 years in all racial and ethnic groups of adults, except non-Hispanic white males. Among hospitalized patients, 65% of those in intensive care, up to 12% on general wards, and 30% of hospitalized alcoholics have hypomagnesemia (1). In 1,033 blood samples from urban primary care hospitals, almost half were low in magnesium (32).
- Signs and symptoms of hypomagnesemia

—Paresthesias (especially numbness or tingling in the face, hands, or feet)
—Trousseau's sign (carpal spasm upon raising sphygmomanometer pressure above systolic)
—Chvostek's sign (twitching facial muscles on tapping of the facial nerve)
—Depressed tendon reflexes
—Muscle spasticity, tremor, myoclonic jerks, athetoid or choreiform movement
—Anorexia, nausea, or vomiting
—Cardiac arrhythmias
—Hypocalcemia and hypokalemia often occur concurrently (2)

- Signs and symptoms of hypermagnesemia

—Hypotension, lethargy, confusion, deterioration in renal function, electro-cardiogram changes (prolongation of P-R and Q-T intervals) tachycardia or bradycardia, muscle weakness, hyporeflexia, complete heart block and cardiac arrest.
—Treatment of severe hypermagnesemia: acute infusion of 5 to 10 mEq calcium, then continuous infusion calcium. Patients with poor renal function should be dialyzed (2).

FACTORS DECREASING AVAILABILITY/ABSORPTION (2)

- Gastrointestinal disorders (motility disorders, inflammatory bowel disease, celiac disease, partial bowel obstruction, radiation enteritis, infections, etc.)
- Renal dysfunction (tubular disorders, metabolic hormonal disorders)
- Drugs (including amphotericin, cisplatin, aminoglycosides, cyclosporine, and pentamidine)
- Endocrine disorders (hyperaldosteronism, hyperparathyroidism with hypercalcemia, post-parathyroidectomy, hyperthyroidism, and diabetes)
- Genetic, congenital, and infectious disorders
- Alcoholism
- Hypercatabolic states (burns, post-surgery)
- Hyperthermia

FACTORS INCREASING AVAILABILITY/ABSORPTION

- Renal insufficiency
- Magnesium-containing antacids or cathartics
- Gastrointestinal disorders (including severe constipation, ulceration, obstruction, or perforation)

LABORATORY TESTS

- Normal serum magnesium: 0.75 to 0.95 mmol/L
- Urine levels will show a reduction in magnesium prior to serum magnesium. The 24-hour magnesium excretion should be more than 10% to 15% of amount ingested. (2)
- The intravenous load or retention test (a high proportion of magnesium retained after intravenous infusion indicates magnesium depletion) can be used if the urine test is equivocal.

Risks

ADVERSE EVENTS

- Diarrhea, gastric irritation
- High doses of magnesium, recommended by a nutritionist, caused fatal hypermagnesemia in a 2.5-year-old neurologically impaired male with normal renal function (33).

Dose

RECOMMENDED DIETARY ALLOWANCE

Infants and children	
0 to 6 months	30 mg/day (adequate intake)
7 to 12 months	75 mg/day (adequate intake)
1 to 3 years	80 mg/day
4 to 8 years	130 mg/day
Males	
9 to 13 years	240 mg/day
14 to 18 years	410 mg/day
19 to 30 years	400 mg/day
31 to 50 years	420 mg/day
51+ years	420 mg/day
Females	
9 to 13 years	240 mg/day
14 to 18 years	360 mg/day
19 to 30 years	310 mg/day
31 to 50 years	320 mg/day
51+ years	320 mg/day
Pregnant	
≤18 years	400 mg/day
19 to 30 years	350 mg/day
31 to 50 years	360 mg/day
Lactating	
≤18 years	360 mg/day
19 to 30 years	310 mg/day
31 to 50 years	320 mg/day

UPPER LIMITS

Infants and children	
0 to 6 months	Not determinable
7 to 12 months	Not determinable
1 to 3 years	65 mg/day
4 to 8 years	110 mg/day
Males	
9 to 13 years	350 mg/day
14 to 18 years	350 mg/day
19 to 50 years	350 mg/day
51+ years	350 mg/day
Females	
9 to 13 years	350 mg/day
14 to 18 years	350 mg/day
19 to 50 years	350 mg/day
51+ years	350 mg/day
Pregnant	350 mg/day
Lactating	350 mg/day

Conversion: mEq/L × 0.41 = mmol/L

Common Questions And Answers

Q: Does magnesium have an anticoagulant effect?
A: Probably not. One double-blind, placebo-controlled study found that infused magnesium inhibited platelet aggregation and fibrinogen binding (34), but another double-blind, placebo-controlled crossover study found no difference between placebo and infused $MgSO_4$ on bleeding time or prostacyclin production (35).

Manganese

 10 Second Take

Manganese deficiency is rare, and neurotoxicity (mostly through inhalation) is well-documented.

 Basics

DESCRIPTION

• Manganese, an essential trace element, is a constituent of metalloenzymes. A hard, brittle, white-gray metal, it is used industrially, mostly in steel alloys.

FOOD SOURCES

• Nuts (18 to 46 ppm), grains (0.4 to 40 ppm), legumes (2.2 to 6.7 ppm), fruits (0.2 to 10 ppm), and vegetables (0.4 to 6.6 ppm). Meat and dairy may contain up to 0.5 ppm (1). Tea is quite high in manganese, but in a form that is not highly bioavailable (2).
• Mean intake of manganese worldwide ranges between 9.5 to 196 μmol (0.52 to 10.8 mg/day) (3).

MECHANISM/PHARMACOKINETICS

• Manganese is a component of many enzymes, including glycosyltransferases, arginase, pyruvate carboxylase, glutamine synthetase, and manganese superoxide dismutase. Although either magnesium or manganese can activate various oxidoreductases, lyases, ligases, hydrolases, kinases, decarboxylases, and transferases, only manganese can activate glycosyltransferases and possibly xylosyltransferase (3).
• Manganese is absorbed poorly (absorption is gastric and intestinal). Absorption is thought to be about 5%, but determination is complicated because endogenous manganese is excreted into the intestine through bile and pancreatic secretions; only traces are found in urine (3).
• The total amount of manganese in the body is 10 to 20 mg. The liver, kidney, and bone retain the highest amount of manganese; the pancreas, pituitary, pineal, and lactating mammary gland also contain high concentrations (2).
• The biologic half-life of manganese in blood ranges from about 12 days (in miners) to about 40 days (in healthy volunteers); animal experiments show that elimination of manganese from the brain is relatively slow compared with the rest of body.

 Evidence

CLINICAL TRIALS

No clinical trials identified.

ANIMAL/IN VITRO

• In animals, deficiency causes impaired growth, skeletal abnormalities, disturbed reproductive function, ataxia in newborns, and defects of lipid and carbohydrate metabolism (3).

OTHER CLAIMED BENEFITS/ACTIONS

• Diabetes
• Osteoporosis
• Seizures
• Menorrhagia
• Wound healing

 Clinical Considerations

DEFICIENCY SIGNS AND SYMPTOMS

• Clinical deficiency is rare and does not appear to have broad effects, probably because magnesium can substitute for manganese in most enzyme-related functions (2). Seven men fed a diet containing only 2.0 μmol (0.11 mg) manganese/day for 39 days showed decreased cholesterol and increased calcium, phosphorus, and alkaline phosphatase activity; five developed fleeting dermatitis (miliaria crystalline) (4). One study compared a low-manganese diet containing 18.2 μmol (1.0 mg) to a diet containing 101.8 μmol (5.6 mg) manganese daily in 14 women for 39 days. The low-manganese diet caused slightly increased plasma glucose concentrations during an intravenous glucose tolerance test and increased menstrual losses of manganese, calcium, iron, and total hemoglobin. Negative manganese balance was not documented (3).
• Manganese deficiency is rare. In one case, a participant in a vitamin K trial who consumed a semipurified formula diet inadvertently devoid of manganese experienced weight loss, depressed hair and nail growth, dermatitis, hypocholesterolemia, and abnormal clotting-protein response to vitamin K, and his black hair turned reddish. He responded to a mixed diet (3).
• Poor growth and extensive bone demineralization in a child on long-term parenteral nutrition was corrected by manganese supplementation (3).

FACTORS DECREASING AVAILABILITY/ABSORPTION

• Calcium
• Phosphate
• Iron
• Phytate
• Epilepsy (low blood levels reported in some epileptics)

• Maple syrup urine disease (4)
• Phenylketonuria (low tissue manganese levels in children) (4)

FACTORS INCREASING AVAILABILITY/ABSORPTION

• Histidine
• Citrate
• Low manganese status (increases absorption)
• Cirrhosis is associated with higher blood levels of manganese (1)
• Iron-deficiency anemia (see questions and answers)

LABORATORY TESTS

• Whole blood: 4 to 15 μg/L, average 9 μg/L (by atomic absorption spectrophotometry)
• Serum: 0.9 to 2.9 μg/L, average 1.8 μg/L (Serum levels are lower than blood because most manganese is bound to hemoglobin.) (1)
• Urine: usually less than 10 μg manganese/L (reflects only very recent exposure)

 Risks

ADVERSE REACTIONS

• Potassium permanganate poisoning

—Orally ingested potassium permanganate (used as a disinfectant, metal cleaner, flower preservative, etc.) can be lethal. Dilute forms (1:10,000 to 1:20,000) are used topically for oozing dermatitis. Solutions stronger than 1:5,000 of potassium permanganate are corrosive and can cause an acid-like coagulation necrosis in the gastrointestinal tract; systemic absorption may cause methemoglobinemia and/or hepatorenal damage. The minimal lethal dose is about 10 g (although one patient survived a 25-g ingestion). No currently available measures effectively increase manganese elimination (1).
—A person who ingested an 8% potassium permanganate solution over 4 weeks suffered abdominal distress, hair loss, paresthesias, loss of concentration, somnolence, and muscle fasciculations; 9 months later a parkinsonian syndrome developed (1).

• Chronic manganese toxicity

—Manganese poisoning, highest among miners, can occur in industrial and agricultural workers and in patients receiving long-term parenteral nutrition (5). One case was associated with a Chinese medication called *Chien Pu Wan* (6).
—Orally ingested manganese may be less toxic than inhaled manganese dust or fumes (the most common route of occupational exposure). Chronic manganese poisoning (manganism) usually requires 2 to 25 years to manifest but occasionally occurs within several months following heavy exposure (1). Early subtle signs include hand tremor, reduced memory, and prolonged reaction time. Workers exposed via inhalation to concentrations near 5 mg Mn/m^3 for more

than 10 years have subtle reductions on hand steadiness and tests of rapid alternating motor movements. Results are mixed on response speed and memory in this group.
—Manganese-related neurotoxicity may occur in stages: Behavioral changes are followed by parkinsonian features, then dystonia with gait disturbances (5). Early symptoms may include fatigue, headache, muscle cramps, insomnia, anorexia, reduced concentration, loss of appetite, emotional lability, and sometimes psychosis (possibly including hallucinations). In Chilean mining villages, this was called *locura manganica* or manganese madness (5).
—Parkinsonian symptoms then develop and later severe dystonia of trunk and extremities (patients at this stage will continue to progress even if removed from exposure). Some have a typical "cock-walk" gait (trunk extended, arms flexed, and toe-walking) (see questions and answers).

• Treatment of chronic poisoning

—Treatment is primarily supportive. Na_2-ethylenediaminetetra-acetic acid (EDTA) chelation increases urinary excretion and may reduce acute psychosis but does not alter chronic neurologic symptoms. Levodopa or levodopa/carbidopa combinations may reverse some neurologic symptoms but are not uniformly effective, especially for dystonias.
—5-Hydroxytryptophan (5-HTP) improved gait and postural reflexes in a hypotonic, hypokinetic patient but only slightly improved a patient with dystonia (5). In two patients with chronic manganism (more than 20 years), para-aminosalicylic acid (PAS) for $3\frac{1}{2}$ months improved parkinsonian symptoms in one and "clinically cured" another, evaluated 19 months later (5).

• Metal fume fever

—Respiratory exposure to high concentrations of manganese oxide may cause metal fume fever (symptoms include cough, thirst, nausea, headache, diaphoresis, fatigue, arthralgias, and dyspnea). Cough or bronchitis is common in those exposed to levels above current standards. Early studies associated manganese with increased pneumonia risk; more recent studies show no excess risk in workers exposed to concentrations close to current standards (1).
—In air: Estimated lowest observed adverse event level (LOAEL) = 150 μg/Mn/m^3
—Occupational Safety and Health Administration (OSHA) permissible exposure limits (PEL) = 5 mg/m^3 as fume
—OSHA PEL-TWA = 1 mg/m^3 as dust
—National Institute of Occupational Safety and Health (NIOSH) recommended exposure–short-term exposure limit (REL-STEL) = 3 mg Mn/m^3.
—Immediately dangerous to life and health (IDLH) level = 500 mg Mn/m^3 (1).

• General population exposure

—Low levels of manganese result from the combustion of unleaded gasoline with the antiknock agent metal cyclopentadienyl manganese tri-carbonyl (MMT) (1).

—Well water contaminated by waste disposal may contain 2,000 μg Mn/L. The Environmental Protection Agency (EPA) limit for manganese in drinking water is 50 μg/L (primarily to avoid discoloration and poor taste) (1).
—Although one cohort study associated chronic neurologic symptoms with ingestion of contaminated well water, a more recent cross-sectional German study found no differences between controls and a population exposed to high levels of manganese in well water (0.3 to 2.16 mg Mn/L over 10 to 40 years) on clinical examination, structured questionnaires, or tests of fine motor coordination (1).

ANIMAL TOXICITY

• Animals exposed to inhaled manganese experience neuropathologic changes, developmental abnormalities, and degenerative changes of the testes (1).

Dose

RECOMMENDED DIETARY ALLOWANCE

Adequate Intakes

Infants and children

0 to 6 months	0.003 mg/day
7 to 12 months	0.6 mg/day
1 to 3 years	1.2 mg/day
4 to 8 years	1.5 mg/day

Males

9 to 13 years	1.9 mg/day
14 to 18 years	2.2 mg/day
19 to 50 years	2.3 mg/day
51+ years	2.3 mg/day

Females

9 to 13 years	1.6 mg/day
14 to 18 years	1.6 mg/day
19 to 50 years	1.8 mg/day
51+ years	1.8 mg/day
Pregnant	2.0 mg/day
Lactating	2.6 mg/day

UPPER LIMITS

Infants and children

0 to 6 months	Not determinable
7 to 12 months	Not determinable
1 to 3 years	2 mg/day
4 to 8 years	3 mg/day

Males

9 to 13 years	6 mg/day
14 to 18 years	9 mg/day
19 to 50 years	11 mg/day
51+ years	11 mg/day

Females

9 to 13 years	6 mg/day
14 to 18 years	9 mg/day
19 to 50 years	11 mg/day
51+ years	11 mg/day

Pregnant

≤18 years	9 mg/day
19 to 50 years	11 mg/day

Lactating

≤18 years	9 mg/day
19 to 50 years	11 mg/day

Common Questions and Answers

Q: How is chronic manganese toxicity distinguished from Parkinson's disease?
A: History of occupational exposure, atypical parkinsonism with dystonia, and infrequent tremor should increase the suspicion of manganism. Behavioral changes may (or may not) precede motor changes; the clinical appearance may be very similar to idiopathic Parkinson's disease. In advanced stages, manganism may cause severe dystonia of trunk and extremities; some develop a "cock-walk" with a toe-walking gait and trunk extended with the arms flexed (5).
Positron emission tomography (PET) scanning with [18F] 6-fluoro-L-dopa is abnormal in idiopathic Parkinson's disease and is normal in patients with manganese neurotoxicity. Most magnetic resonance imaging (MRI) studies of manganese toxicity have shown high signal intensity on T1-weighted images in the globus pallidus; these signals may disappear over time (5).
Manganism causes degeneration of the globus pallidus (and, to a lesser degree, the putamen, caudate nucleus, and the substantia nigra pars reticulata). Parkinson's disease causes neuronal loss and depigmentation of the substantia nigra pars compacta, the locus ceruleus, and the dorsal nucleus of vagus (5).

Q: What is the connection between iron and manganese?
A: Iron-deficiency anemia increases manganese absorption (both use the same divalent metal transporter in the brush border), and iron deficiency upregulates expression of this carrier in enterocytes. A recent 2-month long study of 26 young women fed high- or low-manganese diets found that initial serum ferritin levels influenced manganese absorption more than dietary manganese; women with low ferritin absorbed three to five times more manganese than women with high ferritin (7). Clinical measures of manganese status, however, did not change.

Marshmallow

10 Second Take

Marshmallow has a history of food use and is benign. Its mucilaginous properties make it a logical treatment for stomatitis, dry cough, and pharyngitis, but no clinical trials have been performed.

Basics

FAMILY

Malvaceae

DESCRIPTION

• A perennial plant with lobed, velvety leaves and white to pink flowers, marshmallow grows throughout Europe and western Asia, as well as in the United States. It has been used as a food plant and is approved for use in foods.

PART USED

Root, leaf

KNOWN ACTIVE CONSTITUENTS

• Mucilage polysaccharides (5% to 10%) include galacturonorhamnans, arabinans, glucans, and arabinogalactans. Also contains flavonoid glycosides and tannins (1).

MECHANISM/PHARMACOKINETICS

• Mucilage coats mucosa, which may account for its purported antitussive and gastrointestinal soothing effects. No information on pharmacokinetics is available (1).

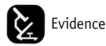

Evidence

CLINICAL TRIALS

No clinical trials identified.

ANIMAL/IN VITRO

• Cough

—In cats, marshmallow extract, syrup, or isolated polysaccharides significantly reduced coughing induced by mechanical irritation (1).

• Hypoglycemic effect

—In mice, intraperitoneal administration reduced plasma glucose levels.

• Immunomodulatory effect

—In mice, intraperitoneal administration doubled the rate of macrophage phagocytosis (1).

OTHER CLAIMED BENEFITS/ACTIONS

• Lung ailments
• Genitourinary ailments, including kidney stones and gonorrhea
• Pharyngitis
• Stomatitis
• Gastroenteritis
• Diarrhea
• Proctitis (enema)
• Dermatitis (ointment or poultice)
• Wounds
• Burns
• Diuretic

Risks

DRUG INTERACTIONS

Marshmallow may inhibit the absorption of other drugs taken simultaneously (1).

 Dose

COMMON DOSAGE FORMS

Oral

- *Dried root*: 2 to 5 g t.i.d.
- *Aqueous macerate*: 0.5 to 3.0 g in cold water, macerated and stirred for 30 minutes before straining, repeated up to a total dose of 6 to 15 g daily.
- *Liquid extract* (root or leaf): 2 to 5 mL (1:1 in 25% ethanol) t.i.d.
- *Syrup*: 2 to 10 mL syrup t.i.d. (3.0 g/5 mL)

Topical

- *Ointment*: 5% powdered leaf applied topically t.i.d.
- *Poultice*

Enema

- 2% to 3% macerate

 Common Questions and Answers

Q: So what part of this plant does one roast over a campfire?
A: The original marshmallow confection, invented by the French, consisted of the peeled root, cooked until spongy with sugar; it was called *pate de guimave*. It is doubtless a far cry from the weightless sweets campers adore; modern marshmallows are made from corn syrup, sugar, albumen, and gelatin. Marshmallow root was also used to thicken dishes, much as gelatin is used today.

Mate

 10 Second Take

Mate is a caffeine-containing herb associated with increased risk of upper gastrointestinal tract and respiratory tract cancers.

 Basics

LATIN NAME

Ilex paraguariensis A. St.-Hil.

FAMILY

Aquifoliaceae

OTHER COMMON NAMES

Mate, yerba mate, yerba, Paraguay tea, St. Bartholomew's tea, and Jesuit's tea

DESCRIPTION

• A species of holly, *Ilex paraguariensis* is an evergreen tree that has small clusters of red, black, or yellow berries and is found in Central and South America. *Ilex* species are found in moderate climates worldwide. Under cultivation it is often maintained as a bush.

PART USED

Leaf (dried and powdered)

KNOWN ACTIVE CONSTITUENTS

• Caffeine 0.56%, theobromine 0.03%, theophylline 0.02% (1). Very high in tannins, mate contains 117 mg tannic acid/g dry herb (2). It is also reported to contain 4% to 16% caffeic acid and chlorogenic acid; the amines trigonelline and choline; amino acids; flavonoids; ursolic acid; and vitamins B_2, B_6, C, niacin, and pantothenic acid (3). Three triterpenoid saponins (mate saponins 2, 3, and 4) have been isolated (4). Mate contains significant amounts of iron, calcium, magnesium, and potassium (5). Mate also contains the carcinogen benzo[a]pyrene; levels are much higher in mate than coffee or tea. One analysis found 0.11 to 1.5 μg/L in mate drink, with ground samples containing 24 to 461 μg/kg (6). Another analysis by the same researcher found 190 to 252 μg/kg benzo[a]pyrene in green mate and 222 to 714 μg/kg in roasted mate; mate drink contained 0.22% to 1.88% benzo[a]pyrene (6,7).

MECHANISM/PHARMACOKINETICS

• Caffeine and other methylxanthines present in mate are stimulants. Benzo[a]pyrene is an aromatic hydrocarbon that is a known local and systemic carcinogen.

 Evidence

CLINICAL TRIALS

• Thermogenesis

—A study of 12 plant preparations on energy expenditure and respiratory quotient in nonobese men and women found that the only herb that had a positive thermogenic effect was mate. Five capsules [Coopération Pharmaceutique Française, each filled with 0.3 g lyophilized hot water extract (21.4%) totaling 1.5 g dry extract] caused a drop in respiratory quotient (signifying an enhancement in proportion of fat oxidized) (8). Mate was tested against placebo in 12 adults; calorimetric measures, heart rate, and blood pressure were measured during five consecutive 45-minute periods after ingestion. Blood pressure was unchanged and heart rate decreased significantly in the mate group.

ANIMAL/IN VITRO

• Antioxidant effect

—*In vitro,* mate shows an antioxidant effect, inhibiting lipid peroxidation in rat liver microsomes; radical scavenging properties were seen with superoxide anion but not hydroxyl radical (9). Water extracts of mate inhibit low density lipoprotein (LDL) oxidation *in vitro* and *in vivo*. Copper-induced oxidation of LDL in whole plasma was inhibited after ingestion of mate (10).

OTHER CLAIMED BENEFITS/ACTIONS

• Reduces fatigue
• Debility
• Diabetes
• Stomach ailments
• Heart conditions
• Rheumatism
• Diuretic

 Risks

ADVERSE REACTIONS

• Oral, esophageal, and pharyngeal cancer

—Several studies show a relationship between mate intake and esophageal cancer. A case-control study of 261 patients with squamous cell carcinoma of the esophagus and 522 hospital controls found a clear dose-response relationship [relative risk (RR) for those drinking more than 2.5 L/day was 12.2] (11). Tobacco and alcohol consumption also were associated with esophageal cancer and appeared to have a synergistic effect on each other.
—Another case-control study of men with oral or pharyngeal cancer (108 cases, 286 controls) in Uruguay found a dose-related increase in risk; heavy consumers had as much as a five-fold increase in risk (12).
—Another case-control study in 226 cases and 469 controls also found a dose-related effect; heavy consumption was associated with an odds ratio (OR) of 6.5 in males and 34.6 in females (13).
—A case-control study of 378 cases and 756 controls in southern Brazil found that both oral (RR 1.9) and laryngeal cancer (RR 2.2) were associated with mate drinking in southern Brazil; the authors estimate that up to 20% of all cases of cancer in southern South America could be related (14). Increased cancer risk in Southern Brazil may also be affected by tannins in red wine made from fox grape (*Vitis labrusca*) (15).

• Renal cell cancer

—Mate (as well as red meat, barbecued meat, and heterocyclic amine consumption) was associated with an increased risk of renal cell cancer (3.0 for heavy drinkers) (16).

• Colorectal cancer

—A case-control study in Argentina (190 cases, 393 hospital controls) indicated that mate was not associated with colorectal cancer (17).

• Lung cancer

—A case-control study in 497 men with lung cancer and 497 controls in Uruguay found no connection with pulmonary adenocarcinoma, but small-cell lung cancer was associated with amount (2.9) and duration (OR 3.6) (18). Smoking and other major variables were controlled for.

- Bladder cancer

—A case-control study of 111 patients with bladder cancer and 222 controls in Uruguay found a significant dose-related effect of mate consumption, with heavy consumers having a seven-fold increase (19). Tobacco and mate had a synergistic effect.

- Esophagitis

—An endoscopy study of 60 males in southern Brazil found that mate drinkers were 2.2 times as likely to develop esophagitis as non-mate drinkers (20). A total of 107 laryngeal cancer and 290 controls found smoking the strongest risk factor, but there was a threefold increase in cancer risk with mate (21).

- Infection

—Infection in neutropenic patients has been traced to bacterial contamination of mate (22).

- Hepatic veno-occlusive disease (probable adulterant)

—A case of hepatic veno-occlusive disease in a 26-year-old woman was attributed to long-term consumption of mate tea, but it is not clear from the report whether the tea was contaminated with another plant (23). Small amounts of pyrrolizidine alkaloids (PAs) (not otherwise characterized) were recovered from the tea, and mate is not known to contain PAs (other locally obtained mate samples did not contain PAs).

- Cholinergic poisoning (adulterant)

—Another case of adulteration occurred in New York City, resulting in an outbreak of cholinergic poisoning in seven people; analysis revealed belladonna alkaloids but neither caffeine nor theophylline (24).

 ## Dose

COMMON DOSAGE FORMS

- Individual intake varies widely. In a typical mate-drinking round, 80 to 120 mg caffeine is ingested (1). It is also available in teabags or extracts used to make instant tea.

 ## Common Questions and Answers

Q: How common is the use of mate?
A: Mate use is common in Uruguay, Paraguay, Argentina, and southern Brazil. A population-based survey of 1,400 adults in southern Brazil found that one third did not drink mate (or drank it less frequently than once a month), another third drank it at least once a month but less than once a day, and one third drank it daily. Daily consumers were more likely to be younger than 60 years, to smoke, and to have migrated from a rural area (25). Males and those who drank alcohol were more likely to consume mate at a higher temperature. Drinking very hot beverages may increase the risk of esophageal cancer. A recent study in southern Brazil tested the temperature of mate infusions prepared in 36 households with 107 mate drinkers; the measured temperature of mate preparations was quite hot ($\geq 60°C$) in 72% of households (26).

Q: How is mate prepared?
A: The word *mate* actually describes the small gourd used to prepare and serve the drink. It is drunk through a filtered straw called a *bombilla* (little pump), which is a straw with a flattened mouthpiece on one end and a teaspoon-shaped filter on the other. The herb (previously blanched, dried, and fragmented) is wet with warm water, the bombilla inserted, and then hot water poured onto the yerba near the bombilla. The drink is sipped, then more water is added. When the drink becomes tasteless, the bombilla is moved to a different part of the gourd (1).

Q: Does mate contain cocaine?
A: No. Cocaine has been identified in a tea called *mate de coca*, a mixture of mate and a species of coca (*Erythroxylum novogranatense* var truxillense; cocaine is usually extracted from *Erythroxylum coca*). Although manufacturers claim that the tea is decocainized, an analysis of the tea in 1991 (it was available commercially in the United States at that time) revealed up to 0.08% cocaine (27). I do not think the tea is still sold in North America; at any rate one cannot really call this a case of adulteration because the tea was honestly labeled!

Melatonin

10 Second Take

Melatonin, N-acetyl-5-methoxytryptamine, may help insomnia and jet lag.

Basics

DESCRIPTION

• Melatonin, the principal secretion of the pineal gland, regulates circadian rhythms. Tryptophan, the main precursor of melatonin, is converted to 5-hydroxytryptophan before being decarboxylated to serotonin, which is then enzymatically converted to melatonin (1).

MECHANISM/PHARMACOKINETICS

• The prevailing light-dark environment affects melatonin synthesis and secretion. Light acts on the neural pathway connecting the retina to the hypothalamic suprachiasmatic nuclei, to preganglionic neurons in the upper thoracic spinal cord, to postganglionic sympathetic fibers from superior cervical ganglia, and finally to the pineal gland (2). Melatonin is also produced in the gut (where its production appears to be controlled by nutritional factors, especially tryptophan availability) (3).
• Peak plasma levels are achieved 1 hour after ingestion; plasma elimination half-life is 30 to 50 minutes. Oral doses of 1 to 5 mg cause plasma concentrations 10 to 100 times the usual nocturnal peak; basal levels are achieved within 48 hours. It is primarily metabolized by the liver to 6-sulphatoxy-melatonin (1).
• Nocturnal secretion of melatonin, highest in young children, decreases with age. In old age, no melatonin rhythm is observed. Melatonin lowers core body temperature, which may be connected to its phase-shifting effects (4). There appears to be a relationship between melatonin and the neuroendocrine-gonadal axis. Although melatonin reduced circulating norepinephrine in young individuals, it did not affect adrenergic activity in 14 healthy postmenopausal women (5).

Evidence

CLINICAL TRIALS

• Sedative/hypnotic

—A double-blind, placebo-controlled trial in 20 healthy males tested daytime doses of melatonin (0.1 to 10 mg orally) on sleep latency and duration, mood, performance, and temperature (6). Compared with placebo, all melatonin doses significantly increased daytime sleep duration and decreased sleep-onset latency; self-reported sleepiness and fatigue increased. With doses of 1.0 or 10 mg of melatonin, oral temperature decreased, as did scores on a vigilance test.
—Schizophrenics have decreased melatonin levels and often report insomnia. In a double-blind, crossover randomized controlled trial (RCT) of 19 schizophrenic patients, melatonin (2 mg controlled-release) or placebo were compared; each was given for 3 weeks (7). Compared with placebo, melatonin significantly improved rest-derived sleep efficiency but not sleep latency or sleep duration.
—A double-blind, placebo-controlled crossover RCT in seven patients with tuberous sclerosis found that melatonin significantly improved total sleep time (mean improvement 0.55 hours) but not sleep-onset time or sleep fragmentation (8).

• Jet lag

—Most studies of jet lag have found benefits for post-flight administration of melatonin (primarily for sleep disturbance); results on pre-flight administration are mixed (4).
—A recent double-blind RCT (not included in the above review) found no difference between placebo and three melatonin regimens (5.0 mg q.h.s., 0.5 mg q.h.s., and 0.5 mg on a shifting schedule) for jet lag in 257 Norwegian physicians returning to Oslo from New York (9).

• Benzodiazepine withdrawal

—A double-blind RCT in 34 participants on benzodiazepines compared melatonin (2 mg controlled-release q.h.s × 6 weeks) to placebo, during which participants reduced benzodiazepines (10). In the second, single-blind part of the study, melatonin was administered for 6 weeks to all participants, with continued attempts to discontinue benzodiazepines. At the end of the first phase, significantly more (4/18) melatonin-treated patients than placebo-treated patients (4/16) discontinued benzodiazepines; sleep quality was also significantly higher in the melatonin group. Six of 12 in the original placebo group who then received melatonin therapy also discontinued benzodiazepine therapy. At 6-month follow-up, 19/24 patients who discontinued benzodiazepines and continued melatonin maintained good sleep quality.

• Phase-shifting

—A double-blind, crossover RCT of 19 emergency medicine residents found no difference in sleep efficiency, sleep latency, Profile of Mood States, or Stanford sleepiness scale.
—Melatonin 1 mg or placebo was used 30 to 60 minutes before a daytime sleep session after a night shift for three consecutive days (11). In 17 police officers, 5 mg melatonin at desired bedtime, compared with baseline or placebo, significantly improved subjective assessment of sleep quality and duration (12).

• Presurgical medication

—A double-blind RCT compared placebo, melatonin 5 mg, and midazolam 15 mg (both sublingual) in 75 women about 100 minutes before receiving anesthesia (13). Compared with placebo, both midazolam and melatonin decreased anxiety and increased levels of sedation before the operation. After surgery, patients in both treatment groups, compared with controls, were more sedated; there were no differences among groups in anxiety.

• Cancer

—Melatonin (40 mg/day for 21 days) did not protect against myelotoxic effects of etoposide or carboplatin in 20 previously untreated patients with inoperable lung cancer (16 had non-small cell lung cancer) (14).
—In one study, 250 patients with metastatic solid tumors were randomized to chemotherapy with or without melatonin 20 mg/day. Adjuvant melatonin was significantly better than chemotherapy alone for tumor regression rate (partial and complete responses 42/124 vs. 19/126), median time to progression (9 months, range 4–14 months vs. 4 months, range 3–6 months), mean time to progression (8.9 ± 1.3 months vs. 4.2 ± 0.8 months), and 1-year survival (63/124 vs. 29/126) (15). Melatonin also was associated with significantly less myelosuppression, thrombocytopenia, neurotoxicity, cardiotoxicity, stomatitis, and asthenia than chemotherapy alone.

• Sunscreen

—A double-blind RCT of the photoprotective effects of different antioxidants compared topical vitamin C, vitamin E, and melatonin, alone or in combination, half an hour before ultraviolet irradiation of the skin (16). Melatonin had a dose-dependent photoprotective effect that was enhanced by combination with vitamins; the best protection was obtained with a combination of all three antioxidants.

• Tardive dyskinesia

—A double-blind, placebo-controlled, cross-over RCT in 19 schizophrenics (mean age 74.0 ± 9.5 years; duration schizophrenia 31.3 ± 7.0 years) tested slow-release melatonin 2 mg/day for 4 weeks (17). There were no beneficial effects on the abnormal involuntary movements scale; the treatment was well-tolerated.

• Cluster headache

—In a double-blind RCT of 20 patients with cluster headaches, participants received a single dose of oral melatonin (10 mg in the evening) or placebo for 2 weeks (1). Two had chronic cluster headache; 18 with episodic headache entered the study after beginning a cluster period. Melatonin, compared with placebo, significantly reduced the mean number of daily attacks during each week. Half of melatonin-treated patients responded.

OTHER CLAIMED BENEFITS/ACTIONS

• Cardiovascular disease
• Cancer prevention
• Antiaging

 ## Risks

ADVERSE REACTIONS

• Sleepiness, headache, nausea, fuzziness, lightheadedness (4).
• Abdominal cramps have been reported with large doses (3 to 6 mg) (18).
• Melatonin taken at the wrong time can destabilize circadian rhythms (19).
• Lowered seizure threshold
• Although melatonin (5 mg p.o. or via g-tube q.h.s.) had a positive effect on sleep-related symptoms in 5/6 children with multiple neurologic deficits and chronic severe sleep complaints, four patients experienced increased seizure activity, which returned to baseline after discontinuing melatonin (20). Three participants rechallenged with 1 mg melatonin experienced increased seizure activity.

DRUG INTERACTIONS

• Nifedipine

—Melatonin may decrease the therapeutic effect of nifedipine. A double-blind crossover study in 47 patients with mild to moderate essential hypertension, who were taking nifedipine, compared placebo with melatonin 5 mg at 11:30 p.m. for 4 weeks. Melatonin significantly increased blood pressure and heart rate throughout a noninvasive 24-hour ambulatory blood pressure monitoring test [Delta systolic blood pressure (SBP) +6.5 mm Hg, Delta diastolic blood pressure (DBP) +4.9 mm Hg, Delta heart rate (HR) +3.9 beats/minute].

• Serotonin reuptake inhibitors

Acute change in mental status
—A 73-year-old women on fluoxetine, conjugated estrogens, beclomethasone nasal inhaler, multivitamins, and melatonin 3 to 6 mg/day was admitted with acute psychosis (21). Computed tomography (CT) scan of the head, complete blood count (CBC), chemistry panel, thyroid-stimulating hormone (TSH), and urinalysis were normal. Although the patient initially reported taking ten 3-mg melatonin tablets on the day of admission, the next day (when her mental status was normal), the patient denied taking more than two melatonin tablets daily. Although this may be a drug interaction effect, this inadequately documented case report is difficult to interpret.
Visual acuity loss
—Possible toxic optic neuropathy was reported in a 42-year-old woman, treated with sertraline for years, who began melatonin and a high-protein diet 2 weeks before developing visual acuity loss, dyschromatopsia, and altered light adaptation (22). Visual acuity and color vision improved within 2 weeks of discontinuing melatonin and the diet. The authors theorize that the combination of melatonin, sertraline, and a high-protein diet may have resulted in a melatonin/dopamine imbalance in the retina, but this case is obviously difficult to interpret.

ANIMAL TOXICITY

• A dose of 800 mg/kg was not lethal in mice; higher doses could not be given because of the limited water solubility of melatonin (11).

 ## Clinical Considerations

LABORATORY TESTS

• Daytime serum concentrations < 20 pg/mL; nocturnal peak levels 40 to 80 pg/mL. Salivary levels range from 27% to 32% of plasma levels.
• Analytical techniques include radio-immunoassay (RIA), high-performance liquid chromatography (HPLC), and gas chromatography-mass spectrometry (GC-MS) (19).

 ## Dose

COMMON DOSAGE FORMS

• Doses of up to 300 mg/day have been tested in clinical trials.
• Physiologic dosing

—A dose of 0.1 to 0.3 mg given in daytime generates peak serum concentrations in the normal nocturnal range (6,19).

• Jet lag

—Traveling east (advanced phase shifting): Pre-flight: 5 mg p.o. × 1 to 3 days in the late afternoon
Post-flight: 5 mg p.o. × 4 days at local bedtime
—Traveling west (advance phase delay): No pre-flight treatment
Post-flight: 5 mg p.o. × 4 days at local bedtime, with second dose if person wakes very early (4)

• Insomnia

—0.3 to 3.0 mg q.h.s. or at 9 p.m.

 ## Common Questions and Answers

Q: Is melatonin in food?
A: Yes, in very small amounts, melatonin occurs in many plants, including rice and bananas. Melatonin is in feverfew (1.37 to 4.45 μg/g); St. John's wort flowers contain 4.39 μg/g (leaves contain 1.75 μg/g); Baikal skullcap (*Scutellaria baicalensis*) contains 7.11 μg/g (23).

Q: How does melatonin figure in forensics?
A: Melatonin measurements have been suggested as a forensic tool to help determine the time of death. Serum and urine analyses are less accurate then melatonin content of the whole pineal body (19).

Q: Why do people think melatonin fights aging?
A: This concept is based on the fallacy that you are as young as your hormones, and that boosting hormones to youthful levels will provide the health or vigor of youth. Long-term effects of taking exogenous melatonin pills are unknown. For those who want to stimulate their natural melatonin, there is certainly no harm in sleeping in a completely dark room or using a sleep mask.

Methionine (Met, M) and SAMe

10 Second Take

Evidence supports the use of methionine or S-adenosyl-L-methionine (SAMe) for depression; it may also be helpful for cholestasis, liver dysfunction, and fibromyalgia. However, long-term use may have an adverse effect on cardiovascular risk factors.

Basics

DESCRIPTION

• Methionine is a sulfur-containing essential amino acid. The methylated form of methionine is SAMe.

FOOD SOURCES

• Most protein-containing foods, especially of animal origin. A normal Western diet provides 15 to 20 mmol (223 g) of sulfur amino acids (methionine and cysteine) per day. The recommended daily allowance (RDA) for sulfur amino acids intake is 13 mg/kg/day (1).

MECHANISM/PHARMACOKINETICS

• SAMe is a methyl group donor that is found in all body tissues and fluids. It is necessary to many transmethylation reactions, including phospholipid synthesis. SAMe is also important to protein structure and function and participates in transsulfuration and polyamine synthesis metabolic pathways.
• There is low bioavailability of SAMe after oral administration. Peak plasma concentration is reached 3 to 5 hours after a single dose of an enteric-coated preparation (400 to 1,000 mg). After administration of an oral 200-mg dose of radioactively labeled SAMe (methyl^{14}C), urinary excretion of radioactivity 48 hours later was 15.5%; feces contained 23.5% at 72 hours. The half-life of SAMe is 80 to 100 minutes in healthy volunteers and 121 minutes in patients with chronic liver disease (2).

Evidence

CLINICAL TRIALS

• Cholestasis of pregnancy

—Three publications by one group reported effectiveness of SAMe for cholestasis of pregnancy (3–5). A dose of 800 mg/day SAMe (orally or intravenously) was given for 2 weeks during the third trimester of pregnancy. Another placebo-controlled trial tested 900 mg/day SAMe intravenously for 20 days for cholestasis of pregnancy; however, no effect was seen (6).

• Liver disease

—A randomized, double-blind trial in 123 patients with alcoholic cirrhosis compared SAMe (1,200 mg per day orally) to placebo for 2 years. There was not a significant difference between the two groups in terms of overall mortality or liver transplantation rates at the end of the trial; there was a statistically significant difference favoring SAMe only if patients in Child C class (most advanced liver disease) were excluded (7).
—In patients with liver cirrhosis, administration of SAMe enhances bile salt conjugation and prevents hepatic glutathione depletion (1). Long-term treatment increased plasma concentrations of cystine and taurine (secondary sulfur-containing amino acids) without changing concentrations of methionine, neutral amino acids, or polyamines (1).
—There are several earlier, small, uncontrolled studies of the efficacy of SAMe in chronic liver disease; most report statistically significant improvement in liver function tests (2).

• Depression

—SAMe appears to be useful in treating depression (2). Most earlier trials of SAMe used intravenous administration; more recent trials have used oral supplementation. A meta-analysis of six placebo-controlled clinical trials (three using oral SAMe, three using parenteral preparations) in a total of 200 patients and seven treatment-controlled trials (two using oral SAMe, five using parenteral preparations) in 201 patients found that oral SAMe (1,600 mg per day) and intravenous SAMe (200 mg/day) were more effective than placebo and about as effective as tricyclic antidepressants for treating major depression (8). Most trials were less than 12 weeks, relatively short-term for a depression trial.

• Fibromyalgia

—A crossover trial in 34 patients with fibromyalgia compared SAMe (600 mg intravenously) to placebo for 10 days. There was no significant difference between the two groups in tender-point change, subjective perception obtained at rest, pain on movement, overall well-being, or other measures (9).
—A double-blind crossover study in 17 patients with primary fibromyalgia evaluated SAMe (200 mg i.m. daily for 21 days) and found that SAMe decreased the number of trigger points and decreased depression (Hamilton rating scale and a self-evaluation questionnaire) (2).

• Fibromyalgia and Sjögren's disease

—A study of 30 patients with Sjögren's disease, fibromyalgia, or both, tested the effect of methionine (200 mg i.m. daily) for 4 weeks. In the 10 patients with Sjögren's, disease symptoms and scores on Zung's Self Rating Scale for Depression did not change significantly; scores on Hamilton Rating Scale for Depression decreased significantly. In the 10 patients with both Sjögren's disease and fibromyalgia, there were no significant changes in symptoms, depression scale scores, or pain and severity scale scores; however, the number of trigger points were reduced significantly. In the 10 patients with fibromyalgia, symptoms, number of trigger points, pain severity, and scores on both depression scales were reduced significantly (10).

• AIDS-associated myelopathy

—A pilot trial in 12 patients with AIDS-associated myelopathy found that seven of the nine patients who finished the study experienced clinical and electrophysiologic improvement (11).

• Lead poisoning

—SAMe may be a useful adjunct in the treatment of lead poisoning. Intravenous administration (12 mg/kg for 22 days) or oral administration (25 to 30 mg/kg daily) improved clinical and biochemical parameters in patients with chronic lead poisoning (2).

• Acetaminophen toxicity

—Methionine has been shown to be effective in the treatment of acetaminophen toxicity (12).

• Pediatrics

—Methionine has been used to treat two cases of infantile porphyria cutanea tarda (1).
—In children, methionine (0.2 g/kg i.v.) increased basal growth hormone levels and potentiated the growth hormone response to 1 μg/kg growth hormone releasing hormone administered intravenously (13).

ANIMAL/IN VITRO

- In baboons, SAMe supplementation attenuates ethanol-induced liver injury. In animals, SAMe protects against intrahepatic cholestasis induced by a variety of agents and reduces the toxic effects of acetaminophen, lead, and alcohol (2).
- In parenteral preparations, SAMe prevents fat accumulation in the livers of rodents (1).
- In animals, methyl deficiency induces preneoplastic or neoplastic lesions, apparently by causing imbalances in deoxynucleotide pools (1).

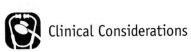 Clinical Considerations

FACTORS DECREASING AVAILABILITY/ABSORPTION

- Betaine supplementation increases methionine transmethylation and transsulfuration (1).

FACTORS INCREASING AVAILABILITY/ABSORPTION

- Chronic alcohol consumption is associated with enhanced methionine use and depletion; circulating methionine levels may be higher in patients with alcoholic liver disease or in patients with other types of liver damage (1).
- Cysteine spares methionine by reducing methionine catabolism through the transsulfuration pathway (1).

LABORATORY TESTS (14)

- Urinary output: 50 μmol/24 hours
- Venous blood: 11 to 30 μmol/L

 Risks

ADVERSE REACTIONS

- Short-term, SAMe is well-tolerated; in clinical trials using doses up to 1,600 mg daily, only mild gastrointestinal effects have been observed. Anxiety, hypomania (in patients with bipolar depression), and one case of a manic episode in a patient with no prior history of mania have been reported (2).
- Homocysteine, endothelial function, and lipid peroxidation

—Two of three studies that examined cardiovascular disease risk factors found an adverse effect of methionine on homocysteine levels and measures of endothelial function (see questions and answers). Although these studies were done on methionine, not SAMe, the results should be the same.

 Dose

RECOMMENDED DIETARY ALLOWANCE (15)

Infants and children

3 to 4 months	58 mg/kg/day
2 to 5 years	27 mg/kg/day
10 to 12 years	22 mg/kg/day
Adults	13 to 15 mg/kg/day

 Common Questions and Answers

Q: What is the difference between administering methionine and SAMe?
A: Administration of SAMe can be more useful than administering methionine because it gets around the issue of enzyme deficiency (if enzymes are deficient it may prevent the conversion of methionine to SAMe) (1).

Q: Is SAMe a good option for treating depression or arthritis?
A: SAMe is available by prescription in Italy, Spain, and Germany for the treatment of these conditions (as well as cholestasis) (16). There is certainly evidence supporting its effectiveness, but long-term safety has not been established; most trials of SAMe have only lasted a few weeks. It is expensive; a month's supply at 1,600 mg/day would cost about $228 (16). Given the availability of numerous effective pharmaceutical antidepressants, I would not recommend long-term use of SAMe at this point.

Q: Can methionine increase the risk of cardiovascular disease?
A: It is theoretically possible. No trials have looked at the long-term effect of methionine on clinical endpoints, but three trials have looked at homocysteine levels and markers of endothelial function, and all found adverse effects of high doses (within the range of what is used therapeutically).

Sixteen healthy volunteers were assessed for endothelial function, plasma homocysteine, and lipid peroxidation after acute methionine (250 mg p.o.), low-dose methionine (250 mg p.o. q.d. × 1 month), or high-dose methionine (100 mg/kg daily for 1 week) (17). Forearm vascular responses, plasma homocysteine levels, and thiobarbituric acid reactive substances were measured. There was no significant difference in endothelial-dependent vascular response or thiobarbituric acid reactive substances. Neither acute nor low-dose methionine increased homocysteine concentrations; however, 1 week of high-dose methionine significantly increased homocysteine.

Another randomized crossover study in 24 healthy volunteers found that an oral methionine load (0.1 g/kg) increased plasma homocysteine and impaired flow-mediated endothelium-dependent vasodilation (18). A third study in patients with arterial or venous disease (17 with hyperhomocysteinemia, 12 without hyperhomocysteinemia) found that a methionine load (100 mg/kg) increased von Willebrand factor (an indication of endothelial dysfunction) (19).

Homocysteine is a known risk factor for cardiovascular disease. Methionine is regenerated from homocysteine through the re-methylation pathway (1). In young men with methionine-replete diets, (approximately 14 mmol/day), about 17 mmol/day of homocysteine was formed; about 38% was re-methylated to methionine, and 62% was catabolized by transsulfuration (1). Vitamin B_{12} and folate are required for the reformation of methionine from homocysteine. (14). In those with high endogenous levels of homocysteine, supplementation with folate or B_{12} lowers homocysteine levels. It would be interesting to see whether B_{12} and folate supplementation given with methionine would reverse adverse effects on homocysteine levels. There is certainly a good rationale for supplementing anyone taking methionine or SAMe with B-complex.

Q: Are vegetarians deficient in methionine?
A: An analysis of long-term vegans found that the intake of sulfur-containing amino acids would meet the average requirements but would be marginal for adults with higher than average requirements (1).

Milk Thistle

10 Second Take

Milk thistle is benign and reduces mortality in *Amanita* mushroom poisoning. Trials on treatment of hepatitis and cirrhosis are mixed.

Basics

LATIN NAME

Silybum marianum (L) Gaertn.

FAMILY

Asteraceae/Compositae

OTHER COMMON NAMES

Wild artichoke, holy thistle, Mary thistle

DESCRIPTION

• Native to Europe and introduced in the United States, milk thistle has spiny, white veined leaves and purple flowers.

PART USED

Dried ripe fruit (also called "seeds")

KNOWN ACTIVE CONSTITUENTS

• Silymarin is a mixture of the isomers silybinin (also called silibinin or silybin), isosilybinin, silydianin (silidianin), and silychristin (silicristin) (1). Silybinin, the most important constituent, composes about half of this complex. Fruits contain 15% to 30% fatty oil and 20% to 30% proteins.

MECHANISM/PHARMACOKINETICS

• After oral administration, 20% to 50% of silymarin is absorbed; 80% is excreted via bile; 10% enters enterohepatic circulation (1). Silybin is rapidly absorbed after an oral dose, with peak plasma concentrations reached after 2 hours.
• The elimination half-life is 6 hours. From an oral dose, 3% to 8% is excreted in urine, with 20% to 40% (as glucuronide and sulfate conjugates) recovered from bile (2).
• In mice, silibinin levels peak in liver, lung, stomach, and pancreas 0.5 hours after administration and in skin and prostate 1 hour after administration (3).
• Silymarin suppresses tumor necrosis factor (TNF)-induced activation of NF-kappa B (a nuclear transcription factor) and TNF-induced activation of several kinases (4).
• Silibinin, an antioxidant, inhibits lipid peroxidation, stimulates ribosomal RNA polymerase, decreases hepatic and mitochondrial glutathione oxidation induced by iron overload, decreases activity of tumor promoters, and stabilizes mast cells (2).
• At 80 μmol/L, silibinin significantly inhibited O_2 and nitric oxide formation of activated Kupffer cells (5). Silibinin also strongly inhibits leukotriene B_4; silibinin concentrations up to 100 mmol/L had no effect on prostaglandin E_2 formation. Free radical scavenging was seen only at very high concentrations unlikely to be achieved *in vivo*. Silibinin inhibits the 5-lipoxygenase pathway and selectively inhibits leukotriene formation by Kupffer cells (5).

Evidence

CLINICAL TRIALS

• Hepatic disease

—A review by the Federal Agency for Health Care Research and Quality (AHRQ) identified six blinded, placebo-controlled randomized controlled trials (RCTs) of milk thistle in chronic alcoholic liver disease (chronicity and severity varied) with a total of 568 patients. All trials used silymarin (Legalon) 280 to 450 mg/day; duration ranged from 28 to 446 days. Confounding effects of alcohol were not controlled for in most trials (6).
—At least one parameter of liver function improved in four trials; two found no benefit of silymarin on any outcome. The largest trial of 200 alcoholics found no benefit for silymarin over placebo in survival or clinical course.
—A double-blind controlled study of 106 patients admitted to a military hospital in Helsinki because of increased liver function tests (LFTs) for more than 1 month found that silymarin (420 mg/day × 4 weeks) improved histology more than placebo (7). A total of 11/15 treated patients and 4/14 controls who underwent before and after liver biopsies showed significantly improved histology. This study was criticized because the groups differed in baseline histology and LFTs (8).
—A French trial in 116 patients with alcoholic hepatitis found no effect of treatment (420 mg/day × 90 days) on histology (6).
—The AHRQ review identified six studies of chronic liver disease of mixed etiology, with a total of 700 patients. Three studies showed improvement in at least one parameter. One of two studies that examined survival found a benefit (6).
—Three trials of milk thistle products for viral hepatitis (two chronic, one acute) were identified in the AHRQ review. A German RCT of 59 subjects with acute viral hepatitis (A or B) found that silymarin (420 mg/day × 25 days) significantly improved aspartate transaminase (AST) and bilirubin but not alanine transaminase (ALT) or alkaline phosphatase (6).
—An RCT of 20 patients with chronic active hepatitis B or C tested placebo against Silipide (containing 240-mg silybin equivalents) daily for 7 days. AST, ALT, and gamma-glutamyl transpeptidase (GGTP) significantly improved; there was no effect on bilirubin, alkaline phosphatase, albumin, or malondialdehyde. Another trial found no effect of silymarin (420 mg Legalon/day × 1 year) over placebo on histology (the only outcome reported) in 24 patients with chronic active hepatitis (CAH) or chronic persistent hepatitis (6).

- Cirrhosis

—Four trials were identified in the AHRQ review; results are mixed. The most recent, a double-blind, multicenter study of 200 patients with alcoholic cirrhosis, found no effect of silymarin (Legalon 450 mg/day); no effect was seen on survival, LFTs, ascites, or clinical course (9).
—A double-blind, placebo-controlled RCT in 172 participants with cirrhosis (alcoholic or nonalcoholic), followed up for approximately 4 years showed no benefit of silymarin 420 mg/day on survival. A three-armed RCT tested Legalon 420 mg/day against aminoimidazolecarboxamial phosphate or placebo in 60 patients with alcoholic cirrhosis for 30 days. Silymarin improved AST, ALT, and GGTP, but not bilirubin.
—The only positive trial identified is a double-blind placebo-controlled RCT of silymarin (140 mg t.i.d.) in 170 patients with cirrhosis (alcoholic and nonalcoholic); mean follow-up was 41 months (10). The 4-year survival rate was 58% ± 9% in silymarin-treated patients and 39% ± 9% in the placebo group ($p = 0.036$). The treatment was most successful in patients with alcoholic cirrhosis and patients initially rated Child A.
—A double-blind, placebo-controlled Italian study of 60 women psychiatric inpatients receiving phenothiazines and/or butyrophenones for at least 5 years divided patients into four groups (11). Two groups continued medication, with adjunctive silymarin (800 mg/day) or placebo. Two groups stopped medication and received either silymarin (800 mg/day) or placebo. Transaminase levels decreased in all groups with no significant difference among groups. Suspending psychotropics reduced serum malondialdehyde significantly. In patients who remained on psychotropics, silymarin significantly decreased malondialdehyde.
—A double-blind placebo-controlled RCT tested placebo versus silymarin (420 mg/ day × 12 weeks) given with tacrine (40 mg/ day × 6 weeks, then 80 mg/day) on liver transaminase elevation in 222 participants; 217 were included in the intent to treat analysis (12). Silymarin did not affect serum ALT levels; however, gastrointestinal and cholinergic side effects were less frequent in the silymarin group.
—In patients with primary biliary cirrhosis and a suboptimal response to ursodeoxycholic acid (UDCA), silymarin (140 mg t.i.d. × 1 year) as an adjuvant to UDCA had no benefit on LFTs (13).
—Silymarin did not improve LFTs in people chronically exposed to malathion (an organophosphate), various solvents, paints, or glue (2).

- *Amanita* mushroom poisoning

—Intravenous silymarin is used in Europe to treat *Amanita phalloides* (deadly angel or death cap fungus) mushroom poisoning. In 220 cases of *Amanita* poisoning in Germany, Switzerland, and Austria, those given intravenous silibinin had a mortality rate of 12.8% (14); lethality in adults is usually more than 20% (15). Sixty consecutive patients

treated with silybinin 20 mg/kg/day (initiated 24 to 36 hours after mushroom ingestion) survived (2).

ANIMAL/IN VITRO

- Hepatotoxicity

—Silymarin protects several species of animals from *Amanita* poisoning (2). One dose of silymarin protected mice from microcystin-LR hepatic damage (16). In lambs, silymarin may be a helpful adjunctive treatment for hepatotoxicity caused by sawfly larvae (17).

- Hypocholesterolemic effects

—Silymarin exhibited anticholesterolemic, dose-dependent effects when given in doses between 0.1% to 1% w/w of a high cholesterol diet in rats (18). This effect was similar to probucol (apparently given in the same doses); silymarin was superior in increasing high density lipoprotein (HDL) and decreasing hepatic cholesterol. Silybinin did not affect any parameters.

- Low density lipoprotein (LDL) oxidation

—Silybin or the silymarin complex inhibits LDL oxidation. Silymarin inhibited copper-induced oxidation of human LDL (silychristin and silydianin, tested separately, had prooxidant effects) (19). In another *in vitro* study, silibinin (5,200 mmol/L) inhibited LDL oxidation (20).

- Cancer

—Silymarin significantly reduced tumor incidence, tumor multiplicity, and tumor volume in a mouse skin tumorigenesis model (21). Topical silymarin [9 mg before ultraviolet B (UVB) exposure] significantly decreased tumor promotion (incidence, multiplicity, and tumor volume) but not UVB-induced tumor initiation (22). However, a protocol using UVB-induced initiation and promotion found that silymarin, compared with controls, decreased tumor incidence, tumor multiplicity, and tumor volume per mouse. In short-term experiments, silymarin significantly inhibited UVB-caused sunburn, apoptotic cell formation, and skin edema; depleted catalase activity; and induced cyclooxygenase and ornithine decarboxylase activities.
—In cell culture, silymarin and silibinin inhibited growth of human prostate, breast, and cervical carcinoma cells (23).
—In a hormone-refractory human prostate carcinoma cell line, silibinin significantly decreased prostate specific antigen and inhibited cell growth via G1 arrest in cell cycle progression (24). Silymarin significantly inhibited both anchorage-dependent and anchorage-independent growth of human prostate carcinoma DU145 cells, apparently through a G1 arrest in cell cycle (25). G1 arrest has also been shown in breast cancer cells (26).

- Other effects

—In rats, silibinin reduced cisplatin-induced decrease in renal glomerular and tubular function (27). Silibinin protected the rat exocrine pancreas from cyclosporine toxicity (28). Silymarin reduced ischemia-reperfusion induced gastric injury, apparently by interfering with neutrophil function (29).

 Risks

ADVERSE REACTIONS

- Milk thistle is quite safe. Side effects are uncommon and include nausea, diarrhea, upset stomach, headache, and pruritus.
- A 57-year-old woman reported intermittent, day-long episodes of sweating, nausea, colicky abdominal pain, diarrhea, vomiting, and weakness, temporally related to ingestion of milk thistle capsules (Microgenics milk thistle Vegicaps) (30). The episodes disappeared on discontinuation of this preparation and recurred on rechallenge. This was probably due to a contaminant or misidentified plant in this preparation. No effort was made to identify components of this preparation.
- A German case report of anaphylactic shock contained inadequate substantiation of causality; a Russian case report noted severe urticaria that resolved with prednisone treatment (6).

 Dose

COMMON DOSAGE FORMS

- Silymarin is poorly soluble in water, so teas are not recommended (14).
- *Dry extract*: 40:1 to 70:1 (w/w) containing 70% to 80% silymarin.
- *Capsules*: one containing 100 to 200 mg silymarin b.i.d.
- *Fruit*: 3 to 5 g fruit as decoction t.i.d. to q.i.d. ½ hour before meals.
- *Amanita* poisoning: Intravenous administration of a silybinin derivative (Legalon SIL) 20 mg silybinin/kg body weight over 24 hours, divided into four doses, each infused over 2 hours.

Molybdenum

 10 Second Take

Molybdenum, an essential trace element, is fairly benign; it may play a role in treating Wilson's disease.

 Basics

DESCRIPTION

• A silver-white metal, molybdenum is a transition element. Molybdate ions are the primary form in blood and urine; enzymatic molybdenum is a small nonprotein cofactor with a pterin nucleus. Soluble molybdenum compounds include ammonium molybdate, ammonium terra paramolybdate, calcium molybdate, and molybdenum trioxide (1).

FOOD SOURCES

• Milk and milk products, legumes, liver, kidney, and whole grain cereals (2). Water contains little molybdenum (less than 2 to 3 μg/L); however, surface water sources close to molybdenum mining areas may be as high as 0.4 mg/L (groundwater levels may reach 25 mg/L).
• The average daily intake may be 0.1 to 0.5 mg (1).

MECHANISM/PHARMACOKINETICS

• Molybdenum, an essential trace element, acts as an electron transfer agent in oxidation-reduction reactions. Molybdenum is part of a complex called molybdenum cofactor, required for the activity of three mammalian enzymes: xanthine oxidase (important in metabolizing purines), aldehyde oxidase (which catalyzes the conversion of acids from aldehyde), and sulfite oxidase (which converts toxic sulfite, generated by sulfur-containing amino acids, to sulfate, and also is necessary for the formation of sulfated compounds necessary for brain function) (3). Molybdenum also may protect steroid hormone receptors against inactivation (2).
• Molybdenum is readily absorbed in the stomach and throughout the small intestine. About 28% to 77% of orally ingested molybdenum is absorbed; urinary excretion is 17% to 80% of total dose (4). Excess molybdate is eliminated renally; significant amounts are excreted in bile (2). Molybdate is bound to α-2-macroglobulins; molybdenum also binds to a protein on the erythrocyte membrane.
• Most molybdenum in the body is found in the liver and kidney, with small amounts found in the adrenal glands and in the long bones (1).

 Evidence

CLINICAL TRIALS

• Cancer

—An uncontrolled Phase 1 clinical trial in 18 metastatic cancer patients (8 women) tested oral tetrathiomolybdate (90, 105, and 120 mg/day) for varying amounts of time (5). Copper is required for angiogenesis, and the goal of the study was to induce copper deficiency. Four patients were removed from the study because of disease progression. Fourteen achieved target copper deficiency; of these, five remained stable (two experienced decreased size and number of lung lesions), eight experienced progression of disease within a month or experienced stable disease for less than 90 days, and one progressed at one site. The five stable patients remained on the therapy for 120 to 413 days after induction of copper deficiency. Several patients received other anticancer therapies, so this study is difficult to interpret. The treatment was nontoxic. Mild reversible anemia occurred in four patients with ceruloplasmin levels 10% to 20% of baseline; several patients also reported sulfuric burping.

• Cancer prevention

—A randomized controlled trial (RCT) of four different nutritional interventions in Linxian, China, where intake of several nutrients is low and rates of esophageal and gastric cancer are high, tested vitamin C (120 mg) and molybdenum (30 μg) as one of four interventions in 29,584 people for 5 years. The vitamin C/molybdenum combination did not affect all-cause mortality rate (6) or the prevalence of esophageal or gastric dysplasia or cancer (7).

• Wilson's disease

—Tetrathiomolybdate can be used for the initial treatment of patients with Wilson's disease. A case series of 33 patients with Wilson's disease and neurologic symptoms tested ammonium tetrathiomolybdate for about 8 weeks. Molybdenum, which complexes copper so that it is not bioavailable, was followed by zinc maintenance therapy. Copper levels were controlled quickly. Only 1/33 patients deteriorated neurologically, and recovery in most patients was good to excellent (8). One patient experienced reversible anemia.

• Dental caries

—Epidemiologic studies in Hungary, New Zealand, and Columbia suggest that molybdenum may decrease the incidence of dental caries (3).

ANIMAL/IN VITRO

• Cancer

—In rats, a high-molybdenum diet (2 ppm) significantly reduced the incidence of esophageal cancer compared with a low-molybdenum (0.032 ppm) diet group (9). Molybdenum reduces the carcinogenic effects of N-nitroso compounds, possibly by preventing disruption of intracellular calcium metabolism and stimulating metabolism of the nitroso compounds via a nontoxic pathway (10).

• Lead poisoning

—In rats, sodium molybdate (1 mg/kg i.p. q.d.) during dietary lead exposure significantly reduced lead uptake in blood, liver, and kidneys (11).

• Dental caries

—In vitro, molybdenum enhances the remineralizing effects of fluoride on bovine enamel (12). In rats, molybdenum (25 or 50 ppm) added to fluoride (50 ppm) reduced dental caries more than fluoride alone (12).

 Clinical Considerations

DEFICIENCY SIGNS AND SYMPTOMS

• Molybdenum deficiency does not occur in free-living humans (3). Sulfur amino acid metabolism can be disrupted by a deficiency of sulfite oxidase (which requires molybdenum for activity) (2).
• There is one known case of total parenteral nutrition (TPN)-induced molybdenum deficiency. After 6 months of total parenteral nutrition, a 24-year-old man with Crohn's disease developed multiple episodes (precipitated by intravenous amino acids) of tachycardia, tachypnea, headache, nausea, vomiting, central scotomas, and night blindness, progressing within 2 days to lethargy, disorientation, and coma (13). Plasma methionine levels were high (250 to 300 μmol/L, normal <55 μmol/L) and serum uric acid levels were low (molybdenum is important in forming uric acid from purines). A reaction to a sulfur load because of sulfite oxidase deficiency was suspected. Ammonium molybdate (300 μg/day) resolved symptoms and normalized laboratory tests.

- Inborn errors of metabolism

—Inborn errors of metabolism involving molybdenum-containing enzymes include hereditary xanthinuria, a benign condition in which xanthine oxidase activity is severely reduced. Most patients are asymptomatic; some infants with the condition are irritable, have intermittent hematuria, and occasional orange-brown discoloration of their diapers (3).
—Hereditary sulfite oxidase deficiency is extremely rare but causes progressive destruction of brain tissue; neurologic problems begin soon after birth and progress to mental retardation, microcephaly, blindness, and spastic quadriparesis (3). Aldehyde oxidase deficiency has not been reported.

- Deficiency in animals

—In goats and minipigs, molybdenum deficiency depresses food intake and growth, impairs reproduction, and elevates copper concentrations in the liver and brain (2).

LABORATORY TESTS

- Neutron activation and atomic absorption are used to determine the concentration of molybdenum; however, the analysis is difficult and subject to contamination.
- Whole blood concentrations of molybdenum in most people are less than 5 ng/mL in whole blood but may be as high as 150 μg molybdenum/mL in those who live in molybdenum mining areas (1).

 Risks

ADVERSE REACTIONS

- Lung cancer/toxicity

—Molybdenum is not considered a suspected carcinogen by either the International Agency for Research on Cancer or the U.S. Toxicology Program. However, a case-control study involving 478 cases (male patients with lung cancer) and 536 controls (male patients without cancer or lung disease) examined exposure to occupational carcinogens and found a significant association between exposure to chromium, mineral oils, and molybdenum with lung cancer (14).
—Pneumoconiosis has been associated with long-term respiratory exposure (4 to 7 years) to high levels of metallic molybdenum and molybdenum trioxide (1 to 19 mg molybdenum/m^3).

- Rheumatologic effects

—Systemic lupus erythematosus temporally associated with a delayed-type hypersensitivity reaction to molybdenum from implanted metal plates was reported in a 24-year-old woman (15).

—Hyperuricemia and low copper levels are associated with high molybdenum intake (1). Arthralgias and hyperuricemia were noted in Armenians consuming 10 to 15 mg molybdenum/day. An epidemiological study in Ankara found a higher incidence of gout in a group with high molybdenum intake, compared with an adjoining settlement (1).

- Exposure standards

—U.S. Environmental Protection Agency (EPA) lowest observable adverse effects level (LOAEL) is 140 μg/kg/day (1).
—U.S. Occupational Safety and Health Administration (OSHA) PEL-TWA for total dust is 5 mg molybdenum/m^3; PEL-TWA for insoluble compounds is 10 mg molybdenum/m^3.
—No observed adverse effect level (NOAEL) for students receiving molybdenum in drinking water was 8 μg/kg/day (1). A dose of 75 μg molybdenum per day was given to 24 girls ages 7 to 9 years; no specific adverse effects were identified (1).
—A tolerable daily intake (TDI) of 0.009 mg molybdenum kg/day has been calculated based on animal studies (4).

- Molybdenum toxicity

—The acute toxicity of molybdenum is low. Treatment for molybdenum toxicity is supportive and may include lavage, emesis, and activated charcoal; it is unknown whether these measures are effective.
—Theoretically, copper sulfate could enhance recovery from chronic molybdenum ingestion, but no data are available to support this (1).

ANIMAL TOXICITY

- Molybdenum toxicity in animals (called teart or molybdenosis) causes anemia, anorexia, severe diarrhea, joint abnormalities, osteoporosis, tear discoloration, reduced sexual activity, and death (1). Toxicity is species-specific. Sheep and cows may have adverse reactions to feed containing as little as 2 ppm molybdenum; horses and pigs can tolerate concentrations over 1,000 ppm. Inorganic sulfate in soil prevents molybdenum intoxication of livestock (16). Animals exposed to molybdenum oxide fumes (53 mg/m^3 for 1 hour daily) developed pulmonary irritation and fatty changes in the liver and kidney (1).

 Dose

RECOMMENDED DIETARY ALLOWANCE

Infants and children	
0 to 6 months	2 μg/day (adequate intake)
7 to 12 months	3 μg/day (adequate intake)
1 to 3 years	17 μg/day
4 to 8 years	22 μg/day
Males	
9 to 13 years	34 μg/day
14 to 18 years	43 μg/day
19 to 50 years	45 μg/day
51+ years	45 μg/day
Females	
9 to 13 years	34 μg/day
14 to 18 years	43 μg/day
19 to 50 years	45 μg/day
51+ years	45 μg/day
Pregnant	50 μg/day
Lactating	50 μg/day

UPPER LIMITS

Infants and children	
0 to 6 months	Not determinable
7 to 12 months	Not determinable
1 to 3 years	300 μg/day
4 to 8 years	600 μg/day
Males	
9 to 13 years	1100 μg/day
14 to 18 years	1700 μg/day
19 to 50 years	2000 μg/day
51+ years	2000 μg/day
Females	
9 to 13 years	1100 μg/day
14 to 18 years	1700 μg/day
19 to 50 years	2000 μg/day
51+ years	2000 μg/day
Pregnant	
≤18 years	1700 μg/day
19 to 50 years	2000 μg/day
Lactating	
≤18 years	1700 μg/day
19 to 50 years	2000 μg/day

 Common Questions and Answers

Q: How is molybdenum used industrially?
A: Molybdenum is used in metallurgy, especially stainless steel and cast iron alloys and for manufacturing ceramic-metal composites. Molybdenum trioxide inhibits corrosion and is also used as a blue dye in ceramic glazes and enamels. Zinc molybdate stabilizes paint. Other molybdenum compounds are used as chemical catalysts and as dry lubricants (1).

Motherwort

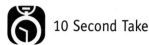 10 Second Take

There are no clinical trials on motherwort. No adverse effects have been reported, but motherwort increased one type of preneoplastic mammary lesion in a mouse study.

 Basics

LATIN NAME

Leonurus cardiaca L.
Chinese Motherwort *Leonurus japonicus* Houtt.
Syn: *Leonurus artemisia* (Lour.) S.Y. Hu

FAMILY

Lamiaceae

OTHER COMMON NAMES

L. cardiaca: common motherwort
L. artemisia: yi mu cao (herb), *chong wei zi* (fruit)

DESCRIPTION

• Motherwort is a dark green, unbranched perennial that grows up to 120 cm tall and in the summer bears aromatic whorls of spotted pink, pale, or purplish flowers. The leaves are cut into five lobes or three-pointed segments. Various species are native to Europe and Asia and the plant has become naturalized in North America.

PART USED

Dried aerial parts

KNOWN ACTIVE CONSTITUENTS

• Motherwort contains the alkaloids L-stachydrine, leonurine, betonicine, turicin, leonurine, leonuridin, and leonurinine; the iridoid glycoside leonuride; bitter glycosides; diterpenoids (including leocardin); triterpenes (ursolic acid); flavonoids; the phenolic glycoside caffeic acid-4 rutinoside; and tannins (5% to 9%), primarily catechin derivatives and pyrogallol (1,2).

MECHANISM/PHARMACOKINETICS

• Leonurine causes central nervous system depression and hypotension in animals (1).

Evidence

CLINICAL TRIALS

No clinical trials identified.

ANIMAL/IN VITRO

• Cancer

—Motherwort enhanced the development of pregnancy-dependent mammary tumors in GR/A mice. These mice have a high level of spontaneous mammary cancers that arise from either pregnancy-dependent mammary tumors or mammary hyperplastic alveolar nodules (3). Motherwort decreased the number of hyperplastic alveolar nodules and the incidence of mammary cancer arising from hyperplastic alveolar nodules; there were no differences between groups in the number of cancers per mouse. The incidence of adenomyosis was lower in treated mice. The authors note that in a previous unpublished study in mice, motherwort did not affect the end bud in the mammary glands but did enhance the growth of ducts.

• Cardiac effects

—In animals, motherwort has sedative, hypotensive, and negative chronotropic effects (1).

• Uterine contraction

—In an *in vitro* experiment, a methanolic extract of *Leonurus artemisia* stimulated uterine contraction in human myometrium (4).

OTHER CLAIMED BENEFITS/ACTIONS

• Heart problems
• Diarrhea
• Sedative
• Palpitations
• Menstrual disorders
• Anxiety
• Laxative

 Risks

PREGNANCY/LACTATION

This herb should be avoided in pregnancy as it causes uterine stimulation.

 Dose

COMMON DOSAGE FORMS

• *Dried herb*: 2 to 4 g t.i.d. or 2 to 4 g as infusion t.i.d.
• *Liquid extract*: (1:1, 25% ethanol) 2 to 4 mL t.i.d.
• *Tincture*: (1:5, 25% ethanol) 4 to 10 mL t.i.d. or (1:5, 45% ethanol) 2 to 6 mL t.i.d.

Mullein

 10 Second Take

There are neither clinical trials of mullein nor reports of adverse events; it has a long tradition of use for respiratory ailments.

 Basics

LATIN NAME

Verbascum thapsus L., *Verbascum densiflora* Bertoloni, *Verbascum phlomoides* L.

FAMILY

Scrophulariaceae

OTHER COMMON NAMES

V. densiflorum Bertol. or *V. thapsiforme* Schrad: large-flowered mullein
V. thapsus L.: great mullein, white mullein, velvet dock, Aaron's rod, gordolobo, punchon
V. phlomoides L.: orange mullein

DESCRIPTION

• Mullein is a biennial plant native to Europe, Egypt, Ethiopia, and temperate Asia that has become naturalized in the eastern United States. The leaves, stems, and calyces are covered with a dense woolly felt of whitish hairs; in its first year only a basal rosette of leaves is produced, whereas in its second year the plant sends up a single, rigid stem, 4 to 8 ft tall, with a flower spike of yellow flowers. It prefers dry slopes.

PART USED

Flowers, leaves (less common)

KNOWN ACTIVE CONSTITUENTS

• Mullein flower contains 3% mucilage polysaccharides, 47% D-galactose, 25% arabinose, 14% D-glucose, 6% D-xylose, 4% L-rhamnose, 2% D-mannose, 1% L-fructose, 12.5% arabinoglycans, flavonoids (1.5% to 4%), triterpene saponins, and sterols (1).

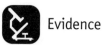 Evidence

CLINICAL TRIALS

No clinical trials identified.

ANIMAL/IN VITRO

• A freeze-dried infusion of mullein flowers (*V. thapsiforme*) has shown antiviral activity against herpes simplex virus 1 (HSV-1), several strains of influenza A and B, and fowl plague virus *in vitro* (2). Another *in vitro* study found that a methanolic extract of *V. thapsus* was active against HSV-1 but not respiratory syncytial virus (RSV), parainfluenza, enteric coronavirus, or rotavirus (3).
• A saponin glycoside and its aglycone from *V. thapsiforme* flowers have been shown to inhibit biosynthesis by inactivating ribosomes (4).

OTHER CLAIMED BENEFITS/ACTIONS

• Asthma
• Cough
• Sore throat
• Congestion
• Otitis media
• Toothache, cramps, convulsions (root)
• Diuretic
• Antirheumatic
• Mucosal inflammation

Risks

No risks identified.

Dose

COMMON DOSAGE FORMS

- *Tea or infusion:* 1.5 to 2.0 g herb in 150 to 250 mL water b.i.d.
- *Decoction:* 1.5 to 2 g in 150 to 250 mL water b.i.d.
- *Fluid extract:* 1:1 (g/mL) 1.5 to 2 mL b.i.d.
- *Tincture:* 1:5 (g/mL) 7.5 to 10 mL b.i.d.
- The herb is sometimes smoked for asthma or coughing

Common Questions and Answers

Q: Is mullein the same as *gordolobo*?
A: Yes, but it is only one of the plants known by that name. *Gordolobo* or *punchon* are Spanish names for *V. thapsus;* it is commonly used for respiratory conditions (5). Cudweed or everlasting (*Gnaphalium conoideum*), another hairy-leafed plant that is a member of the Asteraceae family, is also known as *gordolobo*. There have been no problems associated with either mullein or cudweed, but a dangerous plant has sometimes been mistaken for *Gnaphalium* and sold as *gordolobo*. Groundsel (*Senecio longilobus*) also has hairy leaves (although the flowers are distinctly different) and has been found in *gordolobo* (6). *Senecio longilobus* and several other *Senecio* species contain hepatotoxic pyrrolizidine alkaloids. Two cases of pyrrolizidine poisoning in Mexican-American infants have been reported: a case of hepatitis in a 6-month-old girl and a death in a two-month-old boy (7). In both cases the "*gordolobo*" preparations actually contained *Senecio longilobus.*

Q: Does smoking an herb as a treatment for asthma make sense?
A: Smoking predates inhalers as a way to deliver medication to the lung (it's certainly arguable whether any medication mixed with smoke would be expected to have a net benefit!). Although its use is not common today, the Mohegan and Penobscot Indians smoked dried, often powdered mullein leaves, and the Menominees smoked mullein roots for pulmonary diseases. The treatment was recommended as a home remedy among non-Indians in the 19th century. It is not clear whether the treatment had any efficacy, but another herb smoked for asthma did have a pharmacologic basis for an effect. *Datura stramonium* (jimson weed or thornapple) was the main component of herbal cigarettes sold in the 19th century as a treatment for asthma. This species contains an anticholinergic alkaloid that can decrease bronchial secretions and dilate bronchi (as well as impairing vision through pupil dilation, drying out mucus membranes, and, in high doses, increasing temperature and causing loss of consciousness). Other species of *Datura* (*D. metel* and *D. fastuosa*) have been used in recent times (8).

Q: Where does the name come from?
A: *Verbascum,* the genus name given to the plant by Linnaeus, is assumed to be a variation of barbascum, from the Latin *barba* (a beard) and seems to refer to the plant's hairy leaves. Several of the older common names for *V. thapsus* are interesting; the down is good for tinder when it is quite dry, and one of its old names was candlewick. Another old name was torches; centuries ago the stalks dipped in suet were used as lights in processions (9).

Neem

10 Second Take

Neem, an Indian herb, has antimicrobial, spermicidal, insecticidal, and immune-stimulating effects. Ingestion of the seed oil in children has been linked to a Reye's-like syndrome.

Basics

LATIN NAME

Azadirachta indica

FAMILY

Meliaceae

OTHER COMMON NAMES

Sanskrit—*nimba, arishta*; Bengali—*nim*; Bombay—*Bal-nimb, nim*; Hindu—*nim, nimb*; Tamil—*veppu, vembu, veppam*; Marathi—*nimbay*; Oriya—*nimo, nimba*; Gujerati—*limbado*; Telegu—*nimbamu*; and Urdu—*nim*

DESCRIPTION

• A tall evergreen tree that can grow up to 50 ft tall with rough grayish or brownish bark; white, aromatic flowers; and oblong greenish yellow fruit. It grows throughout most of India and Burma.

PART USED

• Leaves, bark, seed, seed oil (also called Margosa oil). The flowers are used in curries and soups, or fried.

KNOWN ACTIVE CONSTITUENTS

• *Seed oil:* Bitter limonoids (nortriterpenoids) including nimbin, nimbibin, salanin, and the tetranorterpenoid mahmoodin. Also contains sulfur-containing compounds including *cis*- and *trans*-3,5-diethyl-1,2,4-trithiolanes.
• *Leaf extracts:* Sterols, limonoids, flavonoids and their glycosides, and coumarins (1). Aflatoxins (from fungal contamination) have been isolated in some oil samples.

MECHANISM/PHARMACOKINETICS

• Neem oil appears to selectively activate cell-mediated immune mechanisms (2). Neem activates macrophages and induces gamma interferon production by T lymphocytes. Neem oil appears to have immune stimulating effects in mice (2). An aqueous extract of neem inhibits complement and decreases chemoluminescence of activated polymorphonuclear leukocytes (3). The antifertility effect appears to occur at the preimplantation stage (4). The mechanism behind ulcer prevention appears to be due to preventing mast cell degranulation and increasing gastric mucus (5). Neem flowers strongly enhanced glutathione S-transferase activity (2.7 fold higher than controls) (6).
• No information on pharmacokinetics was identified.

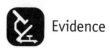

Evidence

CLINICAL TRIALS

• Vaginitis

—A double-blind study of 55 patients with abnormal vaginal discharge assigned 21 patients to placebo cream and 37 women to a mixed herbal cream containing neem seed extract along with reetha saponins (from *Sapindus mukerossi*) and quinine hydro-chloride (7). A dose of 5 mL of each cream was applied vaginally for 14 days. Ten of 12 patients with *Chlamydia trachomatis* achieved clinical and microbiologic cure after 7 to 14 days (2 patients were lost to follow-up). Of 17 patients with bacterial vaginosis, 6 became negative after 2 weeks of application of cream; 5 patients were lost to follow-up. No effect was seen in patients with *Candida albicans* or *Trichomonas vaginalis*. There was no clinical improvement in patients given placebo cream.

• Scabies

—A study of a paste containing neem and turmeric (ground to a paste in a 4:1 ratio) was tested against scabies for 3 to 15 days (successfully treated cases stopped using the cream earlier). Of 824 cases, 97.9% achieved complete cure within 15 days of treatment; cure was faster in those with localized lesions compared with those with secondary infection or widespread lesions (8).

ANIMAL/IN VITRO

- ### Antimicrobial

—Neem sticks from neem bark (used for dental hygiene) reduced bacterial aggregation of oral streptococci (9). Neem extracts inhibit a variety of microorganisms, including *Candida albicans, Candida tropicalis, Neisseria gonorrhea, Staphylococcus aureus, Escherichia coli,* herpes simplex virus 2, and HIV-1 (10). Neem leaf extracts have some antimalarial activity (1). In *Plasmodium falciparum,* trophozoites/schizonts appear to be the susceptible target stage; gametocytes in various maturation stages were also killed by various neem seed fractions (11). Azadirachtin has been shown to have a molluscicidal effect on the snails *Lymneaea acuminata* and *Indoplanorbis exustus* (12). A spermicidal fraction from neem oil, NIM 76, inhibited growth of *E. coli, Klebsiella pneumoniae, C. albicans,* and polio virus (13).

- ### Insecticide/insect repellant effects

—Azadirachtin, found in the seed, leaves, and other parts of the neem tree, is a potent insecticide against mosquitoes and other insects; azadirachtin exhibits several modes of action against insects including growth regulation, sterilization, feeding deterrent, and changes in biologic fitness (14). A 2% neem oil appears to be an effective mosquito repellent (15), and burning 1% neem oil in kerosene lamps repels mosquitoes (this protection is more pronounced against *Anopheles* than *Culex*) (16). Azadirachtin has relatively low stability, and efforts are underway to develop more stable derivatives.

- ### Cancer

—Several limonoids from neem have shown cytotoxic effects to several cell lines *in vitro,* including mouse neuroblastoma (N1E-115) and human osteosarcoma (143B.TK) (17). Neem leaf extracts suppressed DMBA-induced oral carcinogenesis in the hamster buccal pouch (18).

- ### Other

—Neem (10, 30, and 100 mg/kg) had analgesic effects in mice (19). In stressed rats, aqueous leaf extracts (10, 40, or 160 mg leaf/kg in one- or five-dose regimens) dose-dependently reduced gastric ulcer severity in stress-induced ulcers (and reduced ethanol-induced gastric mucosal damage) (6). A neem leaf extract reduced paracetamol (acetaminophen)-induced hepatotoxicity in rats (20).

- ### Antifertility

—Intrauterine neem oil (1 mL) reversibly blocked fertility for 7 to 12 months in bonnet monkeys (21). In rodents and primates, orally administered neem extracts terminate pregnancy at an early postimplantation stage. Neem extracts are also effective spermicides that have been shown to be effective contraceptives in rabbits and baboons (10). A single intra-vas injection of neem oil produced infertility in male rats lasting at least 8 months (22).

OTHER CLAIMED BENEFITS/ACTIONS

- Bark and leaves—fever and tonic
- Leaves—skin diseases, ulcer, and dispelling intestinal parasites
- Oil—chronic skin diseases, ulcers, rheumatism, sprain, leprosy, ear trouble, and gum problems

 Risks

ADVERSE REACTIONS

- Margosa oil (neem seed oil), internally ingested, has been associated with a Reye's-like toxic encephalopathy in infants and young children (23,24). Typical symptoms include vomiting, drowsiness, tachypnea, and recurrent generalized seizures. Leukocytosis and metabolic acidosis may occur; fatalities have been reported.
- Two hours after consumption of 1 L of neem leaf extract, a 24-year-old woman was admitted to the hospital (25). Unconscious, bradycardic, and hypotensive on admission, cardiac and respiratory arrest developed within minutes; the patient was successfully resuscitated, treated with supportive measures, and was discharged a week later. Reasons for ingestion were not provided.

ANIMAL TOXICITY

- A crude extract of neem leaves was tested in guinea pigs and rabbits; adverse cardiovascular effects included hypotension and a dose-related mild negative chronotropic effect; weak antiarrhythmic activity was also demonstrated in rabbits (26). A reproductive toxicological study in rats fed a diet containing 10% debitterized neem oil or groundnut oil did not find any adverse effects on reproductive parameters (27); intrauterine neem treatment did not affect fetal development in the contralateral uterine horn of unilaterally treated rats (5). Aqueous suspensions of neem leaves were fed to goats and guinea pigs in doses of 50 or 200 mg/kg orally for up to 8 weeks. In these doses, neem caused decreased body weight, weakness, loss of appetite, and decreased pulse and respiratory rates. In animals given fresh leaves, diarrhea was observed. In goats, the highest doses of leaves produced tremors and ataxia (28).
- Neem leaf extract at 40 mg/kg for 20 days did not affect thyroid function of mice, but at 100 mg/kg decreased triiodothyronine (T3) levels and increased serum thyroxine concentrations. Increased hepatic lipid peroxidation and decreased glucose-6-phosphatase were noted (29).

Nettle

 10 Second Take

Nettle may benefit benign prostatic hypertrophy; nettle sting may help arthritis.

 Basics

LATIN NAME

Urtica dioica L., *Urtica major* Kanitz, *Urtica gracilis* Ait

FAMILY

Urticaceae

OTHER COMMON NAMES

Common nettle, stinging nettle

DESCRIPTION

- A perennial common throughout temperate zones in Europe, Africa, Asia, Australia, North America, and South America.
- Nettle is covered with stinging hairs, each a sharp, hollow spine containing an irritant fluid.

PART USED

Leaves, roots, or whole herb; occasionally fruit

KNOWN ACTIVE CONSTITUENTS

- *Aerial parts:* Flavonoids (largely kaempferol, isorhamnetin, and quercitin), caffeic acid and esters, up to 20% minerals (calcium, potassium, and silicon), sitosterol, glycoprotein, free amino acids, and chlorophyll (1). Nettle is high in protein (especially aspartic acid and leucine; it is low in histidine, and lacks methionine) (2). Nettle contains vitamin C (20 to 60 mg/100 g dry material), beta-carotene (20 to 30 mg/100 g dry weight), small amounts of xanthophyll, lycopene, and other carotenoids, (3) and alpha-tocopherol (2).
- Essential oil from leaves contains ketones (38.5%); esters (14.7%); free alcohols (2%); and small amounts of phenols, aldehydes, and nitrogenous substances (3).
- *Root:* β-sitosterol and tannins, phenyl propanes, polyphenols, monoterpene diols, lignans, lectins, and polysaccharides (4). *Urtica dioica* agglutinin (UDA) is a mixture of six small isolectins (5).
- *Hairs:* Nettle hair fluid contains acetylcholine, histamine, and serotonin; nettles or nettle hair extracts may contain more than 1 μg/mL histamine and nanogram amounts of leukotrienes (LT) B_4 and LTC/D$_4$ (6). In mast cells and mammalian cells, LTs are usually generated in response to stimuli; nettle LTs appear to be preformed.

MECHANISM/PHARMACOKINETICS

- Several constituents of a methanolic extract of nettle roots inhibit aromatase (7). An aqueous extract of nettle roots inhibits sex hormone binding globulin (SHBG) binding in a dose-related manner (8). Nettle extract did not inhibit α_1 adrenoceptors (9).
- In humans, 30% to 50% of UDA (20 mg) was excreted in the feces; less than 1% was excreted in urine. In mice given radiolabeled UDA, radioactivity was detected in the gut, liver, kidney, blood, and maw (3).
- Nettle sting causes irregular C-fiber discharge that occurs simultaneously with a sensation of pricking and burning; itching does not correlate with discharge frequency (10). Stinging may last 12 hours; in six people, mast cells (but not mononuclear or polymorphonuclear cells) significantly increased at 12 hours (11). A nettle hair with 6.1 ng serotonin contained 33.25 picograms of histamine. Although the immediate pain of a nettle sting is due to histamine, the persistence of the sensation is apparently due to other compounds.

 Evidence

CLINICAL TRIALS

- Osteoarthritis

Nettle stings

—A placebo-controlled double-blind crossover randomized controlled trial (RCT) in 27 patients with osteoarthritic pain at the base of the thumb or index finger tested nettle sting applied to the painful area for about 30 seconds (the leaf was moved twice) daily for 1 week (12). White dead nettle (*Lamium album*), which does not sting, served as placebo. Compared with placebo, nettle significantly decreased visual analog scale pain scores (after day 2) and reduced pain scores and health assessment scores after 1 week. One week into the washout period, the difference was no longer significant. Verbal rating pain scores were lower with stinging nettle only in the group treated with stinging nettle first. Medication use was not affected. The slight itching and rash caused by nettle did not bother 23/27 patients. Fourteen of 27 preferred nettle stings to their usual treatment; 17 wanted to use the treatment in the future.

Stewed nettles

—A randomized pilot study in 40 participants with acute exacerbation of arthritis compared diclofenac 200 mg (with misoprostol) and diclofenac 50 mg with stewed stinging nettles (50 g) for 2 weeks. C-reactive protein and total joint scores improved significantly in both groups, with no difference between groups (13). Side effects were minor, mainly gastrointestinal.

- Allergic rhinitis

—A double-blind RCT of 98 patients (69 completed) with allergic rhinitis compared placebo with freeze-dried *Urtica dioica* (300 mg; two capsules at symptom onset) (14). At 1 hour, patients rated themselves dramatically improved, moderately improved, no change, or worse. The symptom response diary data is difficult to interpret. Apparently 16% of treated subjects and 3% of controls experienced improvement more than 50% of the time; 48% versus 32% experienced moderate improvement; 61% versus 71% had no change; and 0% versus 3% were worse. A total of 52% in the treated group and 79% of controls rated their treatment less effective than previous medications. No statistical assessment is apparent, and it is unclear whether differences between groups were significant. Seven patients taking nettle and five on placebo had side effects, primarily mild gastric discomfort; two individuals apparently had symptom exacerbation (it is not stated which group they were in). The treatment was rated moderately or highly effective in 58% of nettle-treated patients and 37% of controls.

- Benign prostatic hyperplasia

—A double-blind study in 50 patients given placebo or nettle root extract (300 mg b.i.d. × 9 weeks) found that both groups improved symptomatically; only the treated group significantly improved in urine volume, maximum urinary flow and significantly decreased SHBG (15).

—Another double-blind placebo-controlled study in 79 men found that nettle extract (600 mg/day × 6 to 8 weeks) improved mean urinary flow 14%; maximum urinary flow rates improved from 13.8 to 15.4 mL/seconds, and residual urine values decreased by 40% (16). Placebo did not affect urinary parameters.

—A third double-blind placebo-controlled trial in 40 participants (reported in a German book) found that nettle root extract (1,200 mg/day × 6 months) significantly decreased urinary frequency and SHBG levels (1).

—A double-blind controlled trial compared saw palmetto/nettle extract (two capsules daily of PRO 160/120) with finasteride in 543 patients for 48 weeks. Both groups experienced increased urinary flow rates and average flow and decreased micturition time; urinary volume did not change (17). Fewer adverse events occurred in the herb group.

- Gingivitis

—A mouthwash containing nettle, juniper (*Juniperus communis*), and yarrow (*Achillea millefolium*) (1:1:1) was tested in 45 volunteers with moderate gingival inflammation who rinsed with 10 mL of mouthwash b.i.d. for 3 months. There were no differences between groups at 6 weeks or 3 months, measured by plaque index, modified gingival index, and bleeding index (18).

ANIMAL/IN VITRO

• Prostatic effects

—In mice, a polysaccharide fraction of a 20% methanolic root extract reduced induced prostatic hyperplasia 33.8% (19). In dogs, nettle root [90 mg 20% methanolic extract (5:1) per day for 100 days] decreased prostate volume by 30%. In castrated rats, the same extract did not inhibit testosterone-stimulated growth (1).
—In human prostatic tissue, most nettle root extracts, but not UDA, inhibited Na^+, K^+ ATPase activity (20). Nettle extract and UDA decreased cell proliferation in prostate cell cultures from men with benign prostatic hyperplasia (BPH) (1).

• Immunomodulation

—A standardized nettle leaf extract, IDS23, inhibited lipopolysaccharide-stimulated monocyte cytokine expression and inhibited phytohemagglutinin-stimulated production of Th1-specific interleukin (IL)-2 and interferon (IFN)-gamma in peripheral blood mononuclear cells (21). The same extract inhibited NF-kappa B (a nuclear transcription factor) activation (22). UDA stimulates proliferation of murine thymocytes and spleen T lymphocytes. A nettle root extract inhibited human leukocyte elastase (3).

• Diuretic effects

—A diuretic effect of ethanolic nettle whole-plant extract was noted after intraperitoneal (500 mg/kg) but not oral administration (1 g/kg) in rats (23). In rats, an oral aqueous extract of nettle herb (1 g/kg) did not cause diuresis (1).

• Analgesic effect

—No analgesic activity was noted in rats in one study of whole-plant extract (23); however, in mice, nettle herb had an analgesic effect, and in rats, topical application caused local anesthesia (1).

• Antiinflammatory effect

—A nettle leaf extract partially inhibited 5-lipoxygenase-derived synthesis of LTB_4; the same extract reduced lipopolysaccharide-induced secretion of proinflammatory cytokines (tumor necrosis factor-α and IL-1β) in human blood (1). Studies are mixed on whether nettle herb reduces inflammation in the carrageenan rat paw edema test (3,23); nettle root extract and a polysaccharide fraction were effective (1).

• Cancer

—A 20% methanolic root extract (24) and a polysaccharide fraction both inhibited proliferation of prostate carcinoma (LNCaP) cells in vitro in a dose-dependent manner (25). An ethyl acetate root extract induced differentiation in a promyelocytic leukemia line (HL-60) (3).

• Antimicrobial

—UDA strongly inhibits the growth of seven species of chitin-containing fungi (5). UDA inhibited lentivirus, herpes simplex virus 1 (HSV-1), herpes simplex virus 2 (HSV-2), HIV-1 and 2, and cytomegalovirus replication in vitro (26).

OTHER CLAIMED BENEFITS/ACTIONS

• Diuretic
• Arthritis and rheumatism
• Seborrhea
• Diabetes
• Wound healing

 Risks

ANIMAL TOXICITY

• In rats, LD_{50} of nettle intravenous infusion was 1,929 mg dry weight/kg; LD_{50} of extract was 1,721 mg dry weight/kg. A chronic oral toxicity study found that up to 1,310 mg/kg was well tolerated (3). In mice, the intraperitoneal LD_{50} of an aqueous extract of nettle herb was 3.625 g/kg body weight (1).
• In guinea pigs, nettle meal induced hypercholesterolemia; kidney hypertrophy was seen in mice and guinea pigs (2).
• An ethanolic extract of intravenous nettles in rats caused transient hypotension and arrhythmias at doses greater than 500 mg/kg (23).

 Dose

COMMON DOSAGE FORMS

• Dried leaf/herb: 3 to 6 g t.i.d.

—Infusion or decoction: 1.5 to 6 g up to t.i.d.
—Liquid extract: (1:1, 25% ethanol) 2 to 4 mL t.i.d.
—Extract: 0.77 g (7:1) b.i.d.
—Tincture: (1:5, 25% ethanol) 2 to 6 mL t.i.d.
—Fresh juice: 10 to 15 mL up to t.i.d.

• Dried root:

—Infusion made from 1.5 to 4 g root (daily dose)
—Decoction made from 1.5 g root (daily dose; let stand 10 minutes before straining)
—Fluid extract: (1:1, 45% ethanol) daily dose 1.5 to 7.5 mL
—Ethanolic extract: (1:5, 40% ethanol) daily dose 5 mL
—Dried extract: (5:1, 20% methanol) daily dose 600 to 1,200 mg

• Fruit/seed (unusual)

—Decoction: Made with 2 to 4 g—once boiled, let stand 10 minutes before straining (daily dose)

 Common Questions and Answers

Q: Do nettles cause rashes in dead people?
A: Just in case you had any doubt as to whether or not I make up these questions for my own amusement. Nettle wheals could not be induced in dead humans or rats (27). Two of 12 animals stung with nettles immediately before decapitation developed wheals postmortem but these wheals were only a third the size of those produced during life. Okay, maybe this is only of interest to forensic pathologists and murder mystery fans.

Niacin

10 Second Take

High-dose niacin is useful for hyperlipidemia and possibly for insulin-dependent diabetes.

Basics

OTHER COMMON NAMES

Vitamin B_3, nicotinic acid (NA), nicotinamide, nicotinate

DESCRIPTION

• Niacin (pyridine-3-carboxylic acid), a B vitamin, forms part of the cellular electron transport substances NAD^+/NADH and $NADP^+$/NADPH. The predominant form circulating in blood is nicotinamide (niacinamide). Nicotinamide is converted to NA endogenously and vice versa.
• Niacin can be produced endogenously from tryptophan in a vitamin B_6-dependent process. About 1/60 of dietary tryptophan is converted into niacin (1). Niacytin or niacinogen (a bound form of niacin) is common in cereal bran but not highly bioavailable.

FOOD SOURCES

Niacin equivalents (NEs): milk, meat, eggs, corn, nuts, seeds, legumes, whole grains (germ), brewer's yeast, and coffee.

MAIN FUNCTIONS/PHARMACOKINETICS

• Niacin functions in many metabolic pathways, especially anaerobic glycolysis, Krebs cycle-oxidative phosphorylation, and fatty acid synthesis and oxidation.
• Niacin is absorbed by the stomach and small intestine; it is not stored in the body.

Evidence

CLINICAL TRIALS

• Hypercholesterolemia

—NA, in a dosage of 1.5 to 6.0 g/day, lowers serum triglycerides 20% to 50%, lowers low density lipoprotein (LDL) by 10% to 25%, and increases high density lipoprotein (HDL) 15% to 35% (2). Niacin (crystalline NA 3,000 mg/ day or maximum tolerated dosage × 60 weeks) significantly increased HDL, decreased triglycerides, and decreased LDL in the Arterial Disease Multiple Intervention Trial (ADMIT), a prospective, randomized, placebo-controlled multicenter trial of 468 participants with peripheral arterial disease (3).

• Other cardiovascular risk factors

—A double-blind, randomized, placebo-controlled crossover study in seven healthy volunteers (including four females) found no effect of NA (500 mg q.d. × 7 days, then 1 g q.d. × 7 days) on blood pressure (4).
—Niacin treatment decreased fibrinogen in a subset of the ADMIT study (5). Niacin increased plasma homocysteine levels (an undesirable effect) (6).

• Diabetes Mellitus

—Studies are mixed. A 1993 review found that three of six placebo-controlled trials of niacin in patients with recent onset IDDM and residual beta-cell mass showed a benefit in prolonging the non-insulin-requiring interval, lowering insulin requirements, improving metabolic function, and increasing beta-cell function (7).
—More recent studies have not supported a benefit for niacin as an adjunct to intensive insulin therapy. A 1-year study randomized 34 newly diagnosed type I diabetics to intensive insulin therapy + placebo, intensive insulin therapy + nicotinamide (700 mg t.i.d.), or intravenous insulin for 3 days followed by intensive insulin therapy + nicotinamide (700 mg t.i.d.) (8). HbA_{1c} values normalized in all groups; there was no difference among groups in HbA_{1c} or beta-cell function.
—In 84 insulin-dependent diabetics (age 5 to 35), vitamin E (15 mg/kg/day) was compared with NA (25 mg/kg/day) for 1 year; all patients received insulin therapy (9). There were no differences in C-peptide levels, glycosylated hemoglobin, or insulin dose between groups.
—A 1-year study in 74 patients with newly diagnosed IDDM randomized patients to NA 25 mg/kg or 50 mg/kg as an adjunct to intensive insulin therapy (10). There were no significant differences in integrated measures of metabolic control or rates of clinical remission between groups at any time point.
—Niacin treatment caused glucose levels to increase modestly but significantly in patients with noninsulin-dependent diabetes (by 8.7 mg/dL) and nondiabetic patients (by 6.3 mg/dL); levels of HbA_{1c} remained unchanged in niacin-treated diabetics (3).

• Mental functioning

—A review of controlled trials of niacin identified two trials of niacin on hyperactivity and learning disability and one crossover trial in Down's syndrome patients (subjects in both trials also received vitamin B_6 and multivitamins) (11). The authors concluded that there is inadequate support from controlled trials to justify niacin supplementation for mental functioning.

ANIMAL/IN VITRO

Not covered

OTHER CLAIMED BENEFITS/ACTIONS

• Anxiety
• Arthritis
• Asthma

• Bell's palsy (see Questions and Answers)
• Diabetes
• Dysmenorrhea
• Epilepsy
• Hay fever
• Impotence
• Intermittent claudication
• Lupus
• Raynaud's

Clinical Considerations

DEFICIENCY SIGNS AND SYMPTOMS

• Pellagra is caused by lack of niacin. Gross niacin deficiency results in lassitude, ingestion, and anorexia; later effects are the classic "3 Ds": dermatitis (especially in sun-exposed areas), diarrhea (sometimes with vomiting), and dementia.
• Hartnup's disease or syndrome, an inherited autosomal recessive disorder, consists of defective intestinal absorption of tryptophan (a precursor of niacin) and defective renal tubular reabsorption, which leads to aminoaciduria. Interference with tryptophan absorption and utilization causes a pellagra-like rash and cerebellar ataxia. Nicotinamide treatment (40 to 250 mg/day) improves both (12).

FACTORS DECREASING AVAILABILITY/ABSORPTION

• Alcoholism
• Carcinoid syndrome
• Hartnup's syndrome
• B_6, riboflavin, or iron deficiency impedes conversion of tryptophan to niacin.
• An imbalance of amino acids (especially excessive leucine) impedes conversion of tryptophan to niacin (12).

FACTORS INCREASING AVAILABILITY/ABSORPTION

None identified

LABORATORY TESTS

• 24-hour urinary excretion of N1-methylnicotinamide (NMN), a niacin metabolite, is the best method. For adults, NMN < 2.4 mg/day represents low niacin status, and < 0.8 mg/day represents deficiency. Urinary metabolites are more reliable than serum metabolites.
• Random fasting urine samples corrected for creatinine have been used (normal values for adults are > 0.5 mg/g creatinine); these are difficult to interpret because creatinine excretion varies by age.
• Erythrocyte nicotinamide adenine nucleotide (NAD) concentration may serve as a sensitive indicator of niacin depletion; a ratio of erythrocyte NAD to NADP that is less than 1.0 may identify subjects with marginal deficiency (13).

Risks

WARNINGS

• Sustained-release preparations should not be used (see adverse reactions).
• Avoid niacin in patients with hepatic problems or elevated liver enzymes.
• Do not use concurrently with beta-blockers (see drug interactions).

ADVERSE REACTIONS

• Hepatotoxicity

—Sustained-release preparations are associated with hepatotoxicity more commonly than immediate-release preparations (14). In one study, 12 of 23 patients assigned to sustained-release niacin developed elevated liver aminotransferases; five patients were symptomatic for hepatic dysfunction (15). Immediate-release niacin does not cause this effect, even in patients with previous hepatitis resulting from sustained-release niacin (16).

• NIDDM

—High doses used to treat hypercholesterolemia in Type II diabetics may cause deterioration of glycemic control (17).

• Lactic acidosis

—Two cases of lactic acidosis have been reported; one apparently resulting from sustained-release niacin (18) and another, with toxic delirium, attributed to concurrent use of ethanol and niacin (19).

• Rhabdomyolysis

—A case of rhabdomyolysis 11 months after NA 500 mg t.i.d. was combined with lovastatin (40 mg q.d.) has been reported (20).

• Gout

—High doses increase plasma uric acid levels and could theoretically trigger gout (17).

• Ocular effects

—A retrospective survey of hyperlipidemic patients found that those taking niacin were more likely to report sicca syndromes, blurred vision, eyelid edema, and macular edema (21). Spontaneous reporting systems have also noted a possible association of high-dose niacin with decreased vision, discolored eyelids, loss of eyebrows or eyelashes, and superficial punctate keratitis. Both incidence and severity of adverse effects are dose-dependent and reversible on discontinuation of niacin.

• Flushing

—Peripheral vasodilation, flushing, itching, or tingling commonly occurs with high doses of niacin (and occasionally with doses as low as 50 mg/day). These effects usually disappear after several days of use but persist in other patients. A dose of 325 mg aspirin per hour before each niacin dose controls flushing. (Niacinamide does not cause this effect; neither does it lower cholesterol.)

• Other symptoms

—Rashes, facial erythema, hives, dry hair, headaches, or fatigue may occur. Gastrointestinal effects (including soreness or tightness in the mouth, nausea, vomiting, or diarrhea) are common. Acanthosis nigricans that resolved on discontinuation of therapy has been reported (15).

DRUG INTERACTIONS

• Beta-blockers

—Concurrent use can result in life-threatening hypotension resulting from peripheral vasodilation (13).

• Levodopa

—L-dopa, especially when given with decarboxylase inhibitors such as carbidopa, inhibits the production of nicotinamide coenzymes from tryptophan and could predispose to deficiency (22). (Interestingly, in rats, niacin and nicotinamide combined with L-dopa and a dopa decarboxylase inhibitor appeared to extend the period of elevated dopamine levels in the brain) (23).

• Isoniazid

—Isoniazid competes with the cofactor pyridoxal phosphate, required to convert tryptophan to niacin. Prolonged use of isoniazid may, thus, lead to niacin deficiency (12).

• Primidone

—Nicotinamide decreases conversion of primidone to its metabolites (phenobarbital and phenylethylmalonamide) in humans (24). Other epilepsy drugs shorten the half-life of primidone. Theoretically, nicotinamide could be a useful adjunct in primidone-treated patients with poorly controlled seizures or for patients with toxic effects from phenobarbital.

 Dose

NEs take into account both niacin and tryptophan content of foods and constitute a more accurate measure than niacin content alone.

RECOMMENDED DIETARY ALLOWANCES

Infants and children

0 to 6 months	2 mg/day (adequate intake)
7 to 12 months	4 mg/day (adequate intake)
1 to 3 years	6 mg/day
4 to 8 years	8 mg/day

Males

9 to 13 years	12 mg/day
14 to 50 years	16 mg/day
51+ years	16 mg/day

Females

9 to 13 years	12 mg/day
14 to 50 years	14 mg/day
51+ years	14 mg/day
Pregnant	18 mg/day
Lactating	

UPPER LIMITS

Infants and children

0 to 6 months	Not determinable
7 to 12 months	Not determinable
1 to 3 years	10 mg/day
4 to 8 years	15 mg/day

Males

9 to 13 years	20 mg/day
14 to 18 years	30 mg/day
19 to 50 years	35 mg/day
51+ years	35 mg/day

Females

9 to 13 years	20 mg/day
14 to 18 years	30 mg/day
19 to 50 years	35 mg/day
51+ years	35 mg/day

Pregnant

≤18 years	30 mg/day
19 to 50 years	35 mg/day

Lactating

≤18 years	30 mg/day
19 to 50 years	35 mg/day

Correcting deficiency:
Nicotinamide 50 to 500 mg/day p.o. or i.v.

 Common Questions and Answers

Q: Is coffee a good source of niacin?
A: Yes. When coffee is roasted, trigonelline in the beans becomes demethylated and is partially converted to NA (25). American roasts contain only 10 mg niacin/100 g, but dark roasts (such as Italian roasts) can contain 40 mg/100 g. About 85% of the niacin is retained in coffee. So go have an espresso (full-strength; decaffeination decreases niacin).

Q: Is chromium with low-dose niacin effective for hypercholesterolemia?
A: The combination is sometimes promoted by alternative medicine practitioners, apparently based on the incidental finding of reduced cholesterol levels in two hypercholesterolemic subjects during a trial testing the effects of 100 mg NA and 200 μg chromium chloride on glucose levels (26). After a year, total cholesterol decreased in two subjects. No controlled trials have been done. A possible explanation is that the responders were deficient in chromium, which can cause hypercholesterolemia (13).

Q: Is niacin effective for Bell's palsy?
A: There are no controlled trials, but an intriguing case series reported in 1958 claimed successful treatment of 74 patients with Bell's palsy with 100 to 250 mg NA; results were seen in 2 to 4 weeks (27).

Noni

10 Second Take

Noni fruit juice is relatively safe. It has been touted as a panacea despite no clinical evidence of efficacy for any condition. Animal studies to date have not used oral dosing.

Basics

LATIN NAME

Morinda citrifolia

FAMILY

Rubiaceae

OTHER COMMON NAMES

Indian mulberry, morinda, awl tree, limburger tree, hog apple (Cayman Islands); *fromagier, feuille douleur, bois douleur* (Haiti); *bumbo, bungbo* (Africa); *baga, nigua, piñuela, piña de puerco* (Dominican Republic); *bilimbi, pomme macaque, rubarbe caraibe* (French West Indies); *feuille froide* (Dominica); *nhau, nhau lon, nhau nui* (Vietnam); *nho* (Laos); *nhor prey, nhor thom* (Cambodia); *nino* (Philippines); *yor ban* (Thailand); *nona* (Malaysia); and *pain bush* (Trinidad and Tobago).
Bai ji tian or *pa chi tien* (*M. officinalis*) (China)

DESCRIPTION

• Noni is a small evergreen shrub or tree, up to 10 m high, native to southeast Asia. Noni's range is from eastern Polynesia to India, and it has become naturalized in parts of South and Central America and throughout the Caribbean.
• It has large, dark green, deeply veined, leaves; small white flowers; and warty, pitted, 3 to 4 in. long fruits that start out green, turning yellow and then white with ripening.
• The tree fruits year-round; the ripe fruit has a foul "rancid cheese" odor.

PART USED

• Fruit
• Leaf

KNOWN ACTIVE CONSTITUENTS

• Fruits contain 24 to 158 mg ascorbic acid per 100 g dry weight (1).
• According to the United States Department of Agriculture (USDA) Phytochemical Database, *M. citrifolia* root contains morindin, rubichloric acid, rubiadin-1-methyl ether, soranjidiol, asperuloside, nordamnacanthal, and trihydroxy anthraquinones. The ripe fruit contains large amount of fatty acids, primarily hexanoic (caproic) and octanoic (caprylic) acids (2). The fruit also contains asperuloside (3). A commercial juice product was found to be a significant source of potassium (4).

MECHANISM/PHARMACOKINETICS

No information identified (see Questions and Answers)

Evidence

CLINICAL TRIALS

No clinical trials identified.

ANIMAL/IN VITRO

• Anticancer effects

—Noni juice injected intraperitoneally 24 hours after intraperitoneal implantation of Lewis lung carcinoma (noni injections were either daily or q.o.d. for 4 to 5 days) increased the lifespan of C57BL/6 mice, but the effect was not dose-dependent (15 mg per mouse and 6 mg per mouse both increased lifespan 119%, whereas 12 mg per mouse increased lifespan 40%) (5). A precipitate from ethanol fractionation was also active.
—Another experiment by the same investigator found that noni juice 6 to 15 mg per mouse (in four to five injections administered intraperitoneally q.d. or q.o.d.) demonstrated antitumor activity and prolonged lifespan by more than 75% in the Lewis lung carcinoma mouse model (6). An ethanol-insoluble precipitate had a similar effect. A cytotoxicity test of the precipitate found no toxicity to cells in doses below 2 mg/mL; very high doses (more than 6.25 mg/mL) were cytotoxic. The antitumor effect appears to involve the immune system, because an additional experiment in mice found that a macrophage inhibitor (Cl-ade) abolished the effect, and a T-lymphocyte inhibitor (cys-A) attenuated the effect (6).
—An *in vitro* study found that damnacanthal, an anthraquinone compound isolated from a chloroform extract of *Morinda* root, induced normal phenotypes in *ras*-transformed cells, indicating that it is an inhibitor of *ras* function. (7). Damnacanthal appears to inhibit tyrosine kinase and stimulate ultraviolet light-induced apoptosis (8).

• Analgesic effect

—Intraperitoneal administration of a lyophilized aqueous extract of *M. citrifolia* root (800 to 1600 mg/kg) was evaluated in a study that examined analgesic and behavioral effects in mice (9). A dose-related, central analgesic activity was demonstrated in standard writhing and hot plate tests; the effect was reversed by naloxone. A general sedative effect was indicated by decreased behavioral parameters at doses of 500 to 1600 mg/kg.

OTHER CLAIMED BENEFITS/ACTIONS

Cancer, infections, diabetes, hypertension, headaches, arthritis antiaging, asthma, menstrual problems, kidney problems, immune system strengthening, cardiovascular health, injuries, and so forth.

Risks

ADVERSE REACTIONS

• Hyperkalemia

—A patient with chronic renal insufficiency who claimed adherence to a low potassium diet developed hyperkalemia (serum potassium 5.4 to 5.8 mg/dL), elevated blood urea nitrogen, and elevated creatinine after a regimen of noni juice (a shotglass before each meal) (4). The patient refused to stop drinking noni and was lost to follow-up; analysis of a commercial noni juice product revealed 56.3 ±2.5 mEq/L potassium and 122 ±6.3 mEq/L sodium. This level of potassium is similar to orange juice, which contains 51 mEq/L.

DRUG INTERACTIONS

None reported

ANIMAL TOXICITY

No information available

Dose

• Commercial products usually contain noni juice or a juice concentrate; a typical dose is 1 to 4 oz of noni juice before meals.
• Tablets and capsules: liquid concentrates 2 tablespoons daily.
• Powdered extracts: 500 to 1,000 mg daily.
• It is suggested that noni be taken on an empty stomach.

Common Questions and Answers

Q: Why are noni fruit products so popular?
A: Noni fruit juice or extract, often sold in multilevel marketing schemes, has been marketed as a treatment for a plethora of diseases. Noni promoters claim that an alkaloid called "xeronine" is the primary active component (10). However, xeronine appears to exist only in promotional materials for noni; there is no mention of the substance in the chemical literature, and the person credited with discovering xeronine, Dr. Heinicke (11), has no scientific publications on the topic. A widely distributed booklet called "Noni: Polynesia's Natural Pharmacy" looks referenced to the casual reader (12). Through repetition, however, 12 references are made to look like 34. The two primary references are unpublished theses; other references include a newspaper article and a commercial audiotape.

Q: Why would anyone eat a foul-tasting fruit?
A: On its native soil, noni fruit is not generally considered edible, although the unripe fruit (less noxious than the ripe fruit) was used as a famine food in Hawaii and the Marquesas (where noni was much more commonly used to feed hogs than people) (1). The carboxylic acids that give ripe noni fruit its foul smell are not present in sufficient quantities in the marketed products to offend most palates. Also, products often incorporate other fruit juices or flavorings to increase palatability.

Q: Is noni fruit a traditional medicine?
A: Not to the extent one would think from reading promotional materials. The primary indigenous medicinal use is of the leaves, not the fruit, primarily as a topical treatment for conditions including skin inflammations, joint pain, coughs, gout, ulcers, and ringworm (13). The root of another Morinda species (*M. officinalis*) is used in Chinese medicine. Noni fruit is at best a minor medicinal remedy, having been used medicinally for gum disorders in Malaysia, for tuberculosis in the Pacific Islands, and for various ailments in Samoa. The seeds are eaten as an anti-helminthic or purgative in the Philippines, and the juice has been drunk to prevent the adverse effects of kava in the Pacific. But the most popular traditional use of noni was as a dye plant—red, yellow, and purple hues can be obtained depending on the mordants used (13).

Osha

10 Second Take

Osha and *chuan xiong* are benign herbs. Osha is commonly used for colds, allergies, and other conditions. *Chuan xiong*, a Chinese herb, is commonly used for angina.

Basics

LATIN NAME

Osha: *Ligusticum porteri* JM Coulter and JN Rose
Ligusticum: *Ligusticum wallichii* Franch or *Ligusticum chuanxiong* Hort

FAMILY

Apiaceae/Umbelliferae

OTHER COMMON NAMES

Ligusticum porteri: Porter's lovage, Indian parsley, Colorado cough root, and bear medicine
Ligusticum chuanxiong: Hort: Szechuan lovage, chuan xiong

DESCRIPTION

• Osha is found in Idaho, Nevada, Montana, Wyoming, Colorado, New Mexico, and Arizona. It favors high altitudes and is most common above 9,000 feet. The root is hairy and smells of celery.
• Other species of ligusticum that grow on the Pacific Coast, *L. apifolium* and *L. californicum,* are commonly substituted for *Ligusticum porteri.*

PART USED

• *Ligusticum porteri:* roots
• *Ligusticum chuanxiong:* rhizomes

KNOWN ACTIVE CONSTITUENTS

Active alkaloids include tetramethylpyrazine, leucylphenylalanine anhydride, and perlolyrine (1).

MECHANISM/PHARMACOKINETICS

• *Ligusticum porteri:* no information identified
• *Ligusticum chuanxiong:* Tetramethylpyrazine reaches peak levels within 1 to 3 hours after oral administration and its half-life is 29 minutes. Metabolites are excreted in urine and in bile (1).
• Tetramethylpyrazine inhibits superoxide dismutase activity. An extract of this herb inhibits adenosine diphosphate-induced platelet aggregation and thromboxane A_2 synthesis. Tetramethylpyrazine also inhibits endothelin production.

Evidence

CLINICAL TRIALS

• *Ligusticum porteri:* no information identified
• *Ligusticum chuanxiong:* Chinese trials show a beneficial effect of intravenous administration in cerebral ischemia (40 to 80 mg herb, diluted) and angina (100 to 200 mg herb, diluted) (1).

ANIMAL/IN VITRO

• *Ligusticum porteri:* no information identified
• *Ligusticum chuanxiong*

—In rats, tetramethylpyrazine (30 to 50 mg/kg per 12 hours via gastric lavage for 40 days), compared with vehicle, mildly reduced portal venous pressure, mean arterial pressure, and total peripheral resistance in rats that had undergone a partial portal vein ligation and rats that had undergone a bile duct ligation. No effect of tetramethylpyrazine was seen in sham-operated rats (2). Another study found that tetramethylpyrazine reduced portal venous pressure and mean arterial pressure in a dose-dependent manner in cirrhotic rats (3).
—In ischemic rat heart, pretreatment with tetramethylpyrazine (12 mg/kg/day) significantly reduced ischemia-induced and reperfusion-induced ventricular tachycardia and ventricular fibrillation (4).
—Ferulinolol (0.1, 0.5, 1.0 mg/kg intravenously) from *Ligusticum chuanxiong* was shown to have β-1 adrenergic blocking activity and partial β-2 agonist activity in rats (5). No inhibitory effect was noted on α-adrenoceptors. Calcium channel blocking activity has also been demonstrated (6).
—*Ligusticum chuanxiong* increases myocardial contraction, slows the heart rate, improves coronary circulation, dilates coronary vessels and peripheral vessels, and lowers blood pressure. In dogs, tetramethylpyrazine (40 mg/kg) significantly reduces pulmonary artery pressure and pulmonary vascular resistance. Tetramethylpyrazine prevents chronic hypoxic pulmonary hypertension in rats. Tetramethylpyrazine also increases retinal blood flow in guinea pig tissue (1).

OTHER CLAIMED BENEFITS/ACTIONS

- *Ligusticum porteri*

—Allergy
—Colds, flu, upper respiratory infections
—Expectorant
—Antiinflammatory
—Gastrointestinal problems
—Immune system stimulants
—Diuretic

- *Ligusticum chuanxiong*

—Cerebral ischemia
—Stroke
—Headache
—Amenorrhea
—Postpartum pain

 Risks

ADVERSE REACTIONS

Ligusticum chuanxiong may precipitate early menses (1).

DRUG INTERACTIONS

None reported

PREGNANCY/LACTATION

No information available, but the use of either of these herbs is not advised in pregnancy.

ANIMAL TOXICITY

LD_{50} in mice of *Ligusticum chuanxiong* is 65.9 ± 31.3 g/kg intraperitoneally and 66.4 ± 3.2 g/kg intramuscularly. LD_{50} of tetramethylpyrazine in mice is 239 mg/kg intravenously (1).

 Dose

- *Ligusticum porteri*

—Chewed root
—Tea $\frac{1}{2}$ c up to q.i.d.
—Decoction: 2 to 4 oz up to q.i.d.
—Dry root tincture (1:5, 65% alcohol) 30 to 90 drops in hot water (7)

- *Ligusticum chuanxiong* is used as part of Chinese herbal mixtures. Common daily doses: 4 to 11 g as decoctions

Pantothenic Acid

 10 Second Take

Pantothenic acid is a benign vitamin; preliminary evidence indicates promise in treating hyperlipidemia.

 Basics

OTHER COMMON NAMES

Pantethonate, panthenol, pantetheine, pantethine, and vitamin B_5

DESCRIPTION

• Pantothenic acid, a B vitamin, is an important coenzyme involved in energy metabolism and lipid synthesis.
• Panthenol is the alcohol form.
• Pantetheine is a pantothenic acid derivative, of which pantethine is the disulfide form.
• Most vitamin supplements contain calcium or sodium salts of D-pantethonate or panthenol (which is more stable than pantethonate) (1).

FOOD SOURCES

Pantothenic acid is widely distributed in foods. Particularly good sources include yeast, liver, kidney, egg yolk, wheat germ, nuts, beans, avocados, bananas, and broccoli. Cooking destroys 15% to 50% of the vitamin in meat, and the processing of vegetables results in losses of 37% to 78% (1).

MAIN FUNCTIONS/PHARMACOKINETICS

• Pantothenic acid is essential to respiratory metabolism. It is an integral component of coenzyme A and phosphopantetheine and is important as a carrier for acyl groups in various processes, including the first step of the Krebs cycle and the β-oxidation of fatty acids.
• It is also involved in the synthesis of ketones, acetylcholine, and porphyrin (1).

 Evidence

CLINICAL TRIALS

• Ulcerative colitis

—Dexpanthenol enemas administered to three patients in an open-label pilot study (1,000 mg nightly for 4 weeks) had no clinical or histologic benefits (2). Urinary pantothenic acid increased, but there were no significant changes in concentrations of colonic tissue coenzyme A or fecal short-chain fatty acids.

• Radiation-induced skin reactions

—A single-blind controlled study in 86 patients receiving radiation therapy tested topical dexpanthenol cream (Bepanthen, Roche) applied twice daily on randomly selected parts of treatment fields (3). Patients were assessed weekly during radiation treatment, 2 weeks after treatment ended, and 6 to 8 weeks later. This study is notable for the fact that the physicians, but not the patients, were blinded. There was no difference between treated and untreated areas in physician-assessed skin reactions nor was there any difference in itching or pain.

• Hyperlipidemia

—Pantethine may benefit hypercholesterolemia but appropriate controlled trials of reasonable size are lacking. A double-blind crossover study found that administration of 300 mg t.i.d. of pantethine for 8 weeks significantly reduced total and low density lipoprotein (LDL) cholesterol and increased high density lipoprotein (HDL) in 11 subjects with type IIB hypercholesterolemia; there was no effect on total cholesterol, LDL, or HDL in 15 subjects with type IV hypercholesterolemia (4). Both groups experienced a significant decrease in triglycerides.
—A small, controlled crossover study in 10 hyperlipidemic patients tested pantethine 300 mg q.i.d versus placebo (each given for 4 weeks with a 4-week washout period) (5). Total cholesterol, total phospholipids, and the sphingomyelin to phosphatidylcholine ratio decreased significantly during the treatment phase compared with the placebo phase.
—An uncontrolled study of 22 diabetic dialysis patients (8 on hemodialysis, 14 on peritoneal dialysis) found that 300 mg pantethine t.i.d. for 2 months resulted in significant reductions in total and LDL cholesterol as well as triglycerides; HDL was unchanged (6). In this study, total cholesterol was reduced from an average of 275 mg/dL to an average of 231 mg/dL; very low density lipoprotein (VLDL) cholesterol from 66 to 46 mg/dL, and triglycerides from 332 to 227 mg/dL. Additional treatment led to additional benefit with significant improvements at 4 and 6 months; the seven subjects who completed 6 months of treatment had normal cholesterol levels (a mean of 173 mg/dL), triglyceride levels (168 mg/dL), and VLDL levels (30 mg/dL).

—An uncontrolled trial in 31 hemodialysis patients found that 600 to 1,200 mg pantethine daily significantly reduced total cholesterol and triglycerides. There was no effect on levels of HDL or apolipoprotein A (7).
—Another uncontrolled 1-year trial in 24 hyperlipidemic patients, including six diabetics, found significant reductions in total cholesterol, LDL cholesterol, and apolipoprotein B as well as increases in HDL cholesterol and apolipoprotein A (8).

• Wound healing

—In one study, 49 subjects undergoing tattoos were randomized to placebo or a vitamin supplement containing 100 mg vitamin C and 200 mg pantothenic acid for 3 weeks. The supplemented patients showed changes in trace elements but no significant changes in number of fibroblasts or mechanical properties of scar tissue (9). The dose of pantothenic acid was low in this trial.

ANIMAL/IN VITRO EVIDENCE

• Wound healing

—In cell culture, pantothenic acid increases fibroblast growth and proliferation and enhances collagen synthesis and release (9). In rabbits, pantothenic acid appears to aid wound healing (10).

• Endocrinologic effects

—In estrogen-primed hyperprolactinemic rats, orally administered pantethine (up to 1.0 g/kg) had no effect on plasma prolactin levels, but intraperitoneal and intravenous administration markedly decreased serum prolactin levels (11).

OTHER CLAIMED BENEFITS/ACTIONS

• Wound healing
• Immune stimulation

Clinical Considerations

Gross deficiency is extremely rare.

DEFICIENCY SIGNS AND SYMPTOMS

- Vomiting, abdominal distress
- Postural hypotension
- Paresthesias of hands and feet
- Heel tenderness
- Leg cramps and weakness
- Anorexia
- Constipation
- Insomnia
- Fatigue, malaise
- Headache

FACTORS DECREASING AVAILABILITY/ABSORPTION

None known

LABORATORY TESTS

Whole blood pantothenic acid (normal values 100 to 300 μg/dL)

 ## Risks

ADVERSE REACTIONS

Pantothenic acid has very low toxicity. Ingestion of 10 to 100 g resulted only in occasional diarrhea (12).

DRUG INTERACTIONS

None identified

 ## Dose

ADEQUATE INTAKE

Infants and children

0 to 6 months	1.7 mg/day
7 to 12 months	1.8 mg/day
1 to 3 years	2 mg/day
4 to 8 years	3 mg/day

Males

9 to 13 years	4 mg/day
14 to 50 years	5 mg/day
51+ years	5 mg/day

Females

9 to 13 years	4 mg/day
14 to 50 years	5 mg/day
51+ years	5 mg/day
Pregnant	6 mg/day
Lactating	7 mg/day

Correcting deficiency
5 to 20 mg/day
Total parenteral nutrition
15 μg/day

 ## Common Questions and Answers

Q: Is it true that royal jelly is high in pantothenic acid?
A: Yes. The substance fed by bees to larvae that makes them turn into queens contains 511 μg/g pantothenic acid (1).

Passionflower

 10 Second Take

Passiflora incarnata is used as a sedative-hypnotic. Most adverse reactions are due to other *Passiflora* species. However, one case of cardiac arrhythmia has been attributed to *P. incarnata;* this cannot be considered a benign herb.

 Basics

LATIN NAME

Passiflora incarnata L.

FAMILY

Passifloraceae

OTHER COMMON NAMES

Passion vine, apricot vine, granadilla, and maypop

DESCRIPTION

• *Passiflora incarnata,* the species used medicinally, is a perennial climbing vine with intricate yellowish, sweet-scented flowers, three-lobed, finely-serrated leaves, and edible orange fruit.
• *Passiflora caerulea* is an ornamental with blue flowers. Only two species of *Passiflora* are found in North America; the other 430 species occur in the tropical Americas (1).
• The most widely eaten passionfruit is from *Passiflora edulis,* the purple passionfruit (also called purple grenadilla).

PART USED

Aerial parts (stem, leaves, and flowers), usually dried

KNOWN ACTIVE CONSTITUENTS

• Flavonoids (1%), mainly C-glycosides of apigenin and luteolins (vitexin and its 4-O-rhamnoside, isovitexin, isoorientin and their 2-β-D-glucosides, schaftoside, isoschaftoside, swertisin, orientin, and lucenin); maltol (0.05%); essential oil; and gynocardia, a cyanogenic glycoside (0.01%) (2). Maltol may be an artifact produced by heat treatment (3). *P. caerulea* contains cyanogenic glycosides, whereas *P. incarnata* does not (1).
• Harman, a β-carboline alkaloid, has been found in trace amounts in some samples; however, these alkaloids are not found in most commercial material (2). It is unclear which components of passionflower account for its sedative effects.

MECHANISM/PHARMACOKINETICS

• No information on pharmacokinetics is available.
• Chrysin (5,7-dihydroxy flavone), a flavonoid from *P. caerulea,* is a ligand for benzodiazepine receptors, both central (Ki = 3 mM, competitive mechanism) and peripheral (Ki = 13 mM, mixed-type mechanism). Prior administration of a benzodiazepine antagonist abolished the seizure-reducing effect of intracerebroventricular chrysin in mice (4). Chrysin is a partial agonist for benzodiazepine receptors and has a γ-aminobutyric acid (GABA) ratio of 1.4 (compared with diazepam 2.0). The effects of chrysin on sedation, muscle relaxation, or locomotion are much less potent than diazepam (5).

 Evidence

CLINICAL TRIALS

• Sedative/hypnotic effects

—A double-blind randomized treatment-controlled trial study tested *Passiflora* extract 45 drops/day against oxazepam 30 mg/day for 4 weeks in 36 subjects with generalized anxiety disorder (placebo drops were given to the oxazepam group and placebo tablets to the *Passiflora* group to preserve blinding) (6). Both treatments were effective, with no significant difference between groups. Oxazepam was faster acting than *Passiflora;* oxazepam was also associated with significantly more problems relating to impairment of job performance.
—A placebo-controlled crossover study in nine healthy subjects (5 female) tested the hypnotic effects of four capsules of a single dose of an extract of a South American *Passiflora* species (*P. edulis*) (7). No significant hypnotic effect was seen.
—In a double-blind trial in 182 patients with adjustment disorder and anxious mood, a multiherb extract (containing *Passiflora, Crataegus, Ballota, Valeriana, Cola,* and *Paullinia*) was tested against placebo. Hamilton anxiety scale (HAM-A) scores improved in those who took the herbs compared with those who took placebo (8).

• Opiate withdrawal

—A double-blind randomized placebo-controlled trial tested *Passiflora* extract (60 drops/day) as an adjunct to clonidine (0.8 mg/day) in detoxification of 65 opiate-dependent subjects (9). Treatment lasted 14 days; opiate withdrawal symptoms were assessed with the Short Opiate Withdrawal Scale (SOWS). *Passiflora* did not provide additional benefit over placebo as an adjunctive treatment to clonidine for treating physical withdrawal symptoms. However, *Passiflora* plus clonidine was significantly superior to placebo plus clonidine for managing mental symptoms.

ANIMAL/IN VITRO

• Sedation/anxiolytic effect

—A review of seven studies examined the sedative effect of *Passiflora* in rodents (2). Five studies were positive and two were negative. Intraperitoneal administration of an alcohol-free hydroethanolic extract (160 mg/kg) significantly prolonged pentobarbital-induced sleeping time (10). In the same report, a dose of 50 to 400 mg/kg reduced locomotor activity.
—In mice, intraperitoneal administration of extract in a dose of 100 mg/kg, administered before sodium pentobarbital, prolonged sleeping time 40% when compared with the control group. In the same report, *Passiflora* was administered via gastric tube 1 hour before subcutaneous amphetamine. A dose of 50 mg/kg caused a 17% reduction in amphetamine-induced hypermotility (11).
—The other three positive studies included an oral study in mice that found that 25 to 50 mL/kg/day of alcohol-free hydroethanolic extract (equivalent to 1.25 and 2.5 g/kg of dried drug) reduced motor activity, prolonged pentobarbital-induced sleeping time, and inhibited amphetamine-induced aggressiveness and restlessness. Rats given a daily oral dose of 10 mL/kg of extract (equivalent to 5 g/kg) demonstrated reduced activity on a one-arm radial maze. Oral administration of dry extract of *Passiflora* (800 mg/kg containing 2.6% of flavonoids) found a significant prolongation of hexobarbital-induced sleeping time without affecting locomotor activity (2).
—The two negative studies, both in mice, failed to confirm prolongation of sleeping time (hexobarbital-induced) or reduction in exploratory activity. Both studies used an alcohol-free 30% hydroethanolic *Passiflora* extract in a dose of 1.75 and 3.5 mL/kg (2).
—In a study published more recently, 400 mg/kg of hydroalcoholic extract and aqueous extract were shown to have anxiolytic effects in mice; an aqueous extract induced sleep after administration of subhypnotic dose of pentobarbital (12). In another study, three of four *P. edulis* extracts decreased spontaneous motor activity in mice; there were variable effects on pentobarbitone-induced sleeping time. No antiseizure effects were noted (7).
—Compounds from *Passiflora* have been tested as well. Chrysin has anxiolytic activity in mice (in the elevated plus-maze test) without inducing sedation, muscle relaxation, or decreased motor activity (13). Maltol, isolated from *Passiflora,* administered subcutaneously in a dose of 75 mg/kg, inhibited spontaneous motor activity in mice by 50%; at a dose of 135 mg/kg, motor activity was inhibited by 66%. Hexobarbital sleeping time was prolonged in a dose-dependent manner after oral doses of 300 or 500 mg/kg (2). These doses of maltol are far above what would be found in *Passiflora* preparations.

- Analgesic effect

—An alcohol-free hydroethanolic extract in an oral or intraperitoneal dosage of 160 mg/kg increased the threshold to painful stimuli in the tail flick and hot plate tests but not in an electrical stimulation test. The extract also increased onset time of pentylenetetrazole-induced convulsions and prolonged survival in mice (10).

OTHER CLAIMED BENEFITS/ACTIONS

- Antispasmodic (dysmenorrhea, tetanus, pertussis)
- Epilepsy
- Exhaustion
- Insomnia
- Agitation
- Irritability
- Insomnia
- Anxiolytic

 Risks

ADVERSE REACTIONS

- Cardiac arrhythmia

—A 34-year-old woman was hospitalized with vomiting and drowsiness after 2 days treatment with a total of seven tablets of Sedacalm, an extract of *P. incarnata*. Laboratory tests were normal. Electrocardiogram (EKG) showed bradycardia with ventricular bigeminy and episodes of nonsustained ventricular fibrillation. A sample of Sedacalm was compared with another batch as well as samples of *P. incarnata*, digoxin, and digitoxin. The tablets the patient had ingested had similar chromatographic profiles to the second batch of tablets and the sample of herb. No cardiac glycosides were detected (14).

- Change in mental status

—A Norwegian report documented five cases of patients who were hospitalized for reduced consciousness after ingestion of Relaxir, a product sold for insomnia that contains mainly *Passiflora* (15).

- Occupational asthma

—IgE-mediated occupational asthma and rhinitis was associated with *Passiflora alata* in a patient who worked in a compounding pharmacy (16).

- Increased amylase and serum glutamine oxaloacetate transaminase (SGOT)

—A placebo-controlled crossover study in nine healthy subjects (five female) tested the toxicity of four capsules of lyophilized *Passiflora* 10% tea (aqueous solutions of dried powdered leaves of *P. edulis* from northeast Brazil) or four capsules of placebo (brown sugar) administered at 9 p.m. Eleven hours later electroencephalogram (EEG), EKG, and blood tests were performed (7). There was a 1-week interval between tests. After ingestion of *Passiflora*, two volunteers had increased direct bilirubin (0.28 mg% and 0.28 mg%, normal less than 0.25%); one had increased uric acid (8.8%, normal 2.5 to 7 mg%), one, who underwent intense physical exercise the same evening as ingesting the herb, had increased creatine phosphokinase (CPK) (111; normal 10 to 80). Four volunteers had increased amylase 176, 194, 205 and 190 U/L, normal 60 to 160 U/L. No changes were seen after placebo administration. A comparison of mean values found that amylase and SGOT changes were significant.

- Hypersensitivity vasculitis

—An unconvincing case of hypersensitivity reaction with urticaria and a blistering rash that looked like cutaneous vasculitis (no biopsy was done) was reported in a 77-year-old man with rheumatoid arthritis (17). He was taking diclofenac and cyclopenthiazide concurrently. The diagnosis of vasculitis was not proven; also, this may have been an interaction effect.

DRUG INTERACTIONS

None reported (see hypersensitivity vasculitis under adverse reactions)

ANIMAL TOXICITY

- In mice given doses up to 900 mg/kg intraperitoneally, no acute toxicity was observed (2). In rats, 21 days of treatment with 10 mg/kg p.o. (equivalent to 5 g/kg) of a hydroethanolic extract of *Passiflora* had no effect on body weight, EEG, rectal temperature, tail flick, or motor coordination; however, there was a reduction in general motor activity (Sopranzi).
- Rats given access to 1% *P. edulis* herb tea (made from lyophilized extract) instead of water showed no changes in fluid consumption, body weight, electrolytes, liver function tests (LFTs), proteins, lipids, urea, or creatinine after 4 days (7). Two samples were tested for chronic toxicity (90 days) (7). Administration of one sample resulted in increased gamma-glutamyltransferase (GGT) and decreased body weight in rats. The other sample did not cause these effects (however, one rat died on day 40).

 Dose

COMMON DOSAGE FORMS

Adult: 0.5 to 2.0 g of drug t.i.d.
Infusion made from 2.5 g drug t.i.d.
Tincture (1:8) 1 to 4 mL t.i.d.
Children 3 to 12 (under medical supervision): proportion of adult dose by weight

Pau d'arco

 10 Second Take

Lapachol has interesting antimicrobial effects and anticancer effects that should be further investigated; however, high doses in humans can cause nausea, vomiting, and an anticoagulant effect.

 Basics

LATIN NAME

Tabebuia impetiginosa (Mart.) ex DC (Standl.), *T. heptaphylla* (Vell.) Toledo

FAMILY

Bignoniaceae

OTHER COMMON NAMES

Lapacho, taheebo, ipes, ipe roxo, and trumpet bush

DESCRIPTION

Tabebuia is a genus of about 100 hardwood trees (mostly evergreen) native to Central and South America and the West Indies.

PART USED

Inner bark

KNOWN ACTIVE CONSTITUENTS

The heartwood contains 2% to 7% lapachol, a naphthoquinone derivative, and other naphthoquinone derivatives (1). A petroleum extract of *T. impetiginosa* heartwood was found to contain 3.6% lapachol and lesser amounts of β-lapachone, α-lapachone, and dehydro-α-lapachone. Lapachol is not a major constituent of *Tabebuia* barks, and a Canadian survey of 12 commercial taheebo products found that only two contained lapachol (in very low amounts, 0.003% to 0.004%) (1). Two cyclopentene dialdehydes with antiinflammatory activity were recently identified in pau d'arco (2).

MECHANISM/PHARMACOKINETICS

Lapachol appears to be a vitamin K antagonist, and thus may affect the vitamin K-dependent ligand activation of the Ax1 receptor tyrosine kinase (3). β-lapachone activates the DNA-unwinding activity of topoisomerase I (4).

 Evidence

CLINICAL TRIALS

• Cancer

—A phase I toxicology study of lapachol in 19 patients with advanced nonleukemic tumors and two patients with chronic myelocytic leukemia in relapse was sponsored by the National Cancer Institute. Subjects received oral doses of lapachol (250 to 3,750 mg/day) (5). Although this study was a toxicity study, not an efficacy study, one patient with metastatic breast cancer had a regression in one of several bone lesions (other patients did not have objective responses to the drug). Lapachol in doses of 1,500 mg/day or higher caused nausea, vomiting, and prolonged prothrombin time. No hepatic or renal toxicity or myelo-suppression was seen. The Investigational New Drug application (IND) for lapachol was closed in 1970. A later experiment noted that the anticoagulant effects of lapachol could be reversed by the administration of vitamin K. (It is not clear, however, whether or not this would reverse any beneficial effect.)
—An uncontrolled study of nine patients (all previously treated conventionally) found that lapachol (20 to 30 mg/kg/day p.o. × 20 to 60 days or longer) resulted in subjective improvements, including pain reduction, in all patients. Two partial tumor regressions (apparently in a patient with basal cell carcinoma of the cheek metastasized to the cervix and a patient with ulcerated squamous cell carcinoma) and one complete tumor regression (apparently in a patient with hepatic adenocarcinoma) were noted. It is not stated how regressions were measured or how long they lasted.

ANIMAL/IN VITRO

• Cancer

—In animal models, lapachol has cytotoxic effects. It has been found to have antitumor activity in Walker 256 and sarcoma Yoshida ascites cells but did not have significant activity in sarcoma 180, L 1210 leukemia, and adenocarcinoma (5). A crude extract of pau d'arco stimulated macrophages, killed Lewis lung carcinoma cells in culture, and reduced lung metastases in mice after surgery (5). Lapachol had growth inhibitory effects on four melanoma cell lines and a renal cell carcinoma line (6).
—β-lapachone enhances the lethality of x-rays against human laryngeal epidermoid carcinoma cells and enhances the cytotoxic effects of x-rays and other agents that induce DNA strand incisions; it does not appear to create lethal DNA lesions (4).

• Snakebite

—*T. rosea* (a different species than pau d'arco) and several other traditional remedies for snakebite administered orally or intramuscularly significantly reduced the lethal effect of *Bothrops atrox* venom (7).

• Psoriasis

—β-lapachone reduced the growth of human keratinocytes (IC_{50} value of 0.7 mM) to an extent similar to the antipsoriatic drug anthralin, indicating that it may have potential as an antipsoriatic agent.

• Antimicrobial

—Although pau d'arco is reputed to have antimalarial effects, in an *in vitro* experiment, lapachol exhibited only low inhibition of schizogony (reproduction of the malarial parasite) (8). Lapachol and other naphthoquinones reduced skin penetration by *Schisoma mansoni* cercariae (9).

• Ulcers

—Lapachol derived from teak (*Tectona grandis*) (5 mg/kg p.o. b.i.d.) inhibited gastric and duodenal ulcers in rats and guinea pigs (10).

• Analgesia

—Lapachol and an extract from *T. chrysotricha* had analgesic effects in mice (11).

OTHER CLAIMED BENEFITS/ACTIONS

• Cancer
• Rheumatism
• Antibiotic
• Cystitis
• Gastritis
• Prostatitis
• Ulcers
• Liver problems
• Asthma

Risks

ADVERSE REACTIONS

Lapachol in doses of 1,500 mg/day or higher caused nausea, vomiting, and prolonged prothrombin time (5).

DRUG INTERACTIONS

None reported

PREGNANCY/LACTATION

No information available.

ANIMAL TOXICITY

• Injected i.p. into rats, the LD_{50} of lapachol was 1,600 mg/kg, β-lapachone 80 mg/kg, and xyloidine 600 mg/kg. Ten doses of lapachol 500 mg/kg caused death, as did six doses of β-lapachone at 9 mg/kg (12).
• Pregnant Wistar rats were treated with control (water), vehicle (0.5 mL hydro-alcoholic solution), or lapachol (20 mg in 0.5 mL hydroalcoholic solution) by oral gavage from the eighth to the twelfth day of pregnancy. There was no effect on maternal body weight or food intake but there was 100% fetal/embryo mortality (13).

 Dose

• Bark: One cup of a decoction made from 1 tsp bark per 1 cup water two to eight times per day. If lapachol content is 2% to 4%, 15 to 20 g in 500 mL or 1 pint of water as decoction t.i.d. to q.i.d.
• Other forms (aqueous extract, fluid extract, solid extract): based on lapachol content, with daily lapachol intake of 1.5 to 2.0 g.
• Dried inner bark 1.5 to 3.5 g/day.
• Extract (1:2, 45% ethanol) 3 to 7 mL/day.

 Common Questions and Answers

Q: What are lapacho colorado and lapacho morada?
A: Teas sold as lapacho colorado are made from *Tabebuia impetiginosa* (also called *T. avellanedae* in Brazil). Teas sold as lapacho morada are said to be from a high-altitude species called *Tabebuia altissima,* an imaginary species (*Tabebuia* does not grow at high altitude). Some teas sold as lapacho morada or lapacho colorado do not contain *Tabebuia* at all, but contain *Tecoma curialis,* which is closely related (14).

Pennyroyal

10 Second Take

Pennyroyal oil has caused deaths in adults and children; even tea has caused serious poisonings in children.

Basics

LATIN NAME

(*Hedeoma pulegioides* L. Pers.); European pennyroyal (*Mentha pulegium* L.)

FAMILY

Labiatae

OTHER COMMON NAMES

Tick-weed, stinking balm

DESCRIPTION

Part used: leaf

KNOWN ACTIVE CONSTITUENTS

Pulegone and other ketones (L-menthone, D-isomenthone, piperitone) and terpene hydrocarbons. Pulegone levels are highest in the spring (55 mg/g foliage and 3.8 mg/g stem) (1).

MECHANISM/PHARMACOKINETICS

• Pulegone is oxidized by the cytochrome P450 system to the hepatotoxic metabolite menthofuran and possibly other hepatotoxic metabolites. Menthofuran damages hepatic and pulmonary cells; pulegone augments the damage by depleting glutathione (which conjugates many toxins) and thus allowing the buildup of menthofuran (2). Reactive metabolites formed by pulegone apparently form covalent adducts with glutathione (3).
• Menthofuran is metabolized to (R)-2-hydroxymenthofuran. Glutathione-*S*-transferase catalyzes the tautomerization of 2-hydroxymenthofuran to mintlactone and isomintlactone (4).
• In rats, 150 mg/kg intraperitoneally resulted in peak pulegone levels of 13.5 ± 3.0 μg/mL at 15 minutes with a terminal half-life of 1 hour. Menthofuran levels also peaked at 1 hour at 7.0 ± 1.2 μg/mL and had a terminal half-life of about 2 hours (3). In rats, 300 mg/kg i.p. caused hepatocellular damage with necrosis; menthofuran serum level of 250 ng/mL is hepatotoxic in rats (2).

• Little is available on pharmacokinetics in humans. Serum samples collected 26 hours after a death from pennyroyal poisoning revealed pulegone levels of 18 ng/mL and menthofuran levels of 1 ng /mL, but it is unknown whether cellular shifts may have occurred postmortem. In the case of a 20-month-old toddler who had ingested an unknown amount of pennyroyal oil, 10-hour menthofuran serum levels were 40 ng/mL; no pulegone was detected (3). An 8-week-old Hispanic boy given a mint tea containing pulegone had a menthofuran level of 10 ng/mL 3 days after admission; after 24 hours of *N*-acetylcysteine (NAC) the level decreased to 2 ng/mL (2). A 6-month-old Hispanic boy given a pulegone-containing mint tea (2) had pulegone levels of 25 ng/mL and menthofuran levels of 41 ng/mL.

Evidence

CLINICAL TRIALS

No clinical trials identified.

ANIMAL/IN VITRO

No information identified.

OTHER CLAIMED BENEFITS/ACTIONS

• Abortifacient
• Fibroids
• Cramps
• Colds
• Liver and gallbladder ailments
• Gout
• Fainting
• Flatulence
• Insect repellant (topical)

RISKS

ADVERSE REACTIONS

• Pennyroyal oil poisoning

—All severe poisonings in adults have involved pennyroyal oil; however, in infants, fatalities have been reported even with pennyroyal tea. A review identified four fatal cases of pennyroyal oil poisoning in adults reported since 1897 (3). In the most recent case, reported in 1996, a 24-year-old woman with an ectopic pregnancy tried to induce abortion with a pennyroyal alcohol extract and black cohosh extract for 2 weeks, increasing her intake of both herbs shortly before developing abdominal cramps, chills, vomiting and syncope, sustaining a cardiopulmonary arrest 7.5 hours after ingestion. She was resuscitated but developed hemodynamic shock and disseminated intravascular coagulation; an exploratory laparotomy revealed a hemorrhagic ectopic pregnancy with evidence of superinfection; she died after life support was withdrawn 46 hours after ingestion. Autopsy revealed centrilobular hepatic necrosis and degenerative changes in the proximal tubules of the kidney. Bleeding from the ectopic pregnancy and possible sepsis may well have contributed to this death. A letter in response to this report noted that septic shock could also cause hepatic necrosis (5).
—A fatal case of pennyroyal oil poisoning was reported in 1978 in an 18-year-old woman who ingested up to 30 mL pennyroyal oil (about 24 g); she experienced abdominal cramps, nausea, hematemesis, and altered mental status and later developed kidney failure, hepatic necrosis, and disseminated intravascular coagulation. Autopsy showed enlarged pale kidneys and centrilobular hepatic necrosis. In 1955, a case was reported of a 24-year-old woman who ingested two bottles of pennyroyal oil (unknown volume and preparation); an abortion resulted but she later developed malaise, nausea, vomiting, diarrhea, abdominal pain, oliguria, and acute renal failure; she died 14 days after ingestion. Proximal tubule degeneration and slight hepatic centrilobular cloudy swelling were noted. In a case report from 1897, a 23 year old ingested 15 mL pennyroyal oil, developed vomiting and gastritis, and died 8 days after ingestion (3).
—Nine other case reports of moderate to severe outcomes (all involving coma or seizures) were identified. Eight involved pennyroyal oil; this includes three cases involving essence of pennyroyal, which is pennyroyal oil in alcohol (1:7). One case involved pennyroyal tablets. All recovered without sequelae.

—Not all ingestions of pennyroyal oil cause serious adverse effects; for example, a 22 year old ingested 10 mL oil and experienced only an hour of dizziness. A 22-month-old 10-kg girl ingested an unknown amount (up to 20 mL) of pennyroyal oil; gastric lavage was done within 30 minutes of ingestion and she was treated with activated charcoal with sorbitol, and oral N-acetylcysteine (every 4 hours for 17 doses); she experienced no sequelae.

• Pennyroyal tea poisoning

—Pennyroyal tea has not resulted in severe poisonings in adults, but babies are more susceptible. A fatal case of poisoning from a pulegone-containing plant (the report does not specify pennyroyal but other plants contain less pulegone) in an infant was reported in 1996 (2). An 8-week-old Hispanic boy was given 120 mL of a homegrown mint tea 14 hours before being admitted to the hospital with respiratory distress, an elevated white blood cell count, metabolic acidosis, hepatitis, and abnormal coagulation studies. Cytomegalovirus infection was documented and was thought to be a contributing factor. Although treated with N-acetylcysteine, multiple organ failure developed and he died 4 days after admission. Autopsy revealed hepatocellular necrosis, edematous hemorrhagic kidneys, bilateral lung consolidation, and diffuse cerebral edema. No pulegone was detected in samples, but levels of menthofuran were 10 ng/mL on day 3 and 2 ng/mL on day 4 (after treatment with NAC).
—Another 6-month-old Hispanic boy had been given 90 mL homegrown mint tea (from the same unspecified plant species as the previous case) three times weekly for 3 months; he was admitted with seizures, fever, cyanosis, elevated white blood cell count, metabolic acidosis, elevated liver function tests, and coagulopathy (2). Serum levels of 25 ng/mL pulegone and 41 ng/mL menthofuran were documented. Increased intracranial pressure resulting from a sinus hemorrhage was diagnosed on the fourth day. After 2 months the baby was discharged with elevated liver function tests nonspecific myopathic changes, and mild carnitine deficiency (2). Neither infant poisoned by pennyroyal tea had viral hepatitis; it is possible that another concurrent viral infection contributed to these adverse outcomes.

—A woman who drank pennyroyal tea to induce menses (1 tsp herb in 1 cup water) reported dizziness, weakness, and a feeling of impending syncope. She was seen in the emergency department within an hour and her symptoms improved spontaneously; she remained asymptomatic 24 hours later. No other details are given.
—A 24-year-old woman drank two cups of pennyroyal tea (2 tsp herb in 1 pint hot water steeped for 5 to 10 minutes) and then prepared another cup 13 hours later, steeping it for 20 minutes. She developed nausea and abdominal cramping; the cramping persisted for 4 days after which menses began. Assuming that this patient was pregnant, this would be a successful abortion.

• Symptoms of severe poisoning

—Fulminant hepatic failure, acute renal failure, coagulopathy, metabolic acidosis, gastrointestinal hemorrhage, pulmonary congestion with consolidation, mental status changes, and seizures. Hypoglycemia in two infants has also been reported (2).

DRUG INTERACTIONS

None reported. However, any substance with hepatotoxic effects would be expected to amplify toxic effects of pennyroyal.

PREGNANCY/LACTATION

Pennyroyal is an abortifacient but is too dangerous to use for this purpose.

ANIMAL TOXICITY

• In rats given pulegone by gavage, doses of 80 and 160 mg/kg body weight caused atonia, decreased creatinine, lower terminal body weight, and histopathologic changes in the liver and white matter of the cerebellum.
• Topical application of pennyroyal oil to a dog in an effort to repel fleas resulted in vomiting 2 hours later and death within 48 hours (6).

Dose

The use of pennyroyal in any form is not recommended. Typical doses are given for information only.
Infusion: made with 1 to 4 g t.i.d.
Liquid extract (1:1, 45% ethanol): 1 to 4 mL t.i.d.

TREATMENT OF POISONING

Gastric lavage should be done and activated charcoal administered. Pennyroyal oil is rapidly absorbed; ipecac-induced emesis is, thus, less desirable, especially because it increases the risk of aspiration pneumonia. Ingestions of more than 10 mL should also be treated with NAC (140 mg/kg, then 70 mg/kg every four hours for 24 hours) (see questions and answers). Hepatic function, renal function, and coagulation parameters should be monitored in all patients (3).
Because NAC increases glutathione levels and prevents hepatotoxic effects of acetaminophen (the toxic intermediate of which is detoxified by glutathione), NAC is used empirically to treat pennyroyal poisoning. The half-life of pennyroyal metabolites is only a few hours in animals, and it is possible that NAC is only helpful in the first hours after pennyroyal poisoning (3). NAC does not prevent pulegone-induced hepatocellular damage in animals, but the treatment appears to be helpful in humans and should be used (2).

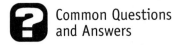

Common Questions and Answers

Q: Why is the effect of pennyroyal oil so variable?
A: Individual susceptibility clearly varies, and a possible factor is individual differences in levels of cytochrome P (CYP) 450 isoenzymes. Inhibitors of CYP 450 lessen pulegone-induced hepatic damage (3). CYP2E, 1CYP1A2, and CYP2C19 oxidize pulegone to menthofuran (7).

Peppermint

 10 Second Take

Evidence supports peppermint oil for irritable bowel syndrome (IBS), spasm during barium enema, and, topically, for headache. It should not be used in babies or small children.

 Basics

LATIN NAME

Mentha x *piperita* L.

FAMILY

Labiatae/Lamiaceae

OTHER COMMON NAMES

Brandy mint, curled mint, and balm mint

DESCRIPTION

• Peppermint is a hybrid of water mint (*Mentha aquatica*) and spearmint (*Mentha* x *spicata*). The latter is a hybrid of two other species, *M. longifolia* and *M. suaveolens*.

PART USED

Essential oil, leaf (dried)

KNOWN ACTIVE CONSTITUENTS

• Volatile oil (1% to 3%), containing principally (−)-menthol (35% to 55%) and its stereoisomers menthone (10% to 40%), (+)-neomenthol (about 3%), and (+) isomenthol (3%). The oil also contains cineol (2% to 13%), limonene (0.2% to 6%), carvone, monoterpenes, and sesquiterpenes (1). Pulegone, the toxic component of pennyroyal, occurs in young plants and may be detected in inferior quality oils; commercial oils do not usually contain pulegone (2).
• Peppermint leaf also contains flavonoids including luteolin, rutin, and hesperidin, as well as phenolic acids and triterpenes (1). Peppermint leaves are high in beta-carotene; retinal equivalents/100 g were found to be 940 by high-pressure liquid chromatography (HPLC) or 1,016 by open-column chromatography (3).

MECHANISM/PHARMACOKINETICS

• In animal models, peppermint oil inhibits muscle contraction induced by serotonin or substance P. Peppermint oil topically applied to the forehead increases skin blood flow (measured by Doppler) (4). Menthol is fat-soluble and quickly absorbed from the small intestine. Peak menthol levels are lower and excretion of menthol metabolites delayed with delayed-release preparations; total urinary excretion of menthol is similar with immediate and delayed-release preparations (1).

 Evidence

CLINICAL TRIALS

• Irritable bowel syndrome (IBS)

—A meta-analysis of peppermint oil for IBS identified eight randomized controlled trials (RCTs) (two parallel group trials and six crossover trials); treatment was administered for 2 weeks to 6 months. Three trials were excluded (two because of insufficient data, one was neither double-blind nor placebo-controlled) (5). The meta-analysis showed that peppermint oil, compared with placebo, significantly improved global symptoms.
—A recent placebo-controlled double-blind RCT (not included in the previous meta-analysis) tested an enteric-coated peppermint oil formulation in 110 patients with IBS (6). Symptoms of abdominal pain, abdominal distension, stool frequency, flatulence, and borborygmi were significantly reduced in the peppermint group, compared with placebo. A double-blind, 2-week RCT in 42 children with IBS found a benefit for enteric-coated peppermint oil capsules (76% improved, compared with 19% of placebo-treated patients) (7).

• Spasm after barium enema

—In one study, 141 patients were randomized either to standard barium suspension or to peppermint oil mixed into the barium suspension (30 mL of a 1 in 125 aqueous solution emulsified with Tween 80) (8). Significantly more of the peppermint-treated patients (60%) experienced no residual spasm compared with 35% of controls. No adverse events were noted. The authors point out that this inexpensive, simple treatment may decrease the need for intravenous spasmolytics.

• Headache

—A crossover RCT compared topical peppermint oil (10% peppermint oil in ethanol) to peppermint-scented placebo for tension headaches in 41 patients; patients also received acetaminophen 1,000 mg or placebo. Each person tried every combination (9). A total of 164 headaches were recorded. The oil was spread across forehead and temples every 15 minutes for 45 minutes; pain intensity was recorded every 15 minutes for 1 hour. Compared with placebo, topical peppermint significantly reduced headache intensity after 15 minutes and throughout the hour. There was no significant difference between acetaminophen and topical peppermint oil; simultaneous administration did not result in a significantly better result than either treatment alone.
—A double-blind placebo-controlled crossover study in 32 healthy men examined topical applications of ethanol and peppermint oil, eucalyptus oil, both oils, and placebo (traces of essential oils were added to some preparations to maintain blinding) (10).

Both peppermint preparations significantly reduced electromyographic (EMG) activity of the temporalis muscle; eucalyptus or ethanol caused no change. Induced pain was generally not different among groups; peppermint reduced pain from ischemic or heat stimulus, but not pressure stimulus; ethanol alone significantly increased pain from heat stimulus. Performance-related activity (a measure of mood state) increased significantly only in the combination group; irritability significantly decreased in both peppermint groups.

• Aromatherapy for postoperative nausea

—In one study, 18 patients who had undergone major gynecologic surgery were assigned to no treatment, inhaled vapors of peppermint oil, or inhaled vapors of peppermint essence (as a placebo) (11). The results did not clearly favor peppermint oil.

• Dyspepsia

—A combination product (peppermint oil 90 mg and caraway oil 50 mg × 4 weeks) was tested against cisapride in 118 patients with functional dyspepsia (12). The primary outcome measure was pain score by visual analog scale. The treatments were similar in reducing frequency of pain and the dyspeptic discomfort score and in improving clinical global impression.
—Another double-blind, placebo-controlled trial in 45 dyspepsia patients (39 completed) tested three enteric-coated capsules daily (each contained 90 mg peppermint oil and 50 mg caraway oil) (13). After 4 weeks, 63.2% of treated patients and 25% of controls were pain-free. Improvement in pain intensity occurred in 89.9% of those treated compared with 45% of controls.
—A commercial combination product containing ethanol-aqueous extracts of peppermint and other herbs [100 mL contained caraway (3.7 g), fennel (8.13 g), peppermint (9.26 g), and wormwood (1.92 g)] was compared with metoclopramide (about 24 mg/day) in 60 participants with upper abdominal complaints (including pain, nausea, heartburn, retching, and gastric cramping) (14). Patients took 25 drops 20 minutes before meals three times daily for their assigned treatment. After 2 weeks, significant differences favoring the herb treatment were seen in epigastric pain, nausea, heartburn, and gastrospasm.

• Decongestant activity

—In 62 volunteers with colds, 30 received a lozenge with 11 mg menthol; in another experiment, 29 healthy participants used an inhaler with 125 mg menthol dissolved in 1 mL paraffin; and in a third experiment, 31 participants inhaled mentholated air for 5 minutes. All of these studies showed a subjective enhancement of nasal air flow; however, none showed any change in nasal airway resistance by rhinomanometry (1).

- Cough

—Inhaled menthol with eucalyptus oil reduced citric acid-induced cough in an experiment involving 20 participants who inhaled air, placebo (pine oil), or menthol dissolved in eucalyptus oil in a 3:1 ratio (15). Because eucalyptus oil is also used to treat cough, it is not possible to separate the effect of menthol from eucalyptus in this experiment.

ANIMAL/IN VITRO

- Peppermint oil inhibits contraction of smooth muscle *in vitro* and reduces morphine-induced spasm in Oddi's sphincter in anesthetized guinea pigs and enhances bile production in dogs. Menthol enhances bile production in rats and dogs (1).
- Peppermint tea (0.4 g/kg body weight) increased bile secretion in cannulated dogs; mixed flavonoids (2 mg/kg) also increased bile secretion in dogs. Intravenous injection of 0.5 mL peppermint tea increased bile acids in cannulated rats. Weak sedative and weak diuretic effects were noted in mice after a single dose (300 mg/kg and 1,000 mg/kg) dried aqueous extract. Menthol inhibits 3-hydroxy-3-methylglutaryl-coenzyme A (HMGCoA) reductase (1).

OTHER CLAIMED BENEFITS/ACTIONS

- Dyspepsia, flatulence, gastritis, colic, biliary disorders, and sedation

 Risks

ADVERSE REACTIONS

- *Menthol:*

—Doses of menthol greater than 2 g could be lethal, but individuals have survived doses as high as 9 g. A review of menthol reactions noted cases of urticaria, allergic cheilitis, and stomatitis; allergic reactions are rare.
—Two cases of fibrillation caused by heavy ingestion of peppermint candy have been reported (no details are reported) (16).
—Mentholated cigarettes have been associated with a case of psychosis and of nonthrombocytopenic purpura (17).
—Bradycardia, ataxia, confusion, and irritability were reported in a 58-year-old woman who smoked 80 mentholated cigarettes daily; electrocardiogram (EKG) showed nonspecific ischemic changes. Discontinuing the cigarettes normalized all symptoms and signs. A rechallenge with menthol (1 g menthol t.i.d. × 1 week) caused anorexia, exhaustion, difficulty concentrating, and bradycardia (17).
—Jaundice in newborns [especially those with glucose-6-phosphate dehydrogenase (G6PD) deficiency] has been associated with menthol (1).

- *Essential oil, ingested:* Heartburn (non-enteric-coated), recurrent muscle pain, gastrointestinal effects include stomatitis, esophagitis, gastritis, diarrhea, and pancreatitis (2)
- *Essential oil (topical):* Skin burns

—A 62-year-old man developed severe necrosis involving deep fasciae and underlying muscle after using a heating pad after topically applying a preparation containing menthol and methyl salicylate (oil of wintergreen) (18). Fever, leucocytosis, metabolic acidosis, abnormal liver and renal function tests, and lung infiltrate were also noted. The authors note that this picture is consistent with chemical and electrical burns with toxic effects from absorption of menthol and methyl salicylate. He was hospitalized for almost a year and received skin grafts; residual renal dysfunction persisted.
—Chemical burns of the hand were reported in a pharmaceutical factory worker exposed to peppermint oil (2).

- Respiratory effects

—Laryngeal and bronchial spasms may occur in babies or small children if peppermint oil is applied to the chest or nasal area (1). Inhalation of menthol may cause apnea or laryngospasm in some individuals (1).

DRUG INTERACTIONS

- None reported. Peppermint oil enhances cyclosporine oral bioavailability in rats (19).
- Patients taking acid blockers or those with achlorhydria should probably use only enteric-coated preparations.

ANIMAL TOXICITY

- Acute oral studies show minimal toxicity of peppermint oil.
- Subchronic and short-term toxicity studies in rats given pulegone, peppermint oil with pulegone, or large doses of menthone found cyst-like cerebellar lesions (20). In rats, 100 mg/kg diluted peppermint oil for 90 days caused nephropathy (1). Pulegone is hepatotoxic (20). In rats, menthofuran (250 mg/kg × 3 days) caused hepatotoxicity (1).
- Peppermint leaf dried aqueous extract given orally to 12 mice (4,000 mg/kg) over 7 days caused no macroscopic signs of toxicity (1).

 Dose

COMMON DOSAGE FORMS

- *Dried leaf:* 2 to 3 g t.i.d.
- *Tea:* 1.5 to 3 g t.i.d.
- *Tincture:* (1:5, 45% ethanol) 2 to 3 mL t.i.d.
- *Oil* (for internal use, pulegone should be limited to less than 1%): Daily dose, 6 to 12 drops
- As an inhalation, 3 to 4 drops in hot water
- For IBS, 0.2 to 0.4 mL t.i.d. in enteric-coated capsules
- *External use:* Dilute preparations, semisolid and oily preparations 5% to 20%, aqueous-ethanol preparations 5% to 10%, nasal ointments 1% to 5% essential oil

—Children 4 to 12 years: Proportion of adult dosage according to body weight or age (see risks).

Phenylalanine (Phe, F)

 10 Second Take

Phenylalanine levels are most important in phenylketonuria (PKU). Limited evidence supports a possible role for phenylalanine in treating vitiligo.

 Basics

DESCRIPTION

Phenylalanine is an essential amino acid.

FOOD SOURCES

Most protein-containing foods. The average intake of phenylalanine and tyrosine by nonvegetarians is 10.4 g/day, among lacto-ovo vegetarians combined intake is 8.8 g daily and among vegans combined intake is 7.0 g daily (1).

MAIN FUNCTIONS/PHARMACOKINETICS

All amino acids are primarily used for protein synthesis; the other important role of phenylalanine is as a precursor of tyrosine (itself a precursor of catecholamines, thyroxine, melanin, and dopa). Phenylalanine hydroxylase is required to convert phenylalanine to tyrosine. The conversion rate depends on intake; a high intake of phenylalanine results in increased conversion to tyrosine. The half-life of phenylalanine in plasma is 2 days (1).

 Evidence

CLINICAL TRIALS

• Vitiligo

—In vitiligo treatment, phenylalanine is thought to inhibit the synthesis of antibodies to melanocyte-associated antigens, thus allowing ultraviolet light to stimulate melanocyte migration from nearby areas. After an open trial showed beneficial effects of combining ultraviolet-A (UVA) treatment and phenylalanine for vitiligo, a small double-blind placebo-controlled trial in 32 patients (24 completed) tested the effect of phenylalanine versus placebo, with or without UVA, in a 2 × 2 design. After 6 months, six of eight patients treated with L-phenylalanine (100 mg/kg/day) and UVA (two to three times/week) showed repigmentation (30% to 60% of affected area); one was stable and one got worse (2). Five received phenylalanine without UVA: one experienced a positive response (25% repigmentation), three were stable, and one deteriorated. Of six receiving placebo plus UVA, four remained stable and two deteriorated. Of five receiving placebo alone, three were stable and two deteriorated.
—An uncontrolled retrospective survey in 193 patients with vitiligo tested oral phenylalanine (50 to 100 mg/kg/day) along with topical phenylalanine (10% gel) in combination with 30 minutes of exposure to sun between 11 a.m. and 3 p.m. (3). Oral phenylalanine was taken 45 minutes before sun exposure and the gel was applied 15 minutes later. In autumn and winter, patients took oral phenylalanine but not gel. Patients were followed every 6 months for up to 3 years. In this study, 56.7% of patients experienced a good response to the treatment (defined as 75% improvement or more). The treatment was most effective for the face and less effective for trunk and limbs. There was no difference between 50 mg and 100 mg or between children and adults.

ANIMAL/IN VITRO EVIDENCE

Not covered

OTHER CLAIMED BENEFITS/ACTIONS

Mood elevation

 Clinical Considerations

• Phenylketonuria

Phenylketonuria (PKU), a group of inherited errors of metabolism that causes excessive accumulation of phenylalanine, affects 1/10,000 Caucasian newborns in the United States and 1/132,000 African American newborns (4). Deficiency of phenylalanine hydroxylase is the most common form, but insufficient amounts of other enzymes or defects in synthesis of tetrahydrobiopterin can also cause PKU. PKU is caused by phenylalanine being converted to phenylpyruvic acid instead of to tyrosine; phenylpyruvic acid is excreted in urine. Expressed before 6 months of age, PKU causes developmental delay, microcephaly, eczema, a musty odor, and abnormal electroencephalogram. Treatment (a low-phenylalanine diet) must begin before 3 weeks of age to prevent mental retardation; early diagnosis and consistent treatment results in normal growth and development.

Those with plasma phenylalanine greater than 250 μmol, plasma tyrosine less than 50 μmol, and normal levels of biopterin and the enzyme DHPR should be treated with a diet that is restricted in phenylalanine and supplemented with tyrosine. Children with biopterin-deficient forms require treatment not only with phenylalanine restriction and tyrosine supplementation but also with administration of levodopa, carbidopa, and tetrahydrobiopterin (4).

In the first year, blood tests should be done twice weekly for the first 3 months and then weekly. The goal is a blood phenylalanine concentration between 120 to 300 mmol as soon as possible but before the infant is 3 weeks old. If phenylalanine levels are greater than 300 mmol (5 mg/dL), more frequent blood tests should be done. Patients with PKU must have some phenylalanine, which is necessary for protein formation for growth and development. Infants with PKU require 15 to 20 mg phenylalanine/kg for growth. At 6 to 12 months, the requirement may decrease to 15 mg/kg/day, but this is variable. Blood phenylalanine concentrations and intake must be monitored; this is especially important in infancy, during growth spurts, and during the latter half of pregnancy. Fetal blood phenylalanine concentrations may be double those of maternal blood. When maternal plasma phenylalanine levels are above 150 μmol, mental retardation in offspring is common.

Natural proteins contain 2.4% to 9% phenylalanine by weight, and one cannot eliminate phenylalanine from the diet while maintaining adequate protein intake. Medical foods must be used for at least part of the diet to supply protein needs. It is best to use a protein supplement containing no phenylalanine so that some phenylalanine can be obtained from regular foods. Serving lists (similar to diabetic exchange lists) are available that group foods of similar phenylalanine content to help parents maintain their children on a low-phenylalanine diet.

It is controversial when or whether the low-phenylalanine diet may be discontinued. Some have suggested discontinuing the diet at age 4, 6, or 12. However, elevated phenylalanine concentrations have been shown to adversely affect neuropsychologic tests and dopamine excretion (4).

DEFICIENCY SIGNS AND SYMPTOMS

Low phenylalanine concentrations (less than 25 mmol) can cause anorexia, decreased growth, and mental retardation (tyrosine can substitute for some of the phenylalanine needed). Decreased phenylalanine levels in blood and urine occurs in the first stage of deficiency; lethargy, anorexia, and failure to grow may or may not occur. Older children may have increased alanine in the blood and β-hydroxybutyric and acetoacetic acidemia. In the second stage, phenylalanine levels may increase (because of degradation of muscle protein) if tyrosine levels are low; the ratio of branched-chain amino acids to other amino acids may also increase. Eczema is often seen; renal tubular malabsorption can occur and cause aminoaciduria. In the third stage of deficiency, levels of amino acids decrease (because of decreased protein synthesis), anemia occurs, hair becomes sparse, and bones become less dense; death may result if deficiency is not corrected (4).

FACTORS DECREASING AVAILABILITY/ABSORPTION

Inadequate dietary intake

FACTORS INCREASING AVAILABILITY/ABSORPTION

- PKU
- Acute infection
- Dietary intake

LABORATORY TESTS

- Average concentration in venous blood is 38 to 73 mmol/L (1)
- Normal urinary output of phenylalanine is 80 mmol/24 hours (1)
- Newborn screening for PKU

—The most common screening test for PKU is the bacterial inhibition assay or Guthrie test, which can detect levels of phenylalanine $\geq$4mg/dL (5). If phenylalanine concentrations in blood are greater than 121 mmol/L (>2 mg/dL), the test should be repeated. Any finding of a level >484 μmol/L (8 mg/dL) requires further workup including quantification of plasma amino acids by ion-exchange chromatography while the infant is on a controlled phenylalanine diet, genotyping of the parents and infant, and biopterin (BH4) and DHPR assays (4).
—The Guthrie test is invalid if antibiotics are used concurrently (4). There are other causes of elevated phenylalanine levels in the blood, including low birthweight, vitamin C deficiency, or high-protein formulas (all of which can cause temporary hypertyrosinemia); liver disease or galactosemia also may elevate levels (4). Fluorometry may also be used for screening but it is more expensive; fluorometric methods are preferred to the Guthrie test for monitoring blood phenylalanine in those who been diagnosed with PKU.
—Urine tests are inadequate for screening because phenylpyruvic acid appears in the urine only after serum levels reach 12 to 15 mg/dL, after damage has probably occurred (5).

 Risks

ADVERSE REACTIONS

No information identified

DRUG INTERACTIONS

No information identified. Theoretically, phenylalanine or tyrosine could induce a sympathomimetic reaction when combined with a monoamine oxidase inhibitor.

ANIMAL TOXICITY

Not covered

 Dose

RECOMMENDED DIETARY ALLOWANCE

Estimates of dietary amino acid requirements (mg/kg/day) by age group (6).

Infants and children

3 to 4 months	125 mg/kg/day
2 to 5 years	69 mg/kg/day
10 to 12 years	22 mg/kg/day
Adults	14 to 39 mg//kg/day

Phosphatidylserine

10 Second Take

Phosphatidylserine appears to help some people with cognitive impairment, but effects are not consistent.

Basics

DESCRIPTION

• Phosphatidylserine is an endogenous, acidic phospholipid that composes 10% to 15% of the lipid bilayer of cell membranes; it is particularly abundant in neuronal cell membranes (1).
• It can be endogenously formed from serine, glycerophosphate, and two fatty acid molecules; some phosphatidylserine comes from dietary sources (2). However, orally ingested phospholipids are partially digested in the small intestine, losing fatty acids, and are unlikely to be absorbed intact (Linder, personal communication, 2001).
• Most currently available supplements are derived from soy; some are combined with other phospholipids.

FOOD SOURCES

Phosphatidylserine is found in small quantities in food plants and animal products but is not very bioavailable.

MAIN FUNCTIONS/PHARMACOKINETICS

• Phosphatidylserine is involved in cell-to-cell communication and protein regulation (including enzymes that mediate signal transduction); activates different protein kinase C isoforms; and affects levels of acetylcholine, dopamine, and norepinephrine (2). Cell membrane experiments have demonstrated an increase in the activity of Na^+-K^+-dependent ATPase, activation of tyrosine hydroxylase, and regulation of calcium uptake. Intravenous injection in mice increases brain glucose and blood glucose and decreases adrenal catecholamines (1).
• Most orally ingested phosphatidylserine is degraded in the gastrointestinal tract; the amount that reaches the central nervous system after oral administration is extremely small, and chronic or repeated administration is necessary to see effects in animal studies (1).

Evidence

CLINICAL TRIALS

Numerous trials have been conducted of phosphatidylserine and dementia, but consistent effects have not been demonstrated. Most experiments have used phosphatidylserine derived from bovine cortex, which is no longer available (see questions and answers).

• Alzheimer's disease

—A 6-month study of 70 patients with probable Alzheimer's disease randomized patients to one of four groups: 17 received social support, 18 cognitive training (twice weekly), 17 cognitive training and pyritinol, and 18 cognitive training and phosphatidylserine (200 mg b.i.d.) (3). Outcome measures included neuropsychologic testing and positron emission tomography scanning for activated glucose pattern in regions typically affected in Alzheimer's disease. At 6 months there were no significant differences between groups in activated glucose pattern or neuropsychologic testing. Scores in the orientation questionnaire were significantly higher at 8 weeks in both the phosphatidylserine and pyritinol groups compared with the other two groups; in addition, the rate of responders (defined as an improvement of 3 or more in the Mini-Mental State Examination score) was significantly higher in both the phosphatidylserine and pyritinol groups compared with the other two groups.
—A double-blind randomized controlled trial in 42 hospitalized Alzheimer's patients (35 completed) tested 100 mg phosphatidylserine t.i.d. against placebo for 6 weeks (4). There was not a significant difference in the Crichton Rating Scale or circle crossing test but there was a significant difference in the Peri test.
—A double-blind crossover study (300 mg/day phosphatidylserine × 8 weeks) in 33 patients with early Alzheimer's found that clinical global improvement was better in treated patients but there was no difference in the Gottfries, Brane and Steen (GBS) dementia scale, psychometric tests, or electroencephalographic mapping (5).

• Age-related cognitive impairment and decline

—A placebo-controlled study of 149 patients 50 to 75 years with age-related cognitive impairment found a significant benefit of 100 mg phosphatidylserine at 3, 6, and 12 weeks in several recall tests, facial recognition, and ability to concentrate (6); patients with initially poor performance were said to benefit the most.
—Another study by the same researcher tested 100 mg phosphatidylserine t.i.d. × 12 weeks against placebo in 51 elderly patients with "probable Alzheimer's disease." The treated group significantly improved on several recall tests (the less impaired did better) (7).
—A double-blind, placebo-controlled study in 494 elderly patients (425 completed) age 65 to 93 with moderate to severe cognitive decline found that 6 months treatment with 300 mg/day phosphatidylserine significantly improved behavior (including motivation, initiative, and socialization) but not behavioral impairment for activities of daily living (self-sufficiency, self care) (8).
—A study of phosphatidylserine 200 mg/day versus placebo in 142 patients with gradual progressive intellectual decline over at least 6 months found no differences in moderately impaired patients. In the subgroup of patients with severe cognitive impairment, significant improvements ($p < 0.05$) in the Blessed dementia scale and the Set test but not the Clifton Assessment scale were demonstrated in the treated group; however this was only a small subgroup of 18 patients that included only 8 treated patients (9).

ANIMAL/IN VITRO EVIDENCE

Phosphatidylserine may decrease severity of several neurochemical and behavioral aging-related changes in rats (1).

Clinical Considerations

DEFICIENCY SIGNS AND SYMPTOMS

None identified

FACTORS DECREASING AVAILABILITY/ABSORPTION

None identified

FACTORS INCREASING AVAILABILITY/ABSORPTION

None identified

LABORATORY TESTS

None identified

 ## Risks

ADVERSE REACTIONS

Stomach upset.
Doses greater than 600 mg near bedtime can cause insomnia.
Doses greater than 300 mg/day lower serum uric acid and alanine aminotransferase (2).

ANIMAL TOXICITY

In rats, the LD_{50} is greater than 5 g/kg body weight (2).

 ## Dose

100 mg t.i.d.

 ## Common Questions and Answers

Q: What is the difference between phosphatidylserine from bovine sources and from soy?
A: There is not much difference; docosahexaenoic acid, an omega-3 fatty acid, is found in the 2 position of bovine but not soy phosphatidylserine. Most clinical trials used phosphatidylserine derived from bovine cortex, no longer considered a safe source. Soybean-derived phosphatidylserine is often sold in a complex containing phosphatidylcholine and phosphatidylethanolamine; no clinical trials have been done on soy preparations.

Phosphorus (Phosphate)

10 Second Take

Phosphorus is widely distributed in foods. In the general population, excess phosphorus intake is common; deficiency is common in hospitalized patients. The ratio of phosphorus to calcium intake is key.

Basics

DESCRIPTION

• Phosphorus is a major mineral intimately involved with calcium and magnesium in bone formation and maintenance; 85% of phosphorus in the body is found in bone.
• Intracellular phosphates are numerous and include adenosine triphosphate (ATP), phosphatidic acid, pyrophosphate, glucose-6-phosphate, inorganic phosphate, phosphoenolpyruvate, phosphoproteins, and, in plants, phytic acid.

FOOD SOURCES

Processed food, colas, other soft drinks, meat, cheese, and other high-protein foods. Whole grains contain mainly the forms phytic acid or phytates, which are not well absorbed (1).

MAIN FUNCTIONS/PHARMACOKINETICS

• Phosphorus plays a main role in bone (and tooth) maintenance as well as in energy metabolism and regulation; it is an integral part of ATP. Phosphorylation of proteins is one of the most common reactions in cells and is important in hormone action and other signaling processes.
• Phosphorus is also part of ribonucleic acid (RNA) and deoxyribonucleic acid (DNA), acts as an intracellular buffer, and composes part of membrane phospholipid.

Evidence

CLINICAL TRIALS

• Osteoporosis, bone fracture, and hypocalcemia

—Excessive intake of phosphorus in relation to calcium has been hypothesized to increase the risk of osteoporosis. Evidence on this is mixed. A study of postmenopausal women found no relationship between soft drink intake and bone density (1a).
—In children, there may be a link between high soft drink intake and bone fracture. One study of 127 children found that intake of cola beverages was strongly correlated with bone fracture in girls (odds ratio 3.59) but not boys (2). Calcium intake was protective. Another case-control study compared 57 children with serum calcium levels less than 2.2 mmol/L with those who had serum calcium levels greater than 2.2 mmol/L and found that consumption of more than 1.5 L of phosphoric acid-containing carbonated beverages was strongly correlated with low serum calcium (OR 5.27) (3).

• Rickets of prematurity

—Phosphate may enhance calcium utilization and prevent rickets in very low birthweight babies. Fifty-three premature babies were randomized to phosphate-supplemented formula (50 mg phosphate/day, in addition to what was contained in the regular milk formula) or regular milk formula. Forty babies completed the trial; of these, 8 of 19 babies in the control group developed rickets but none of the 21 babies who received phosphate-supplemented feeds developed rickets (4). Placental insufficiency appeared to predispose premature infants to the development of rickets, possibly because the transport of calcium and phosphate is affected.

ANIMAL/IN VITRO EVIDENCE

In animals, diets with a high phosphorus to calcium ratio cause hyperparathyroidism and bone loss (5).

OTHER CLAIMED BENEFITS/ACTIONS

None identified

Clinical Considerations

Dietary deficiency is extremely rare in normal patients. However, deficiency is common in alcoholics and in hospitalized patients.

DEFICIENCY SIGNS AND SYMPTOMS

Weakness, acute heart failure, respiratory failure, glucose intolerance, decreased erythrocyte, leukocyte, and platelet function
In children: growth retardation, skeletal deformities, and bone deformities

RISK FACTORS FOR DEFICIENCY

• Cachexia
• Alcoholism (incidence is as high as 50%, resulting from increased urinary excretion)
• Premature birth (see clinical trials)
• Hyperparathyroidism
• Vitamin D deficiency (results in inadequate intestinal absorption of calcium and phosphorus. Parathyroid hormone levels increase, which promotes reabsorption of calcium and renal excretion of phosphorus)
• Chronic acidosis

FACTORS DECREASING AVAILABILITY/ABSORPTION

• Elevated plasma calcium or magnesium
• High dietary ratio of phosphorus to calcium
• Parathyroid hormone
• Estrogen
• Thyroid hormone
• Long-term glucocorticosteroids
• Phosphate-binding antacids
• Sucralfate (see drug interactions)
• Phosphate-deficient total parenteral nutrition (TPN)
• Dextrose or glucose infusions in starved or alcoholic patients (see questions and answers)

FACTORS INCREASING AVAILABILITY/ABSORPTION

• Renal failure (see risks)
• Hypoparathyroidism
• Short-term corticosteroids
• Growth hormone
• Active vitamin D

LABORATORY TESTS

• Serum phosphorus (normal values)
Adults 2.5 to 4.8 mg/dL
Children 4 to 7 mg/dL
• Urinary phosphorus 0.7 to 1.5 g/24 hours
• Levels below 1 mg/dL may presage serious adverse clinical events

Phosphorus (Phosphate)

Risks

- Renal osteodystrophy in patients with chronic renal failure. Patients with chronic renal failure must restrict phosphorus intake because when glomerular filtration of phosphorus is impaired, serum levels increase, which depresses calcium, which in turn stimulates parathyroid hormone. This can lead to renal osteodystrophy, a syndrome of secondary hyperparathyroidism and bone loss. Hyperphosphatemia and hyperparathyroidism may further damage the kidneys.

ADVERSE REACTIONS

- Diarrhea from oral supplementation
- Hypocalcemia from excess supplementation (unlikely except when there is underlying renal disease or hypoparathyroidism)

DRUG INTERACTIONS

- Phosphate-binding antacids (calcium carbonate, aluminum hydroxide) form insoluble complexes in the gastrointestinal tract.
- Sucralfate (forms insoluble complexes in the gastrointestinal tract). Comparable in potency to aluminum hydroxide.

Dose

RECOMMENDED DIETARY ALLOWANCES

- Infants and children

0 to 6 months	100 mg/day (adequate intake)
7 to 12 months	275 mg/day (adequate intake)
1 to 3 years	460 mg/day
4 to 8 years	500 mg/day

Males

9 to 13 years	1,250 mg/day
14 to 18 years	1,250 mg/day
19 to 50 years	700 mg/day
51+ years	700 mg/day

Females

9 to 13 years	1,250 mg/day
14 to 18 years	1,250 mg/day
19 to 50 years	700 mg/day
51+ years	700 mg/day

Pregnant

≤18 years	1,250 mg/day
19 to 50 years	700 mg/day

Lactating

≤18 years	1,250 mg/day
19 to 50 years	700 mg/day

UPPER LIMITS

Infants and children

0 to 6 months	Not determinable
7 to 12 months	Not determinable
1 to 3 years	3,000 mg/day
4 to 8 years	3,000 mg/day

Males

9 to 13 years	4,000 mg/day
14 to 18 years	4,000 mg/day
19 to 50 years	4,000 mg/day
51 to 70 years	4,000 mg/day
71+ years	3,000 mg/day

Females

9 to 13 years	4,000 mg/day
14 to 18 years	4,000 mg/day
19 to 50 years	4,000 mg/day
51 to 70 years	4,000 mg/day
71+ years	3,000 mg/day
Pregnant	3,500 mg/day
Lactating	4,000 mg/day

- Recommended intakes in chronic renal failure

—Before end-stage renal disease (ESRD)

Glomerular filtration rate (GFR) >60 mL/min	no restriction
GFR 25 to 60 mL/min	8 to 12 mg/kg ideal body weight (IBW)/day
GFR 10 to 25 mL/min	5 to 10 mg/kg IBW/day

—Diabetics

GFR 10 to 60 mL/min	8 to 12 mg/kg IBW/day

—Nephrotic syndrome

GFR 10 to 60 mL/min	8 to 12 mg/kg IBW/day

—ESRD

Hemodialysis	<17 mg/kg IBW/day
Peritoneal dialysis	<17 mg/kg IBW/day (with peritonitis, no restriction)

—Post-transplant

First month varies (urinary phosphorus may be high in the first weeks after transplantation)

Subsequent months	17 to 20 mg/kg IBW/day

Conversion: 1 mmol phosphorus = 31 mg

Common Questions and Answers

Q: What is the connection between starvation and hypophosphatemia?
A: Aggressive refeeding of carbohydrates (especially parenterally) in chronically starved patients is dangerous and may precipitate acute hypophosphatemia leading to cardiac failure. During starvation, a lowered metabolic rate reduces the need for phosphorus. Sudden infusions of glucose increase the need for phosphorus and can overwhelm the body's ability to mobilize phosphate from bone. Intracellular phosphate depletion can occur within hours and can result in cardiopulmonary failure and death within days.

Q: Does variable phosphorus intake affect calcium levels?
A: Varying phosphorus levels appear to have no effect on overall calcium balance, at least in those with functioning kidneys. Urinary calcium varies inversely with phosphorus intake, but apparently intestinal absorption of calcium is simultaneously enhanced. The kidney appears to respond to varying phosphorus levels by increasing or decreasing calcitriol levels (5). However, those with limited kidney function or in particularly vulnerable age groups (children, the elderly) are probably at risk of decreased calcium levels from excess phosphorus loss.

Pollen/Bee Pollen

10 Second Take

There is some evidence of efficacy of pollen extract in benign prostatic hyperplasia (BPH). Severe hypersensitivity reactions have been reported.

Basics

OTHER COMMON NAMES

Typha pollen (puhuang), pine pollen, Cernilton, Melbrosia, and NaO Li Su

DESCRIPTION

• Pollen may be harvested from flowers or stolen from honeybees (*Apis mellifera*) through traps placed near beehives; bees returning from pollen-gathering have to clamber through the net-like pollen traps, losing some of the pollen off their hind legs in the process (1).
• *Typha* pollen, from *T. angustata* and other species (also called *puhuang* in Chinese) and pine pollen are collected directly from flowers. Pollen has a long tradition of use in Chinese traditional medicine. Cernilton (or Cernitin) is a Swedish pollen extract of several different plants, including rye-grass (*Secale cereale*), and is a registered pharmaceutical in Switzerland, Austria, Germany, Spain, Greece, Japan, Korea, and Argentina.

KNOWN ACTIVE CONSTITUENTS

• The acetone-soluble fraction of Cernilton contains β-sterols. An active fraction of Cernilton that inhibits the growth of prostate cancer cells has been identified; it appears to be a cyclic hydroxamic acid (2). Nutrient content in pollen varies widely by source; pollen can contain up to 28.3% crude protein, up to 20% lipids, up to 44% carbohydrates, and up to 2.5% flavonoids (1).
• Other constituents include vitamins A, B_1, B_2, C, D, E, K, folic acid, niacin, trace elements, and sterols. β-Sitosterol, rutin, and other constituents have been reported in some types of pollen but not others (1).

MECHANISM/PHARMACOKINETICS

No information identified

Evidence

CLINICAL TRIALS

• Memory

—A traditional Chinese herbal medicine called NaO Li Su contains five herbs and bee pollen and is used for declining memory. The effect of this preparation on memory was tested in 100 elderly Danish volunteers in a 3-month double-blind placebo-controlled crossover trial (3). No positive effects on memory were identified; increased number of red blood cells and increased serum creatinine were seen after active treatment.

• Menopausal symptoms

—A placebo-controlled trial of the effect of a bee pollen product called Melbrosia in women with severe menopausal symptoms was published in German (4). Apparently there were improvements in headache, incontinence, vaginal dryness and "decreasing vitality" in the treatment group (this study was read in abstract).

• Benign prostatic hyperplasia

—A Cochrane review, also published as a paper, identified four controlled trials (three double-blind, two placebo-controlled, two treatment-controlled) that assessed the effects of Cernilton on BPH (5,6). A total of 444 men were enrolled in trails that lasted from 12 to 24 weeks. The treatment controls were natural products not conventionally used in North America: Tadenan (*Pygeum africanum* extract) and Paraprost (a Japanese amino acid product containing 265 mg L-glutamic acid, 100 mg L-alanine, and 45 mg aminoacetic acid). Cernilton was significantly better than placebo and both treatments in self-rated improvement; the weighted relative risk (RR) for self-rated improvement for Cernilton versus placebo was 2.40 (95% CI 1.21 to 4.75), and the weighted RR versus Tadenan was 1.42 (95% CI 1.21 to 4.75). Cernilton reduced nocturia significantly compared with placebo and Paraprost. All treatments were equivalent in improving urologic symptoms based on the International Prostate Symptom Score (IPSS). There was no benefit of Cernilton over placebo or treatment in urinary flow rates, residual volume, or prostate size compared with placebo or other treatments. Cernilton was well tolerated. Methodologic problems included lack of information on doses and formulation and short duration of trials.

• Prostatitis

—Uncontrolled trials have claimed a benefit of Cernilton treatment for chronic prostatitis (7,8).

• Hormone levels

—A double-blind, placebo-controlled, 6-month trial of 60 patients with BPH (included in the previous review) also examined hormone levels; after 6 months treatment with Cernilton (two capsules b.i.d.), levels of luteinizing hormone (LH), follicle-stimulating hormone (FSH), testosterone, and dihydrotestosterone were unchanged (9).

ANIMAL/IN VITRO

• Prostate and urinary tract effects

—Decreased prostate size has been noted in Wistar rats treated with Cernilton (10). Cernilton causes smooth muscle relaxation in mouse and pig urethra and was reported to inhibit the growth of a prostate carcinoma cell line but not cell lines derived from other tissues (11).

• Estrogenic effects

—Estrogenic effects of Melbrosia were tested by examining effects on uterine weight in immature mice (30, 300, or 3,000 mg/kg orally for 3 days) or vaginal smears in ovariectomized rats (3, 30, or 300 mg/kg, injected subcutaneously for 3 days) (12). No estrogenic effect was seen.

• Atherosclerosis

—In rabbits fed a high-fat diet, Cernitin significantly reduced the severity of plaque formation (13).

OTHER CLAIMED BENEFITS/ACTIONS

- Asthma
- Cancer
- Infertility
- Menopausal symptoms
- Lowers cholesterol
- Increases performance
- Antibacterial, antiviral
- Lowers cholesterol
- Laxative
- Fatigue
- Atherosclerosis

 Risks

ADVERSE REACTIONS

- Bee pollen

—There is a case report of hypereosinophilia (13,440 cells/mm^3) after 6 weeks of ingesting bee pollen (14). Symptoms included malaise, headache, nausea, diarrhea, and pruritus. Hypereosinophilia and symptoms resolved after cessation of bee pollen; rechallenge caused eosinophils to increase from 207 to 890 cells/mm^3. Analysis revealed pollens to which the patient was allergic by skin test.
—Eosinophilic gastroenteritis has also been associated with bee pollen. A 34-year-old Spanish women with a history of seasonal rhinoconjunctivitis and honey intolerance began ingesting bee pollen. Three weeks later, she developed anorexia, abdominal pain, diarrhea, hypereosinophilia, and elevated serum IgE levels (15). Duodenal biopsy showed eosinophilic infiltration of the mucosal layer. All signs and symptoms stopped after discontinuation of the bee pollen.
—Hepatitis was reported in a 33-year-old woman who had been taking 2 tablespoons of bee pollen daily for 2 months (16). Tests for hepatitis A, B, C, Epstein-Barr virus, and cytomegalovirus were negative, and the patient denied alcohol use. Other medications included aspirin, butalbital, and erythromycin; symptoms and laboratory tests normalized within 6 weeks with discontinuation of the pollen product (other medications were continued during this time.) This is an unusual case that raises the concern that the product contained other hepatotoxic ingredients; the implicated product was not analyzed to determine whether it contained other substances.

DRUG INTERACTIONS

None reported

ANIMAL TOXICITY

No information identified

 Dose

Powdered or granular forms: usual dose 1/8 to 2 tsp. q.d. to t.i.d.
Extracts (aqueous, hydroalcoholic, and lipoid)
Cernitin pollen extract (63 mg tablets) one to two tablets t.i.d.

Propolis

10 Second Take

Propolis, a resin-derived bee product, is relatively safe and has antimicrobial properties. Primarily used topically, it can cause contact dermatitis, especially in those sensitive to Balsam of Peru.

Basics

DESCRIPTION

Propolis, or "bee glue," is an adhesive, resinous substance used by honeybees in building and sealing a hive. Plant resins are masticated (thus acquiring salivary enzymes) and mixed with beeswax; the resulting mixture is used to repair holes and smooth interior walls. Although the precise composition depends on the source, propolis usually contains 50% resin and vegetable balsam, 30% wax, 10% essential and aromatic oils, 5% pollen, and 5% other (1). The proportion of resins to beeswax varies substantially and may be affected by the use the propolis is put to and the local availability of resins. Propolis contains hydroquinone (0.1%), caffeic acid and its esters (2% to 20%), and quercetin (less than 0.1% to 0.7%) (all of these are in much smaller quantities than in dietary sources). Propolis may be an unintended additive in beeswax and honey.

MECHANISMS/PHARMACOKINETICS

Neither mechanism of action nor pharmacokinetics has been delineated. Flavonoids are the most likely active ingredients in propolis. Flavonoids inhibit a variety of enzymes, and propolis has been shown to inhibit glycosyltransferases, myeloperoxidase, ornithine decarboxylase, lipoxygenase, tyrosine protein kinase, and arachidonic acid metabolism.

Evidence

CLINICAL TRIALS

- Ocular herpes

—One study tested ocular propolis films in 35 patients with postherpetic trophic keratitis and in 20 with postherpetic nebulae (2). Films were applied behind the lower eyelid before bed for 10 to 15 days. Compared with controls, propolis-treated patients recovered nearly twice as fast (7.6 days, compared with 14.1 days in the placebo group).

- Dental plaque inhibition

—A double-blind study comparing a propolis-containing mouthwash with a positive control (chlorhexidine) and a negative control found that the chlorhexidine mouthrinse was significantly better than the others; there was no significant difference between the propolis-containing mouthrinse and the negative control (3).
—Another study tested propolis and honey against oral bacteria in 10 volunteers (an in vitro study was also done). Propolis demonstrated an antibacterial effect on oral streptococci both in vitro and clinically, by reducing salivary bacterial counts (4).

ANIMAL/IN VITRO EVIDENCE

- Anti-tumor effects

—A component of propolis, caffeic acid phenethyl ester (CAPE), applied topically to CD-1 mice, reduced the number and size of chemically-induced skin papillomas in a dose-dependent manner. In an in vitro test, CAPE added to cultured HeLa cells (a cervical cancer line) inhibited the synthesis of deoxyribonucleic acid (DNA) and ribonucleic acid (RNA) in a dose-dependent manner (5). CAPE appears to be selectively cytotoxic to tumor cells and virally transformed cells without being cytotoxic to normal cells. Low doses of CAPE (0.1 to 6.5 nmol/topical treatment) in SENCAR mice inhibit several oxidative tumor-promoting actions, including myeloperoxidase activity (indicative of polymorphonuclear leukocyte infiltration into tissues), hydrogen peroxide production, and formation of oxidized bases in epidermal DNA. At higher doses, edema and ornithine decarboxylase induction was inhibited (6).
—Dietary caffeic acid esters inhibit the growth of cultured colon cancer cells (7) and (in a dietary dose of 600 ppm) inhibited aberrant crypt foci formation in F344 rats (8). Aberrant crypt foci are precursor lesions for colon cancer. A diet containing 750 ppm phenylether-3-methyl caffeate resulted in a significant decrease in adenocarcinomas of the colon as well as a decrease in colon tumor volume (9).

—Two caffeic acid esters were tested on azoxymethane-induced biochemical changes. One of these esters, phenylethyl caffeate (PEC) (present in honey and in propolis and also synthesized), significantly inhibited azoxymethane-induced ornithine decarboxylase and tyrosine protein kinase activities in liver and colon; PEC also suppressed lipooxygenase metabolites but had no effect on cyclooxygenase metabolism (8). The caffeic acid ester methyl caffeate was far less active.

- Antioxidant effects

—CAPE inhibited hydrogen peroxide production in bovine lenses exposed to an oxidizing agent. This effect could theoretically decrease cataract development (6).
—An aqueous extract of propolis as well as propol (a phenolic component), inhibited Cu^{2+} initiated low density lipoprotein (LDL) oxidation; in addition, antiapoptotic action was demonstrated in macrophages exposed to minimally modified LDL (10).

- Antimicrobial effects

—Propolis extracts and constituents have been shown to have antibacterial activity against Staphylococcus aureus, Streptococcus pyogenes, Streptococcus viridans, Corynebacterium diphtheria, Escherichia coli, Salmonella typhi, Salmonella paratyphi, and Toxoplasma gondii (1). An ethanolic extract of propolis was shown to have a marked synergistic effect on antibacterial effects of streptomycin and cloxacillin and a moderate synergistic effect on penicillin G, doxycycline, streptomycin, chloramphenicol, cefradine, and polymixin B; no effect was noted on ampicillin (11).
—Although bactericidal against many strains of Mycobacteria, propolis has no effect on Mycobacterium tuberculosis.
—Propolis appears to have no activity against Entamoeba histolytica in vitro and was effective in vivo against T. gondii and Trichomonas vaginalis only at extremely high doses (in one experiment, survival of trichomonas was extended at lower doses) (1). An in vivo experiment in mice infected with Trypanosoma cruzi found no effect on parasitemia kinetics or survival rate (12).
—Antifungal activity has been demonstrated against species of Candida, Saccharomyces, Cryptococcus neoformans, Histoplasma capsulatum, and several species of Trichosporon and Microsporum (1). An in vitro study that compared different extraction methods found that propolis extracts were particularly effective against Sarcinia lutea, Candida albicans, Rhodotorula glutinis, Schizosaccharamyces pombe and various dermatophytes (13). Solvents made a difference. Edible oil extractions were most active, glycerine solutions were the most variable, and ethanol and propylene glycol solutions afforded long-acting inhibition of affected organisms.

—Propolis also appears to have antiviral activity. *In vitro*, propolis suppresses replication of HIV-1, abolishing syncytium formation at 4.5 μg/mL; p24 antigen production was decreased in a concentration-dependent manner (14). Activity has been demonstrated against herpes simplex virus 1 and 2, adenovirus type 2, vesicular stomatitis virus, and poliovirus type 2. Fractions and isolates of propolis have shown activity against influenza viruses A and B, vaccinia virus, Newcastle disease virus, and a strain of influenza A (1).

—In mice, a water-soluble derivative of propolis was found to induce significant nonspecific host protection against experimental infection with gram-negative pathogens; macrophage activation is suggested as a possible mechanism (15).

• Hepatoprotective effects

—In animals, propolis reduces pathologic liver changes caused by acetaminophen (1). Cuban red propolis protects against galactosamine-induced hepatitis in rats (16). A dose-related effect of aqueous propolis extract was found against hepatotoxicity induced by carbon tetrachloride in liver-cell suspensions (17); a histopathologic study in rats also showed a reduction in carbon tetrachloride-induced hepatotoxicity (18).

• Cardioprotective effects

—In rats, propolis (50 to 100 mg/kg i.p. daily × 5 days) reduced doxorubicin-induced cardiomyopathy, as assessed by histopathology and levels of creatine phosphokinase, malondialdehyde, and glutathione (19).

• Antiinflammatory effects

—An orally administered 13% aqueous extract of propolis (1, 5, and 10 ml/kg) reduced carrageenan-induced rat paw edema and adjuvant-induced arthritis in rats (20). In another experiment, aqueous extract of propolis (5 ml/kg administered orally) reduced carrageenan-induced rat paw edema after whole body gamma irradiation (which exaggerates the inflammatory response) (21). An *in vivo* study showed that dietary propolis suppressed the lipoxygenase pathway of arachidonic acid metabolism during inflammation (22).

OTHER CLAIMED BENEFITS/ACTIONS

• Antiseptic
• Antifungal
• Antiinflammatory
• Antioxidant
• Anesthetic
• Rheumatism
• Sprains
• Topical: wound healing, burns, leg ulcers, herpes ulcers, pruritus ani, antifungal, and beauty creams
• Gingivitis, stomatitis, and cheilitis

 Risks

ADVERSE REACTIONS

Propolis is an allergen and has caused numerous cases of contact dermatitis (23). The allergenic compound may be poplar bud constituents and is most likely the caffeic acid ester, 1,1-dimethylallyl caffeic acid ester (24) (see questions and answers).

CONTRAINDICATIONS

Allergy to Balsam of Peru, which is a resin, similar to benzoin, formed by the Peru balsam tree (*Myroxylon pereirae*); it is used in topical antiseptics and skin protectants.

DRUG INTERACTIONS

None identified

ANIMAL TOXICITY

Oral LD$_{50}$ of propolis extract in the mouse has been reported as greater than 7,340 mg/kg by one researcher and 2,050 mg/kg by another researcher. In mice, 700 mg/kg administered orally was reported to be well tolerated; mice were monitored for 48 hours (1).
In a chronic dosing study, Wistar rats received an alcoholic extract of propolis in drinking water at a dose of 1,875 mg/kg/day for 30 days or 2,470 mg/kg/day for 60 days. Compared with controls, no changes were noted in clinical appearance, behavior, urine output, body weight, or mortality (1). No treatment-related histologic changes were noted in either group. No adverse effects were noted in mice treated with 1,400 mg/kg/day for 90 days (1).

 Dose

No information is available on oral dosing in humans. Burdock notes that if the no-effect level in mice is extrapolated to humans and reduced a thousand-fold to account for the lack of chronic toxicity studies, 1.4 mg/kg/day (approximately 70 mg/day) should be safe in humans (1).

MODE OF ADMINISTRATION

Topical (most popular): ointments, lotions, solutions
Personal products: toothpaste, dental floss, mouthwash, cosmetic products
Oral: capsules, usually 50 mg/capsule, powder, or chewing gum

 Common Questions and Answers

Q: Is there cross-reactivity between pollen allergy and propolis allergy?
A: Most people allergic to propolis are not allergic to pollen. Propolis is gathered from plant resins, not pollen (although propolis may contain some pollen, it is not a large amount). People sensitive to propolis are most commonly sensitive to plant resins, including Balsam of Peru. Some are also sensitive to essential oils, cinnamic acids and aldehydes, or beeswax (1).

Q: Is populus the same thing as propolis?
A: No, but they are similar. Populus is an oleoresin used as a flavoring agent for alcoholic beverages. It comes from resinous material in poplar buds (*Populus* species). The poplar is popular as a resin source for bees, so it is no surprise that populus and propolis are chemically very similar (1).

Q: What else is propolis used for?
A: The use of propolis by humans dates to 300 BC. Stradivari reportedly used propolis as an ingredient in the varnish of his stringed instruments, and it is sometimes used today in the repair of accordions and in rosin for stringed instruments. It has been proposed as a chemical preservative in meat products (1).

Psyllium (Plantain)

 10 Second Take

Psyllium seed or husk is an effective bulk-forming laxative that also may lower cholesterol and blood glucose. Allergic reactions are not uncommon.

 Basics

LATIN NAME

Black psyllium or psyllium may refer to *Plantago indica* L. (also known as *Plantago arenaria* Waldst. & Kit.) or *Plantago psyllium* L. (also called *Plantago afra* L.)
Ispaghula, blond psyllium, psyllium (*Plantago ovata* Forsk, *Plantago ispaghula* Roxb.)
Asian psyllium, *Shazen-shi, Che-quian-zi* (*Plantago asiatica*)
Ribwort plantain (*Plantago lanceolata*)
Plantago major

FAMILY

Plantaginaceae

OTHER COMMON NAMES

Plantain (all species), Spanish psyllium (*Plantago afra*)

DESCRIPTION

• Most *Plantago* species are annual herbs up to 0.5 m tall.
• *Plantago ovata* has white flowers in cylindrical spikes, lanceolate leaves, and oval gray-pink seeds.
• *Plantago indica* has a hairy, frequently branched stem with whorls of linear to filiform leaves.
• *Plantago afra* is an erect herb with whorls of flattened linear or linear-lanceolate leaves (1).
• *Plantago lanceolata* is perennial, with a linear-lanceolate basal rosette of parallel-veined leaves and brownish flowers on long stalks. Psyllium husks are among the best sources of soluble fiber.

PART USED

• Seed or seed husk (most species)
• leaf (*Plantago lanceolata*)

KNOWN ACTIVE CONSTITUENTS

• Seed

—The epidermis is rich in mucilage polysaccharide (10% to 15%), consisting of xylose, galacturonic acid, arabinose and rhamnose (2). The husk of *Plantago* species is easily separated from the seeds and is five times more active than the whole seeds (3).
—Seeds also contain protein (15% to 20%), fixed oil (5% to 13%), planteose (a trisaccharide), triterpenes, phytosterols,

aucubin (an iridoid glucoside), and alkaloids (2).
• Leaf (*Plantago lanceolata*) contains iridoid glycosides including aucubin (0.3% to 2.5%), catalpol (0.3% to 1.1%) and asperuloside, mucilage (6.5%), tannins, phenolic carboxylic acids, the coumarin aesculetin, and flavonoids.

MECHANISM/PHARMACOKINETICS

• Psyllium seeds and husks function as a bulk-forming soluble fiber laxative. It is not absorbed but absorbs fluid within the gastrointestinal tract, increasing the volume and weight of intestinal contents, which in turn accelerates colonic transit. Psyllium husks are resistant to fermentation; its effect is mainly due to the intact material (4). When incubated *in vitro* with gastrointestinal enzymes, *Plantago ovata* seeds and husks had no effect on pepsin, trypsin, or α-amylase and had a stimulating effect on chymotrypsin, lipase, and lactase (5).
• Leaf (*Plantago lanceolata*): Cold aqueous leaf extracts, fluid extracts, and pressed juice have antibacterial activity; aqueous infusions and decoctions do not show activity (6).

 Evidence

CLINICAL TRIALS

• Hypercholesterolemia

—A meta-analysis of cholesterol-lowering effects of dietary fiber identified 17 controlled trials (11 parallel, 6 crossover) with a total of 757 subjects (including 242 women)(7). The analysis found that psyllium lowered cholesterol significantly; each gram of soluble fiber reduced total cholesterol 0.028 mmol/L (1.10 mg/dL); high density lipoprotein (HDL) cholesterol decreased slightly but significantly. None of the soluble fibers affected triglycerides.
—Six normal and five ileostomy subjects received 10 g/day psyllium husk for 3 weeks, and six normal and four ileostomy subjects received 10 g/day psyllium seed. The husk had no effect on cholesterol or triglycerides in either group. In normal subjects treated with psyllium seed, total cholesterol was reduced 6.4% and HDL cholesterol was reduced 9.3%. Seeds increased bile acid in the ileostomy group but did not affect cholesterol levels (8).

• Satiety

—A crossover study in 17 female subjects compared a *Plantago ovata* granular preparation (containing 65 g seeds and 2.2 g husks) with placebo (20 g semolina), both taken with 200 mL water (9). Each was administered 3 hours before meals and immediately before a meal for 3 days. One hour after eating, those receiving plantago were more full (measured by a visual analogue scale); total fat intake was also significantly lower on the day of treatment. The plantago supplement was perceived as less pleasant

than the placebo (the meal eaten afterwards also was perceived as less pleasant, although the meals were identical on both occasions).

• Effects on glucose

—Psyllium can lower peak blood glucose levels, apparently by reducing intestinal absorption. A controlled crossover study in eight diabetics with chronic portal-systemic encephalopathy compared a meat protein diet (0.8 g/kg body weight) with neomycin and laxatives to a vegetable protein diet (0.8 g/kg body weight) with psyllium fiber added to achieve 35 g fiber per day; both diets provided approximately 1,800 kcal/day (10). At the end of the first study period, fasting glucose levels were significantly lower in the vegetable protein diet group. A decrease ≥ 25 mg% of fasting glucose levels was seen in seven of eight patients after the vegetable protein diet and in none after the meat protein diet. The number of bowel movements significantly increased after the vegetable diet. The authors suggest that a vegetable diet with supplemental fiber may be a helpful treatment in patients with diabetes and hepatic encephalopathy.
—In another study, 125 patients with noninsulin-dependent diabetes received 6 weeks of diet counseling followed by a 6-week treatment that compared psyllium (5 g t.i.d.) with placebo, administered before meals (11). Body weight did not change. Following psyllium treatment, HDL cholesterol increased significantly, whereas total cholesterol, low density lipoprotein (LDL) cholesterol, triglycerides, and fasting plasma glucose were significantly reduced. There were no significant adverse effects.

• Constipation and irritable bowel syndrome (IBS)

—A double-blind study in 20 patients with chronic constipation (10 with IBS) compared *Plantago ovata* with placebo and found that frequency of stools increased significantly from 2.5 ± 1 to 8 ± 2.2 stools per week; fecal weight and colonic transit time increased in the treated but not the placebo group (12).
—A study of intestinal transit in 24 healthy volunteers tested the effect of products containing purified sennosides 20 mg, 20 g *Plantago ovata* seeds and husks, and a combination containing 5.4 g plantain seeds and husks and 30 mg sennosides (13). Colonic transit was increased with both products containing senna but was not influenced by plantain alone. Twelve volunteers received loperamide; again both products with senna increased transit time, whereas psyllium alone had no effect.
—An uncontrolled trial in 149 patients with chronic constipation (84% women) treated with *Plantago ovata* seeds 15 to 30 g/day for at least 6 weeks found improvement in 33 patients, cure in 32 patients, and no effect in 84 patients (14).

- Hemorrhoids

—Fifty patients with bleeding internal hemorrhoids were randomized to a commercial preparation of *Plantago ovata* or placebo (15). During the first 15 days of treatment, the average number of bleeding episodes was not different between groups. At 30 and 45 days, however, bleeding episodes were significantly decreased in the treated group compared to the placebo group. The number of congested hemorrhoidal cushions (assessed by endoscopy) diminished from 2.6 ± 1 to 1.6 ± 2.2 after fiber treatment, whereas there were no changes in the placebo group. Hemorrhoids bled on contact in 5 of 22 patients in the fiber group before treatment and in none of the treated patients after treatment; no changes from baseline were seen in the control group. Treatment did not modify the degree of prolapse.

—Another trial of 52 patients with symptomatic hemorrhoids tested placebo against psyllium seed fiber for 6 weeks (20 g daily, mixed in water, in divided doses) (16). Psyllium significantly reduced bleeding and pain on defecation; there was no significant difference between groups in pruritus and anal secretion or prolapse. In the treatment group, 84% were improved or asymptomatic compared with 52% in the placebo group; the difference was significant. Three months after the study ended, the difference between groups was still significant for bleeding.

- Ulcerative colitis

—A randomized open-label trial in 105 patients with ulcerative colitis in remission compared *Plantago ovata* seeds (10 g b.i.d.) with mesalamine (500 mg t.i.d.) or a combination. The primary outcome measure was maintenance of remission for 1-year period. Treatment was successful in 21/35 (60%) of plantago-treated patients, 24/37 mesalamine-treated patients (65%), and 21/30 patients (70%) in the combination group (17). Three patients (all receiving plantago) were withdrawn because of constipation and/or flatulence. Fecal butyrate levels increased significantly in the plantago group.

CASE REPORT

- Plantain leaves for cough

—A 47-year-old woman with lung cancer and intractable cough unresponsive to antitussives, chlorpromazine, morphine, and nebulized lidocaine found that 1 to 2 teaspoons of slippery elm bark and a tea of plantain leaves (2 to 3 g in 150 mL boiling water) drunk in small amounts during the day reduced her cough (18).

ANIMAL/IN VITRO

Not covered

OTHER CLAIMED BENEFITS/ACTIONS

- Seed: diarrhea
- Leaf: mucous membrane inflammation, cough, immune stimulation, wound healing, styptic (6)

 Risks

ADVERSE REACTIONS

—Allergic reactions are not uncommon. Anaphylactic shock resulting from ingestion of a psyllium laxative has been reported (19). Sensitization can occur; in one case a 40-year-old woman who had taken psyllium for 2 years presented with a pruritic, maculopapular and urticarial rash over her entire body except the face and oropharyngeal swelling (20). Symptoms resolved on discontinuation of psyllium and occurred on rechallenge.

—Psyllium seed or husk should always be taken with plenty of water. Intestinal obstruction may occur when bulk-forming laxatives are taken with insufficient fluid. Psyllium should not be used in cases of fecal impaction, ileus, or any condition predisposing to intestinal obstruction.

—Gas and bloating can occur, especially at the beginning of treatment.

—Brittle diabetics may need to adjust insulin.

DRUG INTERACTIONS

- Any bulk-forming laxative can decrease the absorption of drugs or speed intestinal transit; psyllium should not be taken within an hour of other medications.
- Two teaspoons daily of psyllium mucilloid decreased lithium levels in one patient, possibly because the hydrophilic psyllium prevented the lithium from ionizing and being absorbed (21).
- In rabbits, *Plantago ovata* seeds and husks decreased the absorption of ethinylestradiol (22).

PREGNANCY/LACTATION

Psyllium may be used during pregnancy or lactation if no contraindications exist.

ANIMAL TOXICITY

No information identified

 Dose

- *Husk or seed:* For constipation, average daily dose 7 to 30 g in divided doses; for diarrhea, up to 40 g. Whole seed may be presoaked for several hours in 100 to 150 mL warm water.
- *Husk:* Husk may be presoaked for several hours in 150 mL warm water.
- *Powdered husk:* 3 to 5 g stirred into 150 mL *cold* water or fruit juice, drunk immediately and followed with additional liquid up to t.i.d. before meals. For IBS, standard dose may be doubled. For hypercholesterolemia, up to 10 g t.i.d..
- Black psyllium seed: 5 to 10 g whole or ground seed presoaked for several hours in 100 to 150 mL warm water up to t.i.d. For diarrhea, total daily dose may be up to 40 g.
- Children
12 years or older: adult dose
6 to 12 years: half of adult dosage
0 to 6 years: only with medical supervision

 Common Questions and Answers

Q: Does plantain have adverse cardiovascular effects?
A: No, but an accidentally adulterated mixture of herbs meant for "internal cleansing" resulted in two cases of digoxin poisoning; the problem was eventually traced to a supply of plantain contaminated with foxglove (*Digitalis lanata*) (23). (See foxglove for details).

Pygeum

10 Second Take

Pygeum is a well-tolerated herb; clinical trials support its use for reducing symptoms of benign prostatic hypertrophy (BPH).

Basics

LATIN NAME

Prunus africana (Hook. f) Kalkman, *Pygeum africanum* (Hook. f) Kalkman

FAMILY

Rosaceae

OTHER COMMON NAMES

African prune, African cherry, and red stinkwood

DESCRIPTION

• Native to southern and central Africa, *Prunus africana* is an evergreen tree up to 30 m in height with elliptic leaves, small white flowers, and tough red fruit. The tree prefers mountain forests. The bark, fruit, and bruised leaves smell of bitter almonds.

PART USED

Bark

KNOWN ACTIVE CONSTITUENTS

• β-Sitosterol (more than 15%); 3-*O*-glucoside; β-sitostenone; triterpenic acids; oleanolic, ursolic, and crataegolic acids; palmitic acid and other fatty acids; and long-chain fatty alcohols, especially n-docosanol and n-tetracosanol (1).

MECHANISM/PHARMACOKINETICS

• The effect of pygeum is probably multifactorial. It is unclear whether pygeum inhibits 5-α reductase (see questions and answers). In the rat, adrenal androgen secretion is stimulated (the effect is strongest in orchiectomized animals) (2). Pygeum extract inhibits rat prostatic fibroblast proliferation, apparently by inhibiting growth factors (3); inhibition of induced growth of mouse 3T3 fibroblasts has also been demonstrated (2).

Evidence

CLINICAL TRIALS

• A review of nine double-blind placebo-controlled trials of pygeum (75 to 200 mg/day for 6 to 8 weeks) for prostatic hypertrophy found that the treatment was well tolerated and that some outcome measures were significantly improved in almost all trials (4). The largest trial in this review tested the effect of placebo versus pygeum (50 mg b.i.d. × 60 days) on residual urine, uroflowmetry, and nocturia in 263 patients (5). Pygeum was significantly better than placebo on quantitative parameters. Overall assessment showed that micturition improved in 66% of those treated with pygeum, compared with 31% of those in the placebo group.
• Another review identified 12 double-blind controlled trials with a total of 717 patients; most studies found improvements in at least one outcome measure (2).
• A recent randomized double-blind controlled trial of 209 patients with BPH (not included in either review mentioned previously) compared a single versus split dose of pygeum extract (50 mg b.i.d. or 100 mg q.d.) for 2 months. Compared with baseline, both groups experienced significant improvement in the International Prostate Symptom Score (IPSS), nocturia, quality of life, and maximum urinary flow rate; differences between the two groups were not significant (6). Residual volume did not change. The primary outcome measure was a reduction of 40% or greater on IPSS; at the end of the 2 months 42.6% in the split-dose group and 40.7% in the single-dose group achieved this goal. In an open-label extension phase of this trial, 174 patients received 100 mg daily for an additional 10 months. The number of patients achieving the targeted reduction in IPSS score increased over time, achieving 62.8% at the 1-year mark. In addition, prostate volume was reduced slightly but significantly (from 42.0 to 39.9 cm³).

• The Andro review identified 13 open-label studies assessing global outcome with a total of 461 patients (doses ranged from 75 to 150 mg daily) and 19 studies with a total of 849 patients (doses ranged from 75 to 200 mg daily) assessing quantitative outcome measures; all open-label trials showed benefit (2).

• A recent open multicenter trial of 85 men aged 50 to 75 years with prostatic hypertrophy treated with pygeum extract 50 mg b.i.d. found a significant improvement in subjective symptom scores. Nocturnal nocturia was reduced by 32%, a significant change from baseline (7).
• Histologic changes

—In 60 men scheduled for surgery for prostatic adenomas, 28 were pretreated with pygeum and 20 were pretreated with prazosin; the remainder served as controls (8). Histologically, those pretreated with pygeum had a predominance of glandular and fibrotic tissue; smooth muscle constituted the smallest part of the adenomas. In patients who had not been pretreated, focal inflammation predominated. In patients pretreated with prazosin, smooth muscle tissue was predominant and postinflammatory lesions were least common among the group.

• Prostatic acid phosphatase activity

—Administration of pygeum apparently increases prostatic acid phosphatase activity in humans (2).

ANIMAL/IN VITRO

• Urogenital tract effects

—In rabbits, pretreatment with pygeum (1, 10, or 100 mg/kg/day × 3 weeks) did not reduce the hypertrophic effect of the bladder to partial outlet obstruction; compared with oil control, only the 100-mg dose of pygeum had a significant protective effect on induced contractile responses to field stimulation, bethanechol, and potassium chloride (KCl) (9). A subsequent controlled study by the same author found similar results; pretreatment with pygeum (100 mg/kg/day × 3 weeks) had no effect on bladder mass after partial obstruction but protected the bladder from contractile responses to field stimulation, bethanechol, and KCl; in addition, enzyme markers for mitochondrial function (citrate synthase) and sarcoplasmic reticulum [calcium adenosine triphosphatase (ATPase)] rebounded to near-normal levels in the pygeum-treated group while remaining reduced in the vehicle-treated group at 1 and 2 weeks (10).
—Pygeum pretreatment in rats reduced the adverse effect of dihydrotestosterone on micturition frequency and reduced prostate weight in the ventral but not the dorsal lobe of the prostate (11).

• Hormonal effects

—Although pygeum is less effective than saw palmetto (*Serenoa repens*) in inhibiting androgen receptors, inhibition is achieved with pygeum at a concentration of 0.98 mg/mL. A synergistic effect is seen when pygeum is combined with an extract of nettles (*Urtica dioica*) (12).
—An estrogenic effect of pygeum extract was demonstrated by increased uterine weight in 4-week-old ovariectomized and adrenalectomized mice (13).

• Inflammation

—Pygeum extract reduces carrageenan-induced inflammation in the rat paw edema test and reduces histamine-induced vascular permeability (2). Both oral and intra-peritoneally administered extracts reduce edema (1).

OTHER CLAIMED BENEFITS/ACTIONS

• Prostatitis

 Risks

ADVERSE REACTIONS

• Pygeum appears to have an excellent safety profile in humans. Reported side effects have primarily been gastrointestinal (2,4).

ANIMAL TOXICITY

• Single doses of up to 8 g/kg in rats and mice indicated a safety coefficient on the order of 2,000 times the therapeutic dose. Up to 375 mg/kg/day in dogs and up to 750 mg/kg/day in rats for up to 6 months caused no adverse hematologic, biochemical, or pathologic changes. Up to 80 mg/kg/day in male rats and rabbits had no effect on fertility (2).

 Dose

COMMON DOSAGE FORMS

• The usual dose is a single dose of 75 to 150 mg/day of a standardized extract.
• Pygeum products are standardized to contain 14% triterpenes and 0.5% n-docosanol (14).

Common Questions and Answers

Q: Why is it unclear whether or not pygeum affects 5-α reductase?
A: Studies are mixed, possibly because of different solvents used. An *in vitro* study using human prostate cells compared several plant extracts to finasteride as a source of 5-α reductase and found that a pygeum extract did not demonstrate significant 5-α reductase activity (15). However, another study found that a methylene chloride pygeum extract inhibited 5-α reductase activity in a concentration-dependent manner, and a pygeum extract in dimethyl sulfoxide (DMSO) significantly inhibited 5-lipoxygenase metabolites at concentrations as low as 3 μg/mL (a lesser effect was seen in an aqueous solution after alkalinization) (12). In any case, pygeum is far less effective than saw palmetto (*Serenoa repens*) in inhibiting 5-α reductase.

Raspberry

10 Second Take

Raspberry leaf is a benign herb, even in pregnancy. No clinical trials have demonstrated efficacy for any condition.

Basics

LATIN NAME

Rubus idaeus L., *Rubus strigosus* Michx

FAMILY

Rosaceae

OTHER COMMON NAMES

None identified

DESCRIPTION

• A tall, prickly shrub with delicious red or black fruits, raspberry is native to Europe, North America, and temperate Asia.

PART USED

Leaves

KNOWN ACTIVE CONSTITUENTS

• Tannins (gallic and ellagic acids), bioflavonoids (rutin, the glycosides of quercetin and kaempferol), polypeptides, vitamin C, citric acid, oxalic acid, calcium, and ferric iron. (1)

MECHANISM/PHARMACOKINETICS

• Tannins could contribute to antidiarrheal effect. No other information identified.

Evidence

CLINICAL TRIALS

• Raspberry leaf preparations are commonly used in at least some populations; a survey of 172 certified nurse midwives regarding what they used to stimulate labor found that of the 90 midwives who used herbal preparations, 63% used red raspberry leaf (2).
• One randomized, placebo-controlled trial has been done (3). In this study, 240 low-risk, nulliparous women (192 completed) in Sydney, Australia, were given placebo or one raspberry leaf tablet [each contained 1.2 g 3:1 extract (400 mg leaf)] twice daily from 32 weeks gestation until labor. There were no significant differences between groups in blood loss, birth weight, Apgar scores, meconium, length of gestation, likelihood of medical augmentation of labor, emergency Cesarean section rate, need for meperidine or epidural block, artificial rupture of membranes, length of labor, or length of any stage of labor. Side effects, primarily gastrointestinal, were evenly distributed between groups.

• A retrospective record review of women who gave birth at Westmead Hospital in Sydney, Australia, found no safety problems for women or their babies when raspberry leaf products were consumed during pregnancy. Investigators approached women during a postnatal visit and asked whether or not they had consumed raspberry leaf products during their pregnancy. Labor and birth outcomes of 57 women who had consumed raspberry leaf products during their pregnancy were compared with 51 controls (randomly selected from hospital records of women who stated they had not consumed raspberry leaf products). The groups were not significantly different in age, weight, parity, ethnicity, and whether they were receiving public or private care. Of those who used raspberry, 56.1% used raspberry leaf tea, 40.4% tablets, and 3.5% combined products (tea, tablets, and tincture). Dosages varied; 75.1% of tea drinkers consumed between 1 to 3 cups daily; the most common dose of tablets was six tablets daily (43.5%). Thirteen percent began using raspberry products between 8 to 28 weeks gestation, 59% from 30 to 34 weeks, and 28% from 35 to 39 weeks. Duration of consumption ranged from 1 to 32 weeks. Six women discontinued raspberry leaf products; two because they disliked the taste, one experienced diarrhea, one experienced increased Braxton-Hicks contractions, one went into labor, and one stated she "took castor oil instead." Maternal safety outcomes assessed included maternal diastolic blood pressure before labor and blood loss at (vaginal) birth. Infant safety outcomes included duration of gestation, 5-minute Apgar, and likelihood of babies being transferred to neonatal special care or intensive care. Labor outcomes included length of stages of labor, likelihood of medical augmentation, need for epidural, occurrence of meconium, and percentage of normal deliveries (4). There were no differences between groups in any labor (or other) outcomes.

ANIMAL/IN VITRO

• Smooth muscle effects

—A crude aqueous saline extract of raspberry leaves has been reported to inhibit contraction of uteri from pregnant rats but apparently had no effect on uteri from nonpregnant rats (5). In strips of human nonpregnant uterus, no effect of the extract was noted (this finding was qualified by the fact that only pathologic human uteri were available). In strips of normal human pregnant uterus (10 to 16 weeks), however, contractions lasting for a few minutes were noted. In most strips of pregnant human or rat uteri that reacted to the extract, contractions became more regular and less frequent over a 20-minute period, as long as the extract stayed in contact with the tissue.
—A 1954 report found that some aqueous fractions of raspberry leaves appeared to stimulate smooth muscle contraction in guinea pig uterus and ileum (6). Another fraction had a spasmolytic effect on guinea pig ileum; in anesthetized cats, intravenous injection of this spasmolytic fraction caused decreased blood pressure and bradycardia (atropine reversed these effects). Experiments also revealed the presence of an anticholinesterase.

• Antioxidant effects

—In a comparison of the total antioxidant capacity of different berries (blackberry, red raspberry, black raspberry, and strawberry), red raspberry fruits had the highest oxygen radicals absorbance capacity (ORAC), a measure of antioxidant capacity, in the ripe stage; compared with fruits, leaves of species tested generally had even higher ORAC values than fruit (7).

OTHER CLAIMED BENEFITS/ACTIONS

• Sore throat
• Ulcers, wounds, chronic skin conditions, conjunctivitis (topical)
• Gastrointestinal problems
• Respiratory tract problems
• Fever
• Cardiovascular system
• Diarrhea
• Morning sickness
• Preventing miscarriage
• Reducing labor pain
• Dysmenorrhea
• Menorrhagia
• Diabetes

 Risks

ADVERSE REACTIONS

None reported

DRUG INTERACTIONS

None reported

PREGNANCY/LACTATION

Indirect evidence indicates that raspberry leaf products are safe to use during pregnancy (see evidence).

ANIMAL TOXICITY

No information identified

 DOSE

• *Dried leaf:* 4 to 8 g dried raspberry leaf powder or tablets t.i.d.
• *Infusion:* 4 to 8 g as infusion t.i.d.
• *Tea:* 1.5 g (1 to 2 tsp) finely chopped leaf in boiling water, strained after 5 minutes

Red Clover

10 Second Take

Traditionally used for cancer and currently promoted for menopausal symptoms, there is no convincing evidence of efficacy for either claim.

Basics

LATIN NAME

Trifolium pratense L.

FAMILY

Leguminosae

OTHER COMMON NAMES

Purple clover, trefoil, cowgrass, and pavine clover

DESCRIPTION

• Red clover is a nitrogen-fixing perennial that grows up to 2 ft tall. It has red or purple globular "flowers" (actually collections of tiny florets).

PART USED

Flowers

KNOWN ACTIVE CONSTITUENTS

• Red clover contains notable amounts of at least four estrogenic isoflavones: formononetin, biochanin A, daidzein, and genistein. Flowers also contain salicylic acid, *p*-coumaric acid, isorhamnetin glucosides (including trifolianol, a phytosterol glucoside), trifolin, trifolitin, rhamnose, isotrofilin, pratol, pratensol, *trans* and *cis*-cloramide, and phaseolic acid (1).

MECHANISM/PHARMACOKINETICS

• Formononetin, biochanin A, daidzein, and genistein are phytoestrogens, capable of stimulating estrogen receptors and inducing biologic responses.

Evidence

CLINICAL TRIALS

• Hot flashes and other menopausal symptoms

—Two double-blind, placebo-controlled trials of a standardized red clover extract found no benefit of red clover extract on hot flashes. In one crossover trial study of red clover extract, 51 women (whose last menses was at least 6 months past) having at least three hot flashes a day were randomized to one daily tablet of placebo or red clover extract (containing 40 mg total isoflavones, including genistein 4 mg, daidzein 3.5 mg, biochanin 24.5 mg, and formononetin 8.0 mg) (2). The first phase of the trial lasted for 3 months, followed by a 1-month washout period, after which they were crossed over to the other arm for 14 weeks (3 months plus an additional 2 weeks, to accommodate the possibility of change in reporting habits that might occur at the end of a trial). Symptom diaries using the Greene Menopause Score (a validated symptom self-assessment scale) were kept by the participants. At the beginning of the trial, and at the conclusion of each treatment arm, participants underwent a medical examination and blood tests [complete blood count (CBC), liver function tests, and levels of follicle-stimulating hormone (FSH), estradiol, and sex hormone binding globulin (SHBG)]. A 24-hour urine sample was also collected for analysis of genistein, daidzein, formononetin, and biochanin A. A vaginal smear (for vaginal maturation index) was collected, and transvaginal ultrasound was performed to assess endometrial thickness.
Forty-three women completed the study. Hot flush frequency decreased in both placebo and active groups at 12 weeks (about 18% and 20%, respectively), but there were no statistically significant differences between groups in Greene Scores at any timepoint. No significant differences were seen between groups in SHBG levels, blood counts, serum electrolytes, urea, creatinine, or liver function tests. No change in body weight was observed in either group. There were no differences between groups in endometrial thickness or vaginal epithelium in the vaginal maturation index between treatment groups at the beginning and end of the trial. Information on adverse events was not reported.
—In another trial of the effects of red clover extract on menopausal symptoms (3), 37 postmenopausal women having at least three hot flushes per day were randomized to placebo or one of two doses of red clover extract (40 mg or 160 mg) for 12 weeks. Endpoints were similar to the previous trial. Hot flush frequency decreased in all groups over the 12 weeks (35%, 29%, 34%); there was no significant difference among the three groups. There were no significant differences from baseline in any group in FSH, SHBG, vaginal maturation scores, or vaginal pH (the latter two are biologic indicators of

estrogenicity). Serum high density lipoprotein (HDL)-cholesterol levels increased significantly by 18% ($p = 0.038$) in participants taking the 40-mg dose; HDL levels for those taking 160 mg were not different from the placebo group. These data are not possible to evaluate without the total cholesterol levels. The ratio of HDL to total cholesterol is important; if the increase in HDL is due to an increase in total cholesterol, this may not be a benefit. In addition, because the higher dose did not result in a beneficial effect on HDL, it is questionable whether this effect will stand up in future trials. Nowhere in the paper is there a report of adverse events.

• Arterial compliance and lipids

—A third double-blind trial with an unusual design compared the effects of two doses of standardized red clover extract on arterial compliance and plasma lipids in the same group; a much smaller group took placebo. After a 3 to 4 week run-in followed by a 5-week placebo phase, 26 women were randomized either to one tablet of red clover extract (40 mg) or placebo, in a 4:1 ratio (4). After 5 weeks, those on red clover extract had their doses doubled to 80 mg for another 5 weeks, while those receiving placebo continued on placebo. The dropout rate was very high. Nineteen women underwent lipid assessment; 17 underwent measurements of arterial compliance at the end of the first intervention; and only 16 women (including 3 in the placebo group) completed the study. Because the placebo group was so small, those results were not statistically analyzed; comparisons were made among the treatment group at different phases (placebo, 40 mg, 80 mg).
In those who completed the study, a significant increase in arterial compliance was found during the 40- and 80-mg phases, compared with the placebo phase, with no significant difference between 40- and 80-mg doses. There were no significant changes in plasma lipoprotein levels. This trial suffers from problems in blinding and placebo control and, furthermore, had a high dropout rate.

OTHER CLAIMED BENEFITS/ACTIONS

• Cancer treatment
• Cancer prevention
• Heart disease prevention
• Expectorant
• Bronchitis
• Burns, ulcers, sores, athlete's foot (external washes)
• Constipation
• Diuretic
• Rheumatism
• Asthma (smoked)

Risks

ADVERSE REACTIONS

• No adverse reactions have been reported; however, none of the published clinical trials have reported adverse effects (in most studies it is unclear whether this information was gathered). There are theoretical concerns about estrogenic effects on endometrium or breast (see questions and answers).

DRUG INTERACTIONS

• None reported.

ANIMAL TOXICITY

• Clovers may be eaten by grazing animals and can be associated with significant toxicity; white clover (*T. repens*) contains a cyanogenic glycoside and is the species most commonly associated with poisonings (5). Subterranean clover (*T. subterraneum*), like red clover, contains large amounts of phytoestrogens, and its consumption by sheep in Australia in the 1940s resulted in what has come to be known as "clover disease"; infertility, abnormal lactation, dystocia, and prolapsed uterus were attributed to estrogenic effects (6). In ovariectomized sheep, red clover silage causes clear estrogenic effects, including enlargement of the vulva, uterus, udder, and teats, as well as secretion of a milky fluid (6).

 Dose

COMMON DOSAGE FORMS

• Tablets containing solid extract (usually 40 mg)
• *Dried flowerheads:* 2 to 4 g t.i.d.
• *Infusion* made with 2 to 4 g herb taken t.i.d.
• *Fluid extract:* (1:1, 25% ethanol) 1.5 to 4 mL t.i.d.
• *Tincture:* (1:10, 45% ethanol) ½ to 2 mL t.i.d.
• *Topical use:* Infusion, liquid extract, or ointment containing 10% to 15% of flowerheads

 Common Questions and Answers

Q: Does red clover cause estrogenic stimulation of breast or endometrium?
A: Two studies have found no increased endometrial thickness by ultrasound; however, one of these studies was only 8 weeks long (7) and the other 14 weeks long (2). Neither was long enough to adequately assess estrogenic effects on endometrium. This is definitely of concern, especially given known estrogenic effects in grazing animals; admittedly sheep are particularly sensitive to phytoestrogens in fodder, but humans manifest biologic responses to phytoestrogens as well. Breast cancer cell stimulation is also a concern. In one bioactivity assay, red clover was in the top 5% of 150 herbs tested in a binding assay for both estradiol and progesterone binding (8).

Q: Isn't clover used as human food?
A: Clover is edible, but is consumed only in small quantities, and is not commonly eaten. Unlike soybeans (also rich in phytoestrogens), clover has never been a dietary staple of humans. Clovers are occasionally consumed in small quantities as a tea or flavoring, and even that use is among limited populations. In parts of Asia, powdered leaves and flower heads are sprinkled onto rice (9); clover leaves may be put into soups (10). Aztec clover (*Trifolium amabile*) is used in Latin America and mixed with white corn and other herbs by Peruvian Indians, and leaves and stems of *Trifolium ciliatum* are used by the Luisena Indians of California (11). Flower heads and sprouts may be eaten; red clover is considered generally recognized as safe (GRAS). Solid extract may be used in food products, usually at less than 20 ppm, but jams and jellies may contain 525 ppm (1). Most of these uses are uncommon today.

Q: Where do the anticancer claims for red clover come from?
A: It was included in Harry Hoxsey's anticancer formula, a famous cancer remedy popular in the 1940s. The formula contained barberry, buckthorn, burdock, cascara, red clover, licorice, poke, prickly ash, and stillingia (along with topically applied bloodroot). The story goes that the originator of the formula was Hoxsey's great grandfather, who observed a horse with cancer put out to pasture who recovered after eating herbs in the field (Duke, personal communication, 2001). Red clover's anticancer properties are also touted in Jethro Kloss' *Back to Eden,* which states that "Red clover is one of God's greatest blessings to man ... Combined with equal parts of blue violet, burdock, yellow dock, dandelion root, rock rose and goldenseal, it is a most powerful remedy for cancerous growths ... " (12).

Riboflavin (Vitamin B$_2$)

 10 Second Take

Riboflavin is a benign B vitamin that may be helpful in migraine prophylaxis.

 Basics

DESCRIPTION

• Riboflavin is a water-soluble B vitamin that is an enzyme cofactor necessary to all metabolic processes [especially the production of adenosine triphosphate (ATP) through oxidation of glucose and fatty acid] and the support of anabolic processes. Riboflavin is not stored.

FOOD SOURCES

• Milk, eggs, organ meats, nuts, seeds, wheat germ, green vegetables, and yeast. In the United States, major sources are milk products and enriched breads and cereals. Small amounts are found in beer and wine.

MECHANISM/PHARMACOKINETICS

• Riboflavin is involved in various oxidation-reduction reactions as part of two coenzymes, flavin adenine dinucleotide (FAD) and flavin mononucleotide (FMN). Its most important roles are in the succinic dehydrogenase reaction (which links the Krebs cycle to oxidative phosphorylation) and in the pathways necessary to synthesis and oxidation of fatty acids (1).

 Evidence

CLINICAL TRIALS

• Migraine

—A randomized, placebo-controlled trial in 55 patients with migraine found that 400 mg riboflavin daily for 3 months was superior to placebo in reducing attack frequency and headache days (2). The proportion of patients who improved by at least 50% was 59% in the riboflavin group and 15% in the placebo group. Two of three patients who reported mild adverse effects (polyuria and diarrhea) were in the treatment group.
—A previous open-label pilot study by the same investigators compared 26 patients who received 400 mg riboflavin daily for 3 months with 23 patients who received both riboflavin and low-dose (75 mg) aspirin (3). Mean global improvement was 68.2%; there were no significant differences between the groups. One patient in the riboflavin with aspirin group withdrew because of gastric intolerance; otherwise no adverse effects were reported.
—The dose of riboflavin used in these trials is high, about 300 times higher than the recommended daily allowance (RDA). However, riboflavin is extraordinarily benign.

• Sickle cell anemia

—A small trial of riboflavin supplementation (5 mg b.i.d. for 8 weeks) in 30 sickle cell patients did not find a benefit; serum iron and transferrin saturation increased significantly in 18 supplemented patients, compared with 12 unsupplemented patients. Compared with baseline, reduced glutathione levels in supplemented patients also fell significantly. Total iron-binding capacity (TIBC), hemoglobin levels, and serum ferritin levels did not change significantly (4).

• Lactic acidosis

—A case series noted that riboflavin treatment quickly resolved nucleoside analog-induced lactic acidosis in three AIDS patients (5).

• Cataract

—A comparison of various groups with and without cataract found that riboflavin deficiency was significantly more common among older cataract patients than older subjects with clear lenses. However, riboflavin deficiency was not associated with early cataract formation (6).

OTHER CLAIMED BENEFITS/ACTIONS

• Acne
• Muscle cramps
• Anxiety
• Depression
• Carpal tunnel syndrome
• Stress

 Clinical Considerations

Gross riboflavin deficiency is very rare in Western countries. Mild or marginal deficiency may not be uncommon, however, among older adults and among those who do not consume milk products (1). Pregnant women and poor people are also at risk for marginal deficiency. One study of adolescents of low socioeconomic status in New York City found that the prevalence of riboflavin deficiency among those who were not taking vitamin supplements was 26.6% (7).

DEFICIENCY SIGNS AND SYMPTOMS

• Lack of riboflavin causes vascularization of the cornea, photophobia, glossitis, angular stomatitis, and seborrheic dermatitis (especially in the external genital area and nose). Although pellagra is a disease caused by niacin deficiency, riboflavin can relieve some of the symptoms of pellagra.
• Deficiency depresses humoral antibody response to test antigens in animals.
• Deficiency causes cataract in kittens. Studies are mixed on whether deficiency causes cataract in rats.

FACTORS DECREASING AVAILABILITY/ABSORPTION

• Light: Riboflavin is very light-labile; thus, milk should not be stored in glass bottles that are exposed to light.
• Refinement of whole grains removes most of the riboflavin.
• Phenothiazines interfere with riboflavin metabolism.
• Tricyclic antidepressants interfere with riboflavin metabolism.
• Kaolin decreases absorption.
• Negative nitrogen balance (for example, in acute infection) increases urinary losses of riboflavin.

FACTORS INCREASING AVAILABILITY/ABSORPTION

• Food, fiber, phosphates, and lactose all promote riboflavin absorption.

LABORATORY TESTS

- The best indicator of riboflavin status, and the most convenient to measure, is an increase in the erythrocyte glutathione reductase (EGR) activity coefficient. Levels above 1.3 are generally indicative of deficiency. This test is not useful for differentiating levels of deficiency because it plateaus quickly and will not respond to further decreases in tissue reserves of riboflavin (1). Anything that interferes with riboflavin metabolism will interfere with this test.
- Decreased urinary riboflavin levels are also associated with low dietary intake. A 24-hour collection should be done; values of less than 27 μg/g of creatinine are indicative of deficiency in adults. Spurious elevations may be caused by fasting, heat stress, bedrest, or negative nitrogen balance.
- Whole blood, erythrocyte, or plasma levels are not very reliable.

 Risks

DRUG INTERACTIONS

- Phenothiazines, including chlorpromazine, and tricyclic antidepressants interfere with riboflavin metabolism.
- Riboflavin interferes with the TDx drugs-of-abuse assay; B$_2$ is a fluorescent compound that competes with the fluorescein-labeled antibody (8).
- Riboflavin may turn the urine orange (a harmless effect).

ANIMAL TOXICITY

- Toxicity is low to nonexistent. In dogs, 2 g/kg p.o. caused no ill effects; in rats, LD$_{50}$ is 560 g/kg i.p.

 Dose

COMMON DOSAGE FORMS

- The protein complexes of flavin coenzymes include FMN and FAD. FMN is better absorbed than free riboflavin, which is better absorbed than FAD.
- Oral (tablet or liquid) preparations contain free riboflavin; intramuscular or intravenous formulations contain FMN.

RECOMMENDED DIETARY ALLOWANCE

Infants and children

0 to 6 months	0.3 mg/day (adequate intake)
7 to 12 months	0.4 mg/day (adequate intake)
1 to 3 years	0.5 mg/day
4 to 8 years	0.6 mg/day

Males

9 to 13 years	0.9 mg/day
14 to 50 years	1.3 mg/day
51+ years	1.3 mg/day

Females

9 to 13 years	0.9 mg/day
14 to 18 years	1.0 mg/day
19 to 50 years	1.1 mg/day
51+ years	1.1 mg/day
Pregnant	1.4 mg/day
Lactating	1.6 mg/day

- Correcting deficiency

—A dose of 50 to 100 mg p.o. daily or 25 mg i.m. twice weekly for several weeks will correct deficiency.

—For supplementation in at-risk populations, a B-complex preparation containing 25 to 100 mg of riboflavin daily is sufficient.

 Common Questions and Answers

Q: Who should take riboflavin supplements?
A: Supplementation should be considered in older adults, anyone who does not consume dairy products, alcoholics, people with glucose-6-phosphate deficiency, and those taking phenothiazines or tricyclic antidepressants. In the presence of alcohol, riboflavin supplements are better absorbed than dietary riboflavin (9).

Rosemary

10 Second Take

Rosemary is a benign delicious herb with interesting physiologic effects; however, clinical trials of its use for specific conditions are lacking.

Basics

LATIN NAME

Rosmarinus officinalis L.

FAMILY

Labiateae/Lamiaceae

OTHER COMMON NAMES

Rosemarine, romero (Spanish)

DESCRIPTION

• An aromatic, evergreen shrub, about 3 ft high, with pale blue to bluish violet axillary flowers. Creeping rosemary (*R. prostratus*) is a common ground cover in the western United States.

PART USED

Flowering tops (leaves and flowers)

KNOWN ACTIVE CONSTITUENTS

• Rosemary has 1% to 2.5% essential oil containing 1,8-cineole (20% to 50%), α-pinene (15% to 25%), and camphor (10% to 25%); bornyl acetate (1% to 5%), borneol, (1% to 6%), camphene (5% to 10%), and α-terpineol (12% to 24%); smaller amounts of limonene, β-pinene, β-caryophyllene, and myrcene (1). Also contains phenolic acids (including rosmarinic and labiatic acids), caffeic acids, chlorogenic acids, phenolic diterpenes, flavonoids, and triterpenoids (1).

MECHANISM/PHARMACOKINETICS

• In mice, inhalation of rosemary oil results in detectable levels of 1,8-cineole in the blood. Anticarcinogenic effects are thought to involve inhibition of P450 isoenzymes that metabolically activate procarcinogens and induction of the detoxification pathway involving glutathione *S*-transferase and other Phase II enzymes (2). Smooth muscle relaxing effects are thought to be due to inhibiting the increase in intracellular free calcium levels (3).

Evidence

CLINICAL TRIALS

• Alopecia areata

—A study of 86 patients with alopecia areata compared a topical mixture of essential oils including thyme, rosemary, lavender, and cedar wood with placebo oil; each was rubbed into the scalp daily for 7 months. Sequential photographs were rated on an alopecia scale by blinded observers. The primary outcome measure was improvement versus no improvement; 19 (44%) of 43 patients in the essential oil group showed improvement compared with 6 (15%) of 41 patients in the control group. The degree of improvement on photographic assessment was also significant (4).

ANIMAL/IN VITRO

• Anticancer effects

—Topical application of rosemary extract reduced carcinogen-induced skin tumors in mice. In rats, rosemary extract administered for 21 weeks (1% of the diet) reduced 9,10 dimethyl-1,2 benzanthracene (DMBA)-induced mammary tumors; the incidence of mammary carcinoma was 76% in the control group compared with 40% in the treated group (1). In another study of DMBA-induced mammary tumors in rats, rats were fed rosemary extract (0.5% by weight), carnosol (1.0%), or ursolic acid (0.5%) for 2 weeks (5). Rosemary extract, but not carnosol or ursolic acid, significantly reduced the formation of DNA adducts in the mammary glands of DMBA-treated rats, compared with controls. When injected intraperitoneally for 5 days at a dose of 200 mg/kg body weight, rosemary significantly decreased mammary adduct formation by 44%; carnosol reduced adduct formation by 40%, and ursolic acid had no effect. Intraperitoneal injection of the same doses of rosemary and carnosol decreased DMBA-induced mammary adenocarcinomas by 74% and 65%, respectively. Ursolic acid was ineffective at inhibiting mammary adduct formation and for reducing mammary tumors.
—Rosemary oil has cytotoxic effects on leukemia cells (1).
—Rosemary extract, carnosol, or carnosic acid are potent inhibitors of carcinogen-induced DNA adduct formation in human liver and bronchial cells (2).

• Gingivitis

—In a placebo-controlled trial, rosmarinic acid significantly reduced the progression of gingivitis in Rhesus monkeys (6).

• Increased bile flow

—Intravenous injection of a freeze-dried ethanolic tincture of rosemary (equivalent to 5.5 mg dried young shoots) significantly increased bile flow in bile duct-cannulated rats; an extract of young shoots appeared superior to a whole-plant extract.

• Blood sugar levels

—Intramuscular injection of essential oil of rosemary (25 mg/kg) increased plasma glucose levels 2%, 27%, and 55% above that of control animals at 60, 90, and 120 minutes after intraperitoneal administration of glucose. At 30 minutes, insulin levels of treated rabbits were 30% below those of control rabbits. In alloxan-diabetic rabbits, rosemary oil (25 mg/kg) increased fasting plasma glucose levels 17% above levels of control animals 6 hours after administration (3).
—In female mice fed a 2% rosemary diet, the liver microsomal glucuronidation of estradiol and estrone was stimulated, 2-hydroxylation increased 150%, and 16α-hydroxylation of estradiol decreased by 50%. In the same report, a 2% rosemary diet decreased the uterotropic effects of estradiol and estrone on oophorectomized mice by 35% to 50%, compared with controls (7).

• Neurologic effects

—In mice, a 10% extract of rosemary delayed the onset of picrotoxin-induced seizures and reduced mortality in mice (1). In mice, inhalation of 0.5 mL of rosemary oil resulted in increased locomotor activity in mice.

• Inflammation

—Rosmarinic acid reduces rat paw edema. A topically applied methanolic extract reduced induced inflammation and hyperplasia in the skin of mice.

• Hepatotoxicity

—In rats, *R. tomentosus* reduced carbon tetrachloride-induced hepatotoxicity; it reduced alanine transaminase (ALT) and bilirubin, and reduced levels of malondialdehyde (a byproduct of decomposition of lipid peroxides) in the liver (8).

- Smooth muscle relaxation

—An ethanolic extract of rosemary oil inhibited acetylcholine-induced contraction in rabbit trachealis muscle and inhibited histamine-induced stimulation of guinea pig trachealis muscle. An ethanolic extract of rosemary inhibited acetylcholine-induced contraction of guinea pig ileum. In guinea pigs, essential oil of rosemary in a dose of 25 mg/kg counteracted opiate-induced blockage of Oddi's sphincter (1).

- Antimicrobial effects

—Rosemary oil has antibacterial and antifungal effects against a variety of organisms. A dry ethanolic extract of rosemary inhibited the growth of herpes simplex virus type 2 *in vitro*. Carnosolic acid has some activity against HIV-1 viral replication [inhibitory concentration (IC)90 = 0.32 μg/mL] (1).

OTHER CLAIMED BENEFITS/ACTIONS

- Dyspepsia, digestive problems
- Bloating, flatulence
- Biliary problems
- Hepatic problems
- Promotion of wound healing (topical)
- Peripheral vascular disease (topical)

 Risks

ADVERSE REACTIONS

- No adverse reactions associated with consumption of rosemary leaves have been reported. Consumption of essential oil of rosemary can cause gastroenteritis or nephritis (9).

PREGNANCY/LACTATION

- No information available; however, some sources state that it should not be used in pregnancy.

ANIMAL TOXICITY

- In an acute toxicity study, rat and mice were given a single intraperitoneal dose of an alcohol extract of rosemary in a dose of 2 g/kg. No abnormalities were seen in behavior over 15 days nor were there gross abnormalities on autopsy (1).

 Dose

COMMON DOSAGE FORMS

- *Dried leaf:* 2 to 4 g t.i.d.
- *Infusion:* 2 to 4 g as infusion daily t.i.d. (total daily dose less than 6 g)
- *Fluid extract:* (1:1, 45% ethanol V/V) 1.5 to 3 mL daily
- *Tincture:* (1:5, 70% ethanol) 3 to 8.5 mL daily
- *Dry normalized extract:* 4.5 to 5.5:1 (w/w) 0.36 to 0.44 g t.i.d.
- Topical uses include baths, ointments, and fomentations (cloths saturated in hot infusion, then wrung out)
- Topical preparation for alopecia areata: *Rosmarinus officinalis* (3 drops, 114 mg), *Thymus vulgaris* (2 drops, 88 mg), *Lavandula angustifolia* (3 drops, 108 mg), and *Cedrus atlantica* (2 drops, 94 mg) in a carrier oil containing 3 mL jojoba oil and 20 mL grapeseed oil.

Royal Jelly

 10 Second Take

Royal jelly is purported to lower cholesterol and prevent atherosclerosis; credible evidence is lacking. Allergic reactions are not uncommon, especially in atopic individuals.

 Basics

DESCRIPTION

- Royal jelly is a glandular secretion from young honeybees (*Apis mellifera*) used to feed larvae. Those larvae destined to become workers receive royal jelly as part of their diet, whereas larvae destined to become queens are fed exclusively royal jelly (and are provided larger beeswax cells in which to develop).

KNOWN ACTIVE CONSTITUENTS

- Royal jelly contains about 67% water, 12% proteins, 12% sugars, 5% fats, 1% minerals, and 2% other (1). Royal jelly contains vitamin C and most of the vitamin B complex (2). Phytosterol content is high (95 μg/ 100 mg); the dominant phytosterol is β-sitosterol (1). A specific fatty acid is *trans*-10-hydroxy-2-decenoic acid (10-HDA). Royal jelly also contains about 20 mg/kg methyl *p*-hydroxybenzoate (methylparaben) (3).
- Royalisin, a potent antibacterial protein, was purified from royal jelly; it was active against Gram-positive but not Gram-negative bacteria (4).

MECHANISM/PHARMACOKINETICS

- Specific mechanisms have not been well defined. Royal jelly is thought to decrease gastrointestinal absorption of cholesterol and increase its excretion in bile; it may suppress hepatic sterol synthesis (1). In addition, β-sitosterol may block the uptake of cholesterol by competition for sterol binding sites on enterocyte membranes (1).

 Evidence

CLINICAL TRIALS

- Hypercholesterolemia

—Five placebo-controlled studies, none in English, have been published on the use of royal jelly for hypercholesterolemia (1). The total number of patients was 133 (81 treated with royal jelly and 52 treated with placebo). Three trials used injections of royal jelly (10 to 100 mg/day) and two used oral forms (30 to 150 mg/day). A significant effect was found in every trial; the mean decrease in cholesterol was 34 mg/dL. All trials suffered from methodological deficiencies, including poor characterization of disease status and lack of documentation of diet, weight, or concurrent medications (1).

ANIMAL/IN VITRO

- Cardiovascular effects

—In rats and rabbits, royal jelly decreased serum and liver total lipids and cholesterol levels. Royal jelly also decreased the formation of aortic atheromas in rabbits fed an atherogenic diet (1). In rats, royal jelly increased prothrombin time. In dogs, injected royal jelly caused vasodilation of coronary arteries and hepatic veins (1).

- Anti-inflammatory effects

—Oral administration of royal jelly in streptozotocin-diabetic rats showed some antiinflammatory activity and shortened the healing period of desquamated skin lesions. Doses up to 1,000 mg/kg/day did not show any hypoglycemic effects in diabetic rats (5).

- Immunomodulatory effects

—In mice and rats administered royal jelly parenterally and immunized with sheep red blood cells, some immunomodulatory effects were demonstrated but were not consistent. In mice, plaque-forming splenocytes and peripheral blood lymphocytes were increased while neutrophils were decreased; in rats, serum immunoglobulins and total proteins were decreased (6).

OTHER CLAIMED BENEFITS/ACTIONS

- Lowers blood pressure
- Prevents atherosclerosis

Risks

ADVERSE REACTIONS

• Atopy

—A survey of 1,472 hospital employees in Hong Kong found that 461 (31.3%) had used royal jelly. Nine reported atopic reactions including asthma, eczema, rhinitis, and urticaria (7). The 176 respondents underwent skin testing as did 300 consecutive asthma clinic patients; 7.4% of the questionnaire respondents and 7.3% of the asthma clinic attendees had positive skin reactions to pure royal jelly. All but one of the 36 participants with positive royal jelly skin tests were also atopic to other common allergens.
—Immunoassays of sera from seven subjects who experienced asthma or anaphylaxis from royal jelly demonstrated true IgE-mediated hypersensitivity reactions (8). Eighteen different IgE-binding components were found in protein blotting studies.

• Hemorrhagic colitis

—There is a case report of hemorrhagic colitis in a 53-year-old woman who had ingested royal jelly for 25 days (9). A drug-induced lymphocyte stimulation test was slightly positive for royal jelly.

CONTRAINDICATIONS

• Hypersensitivity. Atopic individuals are more likely to be allergic to royal jelly.

 Dose

COMMON DOSAGE FORMS

• *Injections*: 10 to 100 mg/day
• *Oral*: 30 to 150 mg/day
• *Sublingual*: 30+ mg/day

 Common Questions and Answers

Q: What is the quality of marketed royal jelly products?
A: In a study of 39 commercial products analyzed by liquid chromatography, samples labeled as pure royal jelly contained concentrations of 10-HDA, a fatty acid specific to royal jelly, in concentrations ranging from 1.98% to 6.37%. Products labeled as containing royal jelly as an ingredient contained levels of 10-HDA ranging from undetectable to 1.28% (10).

Q: Is there a relationship between allergy to bee venom and to royal jelly?
A: There was no direct relationship between IgE antibody reactivity to bee venom allergens and to royal jelly proteins, although more than a third of the sera reacted to a royal jelly solid phase. More than half of participants with respiratory or food allergies demonstrated IgE antibody reactivity to royal jelly proteins (8).

Sage

 10 Second Take

Sage contains thujone, which is toxic, and in uncooked form should not be consumed chronically.

 Basics

LATIN NAME

Salvia officinalis L.

FAMILY

Labiatae/Lamiaceae

OTHER COMMON NAMES

Garden sage, true sage, broad-leafed sage

DESCRIPTION

A small shrub (up to 70 cm tall), sage has very aromatic leaves and blue-violet flowers arranged in whorls.

PART USED

Leaves

KNOWN ACTIVE CONSTITUENTS

• Up to 2.5% essential oil, consisting of α-thujone (up to 60%) and β-thujone (up to 10%) and other monoterpenoids (particularly cineole and camphor); diterpenoids and triterpenoids (especially oleanolic acid), flavonoids, and phenolic compounds (including rosmarinic, labiatic, and caffeic acids) [1,2]; also contains 3% to 7% tannins [3]. Three phenolic glycosides were recently identified that had moderate antioxidant effects [4].

MECHANISM/PHARMACOKINETICS

• No information available. However, thujone (especially β-thujone) is highly toxic.

 Evidence

CLINICAL TRIALS

• A study of an aqueous extract of fresh sage found that pilocarpine-induced sweating was inhibited by the preparation. In an open, 4-week study of 80 patients with idiopathic hyperhidrosis, two preparations of sage (440 mg dried aqueous extract equivalent to 2.6 g of sage) or an infusion made from 4.5 g of sage reduced sweat secretion (the extract was slightly more effective) [1].

ANIMAL/IN VITRO

• Sage oil has activity against Gram-positive and Gram-negative bacteria, fungi, and yeast and has antiviral activity against vesicular stomatitis virus [1].

OTHER CLAIMED BENEFITS/ACTIONS

• Inflammation of oral mucosa
• Pharyngitis
• Dyspepsia
• Hot flashes
• Night sweats
• Excessive sweating
• Cessation of lactation
• Hypotensive
• Menses induction

Risks

ADVERSE REACTIONS

• No adverse events attributed to sage have been reported. However, sage contains thujone (also found in wormwood), which appears to act as a central nervous system poison.

PREGNANCY/LACTATION

• No information available. However, the use of sage is not recommended during pregnancy or lactation.

ANIMAL TOXICITY

• In rats, intraperitoneal injection of sage oil caused convulsions at doses above 0.5 g/kg; doses above 3.2 g/kg were lethal. In rats, the oral LD_{50} of the essential oil was 2.6 g/kg.
• The oral LD_{50} of mixed α- and β-thujones was 192 mg/kg in rats, 230 mg/kg in mice, and 395 mg/kg in guinea pigs (1).

 Dose

COMMON DOSAGE FORMS

• Regular internal use is not recommended because sage contains thujone.
• *Dried leaf:* 1 to 3 g t.i.d.
• *Infusion:* Made with 1 to 3 g t.i.d.
• *Tincture:* (1:10, 55% ethanol) 1 to 3 mL t.i.d.
• *Extract:* 160 mg dried aqueous extract t.i.d.
• *Fluid extract:* 1:1 (g/mL) 1 to 3 mL t.i.d.
• *Dry aqueous extract:* 1:1 (g/mL) 1 to 3 mL t.i.d.
• Topical uses

—Gargle: Made from an infusion (3 g/ 150 mL) or 2 to 3 drops of essential oil in 100 mL water; or use 5 mL of fluid extract diluted in one glass water, several times daily
—Aqueous or ethanolic extracts are sometimes applied topically.

 Common Questions and Answers

Q: So is it dangerous putting a lot of sage into my turkey stuffing?
A: No, go ahead and enjoy your turkey. It has been in the oven a long time and thujone is inactivated by heat. However, merely pouring boiling water over dried herb to make tea or infusion is not enough to inactivate thujone. Intake of thujone over time causes neurological damage (thujone is the toxin in absinthe that led to its ban in almost every country) (5) (see wormwood entry). Very tiny amounts of thujone are permitted in certain flavoring extracts and liqueurs.

Sarsaparilla

10 Second Take

Sarsaparilla is a benign herb. It does not contain testosterone, and no clinical trials support its use.

Basics

LATIN NAME

Smilax aristolochiifolia Mill., syn. *Smilax medica* Schltdl. & Cham. and other *Smilax* species

FAMILY

Liliaceae (Smilicaceae)

OTHER COMMON NAMES

Mexican sarsaparilla, *zarzaparilla* (Spanish) (*S. medica*)

DESCRIPTION

• Sarsaparilla is a tropical, woody perennial climbing vine native to tropical America and the West Indies. It has small, greenish or yellowish flowers and berries that may be black, blue, or red. It prefers damp forest soil.

PART USED

Root and rhizomes

KNOWN ACTIVE CONSTITUENTS

• Steroidal saponins (1% to 3%) based on the aglycones sarsasapogenin and smilagenin; the major one is parillin (sarsaponin), the 2'6'-diglucosyl-4'-rhamnosyl-3-glucoside of sarsasapogenin, along with desgluco-parillin and desgluco-desrhamnoparillin (1). Also present is sarsaparilloside, a bidesmosidic saponin that can be hydrolyzed to parillin. Phytosterols, including beta-sitosterol and E-sitosterol, sitosterol glucoside, and stigmasterol. Abundant starch (50%), resin (2.5%), sarsapic acid, and potassium (1.25%) (1).

Evidence

CLINICAL TRIALS

No clinical trials identified.

ANIMAL/IN VITRO

• An aqueous extract from *Smilax glabra* inhibits delayed-type hypersensitivity without suppressing humoral immune response and inhibits adjuvant-induced arthritis in rats (2). Smilax also inhibits carrageenan-induced rat paw edema (2,3).
• *Smilax* may increase insulin sensitivity. Four hours after intraperitoneal administration of a methanol extract of *Smilax glabra,* blood glucose of normal mice and KK-Ay mice was reduced; there was no effect on glucose levels in streptozotocin-induced diabetes in mice (4).
• A recently isolated flavanone, smitilbin, reduced alanine transaminase (ALT) release from hepatocytes from mice with immunologic liver injury (5).

OTHER CLAIMED BENEFITS/ACTIONS

• Psoriasis
• Eczema
• Body building
• Rheumatoid arthritis
• Diuretic
• Antiinflammatory

Risks

ADVERSE REACTIONS

- Occupational asthma has been associated with sarsaparilla root dust (6).

 Dose

COMMON DOSAGE FORMS

- *Dried root:* 1 to 4 g t.i.d.
- *Decoction:* made from 1 to 4 g of herb t.i.d.
- *Liquid extract:* (1:1, 50% ethanol) 2 to 4 mL t.i.d.

 Common Questions and Answers

Q: Does sarsaparilla have aphrodisiac properties?
A: Sarsaparilla is a common ingredient in preparations meant to boost male potency. It has been claimed to contain testosterone, but this is not true. Sarsasapogenin, a saponin that occurs in some *Smilax* species, can be converted into testosterone in the laboratory, but there is no evidence that this conversion can take place in the body.

Q: Are there nonmedicinal uses of sarsaparilla?
A: Sarsaparilla is approved as a flavoring extract and has been used to flavor root beer; it has also been used as a foaming agent. The popularity of sarsaparilla has waxed and waned since at least the 16th century when it was most commonly used to treat syphilis. At the turn of the 20th century it was promoted as a panacea (7).

Q: Aren't there other plants called sarsaparilla?
A: Yes, and although sarsaparilla products may contain other species of *Smilax*, they are often adulterated with plants that are not even in the same family. Canadian sarsaparilla (*Aralia nudicaulis*) and Indian or false sarsaparilla (*Hemidesmus indicus*) are not related to *Smilax*, nor do they contain the same saponins. *Hemidesmus indicus* is interesting, though. A constituent of its root extract, 2-hydroxy-4-methoxy benzoic acid, has an adjuvant effect on polyvalent snake venom antiserum (8).

Sassafras

 ## 10 Second Take

Sassafras is an aromatic herb that contains safrole, a procarcinogen. It has no unique medicinal effects.

 ## Basics

LATIN NAME

Sassafras albidum (Nutt.) Nees syn: *Sassafras officinale* Nees & C.H. Eberm, *Sassafras variifolium* (Salisb.) Kuntze

FAMILY

Lauraceae

OTHER COMMON NAMES

Ague tree

DESCRIPTION

• A small tree native to North America, sassafras prefers roadsides and fields and grows up to 30 m in height; it has variable leaves (unlobed, single-lobed, or triple-lobed) and small yellowish flowers; all parts of the plant are aromatic.

PART USED

Roots, root bark

KNOWN ACTIVE CONSTITUENTS

• Essential oil (1% to 2%) containing up to 80% safrole (4-allyl-1,2-methylenedioxy-benzene), as well as other monoterpenes and sesquiterpenes and phenylpropanes. A recent analysis of essential oil found that it contained 85% safrole, 3.25% camphor, and 1.10% methyleugenol, as well as 10 sesquiterpenes and 9 compounds not previously identified in sassafras (1). Also contains small amounts of lignans, tannins, phytosterols, and other sterols (2). Aporphine and benzylisoquinoline alkaloids have been identified in the root bark.

MECHANISM/PHARMACOKINETICS

• Safrole is metabolically activated into a highly electrophilic sulfuric acid monoester carcinogen through a two-step process involving enzymatic oxidation at the secondary benzylic/allylic position; sulfate donation creates 1-sulfooxysafrole, a metabolite that can form DNA adducts, initiating chemical carcinogenesis (3).

 ## Evidence

CLINICAL TRIALS

No clinical trials identified.

OTHER CLAIMED BENEFITS/ACTIONS

• Tonic
• Colds
• Flu
• Arthritis
• Acne

Risks

ADVERSE REACTIONS

- One fatal poisoning from ingestion of 5 mL sassafras essential oil was reported in a child (4).
- In another poisoning case, a 47-year-old woman accidentally ingested a teaspoonful of sassafras essential oil (5). She experienced shakiness and vomiting and presented to the emergency department, where examination revealed only flushing, tremulousness, and tachycardia. She was treated with activated charcoal with sorbitol and intravenous electrolyte solution and discharged the next day. Liver and kidney function tests were normal.
- A case of daily episodes of diaphoresis resembling hot flashes was reported in a 72-year-old hypertensive woman who had recently begun drinking up to 10 cups of sassafras tea daily. Symptoms resolved on cessation of sassafras (6).

PREGNANCY/LACTATION

- Transplacental transport of safrole has been demonstrated in mice. Safrole is bound primarily to liver; fetal adduct levels were lower than maternal adduct levels (7). Another study by the same researcher compared the effects of safrole and 1'-hydroxysafrole in pregnant and non-pregnant mice; pregnancy increased the binding of safrole and 1'-hydroxysafrole to liver and kidney DNA 2.3- to 3.5-fold, suggesting that these compounds are more hazardous during pregnancy (8).

ANIMAL TOXICITY

- Safrole is a hepatocarcinogen; an aqueous safrole-free fraction produced malignant mesenchymal tumors in 66% of rats (9). Isosafrole is a weak carcinogen, but dihydrosafrole is moderately active in producing hepatic and esophageal tumors in mice (10).
- In animals, the oral LD_{50} of essential oil of sassafras is 1.9 g/kg (11).

 Dose

COMMON DOSAGE FORMS

- Sassafras use is not recommended.
- *Dried bark:* 2 to 4 g t.i.d.
- *Infusion:* made from 2 to 4 g t.i.d.
- *Liquid extract:* (1:1, 25% ethanol) 2 to 4 mL t.i.d.

 Common Questions and Answers

Q: So is gumbo carcinogenic?
A: Probably not. Although filé, a vital part of gumbo, is made from dried powdered sassafras leaves, the leaves do not contain significant amounts of safrole, and the amount of filé in a serving of gumbo is quite small. Besides, safrole occurs in small amounts in anise, basil, nutmeg, mace, cinnamon, cocoa, anise, and black pepper (10). Avoiding dietary safrole completely would eliminate pesto, eggnog, apple pie, steak au poivre ... life would hardly be worth living.

Q: What about the sassafras tea available at the health food store?
A: It is anything but a health food; sassafras tea may contain significant amounts of safrole. Eight tea samples (ground, unbrewed) contained from 299 to 17,400 mg/kg safrole (10). Another study examined brewed teas made from sassafras root bark powders and tinctures and found that safrole ranged from 0.09 to 4.66 mg/cup (so a cup of sassafras tea could contain up to 200 mg safrole).

Q: But isn't sassafras used as a food flavoring?
A: Not any more. Sassafras was used as a flavoring in root beer and other soft drinks and toothpaste before 1961. In 1960, after the Food and Drug Administration conducted studies showing that safrole is a weak liver carcinogen in rats and found that root beer samples contained safrole in levels of 8 to 26.7 ppm, sassafras oil and safrole were banned as flavoring agents (3). Safrole adds a distinctive flavor, so modern root beer tastes different than root beer made with sassafras. Safrole is still used to scent soaps and cleansers, as well as an economical starting ingredient to manufacture piperonal, used in perfumery (3).

Q: Is sassafras used as a recreational drug?
A: As a starting material, yes. Sassafras oil, safrole, and isosafrole have been used in the illegal production of methylenedioxy-methamphetamine (MDMA) (3).

Saw Palmetto

 10 Second Take

Saw palmetto fruits, once used as food, are benign. Clinical trial evidence supports its efficacy for treating benign prostatic hyperplasia (BPH); prostate-specific antigen (PSA) is not affected.

 Basics

LATIN NAME

Serenoa repens [Bartr.] Small, syn. *S. serrulata* [Mich.] Hook f., *Sabal serrulata* [Mich.] Nuttall ex Schult.

FAMILY

Palmae/Arecaceae

OTHER COMMON NAMES

Dwarf American palm

DESCRIPTION

• Saw palmetto, the most common palm in the United States, is 6 to 10 ft tall and has fan shaped, deeply divided leaves up to 1 m in width, and black fruits. Its branching stems are unusual in a palm (1). Saw palmetto grows throughout Florida, north to South Carolina, and west to Texas. It provides food or cover for more than 100 bird, 27 mammal, 25 amphibian, and 61 reptile species (1).

PART USED

Dried ripe fruit

KNOWN ACTIVE CONSTITUENTS

• β-Sitosterol and its glucoside, stigmasterol, and campesterol are thought to be the most important constituents (2). High molecular weight fatty alcohols (especially docosanol, hexacosanol, octacosanol, and triacontanol) also appear to be important (2). The purified lipid extract contains 85% to 95% fatty acids and sterols (including β-sitosterol, stigmasterol, cycloartenol, lupeol, lupenone, and methylcycloartenol) (3). Free fatty acids (including capric, caprylic, caproic, lauric, palmitic, and oleic acids) compose nearly two thirds of the oil (1).

MECHANISM/PHARMACOKINETICS

• The mechanism of *Serenoa repens* has not been well established. *In vitro* and *in vivo* studies indicate that saw palmetto inhibits binding of dihydrotestosterone (DHT) to androgen receptors.
• An antiestrogenic effect of saw palmetto was noted in a placebo-controlled trial of 35 men with BPH who received *Serenoa repens* 160 mg b.i.d. (4). Prostate cell nuclear fraction was positive for estrogen receptors in only 1 of 18 men receiving active therapy versus 14 of 17 men on placebo (the cytosolic fraction was estrogen receptor positive for 12 men in each group).
• Saw palmetto may competitively block translocation of estrogen receptors from the cytosol to the nucleus.
• *In vitro* studies are mixed on whether or not saw palmetto extracts inhibit 5 α-reductase (5,6), but no evidence of 5-alpha-reductase inhibition was noted in 32 healthy men treated with 320 mg Permixon for 1 week (7).
• A potent α_1-adrenoceptor effect of saw palmetto extract was noted *in vitro* (8).
• In rats, saw palmetto concentrates to a higher extent in the prostate than in other genitourinary tissues or liver (4).

 Evidence

CLINICAL TRIALS

• A systematic review of randomized trials of *Serenoa repens* in symptomatic BPH identified 18 randomized controlled trials (16 double-blind) that included a total of 2,939 men (9). Trials were 4 to 48 weeks in duration; the average study duration was 9 weeks. Ten trials were placebo-controlled, two drug-controlled, one compared *Serenoa repens* with another herb and active control, one compared active control with a mixture containing *Serenoa repens,* and one bioequivalence study compared an oral formulation with a rectal suppository. Compared with placebo, those treated with saw palmetto experienced decreased urinary tract symptom scores (weighted mean difference 1.41 points), decreased nocturia (weighted mean difference 0.76 times for evening), improvement in self rating of urinary tract symptoms (risk ratio for improvement 1.72), and improved peak urine flow (weighted mean difference 1.93 mL/second).
• A meta-analysis of all published clinical trial data on Permixon (a standardized lipid-sterolic extract) in patients with BPH identified 11 randomized clinical trials and two open-label trials that enrolled a total of 2,859 patients and lasted from 21 to 180 days (10). Nine of these trials are covered in the Wilt systematic review discussed previously. Seven trials were placebo-controlled, three compared Permixon with pharmaceutical drugs (finasteride, prazosin and alfuzosin), and one three-armed trial compared Permixon with *Pygeum africanum* extract (Tadenan) and placebo. Common endpoints were peak urinary flow rate and nocturia. Compared with placebo, Permixon caused a significantly higher improvement in peak flow rate, increasing flow rates by 2.2 mL/second [95% confidence interval (CI) 1.2 to 3.2] and reducing nocturia by 0.50 episodes (95% CI 0.40 to 0.52).
• Drug-controlled trials included in the reviews above are summarized in the questions and answers section.
• A recent double-blind study, not included in the previous reviews, randomized 44 men with symptomatic BPH to placebo or a saw palmetto herbal blend. Each capsule contained saw palmetto lipoidal extract 106 mg, nettle root extract 80 mg, pumpkin seed oil extract 160 mg, lemon bioflavonoids extract 33 mg, and vitamin A as beta-carotene 190 IU for 6 months (11). Clinical parameters improved in both groups, with no difference between groups. However, in the saw palmetto group, prostate epithelial contraction in the transitional zone decreased significantly from 17.8% percent epithelium to 10.7%. The percent of atrophic glands increased from 25.2% to 40.9% after treatment, also a significant difference. No adverse effects were noted.

ANIMAL/IN VITRO

- *In vitro,* a liposterolic extract of *Serenoa repens* inhibits both type I and type II isoenzymes of 5α-reductase, inhibits binding of DHT to androgen receptors in prostate cells (specifically the cytosol), and inhibits binding of [3H] DHT to its receptor in human foreskin fibroblasts (4).
- In hormone-treated castrated rats, a liposterolic extract of *Serenoa repens* inhibited the increase in prostate wet weight (12).
- Phytosterols (a mixture of β-sitosterol, campesterol, and stigmasterol) do not appear to bind to estrogen receptors and do not stimulate transcriptional activity of human estrogen receptors in a recombinant yeast strain (13).

OTHER CLAIMED BENEFITS/ACTIONS

- Hirsutism (in women)
- Aphrodisiac
- Diuretic
- Renal and bladder disorders
- Stimulate breast growth
- Digestion
- Ergogenic
- Lung disorders

 Risks

ADVERSE REACTIONS

- Saw palmetto is well tolerated; the most common adverse effects are minor gastrointestinal complaints including nausea and abdominal pain (4).

PREGNANCY/LACTATION

- No information available. However, pregnant women should avoid saw palmetto.

 Dose

COMMON DOSAGE FORMS

- *Liposterolic extract* [soft native extract 10:1 to 14:1 (w/w)] standardized to contain 85% to 95% fatty acids, 160 mg b.i.d. with meals
- *Dried fruit:* 0.5 to 1.0 g t.i.d.
- *Decoction:* made with 0.5 to 1.0 g t.i.d.
- *Fluid extract:* 1:1 (g/mL) 1 to 2 mL b.i.d.
- *Fluid extract:* 1:2 (g/mL) 2 to 4 mL b.i.d
- *Dry normalized extract:* 4:1 (w/w) (approximately 25% fatty acids) 400 mg b.i.d.

 Common Questions and Answers

Q: Does saw palmetto affect tests for prostate specific antigen?
A: No. PSA levels were assessed in at least three trials (11,14,15), none of which found an effect of saw palmetto on PSA.

Q: How does saw palmetto compare to drugs used to treat BPH?
A: No trials have compared saw palmetto to terazosin to date, but the herb has been compared with two other alpha-blockers and finasteride. A 3-week study in 63 patients with BPH compared saw palmetto (160 mg b.i.d.) to alfuzosin (2.5 mg t.i.d.) (16). Clinical symptoms, urinary flow rates, and residual urinary volume by transabdominal ultrasound were assessed. Both treatments significantly improved nocturia, daytime frequency, peak flow rates, mean flow rates and residual urinary volume, with no significant difference between groups. However, alfuzosin was significantly more effective than saw palmetto for total symptom score on Boyarsky's scale, visual analog scale and on overall clinical impression.
A 12-week trial compared Permixon (2 tablets daily) to prazosin (4 mg/day) in 42 men; peak flow increased from 9.75 ± 7.29 mL/s to 11.25 ± 8.77 mL/s in the Permixon group, compared with 10.36 ± 7.86 mL/s to 10.83 ± 11.07 mL/s in the prazosin group. Episodes of nocturia decreased from 2.5 ± 1.17 to 2.3 ± 1.39 in the Permixon group compared with a change from 2.1 ± 1.61 to 1.7 ± 1.76 in the prazosin group (17). Results apparently favored prazosin, but no statistical analysis was done (4).
A double-blind randomized study compared 5 mg finasteride to Permixon 320 mg for 6 months in 1,098 men with moderate BPH (14). Permixon and finasteride were equivalent in decreasing the International Prostate Symptom Score, improving quality of life, and increasing peak urinary flow. Finasteride decreased prostate volume and serum PSA levels, whereas Permixon had no effect on either. Permixon was less likely to cause complaints of decreased libido and impotence.

Q: What other uses are there for saw palmetto?
A: Saw palmetto stems were once used as a starch, and the fruits were an important food for pre-Colombian people and Creek immigrants in Florida, although they are not uniformly popular. One correspondent described the taste as "rotten cheese steeped in tobacco" (1). Fibers have been used to make scrubbing brushes, roots were used for paper manufacture, leaves and stem fibers have been used as upholstery fill, and the stem was once used as a cork substitute. The fibers are also widely used in Seminole and Miccosukee crafts. Leaves are sometimes used as roof thatch.

Selenium

10 Second Take

Selenium deficiency and toxicity are associated with severe adverse effects. Selenium may be important in cancer prevention.

Basics

DESCRIPTION

• Selenium is an essential trace mineral. Inorganic forms, including selenite or selenate, are more toxic than organic forms, which include selenomethionine and selenocysteine. Daily selenium intake in the United States is 60 to 216 μg, in Canada 113 to 220 μg, in Spain 60 to 106 μg, and in Greece 95 to 110 μg. Total amount of selenium in the body is 3 to 20 mg (1).

FOOD SOURCES

• Brazil nuts (2.54 ppm), kidney, liver, fish, crab, and other shellfish. Although animal products provide a significant proportion of selenium, plants and selenium-enriched yeast contain more bioavailable forms (1). The most common form of selenium in plants is L (+)-selenomethionine; very low levels of Se-methylselenocysteine and selenocystathi-onine are found in most plants (selenium-accumulating plants and broccoli, garlic, and onions grown in selenium-rich soil may have higher levels) (2). Most crops contain less than 1 mg selenium/kg; root vegetables contain more. Concentrations in grain vary considerably depending on soil (1). Garlic and mushrooms can be high in selenium (3).
• Organ meats and seafood contain 0.4 to 1.5 μg/g selenium, muscle meats 0.1 to 0.4 μg/g, cereals and grains less than 0.1 μ/g to more than 0.8 μg/g (4). Selenium in water (predominantly selenate) is less bioavailable than selenium in foods.

MECHANISM/PHARMACOKINETICS

• Selenium is a component of at least 35 selenoproteins that are crucial in oxidation-reduction reactions. Selenium-dependent glutathione peroxidase destroys hydrogen peroxide, and the iodothyronine deiodinases are all selenoproteins (5). Selenium stimulates the immune system, specifically enhancing the proliferation of activated T cells (6), and may protect against heavy metal toxicity (5).
• Selenium binds to plasma proteins and distributes largely to liver and kidney, as well as spleen, pancreas, heart, brain, and skeletal muscle. Of the total body pool, 40% to 50% is in skeletal muscle as selenomethi-onine. Kidneys and intestine are both involved in excretion (1). Elimination of selenite in humans involves three phases: a rapid phase (1 day), second phase (8 to 20 days), and a third phase (65 to 116 days). Selenium crosses the placenta and is secreted into breast milk.

Evidence

CLINICAL TRIALS

• Cancer

—Numerous epidemiologic studies have found an inverse relationship between selenium intake and cancer mortality. Few supplementation trials exist. In the Nutritional Prevention of Cancer trial, a double-blind, placebo-controlled randomized controlled trial (RCT) in 1,312 people with a history of nonmelanoma skin cancer, participants received placebo or selenium (200 μg/day selenium as brewer's yeast) for a mean of 4.5 years (7). There was no effect on the primary endpoint of nonmelanoma skin cancer, but compared with placebo, selenium appeared to reduce total cancer mortality [relative risk (RR) .50, 95% confidence interval (CI) 0.31 to 0.80], as well as risk of prostate cancer (RR 0.37, 95% CI 0.18 to 0.71), colorectal cancer (RR 0.42, 95% CI 0.18 to 0.95), and lung cancer (RR 0.54, 95% CI 0.30 to 0.98).
—In China's Qidong county (which has a high rate of hepatocellular carcinoma) an RCT in 226 hepatitis B antigen carriers compared placebo with 200 μg selenium (as brewer's yeast) (6). None of the selenium group and seven in the placebo group developed hepatocellular carcinoma.
—In another study of 130,000 people in five townships in Qidong, salt fortified with sodium selenite (15 mg/kg) reduced hepatocellular carcinoma incidence by 35%, compared with townships receiving unfortified salt (6).

• Cardiovascular disease

—Although at least nine epidemiologic studies have examined possible connections between cardiovascular risk and low selenium, studies have been mixed (6). No supplementation trials were identified.

• Pancreatitis

—A small controlled trial of intravenous selenium in patients with acute necrotizing pancreatitis found that selenium reduced mortality from 89% in controls to zero in the treated group (6).

• Fertility

—One study in subfertile Norwegian men found that sperm concentration was related to selenium concentration in seminal plasma. Supplementation of subfertile men with selenium (100 μg/day × 3 months) increased sperm motility. None in the placebo group achieved pregnancy, whereas 11% of the supplemented group achieved pregnancy.
—In another trial, however, 200 μg selenium given to subfertile Polish men for 3 months did not benefit sperm motility (6).

• Asthma

—A small double-blind placebo-controlled study in 24 asthmatics (19 completed) tested sodium selenite (100 μg/day × 14 weeks); significantly more treated patients reported subjective improvement, but there were no significant differences between groups on measures of lung function or airway responsiveness (8).

• Rheumatoid arthritis

—A double-blind trial in 40 patients treated for 6 months with 256 μg yeast selenium found no clinical or laboratory improvement; another double-blind placebo-controlled trial in 47 patients found no clinical benefit of selenium 600 μg × 4 months (9).

• Other

—Selenium deprivation causes depression and hostility; in two studies, selenium supplementation (100 μg daily selenium in one, 226.5 μg selenium in the other) improved mood (6).
—Selenium supplementation decreased plasma thyroxine (T_4) in older individuals [probably by enhancing conversion to triiodothyronine (T_3)] (6).
—Cretinism in newborns may be more likely when mothers are deficient in both iodine and selenium (combined deficiency causes more severe hypothyroidism than iodine deficiency alone in animals) (4).

Clinical Considerations

DEFICIENCY SIGNS AND SYMPTOMS

• Selenium deficiency can predispose a host to viral infection. Selenium may be especially important for HIV-infected patients; loss of CD4 T cells appears to parallel decline in plasma selenium. In 95 HIV-positive subjects, serum selenium correlated with CD4 cell count, p24 antigenemia, and decreased risk of death (10). Selenium may also help to protect patients with viral hepatitis from progressing to liver cancer (6).
• Selenium is clearly important to sperm function (6).
• Selenium is important to the brain; selenium deficiency affects the turnover rate of some neurotransmitters (6).
• Selenium deficiency is endemic in parts of China and results in two deficiency diseases, Keshan disease and Kashin-Beck disease. Keshan disease, a cardiovascular disease associated with congestive heart failure, cardiogenic shock and death, affects primarily women and children. Although selenium supplementation dramatically reduced acute and subacute cases of Keshan disease, chronic cases still exist, indicating the possibility that selenium deficiency predisposes to rather than causes the disease.
• Kashin-Beck disease, a chronic osteoarthropathy seen in Russia, Korea, and especially China, involves atrophy, degeneration, and necrosis of cartilage, causing short stature in children (1).

FACTORS DECREASING AVAILABILITY/ABSORPTION

• Dietary intake

FACTORS ENHANCING EXCRETION

• Duchenne's muscular dystrophy (3)

FACTORS INCREASING AVAILABILITY/ABSORPTION

• Dietary intake

LABORATORY TESTS

• Blood levels are usually less than 0.2 mg/L (newborns 0.03 mg/L, increasing to 0.1 mg/L at 1 year).
• Less than 0.1 mg selenium/L indicates marginal dietary intake.
• Less than 0.05 mg/L indicates deficiency.
• More than 0.6 mg/L indicates overexposure.
• Plasma levels of selenium are about 70% of whole blood (1).
• Hair and nails concentrate selenium. Toenail clippings may be used to determine selenium status; hair is not reliable because shampoos contain selenium (11).
• Random urine tests are unreliable because urine is affected by dilution and content of the last meal (12).

 ## Risks

• Lowest observed adverse effects level (LOAEL): 1570 ± 653 μg selenium/day
• No observed adverse effect level (NOAEL): 819 ± 126 μg selenium/day
• Maximum safe dietary intake: 400 μg selenium/day
• World Health Organization (WHO) standard for drinking water: 10 μg selenium/L

ADVERSE REACTIONS

• Ingestion up to 200 μg selenium/day does not produce adverse effects.
• During a severe drought in China, people who ingested an average of 5,000 μg selenium/day over 10 years experienced alopecia, skin lesions, nail deformities, tooth decay, paresthesias, and hyperreflexia (1). Chronic toxicity causes brittle hair, pruritic rash on the scalp, and yellowish white or red longitudinal streaks or transverse lines on the nail. Skin lesions may include erythema, vesiculation, or secondary infection.
• Usually, doses $\geq$900 μg/day are needed to induce selenium toxicity; some can ingest 1,500 μg selenium/day without developing selenosis.
• Inorganic selenium is more toxic than organic selenium (of the organic selenium compounds, selenocysteine is the most toxic). High-selenium brewer's yeast has caused mostly gastrointestinal complaints in clinical trials.
• Inhaled selenium dust can cause respiratory tract irritation; selenium dioxide exposure can cause metal fume fever (headache, chills, bronchitis, and pulmonary infiltrates, all of which resolve within 1 week). Chronic exposure to more than 0.2 to 0.4 mg selenium/m^3 causes garlic odor of the breath (resulting from expired dimethyl selenide), gastrointestinal discomfort, skin lesions, metallic taste, and psychologic changes. Acute inhalation of hydrogen selenide causes upper respiratory tract irritation, metallic taste, bronchopneumonia, and pulmonary edema.
• Ingestion of large doses of selenious acid causes stupor, respiratory depression, hypotension, and almost invariably death. A garlic odor is characteristic of selenium poisoning, and nails, hair, or teeth may have a red pigmentation. There is no antidote to selenium poisoning; in animals, dimercaprol (BAL) slows recovery from selenium poisoning and calcium disodium ethylenediaminetetraacetate (CaNa$_2$EDTA) does not improve survival rates (1).
• Teratogenicity is low in humans (1).

ANIMAL TOXICITY

• High levels of selenium concentration in water (average 300 μg/L, with levels as high as 1.35 mg/L) was associated with deaths and deformities in fish and waterfowl in the Kesterson wildlife refuge. A community health survey did not reveal adverse health effects in the local human population. In animals, vitamin E deficiency and low dietary sulfate enhances selenium toxicity, and protein, methionine, and zinc reduce toxicity (1).

 ## Dose

RECOMMENDED DIETARY ALLOWANCE

Infants and children

0 to months	15 μg/day (adequate intake)
7 to 12 months	20 μg/day (adequate intake)
1 to 3 years	20 μg/day
4 to 8 years	30 μg/day

Males

9 to 13 years	40 μg/day
14 to 18 years	55 μg /day
19 to 50 years	55 μg/day
51+ years	55 μg/day

Females

9 to 13 years	40 μg/day
14 to 18 years	55 μg/day
19 to 50 years	55 μg/day
51+ years	55 μg/day
Pregnant	60 μg/day
Lactating	70 μg/day

UPPER LIMITS

Infants and children

0 to 6 months	45 μg/day
7 to 12 months	60 μg/day
1 to 3 years	90 μg/day
4 to 8 years	150 μg/day

Males

9 to 13 years	280 μg/day
14 to 18 years	400 μg/day
19 to 50 years	400 μg/day
51+ years	400 μg/day

Females

9 to 13 years	280 μg/day
14 to 18 years	400 μg/day
19 to 50 years	400 μg/day
51+ years	400 μg/day
Pregnant	400 μg/day
Lactating	400 μg/day

• *Quality note:* Yeast-based selenium supplements may contain selenomethionine or inorganic selenium (selenite or selenite); only selenomethionine-containing yeast has been tested in cancer prevention trials (2).

Senna

10 Second Take

Senna is an anthranoid-containing herb with laxative effects. Too high a dose can cause diarrhea and electrolyte loss; chronic use can cause laxative dependence or pseudomelanosis coli.

Basics

LATIN NAME

Cassia angustifolia Vahle, *C. acutifolia* Delile, and *C. senna* L are all the same species

FAMILY

Fabaceae (Leguminosae)

OTHER COMMON NAMES

Alexandrian senna, Indian senna

DESCRIPTION

• Senna is a low shrub up to 1.5 m high, with leaves composed of three to seven pairs of leaflets, with pod-like fruit.

PART USED

Leaf, dried ripe fruit

KNOWN ACTIVE CONSTITUENTS

• Sennosides (especially sennosides A and B), which are hydroxyanthracene glycosides (usually more than 2.5%).

MECHANISM/PHARMACOKINETICS

• Anthranoids are compounds based on anthraquinone, dianthrone, or anthrone structures. Most anthranoids in plants are found in the glycoside form; these hydrophilic molecules pass unabsorbed through the stomach and large intestine, requiring the intervention of intestinal bacteria to split off the sugar and release the active aglycone anthrone. Aglycone anthrones include rhein, aloe-emodin, emodin, alizarin, chrysophanol, and lucidin. Anthrones are highly reactive (anthrones are 100-fold more cytotoxic than anthraquinones) and are primarily responsible for the laxative effect of anthranoid-containing plants (1).
• It is believed that only anthrones, not anthraquinones, increase peristalsis (in colostomy patients, peristalsis can be induced with rhein anthrone but not with rhein anthraquinone). Anthraquinones affect secretory and absorption mechanisms; mechanisms are believed to include inhibition of the sodium-potassium pump, increased mucosal permeability of the colonic mucosa, possible effects on Meissner's plexus, or prostaglandin-mediated effects (2).
• In humans, an unknown but probably small amount of aglycone anthrones is absorbed; after absorption, anthranoids are converted primarily to corresponding glucoronide and sulfate derivatives, excreted mainly in urine and bile (the kidneys retain some anthranoid derivatives) (2). Sennosides are converted to the active metabolite (rhein-anthrone) by bacteria in the large intestine (3). After oral administration of sennosides, about 90% are excreted in feces; 3% to 6% of sennoside metabolites are excreted in urine. Pharmacokinetic studies of senna pod powder equivalent to 20 mg sennosides (p.o. × 7 days) resulted in a maximum concentration of 100 ng/mL rhein in blood (3). Another pharmacokinetic study of therapeutic doses of senna given to 10 healthy participants found that rhein concentrations were as high as 150 ng/mL, with peaks at 3 to 5 hours and 10 to 11 hours after administration (an effect most likely due to initial effects of free rhein and then rhein released from sennosides) (4). This study found no detectable levels of aloe-emodin.

Evidence

CLINICAL TRIALS

• Constipation

—In an open controlled 7-day trial in 91 terminal cancer patients with opiate-induced constipation, senna [0.4 to 1.6 mL (12 to 48 mg)] was as effective as lactulose [15 to 60 mL (10 to 40 g)] in improving defecation-free intervals of 72 hours and days with defecation (5). Senna is less expensive than lactulose.

• Surgical preparation

—A randomized, single-blind multicenter study of 523 preoperative patients with colonic or rectal carcinoma or sigmoid diverticular disease scheduled for resection and immediate anastomosis compared senna (one package in a glass of water) to polyethylene glycol (two packages in 2 to 3 L of water) administered the evening before surgery (6). Senna was significantly better than polyethylene glycol in terms of better colonic cleanliness and less fluid fecal matter in the colonic lumen; there was no difference in postoperative infections, anastomotic leakage, or intraoperative fecal soiling.

ANIMAL/IN VITRO

• *In vitro* experiments demonstrate the ability of human gut flora, including *Streptococcus faecalis, Streptococcus faecium,* and *Bacteroides fragilis,* to reduce sennosides A/B to rhein. *S. faecalis* and *S. faecium* lacked hydrolyzing characteristics.

Risks

ADVERSE REACTIONS

- Fluid and electrolyte loss (potassium loss may be clinically significant)
- Abdominal spasms and pain (see questions and answers)
- Diarrhea
- Decreased peristalsis (chronic use can cause damage to the smooth muscles and myenteric plexus)
- Toxic hepatitis was reported in a 26-year-old nurse 1 month after she added a daily dose of senna extract (containing 100 mg sennosides B) to a chronically ingested twice-weekly tea containing 10 g senna leaf (7).
- A case report of digit clubbing and hypertrophic osteoarthropathy was associated with 3 years of senna tablet abuse (Senokot, three tablets daily, tablet dose not given). Within 6 months of discontinuing senna, finger and toe clubbing disappeared and rheumatic symptoms were less severe, although still present (8).
- Anthranoid-containing laxatives should not be used in intestinal obstruction or ileus.

DRUG INTERACTIONS

- Senna has the potential to interfere with many concomitantly administered oral drugs by increasing intestinal transit time.
- Potassium loss from anthranoid-containing laxatives may predispose those on cardiac glycosides to cardiac arrhythmias.

HARMLESS EFFECTS

- Pseudomelanosis coli (see questions and answers)
- Discolored urine or feces (yellowish brown or red discoloration—the color is pH-dependent).

ANIMAL TOXICITY

- A review of the genotoxic risk from senna products concluded that there is no genotoxic effect under normal conditions of use (9).
- In mice and rats, the acute oral toxicity of senna pods, senna pod extracts, and sennosides is low. In mice, acute toxicity of sennosides A and B LD_{50} was 4,100 mg/kg intravenously and more than 5,000 mg/kg orally. A 4-week study of sennosides in dogs (up to 500 mg/kg) and a 6-month chronic toxicity study in rats (100 mg/kg/day) demonstrated no specific toxicity (3).

 Dose

COMMON DOSAGE FORMS

- Daily dose may be taken in a single dose or divided into two doses. A total daily dose should contain 10 to 30 mg (maximum 60 mg) of hydroxyanthracene glycosides. Time of action is 8 to 12 hours. Laxatives should only be taken longer than 1 to 2 weeks under medical supervision.
- *Senna pods:* 0.6 to 2.0 g dried pod "powdered or whole."
- *Dried leaf:* 0.5 to 2 g finely chopped herb as infusion, decoction, or cold macerate (macerated for 2 to 3 hours).
- *Fluid extract* 1:1 (g/mL): 0.6 to 2.0 mL.
- *Dry hydroalcoholic extract* (5.5%–8.0% hydroxyanthracene glycosides): 0.25–0.55 g.
- Lower doses of Alexandrian senna fruit should be used, because Alexandrian fruit has a higher (5%) content of hydroxyanthracene derivatives.
- Children

—10 years and older: As for adults
—Younger than 10 years: Not recommended

 Common Questions and Answers

Q: Should anthraquinones be used for chronic constipation?
A: No. Bulk-forming agents are preferable for chronic constipation. Chronic use of anthraquinones can damage the myenteric plexus and lead to laxative dependence.

Q: Is there a way to decrease cramping with senna preparations?
A: Yes. Cramping appears to occur less often with senna fruit than senna leaf preparations, despite the lower anthracene glycoside content of the leaf. Cold macerates of senna leaf extract fewer resins and, thus, cause fewer colicky pains. The addition of some coriander or fennel seeds to teas or infusions also will decrease cramping and gas.

Q: Is it really acceptable to use senna in lactating women?
A: Yes. Although anthraquinones are partially excreted into milk, the risk of the infant developing diarrhea is apparently minimal (1). Although some sources (3) recommend against breastfeeding while using anthraquinones, senna and cascara are two of only seven drugs that the American Academy of Pediatrics considers compatible with breast feeding (the other five are cimetidine, atropine, cascara, cisapride, loperamide, and magnesium sulfate) (10). Some anthra-quinones, however, including aloe-emodin and emodin, are genotoxic, so some question the use of anthraquinone in breast-feeding mothers (1). Apart from effects on infants, anthraquinone laxatives are not completely benign and should be reserved for cases in which bulk-forming agents with adequate hydration have failed.

Q: What is pseudomelanosis coli?
A: Pseudomelanosis coli is a harmless, abnormal discoloration of the colonic mucosa (typically a reticular pattern of dark lines resembling alligator skin; histologically, dark granules are noted in the macrophages of the lamina propria). Seventy-three percent of chronic anthraquinone users manifest it, rendering it a reliable marker for chronic laxative abuse (11). Melanosis has also been reported in the gastric mucosa, but this is unusual (11). Pigmentation is reversible within 4 to 12 months after cessation of laxative use.

Q: Isn't there a link between colon cancer and anthranoid laxatives?
A: It is not clear whether anthranoid laxatives increase the risk of colorectal cancer in humans. Two case control studies published in German found no link between anthranoid laxative use and colorectal cancer (3). A prospective study of 1,095 patients found that pseudomelanosis coli (a marker of recent chronic anthranoid laxative use) was more common in patients with colorectal carcinomas; pseudomelanosis coli was found to be 6.9% for patients with no abnormality, 9.8% for patients with adenomas, and 18.6% for patients with colorectal carcinomas (12). A retrospective study of 3,049 patients who underwent colorectal endoscopy was less clear: In patients without pathologic changes, the incidence of pseudomelanosis coli was 3.13%, in those with colorectal adenomas 8.64%, and in those with colorectal carcinomas 3.29%. Because pseudomelanosis coli resolves within 4 to 12 months, studies can only pick up relatively recent chronic use. Those with colon cancer may be more likely to use laxatives, which would render these findings spurious.

In rats, senna and cascara glycosides may be weak promoters of colon carcinogenesis (13). On their own, these glycosides did not increase preneoplastic lesions called aberrant crypt foci (ACF). However, rats treated with a carcinogen and the highest dose of glycosides had more ACF than those treated only with the inducer.

Serine

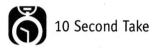 10 Second Take

L-serine is a nonessential amino acid; D-serine has been tested as an adjunct to schizophrenia treatment with mixed results.

 Basics

DESCRIPTION

- L-serine is a nonessential amino acid.

FOOD SOURCES

Most protein-containing foods

MAIN FUNCTIONS/PHARMACOKINETICS

- Amino acids are used for protein synthesis and energy production. Serine is also a constituent of phospholipids, a precursor of ethanolamine and choline, and a precursor of sphingolipids (1). Serine acts as an agonist at the glycine site on the N-methyl-D-aspartate (NMDA) receptor.
- Free serine concentration in blood plasma is 76 to 164 μmol/L in venous blood, 132 μmol/L in arterial blood. Urinary output is 400 μmol/24 hours. Plasma clearance half-life is 17 hours.

Evidence

CLINICAL TRIALS

No trials were identified for L-serine, the normal dietary form.

• Schizophrenia

—D-serine may be a useful adjunctive treatment in schizophrenia but does not add to the effect of clozapine. A study of 31 Taiwanese schizophrenic patients compared D-serine (30 mg/kg/day) as adjunctive treatment to non-clozapine antipsychotic drugs. Twenty-eight patients completed the trial. Serine-treated patients had significant improvements in positive, negative, and cognitive symptoms (2).
—The same investigators compared placebo with D-serine (30 mg/kg/day) as an adjunctive treatment to clozapine in a double-blind, placebo-controlled, 6-week trial of 20 schizophrenic patients. Biweekly assessments (Clinical Global Impression, Positive and Negative Syndrome Scale, Scale for the Assessment of Negative Symptoms, and Hamilton Depression Rating Scale) showed no additional improvement or worsening of symptoms with D-serine (3). The authors postulate that perhaps clozapine maximally enhances NMDA neurotransmission and that this cannot be improved on by serine.

ANIMAL/IN VITRO

• Hyperactivity

—In mice, intraventricularly administered glycine and D-serine reduced chemically induced hyperactivity (4).

• Ulcers

—L-serine produces a dose-dependent inhibition of gastric acid secretion in pylorus-ligated rats and attenuates the formation of gastric ulcers induced by stress, indomethacin, and necrotizing agents (5).

• Teratogenicity

—In rats, serine attenuates teratogenicity induced by 2-methoxyethanol (6).

 Risks

No risks identified.

 Dose

• Serine is nonessential. The dose used in clinical trials has been 30 mg/kg/day.

Silicon

10 Second Take

Silicon is relatively harmless ingested orally, but no clinical trials support its therapeutic use for any condition.

Basics

DESCRIPTION

• Only recently identified as essential, silicon is a trace element important in the formation of glycosaminoglycans. Found mainly in skin and cartilage, the highest concentrations of silicon are found in the skin, tendons, bone epiphyses, and arterial walls (1). Silica crystals are also found in the lymph nodes. Silicic acid (apparently the free form) is freely diffusable and is the form excreted in urine (the primary elimination route) (1).
• The average daily intake of silicon apparently ranges between 0.71 to 1.79 mmol (20 to 50 mg) (2).

FOOD SOURCES

• Unrefined, high-fiber grains, cereals, and root vegetables (2). Intake is estimated to be 20 to 46 mg/day of which 30% to 50% may be absorbed (1). Water (which contains 2 to 12 μg/mL), with highest amounts in "hard" water, may also be a significant source. In addition, beer is a significant source of silicon, most of which is rapidly absorbed and excreted within 8 hours (3).

MAIN FUNCTIONS/PHARMACOKINETICS

• Silicon influences cartilage formation and calcification, thus affecting bone formation (2). Silicon appears to have a role in decreasing the absorption of aluminum (3).
• Little is known about silicon metabolism. Different forms of silicon are absorbed to different extents (10% to 70%) (2). Aluminosilicates and silica are less bioavailable than sodium metasilicate.
• Silicate food additives are not very bioavailable (4).

Evidence

CLINICAL TRIALS

No clinical trials identified.

Other Claimed Benefits/Actions

• Prevention of cardiovascular disease
• Hair growth
• Skin quality
• Osteoarthritis
• Osteoporosis
• Hypertension
• Alzheimer's disease

Clinical Considerations

DEFICIENCY SIGNS AND SYMPTOMS

• Silicon deficiency signs are not established in humans. In chickens and rats, silicon deficiency causes defects in connective tissue and bone. In silicon-deficient animals, hexosamine (glycosaminoglycan) and collagen concentrations in bone are depressed, but mineral composition does not appear to be affected. Rats fed a low-calcium, low-silicon, high-aluminum diet accumulated large amounts of aluminum in the brain (4).

FACTORS DECREASING AVAILABILITY/ABSORPTION

Dietary intake

FACTORS INCREASING AVAILABILITY/ABSORPTION

Dietary intake

LABORATORY TESTS

• Whole blood: approximately 1 μg/mL
• Plasma: approximately 0.5 μg/mL

Risks

• Silicon is nontoxic orally and is used as an anticaking or antifoaming agent in foods, as well as in the antacid magnesium trisilicate (2). Inhaled silica dust increases the risk of silicosis and lung cancer (5), as well as silica-induced systemic sclerosis (6). The current Occupational Safety and Health Administration (OSHA) standard is 0.1 mg/meter^3; a recent review recommends lowering exposure to 0.05 mg/meter^3 (5).

ANIMAL TOXICITY

• Ruminants that consume plants with high silicon content can develop siliceous renal calculi (renal calculi in humans may also contain silicates) (4). In rats fed high amounts of sodium metasilicate, antioxidant enzymes (superoxide dismutase, catalase, and glutathione peroxidase) were reduced (2).

 Dose

COMMON DOSAGE FORMS

• The requirement for silicon is probably in the range of 0.07 to 0.18 mmol (2 to 5 mg/day); however, because much ingested silicon is not absorbed (10% to 70%, depending on the compound), dietary intake should be higher. Suggested intake is 5 to 10 mg/day (2).

 Common Questions and Answers

Q: Why do people think that silica is good for cardiovascular disease?
A: The intimal layer of arteries contains very high amounts of bound silicon, and several reports from the 1970s found an inverse relationship between the amount of silicon in arterial walls and the presence of atherosclerosis (1). In rabbits, silicon intake appears to reduce formation of atheromatous plaque, and one epidemiological study provides indirect support for this hypothesis. In Finland, one population with a rate of cardiovascular disease half that of another population was found to drink water that was almost twice as high in silicon as the high-risk group (apparently other risk factors were controlled for). High-fiber diets and consumption of hard (mineral-rich) water have been associated with lower rates of cardiovascular disease, and silicon may play a role (1). This is all intriguing but does not constitute hard evidence. Observational studies have led us astray previously, and no prospective studies of silicon supplementation exist.

Silver (Ag), Colloidal Silver

 10 Second Take

Silver is a nonessential mineral; although it has antibiotic properties, it has no advantage over pharmaceutical antibiotics and can cause toxic effects.

 Basics

DESCRIPTION

- A white, lustrous, transition metal
- Many silver salts are irritants and light-sensitive; silver nitrate, for example, is used in photography (as well as for various other industrial uses). Silver nitrate, a powerful oxidizing agent, is very toxic.

FOOD SOURCES

- Small, harmless amounts of silver are found in many foods; mushrooms and milk are particularly high in silver. Wheat flour contains 0.3 μg/g and mushrooms contain up to several hundred μg/g. Milk contains 27 to 54 μg/L. The metallic sugar balls used to decorate cakes are coated with real silver, and bits of silver foil are sometimes used to decorate desserts, especially in India. Silver acetate is also used in some smoking-deterrent lozenges and chewing gums.

MAIN FUNCTIONS/PHARMACOKINETICS

- Silver is not an essential trace element and has no known function in humans. Inorganic silver compounds are microbicidal because they readily denature and precipitate proteins. Silver compounds inactivate enzymes by forming hemisilver sulfides with sulfhydryl groups; silver can also bind amino, carboxylic, phosphate, and imidazole groups and reduce the activity of lactate dehydrogenase and glutathione peroxidases. Although the biologic half-life ranges from days to months, absorbed silver is deposited in skin, where it has a significantly longer half-life. Up to 10% of silver salts are absorbed (absorption is increased in disrupted mucus membranes, a situation worsened because soluble silver salts may corrode gastrointestinal mucosa). Excretion is primarily via fecal elimination with active biliary excretion (1).

 Evidence

CLINICAL TRIALS

No clinical trials identified.

OTHER CLAIMED BENEFITS/ACTIONS

- Antibiotic
- Smoking deterrent
- Immune system stimulant
- Fungal infections
- Tuberculosis
- Malaria
- Preventing cancer
- Preventing AIDS
- Preventing diabetes

 Risks

ADVERSE REACTIONS

- Silver accumulates widely in the body, with the highest concentrations found in the skin, liver, spleen, and adrenals. Smaller amounts are deposited in muscle and brain. Silver salts can penetrate the blood–brain barrier and accumulate in neurons and glial cells of the brain and spinal cord (1).
- Silver poisoning

—The average fatal dose of silver is about 10 g, although some people have apparently survived doses of 30 g (1). There is no specific antidote; treatment is supportive.
—Symptoms of severe silver nitrate poisoning include pain and burning in the mouth, blackening of skin and mucous membranes, salivation, black vomitus, diarrhea, shock, convulsion, coma, and death.

- Argyria (also called argyriasis or argyrosis)

—Chronic use of silver-containing products can cause deposition of silver in the skin and internal organs. The average amount of exposure required to develop argyria is about 3.8 g of elemental silver. The first sign of argyria is often a slate-blue or silver line in the gingiva. In the skin, the grayish hue that characterizes argyria is a combination of silver deposits and melanin pigmentation; silver stimulates melanocytes. Discoloration is often more pronounced in sun-exposed areas, because light reduces silver. Argyria, although generally harmless, is irreversible and unattractive. Chelation therapy with dimercaprol (BAL) or D-penicillamine has been ineffective. Intradermal injection with 6% sodium thiosulfate or 1% potassium ferrocyanide has occasionally resulted in successful local reversal, but this is not practical for large areas of discoloration.
—Silver acetate is used in some smoking-deterrent lozenges and chewing gums, and several cases of argyria have been reported in heavy users of these preparations. About 10 cases of argyria were reported in Japan due to breath fresheners (Jintan brand) that contained silver (2). In a recent case, a 79-year-old man consumed silver sugar cake decorations for 15 years in an effort to stop smoking. Over 3 years, he developed blue lunulae and a gray-brown discoloration over his skin, particularly prominent in the sun-exposed parts of his face, neck, and hands (2).
—Recent cases of argyria have been linked with colloidal silver products promoted as natural antibiotics (see questions and answers). A 35-year-old woman presented with typical blue-gray discoloration of skin and nail beds after ingesting mild colloidal silver protein (25 μg/tsp) for 1 year (3).
—In another case, a 38-year-old woman presented with a gray-blue facial discoloration after ingesting an unspecified form of colloidal silver (1/4 cup t.i.d. for 8 months) in an effort to treat Lyme disease with this "natural" antibiotic (4). Neither patient had other complications.
—A 55-year-old man who had been taking a teaspoon of colloidal silver three times daily for 3 years in an effort to treat allergies also developed argyria (5).

• Localized argyria

—A case of localized argyria with chrysiasis (gold deposition) caused by implanted acupuncture needles in a 41-year-old Japanese woman has been reported (6).
—The use of topical silver products on mucus membranes may result in localized argyria of the oral or nasal mucosa. In ocular argyria (caused by silver-containing eye drops or occupational exposure), the affected eye turns bluish gray or brownish black.

• Generalized argyrosis

—Although argyria was much more common before 1951, several recent cases of generalized argyrosis have been reported associated with the oral ingestion of silver preparations, including a 52-year-old man who had treated a duodenal ulcer with a silver preparation for 18 years. He died of cardiac failure and autopsy showed dense silver deposits in most blood vessels, renal glomeruli, choroids plexus, seminiferous tubules, and liver portal fields (1).
—In rare cases, neurological deficits may result. In one case a 55-year-old woman had treated her oral mucosa with one stick of silver nitrate daily for what she thought was oral mycosis. She had a gray-green discoloration of the skin and reduced iron and copper levels. Her symptoms included gait disturbance, weakness, hypogeusia, hyposmia, dizziness, and generalized skin hypesthesia. Microscopy of tissue samples revealed silver deposits in basal membranes, macrophages, perineurium of peripheral nerves, and along elastic and collagenous fibers and necrotic cells of the oral submucosa (7).
—In another case, a schizophrenic patient who consumed silver antismoking pills for 40 years developed seizures; an extremely high serum concentration of silver was detected (8).
—Silver exposure has been associated with glomerular damage and proteinuria; abdominal pain has been associated with elevated silver levels in those occupationally exposed (1).

• Other effects

—Topical use of silver nitrate in burn treatment may cause methemoglobinemia, hypochloridemia, hyponatremia, and eschars that adhere to dressings. Silver sulfadiazine, although much safer than silver nitrate, can cause leukopenia and nephritic syndrome (these cases are rare).
—Inhaled silver may cause chemical pneumonitis (1).
—There is a possible association with birth defects (see questions and answers).

• Silver may interfere with aspects of copper metabolism (9).

Dose

COMMON DOSAGE FORMS

• Dietary and safe limits

—A normal diet may contain up to 990 μg of silver daily.
—The Environmental Protection Agency (EPA) reference dose (a dose unlikely to be associated with significant deleterious effects during a lifetime) is 5 μg/kg/day with a critical dose estimated at 14 μ/kg/day.
—The maximum contaminant level goal proposed by the EPA for silver in the drinking water is <100 μg/L.

• Over-the-counter products

—Colloidal silver proteins are made by mixing silver nitrate, sodium hydroxide, and gelatin, then diluting this mixture to form a complex colloidal aggregate. Mild silver protein contains 19% to 23% silver, and strong silver protein contains 7.5% to 8.5%. Currently available colloidal silver products (usually a dilution of mild silver protein or strong silver protein) are reported to have an active silver ion concentration of about 1 to 6 ppm (5 to 30 μg per dose). However, the concentration of silver in currently available products varies widely (1).

Common Questions and Answers

Q: What is the possible connection between silver and birth defects?
A: There may be some association between maternal exposure to silver in drinking water and some fetal developmental anomalies. A case-control study of women that examined the relationship between community drinking water quality and occurrence of adverse pregnancy outcomes suggested an association between maternal exposure to 0.001 mg/L of silver in drinking water and increased fetal developmental anomalies of the ear, face, and neck (10).

Q: Isn't silver present in several burn creams?
A: Yes. Mild silver protein is used in ophthalmic and other topical silver nitrate and silver sulfadiazine preparations, available by prescription. Mild silver protein was once reviewed by the Food and Drug Administration (FDA) as a potential antiseptic; an FDA advisory expert panel noted a lack of human efficacy data and recommended that efficacy studies be conducted. Because no further data were received, silver was removed from the over-the-counter monograph in 1992 (1).

Q: Colloidal silver is being heavily marketed as a "natural, safe" antibiotic. Is there any truth to this?
A: Silver medicinals have a long history of use in both conventional and unconventional medicine. Lunar Caustic (silver nitrate) was used for nervous disorders in the Middle Ages, silver nitrate for epilepsy in the 19th century, and silver arsphenamine for syphilis in the early 20th century. Colloidal silver proteins were used in cold remedies in the early part of the 20th century. Silver nitrate has been used in conventional medicine as a cauterizing agent for uncontrolled epistaxis or to treat warts and corns. There is truth in the statement that silver has antibacterial properties; in fact, colloidal silver proteins have been used in conventional medicine to treat or prevent gonorrhea and gonorrheal conjunctivitis. However, safer and more effective antibiotics have replaced these treatments. Silver can be toxic and has no demonstrated advantage over other antimicrobials. There is no evidence that the colloidal silver products currently marketed are effective for the claims being made for them.

Skullcap

10 Second Take

There are no clinical trials of skullcap herb; skullcap root components have antimicrobial properties *in vitro*. Hepatotoxicity associated with skullcap is most likely due to adulteration with germander.

Basics

LATIN NAME

Scutellaria laterifolia L.; Baikal skullcap, *Scutellaria baicalensis* Georgi

FAMILY

Labiatae

OTHER COMMON NAMES

Huangqin (*Scutellaria baicalensis, Scutellaria barbata,* and other species of *Scutellaria*) (China), *ogon,* and *wogon* (Japan)

DESCRIPTION

• Skullcap is a perennial mint that grows 1 to 3 ft in height; it has a striated stem and violet-blue flowers with a typical hooded calyx. The plant favors rich woods and grows throughout much of eastern North America.

PART USED

Aerial part (United States and Western countries), root (Asia)

KNOWN ACTIVE CONSTITUENTS

• *Root:* Sterols and many different flavonoids, including the aglycone baicalein (scutellarein) (less than 0.1% to 5.2%), baicalin (0.1% to 20.6%), baicalein-7-*O*-β-D-glycopyranoside, wogonin (0.1% to 2.1%), wogonin-7-*O*-glucoronide (less than 0.1% to 5.4%), oroxylin A, oroxylin A 7-*O*-glucoronide (less than 0.1% to 4.1%), dihydrooroxylin A, scullcapflavone I, scullcapflavone II, and chrysin (1).
• *Leaf:* The flavonoids carthamidin, isocarthamidin, and isoscutellarein-8-*O*-glucoronide. Although neither flower nor leaf contain the major flavonoids found in the root, small amounts of baicalin and wogonin-7-*O*-glucoronide are found in the stem (higher amounts in the lower compared with the upper stem).
• *S. baicalensis* contains substantial amounts of melatonin (7.11 μg/g); *S. laterifolia* contains less (0.09 μg/g) (2).

MECHANISM/PHARMACOKINETICS

• No information on pharmacokinetics identified in humans. In rats, after oral administration of baicalin, approximately half of metabolites were excreted in bile. The administration of baicalein results in recovery of the same metabolites, and it is thought that baicalin is hydrolyzed in the gastrointestinal tract to baicalein.
• Antimicrobial activity of *Scutellaria* may be due to stimulation of nitric oxide production from macrophages (3). Baicalein (5 to 25 mM) and wogonin (5 to 50 mM) inhibit lipopolysaccharide-induced nitric oxide generation, which may be involved in antiinflammatory effects (4).
• Several components of *Scutellaria* bind to the benzodiazepine site of the γ-aminobutyric acid$_A$ (GABA$_A$) receptor; the order of affinity is wogonin > baicalein > scuttelarein > baicalin (5).
• Baicalein and baicalin were shown to have free radical scavenging and antioxidant effects (6).

Evidence

CLINICAL TRIALS

No clinical trials identified.

ANIMAL/IN VITRO

• No studies were identified with skullcap aerial parts; all studies identified used *Scutellaria* root extract or baicalein.
• Antimicrobial effects

—Baicalin may be potentially useful as an adjunct to beta-lactam treatments against resistant microorganisms. Baicalin (16 μg/mL) decreases the minimum inhibitory concentration of benzyl penicillin against methicillin-resistant *Staphylococcus aureus* from 125 μg/mL to 4 μg/mL and against penicillin-resistant *S. aureus* from 250 μg/mL to 16 μg/mL (7). Baicalin inhibits HIV infection and replication *in vitro* (8) and also inhibits human T cell leukemia virus type 1 with no loss of cell viability (9).
—Several flavones from *S. baicalensis* roots were found to inhibit Epstein-Barr virus early antigen activation (10). A lyophilized tea of *Scutellaria* was found to inhibit *Klebsiella pneumoniae, Proteus vulgaris* and *Candida albicans* at 200 μg/mL, and *Mycobacterium smegmatis* at less than 100 μg/mL (11).
—A decoction of *S. baicalensis* was tested against oral bacteria; a concentration of 3.13% was required for bactericidal effect. Tetracycline, alexidine, and stannous fluoride were much more effective (12).
—Antimicrobial activity may be due to stimulating nitric oxide production from macrophages; stimulation of recombinant interferon-gamma-primed mouse peritoneal macrophages with *S. baicalensis* resulted in increased nitric oxide production (*Scutellaria* on its own did not affect nitric oxide production) (3).
—Sho-saiko-to, a seven-herb mixture, induced interleukin-10 production in mononuclear cells from patients with hepatitis B or hepatitis C; the effect was found to be due mainly to *Scutellaria* root and licorice root (13).

• Cardiovascular

—An extract of *S. baicalensis* reduced cell death in a cardiomyocyte model of ischemia and reperfusion (14). In cultured human umbilical vein endothelial cells, baicalein prevents trypsin-induced thrombotic tendencies (15). Another experiment, also using cultured human umbilical vein endothelial cells, found that baicalein inhibited thrombin induced plasminogen activator inhibitor-1, possibly by reducing elevation of intracellular calcium (16). In rat mesenteric artery, baicalein had a contracting effect at low concentrations and relaxed arterial smooth muscle at higher concentrations (17).

- Anticancer

—Several flavones from *Scutellaria baicalensis* roots were found to inhibit mouse skin tumor promotion in a two-stage carcinogenesis test (10).

OTHER CLAIMED BENEFITS/ACTIONS

- *Leaf*

—Tonic
—Sedative
—Antispasmodic
—Anticonvulsant

- *Root*

—Diuretic
—Sedative
—Antihypertensive
—Antiviral
—Antibacterial
—Anticancer
—Antiinflammatory

 Risks

ADVERSE REACTIONS

- Hepatotoxicity

—Hepatotoxicity has been attributed to skullcap, but all of these cases are likely due to mistaken identity; skullcap is commonly adulterated with common germander (*Teucrium chamaedrys*), which is known to be hepatotoxic. The common names can be confusing; material known as "pink skullcap" is actually wild germander (*Teucrium canadense*) (18). In all cases of hepato-toxicity, combination herbal products were used, and none of the reports include analyses of the herbs, so the actual identity of the plant material was never established.
—Four cases of acute hepatitis in the United Kingdom were attributed to the use of stress-reducing tablets (three used the preparation called Kalms, which purportedly contains valerian, asafetida, hops, and gentian), and one used a preparation called Neurelax (other ingredients are not listed in the case report) (19). Although skullcap and valerian were common to both preparations, numerous other herbs were present in these tablets.
—Another case of hepatitis occurred in a 49-year-old woman taking herbal tablets that contained mistletoe, motherwort, kelp, wild lettuce, and skullcap (20); as the authors point out, mistletoe has known hepatotoxic effects.
—A 56-year-old woman in Australia developed hepatitis after taking a variety of herbal products that included mistletoe, celery fruit, guaiacum, burdock root, sarsaparilla, valerian, skullcap, and passion flower (1).

—In a fatal case, a 28-year-old man presented with jaundice after treating mild multiple sclerosis with zinc, skullcap (six tablets daily, no other information given), and p'au d'arco (21). The patient tested negative for HIV and hepatitis virus A, B, and C; toxicology screens were negative, and antinuclear antibodies were positive. On autopsy, hepatic venoocclusive disease with associated hepatic necrosis was noted. The herbal compounds were not analyzed, but the authors conjecture that the mixture was adulterated with an herb containing pyrrolizidine alkaloids.

- *Scutellaria* is commonly used in traditional Chinese medicine, and normally neither administration of root preparations nor injection of baicalin or baicalein have been associated with adverse effects beyond rare gastrointestinal symptoms (1). However, an unreferenced statement in a pharmacology text states that 150 mg baicalin given by intramuscular injection can cause fever and muscle aches; 27 mg baicalin administered intravenously can cause fever and decreased leukocytes (22).

DRUG INTERACTIONS

- None reported. In rats, *S. baicalensis* root decoction administered for 5 days had no effect on cytochrome P450 levels or bilirubin metabolizing enzymes (23).

ANIMAL TOXICITY

- Baicalin administered intraperitoneally was reported to have an LD_{50} of 3 g/kg in mice.
- Chinese studies of *Scutellaria* root have found low toxicity when administered orally (1).
- Female mice treated subcutaneously with an aqueous extract of *S. baicalensis* for 5 days did not experience decreased fertility. Rats treated with aqueous extract concentrates of *Scutellaria* root in oral doses up to 25 g/kg/day from day 7 to day 17 of pregnancy were observed to have offspring with an increased incidence of lumbar rib and abnormalities of the urinary system (1).

 Dose

COMMON DOSAGE FORMS

- *Dried herb:* 1 to 2 g t.i.d.
- *Infusion:* 1 to 2 g t.i.d.
- *Liquid extract:* (1:1, 25% ethanol) 2 to 4 mL t.i.d.
- *Tincture:* (1:5, 45% ethanol) 1 to 2 mL t.i.d.

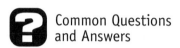 Common Questions and Answers

Q: Wasn't skullcap once used to treat rabies?
A: Yes, which explains its 18th century name of mad-dog skullcap. Popular in the late 18th and early 19th centuries, skullcap was considered a quack remedy by the 1820s (18).

Slippery Elm

10 Second Take

Slippery elm bark is a harmless herb used for sore throat and gastrointestinal irritation; no clinical trials were identified.

Basics

LATIN NAME

Ulmus rubra Muhl., syn. *Ulmus fulva* Michx.

FAMILY

Ulmaceae

OTHER COMMON NAMES

Red elm, Indian elm

DESCRIPTION

• A tree that grows up to 60 ft in the northern and eastern United States, slippery elm has deeply furrowed bark and toothed leaves, which are fuzzy on the underside. The inner bark is pinkish.

PART USED

Inner bark

KNOWN ACTIVE CONSTITUENTS

• Mucilage contains D-galacturonic acid, L-rhamnose, and D-galactose (1). 3-*O*-methyl-D-galactose, the methylated polysaccharide, yields 3-*O*- and 4-*O*-methyl-L-rhamnose, 2,3,4,6-tetra- and 2,3,6-tri-*O*-methyl-D-galactose, and 2,3,4 tri- and 2,3-di-*O*-methyl-D-galacturonic acid (2). Three oligosaccharides have also been isolated from the mucilage (3).

MECHANISM/PHARMACOKINETICS

• No information identified. Therapeutic effects are attributed to the emollient effect of mucilage in the herb.

Evidence

CLINICAL TRIALS

• None identified.
• A case report noted that a 47-year-old woman with lymphangitic lung adenocarcinoma and intractable cough resistant to lidocaine, morphine, chlorpromazine, and carbamazepine found that a teaspoon of slippery elm bark added to cereal or pudding in the morning reduced her cough considerably (4).

OTHER CLAIMED BENEFITS/ACTIONS

- Laxative
- Hemorrhoids
- Gastritis/gastroenteritis
- Upper respiratory infection (URI)
- Sore throats
- Skin problems
- Toothache
- Worms
- Diarrhea
- Ulcers
- Easing childbirth
- Abortion (see questions and answers)
- Wounds, burns (topical)
- Mastitis (topical)

 Risks

No risks identified.

 Dose

COMMON DOSAGE FORMS

- Tablets or lozenges taken ad lib
- *Powdered bark:* One part herb to 10 parts hot water, 5 to 20 mL ad lib
- *Decoction:* One part herb to eight parts water, 4 to 16 mL t.i.d.
- *Liquid extract:* (1:1, 60% ethanol) 5 mL t.i.d.
- *Topical application:* Poultices have been made of powdered bark mixed with boiling water and cooled.

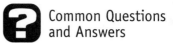 Common Questions and Answers

Q: How was slippery elm used in abortion?
A: Sticks of slippery elm were once inserted into the uterus as a home abortifacient technique. Absorption of fluid would cause swelling and, thus, cervical dilation. (*Laminaria* tents are used in a similar manner today.) To prevent its use for this purpose, several state legislatures apparently passed laws prohibiting the sale of slippery elm pieces more than $1\frac{1}{2}$ in long (5).

Q: What are other uses of slippery elm?
A: Powdered bark (mixed into paste with cold water, then thinned gradually with hot water) was made into a gruel to be fed to infants and sick people. The bark once was used to wrap meats to deter rancidity and was once molded into bandages for covering wounds (5). An old miner's remedy consisted of sucking bark with a little kerosene to prevent coal dust from sticking to the throat (the kerosene sounds like a particularly bad idea) (6).

Spirulina

 10 Second Take

Spirulina is a harmless alga with some nutritional value; it is especially high in vitamin A and carotenoids. There is no good evidence that it decreases cholesterol or combats obesity in humans.

 Basics

LATIN NAME

Spirulina platensis or *Arthrospira platensis, Spirulina maxima, Spirulina fusiformis*

FAMILY

Oscillatoriaceae

DESCRIPTION

• Spirulina is a microscopic filamentous blue-green alga (*Cyanobacterium*), which is not a true alga. Blue-green algae have traditionally been used as food on Mexico (*Spirulina platensis*) and Chad (*Spirulina maxima*) (1).

PART USED

Entire plant

KNOWN ACTIVE CONSTITUENTS

• Protein 60% to 70% by weight (including about 41.5% essential amino acids), vitamin B_{12}, thiamine, riboflavin, vitamin A, and iron (2). Spirulina is an extremely good source of vitamin A and carotenoids, and it is claimed to be an effective means of supplementation in children (3) and rats (4). Spirulina also contains gamma-linolenic acid (GLA) (1% to 1.5% of dry weight) (5).
• One analysis of spirulina found the following (2):

	% US RDA
Protein	3%
Vitamin A	187%
Vitamin E	3%
Vitamin C	<2%
Thiamine	11%
Riboflavin	7.5%
Niacin	1.8%
Vitamin B_{12}	80% (see questions and answers)
Iron	8%
Zinc	0.6%
Calcium	0.5%

• Its essential amino acid content as a percentage of total protein is:

Isoleucine	5.7%
Leucine	8.7%
Lysine	5.1%
Methionine	2.6%
Phenylalanine	5.0%
Threonine	5.4%
Tryptophan	1.5%
Valine	7.5%

 Evidence

CLINICAL TRIALS

• Oral leukoplakia

—A placebo-controlled trial of 87 tobacco chewers with oral leukoplakia tested 1 g daily of *Spirulina fusiformis* against placebo for 12 months (6). Complete regression of lesions was noted in 20/44 (45%) of the spirulina-treated group compared with 3/43 (7%) of the placebo group ($p < 0.0001$). No effect was seen in those with ulcerated or nodular lesions. Within 1 year of discontinuation, 9/20 complete responders developed recurrent lesions. No toxicity was noted. These results could be explained by spirulina's high vitamin A content, but no increase in serum concentrations of retinol or beta-carotene was seen.

• Hypercholesterolemia

—In an inadequately reported study, 30 men were divided into two groups. Both groups received 4.2 g/day spirulina (divided into three doses taken after meals); one group was treated for 8 weeks and the second group treated for 4 weeks (7). The report states that participants had "one or more of the following conditions": total cholesterol > 220 mg/dL, serum triglycerides > 150 mg/dL, or diastolic blood pressure > 90 mm Hg. Nowhere is it stated how many participants were actually hypercholesterolemic (individual data is not presented; only group means are provided). Serum cholesterol decreased significantly in the group treated for 8 weeks, with a difference apparent at 4 weeks; however, there was no significant change in total cholesterol in the second group at 4 weeks. Neither group experienced changes in serum triglyceride, high density lipoprotein (HDL)-cholesterol, or low density lipoprotein (LDL)-cholesterol. It is stated that diastolic blood pressure was reduced in both groups at 8 weeks (with no difference between groups), but these data are not presented. This is not a convincing study.

• Obesity

—In a double-blind placebo-controlled study of the effect of spirulina in 16 overweight participants (15 female), participants consumed 2.8 g (fourteen 200-mg tablets) of spirulina or spinach before meals three times daily for 4 weeks (8). After a 2-week washout period they were crossed over to the other group. Although this study is reported as showing "a small but statistically significant reduction of body weight in obese outpatients," in fact there was no difference in weight loss between the active and placebo phases (body weight decreased by an average of 1.4 kg during the active phase and 0.7 kg during the spirulina phase).

ANIMAL/IN VITRO

• Lipids

—In rats, spirulina as 5% to 16% of the diet has been reported to decrease total and HDL-cholesterol and triglycerides (4).

• Anticancer/immune system effects

—In hamsters, an extract of spirulina and *Dunaltella* prevented tumor development in hamster buccal pouch; the immune response of mice was enhanced in those fed spirulina-enhanced feeds.
—Calcium spirulan, a novel sulfated polysaccharide isolated from *Spirulina platensis,* inhibited tumor invasion of basement membrane of several types of cancer cells in an *in vitro* model (9).

• Renal toxicity

—In rats, a 30% spirulina diet appears to have a protective effect against renal toxicity induced by a number of agents (4).

• Antiviral effects

—*In vivo,* an aqueous extract of *Arthrospira platensis* (*Spirulina platensis*) inhibited HIV-1 replication in human T-cell lines, peripheral blood mononuclear cells, and Langerhans cells (10). Extract concentrations between 0.3 and 1.2 μg/mL reduced viral production by about 50%.
—Calcium spirulan, a novel sulfated polysaccharide isolated from *Spirulina platensis,* has demonstrated antiviral effects against HIV in three different assays and also demonstrated activity against herpes simplex virus type 1 (11). Compared with dextran sulfate, another sulfated polysaccharide, calcium spirulan showed a longer half-life in mice.

OTHER CLAIMED BENEFITS/ACTIONS

• Tonic

 Risks

ANIMAL TOXICITY

• A 13-week subchronic toxicity study of *Spirulina maxima* found that in mice, spirulina in doses up to 30% of the diet had no effect on growth; survival; food intake; or behavior, hematology, or clinical chemistry tests (12).

• Reproductive effects

—A toxicology study in mice tested spirulina in doses up to 30% of the diet and found no effect on fertility, number of abnormal pups, or developmental markers (nor were there any signs of toxicity) (13). A similar study found no adverse effects on fertility, pregnancy rate, number of fetuses, number of abnormal pups, length of gestation, parturition status, or litter values. There was a significant reduction in body weight and survival rate on postnatal days 0 to 4 in the high-dose group (14).

 Dose

COMMON DOSAGE/FORMS

• Typically taken in powder form or in capsules (300 to 500 mg) for a total daily dose of 1,800 to 4,000 mg daily.

 Common Questions and Answers

Q: Are all blue-green algae alike?
A: No, some are harmful. See *Aphanizomenon flos-aquae.*

Q: What about spirulina as a food source?
A: In the 1970s there was talk of growing spirulina as an alternative protein source for humans, because large amounts can be grown in a relatively small amount of space. As a cure for world hunger, spirulina did not catch on, but the use of spirulina as a dietary supplement (usually in capsule form) did become popular.
Although it is true that spirulina is a decent source of nutrients by weight, it would strain most people's palates to eat enough to matter. It would be difficult to consume enough in pill form to be a good nutritional source.
As shown by the analysis above (see section on known active constituents), a multivitamin supplies more of most nutrients and also costs far less (2).

Q: Is spirulina gathered in the wild or cultivated?
A: It is generally cultivated in long, open ponds, then harvested by pumping the algae and water through a series of screens and filters, after which it is washed and then dried into powder.

Q: Is spirulina a good source of vitamin B_{12}?
A: Spirulina is touted as a vegetarian source of B_{12} (which occurs mainly in animal products), and some testing procedures have shown the presence of this vitamin in significant amounts. However, more sophisticated testing has revealed that there are more B_{12} analogs in spirulina then there is B_{12}. By microbiologic assay, a 500-mg tablet of spirulina contains 0.25 to 1 μg of vitamin B_{12}, but radioassays reveal that more than 80% of this amount is actually analogs (15).

Q: Don't algae concentrate heavy metals?
A: Yes. An analysis of eight commercial samples of spirulina from Thailand, Mexico, the United States, Israel, and Taiwan in 1982 found that samples contained high concentrations of mercury (9.1 to 24.4 μg/g) and lead (1.3 to 6.7 μg/g), as well as copper (2.6 to 12.4 μg/g), iron (220 to 690 μg/g), manganese (13 to 205 μg/g), and zinc (7.4 to 106.1 μg/g) (16). Concentrations of all minerals varied widely among samples. The researchers point out that intake of 10 to 20 g/day of spirulina could result in mercury exposures above the "prudent" level set by the Food and Drug Administration.

Stevia

 10 Second Take

Stevia, a noncaloric sweetener, may have antihypertensive effects; possible effects on fertility are of concern.

 Basics

LATIN NAME

Stevia rebaudiana (Bertoni) Hemsl.

FAMILY

Compositae

DESCRIPTION

• There are at least 300 species of stevia; *Stevia rebaudiana* is native to high altitude regions of Brazil and Paraguay; it is also cultivated in Brazil, Israel, Japan, Korea, and China. Stevioside is currently marketed in Brazil, Paraguay, and Japan as a sweetener (1).

PART USED

Leaves

KNOWN ACTIVE CONSTITUENTS

• Stevioside, rebaudioside A, rebaudioside C, and other diterpene glycosides. Eight different ent-kaurene glycosides have been isolated; the common aglycone is steviol, chemically ent-13-hydroxy-kaur-16-en-19-oic acid.
• Dried stevia leaves contain 6% to 8% stevioside, which has little caloric value and is 300 times sweeter than sucrose (0.4% concentration) and 100 times sweeter than sucrose (10% concentration) (2). Stevia's sweetness is stable to heat and yeast fermentation; however, stevioside has a persistent bitter, metallic astringent aftertaste, and many processes have been used to decrease the aftertaste.

MECHANISM/PHARMACOKINETICS

• In rats, stevioside and the rebaudiosides are degraded to steviol by rat cecal flora; it is unclear whether this can be extrapolated to humans, who have different intestinal flora (2).

 Evidence

CLINICAL TRIALS

• Hypertension

—A randomized, double-blind, placebo-controlled study in 106 Chinese hypertensive patients (including 26 women) compared placebo with stevioside (250 mg t.i.d.) for 1 year (3). Participants, who were not on other antihypertensive medications, were assessed monthly. One hundred participants completed the trial. After 3 months, both systolic and diastolic blood pressure in the treated group decreased significantly, an effect that persisted throughout the year. No changes were seen in lipid levels or glucose levels, and no significant adverse effects were observed.

• Hypoglycemic effect

—Several studies, reported only in abstract form, claim a hypoglycemic effect of dried aqueous stevia extract (2). In a clinical trial reported as a letter to the *Brazilian Journal of Medical and Biological Research,* 16 healthy adults underwent a glucose tolerance test (GTT) after receiving an aqueous extract of stevia (each dose consisted of 5 g stevia dry leaves immersed in boiling water for 20 minutes) (4). Six controls received arabinose (250 mg) over the same schedule (arabinose was chosen because stevia contains large amounts of arabinose). The second GTT was done 2 hours after the first dose of stevia (and 21 hours after the baseline GTT). Compared with baseline GTT, plasma glucose levels after stevia ingestion were significantly lower at each timepoint tested (basal, 30, 60, 90, 120, 150, and 180 minutes). There was no difference between the first and second GTT in the arabinose controls. Apparently 13 doses of stevia or arabinose were administered at 6-hour intervals, but glucose levels are reported only after the first dose of stevia. Mysteriously, no information is given about results over the next 3 days, which renders the reported results of this study uninterpretable.

ANIMAL/IN VITRO

• Hypertension

—In spontaneously hypertensive rats, intravenous stevioside (50, 100, and 200 mg/kg) had a dose-related hypotensive effect on both systolic and diastolic blood pressure; the effect lasted for more than an hour at a dose of 200 mg/kg (5). In the same report, there were no changes in serum dopamine, norepinephrine, and epinephrine after stevioside 100 mg/kg was administered to anesthetized rats.

• Effects on blood sugar

—Feeding studies show no changes in glucose levels in rats consuming 0.5 to 1.0 g stevia extract or stevioside as 7% of the diet for 56 days (2). Rats fed 0.1% stevioside with a high-fat diet had no change in blood glucose or liver glycogen levels compared with rats fed only a high-fat diet. Rats fed the same amount of stevioside with a high-carbohydrate diet had decreased liver glycogen; blood glucose was not affected (2).
—A topical product called SUNCARE, which apparently contains *Stevia rebaudiana* and chrysanthemum flowers, has been used orally by diabetics; a study of escalating doses of this preparation [3 drops (3 mL) for 3 days, then a single 6-mL dose] in nondiabetic dogs resulted in no reductions in blood glucose and no changes in complete blood count (CBC) or blood chemistries (6).
—Intravenous stevioside only transiently lowers the level of blood glucose in alloxan-treated diabetic rabbits (2). In rat pancreas, stevioside 15 μM did not affect arginine-induced insulin or glucagon secretion (2). In incubated mouse islets, stevioside and steviol (1 nmol to 1 mmol/L) enhanced insulin secretion in the presence of glucose in a dose-dependent manner (7). Further investigation showed that stevioside and steviol stimulate insulin secretion through a direct effect on beta cells.

• Reproductive effects/contraception

—Stevia may reduce fertility. Two studies found that a diet that included 5% aqueous extract of stevia reduced fertility in female rats; however, a third study did not confirm this effect (8).

—Stevia appears to lower fertility in male rats. Twenty male Wistar rats were given an aqueous extract of stevia (66.7 g dried leaves/100 mL) b.i.d. for 60 days. There was a significant decrease in concentration of spermatozoa in the cauda epididymis and the weights of cauda epididymis, seminal vesicle, and testes were decreased (8). There was a significant decrease in plasma testosterone levels but not luteinizing hormone (LH) levels. Administration of stevia did not cause any significant change in food consumption, body weight, or blood glucose levels. The authors theorize that stevia may have a direct action on testosterone synthesis, possibly by interference with enzymes involved in testosterone synthesis or interference with LH receptors on Leydig cells.
—See also animal toxicity for reproductive toxicology studies.

- Effect on caries

—Stevioside and rebaudioside A do not appear to be cariogenic. Stevioside and rebaudioside A were tested in 60 rat pups colonized with *Streptococcus sobrinus*. One group of rats received a 30% sucrose diet, another group 0.5% stevioside, a third group 0.5% rebaudioside A, and the fourth group received a normal diet (9). The group receiving a 30% glucose diet had significantly more caries than other groups; there were no significant differences among the other three groups.

- Antimicrobial effect

—A fermented hot water extract of stevia was strongly bactericidal toward a variety of food-borne pathogenic bacteria, including enterohemorrhagic *Escherichia coli* 0157:H7. Secretion of verocytotoxin 1 and 2 was also diminished at a concentration of $\geq$10% (v/v) (10). Bifidobacteria and lactobacilli were not significantly killed by the fermented extract.

- Renal effects

—A crude extract of stevia administered intravenously (0.05 mg/minute/100 g) did not cause any significant changes in mean arterial pressure or renal hemodynamics in Wistar rats (11). The extract significantly increased reabsorption of water by the collecting duct under antidiuresis conditions; under conditions of water diuresis the extract increased free water clearance, suggesting that the extract preferentially acts in proximal tubular cells involved with salt transport (11).

OTHER CLAIMED BENEFITS/ACTIONS

- Contraception
- Diabetes
- Burns
- Wounds
- Eczema
- Acne, other skin conditions (topical)

 Risks

ADVERSE REACTIONS

- No significant adverse reactions reported. However, fertility may be affected (see reproductive effects).

PREGNANCY/LACTATION

- No information on humans identified. (See animal toxicity.)

ANIMAL TOXICITY

- Orally administered stevioside and stevia extract are not toxic in mice, rats, hamsters, and guinea pigs. However, doses administered intraperitoneally or intravenously can cause acute toxicity and fatalities (12). LD_{50} doses of stevioside administered intraperitoneally or intravenously are between 1 and 34 g/kg body weight. Long-term feeding studies for 2 years in rats and for 6 months in hamsters did not result in any carcinogenicity (12).
- The LD_{50} of intraperitoneally administered stevia extract containing 50% stevioside in rats is 3.4 g/kg; the oral LD_{50} of stevioside in rats is reportedly 8.2 g/kg (2). High doses of orally administered stevioside (2.0 g/kg), rebaudiosides A-C, steviolbioside, or dulcoside are acutely toxic in mice. Up to 7% stevioside fed to rats for 3 months produced no remarkable toxic effects.

- Reproductive effects

—A study found that up to 3.0% dietary stevioside caused no fertility problems or teratogenic effects (2).
—Stevioside in doses up to 2.5 g/kg body weight/day affected neither growth nor reproduction in hamsters (13). Orally administered stevioside and stevia extract are not teratogenic in mice, rats, hamsters, or guinea pigs (12).
—In pregnant hamsters, steviol in doses up to 0.25 g/kg/body weight/day had no observable effect. This dose of steviol is equivalent to a dose of stevioside approximately 80 times higher than suggested acceptable daily intake of stevioside for humans (7.938 mg/kg body weight/day). Very high doses of steviol (0.75 and 1.0 g/kg body weight) were highly toxic to both dams and fetuses; the same dose also reduced both the number of live fetuses and mean fetal weight (14).
—Neither stevioside nor steviol affected chromosomes in an *in vitro* study of cultured human lymphocytes from five healthy donors (12).
—An *in vitro* study found that purified stevioside displaced 5α-dihydrotestosterone bound to prostate androgen receptors; however, chronic administration of stevia to male rats did not change the number of androgen binding sites (8).

 Dose

COMMON DOSAGE FORMS

For sweetening, $1\frac{1}{2}$ to 2 tablespoons can be substituted for 1 cup of sugar, or 2 to 3 leaves to sweeten one cup of beverage. Stevia may have a slightly bitter aftertaste.

Taurine

 10 Second Take

Taurine is benign; preliminary evidence supports cardiovascular benefits. It deserves further study.

 Basics

DESCRIPTION

• Taurine is one of three important sulfur-containing compounds [the others are the amino acids methionine and cyst(e)ine]. Taurine is an end product of cysteine catabolism, formed by removing a carboxyl group and formation of the sulfonic acid group (1). It is found in high concentrations in the retina and platelets and is a conditionally essential sulfur amino compound in neonates.

FOOD SOURCES

• Most taurine is derived from the diet. Most animal foods contain taurine; eggs and most plant foods, with the exception of seaweed, lack taurine. Omnivorous adults in the United States consume 1,000 to 1,200 μmol taurine/day. In England omnivores consume about 463 μmol/day, and Chinese men consume 34 to 80 mg/day (2).
• Per 100 g, poultry contains 89 to 2,445 μmol, beef and pork 307 to 489 μmol, processed meats 251 to 981 μmol, seafood 84 to 6,614 μmol, and seaweed 1.5 to 100 μmol (1). In Chinese food, the highest concentration of taurine was found in crustaceans and mollusks (300 to 800 mg/100 g) (2).
• Breast milk contains 33.7 $\pm$ 2.8 μmol taurine/100 mL (1). Although the milk of vegan mothers is lower in taurine than that of omnivorous mothers (strict vegans may consume almost no taurine), taurine levels in breast milk of vegan mothers is still about 30 times the level of unsupplemented cow's milk, which contains 18 to 20 μmol taurine/100 mL. Cow's milk-based infant formulas have been supplemented with taurine since the 1980s (1).

MECHANISM/PHARMACOKINETICS

• Taurine is a breakdown product of cyst(e)ine. Taurine has a possible role in growth and development; in cats, deficiency causes retinal degeneration, but there is no evidence that this occurs in humans (1). Taurine may have antioxidant effects (this is controversial; it may be only the precursor of taurine, hypotaurine, that is an antioxidant) (3). Although taurine is not completely reabsorbed by the kidney (in contrast, cysteine and methionine are almost completely reabsorbed), the kidney is still involved in regulating taurine body stores by regulating the proximal tubule brush-border membrane transporter for taurine (beta system) (1). Taurine is excreted as a conjugate with bile acids (4).

 Evidence

CLINICAL TRIALS

• Congestive heart failure

—A double-blind randomized crossover trial of 62 patients (58 completed) with congestive heart failure tested placebo against taurine (2 g t.i.d.) for 4 weeks. Compared with placebo, the taurine-treated group experienced significant improvements in physician assessment (dyspnea, palpitations, crackles, edema, and cardiothoracic ratio on chest x-ray film) and New York Heart Association functional class (5). Subjective symptoms decreased significantly from baseline in both groups during the first month; neither group experienced further decreases in symptoms during the second month. The treatment was well tolerated; 11.9% of those receiving taurine reported (primarily gastrointestinal) side effects, compared with 6.6% of those receiving placebo.
—A placebo-controlled study of intravenous taurine in 12 patients undergoing coronary bypass surgery found that 5 g taurine administered 1 to 3 hours before surgery reduced reperfusion lipoperoxidation and decreased cell damage by electron microscopy (6).

• Hypertension

—A double-blind placebo-controlled trial in 19 men with borderline hypertension compared placebo with taurine (6 g/day $\times$ 1 week) and found that taurine significantly decreased both diastolic and systolic blood pressure; plasma epinephrine also decreased significantly. In another experiment that included 12 men with borderline hypertension, taurine reduced blood pressure and attenuated increased response to intravenous glucagon; there was no effect on blood pressure or glucagon response in 9 age-matched normotensive subjects (7).

• Platelet aggregation

—Taurine decreases platelet aggregation. Two doses of taurine (400 mg and 1,600 mg $\times$ 8 days each, with a month washout between doses) were tested in five healthy men (8). Platelets from the taurine-supplemented participants resisted collagen-induced platelet aggregation; the effect was dose-dependent. Serum taurine levels increased about 40% with both doses.
—After demonstrating that doses of arachidonic acid required for platelet aggregation were significantly lower in diabetic patients than controls, another study found that taurine supplementation (1.5 g/day for 90 days) caused values in diabetics to be equivalent to controls (9). *In vitro* experiments found that taurine reduced aggregation in platelets from diabetic patients in a dose-dependent manner; platelet aggregation in healthy participants was not affected.

• Lipid effects

—A single-blind Japanese study tested the effect of taurine 6 g/day versus placebo in 22 healthy males fed diets containing 40% fat for 3 weeks (10). Although the authors conclude that taurine attenuated increases in total cholesterol (TC) induced by a high-fat (by Japanese standards) diet, the difference between groups is unimpressive. In the placebo group, TC increased from 169.7 $\pm$ 26.3 mg/dL to 195.1 $\pm$ 24.7 mg/dL (a significant difference) and TC increased from 195.3 $\pm$ 37.7 mg/dL to 217.4 $\pm$ 33.4 mg/dL in the taurine group (not a significant difference from baseline). The taurine group also experienced significant increases in very low density lipoprotein (VLDL) and triglycerides; the placebo group experienced a significant increase in low density lipoprotein (LDL).

ANIMAL/IN VITRO

• Cats cannot synthesize taurine and suffer retinal degeneration without it.
• Anticancer adjuvant

—Because taurine is abundant in lymphocytes and may modulate lymphocyte function, its effect was studied on interleukin-2 (IL-2)-activated, lymphocyte-mediated endothelial cell and tumor cell cytotoxicity (11). IL-2 immunotherapy is limited by its cytotoxic effects on endothelial cells. The addition of taurine reduced IL-induced cytotoxicity and did not reduce antitumor response mediated by natural killer cells. Taurine also apparently increased tumor cytotoxicity.

• Cardiovascular effects

—Taurine reduces blood pressure in hypertensive but not normotensive rats (3). Taurine appears to lower lipid levels in animal studies (3). In rats, taurine appears to lower blood lipids and have antiatherosclerotic effects (1).
—Taurine reduces hyperglycemia-induced human umbilical vein endothelial cells apoptosis, apparently through the lowering of reactive oxygen species and elevation of intracellular calcium levels (12).

• Hepatic effects

—In rats, hepatic steatosis and lipid peroxidation induced by chronic alcohol consumption can be reversed by administration of taurine; the authors suggest that increased bile flow may help to remove lipid peroxides (13).

OTHER CLAIMED BENEFITS/ACTIONS

• Cardiovascular diseases

Clinical Considerations

There are no specific recommendations for taurine intake. The recommended daily allowance (RDA) for sulfur amino acid intake is 13 mg/kg/day (14).
Plasma taurine is somewhat lower in females and in vegans. Although vegans consume little or no preformed taurine, this does not appear to be associated with any adverse health effects in vegans or their children (1).

DEFICIENCY SIGNS AND SYMPTOMS

• Taurine is considered conditionally essential during infant development and may be conditionally essential for adults in some circumstances. Since the 1980s, taurine has been added to infant formulas and pediatric parenteral solutions.
• Neonates fed breast milk, infant formula with taurine, or infant formula without taurine were studied up until 12 weeks of age (15). Whole blood taurine levels dropped in all three groups over the first 4 weeks. Auditory brainstem responses (ABR) wave latency was shorter in the nonsupplemented group (wave V showed the greatest reductions) than the other groups. Transient evoked otoacoustic emissions were larger in low to middle frequencies in the breast-fed group (possibly suggesting improved middle ear function).

FACTORS DECREASING AVAILABILITY/ABSORPTION

• Prematurity is associated with lower stores of taurine and causes a conditional requirement for taurine and cysteine, possibly because the capacity for transsulfuration is insufficient (even term infants appear to have only a limited capacity for transsulfuration). In addition, the beta-amino acid transport system in an immature kidney does not increase absorption of taurine in response to poor taurine status (1).
• Fetuses with intrauterine growth retardation have low plasma levels of taurine; this may be caused by reduced activity of placental taurine transporters (16).
• Diabetics have reduced levels of plasma and platelet taurine concentrations, compared with controls (65.6 $\pm$ 3.1 μmol/L vs. 93.3 $\pm$ 6.3 μmol/L) (9).
• Hepatic dysfunction can lower taurine levels (as well as other sulfur-containing amino acids).
• Total parenteral nutrition (TPN) can result in lower sulfur amino acid status; TPN solutions do not routinely contain taurine. Although taurine can be synthesized from methionine, which is included, synthesis is limited.

FACTORS INCREASING AVAILABILITY/ABSORPTION

• In athletes, levels of taurine increase significantly after endurance exercises; increases are even greater with higher intensity exercise versus longer duration (17).

LABORATORY TESTS

• Measures of nitrogen balance or growth are usually used to assess whether sulfur amino acids are adequate.
• Plasma concentration 39 to 116 μmol/L.
• Whole blood taurine 160 to 320 μmol/L (mean = 225 μmol/L). Plasma taurine concentrations are more responsive to changes in dietary taurine than are whole blood concentrations (plasma and whole blood concentrations correlate poorly except during periods of depletion or excess) (1).
• Hemolysis or contamination of plasma with platelets or white cells interferes with analysis of plasma but not whole blood taurine.

 ## Risks

ANIMAL TOXICITY

• No adverse effects were seen in cats fed up to 1 g (88 mmol)/100 g diet taurine (1).

Tea Tree

10 Second Take

Tea tree essential oil has antibacterial and antifungal effects; clinical trials support topical use for acne, onychomycosis, and possibly tinea pedis. Topical use is benign (although sensitization can occur); essential oils should not be used internally.

Basics

LATIN NAME

Melaleuca alternifolia

FAMILY

Myrtaceae

DESCRIPTION

• A small tree with narrow, needle-like leaves, tea tree is native to the northeast coastal region of New South Wales and southern Queensland, Australia.

PART USED

Leaves (usually as essential oil)

KNOWN ACTIVE CONSTITUENTS

• *Melaleuca* contains a complex mixture of about a hundred constituents, predominantly hydrocarbons and terpenes. Terpinen-4-ol, 1,8-cineole, α-terpineol, terpinolene, and α- and γ-terpinene comprise up to 90% of the oil. Terpinen-4-ol is thought to be the most active antimicrobial constituent; cineole probably has little antimicrobial activity, although there are reports of antihelminthic and antifungal activity (1).

Evidence

CLINICAL TRIALS

• Tinea pedis

—A randomized controlled trial in 104 patients compared a 10% tea tree oil topical cream with 1% tolnaftate and placebo (2). Only tolnaftate was better than placebo in achieving negative cultures; 85% of those treated with tolnaftate, 30% of those receiving tea tree, and 21% of those on placebo achieved culture cure. Both treatments were significantly better than placebo in treating symptoms; 24/37 in the tea tree oil group, 19/33 in tolnaftate, and 14/34 of those in placebo group improved in scaling, itching, burning, and inflammation.

• Acne

—A single-blind randomized trial in 124 participants with mild to moderate acne compared 5% tea tree oil with 5% benzoyl peroxide (3). Both treatments were effective in reducing the number of open and closed comedones; tea tree was slower in onset but was associated with fewer side effects. Benzoyl peroxide was more effective than tea tree oil at all timepoints (1, 2, and 3 months). In the benzoyl peroxide group, 79% reported side effects compared with 44% of the participants in the tea tree oil group (dryness was the most common symptom in both groups).

• Oral candidiasis

—A small open pilot trial tested tea tree oil oral solution for refractory oral candidiasis in AIDS patients (4). Thirteen patients with oral candidiasis clinically refractory to fluconazole [*in vitro* resistance was also demonstrated by a minimum inhibitory concentration (MIC) of ≥ 20 μg/mL] were given 15 mL of a *Melaleuca*-containing commercial mouthwash (concentration not specified) q.i.d. to swish and expel. Weekly evaluations consisted of evaluation of signs and symptoms, as well as quantitative yeast cultures. Twelve patients were evaluable at 4 weeks. Two were cured, six improved, four had no response, and one patient was worse. Mycologic response was seen in 7 of 12 patients. At follow-up 2 to 4 weeks after the therapy ended, no clinical relapse was seen in the two patients who were cured.

• Onychomycosis

—A double-blind, randomized controlled trial of 117 patients with distal subungual onychomycosis compared 1% clotrimazole with 100% tea tree oil (applied topically b.i.d.) for 6 months (5). Debridement and assessment were performed at baseline and after 1, 3, and 6 months. At the end of the trial, 11% of the clotrimazole group and 18% of the tea tree oil were cured by culture; clinically 61% of the clotrimazole group and 60% of the tea tree oil group were partially or fully resolved clinically. Three months later,

about half of each group reported continued improvement or resolution. There were no significant differences between treatments. —A randomized, double-blind trial of cream containing 5% *Melaleuca alternifolia* oil and 2% butenafine in 60 adults who had had onychomycosis for 6 to 36 months assigned 40 participants to active treatment and 20 to placebo (6). After 16 weeks, 80% of patients using tea tree oil cream were cured, compared with none in the placebo group. Four patients experienced mild inflammation that did not cause them to drop out of the trial.

• Vaginal infections

—A case series published in 1962 found that tea tree oil was effective in trichomonal vaginitis (7). However, this required quite a bit of effort. The vagina was first washed with pHisoHex, then washed with 0.4% tea tree oil, then a tampon saturated in an emulsified 40% solution of tea tree oil and alcohol was inserted and left in place. In addition, participants administered daily vaginal douches containing 0.4% tea tree oil. Clinical cure was achieved after an average of six office visits and 42 vaginal douches. (Such repeated ablutions with tap water may have worked just as well.) —A case report of a 40-year-old woman with bacterial vaginosis found a 5-day course of tea-tree oil suppositories (containing 200 mg tea tree oil in a vegetable oil base) successful (8).

• Topical decolonization of methicillin-resistant *Staphylococcus aureus* (MRSA)

—A randomized controlled trial tested a tea tree oil preparation for eradication of MRSA carriage (9). The combination of a 4% tea tree oil nasal ointment and 5% tea tree oil body wash was found to be equivalent to a 2% mupirocin nasal ointment and triclosan body wash (see also *in vitro*).

OTHER CLAIMED BENEFITS/ACTIONS

• Boils
• Skin infections
• Burns
• Wound healing
• Gum disease
• Body odor

ANIMAL/IN VITRO

• Antimicrobial effects

—An *in vitro* study of tea tree oil and mupirocin in 100 clinical isolates of MRSA found that 23% of the MRSA strains were susceptible to mupirocin, 45% exhibited low-level resistance, and 32% were highly resistant (10). All strains were susceptible to tea tree oil (although the authors note that its common use in topical products could change this). The MIC range for tea tree oil was 0.16% to .32%, and minimum bactericidal concentration (MBC) range was 0.32 to 1.25.

—In an *in vitro* study of skin flora susceptibility, *S. aureus* and most of the Gram-negative bacteria tested (including *Acinetobacter baumannii, Klebsiella pneumoniae,* and *Serratia marcescens*) were more susceptible to tea tree oil than the coagulase-negative staphylococci and micrococci (1).

—A commercial tea tree preparation (containing 40 mg/g tea tree oil and 1 mg/g triclosan in a sorbalene base) was tested against *Enterococcus faecalis, S. aureus, Escherichia coli,* and *Pseudomonas aeruginosa.* Only *S. aureus* and *E. coli* showed zones of growth inhibition, and these zones were similar to the sorbalene base alone (11). This commercial preparation is marketed for burns; given the lack of efficacy against organisms that commonly infect burns, the investigators recommended against its use.

—An antimicrobial activity test of eight components revealed that terpinen-4-ol was active against all test organisms; ρ-cymene had no antimicrobial activity; linalool and α-terpineol were active against all but *P. aeruginosa* (12). Sixty-six isolates of *S. aureus* (including 64 methicillin-resistant strains and 33 mupirocin-resistant strains) were all susceptible to tea tree oil in disc diffusion and modified broth microdilution methods; MIC was 0.25% and MBC was 0.5% (12).

• Head lice

—*In vitro,* tea tree oil (as well as numerous other essential oils including thyme, rosemary, and pine) was effective against head lice; the oils were applied in an alcohol solution and followed the next day with a rinse of the essential oil in a vinegar water solution (13).

• Vaginal organisms

—An *in vitro* test of tea tree oil against organisms associated with bacterial vaginosis found that most pathogens were sensitive but that *Lactobacilli* were relatively resistant (14). In an agar dilution assay, tea tree oil MICs for five *Gardnerella vaginalis* isolates were all 0.06%, and for three of four *Mobiluncus* isolates the MICs were 0.03% (it was 0.06% for the fourth). The minimum inhibitory concentration for 90% of organisms (MIC$_{90}$) was 0.5% for *Bacteroides* (12 isolates); 0.25% for *Prevotella* (24 isolates), *Fusobacterium* (10 isolates), and *Peptostreptococcus anaerobius* (12 isolates); and 0.12% for other Gram-positive anaerobic cocci (12 isolates). By broth macrodilution, MICs for all six *Bacteroides* species was 0.06% (the MBCs for five isolates was 0.06%, whereas the MBC for the last isolate was 0.12%). In contrast, MICs for the lactobacilli ranged from 0.12% to 2.0% and the minimum bactericidal concentration for 90% of organisms (MBC$_{90}$) was 2.0%. Tea tree oil also inhibits the growth of many fungi, including 32 strains of *Candida* (15).

Risks

ADVERSE REACTIONS

• Terpenes can produce central nervous system (CNS) depression and gastrointestinal and dermal irritation. There are a few case reports of tea tree oil poisonings in humans, primarily in children.

—In one case, a 23-month-old boy ingested 10 mL of tea tree oil. Initially confused and unable to walk, the child was treated with activated charcoal with sorbitol and became asymptomatic within 5 hours of ingestion (16).

—In another case, a 17-month-old boy who ingested less than 10 mL tea tree oil also developed ataxia and drowsiness (17).

—Half a teaspoon of tea tree oil ingested by a 60-year-old man resulted in a nonpruritic rash; swelling of the hands, feet, and face; and feeling of unwellness. The patient had previously ingested similar doses without symptoms (18).

—In another case a patient ingested half a cup of tea tree oil and was comatose for 12 hours and semicomatose for 36 hours; abdominal pain and diarrhea persisted for 6 weeks (19).

• Topically applied tea tree oil has been associated with dermatitis or skin dryness. Eight of 12 patients in the oral candidiasis trial (4) noted mild to moderate oral mucosal burning on contact with the solution (primarily during the first week of therapy; this symptom improved with improvement of the candidiasis).

• Several studies have been done using patch tests with 1% and 5% tea tree oil; in three tests totaling 85 patients, no adverse events were seen. In another patch test of 25% tea tree oil in 28 participants over 21 days, no sensitivity was seen in 25 participants; however, three participants experienced severe allergic responses (20). The degradation products of tea tree oil appear to be the most sensitizing (21).

ANIMAL TOXICITY

• Acute lethal dose of tea tree oil in rats is 1.9 to 2.6 g/kg body weight (20). Animals appear to be especially susceptible to CNS effects; high doses of topically applied tea tree oil can cause depression, weakness, incoordination, and muscle tremors. Supportive care usually results in recovery within 2 to 3 days (22).

Dose

COMMON DOSAGE FORMS

• Essential oils should never be ingested internally. Topical preparations may contain from 1% to 100% tea tree oil.
• *Quality Note:* Under the Australian standard, commercial tea tree oil must contain more than 30% terpinen-4-ol (thought to be the most active antimicrobial constituent) and less than 15% 1,8 cineole (a skin irritant) (23). The best-quality oils contain 40% to 47% terpinen-4-ol and 2.5% cineole (24).

Common Questions and Answers

Q: Where does tea tree get its name?
A: It is said that Captain Cook is responsible for the misleading common name of this plant: After observing aborigines brewing the leaves of this plant into a medicinal tea, he gave the plant its common name—the *tea tree.* It is no relation to the varieties of *Camellia* used to brew regular tea. Its camphor smell would not encourage anyone to consume it for enjoyment: It is one of the most "medicinal" smelling herbs.

Thiamin, Thiamine (Vitamin B$_1$)

10 Second Take

Thiamin is a benign vitamin. Deficiency is common, especially among older adults and alcoholics. Patients who present with acute alcohol toxicity should receive intravenous thiamin before intravenous glucose to avoid lactic acidosis.

Basics

DESCRIPTION

• A water-soluble, heat-labile B vitamin required in the metabolism of all cells, thiamin is a crucial coenzyme in three enzyme reactions: pyruvate decarboxylase, α-ketoglutarate decarboxylase (in the Krebs cycle), and transketolase (in the pentose-phosphate shunt).

FOOD SOURCES

Seeds, nuts, whole grains, brewer's yeast, wheat germ, legumes, and lean meat

MECHANISM/PHARMACOKINETICS

• Thiamin is necessary for energy metabolism and nerve cell function. Thiamin is crucial to the breakdown of branched-chain amino acids and is a coenzyme in decarboxylation and transketolase reactions necessary for intermediate metabolism of all cells. Pyruvate cannot enter the Krebs cycle in the absence of thiamin. Thiamin is also necessary for the formation of acetylcholine. A metabolite, thiamin triphosphate, may have an important separate role in brain cell function.

Evidence

CLINICAL TRIALS

• Congestive heart failure (CHF)

—Thiamin deficiency is common in CHF patients on loop diuretics (1).
—In a double-blind placebo-controlled trial of 30 CHF patients receiving long-term furosemide, 15 received 200 mg thiamin i.v., and 15 patients received placebo. Thiamine repletion increased left ventricular ejection fraction, diuresis, and sodium excretion (2).

• Working memory in alcoholics

—A randomized, double-blind study in 169 (107 included in final analysis) alcohol-dependent participants without acute Wernicke-Korsakoff syndrome (WKS), who were undergoing detoxification tested five different doses of intramuscular thiamin (5, 20, 50, 100, or 200 mg) for two consecutive days on delayed alternation, a learning test sensitive to cognitive impairment associated with WKS. The 200-mg group had significantly higher posttreatment scores on the delayed alternation task (3). Thiamin status was not determined, but thiamin deficiency is common among alcoholics.

• Mood and memory

—A double-blind trial of 120 thiamin-replete female college students tested the effects of thiamin 50 mg/day for 2 months on mood, memory, and reaction time (4). Compared with placebo, thiamin had no effect on memory or general health but increased reaction times and resulted in significantly better mood, assessed by the profile of mood states ($p < 0.05$) compared with placebo. Positive changes in mood were correlated with thiamin (but not riboflavin or pyridoxine) status. This study is notable for finding a benefit of supplementation in nondeficient participants.

• Alzheimer's disease

—High-dose thiamin may have a mild beneficial effect in Alzheimer's disease. In a randomized, double-blind, placebo-controlled crossover trial of 18 patients (including 13 women), patients received thiamin (3 g/day) or placebo for 1 month each (with no washout period) (5). Alzheimer's Disease Assessment Scale (ADAS) scores were better during the thiamin phase than the placebo phase in 13 of 17 patients ($p \le 0.03$). There was, however, no significant improvement over baseline scores. Thiamin status was not determined.
—In a second trial reported in the same paper, 17 participants (including 6 from the previous trial) were administered up to 8 g thiamin/day for 5 to 12 months in a partially open phase, partially crossover, single-blind study (5). Although significant improvement in ADAS scores compared with baseline were seen at 4/11 timepoints, there was no consistent dose or duration effect.

• Peripheral neuropathy

—In Tanzania, diabetic peripheral neuropathy is associated with thiamin deficiency; in a controlled study comparing thiamin 25 mg q.d. and pyridoxine 50 mg q.d. to placebo (containing thiamin 1 mg and pyridoxine 1 mg), significant improvement in pain, numbness, paresthesia, and impairment of sensation in the legs was noted in the treatment group (5a). The severity of peripheral neuropathy decreased in 48.9% of the treatment group compared with 11.4% in the placebo group.

• Fibromyalgia

—No controlled trials were identified. Small, uncontrolled pilot studies claim a benefit of thiamin treatment of fibromyalgia, with thiamin pyrophosphate appearing to be more successful than thiamin hydrochloride (both 50 mg i.m. three times weekly × 6 weeks) (6).

ANIMAL/IN VITRO

• In dogs with induced heart attacks, intravenous injections of thiamin pyrophospate (cocarboxylase) decreased heart rate, increased stroke volume, decreased systemic vascular resistance, and decreased myocardial oxygen consumption in the injured hearts (7).

OTHER CLAIMED BENEFITS/ACTIONS

• Depression
• Anxiety
• Schizophrenia
• Alzheimer's disease, other dementias
• Flea repellant

Clinical Considerations

DEFICIENCY SIGNS AND SYMPTOMS

• Marginal deficiency may occur in 17% to 27% of Americans and is especially common among alcoholics and older adults. AIDS patients are also at risk of thiamin deficiency, and several reports have noted neuropathologic changes characteristic of Wernicke's encephalopathy in patients with AIDS.

• Vitamin B$_1$ is not stored in the body, and deficiency symptoms may occur within a week of thiamin deprivation. Within a month of being fed a thiamin-deficient diet, participants experienced generalized weakness, paresthesias, and marked irritability and depression (8).

• Beriberi

—"Dry" beriberi or thiamin deficiency neuropathy are terms used for neurologic manifestations, which usually present as a motor disability. Signs are bilateral and worse in the lower extremities; thigh muscles are often affected and footdrop or wristdrop may occur. Tendon reflexes are reduced. Pain and paresthesia are the main complaints in 25% of patients with thiamin deficiency neuropathy. Legs are generally affected earlier and more severely than arms; manifestations begin in distal dermatomes and progress proximally. Paresthesias may include a burning sensation of the feet or a constant dull aching, cramping, or tightness in the feet or legs (9). Affected areas are often exquisitely tender, and atrophy of muscles may occur. Other symptoms may include fatigue, amnesia, and decreased attention span.
—"Wet" beriberi connotes cardiovascular manifestations, including cardiomegaly and tachycardia on mild exertion. Thiamine supplementation can cause dramatic cardiovascular improvement.

- Wernicke-Korsakoff syndrome

—A thiamin deficiency disease seen mainly in chronic alcoholics, features of WKS include confusion, memory impairment, loss of appetite, vomiting, nystagmus, diplopia, ocular muscle paralysis, and possibly coma. (Patients who present with acute alcohol toxicity should receive 100 to 250 mg thiamin i.v. before receiving intravenous glucose; see lactic acidosis).

- Lactic acidosis

—Thiamin-deficient patients given glucose may develop life-threatening lactic acidosis (10). Pyruvate cannot enter the Krebs cycle in the absence of thiamin, and lactic acidosis may result from pyruvate accumulation. Patients who present with acute alcohol toxicity should receive 100 to 250 mg thiamin i.v. before receiving intravenous glucose.
—During a nationwide shortage of intravenous multivitamins in 1988, 3 of 59 patients receiving total parenteral nutrition without thiamin at a large university medical hospital died of refractory lactic acidosis after clinical courses suggestive of acute beriberi. Autopsies on two of these cases showed brain lesions diagnostic for acute thiamin deficiency (11).

- Thiamin-responsive anemia

—A syndrome that includes megaloblastic anemia responsive only to thiamin has been reported. The disorder occurs with diabetes mellitus and sensorineural deafness and may be genetic in origin. The syndrome occurs without laboratory evidence of thiamin deficiency (12).

- Postoperative confusion

—Thiamin levels may drop postoperatively even in those who are not deficient preoperatively. A study of 64 older orthopedic patients found that those patients who were notably confused after surgery were found to have had a considerable drop in their thiamin status (13).

FACTORS DECREASING AVAILABILITY/ABSORPTION

- Loop diuretics: Long-term furosemide therapy in patients with CHF can cause subclinical thiamin deficiency. In 38 patients with CHF treated with loop diuretics, biochemical evidence of deficiency was seen in 8 (21%), evidence for risk for dietary thiamin inadequacy was seen in 10 (25%) (1).
- Ethanol interferes both with the gastrointestinal absorption and the utilization of thiamin.
- Raw fish and shellfish contain thiaminases, which destroy thiamin.
- Tea and coffee contain tannins, which oxidize thiamin.
- The refinement of whole grains removes most thiamin.
- Heat destroys thiamin.

DIAGNOSTIC TESTS

- Whole blood erythrocyte transketolase activity involves the stimulation of red blood cell (RBC) transketolase activity *in vitro* by the addition of thiamin pyrophosphate. This is referred to as the TPP effect; if the increase is more than 15%, then deficiency is likely.
- Urinary thiamin excretion or RBC thiamin diphosphate levels may also be used, but are considered less reliable.
- Electrophysiologic studies are not specific but may support the diagnosis of thiamin deficiency; nerve conduction studies may show mild slowing; evoked potential amplitudes may be reduced; electromyograms may show signs of degeneration.

 Risks

ADVERSE REACTIONS

- No ill effects have been noted in humans in doses up to 200 times the recommended daily allowance (RDA).
- Animal Toxicity

—The LD_{50} in mice and dogs is 125 to 350 mg/kg i.v. (14).

 Dose

MODE OF ADMINISTRATION

- Vitamin B_1 is usually administered as thiamin hydrochloride or thiamin mononitrate. It may be given p.o., i.m., or i.v.

RECOMMENDED DIETARY ALLOWANCE

- Depends on energy expended: 0.5 mg/ 1,000 kcal expended per day

Infants and children

0 to 6 months	0.2 mg/day (adequate intake)
7 to 12 months	0.3 mg/day (adequate intake)
1 to 3 years	0.5 mg/day
4 to 8 years	0.6 mg/day

Males

9 to 13 years	0.9 mg/day
14 to 50 years	1.2 mg/day
51+ years	1.2 mg/day

Females

9 to 13 years	0.9 mg/day
14 to 18 years	1.0 mg/day
19 to 50 years	1.1 mg/day
51+ years	1.1 mg/day
Pregnant	1.4 mg/day
Lactating	1.4 mg/day

- *Correcting deficiency*: Thiamin deficiency is best treated with 50 mg thiamin i.m. three times weekly or 100 mg thiamin p.o. q.d. In patients with malabsorption problems, 100 mg i.m. may be given weekly.

 Common Questions and Answers

Q: How much heat does it take to affect thiamin content?
A: Thiamin is extremely heat-labile; toasting bread lowers its thiamin content considerably. Even 60 seconds of toasting lowers the thiamin in whole wheat bread by 15%, enriched white bread by 15%, and unenriched white bread by 27% (14). Our older adult "tea and toast" patients are at particular risk of thiamin deficiency because tea contains tannins, which oxidize thiamin.

Q: Who should take thiamin supplements?
A: It is particularly important to consider supplementation in older adults, patients with AIDS, alcoholics, and patients with CHF on loop diuretics. Given the results of the Benton study, perhaps teenage girls should be supplemented as well. An oral B-complex supplement containing 50 to 100 mg/day is adequate.

Threonine (Thr, T)

 10 Second Take

Threonine is a harmless amino acid; clinical trials have demonstrated a modest reduction in spasticity that does not appear to be clinically significant.

 Basics

DESCRIPTION

Threonine is an essential neutral (aliphatic) amino acid.

FOOD SOURCES

Most protein-containing foods

MECHANISM/PHARMACOKINETICS

• Threonine is a part of most proteins and is one precursor of glycine; administration of L-threonine increases glycine levels in rat spinal cord (1). Plasma half-life is 2 days (2).

 Evidence

CLINICAL TRIALS

• Familial spastic paraparesis

—A double-blind, placebo-controlled crossover study in 18 patients with familial spastic paraparesis (FSP) tested the effects of L-threonine (4.5 or 6.0 g/day, each for 2 weeks). Outcome measures included physician global impression; patient global impression; and semiquantitative ratings of strength, muscle tone, deep tendon reflexes, walking, hopping, and running. There was a statistically significant decrease in motor impairment and spasticity; however, neither physician nor patient global impressions noted significant treatment effects (1).

• Spinal spasticity

—A double-blind, placebo-controlled, crossover study of oral L-threonine (6 g/day × 2 weeks, with a 2-week washout between phases) in 33 patients with spinal spasticity (29 completed) found a modest benefit of L-threonine over placebo (3). A sequential analysis was used (in which patients were enrolled until patient preferences reached significance at the 5% level); this level was reached for threonine after 33 patients were enrolled. As measured by the Ashworth scale, which assesses lower limb spasticity, 16 patients responded to threonine, 3 to placebo, 2 to both and 8 responded to neither. Symptomatic improvement was reported by six patients receiving threonine and two patients receiving placebo. One treated patient reported diarrhea, and one reported indigestion.

- Multiple sclerosis

—A randomized, placebo-controlled crossover trial tested threonine (7.5 g/day in divided doses) in 26 ambulatory patients with multiple sclerosis (21 completed both phases). Each phase lasted 8 weeks, and there was a 2-week washout between phases. Threonine significantly reduced signs of spasticity on clinical examination (Clinician Spasticity Scale); however, neither physician nor patient noted any symptomatic improvement. Neurophysiologic measures did not differ between phases. No side effects of threonine were seen (4).

- Amyotrophic lateral sclerosis

—A randomized year-long trial of 30 patients with amyotrophic lateral sclerosis compared L-threonine with vitamin B complex or carnitine. Only 13 patients (including 9 patients taking threonine and 4 controls) completed the trial. There were no significant differences between the threonine-treated group and the control participants in decreased clinical assessment scores (5). A randomized, double-blind, placebo-controlled trial of L-threonine (2 g daily) in 15 patients with amyotrophic lateral sclerosis found no significant differences between the two groups (6).

OTHER CLAIMED BENEFITS/ACTIONS

- Neurologic diseases

 Clinical Considerations

LABORATORY TESTS

- Free amino acid concentration in venous blood: 76 to 194 μmol/L
- Urinary output: 150 μmol/24 hours

 Risks

No risks identified.

 Dose

RECOMMENDED DIETARY ALLOWANCE

Estimates of Dietary Amino Acid Requirements (7)

Infants and children
3 to 4 months	87 mg/kg/day
2 to 5 years	37 mg/kg/day
10 to 12 years	28 mg/kg/day
Adults	7 to 15 mg/kg/day

Thyme

 10 Second Take

Thyme is a safe herb for culinary or medicinal use; it has some antimicrobial properties but clinical trials are lacking.

 Basics

LATIN NAME

Thymus vulgaris

FAMILY

Lamiaceae

OTHER COMMON NAMES

Common thyme, garden thyme, and French thyme

DESCRIPTION

• Thyme is a dwarf shrub with aromatic leaves and whorls of pale violet flowers. It is native to southern Europe, the Balkans, and the Caucasus; it is now widely cultivated in many parts of the world. The culinary herb is often imported from Spain, Morocco, France, Bulgaria, and Hungary.

PART USED

Leaves, flowers

KNOWN ACTIVE CONSTITUENTS

• Thyme contains 1.0% to 2.5% essential oil, the main constituents of which are the monoterpenes thymol (30% to 70%) and carvacrol (3% to 15%). Other monoterpenes include *p*-cymene, terpinene, and limonene; also contains small amounts of tannins, flavonoids, and triterpenes.

 Evidence

CLINICAL TRIALS

• Alopecia areata

—A study of 86 patients with alopecia areata compared a topical mixture of essential oils including thyme, rosemary, lavender, and cedar wood with placebo; each was rubbed into the scalp daily for 7 months. Sequential photographs were rated on an alopecia scale by blinded observers. The primary outcome measure was improvement versus no improvement; 19 (44%) of 43 patients in the essential oil group showed improvement compared with 6 (15%) of 41 patients in the control group. The degree of improvement on photographic assessment was also significant (1).

• Cough

—A double-blind, randomized study compared the effect of thyme syrup to bromhexine to treat coughing in 60 patients. Treatment was given for 5 days; both groups improved with no difference between groups (2).

• Insect repellent

—Essential oil of thyme in concentrations 25% to 100% repelled mosquitoes from human skin (duration ranged from 90 minutes to 3½ hours, depending on concentration); however, the two participants in this trial found the odor of essential oils unacceptable at concentrations greater than or equal to 25% (3).

ANIMAL/IN VITRO

• Antimicrobial effects

—Essential oil of thyme has antibacterial effects; carvacrol and thymol are the most active compounds against food-derived spoilage bacteria and pathogenic bacteria (4). Thyme oil or its components have been proposed as a food additive to extend shelf life of processed foods. An investigation of 52 plant oils and extracts against a variety of organisms found that the lowest minimum inhibitory concentrations against *Candida albicans* and *Escherichia coli* were achieved with essential oil of thyme 0.03% (v/v) (5). —Vapor contact with essential oil of thyme (1 to 4 μg mL-L air) killed *Trichophyton* conidia, inhibited germination, and inhibited hyphal elongation; an *in vivo* study found a beneficial effect in guinea pigs infected with *Trichophyton mentagrophytes* (6). Vapor contact with essential oil of thyme retarded growth of *Aspergillus fumigatus* at 6.3 μg mL-L air and stopped growth at 63 μg mL-L air (7).

• Antispasmodic and respiratory tract effects

—An ethanolic extract of thyme antagonizes contraction of isolated guinea pig trachea (8). Essential oil of thyme appears to improve increased secretions in the upper respiratory tract and enhance movement of the cilia in the bronchi (9).

• Antioxidant effects

—In the rat, thyme oil tended to maintain higher polyunsaturated fatty acid levels in several tissues studied, including brain, kidney, and heart. Thymol appeared to be responsible for this effect, but thymol alone was not more effective than thyme oil (10).

OTHER CLAIMED BENEFITS/ACTIONS

• Bronchitis
• Whooping cough
• Expectorant
• Bronchospasm
• Antibacterial
• Gastrointestinal
• Diuretic
• Laryngitis
• Diarrhea

 Risks

ADVERSE REACTIONS

• Thyme dust can cause occupational airborne contact dermatitis. A study in 46 farmers during threshing of dried thyme found that four showed skin symptoms after less than or equal to 30 minutes of exposure to thyme dust (11). The reaction may be due to an irritant effect; it does not appear to be IgE mediated as thyme-specific IgE was noted in one symptomatic farmer and two asymptomatic farmers.

 Dose

COMMON DOSAGE FORMS

• *Dried herb:* 1 to 4 g t.i.d.
• *Infusion* made from 1 to 2 g b.i.d. to t.i.d.
• *Fluid extract:* 1/1 (g/mL) 1 to 2 mL q.d. to t.i.d.
• *Tincture:* (1:10, 70% ethanol) 40 drops q.d. to t.i.d.
• Children:

—Age 0 to 1 year: 0.5 to 1 g dried herb in infusion b.i.d. to t.i.d.
—1 year and older: 1 g herb in infusion b.i.d. to t.i.d.

• Topical uses include gargle or mouthwash (5% infusion) and compresses (cloths saturated in 5% infusion).

Tryptophan (Trp, W) and 5-hydroxytryptophan (5-HTP)

 10 Second Take

Tryptophan is not commercially available in the United States because of its link to eosinophilia-myalgia syndrome. 5-Hydroxytryptophan (5-HTP) is available but is not necessarily safe.

 Basics

DESCRIPTION

• Tryptophan, an essential amino acid, is converted to 5-hydroxytryptophan (5-HTP), the intermediate metabolite in the serotonin pathway, by tryptophan hydroxylase. 5-HTP is commercially produced from the seeds of an African herb, *Griffonia simplicifolia*.

FOOD SOURCES

• Many protein-containing foods. Average daily intake of tryptophan among nonvegetarians is 1.5 g/day, among lacto-ovo vegetarians 1.2 g/day, and among vegans 1.1 g/day (1).

MECHANISM/PHARMACOKINETICS

• Tryptophan, a precursor of serotonin and nicotinamide, is a major dietary source of niacin; the term *niacin-equivalents* takes tryptophan ingestion into account. The conversion of tryptophan to 5-HTP by tryptophan hydroxylase is the rate-limiting step in serotonin synthesis. Normal levels of 5-HTP are ≤ 1 ng/mL; after carbidopa pretreatment and administration of 50 to 100 mg 5-HTP, serum levels can reach 1,000 ng/mL; levels above 100 ng/mL are maintained for least 8 hours. Half-life of 5-HTP is between 2½ to 7 hours after a single oral dose of 200 mg in participants pretreated with carbidopa (2).

 Evidence

CLINICAL TRIALS

• Mood disorders

—Tryptophan has been used since the 1970s in an effort to increase serotonin levels, but controlled trials are lacking. A review of small, mostly uncontrolled studies concluded that tryptophan alone has not been demonstrated to be effective for depression (3). Tryptophan depletion can increase depressive symptoms in patients with major depression (4), seasonal affective disorder (5,6), and bulimia nervosa (7) and significantly increases anxiety in patients with panic disorder (8).
—In an open crossover study, tryptophan × 4 weeks was compared with light therapy × 2 weeks in 13 patients with seasonal affective disorder (including 11 women) (9). Both treatments improved scores on a modified Hamilton depression rating scale. Four patients did not respond to either therapy, four responded only to light therapy, and one responded only to tryptophan.

• Premenstrual syndrome

—A randomized controlled trial (RCT) in 71 women (63 completed) with premenstrual syndrome tested the effects of L-tryptophan 6 g/day for the latter half of the cycle (and for the first three days of menses) (10). L-tryptophan, compared with placebo, decreased mood symptoms (dysphoria, mood swings, tension, and irritability). Compared with baseline, maximum luteal phase mood scores decreased 34.5% with L-tryptophan compared with 10.4% with placebo. There were no differences between groups for headache, edema, or breast sensitivity.

• Fatigue

—A crossover trial in six participants tested a soft drink with or without L-tryptophan (30 mg/kg) on fatigue (11). Tryptophan significantly increased subjective and objective measures of central fatigue. Tryptophan did not affect grip strength but significantly increased ergometric work output.

• 5-HTP and mood disorders

—A review of 5-HTP identified seven double-blind controlled trials of 5-HTP for depression (2). Five small trials (three placebo-controlled, one imipramine-controlled, and one that tested 5-HTP against placebo as an adjunct to nialamide) reported in the 1970s claimed improvement with 5-HTP, but crucial information appears to be missing. A 1980 trial compared placebo with 5-HTP (300 mg 5-HTP/dose with carbidopa pretreatment for 32 days) or a 5-HTP-deprenyl combination in 58 patients with unipolar or bipolar depression. 5-HTP and deprenyl, but not 5-HTP alone, was significantly better than placebo. Another three-armed trial in 45 depressed patients compared tryptophan (5 g/day) with 5-HTP (200 mg with

carbidopa) and placebo for 20 days. 5-HTP was statistically superior to placebo.

• 5-HTP for headaches

—A double-blind RCT in 78 patients (65 completed) with chronic tension-type headaches compared L-5-hydroxytryptophan (300 mg/day × 8 weeks) to placebo (12). Neither group improved in number of days with headache or in headache intensity; however, analgesic consumption was significantly less in the treated group. During the 2 weeks after treatment ended, participants treated with 5-HTP had fewer days with headache.

• 5-HTP in Friedreich's ataxia

—A double-blind placebo-controlled study in 26 patients (19 completed) with cerebellar symptoms of Friedreich's ataxia found a significant, but clinically unimportant, benefit of L-5-HTP on coordination (13).

OTHER CLAIMED BENEFITS/ACTIONS

• Insomnia
• Pain
• Mood disorders

 Clinical Considerations

DEFICIENCY SIGNS AND SYMPTOMS

• None identified (would be the same as for protein deficiency)

FACTORS DECREASING AVAILABILITY/ABSORPTION

• None identified for tryptophan.
• Hyperphenylalaninemia due to dihydropteridine reductase deficiency or problems with biopterin synthesis require 5-HTP as part of treatment (14).

FACTORS INCREASING AVAILABILITY/ABSORPTION

• Hyperammonemia or a high carbohydrate, low-protein diet may stimulate tryptophan transport into the brain, possibly causing anorexia (14).
• Pretreatment with carbidopa increases the absorption of 5-HTP (2).

Tryptophan (Trp, W) and 5-hydroxytryptophan (5-HTP)

 Risks

ADVERSE REACTIONS

• Tryptophan and eosinophilia-myalgia syndrome (EMS)

—Contaminated tryptophan caused an epidemic of EMS that peaked in 1989 (15). More than 1,500 cases were reported by 1998, including 27 deaths (16). Most patients had arthralgia (73%), rash (50%), cough or dyspnea (59%), peripheral edema (59%), elevated aldolase levels (46%), and elevated liver function tests (43%). Neuropathy or neuritis was seen in 27%.
—Almost all cases for whom information was available had consumed tryptophan manufactured by Showu Denko, a company that had recently changed both its manufacturing process and the strain of *Bacillus* used to manufacture tryptophan (17). It is not clear that uncontaminated tryptophan is safe (see questions and answers).

• 5-HTP and EMS

—Although 5-HTP has so far not been associated with the same magnitude of problems as L-tryptophan, it cannot be presumed safe. Several cases of EMS-like syndromes have been reported in people ingesting L-5-HTP (in only one of these was the substance analyzed). In 1994, a typical case of EMS was reported in a 28-year-old woman who was exposed to 5-HTP by handling powder fed to her two children (who were being treated with 5-HTP for a defect in tetrahydrobiopterin synthesis) (18). The children's father, also exposed, manifested no signs or symptoms. Although both children were asymptomatic, both had increased white blood cell (WBC) counts and mild eosinophilia that resolved after they were switched to a different lot of 5-HTP. Subsequent high-pressure liquid chromatography (HPLC) analysis of the case-associated lot found a minor peak (dubbed peak X) that may represent a contaminant (examination of multiple lots revealed the presence of peak X in one of nine other lots sampled).
—In 1998, peak X was reported to be a beta-carboline derivative (6-hydroxy-1,2,3,4,4a, 9a-hexa-hydro-β-carboline-3-carboxylic acid), similar in structure to two contaminants in EMS-associated tryptophan (19). Later work found that peak X actually was a group of related compounds. An analysis of eight over-the-counter (OTC) 5-HTP products found that all contained three or more contaminants of the peak X family (20). Another analysis of six OTC samples also found low levels of peak X compounds (19). Although peak X consti-tuted only 3% to 15% of levels found in case-implicated 5-HTP, investigators pointed out that consuming 300 to 900 mg/day could bring intake into case-implicated levels. An ataxia study in which 28 patients received L-5-HTP and carbidopa was halted because of eosinophilia in three patients (18). Two

participants had mild eosinophilia; the third [concurrently exposed to mace (1-chloroacetophenone)] had marked eosino-philia (36%, or 5,500 eosinophils/mm^3).

• 5-HTP: other adverse effects

—Abdominal cramping, nausea, and diarrhea are common; insomnia, headache, and palpitations have been associated with 5-HTP. Hematologic tests and liver function tests do not appear to be affected. Very large doses of 5-HTP (2,500 to 9,000 mg/day with carbidopa) in schizophrenic patients caused transient increased psychosis, motor activity, and mild hypotension when doses were increased more than 2,000 mg in a day (2).
—Two participants suddenly discontinued from high doses had grand mal seizures.
—Another study of high-dose 5-HTP (400 to 2,000 mg/day up to 3 years, with carbidopa) found that 10/18 participants experienced stimulatory effects, including rapid speech and agitation; 2 required antipsychotics, and 1 developed a dermatomyositis-scleroderma like illness (2).
—Intravenous 5-HTP (200 to 300 mg) can cause confusion, memory impairment, rapid change in affect, pupillary dilation, hyperreflexia, ataxia, and dysarthria.
—Hypomania or mania has been reported after 5-HTP administration (2).

DRUG INTERACTIONS

• Monoamine oxidase inhibitors (MAOIs)

—Combining tryptophan with MAOIs (including phenelzine and tranylcypromine) has been associated with more than 10 cases of behavioral or neurologic toxicity. Symptoms included hypomania, agitation, delirium, and myoclonus (21).
—Combining lithium, phenelzine, and L-tryptophan has resulted in fatalities (22,23).

• Fluoxetine

—Five cases of toxicity have been reported when high-dose fluoxetine (50 to 100 mg daily) and L-tryptophan (2 to 4 g daily) were combined in patients with obsessive-compulsive disorder (OCD) (24). Symptoms (most typical of excessive serotonin levels) included worsened OCD symptoms, agitation, insomnia, aggression, headaches, palpitations, nausea, cramping, and diarrhea. These symptoms are typical of serotonin syndrome resulting from excessive serotonin levels (25).

• Electroconvulsive therapy

—When tryptophan is administered to patients receiving electroconvulsive therapy, seizure duration but not treatment effectiveness is increased (26).

• 5-HTP

—Although the same potential may exist for 5-HTP to interact with MAOIs and serotonin reuptake inhibitors (SRIs), there are many studies in which 5-HTP has been used adjunctively to enhance therapeutic effect (27,28).

ANIMAL TOXICITY

• Of 21 dogs who accidentally ingested 5-HTP, 3 died and 19 developed toxicosis; the most common symptoms were vomiting and/or diarrhea, seizures, hyperthermia, depression, and tremors (29). The minimum toxic dose was 23.6 mg/kg, and minimal lethal dose was 128 mg/kg (see questions and answers).

 Dose

RECOMMENDED DIETARY ALLOWANCE

Estimates of Dietary Amino Acid Requirements by Age Group (17)

Infants and children

3 to 4 months	17 mg/kg/day
2 to 5 years	12 mg/kg/day
10 to 12 years	3 mg/kg/day
Adults	4 to 6 mg/kg/day

 Common Questions and Answers

Q: Is uncontaminated tryptophan safe?
A: Probably, but it is not entirely clear. Although no human cases of EMS have been linked to uncontaminated tryptophan, abnormal tryptophan metabolism has been noted in scleroderma, and animal studies suggest that excess tryptophan or tryptophan metabolites could amplify some pathologic features of EMS (30). Lewis rats treated with contaminated L-tryptophan develop fasciitis and perimyositis, but animals receiving uncontaminated L-tryptophan show a mild but significant increase in myofascial thickness (31). It has been suggested that EMS may be a form of allergic reaction to L-tryptophan preparations in patients primarily suffering from fibromyalgia (32).

Turmeric

 10 Second Take

Turmeric, a common spice, has promising antioxidant effects and chemoprotective effects in animals; no clinical chemoprevention trials have been performed.

 Basics

LATIN NAME

Curcuma longa L.

FAMILY

Zingiberaceae

OTHER COMMON NAMES

Indian saffron

DESCRIPTION

• Turmeric is a perennial shrub native to southern Asia and cultivated in other parts of Asia, as well as Africa. Related to ginger, its yellow, fleshy rhizome is extensively used as a spice (it is an integral part of curry powder).

PART USED

Rhizomes

KNOWN ACTIVE CONSTITUENTS

• Curcumin, a curcuminoid, is the most active component of turmeric. The essential oil of turmeric (3% to 7.2%) contains sesquiterpenes (α- and β-turmerone, αr-turmerone, α-curcumen and zingiberene); minor amounts of monoterpenes (including cineole); and curcuminoids, predominately curcumin. Turmeric also contains 45% to 55% polysaccharides and contains potassium, carotenoids, and vitamin C.

MECHANISM/PHARMACOKINETICS

• Curcumin has antioxidant effects, inhibits arachidonic acid metabolism, and has antiinflammatory effects (1). In rats, 60% to 65% of curcumin is absorbed from the gastrointestinal tract after a single oral dose of 400 mg/kg (2).

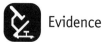 Evidence

CLINICAL TRIALS

• Ulcers

—A double-blind placebo-controlled trial tested turmeric in 118 patients with endoscopy-verified single duodenal ulcers $\geq$ 5 mm in diameter. Participants were treated with turmeric (6 g q.d. $\times$ 8 weeks) (3). Endoscopy was performed at 4 and 8 weeks. There was no benefit of turmeric over placebo in healing ulcers at either 1 or 2 months; at the end of the study 27% of ulcers were healed in the turmeric group versus 29% in the placebo group. A burning sensation was reported by 15 in the turmeric group and 8 in the placebo group. Side effects (most commonly burning sensation or constipation) were reported in 36.9% of the turmeric group and 20% of the placebo group.

• Oral submucous fibrosis

—An open study of 58 patients with oral submucous fibrosis compared three turmeric regimens (4). Each regimen included 3 g turmeric extract/day. One regimen added 600 mg turmeric oil, and the second regimen added 600 mg turmeric oleoresin/day. Thirty-nine completed all of the different regimens. Compared with baseline, all treatments decreased the number of micronucleated cells in oral mucosal cells and in circulating lymphocytes.

• Postoperative inflammation

—A study of 45 patients compared the effects of curcumin (400 mg), phenylbutazone (100 mg), or placebo, each t.i.d. for 5 days starting on the first postoperative day after surgery for hernia or hydrocele (5). Total pain and tenderness scores were higher in the curcumin group initially; on the sixth day both curcumin and phenylbutazone groups had a significant reduction in total intensity score (pain at site, edema, and tenderness). There was no change in the placebo group.

• Scabies

—A case series of 824 patients with scabies tested the effects of a topically applied paste made from neem (Azadirachta indica) and turmeric in a 4:1 ratio (6). After a scrub bath, the paste was applied over the body and left to dry; the treatment was repeated daily. Patients were treated until cured or 15 days, whichever came first; 97% of cases were cured within 15 days. No adverse reactions were noted.

• Lipid peroxides

—Oral ingestion of a hydroethanolic extract of turmeric (equivalent to 20 mg of curcumin daily) significantly decreased serum lipid peroxides, LDL, and apolipoprotein B, and increased HDL and apolipoprotein A (7).

ANIMAL/IN VITRO

• Antifertility effect

—Washed sperm from seven humans was exposed to curcumin (1 to 100 μg/mL for 0, 30, and 60 minutes) (8). Sperm motion decreased fivefold within 60 minutes of exposure to 100 μg/mL; the effect appeared to be time- and dose-dependent. Sperm viability or membrane integrity was not affected.

• Anticancer effects

—Turmeric, or an ethanolic turmeric extract, decreased DMBA-induced mammary tumors in rats; effects were seen either during or after initiation (9). A curcumin-free aqueous turmeric extract had only weak effects, and only when administered postinitiation.
—Two percent dietary curcumin given to female mice for 14 days decreased benzo[a]pyrene-induced forestomach cancer (10). Increased hepatic glutathione S-transferase and epoxide hydrolase levels were noted.
—Curcumin decreased the incidence and number of adenomas induced by azoxymethane but did not significantly decrease adenocarcinomas; the investigators note that few adenocarcinomas occurred (11). In the same report, only weak effects of curcumin were seen in the mammary model. Curcumin, especially in combination with genistein, inhibited growth of estrogen receptor (ER)-positive and ER-negative breast cancer cells induced by o,p-DDT,4-nonylphenol and 4-octylphenol (12).
—In the skin of mice, curcumin inhibits phorbol ester-induced tumor promotion (1). Three compounds isolated from curcumin increased the lifespan of animals with Ehrlich ascites tumor; intraperitoneal administration reduced the volume of solid tumors in mice; mortality rates were not affected (1).
—Curcumin weakly stimulates differentiation in human promyelocytic leukemia HL-60 cells; it appears to have a synergistic effect when combined with all-trans-retinoid acid or vitamin D_3 (13).
—Dietary or topically applied turmeric significantly reduced DNA adducts, tumor number, and tumor burden in DMBA-induced buccal pouch tumors in Syrian golden hamsters (14).
—Curcumin induces apoptosis in both androgen-dependent and androgen-independent prostate cancer cells (15). Turmeric also appears to have antiangiogenesis activity, inhibiting basic fibroblast growth factor-induced neovascularization in mouse cornea (16).

- Antimicrobial effects

—In guinea pigs with stable *Trichophyton*-induced dermatophytosis, a topical preparation of turmeric oil (dilution 1:80) improved scale and erythema within 5 days; lesions disappeared within 7 days (17). Turmeric oil at dilutions of up to 1:320 inhibited 15 isolates of dermatophytes including *Trichophyton rubrum*, *Trichophyton mentagrophytes*, *Epidermophyton floccosum*, and *Microsporum gypseum* (17). Curcumin, however, had no effect. Neither turmeric oil nor curcumin affected any of six isolates of *Candida*. Turmeric oil at dilutions of 1:40 to 1:80 inhibited four species of pathogenic molds (*T. rubrum*, *T. mentagrophytes*, *E. floccosum*, and *Sporothrix schenckii*); curcumin had no effect.

—Curcumin is a potent, selective inhibitor of HIV-1 long terminal repeat-directed gene expression at noncytotoxic levels (18).

- Miscellaneous effects

—In rat lenses, curcumin protected against cataract induced by 4-hydroxy-2-*trans*-nonenal (19). Dietary curcumin also mitigated ocular toxicity of naphthalene in rats (20).

—Pretreatment of rats with turmeric mitigated the hepatotoxic effects of carbon tetrachloride (21). In rats, curcumin (200 to 600 mg/kg/day) suppressed diethylnitrosamine-induced liver inflammation (22). In rats, curcumin treatment mitigated the toxic effects of paraquat (23).

—A dose of 500 mg/kg of an ethanol extract of turmeric decreased ulcers caused by hypothermic-restraint stress, pyloric ligation, indomethacin, or reserpine, but not cysteamine (24).

—In rats receiving curcumin as 0.5% of their diet and a high cholesterol diet for 8 weeks, the low density and very low density lipoprotein (LDL-VLDL) fraction and total cholesterol were significantly less than those fed a high cholesterol diet alone (25). In diabetic rats, dietary curcumin was associated with significantly lower LDL-VLDL fractions and total cholesterol in rats fed both a normal diet and a high cholesterol diet.

OTHER CLAIMED BENEFITS/ACTIONS

- Cancer
- Skin conditions
- Flatulence, bloating, appetite loss, digestive disorders
- Stimulates bile flow
- Wounds, eczema, inflammation
- Arthritis
- Amenorrhea

 Risks

ANIMAL TOXICITY

- Turmeric in doses of 0.2%, 1.0%, or 5.0% was hepatotoxic in mice (26).
- A subchronic oral toxicity study administered turmeric (0%, 1%, and 5%) and an ethanolic extract of turmeric (0%, 0.05%, and 0.25%) to female Swiss mice and Wistar rats for 14 or 90 days (27). In mice, even low doses of turmeric (0.2% to 1%) for 2 weeks caused hepatotoxicity; a 5% dietary dose for 90 days caused hepatotoxicity, altered liver weights, and reduced body weight gain in both mice and rats.
- An earlier review found that turmeric or its oleoresin did not cause major pathologic effects in rats, mice, guinea pigs, dogs, and monkeys. A study with oleoresin in the pig caused changes in the liver, thyroid, bladder, and kidney. Limited feeding studies in rats did not show carcinogenic effects; however, oral administration of turmeric or its oleoresin has caused chromosome damage in rodents (28).

 Dose

COMMON DOSAGE FORMS

- *Dried root:* 0.5 to 4 g cut root or powder t.i.d.
- *Fluid extract:* 1:1 (g/mL) 1.5 to 3 mL daily in divided doses.
- *Tincture:* 1:5 (g/mL) 10 mL daily in divided doses.
- A paste may be made with water for topical application.
- Preparations should contain not less than 3% dicinnamoylmethane derivatives, calculated as curcumin, and not less than 3% volatile oil.

Tyrosine (Tyr, Y)

 10 Second Take

Tyrosine is a benign amino acid; there is little evidence for efficacy in mental illness, but it may improve performance under stressful conditions.

 Basics

DESCRIPTION

• Tyrosine is a conditionally essential, large neutral amino acid that is a precursor of thyroid hormones; melanin; and the catecholamine neurotransmitters dopamine, norepinephrine, and epinephrine.

FOOD SOURCES

Most protein-containing foods

MECHANISM/PHARMACOKINETICS

• Tyrosine is essential for the synthesis of protein, catecholamines, melanin, and thyroid hormone. It is formed from the amino acid phenylalanine and also provides energy when catabolized through p-hydroxyphenylpyruvate to fumarate and acetoacetate.
• After a large dose, plasma tyrosine levels peak about 2 hours after oral ingestion and remain elevated for about 7 hours.

 Evidence

CLINICAL TRIALS

• Phenylketonuria

—Tyrosine does not seem to benefit the cognitive function of phenylketonurics. A double-blind, placebo-controlled crossover study tested the effect of oral high-dose tyrosine therapy (100 mg/kg body weight per day) in 24 phenylketonurics and 24 controls. Although plasma tyrosine concentrations increased during supplementation, no beneficial effects were seen in the brain function of adults with phenylketonuria (1). Another randomized controlled crossover trial in 21 children and adults with phenylketonuria tested 100 mg/kg body weight per day of L-tyrosine or L-alanine (placebo); although baseline testing showed a correlation of several of the neuropsychologic tests with tyrosine levels, this study found no differences in neuropsychologic test performance with tyrosine supplementation in phenylketonurics (2).

• Cognitive task performance

—Tyrosine may reduce the effects of stress and fatigue on cognitive task performance. In a placebo-controlled trial, the effects of tyrosine (10 g per day) on cognitive task performance, mood, blood pressure (BP), and MHPG (a norepinephrine metabolite) were studied in 21 cadets assessed immediately before and on the sixth day of a military combat training course (3). The group receiving tyrosine performed significantly better on a memory task and a tracking task than the group given placebo. There were no significant effects on mood; however, tyrosine did decrease systolic BP.

• Cocaine dependence

—Because chronic cocaine use depletes catecholamines, tyrosine (2 g q 8h) was tested in an open-label trial in 49 cocaine-dependent people, as an adjunct treatment to outpatient drug abuse counseling (4). No side effects were reported. Retention in treatment at 90 days was apparently an endpoint; median retention in the trial was 17 days, which does not support a beneficial effect of tyrosine.

• Response to stress

—A double-blind, placebo-controlled trial tested the behavioral effects of tyrosine (115 mg/kg in a split dose) during an episode of continuous nighttime work involving one night's sleep loss (5). Tyrosine administration lessened the usual performance decline on a psychomotor task and significantly reduced lapse probability on a high-event-rate vigilance task. Improvements lasted about 3 hours.

—A placebo-controlled crossover study found that tyrosine (100 mg/kg) in 16 healthy young participants improved the performance on stress-sensitive cognitive tasks after a noise stressor, and also decreased diastolic BP transiently (this effect was seen 15 minutes after ingestion, but at 1 hour there was no difference between tyrosine and placebo). No effects on mood, systolic BP, or heart rate were found (6).
—Another placebo-controlled study of eight male volunteers found that tyrosine (150 mg per kg) improved performance on a memory test after exposure to cold stress (which normally impairs short-term memory) (7).

• Schizophrenia

—A placebo-controlled, double-blind crossover trial of L-tyrosine as an adjunct to molindone treatment for schizophrenia found no improvements as measured by weekly Brief Psychiatric Rating Scale (BPRS), Schedule for the Assessment of Negative Symptoms (SANS), or Clinical Global Impressions (CGI) scales; Smooth Pursuits Eye Movement Performance (SPEM) showed increased saccades, suggesting that tyrosine may have some central effect (8).

• Cardiovascular stress

—A double-blind, placebo-controlled crossover study tested the effects of tyrosine (50 mg/kg) in reducing the effects of cardiovascular stress as measured by Lower Body Negative Pressure (LBNP) (which simulates a gravitational load by exposing the lower body to subatmospheric pressure) in 22 healthy adult men (9). LBNP usually decreases pulse pressure. Following tyrosine treatment, mean pulse pressures increased significantly more than following placebo treatment; there were no significant differences between placebo and tyrosine treatment in terms of event related potentials, cortisol levels, performance tasks, or profile of mood states (POMS). There were no differences in terms of LBNP tolerance, although tyrosine treatment significantly increased the LBNP tolerance of participants receiving placebo followed by tyrosine and decreased the LBNP tolerance of participants receiving tyrosine followed by placebo.

ANIMAL/IN VITRO

• Animal studies demonstrate that tyrosine reduces adverse reactions to acute stress and restores normal levels of aggression in animals subjected to cold-water stress. It improves performance in rats subjected to cold stress, lowers BP in hypertensive rats that are stressed, and decreases the vulnerability of the dog heart to ventricular fibrillation (9).

OTHER CLAIMED BENEFITS/ACTIONS

• Depression
• Addiction

Clinical Considerations

 ## Risks

 ## Dose

FACTORS DECREASING AVAILABILITY/ABSORPTION

• Phenylketonuria: These patients must be treated not only with phenylalanine-restricted diets but must also be supplemented with tyrosine.

FACTORS INCREASING AVAILABILITY/ABSORPTION

• There are seven clinical forms of hereditary tyrosinemia. Type 1 is most serious, causing both hepatic and renal complications. Phenylalanine and tyrosine restriction is necessary for treatment of all tyrosinemias; however, restriction is less severe for types II and III (for which the prognosis is excellent) (10).

• Type 1a

—Hepatorenal tyrosinemia, which involves a defect in fumarylacetoacetate hydrolyase, is characterized by renal tubular impairment and progressive liver failure; it can cause cirrhosis, renal Fanconi syndrome, and porphyria, and is a risk factor for hepatocellular carcinoma.

• Type 1b

—Hepatorenal tyrosinemia, which involves a defect in maleylacetoacetate isomerase, can result in liver failure, Fanconi syndrome, and psychomotor retardation.

• Type II

—Oculocutaneous tyrosinemia involves a defect in hepatic cytosol tyrosine aminotransferase; it characteristically causes greatly elevated levels of tyrosine in blood and urine and also increases urinary tyramine and N-acetyltyrosine. It typically causes skin and eye disorders with variable mental retardation.

• Type III

—There are three subsets of type III tyrosinemia, all of which result from dysfunction of the enzyme p-hydroxy-phenylpyruvate dioxygenase (p-OHPPAD). Primary p-OHPPAD deficiency (type IIIa) causes neurologic abnormalities and mental retardation; Hawkinsinuria (type IIIb) causes metabolic acidosis, microcephaly, and failure to thrive with a chlorine odor. Transient neonatal (type IIIc) occurs in 0.2% to 10% of neonates and may be linked with prematurity. It is associated with increased plasma and urine tyrosine and its metabolites. Short-term protein restriction (less than 2.0 g/kg/day) is effective in lowering plasma tyrosine concentrations in most patients (10). Ascorbate, a cofactor for p-OHPPAD, may have a role in stabilizing this condition (11).

LABORATORY TESTS

• Free amino acid concentration of tyrosine in venous blood is 22 to 83 μmol/L. Urinary output of tyrosine is 110 μmol/24 hr (12).

ADVERSE REACTIONS

Tyrosine is nontoxic and has not been associated with adverse events (9).

Tyrosine is conditionally essential, because phenylalanine intake supplies part of daily requirements. Phenylalanine plus tyrosine constitutes about 8% of protein intake (11). Supplemental doses used in clinical trials have ranged from 10 g/day to 100 mg/kg/day.

Valerian

 10 Second Take

Valerian is a benign sedative-hypnotic; clinical trials support its use.

 Basics

LATIN NAME

Valeriana officinalis L., *V. edulis* Meyer, *V. jatamansi* Jones (syn *V. wallichii* DC)

FAMILY

Valerianaceae

OTHER COMMON NAMES

Indian valerian (*V. wallichii*), kesso (Japan, for *V. officinalis* var *latifolia*)

DESCRIPTION

• Valerian, a perennial, has white to pale pink, scented flowers. It grows in meadows or woods in Europe and North America and is cultivated in Europe, Japan, and Russia. Used medicinally for at least 2,000 years, it was known to Dioscorides and Galen (1).

PART USED

Root, rhizome

KNOWN ACTIVE CONSTITUENTS

• Essential oil containing monoterpenes (including bornyl esters, camphene, and pinenes), sesquiterpenes (including valerenal and valeranone), sequiterpene carboxylic acids, gamma-aminobutyric acid (GABA), glutamine, and arginine. Commercial preparations contain 67 to 322 mg sesquiterpenes per 100 g (2). Valepotriates, highest in *V. edulis,* vary from 0.5% to 8.0% among different species (2). Diene valepotriates (valtrate, isovaltrate, acevaltrate) are quite labile, quickly yielding baldrinals in water (3). Monoene valepotriates (didrovaldrate and isovaleroxyhydroxy-didrovaldrate) are more stable. Valepotriates and decomposition products (chiefly baldrinals) are present in fresh but not dried root.

MECHANISM/PHARMACOKINETICS

• Mechanism has not been definitively established. Both alcohol and aqueous extracts show affinity for the $GABA_A$ receptor in the rat brain (4). Although GABA concentration is quite high in valerian extract, GABA does not cross the blood–brain barrier. In very high doses, hydroxyvalerenic acid and acetoxyvalerenic acid can inhibit the breakdown of GABA (4). A lipophilic fraction of a hydroalcoholic extract bound to barbiturate receptors and (to a lesser extent) mitochondrial benzodiazepine receptors (5). In addition, valerian extract displaces radiolabeled melatonin from binding sites in human cerebellum in a dose-dependent manner (6,7). Valerian does not interact significantly with benzodiazepine and gamma-opiates receptors (7). A valerian root extract high in valtrate interacted with adenosine receptors; however, valtrate decomposes quickly and is not expected to be in finished products. Glutamine may also contribute to valerian's sedative effect (4).

 Evidence

CLINICAL TRIALS

• A placebo-controlled study examined next-morning alertness in volunteers treated with valerian syrup, tablets containing valerian and hops, or flunitrazepam 1 mg. Only flunitrazepam impaired performance on the morning after treatment (1).

• Insomnia

—A double-blind crossover randomized controlled trial (RCT) in 16 patients with insomnia tested valerian root (600 mg 5:1 dry extract, 1 hour before bedtime) versus placebo, each for 14 days, on subjective sleep quality and changes in polysomnography (8). Valerian, compared with placebo, significantly reduced slow-wave sleep latency (21.3 vs. 13.5 minutes) and increased slow-wave sleep latency percentage of time in bed. Other measures did not change.

—A double-blind, placebo-controlled RCT tested a mixture of 360 mg of valerian extract and 240 mg of lemon balm extract in 98 healthy volunteers (including 58 women) for 30 days (9). The treatment was well tolerated; sleep disturbances, tiredness, and other side effects were similar between groups. Blood pressure, pulse, body weight, hematology tests, and liver function tests (LFTs) [alkaline phosphatase, alanine transaminase (ALT), aspartate transaminase (AST), and γ-glutamyltransferase (GGT)] were measured. Significantly more treated participants (33.3% vs 9.4%) reported improved sleep quality; however, there were no differences in a visual analog scale of sleep quality.

—A pure valerian extract (400 mg) was compared with a commercial mixed herbal preparation [containing valerian 60 mg and hops flower (*Humulus lupulus*) extract 30 mg] and placebo in 128 participants with a range of sleep quality. Three of each pill were taken in random order on nonconsecutive nights. Both valerian preparations significantly decreased subjective sleep latency scores and sleep quality. Valerian did not affect night awakenings, dream recall, or morning alertness (10).

—One dose of valerian freeze-dried aqueous extract (450 mg or 900 mg) was given to 10 normal participants to take at home and to 8 in a sleep laboratory. At home, both doses reduced perceived sleep latency and wake time after sleep onset (11). In the sleep lab, there was no difference between 900 mg valerian and placebo.

—A small study of 14 older adult poor sleepers found no difference between placebo and dried aqueous valerian extract (405 mg) on sleep onset time or time awake after sleep onset (12). Valerian did, however, increase slow-wave sleep and decrease sleep stage I.

—Twenty-seven patients with sleep difficulties took two different hops and lemon balm preparations on consecutive nights. One pill contained 4 mg of valerian, the other a full 400-mg dose. (Valerian is a much stronger sedative than lemon balm.) A total of 78% of the participants preferred full-dose valerian, 15% preferred the low-dose valerian, and 7% had no preference (2).

—A double-blind placebo-controlled trial in 182 patients (all completed) with adjustment disorder and anxious mood tested a multiherb extract (containing *Passiflora, Crataegus, Ballota, Valeriana, Cola,* and *Paullinia*). After 28 days, significantly more treated patients (42.9%) than placebo-treated participants (25.3%) had a Hamilton Anxiety (HAM-A) score less than 10 (13).

• Physiologic activation

—A study of valerian and propranolol on activation, performance, and mood under social stress found that propranolol prevented physiologic activation, whereas valerian decreased subjective feelings of somatic arousal without affecting physiologic activation. No interaction was observed (14).

• Attention impairment

—A placebo-controlled, double-blind study of 54 participants found no effect of valerian root/lemon balm extract on reaction time, concentration, or attention span or on alcohol-induced impairment. However, another report found significant impairment of vigilance and complex information processing in participants consuming 4 g valerian (1).

ANIMAL/IN VITRO

• Sedative/anticonvulsant

—In mice, valerian extracts exhibit sedative effects and mild anticonvulsant effects. Intraperitoneal injection of valerian (4.5 to 6 mg/kg) prolonged thiopental anesthesia in mice and was anticonvulsant against one of three agents (15). Valerian extract administered by gavage (2 mg/kg) increased thiopental-induced sleeping time by a factor of 1.6 (16).

• Cytotoxicity (see questions and answers)

—Valepotriates are cytotoxic *in vitro*; valtrate inhibits incorporation of thymidine into DNA (7). In human small cell lung cancer (GLC-4r) and colorectal cancer (COLO 320) cell lines, diene valepotriates (valtrate, isovaltrate, and acevaltrate) were the most toxic, with inhibitory concentration $(IC)_{50}$ values slightly higher than cisplatin (3). Monoene type valepotriates (didrovaldrate and isovaleroxyhydroxydidrovaltrate) were two- to threefold less toxic. Baldrinal and homobaldrinal (decomposition products), were 10- to 30-fold less toxic. However, isovaltral, another decomposition product, was even more cytotoxic than its parent compound isovaltrate. Valerenic acid and its derivatives had low toxicity, with IC_{50} values between 100 to 200 μmol.

 Risks

ADVERSE REACTIONS

• Overdose

—In a suicide attempt, an 18-year-old student ingested 18.8 to 23.5 g valerian root and developed fatigue, crampy abdominal pain, chest tightness, tremor, and lightheadedness. Physical examination revealed only mydriasis and a fine hand tremor. The patient was treated with activated charcoal; all symptoms resolved within 24 hours (17).
—Twenty-three patients in Hong Kong who deliberately consumed overdoses of Sleep-Qik (valerian dry extract 75 mg, hyoscine hydrobromide 0.25 mg, and cyproheptadine hydrochloride 2 mg) developed signs of central nervous system (CNS) depression and anticholinergic poisoning including drowsiness, mydriasis, tachycardia, nausea, confusion and urinary retention (all attributable to the antimuscarinic effects of the two drugs; cyproheptadine also antagonizes histamine and serotonin) (18). Valerian ingestion ranged from 0.5 to 12 g; LFTs showed no abnormalities.

• Valerian root withdrawal

—A case of possible valerian root withdrawal was described in a 58-year-old hypertensive man with coronary artery disease and congestive heart failure (CHF), on multiple medications, who had multiple episodes of oxygen desaturation during a biopsy and developed high-output cardiac failure (19). The patient had taken valerian root extract (530 mg to 2 g/dose) five times daily. Midazolam improved signs and symptoms. This case is interesting but difficult to interpret, because no compounds have been found in valerian that are similar to benzodiazepines (although both may affect GABA transmission).

• Hepatotoxicity

Four cases of hepatitis in women were attributed to Neurelax or Kalms tablets, which apparently contain numerous herbs (20), including, purportedly, skullcap and valerian. Considering that hepatotoxic germander is often substituted for skullcap (see skullcap topic), valerian is probably not a factor. A month-long valerian trial found no adverse effects on LFTs (9).

DRUG INTERACTIONS

• Valerian may reduce the effects of alcohol. A double-blind study found that mixed valepotriates from valerian increased the ability to concentrate in a dose-dependent manner, and the addition of alcohol did not prevent this effect (3).

ANIMAL TOXICITY

• The LD_{50} of an alcoholic extract of valerian in mice was reported to be 3.3 g/kg i.p. (4). Repeated dosing with 300 and 600 mg/kg for 30 days in rats caused no changes in body or organ weights, hematology, or blood chemistry (21). In mice, no carcinogenic effects were seen in doses up to 1,350 mg/kg i.p. (7).

 Dose

COMMON DOSAGE FORMS

• Adults: 1 to 3 g of drug as infusion or equivalent dry extract p.o. q.d. to t.i.d. (for insomnia, a single dose 30 minutes before bedtime, with an additional dose earlier in the evening if necessary).

—*Tincture:* (1:5 ethanol 70% V/V) 1 to 5 mL q.d. to t.i.d.
—*Liquid extract:* 0.3 to 1.0 mL
—*Topical use:* Occasionally used externally in baths

• Children 3 to 12 (under medical supervision)

—Proportion of adult dose by body weight, as tea, infusion, or dry extract
—Should not be used by children under 3

• *Quality note:* High-quality material reportedly contains from 1.0% to 1.5% essential oil and more than 0.5% valerenic acid (1).

 Common Questions and Answers

Q: Why aren't valepotriates a safety issue?
A: Valepotriates are poorly absorbed orally. Besides, the most cytotoxic ones are so unstable that they do not appear in commercial products (this is an instance in which fresh is not best!). Diene valepotriates (valtrate, isovaltrate, and acevaltrate) are primarily responsible for the cytotoxicity of valerian preparations. One study found that isovaltrate was not detected even in fresh tinctures; other valepotriates decomposed in tinctures that had been stored for at least 2 months. Interestingly, there was no concurrent increase in baldrinal, which may break down into unknown products (3). The authors recommend that valerian tinctures be stored for at least 2 months.

Q: Why do valerian products smell like dirty sneakers?
A: Fresh valerian does not have the characteristic smell associated with valerian; enzyme hydrolysis of some essential oil components over time results in the release of isovaleric acid, the source of the smell (22).

Valine (Val, V)

10 Second Take

Valine is an essential amino acid; there is limited evidence that combined branched-chain amino acids (BCAAs) improve appetite. Supplemental valine may increase the risk of depression.

Basics

DESCRIPTION

Valine is an essential branched chain amino acid (BCAA); the others are leucine and isoleucine.

FOOD SOURCES

Most protein-containing foods

MECHANISM/PHARMACOKINETICS

- The hydrophobicity of BCAAs make them important to protein formation; BCAAs also affect response to infection (1). BCAAs make up about a third of muscle protein and are an important constituent of other tissues (2). The plasma half-life of valine is 9 days.

Evidence

CLINICAL TRIALS

- Depression

—Supplemental valine may increase depression; it inhibits tryptophan transport across the blood–brain barrier and, thus, may decrease brain serotonin [5-hydroxytryptophan (5-HT)]. In healthy participants, a single dose of valine (30 g) significantly decreased the prolactin response to D-fenfluramine (a 5-HT releasing agent), administered an hour later (3). In 12 remitted, asymptomatic, treated patients with depression, a single dose of valine (30 g) caused transient depressive symptoms in four participants, all of whom were taking selective serotonin reuptake inhibitors (SSRIs) (3).

- BCAAs and phenylketonuria

—A mixture of valine, isoleucine, and leucine was administered to 16 adolescents and young adults with phenylketonuria in a double-blind crossover study comprising four 3-month periods (4). Time to completion of the Attention Diagnostic Methods (which requires substantial attention with mental processing) was significantly faster during the period in which the amino acid mixture was administered. There was not a significant change seen on the Continuous Performance Test.

- BCAA in amyotrophic lateral sclerosis (ALS)

—A double-blind, placebo-controlled trial compared BCAAs (L-leucine 12 g, isoleucine 8 g, and L-valine 6.4 g with pyridoxal phosphate 160 mg daily) to L-threonine (4 g daily) or placebo for 6 months in 95 patients with ALS. Every 2 months, muscle strength, muscle torque, forced vital capacity (FVC), activities of daily living involving upper and lower limbs, and timed tasks were tested. Both the placebo group and the threonine group lost weight, whereas the BCAA-supplemented group gained weight; the difference was significant. Estimated decline in FVC was 2.5 times greater in both groups supplemented with amino acids, compared with placebo. No other significant differences were seen among treatment groups. The amino acids were well tolerated, but the authors point out that adverse effects of these amino acids on pulmonary function could not be ruled out (5). Long-term effects of this mixture also are unknown. Another trial of BCAAs for ALS was halted after 126 participants were recruited because of what appeared to be excess mortality among those randomized to active treatment (24 BCAA, 13 placebo); there was also no evidence of difference in disability scales between the two groups (6).

- BCAAs and tardive dyskinesia (TD)

—An uncontrolled 2-week trial in nine men with neuroleptic-induced TD tested administration of a BCAA medical food three times a day for 2 weeks (7). Compared with baseline, frequency of TD movements (collected by videotape and analyzed in blinded random sequence) decreased significantly; movements decreased at least 38% in all participants.

- BCAAs and appetite

—A double-blind study in 28 cancer patients compared BCAAs (4.8 g daily) with placebo; improvements in appetite were seen in 55% of the treatment group compared with 16% of those in the placebo group (8).

- BCAAs in protein wasting associated with bedrest

—Nineteen healthy participants were randomized into two groups; one group received 30 μmol/day of BCAAs, whereas the other received the same amount of nonessential amino acids. BCAAs supplementation attenuated nitrogen loss during short-term bedrest (9).

ANIMAL/IN VITRO

- In animals, valine appears to decrease serotonin levels by inhibiting tryptophan transport.

OTHER CLAIMED BENEFITS/ACTIONS

- Muscular dystrophy
- Improves healing
- Improves athletic performance

 Clinical Considerations

FACTORS INCREASING AVAILABILITY/ABSORPTION

- Maple syrup urine disease (MSUD) or branched chain α-ketoaciduria is the group of inherited disorders of leucine, isoleucine, and valine metabolism. Infants do not manifest symptoms until they start eating protein-containing food; the most deficient in enzymes may die within 10 days of birth. Progressive neurologic dysfunction and urine and ear wax that smells of caramel or maple syrup characterize this disease. Screening should be done in the first week of life. Long-term management of MSUD involves dietary manipulation designed to maintain plasma concentrations of BCAAs 3 to 4 hours after a meal in a specific range (isoleucine, 40 to 90 μmol; leucine, 80 to 200 μmol; and valine, 200 to 425 μmol).

LABORATORY TESTS

- Free amino acid concentration is 168 to 317 μmol/L in venous blood
- Urinary output is 90 μmol per 24 hours

 Risks

ADVERSE REACTIONS

- Possible increase in depression

 Dose

RECOMMENDED DIETARY ALLOWANCE (10)

Infants and children

3 to 4 months	93 mg/kg/day
2 to 5 years	38 mg/kg/day
10 to 12 years	25 mg/kg/day
Adults	10 to 20 mg/kg/day

Vanadium

10 Second Take

Vanadium, a potentially beneficial adjunctive treatment in diabetes, causes nausea and diarrhea, and its oxidant effects are worrisome.

Basics

DESCRIPTION

• Probably an essential trace mineral, vanadium is a steel-gray metal, a widely distributed transition element that exists in at least six different oxidation states (and can form polymers). Pentavalent salts include metavanadate (VO_3^-) and orthovanadate ($H_2VO_4^-$) (1). The tetravalent vanadyl cation (VO^{2+}) and the pentavalent forms are the most important forms in higher animals (2).

FOOD SOURCES

• Foods high in vanadium include black pepper, dill seed, mushrooms (0.05 to 2 μg/g), parsley (1.8 μg/g), shellfish, and spinach (0.5 to 0.8 μg/g) (1). Estimated daily intake ranges from 10 to 60 μg. Food processing increases vanadium levels.
• Other sources

—Tobacco smoke contains high concentrations of vanadium (1 to 8 ppm). Air is also a significant source of the mineral, especially near metallurgical industries or in areas where coal, petroleum, and heavy oils are used to generate electricity or heat (1).

MECHANISM/PHARMACOKINETICS

• Vanadium does not have a defined biochemical function in humans; it is arguable whether or not it is an essential trace element (1). At high concentrations, vanadium inhibits adenosine triphosphate (ATP)-hydrolyzing enzymes, glucose-6-phosphatase, alkaline phosphatase, and several enzymes involved in glycolysis (3). Vanadium also has insulin-like effects and stimulates several growth factors. The pentavalent form is most common in extracellular body fluids; the quadrivalent form is most common intracellularly (1). The vanadate ion inhibits the sodium potassium ATPase pump.
• Vanadium salts are poorly absorbed gastrointestinally, but the lungs absorb vanadium pentoxide (V_2O_5) very well. Most ingested vanadium is eliminated unabsorbed in feces; 40% to 60% of absorbed vanadium is excreted by the kidney within 1 to 3 days. Less than 10% is excreted in bile (1).

• The half-life in blood is about 1 hour (1). Vanadate in the blood is converted into the vanadyl cation, which, via transferrin, enters intracellular ferritin (however, it is not incorporated into heme) (3). Ingested vanadium is probably transformed to tetravalent vanadyl (VO^{2+}) in the stomach; however, vanadate can also enter cells (2).

Evidence

CLINICAL TRIALS

• Depression

—Early reports suggested that blood vanadium concentrations are lower during recovery from manic-depressive illness; however, recent reports have not confirmed a correlation between vanadium levels and depression (1).

• Diabetes

—Four small studies on the effect of vanadium compounds in diabetics are not entirely consistent.
—In the most recent study, 16 Type II diabetics were given vanadyl sulfate ($VOSO_4$ 25 to 100 mg t.i.d.) for 2 weeks (4). Fasting glucose and total cholesterol decreased significantly [high density lipoprotein (HDL) decreased as well] only in the group receiving 300 mg/day. HbA_{1c} decreased significantly in the 150 mg/day and the 300 mg/day group. There were no changes in basal hepatic glucose production (HGP) or insulin-induced suppression of HGP. Glucose metabolism during euglycemic insulin clamp (insulin is infused, then glucose levels are maintained at a constant level by feedback-controlled infusion) improved in 3/5 participants receiving 150 mg/day and 4/8 receiving 300 mg/day; there was no effect at 75 mg/day.
—Eight patients (including four women) with Type II diabetes received vanadyl sulfate (50 mg b.i.d.) for 4 weeks (5). Six participants received placebo for an additional 4 weeks. Vanadium was associated with decreased hepatic glucose output during hyperinsulinemia (from 5.0 $\pm$ 1.0 pretreatment to 3.1 $\pm$ 0.9 μmol/kg/minute posttreatment). Vanadium did not affect rates of total body glucose uptake, glycogen synthesis, glycolysis, carbohydrate oxidation, or lipolysis during euglycemic-hyper-insulinemic clamps. Side effects included diarrhea, abdominal cramps, flatulence, and nausea. Most symptoms resolved within the first week.
—In 10 diabetics (5 Type I and 5 Type II), sodium orthovanadate ($NaVO_3$ 125 mg/day × 2 weeks) significantly lowered insulin requirements in patients with Type I, but not Type II, diabetes (6). Type II (but not Type I) diabetics showed improved insulin sensitivity; cholesterol levels in Type II diabetics also significantly decreased (from 6.92 $\pm$ 0.75 to 5.28 $\pm$ 0.46 mmol/L). There was no effect on

basal C-peptide levels or HGP. Nausea and vomiting were reported.
—In another study, vanadyl sulfate was tested in six people with Type II noninsulin dependent diabetes mellitus (NIDDM) on sulfonylurea drugs, who received placebo for 2 weeks, vanadyl sulfate (100 mg/day) for 3 weeks, and then placebo again for 2 weeks. Significant improvements were seen in fasting plasma glucose (210 $\pm$ 19 mg/dL to 181 $\pm$ 14 mg/dL) and HbA_{1c} (9.6% $\pm$ 0.6% to 8.8% $\pm$ 0.6%). The glucose infusion rate during euglycemic-hyperinsulinemic clamps increased significantly from 1.80 to 3.38 mg/kg/minute, an increase of approximately 88%. Both hepatic and peripheral insulin sensitivity improved in insulin-resistant patients; improvement persisted up to 2 weeks (7).

• Ergogenics

—Vanadyl sulfate was ineffective in changing body composition in weight-training athletes (8). A 12-week, double-blind, placebo-controlled trial of oral vanadyl sulfate (0.5 mg/kg/day) in 31 weight-training volunteers found no benefit for vanadium in improving performance.

ANIMAL/IN VITRO

• Bis-cyclopentadienyl (Cp) complexes of vanadium (IV) (vanadocenes) are potent spermicidal agents (9).
• Vanadium (IV)-containing metallocenes were toxic against two testicular cancer cell lines (Tera-2 and Ntera-2) and induced apoptosis within 24 hours (10).
• In diabetic animals, vanadium normalized hyperphagia (11).
• Although early studies showed that V_2O_3 protected several species of animals from dental caries, later work did not confirm this (3).

OTHER CLAIMED BENEFITS/ACTIONS

• Hypercholesterolemia

Clinical Considerations

DEFICIENCY SIGNS AND SYMPTOMS

- Vanadium deficiency signs in humans have not been described. In goats, vanadium deprivation increases the mortality of kids and is associated with skeletal deformations. In rats, vanadium deprivation increases thyroid weight and decreases growth.

LABORATORY TESTS

- Urine: 0.1 to 0.2 μg vanadium/L in the general population (and usually less than 1 μg vanadium/g creatinine). Urine vanadium is a more reliable measure of exposure (after adjusting for creatinine) than blood vanadium levels.
- No reference values for vanadium are established; however, levels of about 1.0 nmol/L for blood and serum and about 10 nmol/L for urine are considered tentative normal values (12).

Risks

ADVERSE REACTIONS

- Poisoning

—Vanadium is eliminated fairly quickly, and there are few data on the effectiveness of methods to enhance elimination. Substances that can mitigate vanadium toxicity include ethylenediaminetetraacetic acid (EDTA), chromium, protein, ferrous iron, chloride, and aluminum hydroxide. In animals, ascorbic acid is the most effective agent for preventing vanadium poisoning (ascorbic acid reduces the pentavalent vanadate ion to the quadrivalent vanadyl ion, which is less toxic). However, ascorbic acid is apparently ineffective for treating vanadium poisoning; in mice, deferoxamine and tiron are more effective chelating agents then EDTA or diethylenetriamine pentaacetic acid (DPTA).
—Hemodialysis would not be expected to increase clearance because vanadate is 90% protein-bound (1).
—U.S. Occupational Safety and Health Administration (OSHA) permissible exposure limit-time weighted average (PEL-TWA) for vanadium dust and fume (V_2O_5) is 50 μg/m. Biologic threshold level in urine collected at the end of the work week is 50 μg vanadium/g creatinine, according to the American Conference of Governmental and Industrial Hygienists (1).

- Vanadium is used in steel production and the production of non-ferrous alloys; as a catalyst in the manufacture of plastics; in the manufacturing of semiconductors, photographic developers, and coloring agents; and in the production of yellow pigments and ceramics. Vanadium occurs naturally in fuel oils, and cleaning oil- or gas-fired boilers is a risk factor for vanadium poisoning.

—Vanadium dust exposure can cause "boilermakers bronchitis," an upper respiratory tract irritation, especially rhinitis and cough. A metallic taste along with a green discolored tongue can indicate vanadium exposure; this usually resolves within a week. At high concentrations, vanadium can be a weak sensitizing agent (1).
—In two healthy volunteers exposed to V_2O_5 (0.08 mg/m^3), no irritation resulted; 1 mg/m^3 produced a cough that lasted 8 days but no alterations in x-ray films or pulmonary function tests. Twenty-four workers exposed to an average of 0.3 mg/m^3 developed a productive cough; irritation of the nose, throat, and eyes; rhinitis; and green tongue; all symptoms resolved within several days following exposure.
—A report from 1915 noted that patients with syphilis tolerated intravenous doses of V_2O_5 600 mg over 13 to 23 days. A dose of 20 mg sodium tetravanadate caused lacrimation, hypotension, throat constriction, vomiting, and apnea (1).
—A 1963 report about the effect of vanadium on lipid levels found that ammonium vanadyl tartrate 50 to 100 mg/day for 6 to 9 weeks did not significantly change lipid levels. All participants experienced abdominal cramps and diarrhea; transient purple-green tint of the tongue was also noted (13).
—Workers occupationally exposed to vanadium have reported nonspecific symptoms including headache, weakness, tinnitus, dizziness, and palpitations (1).

ANIMAL TOXICITY

- In rats, acute sodium vanadate poisoning causes desquamative enteritis, mild congestion of the liver with fatty changes, and mild parenchymal degeneration of renal tubules (1). In monkeys, airflow limitation, apparently resulting from pulmonary inflammation, develops after exposure to V_2O_5 5 mg/m^3. In mice, high doses (20 mg/kg) of ammonium metavanadate cause renal tubular necrosis, lymphoid tissue necrosis, and pulmonary hemorrhage (1). Systemic effects are thought to be due to the oxidizing effect of vanadium. Possible mechanisms include inhibition of oxidative phosphorylation, interference with phosphate-containing enzymes, or competitive inhibition of Na,K-ATPase.

- Reproductive effects

—Vanadium does not accumulate in the reproductive tract; in animals, maternal toxicity precedes teratogenicity (1).

Dose

RECOMMENDED DIETARY ALLOWANCE

It is unknown how much (or even whether) vanadium is necessary; it is thought that 196 nmol (10 μg) daily is adequate (2).

UPPER LIMITS

Infants and children

0 to 6 months	Not determinable
7 to 12 months	Not determinable
1 to 3 years	Not determinable
4 to 8 years	Not determinable

Males

9 to 13 years	Not determinable
14 to 18 years	Not determinable
19 to 50 years	1.8 mg/day
51+ years	1.8 mg/day

Females

9 to 13 years	Not determinable
14 to 18 years	Not determinable
19 to 50 years	1.8 mg/day
51+ years	1.8 mg/day
Pregnant	Not determinable
Lactating	Not determinable

Vitamin A (See Also Carotenoids)

 10 Second Take

Vitamin A deficiency is a serious public health concern globally (although not in North America). Excessive vitamin A intake can be toxic.

 Basics

DESCRIPTION

• Vitamin A exists in three oxidation states: the alcohol, retinol; the acid, retinoic acid; and the aldehyde, retinal. The term *retinoids* includes natural forms, synthetic forms, and metabolites of vitamin A. Animal products contain retinol (preformed vitamin A); plants contain provitamin A carotenoids (1). About 50 of over 600 carotenoids (including beta-carotene, alpha-carotene, gamma-carotene, and lutein) can act as precursors to vitamin A (2). Vitamin A is stored in the liver, which can hold an entire year's supply.

FOOD SOURCES

• *Retinol:* liver, fish oils, egg yolk, and milk fat
• *Carotenoids:* Yellow-orange or red fruits (cantaloupe, peaches, mangoes, strawberries) and vegetables (carrots, sweet potatoes, tomatoes), dark green vegetables (kale, collards, spinach)

MECHANISM/PHARMACOKINETICS

• Seventy percent to 90% of ingested vitamin A is absorbed (dietary fat is necessary for absorption). Absorption occurs through the small intestine, after which vitamin A is packaged into chylomicrons and transported to the liver, which stores 50% to 85% of total body retinol and regulates secretion of retinol (bound to retinol-binding protein).
• All-*trans*-retinol is the primary form found in plasma; most tissues contain esterified retinol (3).
• Main functions: vision (phototransduction and maintaining normal differentiation of cells in the cornea and conjunctiva), integrity of epithelial tissues, immunity (both cell-mediated and antibody-mediated), growth, and development (3).

 Evidence

CLINICAL TRIALS

• Child health

—Vitamin A deficiency is very common in many parts of the world; it has been estimated that 3.3 million children worldwide are deficient. Most but not all community-based trials in children have found that vitamin A supplementation reduces overall mortality; pooled results from eight trials indicate that total mortality is reduced by about 34% (4).
—In hospitalized children, vitamin A supplementation reduces mortality from measles infection by about 60% (4). There is little evidence of benefit in children hospitalized for nonmeasles pneumonia; among well-nourished children, supplementation may be associated with adverse effects (4).
—Most trials of vitamin A found that supplementation reduced severity of diarrhea in children (4).
—A Cochrane meta-analysis of six randomized controlled trials of supplemental vitamin A in very low birthweight infants (≤ 1,500 g) found that vitamin A reduced oxygen requirements at 36 weeks postmenstrual age [relative risk (RR) 0.85 (0.73, 0.98)].

ANIMAL/IN VITRO

• Induction of skin, lung, bladder, colon, and mammary tumors can be inhibited by high doses of vitamin A.

OTHER CLAIMED BENEFITS/ACTIONS

• Cancer
• Dry skin
• Eye problems
• Lung disease
• Skin papillomas
• Vocal cord papillomas
• Wrinkles
• Wound healing

 Clinical Considerations

DEFICIENCY SIGNS AND SYMPTOMS

• Vitamin A deficiency is unusual in the United States and Canada, and supplementation is rarely indicated; exceptions include malnourished children, patients with cystic fibrosis, and alcoholics.
• Vision

—Globally, vitamin A is the leading cause of blindness among children. Deficiency may cause night blindness, Bitôt's spots (small, triangular, gray deposits on the bulbar conjunctiva adjacent to the cornea, near the palpebral fissure), xerophthalmia, keratomalacia (the most severe stage of xerophthalmia, sometimes with corneal ulceration), and blindness.

• Infectious disease

—Vitamin A deficiency is associated with increased susceptibility to chicken pox, diarrhea, malaria, measles, pneumonia, respiratory syncytial virus, and HIV. Vitamin A deficiency compromises mucosal immunity, causing epithelial changes, decreased goblet cells, and decreased secretory IgA, as well as alterations in the number of CD4 cells. Acute phase response may cause abnormal urinary loss of vitamin A, thus decreasing serum levels. Acute infectious disease appears to reduce vitamin A levels. Low serum levels of serum vitamin A (whether resulting from acute phase response or insufficient hepatic stores) are associated with decreased survival in adults with HIV, measles, respiratory syncytial virus infection, and meningococcal disease. In addition, vitamin A deficiency is associated with increased maternal-fetal transmission of HIV (2).

• Other effects

—Vitamin A deficiency can cause stunting and wasting in children, decreased fertility (in males and females), chorioamnionitis, low birthweight, anemia, and increased plasma thyroxine concentrations (without symptoms of hyperthyroidism).

RISK FACTORS FOR DEFICIENCY

• Alcoholism, poor nutrition, cystic fibrosis, pancreatic disease, and infectious disease.

FACTORS DECREASING AVAILABILITY/ABSORPTION

• Gastrointestinal malabsorption, gastrectomy/gastrotomy, cholestyramine, colestipol, and mineral oil

FACTORS INCREASING AVAILABILITY/ABSORPTION

• Hepatic disease, chronic renal failure

LABORATORY TESTS

• Deficiency serum retinol level: < 0.35 μmol/L
• Marginal: 0.35 to 0.7 μmol/L
• Adequate: 0.7 to 3.0 μmol/L
• Excessive: > 3.0 μmol/L (5)
• Other tests include dark adaptation or conjunctival impression cytology (both of which measure end-organ effects) or relative or modified relative dose response (which are indirect measures of hepatic vitamin A stores). Serum vitamin A concentrations greater than 1.4 μmol/L predicts normal dark adaptation 95% of the time (6).

 Risks

ADVERSE REACTIONS

• Most likely to occur in adults taking more than 25,000 IUs daily or children taking more than 18,000 IUs daily over many months. Supplementation should be avoided in those with hepatic disease (excess vitamin A can damage hepatic cells) or renal failure (malfunctioning kidneys can excrete retinol-binding protein, which is not normally excreted).
• Symptoms of vitamin A toxicity include headache, vomiting, diplopia, alopecia, dry mucous membranes, desquamation, bone pain, joint pain, liver damage, hemorrhage, and coma. Infants may have a bulging fontanelle.

Vitamin A (See Also Carotenoids)

DRUG INTERACTIONS

• Cholestyramine, colestipol, other cholesterol-adsorbing resins, and mineral oil reduce absorption of vitamin A.

PREGNANCY/LACTATION

• High doses of vitamin A have been linked with congenital malformations (see questions and answers).

 Dose

RECOMMENDED DIETARY ALLOWANCE (IN RETINOL ACTIVITY EQUIVALENTS) (7)

Infants and children

0 to 6 months	400 μg/day (adequate intake)
7 to 12 months	500 μg/day (adequate intake)
1 to 3 years	300 μg/day
4 to 8 years	400 μg/day

Males

9 to 13 years	600 μg/day
14 to 50 years	900 μg/day
51+ years	900 μg/day

Females

9 to 13 years	600 μg/day
14 to 50 years	700 μg/day
51+ years	700 μg/day

Pregnant

≤18 years	750 μg/day
19 to 50 years	770 μg/day

Lactating

≤18 years	1,200 μg/day
19 to 50 years	1,300 μg/day

UPPER LIMITS

Infants and children

0 to 6 months	600 μg/day
7 to 12 months	600 μg/day
1 to 3 years	600 μg/day
4 to 8 years	900 μg/day

Males

9 to 13 years	1,700 μg/day
14 to 18 years	2,800 μg/day
19 to 50 years	3,000 μg/day
51+ years	3,000 μg/day

Females

9 to 13 years	1,700 μg/day
14 to 18 years	2,800 μg/day
19 to 50 years	3,000 μg/day
51+ years	3,000 μg/day

Pregnant

≤18 years	2,800 μg/day
19 to 50 years	3,000 μg/day

Lactating

≤18 years	2,800 μg/day
19 to 50 years	3,000 μg/day

One retinol activity equivalent (RAE)

= 1 μg all-*trans* retinol
= 12 μg all-*trans*-β-carotene
= 24 μg other provitamin A carotenoids

One IU Vitamin A activity

= 0.3 μg all-*trans* retinol
= 3.6 μg all-*trans*-β-carotene
= 7.2 μg other provitamin A carotenoids

• *Correcting deficiency:* Deficiency can generally be corrected by giving 30,000 IUs or more of retinol daily (with some dietary fat) for several days.
• In children older than 1 year, World Health Organization (WHO) recommends that vitamin A deficiency should be treated with 110 mg retinol palmitate p.o. (or 55 mg i.m.) plus two additional doses of 110 mg p.o. over the next week.
• A prophylactic regimen used for children 1 to 6 years in developing countries is a single capsule containing 200,000 IUs of vitamin A every 3 to 6 months (2).

 Common Questions and Answers

Q: What dose of vitamin A is teratogenic in pregnancy?
A: It is not clear. Case-control studies and cohort studies have linked high doses of vitamin A with congenital malformations. However, a large prospective study conducted by the European Network of Teratology Information Services of 423 pregnancies exposed during the first 9 weeks of gestation to vitamin A greater than 10,000 IU/day found no association of high vitamin A intake during the organogenetic period with malformations (8). Daily doses greater than 25,000 IU may be teratogenic, 5,000 IU/day is not associated with teratogenicity, and there are insufficient data available to determine whether or not doses between 5,000 IU and 25,000 IUs are teratogenic. There is no reason to supplement with more than 5,000 IU during pregnancy and that dose seems to be safe.

Q: Is it true that although vitamin A is toxic, beta-carotene is not?
A: Vitamin A is stored in the liver; although a small amount of carotenoids are stored in the liver, most are stored in fat tissue. Although it has long been thought that the body is not capable of converting enough beta-carotene (or other carotenoids) to reach toxic amounts of vitamin A, recent studies showed swollen mitochondria in the livers of animals fed alcohol in combination with beta-carotene. This may be an interaction effect.

There are other problems with beta-carotene. Two supplementation trials found that beta-carotene was associated with a higher rate of lung cancer in smokers and asbestos-exposed workers. This may be due to displacement of other carotenoids by beta-carotene. Smoke and beta-carotene may be a particularly bad combination. Experiments with ferrets found far lower levels of beta-carotene in the blood of smoke-exposed ferrets (whether or not they were beta-carotene supplemented); lower levels were correlated with increased breakdown of beta-carotene into eccentric cleavage oxidation products (6). Necropsy showed alveolar cell proliferation and squamous metaplasia in ferrets supplemented with beta-carotene and exposed to smoke. Excess dietary or supplemental β-carotene (usually more than 30 mg beta-carotene/day over an extended period) can cause hypercarotenemia and carotenodermia, a yellowish tint to the skin most easily seen on the palms and soles (β-carotene is stored in adipocytes). Carotenodermia may be distinguished from jaundice because it does not involve sclerae or nails.

Q: Is it possible to overdose on vitamin A from dietary sources?
A: There is no need to worry about this in a normal diet; it is theoretically possible if someone is subsisting solely on liver. We were taught in medical school that polar bear liver contains toxic amounts of vitamin A. Although this is true (polar bear liver contains 2 million IUs vitamin A/100 g), this hardly constitutes a public health problem.

Q: Can vitamin A derivatives cause toxicity?
A: Yes. Oral forms of vitamin A derivatives such as isotretinoin (13-*cis* retinoic acid), tretinoin (all-*trans* retinoic acid), or etretinate are used to treat acne and psoriasis; isotretinoin, which is not stored, is also used to treat certain epithelial cell cancers. Although generally safer than megadoses of vitamin A, these derivatives are teratogenic and long-term oral intake can result in typical retinoid toxicity.
Topical derivatives have been used to treat acne and wrinkles; far less toxic than oral dosage forms, the main side effects with topical preparations are photosensitivity, erythema, and desquamation.

Vitamin B$_6$ (Pyridoxine)

 10 Second Take

B$_6$ may benefit premenstrual syndrome (PMS), pediatric seizures, and morning sickness; high chronic doses may cause neuropathy.

 Basics

DESCRIPTION

• Vitamin B$_6$ is a collective term for nitrogen-containing compounds including pyridoxine (most commonly found in plants) and pyridoxal and pyridoxamine phosphate (phosphorylated forms are most common in animal tissues) (1).

FOOD SOURCES

Liver, meat, fish, whole grains, soybeans, peanuts, other legumes, nuts, bananas, and avocados

MAIN FUNCTIONS/PHARMACOKINETICS

• Vitamin B$_6$ is especially important in amino acid synthesis, catabolism, and transport; phospholipid and sphingolipid synthesis; and porphyrin synthesis.
• After intestinal absorption, the liver converts the three vitamers to pyridoxal 5'phosphate (PLP), a cofactor for over 100 enzymes. PLP is involved in gluconeogenesis, niacin formation, lipid metabolism, cell-mediated immunity, and steroid hormone modulation (2).
• B$_6$ is needed for transamination, in the synthesis of nonessential amino acids; decarboxylation, in the synthesis of neuroactive amines including serotonin, histamine, and GABA; in the dehydratase reaction by which serine and threonine are converted to their α-keto acids; and in side-chain cleavage reactions.
• B$_6$ may influence glucose/glycogen metabolism; about half of endogenous B$_6$ is attached to glycogen phosphorylase (which catalyzes carbohydrate breakdown) (1).
• Excess B$_6$ is metabolized to 4-pyridoxic acid and excreted in urine. Most B$_6$ in the body is in muscles bound to glycogen phosphorylase. Pyridoxine is not stored in appreciable amounts (2).

 Evidence

CLINICAL TRIALS

• Carpal tunnel syndrome

—A review of vitamin B$_6$ and carpal tunnel syndrome noted that most supportive studies of B$_6$ were from the same investigators and were methodologically poor; studies refuting the value of B$_6$ were methodologically better. B$_6$ may be useful as adjunctive therapy (3).

• Premenstrual syndrome (PMS)

—A systematic review of B$_6$ for PMS analyzed nine randomized, placebo-controlled, double-blind, parallel, or crossover studies with a total of 940 women (4). Most trials were methodologically poor. B$_6$ (50 to 600 mg/day) was superior to placebo. The overall odds ratio (OR) was 2.32 [95% confidence interval (CI) 1.95 to 2.54] and for depression, evaluated in five trials, the OR was 2.12 (95% CI 1.80 to 2.48; $p < 0.001$). No dose-response effect was seen.

• Nausea and vomiting

—A study in Thailand randomized 342 pregnant women with morning sickness to pyridoxine (10 mg t.i.d.) or placebo. Mean nausea (but not vomiting) scores decreased significantly more in the pyridoxine group than in the placebo group (5).
—Another randomized, double-blind, placebo-controlled study of 59 women with morning sickness tested vitamin B$_6$ (25 mg t.i.d. × 3 days). Compared with placebo, B$_6$ benefited only patients with severe nausea; there was no difference between groups in those with mild to moderate nausea or overall. Significantly fewer B$_6$-treated patients (8/31) vomited than placebo-treated patients (15/28) (6).
—A randomized trial in 104 patients found no benefit of adjunctive controlled-release pyridoxine (100 mg/day, 1 hour before radiation therapy for 1 week) in preventing radiation-induced sickness (7).

• Pediatric seizures (see questions and answers for pyridoxine-dependent seizures)

—A controlled study of 90 infants and children with recurrent seizures (most resulting from infectious disease) tested adjunctive high-dose pyridoxine (30 or 50 mg/kg/day intravenously) against conventional treatment alone (8). Seizures resolved significantly earlier (2.4 ± 1.4 days) in the pyridoxine group, compared with controls (3.7 ± 2.0 days).

• Autism

—Although open-label studies have claimed benefit for administration of pyridoxine and magnesium to autistic children, a small, double-blind, placebo-controlled trial found that pyridoxine (average dose 638.9 mg) and magnesium oxide (216.3 mg) in 12 patients (10 completed) had no effect on three scales used to assess autism (9).

• Atopic dermatitis

—A double-blind, placebo-controlled study of 20 patients with atopic dermatitis tested pyridoxine (1.5 mg/kg/day × 1 month). Significantly more pyridoxine-treated patients (6/10) improved, compared with 1/10 patients on placebo. However, a randomized, double-blind, placebo-controlled trial in 48 children (41 completed) with moderate or severe atopic dermatitis found no significant difference in clinical severity scores or symptom scores between groups given placebo or pyridoxine (15 mg/day × 4 weeks) (10).

• Alcohol intoxication

—A randomized double-blind controlled study of 108 patients with acute alcohol intoxication compared intravenous pyridoxine (1 g) to saline placebo (11). After 1 hour, there was no difference in the mean decrease in blood alcohol concentration or level of consciousness.

• Side effects of drugs

—A randomized controlled trial in 124 symptomatic women on low-dose combined oral contraceptives tested vitamin B$_6$ (150 mg daily × 1 month) on nausea, headache, vomiting, dizziness, depression, and irritability. There were no differences between the vitamin B$_6$ group and the placebo group (12).
—A randomized, double-blind placebo-controlled crossover study of 20 (15 completed) participants tested pyridoxine 15 mg on theophylline-induced hand tremor; pyridoxine significantly reduced tremor after a single theophylline dose but not repeated doses (13). There were no differences between groups in psychomotor tests, electrophysiologic tests, or sleep quality.

OTHER CLAIMED BENEFITS/ACTIONS

• Depression
• Asthma
• Cardiovascular disease

 Clinical Considerations

DEFICIENCY SIGNS AND SYMPTOMS

• Stomatitis, cheilosis, glossitis, irritability, confusion, seizures (in infants), nephrolithiasis (calcium oxalate stones from hyperoxaluria), and homocysteinemia

Vitamin B₆ (Pyridoxine)

FACTORS DECREASING AVAILABILITY/ABSORPTION

- Bioavailability varies among foods. Increased protein intake, asthma, renal disease, alcoholism, coronary heart disease, breast cancer, Hodgkin's disease, sickle cell anemia, and diabetes can lower plasma PLP concentrations (2). Smoking can lower plasma PLP concentrations (2). Genetic defects of PLP-dependent enzymes (homocystinuria; cystathionuria; xanthurenic aciduria, a defect in ornithine aminotransferase) can mimic B₆ deficiency. Dialysis patients often manifest vitamin B₆ deficiency (14). B₆ metabolism is impaired in premature infants (15).

LABORATORY TESTS

- Tissue reserves are best estimated by functional measures of B₆ status. In the tryptophan load test, subjects are given 5 to 10 g tryptophan. B₆ deficient patients will excrete more than 250 mg xanthurenic acid in a 24-hour urine collection (1).
- In the PLP stimulation test, B₆ dependent transaminases are measured before and after PLP stimulation. Erythrocyte glutamate-oxaloacetate transaminase (EGOT) and erythrocyte glutamate-pyruvate transaminase (EGPT) are the most commonly used enzyme systems (1).
- For adults, urinary excretion of vitamin B₆ of less than 35 μg/day (or 20 μg/gm creatinine) indicates inadequate intake; urinary B₆ excretion reflects only recent dietary intake.

 Risks

ADVERSE REACTIONS

- Acute toxicity is low; 1 g/kg is well tolerated (1).
- Peripheral neuropathy

—Chronic daily doses of 500 to 6,000 mg can cause peripheral neuropathy and possibly central neurologic toxicity. Signs may include gradually progressive sensory ataxia and impairment of position and vibration sense in distal limbs. These effects usually take years to develop, but some may develop mild neuropathy with chronic doses as low as 50 mg/day.

- Other

—Skin changes resembling porphyria cutanea tarda were reported in two people who had ingested 2 to 4 g/day of pyridoxine for 2 to 4 years (16). Large acute doses can reduce prolactin secretion and, thus, lower milk production in lactating women (1).

DRUG INTERACTIONS

- Many drugs interfere with B₆ metabolism. When a drug interacts directly with PLP, pyridoxine intake of more than 10 mg/day could affect drug efficacy (2).

- Isoniazid interacts with PLP (pyridoxine 5 g parenterally is used to treat isoniazid-induced seizures) (17).
- Iproniazid interacts with PLP.
- Cycloserine interacts with PLP.
- Penicillamine interacts with PLP.
- L-3,4-dihydroxyphenylalanine interacts with PLP.
- Ethanol increases catabolism of PLP.
- Theophylline and caffeine inhibit pyridoxal kinase.
- Oral contraceptives (ethinylestradiol, mestranol) increase PLP enzyme levels and tissue retention of PLP (2).
- Case reports of interactions include

—Amiodarone: Photosensitivity reactions were enhanced (16).
—Barbiturates: Pyridoxine decreases barbiturate effect, possibly by increasing metabolism (18).
—Phenytoin: Pyridoxine occasionally decreases phenytoin effect, possibly by increasing metabolism (18).

ANIMAL TOXICITY

- Doses of more than 150 mg/kg/day of pyridoxine in dogs caused neurologic impairment and nerve degeneration (16).
- Rats and dogs given 200 mg/kg to 1 g/kg/day pyridoxine acquired progressively unsteady gait.
- Histopathologic studies in dogs have shown degeneration of sensory neurons in the dorsal roots and central and peripheral processes, as well as nerve fiber degeneration in the distal portions of sensory axons (19). In rats, pyridoxine (20 to 80 mg/kg) did not affect offspring (16).

 Dose

RECOMMENDED DIETARY ALLOWANCE

Infants and children

0 to 6 months	0.1 mg/day (adequate intake)
7 to 12 months	0.3 mg/day (adequate intake)
1 to 3 years	0.5 mg/day
4 to 8 years	0.6 mg/day

Males

9 to 13 years	1.0 mg/day
14 to 50 years	1.3 mg/day
51+ years	1.7 mg/day

Females

9 to 13 years	1.0 mg/day
14 to 18 years	1.2 mg/day
19 to 50 years	1.3 mg/day
51+ years	1.5 mg/day
Pregnant	1.9 mg/day
Lactating	2.0 mg/day

Note: The recommended daily allowance (RDA) for older adults should probably be increased by at least 15% (1).

UPPER LIMITS

Infants and children

0 to 6 months	Not determinable
7 to 12 months	Not determinable
1 to 3 years	30 mg/day
4 to 8 years	40 mg/day

Males

9 to 13 years	60 mg/day
14 to 18 years	80 mg/day
19 to 50 years	100 mg/day
51+ years	100 mg/day

Females

9 to 13 years	60 mg/day
14 to 18 years	80 mg/day
19 to 50 years	100 mg/day
51+ years	100 mg/day

Pregnant

≤18 years	80 mg/day
19 to 50 years	100 mg/day

Lactating

≤18 years	80 mg/day
19 to 50 years	100 mg/day

 Common Questions and Answers

Q: What are pyridoxine-dependent seizures?
A: Inherited as an autosomal recessive trait, pyridoxine-dependent seizures may begin before birth, after birth, or up to 2 years of age (20). Prenatal diagnosis can sometimes be achieved by close questioning of the mother about rhythmic movements *in utero,* (distinct from usual fetal movements). Pyridoxine treatment during pregnancy increases the chance of normal neurodevelopmental outcome (21). Pyridoxine-dependent seizures (usually generalized) may be preceded by irritability, restlessness, crying, and vomiting. Anticonvulsants are usually ineffective (20). Possible causes include defective binding of pyridoxine to its apoenzyme, preventing conversion of glutamic acid to GABA, or possibly inability to maintain normal levels of pyridoxal phosphate. Treatment is pyridoxine, usually 50 mg/day (very high doses have been associated with severe hypotonia or sensory neuropathy) (20).

Vitamin B₁₂ (Cobalamin)

 10 Second Take

Vitamin B_{12} is nontoxic. Deficiency is not uncommon, especially among older adults.

 Basics

DESCRIPTION

• Cobalamin, a water-soluble vitamin, is almost completely absent in plants. A cobalt-containing coenzyme, cobalamin functions closely with folic acid. In humans, 50% to 90% of the body's stores are in the liver; it takes years to deplete bodily stores.

FOOD SOURCES

• Meats (especially liver and kidney), poultry, dairy products, eggs, and seafoods (especially bivalves). Trace amounts in legumes, soybeans, seaweed, and blue-green algae, including spirulina

MECHANISM/PHARMACOKINETICS

• Involved in methylation reactions; required for methylmalonyl-CoA mutase (which transforms methylmalonyl to succinyl-CoA for degradation of odd-numbered carbon fatty acids) and methionine synthetase, which interacts with methyltetrahydrofolic acid to form *trans*-homocysteine into methionine.
• Orally ingested cobalamin binds to a carrier protein in saliva and gastric juices and then is released to intrinsic factor, secreted by stomach cells. This complex binds to the brush border of ileal mucosal cells, where it is absorbed.

 Evidence

CLINICAL TRIALS

• Osteoarthritis

—A double-blind crossover study in 26 participants (including 23 women) with osteoarthritis of the hands compared placebo with folate (6,400 mcg) or a combination of folate (6,400 mcg) and a very low dose of cobalamin (20 μg) for 2 months each (1). There were no clear differences among groups in grip strength, tender joints, acetaminophen use, or other measures; mean patient assessments did not change from baseline.

• Diabetic neuropathy

—A randomized placebo-controlled double-blind study of 50 patients with diabetic neuropathy (36 completed) tested the effects of methylcobalamin 500 mg t.i.d. × 4 months on nerve conduction studies and a peripheral neurology score that included somatic symptoms, autonomic symptoms, and clinical signs (2). Compared with baseline, peripheral neurology scores improved significantly in the treated, but not the placebo, group ($p < 0.05$). Nerve conduction studies did not change.

• Seasonal affective disorder

—A double-blind, randomized study tested cyanocobalamin in 27 patients with seasonal affective disorder (3). After a 2-week placebo washout, participants received 1.5 mg cyanocobalamin t.i.d. or placebo for 2 weeks. No significant differences were seen between groups in a structured depression rating.

EPIDEMIOLOGIC STUDIES

• Incontinence

—A case-control study of 104 matched pairs found that those with B_{12} deficiency (serum levels less than 250 pg/mL) were 2.63 times as likely to be incontinent than matched controls [$p = 0.026$, 95% confidence interval (CI) 1.11, 6.44] (4).

• Depression

—Among 700 disabled, nondemented women older than 65 years, participants with B_{12} deficiency were 2.05 times as likely to be severely depressed than nondeficient participants (assessed by the geriatric depression scale) (5).

• Impaired hearing/tinnitus

—In 55 women aged 60 to 71 years, pure-tone averages were inversely correlated with serum B_{12} and red blood cell folate; participants with impaired hearing had significantly lower serum B_{12} (38%) and lower red blood cell folate (31%) than women with normal hearing (6).
—In 113 army personnel, B_{12} deficiency was significantly more common in those with tinnitus and noise-induced hearing loss (47%) than in those with noise-induced hearing loss only (27%) or in normal subjects (19%) (7).

ANIMAL/IN VITRO

• Hydroxycobalamin inhibits HIV-1 infection of human blood monocytes and lymphocytes *in vitro* (8).

OTHER CLAIMED BENEFITS/ACTIONS

• Asthma
• Bursitis
• Dementia
• Depression
• Diabetic neuropathy
• Multiple sclerosis
• Osteoporosis

 Clinical Considerations

DEFICIENCY SIGNS AND SYMPTOMS

• Macrocytic anemia [mean corpuscular volume (MCV) greater than 100 μ^3, hypersegmented neutrophils] (most commonly pernicious anemia), leukopenia, thrombocytopenia, stomatitis, and glossitis (9). Neurologic manifestations may include peripheral neuropathy (often beginning with symmetrical paresthesias of the lower extremities; may include hyporeflexia), spinal cord involvement (resulting in loss of position and vibratory sense, ataxia, weakness, spasticity, urinary and fecal incontinence, impotence, hyperreflexia, clonus, and positive Babinski reflex), autonomic neuropathy (which may present as orthostatic hypotension), and visual impairment (retrobulbar neuritis, optic atrophy, pseudotumor cerebri). Psychiatric manifestations may include dementia, hallucinations, psychosis ("megaloblastic madness"), paranoia, depression, and personality changes (10).
• Risk factors for deficiency

—Age (deficiency is common in older adults, who should take 3 μg B_{12} daily)
—B_{12} metabolic defect (homocystinuria, B_{12}-responsive methylmalonic acidemia)
—Partial gastrectomy (decreases intrinsic factor)
—Ileal resection
—Pancreatectomy
—Inflammatory bowel disease
—Sprue
—Alcoholism
—Vegan diet
—Parasites

FACTORS DECREASING AVAILABILITY/ABSORPTION

• Liver disease, severe pancreatic disease, hyperthyroidism, increased hematopoiesis, bacterial overgrowth in the small intestine, excessive soluble fiber intake, anticonvulsants, biguanides, methotrexate, neomycin, *para*-aminosalicylic acid (PAS), tetracycline, sodium nitroprusside, potassium chloride (slow-release), cimetidine, cholestyramine, and colchicine

FACTORS INCREASING AVAILABILITY/ABSORPTION

• Nonionic surfactants (polyoxyethylene sorbitans)

LABORATORY TESTS

- Samples should be collected fasting.
- Plasma B$_{12}$: normal values 200 to 700 pg/mL; levels less than 150 pg/mL indicate deficiency.
- Competitive binding assays are preferred. Either serum or plasma may be used, but blood tubes containing heparin or fluoride should be avoided (both degrade B$_{12}$) (11). Falsely low serum B$_{12}$ levels may be seen with multiple myeloma, malignancy, aplastic anemia, transcobalamin I deficiency recent radioisotope studies, or high dose vitamin C. Falsely normal levels (in the presence of deficiency) may be seen in severe liver disease, chronic granulocytic leukemia, transcobalamin II deficiency, congenital cobalamin coenzyme deficiency, or recent nitrous oxide inhalation (10). Methylmalonic acid and homocysteine levels may be earlier indicators of marginal B$_{12}$ status. Normal homocysteine range is 7 to 22 μmol/L.
- Schilling test

—A Schilling test differentiates between B$_{12}$ deficiency caused by pernicious anemia or intestinal malfunction. After intramuscular administration of 1,000 μg of B$_{12}$, intestinal absorption of unbound B$_{12}$ and bound B$_{12}$ are compared. With intestinal dysfunction, neither isotope is absorbed normally. In pernicious anemia, bound, but not unbound, B$_{12}$ is well absorbed. Some patients with pernicious anemia can absorb crystalline B$_{12}$ but not protein-bound B$_{12}$; these people will have normal Schilling tests unless a "food" Schilling test is done.

Risks

ADVERSE REACTIONS

B$_{12}$ is very safe.

DRUG INTERACTIONS

- Biguanides: reduce absorption of B$_{12}$
- Cimetidine: decreases absorption of protein-bound vitamin B$_{12}$
- Cholestyramine: decreases absorption by binding intrinsic factor
- Colchicine: decreases absorption through disturbing intestinal mucosal function
- Methotrexate: possibly impairs absorption
- Neomycin: decreases absorption
- PAS: decreases absorption
- Potassium chloride (slow-release): inhibits intrinsic factor activity by lowering ileal pH
- Sodium nitroprusside: decreases serum B$_{12}$ temporarily

Dose

MODE OF ADMINISTRATION

- Vitamin B$_{12}$ may be administered p.o., i.m., i.v., sublingually, or as an intranasal gel.
- Different forms include cyanocobalamin; hydroxocobalamin; and two coenzyme forms, methylcobalamin and adenosylcobalamin. Methylcobalamin may be more effective than cyanocobalamin. Hydroxycobalamin is best for those with tobacco amblyopia or tropical nutritional amblyopia (12) (see questions and answers).

RECOMMENDED DIETARY ALLOWANCE

Infants and children

0 to 6 months	0.4 μg/day (adequate intake)
7 to 12 months	0.5 μg/day (adequate intake)
1 to 3 years	0.9 μg/day
4 to 8 years	1.2 μg/day
Males	
9 to 13 years	1.8 μg/day
14 to 50 years	2.4 μg/day
51+ years	2.4 μg/day
Females	
9 to 13 years	1.8 μg/day
14 to 50 years	2.4 μg/day
51+ years	2.4 μg/day
Pregnant	2.6 μg/day
Lactating	2.8 μg/day

CORRECTING DEFICIENCY

- A dose of 100 to 1,000 μg cyanocobalamin or hydroxycobalamin i.m. × 1, then 100 μg q.d. × several days; 1,000 μg cobalamin p.o. q.d. is also effective.
- For chronic therapy, 1 mg p.o. q.d. or 100 μg i.m. monthly.

Common Questions and Answers

Q: What is the connection between nitrous oxide and vitamin B$_{12}$?
A: Nitrous oxide inactivates cob(I)alamin, and in vitamin B$_{12}$-deficient patients may cause demyelination, spastic paresis, subacute combined degeneration of the spinal cord, and encephalopathy (13). Debilitated, B$_{12}$-deficient and possible folate-deficient patients may experience major problems from nitrous oxide; prophylactic supplementation is advised (14).

Q: Are all vegetarians deficient in B$_{12}$?
A: No. Ova-lacto vegetarians, who consume eggs and dairy products, are not at increased risk of B$_{12}$ deficiency. Vegans (who consume no animal products) are at higher risk, although adequate B$_{12}$ may be obtained from a vegan diet if enough sea vegetables and/or fermented products are consumed. In 21 long-term adherents of a strict uncooked vegan ("living food") diet, serum B$_{12}$ levels were significantly lower than matched controls; more than half fell below the lower reference limit (15).
Vegans consuming nori and/or *Chlorella* seaweeds had B$_{12}$ levels twice as high as vegans who did not consume seaweed. Six of nine vegans showed a slow but significant decline in B$_{12}$ levels over a 2-year observation period.

Q: Is injected B$_{12}$ more effective than oral or sublingual B$_{12}$?
A: In some cases, but for most cases of nutritional deficiency, injected B$_{12}$ is more effective only at low doses. Although B$_{12}$ injections are more commonly used than oral replacement in the United States, oral cobalamin is just as effective and certainly more convenient. Distrust of oral B$_{12}$ stems from early studies that showed variable absorption of orally administered B$_{12}$ (100 to 250 μg). This can easily be resolved, however, by giving higher oral doses of 1,000 μg/day. Some recommend that deficient patients should receive 2,000 μg b.i.d. for the first month to rapidly replenish liver stores.
High doses of sublingual B$_{12}$ (2,000 μg/day × 7 to 12 days) have been shown to normalize cobalamin concentration in deficient subjects, but there is no proven advantage of this form of administration (16). There are several cases in which hydroxycobalamin is preferred, although it is available only in parenteral forms. Hydroxocobalamin is a cyanide antagonist (and has been used as an antidote to cyanide poisoning in fire victims) (17). Cyanocobalamin does not bind cyanide. Cyanocobalamin is ineffective for those with tobacco amblyopia or in smokers with pernicious anemia; hydroxycobalamin must be used in these cases (12).

Q: What is the connection between B$_{12}$ and homocysteinemia?
A: Elevated levels of homocysteine are associated with increased risk of cardiovascular disease (18), stroke (19), deep vein thrombosis (20), and neural tube defects (21). Folic acid is more effective than B$_{12}$ in lowering homocysteine levels, except when homocysteinemia is due to B$_{12}$ deficiency. Those with low normal B$_{12}$ levels may derive maximum benefit from combined therapy. In one trial, 0.4 mg of cyanocobalamin lowered homocysteine concentrations 14.8%; folic acid, however, reduced concentrations by 41.7% (22).

Vitamin C (Ascorbic Acid, Ascorbate)

 10 Second Take

Vitamin C is benign; clinical trials do not support its use in colds or cancer.

 Basics

DESCRIPTION

• Ascorbic acid (2,3-didehydro-L-threo-hexano-1,4-lactone) is a partially oxidized form of glucose; a potent reducing agent, it is an important antioxidant (1). Although most mammals can synthesize ascorbate from glucose, primates, flying mammals, fish, guinea pigs, and most birds cannot (1).

FOOD SOURCES

• Many fruits and vegetables, especially citrus fruits, rose hips, black currant, cranberries, melons, mango, strawberries, kiwi, tomatoes, asparagus, cruciferous vegetables, peppers, snow peas, and sweet potatoes.
• In the U.S., adult males consume 84 mg/day and females 73 mg/day. Vitamin C is stable in acid, but not heat, neutral pH, or alkaline pH. Vitamin C content in food varies with season, transport, processing, and cooking. Boiling vegetables can reduce levels 50 to 80% (2).

MECHANISM/PHARMACOKINETICS

• Ascorbate is a cofactor or co-substrate for eight enzymes. An antioxidant, ascorbate keeps functional groups on enzymes reduced, and reduces superoxide, hydroxyl and peroxyl radicals. Necessary for the synthesis of carnitine, neurotransmitters, and collagen, vitamin C is important in the mixed function oxidase system and enhances iron absorption by keeping iron reduced (3). Vitamin C increases prostacyclin production by aortic vascular wall endothelium and protects prostacyclin synthetase from inhibitors (4). High doses (>1 g/day) decrease blood histamine levels and leukotriene B_4 and 5-lipoxygenase activity (1).
• Ingesting 200 mg/day or 2500 mg/day results in similar mean steady-state plasma concentrations (approximately 12 to 15 mg/L) (5). Ascorbate is partially reabsorbed renally and excreted in the urine.

 Evidence

CLINICAL TRIALS

• Colds

—Most trials of vitamin C for colds, done in the 1970s, are flawed. One analysis found that 6 of 8 double-blind controlled trials of vitamin C (250 mg to 1 g q.d.; some studies increased the dose to 1.5 g to 5 g if a cold occurred) found no difference in incidence or duration of colds (1). Two prophylaxis trials in children (1 to 2 g/day) noted decreased duration of colds. Three negative trials noted a significant decrease in "days at home" (1). A meta-analysis of seven studies published before 1975 (including three in the Linder review) concluded that the difference in duration of colds was clinically insignificant (6). Another analysis of the six largest placebo-controlled trials utilizing doses equal to 1,000 mg found no benefit for vitamin C in reducing incidence of colds (7).

• Dermatology

—Topical 10% L-ascorbic acid reduced UVB radiation-induced erythema compared to control. A similar regimen attenuated UVA-mediated phototoxic response (8). A double-blind, placebo-controlled, eight day trial found no benefit for vitamin C (3 g/day) with vitamin E (1,500 IU/day) in photo-provocation tests in nine patients with polymorphous light eruption (a common, often transient photosensitivity disease) (9).
—A double-blind, placebo-controlled study found that oral vitamin C (2 g) with vitamin E (1,000 IU) reduced sunburn reaction significantly more than placebo (10).
—A double-blind RCT of 19 subjects with mild to moderately photodamaged facial skin found a benefit for a commercial topical ascorbic acid formulation, compared to vehicle (applied to different sides of the face for 3 months) (11).

• Radiation dermatitis

—In a study of 84 patients undergoing radiation for brain tumors, patients did not prefer topical vitamin C over placebo (on opposite sides of the head) for preventing radiation dermatitis (12).

• Pressure sores

—In 20 patients, ascorbic acid 500 mg/day for 1 month significantly reduced pressure sore area (84%, compared with 42.7% in the placebo group) (13).

• Asthma

—Asthmatic patients have lower vitamin C concentrations in plasma and leukocytes (14). A review found that 7 of 11 studies of vitamin C (1 to 2 g/day) showed significantly improved respiratory measurements in asthmatics.
—Another study, not included above, found that vitamin C (2 g, one hour before exercise), compared to placebo, prevented exercise-induced asthma in 9 of 20 subjects; in two others airway hyperreactivity was reduced (15). Pulmonary function tests after one hour were unaffected.

• Cardiovascular disease

—A review of vitamin C and cardiovascular disease found no conclusive evidence that vitamin C benefits cardiovascular disease (4). Studies are mixed on whether vitamin C affects clotting factors. A study of 84 hospitalized subjects given 1 g/day vitamin C found a 27% reduction in deep venous thrombosis; another study in 538 institutionalized elderly found no benefit of vitamin C (200 mg/day for 6 months) over placebo (4).

• Hypertension

—A short review of four studies on ascorbic acid in hypertension concluded that an effect, if present, was small (16).

• Reflex sympathetic dystrophy (RSD)

—A double-blind trial tested vitamin C (500 mg) or placebo for 50 days in 123 adults with 127 wrist fractures (115 patients completed) (17). The relative risk of RSD in the placebo group was 2.91 (95% confidence interval of 1.02 to 8.32) compared to the treated group.

• Preeclampsia

—In one study, 283 women at increased risk of preeclampsia were randomized to placebo or vitamin C (1,000 mg/day) and vitamin E (400 IU/day) at 16 to 22 weeks gestation (18). In the intention-to-treat cohort, preeclampsia occurred in 24 of 142 women (17%) in the placebo group and 11 of 141 (8%) in the vitamin group (adjusted odds ratio 0.39 [0.17–0.90], p = 0.02).

• Cancer

—A study of 150 patients with advanced cancer were randomized to placebo or vitamin C (10 g/day) (19). There was no significant difference in survival or symptoms between the two groups.

OTHER CLAIMED BENEFITS/ACTIONS

• Cancer, infection, cardiovascular disease prevention, and wound healing.

Clinical Considerations

DEFICIENCY SIGNS AND SYMPTOMS

• Scurvy, rare in developed countries, may occur in substance abusers or those on very restricted diets. Symptoms include lassitude, petechiae, ecchymoses, follicular hyperkeratosis (especially in the lower extremities), bleeding gums, ocular hemorrhage in the bulbar conjunctiva, arthralgias, Sjogren's syndrome, and depression.

FACTORS DECREASING AVAILABILITY/ABSORPTION

• Smoking (RDA 100 mg/day), pregnancy, lactation, oral contraceptives (possibly, results are mixed), and dialysis (ascorbate is freely dialyzed; patients must be supplemented).

LABORATORY TESTS

• Adequate intake: plasma >23 μmol/L (0.4 mg/dL) or mixed leukocytes >114 nmol/10^8 cells (>20 μg/10^8 cells) or mononuclear leukocytes >142 nmol/10^8 cells (>25 μg/10^8 cells)
• Deficient: plasma <11.4 μmol/L (<0.2 mg/dL); mixed leukocytes <57 nmol/10^8 cells (<10 μg/10^8 cells) mononuclear leukocytes <114 nmol/10^8 cells (<20 μg/10^8 cells)

 Risks

ADVERSE REACTIONS

• Diarrhea and abdominal bloating can occur with large (usually >5 g) dosages.
In patients with iron overload conditions, ascorbate enhances iron absorption and possibly enhances oxidative damage. There is no evidence that vitamin C causes iron overload in normal subjects or those heterozygous for hemochromatosis (2).
• Hemolysis was reported after a patient with glucose-6-phosphate dehydrogenase deficiency was given intravenous ascorbate and in one case where a patient ingested >6 g ascorbate in a single dose (2).
• Hyperoxalemia occurred in dialysis patients given repeated intravenous doses of 1 g vitamin C.
• Data are mixed on whether ascorbate affects urate and oxalate excretion (2) (see common questions and answers).

DRUG INTERACTIONS

• Vitamin C intake >250 mg/day can cause false-negative results for occult blood in stool.
• Aluminum-containing antacids: Ascorbic acid may increase gastrointestinal aluminum absorption (20).

• Warfarin: Rare cases of decreased anti-coagulant effect have been reported (21,22).
• Estrogens: >1 g/day vitamin C may decrease metabolism and increase serum concentrations of estrogen (23).
• Levonorgestrel: Gram doses of vitamin C had no effect on levonorgestrel metabolites (24).
• Propranolol: Vitamin C (2 g) given with 80-mg propranolol decreased C_{max}, T_{max}, and AUC (25).

 Dose

RECOMMENDED DIETARY ALLOWANCE

Infants and children	
0 to 6 months	40 mg/day (adequate intake)
7 to 12 months	50 mg/day (adequate intake)
1 to 3 years	15 mg/day
4 to 8 years	25 mg/day
Males	
9 to 13 years	45 mg/day
14 to 18 years	75 mg/day
19 to 50 years	90 mg/day
51+ years	90 mg/day
Females	
9 to 13 years	45 mg/day
14 to 18 years	65 mg/day
19 to 50 years	75 mg/day
51+ years	75 mg/day
Pregnant	
≤18 years	80 mg/day
19 to 50 years	85 mg/day
Lactating	
≤18 years	115 mg/day
19 to 50 years	120 mg/day

UPPER LIMITS

Infants and children	
0 to 6 months	Not determinable
7 to 12 months	Not determinable
1 to 3 years	400 mg/day
4 to 8 years	650 mg/day
Males	
9 to 3 years	1,200 mg/day
14 to 18 years	1,800 mg/day
19 to 50 years	2,000 mg/day
51+ years	2,000 mg/day
Females	
9 to 13 years	1,200 mg/day
14 to 18 years	1,800 mg/day
19 to 50 years	2,000 mg/day
51+ years	2,000 mg/day
Pregnant	
≤18 years	1,800 mg/day
19 to 50 years	2,000 mg/day
Lactating	
≤18 years	1,800 mg/day
19 to 50 years	2,000 mg/day

 Common Questions and Answers

Q: Isn't vitamin C pro-oxidant?
A: Most antioxidants have the capacity to become prooxidant at very high doses. While high doses of vitamin C have prooxidant activity in some *in vitro* systems, there is little evidence for such activity *in vivo* (2). A study of 30 healthy volunteers found that supplementation with 500 mg/day ascorbic acid for 6 weeks resulted in significant increases in 8-oxoadenine levels (and significant decreases in 8-oxoguanine levels) in DNA isolated from lymphocytes (both are markers of oxygen radical-mediated DNA damage) (26).

Q: Does vitamin C increase the risk of kidney stones?
A: Probably not. Ascorbate is commonly catabolized to oxalate (17% to 40% of ascorbate is excreted as oxalate) but excessive ascorbate intake simply decreases intestinal absorption and increases urinary excretion (1).
Although early studies reported that high doses of ascorbic acid elevated urinary oxalate, ascorbic acid interferes with the test for oxalate (27). An analysis utilizing ion chromatography found that the statistically significant but small increase in oxalate in subjects ingesting 5-g to 10-g ascorbate/day could be explained by oxalate production from ascorbate during analysis.
A prospective study in 45,251 men 40 to 75 years old, found that at six years, the age-adjusted relative risk of symptomatic kidney stones for men consuming ≥1,500 mg vitamin C daily (compared to <250 mg) was 0.78 (95% CI 0.54 to 1.11) (28). A similar analysis in 85,557 women found that vitamin C intake did not affect risk; the multivariate relative risk for women in the highest category of vitamin C intake compared to the lowest category was 1.06 (95% CI 0.69 to 1.64) (29).

Q: Are some types of vitamin C better than others?
A: No. A crossover study in nine subjects (including two smokers) of the relative bioavailability of ascorbic acid, Ester-C and a combination of ascorbic acid with hesperidin-rutin-buckwheat citrus bioflavonoids found the three preparations bioequivalent (30). Ester-C and bioflavonoid preparations cost more.

Q: Isn't vitamin C associated with hemolysis in premature infants?
A: Heinz body hemolytic anemia developed in a premature neonate after receiving a multivitamin; a subsequent study in guinea pigs demonstrated that vitamin C hemolyzed erythrocytes. However, a double-blind, placebo-controlled RCT of vitamin C (50 mg/day for 14 days) in premature neonates found no evidence of hemolysis (31).

Vitamin D (Calciferol, Cholecalciferol)

 10 Second Take

Vitamin D deficiency is common among exclusively breast-fed babies and older adults. High doses are potentially toxic.

 Basics

DESCRIPTION

- Vitamin D, a fat-soluble vitamin, is the only vitamin that humans can produce endogenously, with the aid of ultraviolet light. It functions as a steroid hormone. Stored in the liver, it is released as 25-hydroxyvitamin D and undergoes further hydroxylation in the kidney.
- Vitamin D_2 = ergocalciferol (plant sources; also added to milk)
- Vitamin D_3 = cholecalciferol (animal sources; also made in our skin)
- 25-OH-D_3 = 25-hydroxyvitamin D (hydroxylated and released from the liver)
- 1,25-diOHD = 1,25(OH)$_2$D = 1,25(OH)$_2$D$_3$ = 1,25-dihydroxyvitamin D = "active vitamin D" (hydroxylated and released from the kidney)

FOOD SOURCES

Liver (animal and fish), egg yolk, and fortified milk

MECHANISM/PHARMACOKINETICS

- Necessary for regulating plasma calcium levels, vitamin D also has direct effects on osteoclasts. Vitamin D receptors are found in most tissues, including the heart, pancreas, and cells of the immune system. 1,25-diOHD appears necessary for normal cardiac muscle contraction and, via effects on calcium homeostasis, for regulating blood pressure (1).
- Ultraviolet light catalyzes the formation of the provitamin in skin from 7-dehydrocholesterol. The provitamin rearranges to D_3 (cholecalciferol), which then binds to the vitamin D binding protein (DBP) in serum. A portion of liver stores of vitamin D is 25-hydroxylated and released for circulation. Low serum calcium triggers the release of parathyroid hormone, triggering a second hydroxylation in the kidney; this creates the active form, 1,25-dihydroxyvitamin D.

 Evidence

CLINICAL TRIALS

Numerous analogs of vitamin D are used to treat renal osteodystrophy, postmenopausal osteoporosis, hypocalcemia, and psoriasis; others are under investigation for use in leukemia, breast, prostate, and colon cancer (2).

- Seasonal affective disorder (SAD)

—A small, randomized controlled trial in 15 patients with SAD compared phototherapy in seven participants with administration of a single dose of vitamin D 100,000 IU (3). After 1 month, all participants who received vitamin D improved on the Hamilton Depression scale, the SIGH-SAD, and the SAD-8 depression scales; the phototherapy group did not improve significantly in any measure. Vitamin D status increased significantly in both groups (74% in the vitamin D group and 36% in the phototherapy group); improved outcomes were significantly associated with serum 25-hydroxyvitamin D levels.

 Clinical Considerations

Marginal deficiency is common among older adults, who may have less sun exposure, reduced dietary intake, reduced absorption, reduced vitamin D synthesis in the skin, and impaired renal hydroxylation.

DEFICIENCY SIGNS AND SYMPTOMS

- *In children:* Rickets, resulting in stunted growth and bony deformities because of enlarged epiphyseal growth plates. Bowed legs and the beaded appearance of enlarged epiphyseal plates at the costochondral junctions (the "rachitic rosary") may be apparent.
- *In adults:* Osteomalacia and pathologic fractures may be presenting signs. Occult vitamin D deficiency has been associated with increased risk of hip fracture (4).
- Laboratory findings in deficiency states may include hypocalcemia, hypophosphatemia, high alkaline phosphatase, increased parathyroid hormone, and decreased plasma citrate.

FACTORS DECREASING AVAILABILITY/ABSORPTION

- Chronic fat malabsorption, cystic fibrosis, renal failure, lack of sunshine, northern climates, dark skin, disability, ozone air pollution, sunscreen (see questions and answers), mineral oil (ingested), and insufficient vitamin production with insufficient dietary intake of vitamin D or fat

- Risk factors for babies include

—Exclusive breast-feeding (human milk is very low in vitamin D)
—Birth in northern climes
—Birth in the late summer, with little exposure to sunshine in fall and winter
—Maternal vitamin D deficiency (congenital rickets)

FACTORS INCREASING AVAILABILITY/ABSORPTION

- Increased dietary or supplemental intake
- Oral contraception use increases serum levels (see questions and answers)
- Sarcoidosis and other granulomatous disease
- Hypercalcemia occurs in 10% to 20% of patients with sarcoid, who manifest elevated serum levels of 1,25-diOHD during hypercalcemic episodes. Elevated levels of 1,25-diOHD with hypercalcemia have been reported in leprosy, disseminated candidiasis, silicone-induced granuloma, and plasma-cell granuloma. Abnormally high levels of 1,25-(OH)$_2$D$_3$ have been noted in several patients with tuberculosis (5).

LABORATORY TESTS

- 25-OH-D_3 in serum, the best index of vitamin D stores in the liver, is useful for assessing both deficiency and toxicity. The ligand-binding assay is recommended; normal reference range is 8 to 55 ng/mL. Signs of toxicity are usually seen with levels greater than 400 hg/mL.
- Laboratory measures of 1,25-diOHD are not useful for measuring dietary status and are only recommended for patients with hypocalcemic and hypercalcemic disorders.
- For high sensitivity and specificity, a combination of tests is usually used: first column chromatography or high-pressure liquid chromatography (HPLC) as separative techniques, then competitive protein binding (CPB), radioimmunoassay (RIA), or mass spectrometry as detection techniques.

 Risks

ADVERSE REACTIONS

- Daily doses greater than 1,000 IU (or 25 μg) are not recommended; doses greater than 2,000 IU daily are toxic. Hypervitaminosis D causes weakness, fatigue, headache, nausea, vomiting, hypercalcemia (calcium greater than 12 mg/dL), hypercalciuria, and impaired renal function. Deposition of calcium in soft tissues may cause cardiac myopathy, atherosclerotic lesions, and nephrolithiasis. In children, high doses can cause growth arrest.

- The no adverse effect level (NOAEL) set by the Food and Nutrition Board is 50 μg/day; the lowest observed adverse effect level (LOAEL) for prolonged intake, 95 μg vitamin D/day, may cause hypercalcemia in healthy adults. However, in 61 healthy men and women, 25 μg (100 IU) or 100 μg (4,000 IU)/day for 2 to 5 months increased 25-OH-D$_3$ levels only to high normal concentrations; neither serum nor urinary calcium levels changed significantly (6).

DRUG INTERACTIONS

- Cholestyramine decreases absorption from dietary sources.
- Oral contraception increases 25-OH-D$_3$ (see questions and answers).

 ## Dose

ADEQUATE INTAKE

Infants and children

0 to 6 months	5 μg/day
7 to 12 months	5 μg/day
1 to 3 years	5 μg/day
4 to 8 years	5 μg/day

Males

9 to 13 years	5 μg/day
14 to 50 years	5 μg/day
51 to 70 years	10 μg/day
71+ years	15 μg/day

Females

9 to 13 years	5 μg/day
14 to 18 years	5 μg/day
19 to 50 years	5 μg/day
51 to 70 years	10 μg/day
71+ years	15 μg/day
Pregnant	5 μg/day
Lactating	5 μg/day

UPPER LIMITS

Infants and children

0 to 6 months	25 μg/day
7 to 12 months	25 μg/day
1 to 3 years	50 μg/day
4 to 8 years	50 μg/day

Males

9 to 13 years	50 μg/day
14 to 50 years	50 μg/day
51 to 70 years	50 μg/day
71+ years	50 μg/day

Females

9 to 13 years	50 μg/day
14 to 18 years	50 μg/day
19 to 50 years	50 μg/day
51 to 70 years	50 μg/day
71+ years	50 μg/day
Pregnant	50 μg/day
Lactating	50 μg/day

1 μg calciferol = 40 IU vitamin D

- Correcting deficiency

—400 to 5,000 IU p.o. q.d. or 50,000 IU once weekly for 8 weeks
—Rickets: 1,000 IU daily
—Prevention of deficiency in nursing home residents: 50,000 IU once monthly (7)

- Treatment of hypervitaminosis D

—Mild hypervitaminosis: Discontinuing supplements, avoiding dietary sources
—Severe hypervitaminosis: Treated with glucocorticosteroids or calcitonin to decrease plasma calcium levels

 ## Common Questions and Answers

Q: What dose of vitamin D does sunlight provide?
A: Exposure of 10% of the body until minimal erythema [one minimal erythemal dose (MED)] provides about 100 IU. Thrice-weekly exposure of hands, arms, and face for half of a MED (in Boston, about 5 minutes at noon in July) is probably enough to prevent deficiency (8).

Q: Does sunscreen affect vitamin D conversion?
A: Yes. Wearing sunscreen with a sun protection factor of 8 can completely prevent cutaneous production of provitamin D$_3$. One study in Illinois found that almost half of adults who always wore sunscreen had overt vitamin D deficiency (8).

Q: What other factors affect cutaneous production of D$_3$?
A: Age decreases efficiency of cutaneous production of D$_3$. Geographic location is important; in Los Angeles and Puerto Rico, sunlight allows cutaneous conversion all year, but in Boston, cutaneous photosynthesis cannot occur between November and February. Just 10 degrees north, in Edmonton (Alberta), Canada, this period lasts from mid-October to mid-March (8). People who live at latitudes greater than or equal to 40 degrees north (New York City, Beijing) or south (Buenos Aires, Auckland) produce little vitamin D in the winter (9).

Q: Does oral contraceptive use improve vitamin D nutriture?
A: No, but oral contraceptive use does increase serum levels of 25-OH-D$_3$, possibly by affecting DBP and altering the ratio of free to bound 25-OH-D$_3$ (10). This effect may confound determination of vitamin D sufficiency in women on oral contraceptives.

Q: Does vitamin D increase atherosclerotic disease?
A: Probably not. Hypervitaminosis D does cause cardiac myopathy and atherosclerosis, but it would be very difficult to derive excessive D from a normal diet. In monkeys, chronic intake of vitamin D$_3$ at levels 5 to 10 times the recommended daily allowance (RDA) induces arterial damage and atherosclerosis. Vitamin D$_2$ (the form added to milk) does not have the same effect, at least in squirrel monkeys.

Q: Who should take vitamin D supplements?
A: People with fat malabsorption, renal failure (kidney function is necessary to activate the active hormone), or familial hypophosphatemia should be supplemented. Exclusively breast-fed infants should be supplemented (formula and cow's milk is fortified, but human milk is deficient in vitamin D). Although milk fortification has reduced the incidence of rickets in North American children, the disease is reappearing, especially in dark-skinned and/or exclusively breast-fed children (11). A vitamin D-resistant form of rickets exists; it is characterized by a disturbance of phosphate transport and resorption. Children who neither drink fortified milk nor receive much sunshine should be supplemented. Supplementation should be considered in older adults.

Q: Is there a link between sunshine and breast cancer?
A: A controversial theory holds that geographic variation in breast cancer mortality is linked to sun exposure. A study of 87 counties of the United States found an inverse relationship between breast cancer mortality and exposure to solar radiation (12). The authors postulate that endogenous vitamin D production reduces the risk of breast, and possibly colon, cancer. This is not a generally accepted view, but the issue certainly deserves further study.

Q: How common is vitamin D toxicity?
A: Reports of vitamin D intoxication from dietary sources are rare, although eight cases were recently linked to a dairy that had overfortified milk for at least 4 years, adding 70 to 600 times the recommended 400 IU/quart (13). A study of 72 exposed households found that although increased milk consumption was associated with increased serum 25-OH-D$_3$ and urinary calcium, findings were within normal range. Participants were asymptomatic and renal function tests were normal (14).
Vitamin D analogs are more toxic than vitamin D dietary supplements; 25-OH-D$_3$-1-hydroxylase in the kidney is normally a rate-limiting step for vitamin D conversion; analogs bypass this step, making it easier to overdose than with dietary supplements.

Vitamin E

10 Second Take

Vitamin E is benign and may benefit diabetes, intermittent claudication, and tardive dyskinesia.

Basics

DESCRIPTION

- Vitamin E, a collective term, comprises four tocopherols (α-, β-, γ-, and δ-tocopherol) and four tocotrienols. RRR α-tocopherol (formerly D-α-tocopherol) is the naturally occurring, most biologically active form. Synthetic vitamin E is all-rac-α-tocopherol (formerly D,L-α-tocopherol) (1). Most supplements contain only D- or D,L-α-tocopherol. Americans consume 4 to 13 mg (7 to 9 IU) daily (2).

FOOD SOURCES

- Vegetable oils, nuts, whole grains, seeds, and egg yolks. γ-Tocopherol is the principal form of dietary vitamin E. Processing vegetable oils destroys up to two thirds of vitamin E (2).

MECHANISM/PHARMACOKINETICS

- An antioxidant, vitamin E protects polyunsaturated fatty acids (PUFAs) in cell membranes and plasma lipoproteins, regulates vascular smooth muscle cell proliferation and protein kinase E activity, suppresses arachidonic acid metabolism through phospholipase A_2 inhibition, inhibits low density lipoprotein (LDL) oxidation, and inhibits platelet aggregation. Large doses of α-tocopherol displace γ-tocopherol in tissues (3).

Evidence

CLINICAL TRIALS

- Neurology

—A Cochrane review identified eight studies of vitamin E for neuroleptic-induced tardive dyskinesia. Overall, vitamin E was superior to placebo [odds ratio (OR) 0.16, confidence interval (CI) 0.04 to 0.7] for clinically relevant improvements and OR 0.23 (CI 0.10 to 0.55) for any improvement (4). DATATOP, a double-blind, placebo-controlled study in 800 patients with Parkinson's disease, tested vitamin E (2,000 IU/day), deprenyl 10 mg/day, or both; there was no benefit for vitamin E (5).

—A double-blind, placebo-controlled multicenter randomized controlled trial (RCT) of 341 patients with Alzheimer's disease tested vitamin E 2,000 IU/day, selegiline, both, or placebo for 2 years. All treatments benefited the primary endpoint [time to death, institutionalization, severe dementia, or loss of ability to perform basic activities of daily living (ADL)] (6).

- Diabetes

—A double-blind crossover RCT of 36 Type I diabetic and nine nondiabetic participants found that 1,800 IU vitamin E/day × 4 months, compared with placebo, significantly improved retinal blood flow and normalized elevated creatinine clearance (7).
—A placebo-controlled RCT in 40 Type II diabetics found that vitamin E (600 mg/day × 8 weeks) significantly improved the percent change in brachial artery diameter and oxidative stress indices (8).
—A double-blind RCT of 21 Type II diabetics with neuropathy found that vitamin E (900 mg/day × 6 months), compared with placebo (9), significantly improved 2/12 electrophysiologic parameters.

- Retinopathy of prematurity (ROP)

—A meta-analysis of published RCTs of vitamin E prophylaxis of severe ROP in infants who weighed less than 1,500 g identified six trials with 1,418 infants (1,087 completed). Overall incidence of ROP was similar between groups; however, vitamin E significantly reduced the risk of developing stage 3+ ROP (pooled odds ratio 0.44, 95% CI 0.21 to 0.81, $p < 0.02$) (10).

- Cardiovascular and cerebrovascular disease

—Observational studies have linked dietary or supplemental vitamin E with reduced risk of coronary heart disease (11–14), but controlled trials are not impressive. The placebo-controlled Heart Outcomes Prevention Evaluation study in 2,545 women and 6,996 men 55 years or older at high risk of cardiovascular events tested vitamin E 400 IU daily (for a mean of 4.5 years) with or without ramipril (15). Vitamin E did not affect cardiovascular outcomes [myocardial infarction (MI), stroke, or cardiovascular death]. The Alpha Tocopherol Beta Carotene (ATBC) Cancer Prevention Study, a placebo-controlled RCT, tested vitamin E (50 mg), beta-carotene (20 mg), or both for 5 to 8 years in 29,133 male Finnish smokers (16). Primary major coronary events increased slightly in the beta-carotene group but decreased 4.0% (95% CI −12% to 4%) in the vitamin E group. There was no benefit in major coronary events among 1,862 men with a previous MI (17). In male smokers at high risk of stroke, vitamin E increased the risk of subarachnoid hemorrhage [relative risk (RR) 2.45, 95% CI 1.08 to 5.55] but decreased risk of cerebral infarction (RR .70, 95% CI 0.55 to 0.89) among hypertensive men (18).

—In the Cambridge Heart Antioxidant Study, an RCT in 2,002 patients with coronary artery disease, α-tocopherol (400 or 800 IU), compared with placebo, reduced non-fatal MI by 77% but did not affect cardiovascular deaths or all-cause mortality (19).
—In another study, 11,324 patients with recent MIs received omega-3 PUFAs (1 g/day), vitamin E (300 mg/day), both, or placebo for up to 2 years (20). Vitamin E did not affect the primary endpoint (death, nonfatal MI, or stroke).
—A double-blind RCT in 56 participants with heart failure found no benefit of RRR-α-tocopherol 500 IU × 12 weeks (21).
—In the ATBC study, vitamin E 50 mg did not reduce new incidence of angina in 22,269 men (22). Another placebo-controlled trial in 60 patients found that α-tocopherol acetate 300 mg/day did not reduce number of anginal attacks (23).

- Nitrate tolerance

—A double-blind trial in 48 participants (24 with ischemic heart disease) found that, compared with placebo, vitamin E (200 mg t.i.d.) significantly attenuated the development of nitrate tolerance (24).

- Intermittent claudication

—A Cochrane review of vitamin E identified five placebo-controlled studies with 265 (mostly male) participants followed for 3 to 18 months. All trials (generally small, poor quality, and heterogeneous) showed positive effects. When two trials that lasted about 8 months and used similar doses were combined, the relative risk was 0.57 (95% CI 0.28 to 1.15) (25).

- Cancer prevention

—In the ATBC trial, vitamin E did not affect incidence or mortality from pancreatic cancer (26) but reduced prostate cancer incidence 32% and mortality 41% (27).

- Hot flashes

—In a placebo-controlled crossover RCT of vitamin E (400 IU b.i.d.) in women with breast cancer, hot flash frequency decreased in both groups with no differences between groups after 4 weeks (28). Vitamin E decreased overall hot flash scores and frequency significantly but slightly; participants did not prefer vitamin E to placebo.

- Arthritis

—In a double-blind RCT of 42 patients with rheumatoid arthritis, participants received placebo or 600 mg α-tocopherol b.i.d. × 12 weeks (29). Clinical and laboratory measures were unaffected by vitamin E, but pain parameters decreased significantly.
—A double-blind placebo controlled RCT of 77 osteoarthritis patients found no benefit of 500 IU/day Vitamin E at 1, 3, or 6 months (30).

• Hepatitis B

—A RCT in 32 patients with chronic hepatitis B found that vitamin E (300 mg b.i.d. × 3 months), compared with no treatment (31), was associated with normalized alanine transaminase (ALT) in more participants (47% vs. 6%) and negative HBV-DNA tests (53% vs. 18%).

• Dysmenorrhea

—A double-blind RCT found that vitamin E (500 IU for 5 days a month, beginning 2 days before expected menses) was significantly better than placebo at 2 months (32).

• Male infertility

—A controlled trial in 110 men (87 completed) with impaired sperm motility found that vitamin E (100 mg t.i.d. × 6 months), compared with placebo, significantly increased sperm motility (60% of treated subjects vs. 15% of controls improved) and pregnancy rates (11 vs. 0) (33).
—In a 2-year crossover trial, vitamin E 600 mg/day, compared with placebo, significantly improved human sperm function in zona binding tests (34).

• Dermatology

—A double-blind study in 10 participants found that oral vitamin C 2 g with d-α-tocopherol 1,000 IU, compared with placebo, reduced sunburn (35).
—A double-blind trial found no benefit of topical cream (d-α-tocopherol 320 IU/g) versus vehicle in cosmetic appearance of scars in 15 patients (33% developed contact dermatitis with the vitamin E cream) (36).
—A single-blind randomized study in 80 patients with hypertrophic scars and keloids found that Vitamin E added to topical silicone gel sheets (worn overnight × 2 months) significantly improved more patients than the silicone sheets alone (95% vs. 75%) (37).

• Oral mucositis (topical)

—A double-blind RCT of 18 patients found that vitamin E (1 mL, with 400 mg/mL b.i.d. × 5 days), compared with placebo, resolved oral mucositis lesions in significantly more patients on chemotherapy (6/9 vs. 1/9) (38).

 ## Clinical Considerations

DEFICIENCY SIGNS AND SYMPTOMS

• Spinocerebellar ataxia
• Skeletal myopathy
• Pigmented retinopathy
• Decreased or absent reflexes, then progressive peripheral neuropathy

FACTORS DECREASING AVAILABILITY/ABSORPTION

• Genetic abnormalities [ataxia with vitamin E deficiency (AVED), homozygous], hypobetalipoproteinemia, fat malabsorption syndromes, cystic fibrosis, pancreatic insufficiency, short bowel syndromes, inflammatory bowel disease, chronic steatorrhea, and total parenteral nutrition

FACTORS INCREASING AVAILABILITY/ABSORPTION

• Fat intake is necessary for absorption.

LABORATORY TESTS

• Plasma normal value greater than 10 nmol α-tocopherol/mL (or mmol) or 5 μg/mL [high-pressure liquid chromatography (HPLC) reverse phase].
• Lipid: greater than 0.8 mg α-tocopherol/g total lipid or 2.8 mg/g cholesterol
• Adipose tissue: greater than 100 μg α-tocopherol/mg triglyceride (39)
• Hypertriglyceridemia may falsely elevate values (2)

 ## Risks

ADVERSE REACTIONS

• In humans, doses up to 800 IU α-tocopherol for 3 years caused no changes in blood chemistry or adverse effects (2).
• Bleeding risk

—Studies designed to examine bleeding risk have found no effect. High doses could increase bleeding in people with suboptimal vitamin K status (vitamin E decreases prothrombin levels in warfarin-treated rats with mild vitamin K deficiency) (2).
—A warfarin-treated patient developed ecchymoses and elevated prothrombin time while taking vitamin E 1,200 IU/day; rechallenge confirmed an association (40).
—A substudy of 409 male smokers in a vitamin E trial found that α-tocopherol 50 mg (especially combined with aspirin) increased gingival bleeding on probing (41).
—However, a double-blind, placebo-controlled study found no effect of all-rac-α-tocopherol (60, 200, or 800 IU × 4 months) on bleeding time in 88 healthy participants older than 65 years (42).
—Another study randomized 12 patients on chronic warfarin (11 completed) to placebo or vitamin E (800 IU or 1,200 IU × 4 weeks); international normalized ratio (INR), taken twice weekly, was unaffected (43).

DRUG INTERACTIONS

No effect on warfarin (see adverse effects)

 ## Dose

RECOMMENDED DIETARY ALLOWANCE

Infants and children

0 to 6 months	4 mg/day (adequate intake)
7 to 12 months	5 mg/day (adequate intake)
1 to 3 years	6 mg/day
4 to 8 years	7 mg/day

Males

9 to 13 years	11 mg/day
14 to 50 years	15 mg/day
51+ years	15 mg/day

Females

9 to 13 years	11 mg/day
14 to 50 years	15 mg/day
51+ years	15 mg/day
Pregnant	15 mg/day
Lactating	19 mg/day

UPPER LIMITS

Infants and children

0 to 6 months	Not determinable
7 to 12 months	Not determinable
1 to 3 years	200 mg/day
4 to 8 years	300 mg/day

Males

9 to 13 years	600 mg/day
14 to 18 years	800 mg/day
19 to 50 years	1,000 mg/day
51+ years	1,000 mg/day

Females

9 to 13 years	600 mg/day
14 to 18 years	800 mg/day
19 to 50 years	1,000 mg/day
51+ years	1,000 mg/day

Pregnant

≤18 years	800 mg/day
19 to 50 years	1,000 mg/day

Lactating

≤18 years	800 mg/day
19 to 50 years	1,000 mg/day

• One IU = 1 mg all-rac-α-tocopherol acetate = 0.67 mg RRR-α-tocopherol = 0.74 mg RRR α-tocopherol acetate (1)
• γ-Tocopherol is considered to substitute for α-tocopherol at 10% efficiency, β-tocopherol 50%, and α-tocotrienol 30% (however, there are functional differences among these forms) (2).

Vitamin K

10 Second Take

Vitamin K, involved in clotting, is benign. An effective treatment for hemorrhagic disease of the newborn and warfarin coagulopathy, limited evidence supports a role for vitamin K in bone strength.

Basics

DESCRIPTION

- Vitamin K_1, or phylloquinone (2-methyl-3-phytyl-1,4-napthoquinone) is the only form of vitamin K found in plants. Menaquinones have unsaturated isoprenyl side chains and are the form produced by gut bacteria. They are numbered by the number of isoprenoid groups in the side chain; vitamin K_2 is menaquinone-7. Menadione (2-methyl-1,4-napthoquinone) is a synthetic form that is alkylated to menaquinone-4 in the liver of mammals. All vitamin K compounds contain a 2-methyl-1, 4-napthoquinone nucleus with a lipophilic side chain at position 3 (1).

FOOD SOURCES

- Leafy vegetables, broccoli, cabbage, alfalfa and green tea contain large quantities of phylloquinone (vitamin K_1). Dry green tea contains 712 μg/100 g, turnip greens contain 650 μg/100 g, broccoli and cabbage contain 125 to 200 μg/100 g, lettuce contains 120 μg/100 g, and spinach contains 89 μg/100 g (1). Meats, cheese, and other fermented foods provide menaquinone (which is also synthesized by endogenous gut bacteria). Liver contains 13 μg/100 g menaquinone; natto, a fermented soybean product, can contain up to 2 mg/100 g menaquinone-7 (2). Tobacco is very high in phylloquinones, containing 5,000 μg/100 g. Smoking causes a very small percentage to volatilize; this can be absorbed through the respiratory tract. Human milk is quite low in vitamin K, containing 2 to 3 μg/L phylloquinones. Commercial infant formula is supplemented with vitamin K.

MECHANISM/PHARMACOKINETICS

- Vitamin K is a fat-soluble vitamin necessary for blood clotting and important in converting protein-bound glutamate residues to gamma-carboxyglutamate (Gla), which is necessary for calcium binding. Proteins containing Gla are found in bone, kidney, placenta, pancreas, spleen, and lungs (3). Seven coagulation proteins are dependent on vitamin K. Two bone proteins are vitamin K-dependent: These are osteocalcin (also called bone GLA protein), secreted by osteoblasts; and matrix GLa protein that exists in bone, dentin, and cartilage (2).

- The vitamin K cycle, a salvage pathway, occurs in the hepatic endoplasmic reticulum; a carboxylation reaction creates K-2,3-epoxide, which is converted to vitamin K hydroquinone, which is then available for carboxylation (2).
- The absorption of vitamin K ranges from 10% to 80% depending on fat in the diet and presence of bile acids. Absorbed in the small bowel, vitamin K is incorporated into chylomicrons and enters the lymph. Orally administered vitamin K appears in the plasma within 20 minutes, peaks at 2 hours, and diminishes rapidly within 48 to 72 hours, when fasting levels of 1 to 2 nM are reached. Over 5 days, 45% to 60% of vitamin K is excreted in the feces; 8% to 30% is excreted renally (2). Only a small amount of vitamin K (about 1.4 μg/kg or 3.1 nmol/kg) is present in the body pool; turnover is high.
- The liver contains both phylloquinone (2 to 20 mg/g liver) and menaquinone (in levels about 10-fold higher than phylloquinone) (4). Only phylloquinones are found in the blood; about half of plasma phylloquinone is in very low density lipoprotein (VLDL), and the rest is split between low density lipoprotein (LDL) and high density lipoprotein (HDL).

Evidence

CLINICAL TRIALS

- A Cochrane review of vitamin K administered before preterm birth in an attempt to prevent neonatal periventricular hemorrhage identified five trials that included more than 420 women (5). Antenatal vitamin K administered to women before preterm birth did not significantly prevent periventricular hemorrhage in preterm infants.
- A Cochrane review of prophylactic vitamin K for vitamin K deficiency bleeding in neonates identified two randomized trials that assessed the effect of a single dose of intramuscular vitamin K on clinical bleeding and 11 randomized trials of oral doses of vitamin K (none of which assessed clinical bleeding) (6). The authors concluded that a single intramuscular dose (1.0 mg) is effective in preventing hemorrhagic disease of the newborn. Vitamin K administered either orally or intramuscularly (1.0 mg) improves coagulation status at 1 to 7 days. The effect of vitamin K on late hemorrhagic disease of the newborn (3 to 8 weeks) has not been tested in randomized trials.

- Warfarin coagulopathy

—Coumarin anticoagulants inhibit the hepatic production of vitamin K dependent factors, including prothrombin. Intravenous administration of vitamin K_1 can reinitiate prothrombin synthesis in the liver within minutes. A randomized controlled double-blind multicenter trial found that low-dose oral vitamin K (1 mg) was significantly more effective than placebo in rapidly lowering abnormally high international normalized ratio (INR) levels (4.5 to 10.0) in patients taking warfarin (7). Warfarin was withheld and patients were treated with placebo or vitamin K. Twenty-five of 45 (56%) in the treated group, compared with 9 of 44 (20%) of patients' achieved INR value of 1.8 to 3.2 on the day after treatment.

- Bone

—Vitamin K may be important to bone strength; levels are lower in patients with bone fractures, and vitamin K supplementation reduces bone loss and reduces calcium excretion. Anticoagulant use is associated with decreased bone density, also circulating osteocalcin levels decrease with age (8). A prospective analysis of women in the Nurses Health Study found that low intake of vitamin K appears to increase the risk of hip fracture. Women in the second to fifth quintile of vitamin K intake had a relative risk of 0.70 [95% confidence interval (CI) 0.53 to 0.93] for hip fracture compared with women in the lowest quintile (9). The effect was not dose-related. The risk of hip fracture was inversely associated with lettuce consumption (lettuce was the most common dietary source of vitamin K).
—In 20 patients with chronic glomerular nephritis who were starting prednisolone treatment, the effect of vitamin K treatment (menatetrenone 15 mg t.i.d.) on bone mineral (10). Lumbar bone decreased significantly in the group treated with prednisolone alone; lumbar bone mineral density (BMD) did not change in the vitamin K treated group.
—In 108 hemiplegic stroke patients, the effects of menatetrenone 45 mg/day × 1 year were tested on metacarpal bone and markers of bone metabolism (11). BMD on the hemiplegic side decreased by 4.7% in the untreated group and increased by 4.3% in the treated group; BMD on the intact side decreased in both groups, but the decrease was significantly less in the treated group (0.9%) than in the untreated group (2.7%).

OTHER CLAIMED BENEFITS/ACTIONS

- Cancer

Clinical Considerations

DEFICIENCY SIGNS AND SYMPTOMS

• Deficiency is uncommon in healthy adults. Vitamin K is common in foods, the vitamin K cycle conserves the vitamin, and gut flora synthesize menaquinones. The most common manifestation of deficiency is bleeding. Vitamin K deficiency, however, is common in newborns, especially if breast-fed. Newborns are at special risk because their immature livers do not synthesize adequate prothrombin, the infant gut is sterile, and human breast milk is quite low in vitamin K (2).

FACTORS DECREASING AVAILABILITY/ABSORPTION

• Drugs

—Hydroxycoumarins (block vitamin K epoxide and vitamin K reductase); salicylates (large doses may inhibit vitamin K epoxide reductase)
—Broad-spectrum antibiotics including neomycin, sulfaquinoxaline, cefamandole, and moxalactam (which sterilize the bowel)

• Malabsorption syndromes (biliary obstruction, cystic fibrosis, sprue, celiac disease, ulcerative colitis, etc.)
• Ileojejunostomy
• Parenchymal liver disease (may result in an inability to use vitamin K to synthesize clotting factors)
• High intake of supplemental vitamin A
• High intake of supplemental vitamin E
• Surgery
• Debilitation
• Low dietary intake (usually combined with another risk factor)
• Dietary restriction (rare)
• Low fat intake

FACTORS INCREASING AVAILABILITY/ABSORPTION

• Hyperlipidemia
• Apolipoprotein E genotype

LABORATORY TESTS

• Greater than 50% reduction in vitamin K-dependent clotting factors (prothrombin, factor X, factor IX, factor VII, and protein C) indicates vitamin K deficiency.
• An antibody test for des-gamma-carboxyprothrombin (DCP) in plasma is a sensitive test; DCP is not seen in healthy people but can be as high as 30% of total prothrombin (approximately 0.5 μmol) in those with vitamin K deficiency and/or liver disease (2).
• Under-gamma-carboxylation of circulating osteocalcin is a sensitive indicator of insufficient vitamin K that may become an important indicator of vitamin K status (4).
• The range of phylloquinone concentrations in fasting adults is 0.29 to 2.64 μmol or 0.15 to 1.0 ng/mL (2).

Risks

Phylloquinones are nontoxic even at 500 times their recommended daily allowance (RDA). Menadione, however, can be quite toxic; it can bind to sulfhydryl groups in membranes and cause hemolytic anemia, hyperbilirubinemia, and kernicterus. Its use is not recommended (2).

DRUG INTERACTIONS

• Warfarin, other hydroxycoumarins, other drugs, and megadoses of vitamin A and E (see factors that decrease availability)

Dose

RECOMMENDED DIETARY ALLOWANCE

Adequate Intake

Infants and children

0 to 6 months	2.0 μg/day
7 to 12 months	2.5 μg/day
1 to 3 years	30 μg/day
4 to 8 years	55 μg/day

Males

9 to 13 years	60 μg/day
14 to 18 years	75 μg/day
19 to 50 years	120 μg/day
51+ years	120 μg/day

Females

9 to 13 years	60 μg/day
14 to 18 years	75 μg/day
19 to 50 years	90 μg/day
51+ years	90 μg/day

Pregnant

≤18 years	75 μg/day
19 to 50 years	90 μg/day

Lactating

≤18 years	75 μg/day
19 to 50 years	90 μg/day

• The usual dose of vitamin K given to newborns is 1 mg (2.2 μmol) intramuscularly.

Common Questions and Answers

Q: Why is it called vitamin K?
A: Discovered by Henrik Dam in Copenhagen in 1929, vitamin K was named in 1934 and isolated in 1939 (K_1 was isolated from alfalfa; K_2 was isolated from putrefied fish meal). It was named K for "koagulation" (2).

Q: Isn't there a link between vitamin K supplementation and childhood cancer?
A: An epidemiologic study in the United Kingdom suggested that intramuscular but not oral vitamin K prophylaxis was associated with an increased risk of childhood cancer. However, other epidemiologic studies have not confirmed this (3).

Vitex

10 Second Take

Vitex is benign, but can cause an acneiform rash or urticaria in some users. Evidence supports its use for premenstrual syndrome.

Basics

LATIN NAME

Vitex agnus-castus L.

FAMILY

Verbenaceae

OTHER COMMON NAMES

Chaste-tree berry, Monk's pepper

DESCRIPTION

• Vitex is a deciduous shrub, up to 6 m (18 ft) high, with twigs covered in gray down; spikes of violet flowers; and reddish black, aromatic fruit. Indigenous to the Mediterranean region and central Asia, vitex is cultivated as an ornamental in temperate climates.

PART USED

Dried ripe fruit

KNOWN ACTIVE CONSTITUENTS

• It is unclear what constituents of vitex are most active. It contains iridoids (aucubin and agnuside); flavonoids, primarily casticin (0.01% to 0.25%); monoterpenes; diterpenoids; and sesquiterpenoids. Diterpenoids include vitexilactone, rotundifuran, and $6\beta,7\beta$-diacetoxy-13-hydroxylabda-8,14-diene. The volatile oil contains primarily bornyl acetate and 1,8-cineole. The fruits contain fatty acids [5.5%, mainly α-linolenic acid (75%)] (1).

MECHANISM/PHARMACOKINETICS

• Vitex may inhibit prolactin activity and appears to have dopaminergic effects. No data are available on pharmacokinetics in humans. The bioavailability of aucubin (100 mg/kg) in rats is 83.5% after hepatoportal administration, 76.8% after intraperitoneal administration, and 19.3% after oral administration (low oral bioavailability is thought to be due to metabolism by gut flora) (1).

Evidence

CLINICAL TRIALS

• Premenstrual syndrome (PMS)

—A randomized, double-blind, placebo-controlled trial of vitex (ZE 440, one tablet daily) in 170 women with PMS (23 on oral contraceptives) for three cycles assessed irritability, mood changes, anger, headache, breast fullness, and other symptoms, including bloating, by visual analog scale (2). Compared with the placebo group, improvements in symptom score were significantly higher in the vitex-treated group. Assessed individually, all symptoms except "other symptoms and bloating" improved more in the treated group than in the placebo group. Four women in the treated group experienced mild adverse effects including acne, urticaria, intermenstrual bleeding, and "multiple abscesses."

—A randomized controlled trial compared vitex (one capsule daily of Agnolyt, a commercial dried extract) to pyridoxine (100 mg b.i.d.) in 175 women with PMS on days 16 to 35 of the menstrual cycle for three cycles (3). Both vitex and Vitamin B_6 reduced Premenstrual Tension Syndrome Scale (PTMS) scores significantly (from 15.2 to 5.1 in the vitex group and from 11.4 to 5.1 in the B_6 group). Vitex was superior in relieving breast tenderness, edema, headache, constipation, and depression. More than a third (36.1%) of those in the vitex group became asymptomatic, compared with 21.3% in the pyridoxine group. Although not an endpoint of the trial, it is notable that five patients in the vitex group became pregnant, whereas none in the B_6 group did. There were more adverse events in the vitex group, including gastroenteritis, nausea, and rashes.

—In 217 women given soy placebo or vitex powder (1,800 mg/day in divided doses) for 3 months, a modified Moos Menstrual Distress Questionnaire (MMDQ) showed no difference in symptoms (4). Soy may not have been an inactive placebo in this trial.

• Mastalgia

—A randomized double-blind placebo-controlled trial tested Mastodynon liquid (30 drops b.i.d.) or tablets (one tablet b.i.d.) (Mastodynon contains chaste-tree berry extract and homeopathic dilutions of several other herbs) in 104 women with mastalgia for three cycles. Both active preparations decreased breast pain by visual analog scale (5).

—Another randomized double-blind placebo-controlled trial tested Mastodynon liquid (30 drops b.i.d.) for three cycles in 97 women (86 completed); the treatment group had lower pain intensity scores than the placebo group at 1 and 2 months, but not at 3 months (6).

—A third randomized controlled trial compared Mastodynon liquid (30 drops b.i.d.) with placebo or the progestin gestagen in 160 women; both treatments were significantly more effective than placebo, with no difference between treatments (7).

• Fertility disorders

—A double-blind, placebo-controlled trial in 96 women with fertility disorders (31 luteal insufficiency, 38 secondary amenorrhea, and 27 idiopathic) tested Mastodynon (8). Only 66 were evaluated. Outcomes varied by group: pregnancy or menstrual bleeding in amenorrhea; pregnancy or improved luteal hormone levels in the two other groups. These outcomes were achieved by 54.5% of those treated with Mastodynon and 36.4% in the placebo group ($p = 0.05$).

—A double-blind placebo-controlled trial was done of vitex (Strotan, containing 20 mg drug, q.d. for 3 months) in 52 women with luteal phase defect and high prolactin levels [120 ng/mL at 30 minutes and 70 ng/mL at 15 minutes after thyrotropin-releasing hormone (TRH) challenge] (9). Thirty-seven case reports were complete enough for analysis. Vitex reduced prolactin levels, lengthened luteal phases significantly (by an average of 5 days), and increased midluteal phase progesterone levels to normal levels at 3 months. 17β-estradiol levels were also higher in the treatment group during the luteal phase. Two women, both in the vitex group, became pregnant. No side effects were noted.

• Prolactin levels

—A randomized double-blind placebo-controlled trial tested Mastodynon liquid (30 drops b.i.d.) or tablets (one tablet b.i.d.) in 104 women with mastalgia for three cycles. Basal prolactin levels, but not metoclopramide-stimulated prolactin levels, were significantly reduced by the active treatments (10).

—A placebo-controlled crossover study tested three doses of the vitex extract BNO 1095 in 20 healthy males for 14 days; 120 mg and 480 mg, but not 240 mg, significantly increased the area under the curve for TRH-stimulated prolactin levels (11).

• Other hormone levels

—Vitex does not appear to affect luteinizing hormone (LH) or follicle-stimulating hormone (FSH) levels. Effects on progesterone and estradiol levels are not consistent (12).

ANIMAL/IN VITRO

- Extracts of vitex inhibit prolactin secretion of rat pituitary cells *in vitro*. In cultured anterior pituitary cells from male rats, an aqueous extract of vitex reduced both basal prolactin release by 80% and TRH-induced prolactin release by 65% (13). A later experiment in cultured anterior pituitary cells from female rats found that vitex extract inhibited both basal and TRH-induced prolactin release in a dose-dependent manner (maximum inhibition was achieved at 460 μg/mL). This effect could be blocked by haloperidol, a dopamine receptor blocker (14). *In vitro,* vitex affects prolactin release but not LH or FSH. Vitex extract binds to D2 receptors in the corpus striatum membrane dopamine receptor binding assay (15). In animals, high doses are necessary to inhibit prolactin; one experiment found that 60 mg intravenously was necessary to achieve significant results (16).

OTHER CLAIMED BENEFITS/ACTIONS

- Menopausal symptoms
- Irregular cycles
- Menometrorrhagia
- Acne
- Lactation stimulant
- Mastalgia
- Antibacterial

 Risks

ADVERSE REACTIONS

- Symptoms reported in clinical trials include gastrointestinal symptoms, dermatologic reactions (acne, skin rashes, urticaria), and menstrual cycle changes. A 14-day study in males showed no effect on blood chemistry or liver function tests (12).
- Ovarian hyperstimulation

—A case of ovarian hyperstimulation apparently resulting from ingestion of vitex has been reported (17). A 32-year-old woman with tubal infertility who had developed single follicles with gonadotrophin stimulation in three cycles took vitex before and during the early follicular phase of the fourth cycle (no other medications were taken during this cycle). Vaginal ultrasonography on day 6 revealed three developing follicles on the right ovary and one on the left.

DRUG INTERACTIONS

- No drug interactions have been reported. However, dopaminergic drugs and dopamine antagonists may interact with vitex. It is also theoretically possible that vitex could diminish the efficacy of oral contraceptives, especially low-dose pills (see questions and answers).

PREGNANCY/LACTATION

- Vitex should not be used in pregnancy. It should not be used during lactation; although it is sometimes used to stimulate milk production, it may actually decrease milk production.

ANIMAL TOXICITY

- In rats and mice given the chaste-tree extract BNO 1095, no deaths occurred after oral or intraperitoneal doses up to 2,000 mg/kg. A 28-day subacute study of BNO 1095 found the no-effect level to be 50 mg/kg; a chronic toxicity study for 26 weeks found a no-effect level of 40 mg/kg.
- In Wistar rats given Mastodynon in doses up to 80 times the recommended dose, there were no problems in mating, fertility, pregnancy, or lactation and no fetal malformations; offspring were normal. One animal lactation study indicated decreased milk consumption in offspring of animals given chaste-tree fruits (12).

 Dose

COMMON DOSAGE FORMS

- The usual dose is 0.5 to 1.0 g of the fruit three times a day.
- Aqueous-alcohol extracts corresponding to 30 to 40 mg drug.
- Mastodynon contains chaste-tree berry extract and homeopathic dilutions of *Caulophyllum thalictroides* D4, *Cyclamen purpurascens* D4, *Strychnos ignatii* D6, *Iris versicolor* D2, and *Lilium tigrinum* D3. One g tincture contains 200 mg crude drug; 60 drops/day is equivalent to 32 mg drug.
- Agnolyt capsules contain 3.5 to 4.2 mg dry extract (9.58:1 to 11.5:1 extract) equivalent to 41 mg drug; solution (1:5 extract) contains 36 mg drug/40 drops.
- BNO 1095 20 mg native extract (6:1 to 12:1) contains 120 to 240 mg drug.
- Ze 440 tablets contain 20 mg native extract (0.6% casticin), with 120 to 240 mg drug/tablet.
- Strotan capsules contain 3 mg dry extract (6:1 to 16:1) containing 20 mg drug/capsule.

 Common Questions and Answers

Q: Where does the name chaste-tree berry come from?
A: Vitex has been reputed to lower libido in both women and men; and both its common and species names reflect this. Common names include chaste-tree berry and monk's pepper. *Agnus-castus* comes from the Latin, *agnus* meaning lamb (innocence), and *castus,* chaste. It is also possible that agnus comes from *agono,* the Greek word for chaste, although this would be rather repetitious.

Q: Is it safe to combine Vitex with hormonal treatment?
A: Most herbalists note that vitex should not be combined with birth control pills or hormone replacement therapy. The modes of action seem quite distinct, and combined use is probably not harmful. Still, there is a theoretical risk that the stimulating effect vitex has on the ovaries could increase the chance of breakthrough ovulation and, thus, pregnancy with low-dose oral contraceptives.

Willow

10 Second Take

Willow bark has analgesic effects but lacks antithrombotic effects. It should not be used in salicylate-sensitive individuals.

Basics

LATIN NAME

Salix alba L. (white willow) and other species

FAMILY

Salicaceae

OTHER COMMON NAMES

None identified

DESCRIPTION

• Willows encompass woody trees, stemmed shrubs, and creeping shrublets; there are about 400 species worldwide, including about 150 in the Western hemisphere. It is often difficult to identify individual species because of variability and hybridization.

PART USED

Bark (trunk or branch) or young twigs. The outer bark is removed in older trees.

KNOWN ACTIVE CONSTITUENTS

• Willow contains phenolic glycosides including salicin (usually less than 1%). This is the basis for aspirin and salicin esters (salicortin 0.03% to 4% or 2′-*O*-acetlysalicortin 0.5% to 10%); 2′-*O*-acetylsalicin, also called fragilin (0.03% to 4%); and tremulacin (0.12% to 2%). Total salicin content varies; species rich in salicin include *S. daphnoides, S. purpurea,* and *S. fragilis,* which may contain up to 10%. Other phenolic glycosides vary by species.
• Willow also contains flavonoid glycosides including (+)- and (−)-naringenin-5-glucoside, naringenin-7-glucoside, eriodictyol-7-glucoside, polyphenols, and chalcone glycosides, biflavones, flavanones, and condensed flavanones (1).

MECHANISM/PHARMACOKINETICS

• Salicortin is hydrolyzed in the small intestines into salicin and esters (which are subsequently hydrolyzed to saligenin and glucose). Saligenin is oxidized to salicylic acid.
• In a pharmacokinetic study in 10 participants, 1,360 mg extract (containing 240 mg total salicin) was administered in two doses 2 hours apart. The half-life was 2.45 hours; peak levels were reached at 4 to 6 hours, and the C_{max} was 10 mmol/L (this is less than 10% of salicylate levels after administration of 500 mg aspirin). A 24-hour urine collection showed that 16% of administered salicylate was excreted in urine (71% as salicyluric acid).
• Administration of salicin (4 g, equivalent to 1,730 mg saligenin) to a single individual resulted in a C_{max} of 100 μg/mL (2). The bioavailability of salicylic acid from salicin is estimated to be less than 20% (1).

Evidence

CLINICAL TRIALS

• Pain

—A randomized, double-blind trial of willow bark in 210 participants (191 completed) with chronic low back pain tested two doses (60 mg b.i.d. or 120 mg b.i.d.) for 4 weeks (3). Use of tramadol was allowed. The primary endpoint was being pain-free without tramadol for 5 days in the last week of the trial. Willow bark was significantly more effective than placebo; the primary endpoint was achieved by 7% of the placebo group, 25% of the group treated with 120 mg/day willow bark, and 41% of the group treated with 240 mg/day. One treated patient experienced an allergic reaction (rash, swollen eyes, pruritus) that resolved within 2 days of discontinuing treatment.
—A proprietary willow bark extract (Assalix, containing 240 mg salicin/day) was compared with rofecoxib (12.5 mg/day) for 4 weeks in an open, randomized trial in 228 participants (183 completed) with low back pain (4). Participants were allowed to use other analgesics or treatments (most did not, and there were no significant differences between groups in this respect). After 4 weeks, treatments were equivalent, as assessed by a modified Arhus index and the Total Pain index.
—A randomized, placebo-controlled double-blind study of 78 patients with osteoarthritis of the knee and hip compared placebo with coated tablets containing 1,360 mg willow bark extract (in divided doses) for 2 weeks. There was a significant difference between the groups receiving willow and placebo on a visual analog scale, a pain index, and patient assessment (5).

• Platelet aggregation (see questions and answers)

—Willow bark has a mild effect on platelet aggregation but is not equivalent to aspirin. In 35 patients randomized to white willow extract (containing 240 mg salicin/day) or placebo, the mean maximal arachidonic acid-induced platelet aggregation was 61% in the willow-treated group and 78% in the placebo-treated group (6). In a separate group of patients with heart disease, given 100 mg/day acetylsalicylate, the mean maximal arachidonic acid-induced platelet aggregation was 13%. Compared with placebo, willow bark significantly reduced arachidonic acid-induced and adenosine diphosphate (ADP)-induced (but not collagen-induced) platelet aggregation.

ANIMAL/IN VITRO

• Tremulacin administered subcutaneously exerts an antiinflammatory effect in two animal models: the carrageenan-induced rat paw edema test and the croton oil-induced mouse ear edema test.
• *In vitro* tests did not show prostaglandin inhibition with salicin, salicortin, or crude extracts; salicin and salicortin marginally inhibited 5-lipoxygenase. Tremulacin inhibited leukotriene production by 30% in a test of stimulated rat pleural leukocytes.
• Antifungal effects *in vitro* have been demonstrated against *Penicillium digitatum, Botrytis cinerea,* and three species of *Aspergillus* (1).

OTHER CLAIMED BENEFITS/ACTIONS

• Antiseptic
• Antiinflammatory
• Antipyretic
• Antifungal
• Plantar warts (topical)
• Burns and wounds (topical)

Risks

ADVERSE REACTIONS

• Willow contains significant amount of tannins that may cause upset stomach or constipation. In participants treated with three different willow preparations, mild adverse effects (not otherwise described) were reported in 3.7% of 733 participants. In studies of willow mixed with kola nut or passionflower, reported adverse events were uncommon, primarily consisting of gastrointestinal symptoms.
• *Salix caprea* and hemolysis in glucose-6-phosphate dehydrogenase (G6PD) deficiency

—A 64-year-old woman with G6PD deficiency suffered massive intravascular homolysis with acute renal failure after ingesting about 5 mL of an Ayurvedic medicine for constipation (7). Her only concurrent medicine was amiloride/hydrochlorothiazide. This is not a very convincing report; although the episode was attributed to *Salix caprea,* the preparation also contained other ingredients not identified in this report.

DRUG INTERACTIONS

None reported

 Dose

COMMON DOSAGE FORMS

• Recommended daily dose is 60 to 120 mg total salicin; 4 mg salicin is equivalent to 2.52 mg aspirin.
• *Dried bark:* 1 to 4 g t.i.d.
• *Infusion* or *decoction* made from 2 to 3 g chopped dried bark in 150 to 250 mL water.
• *Liquid tincture:* (1:5 wt/V, 25% ethanol) 5 to 8 mL t.i.d.
• *Fluid extract:* (1:1 g/mL, 25% ethanol) 1 to 2 mL t.i.d.
• *Dry extract:* (standardized to 20 to 40 mg salicin) t.i.d.
• Topical preparations include fomentation (cloth soaked in decoction, applied as a compress).
• Children

—Age 4 to 10: preparations equivalent to 30 60 mg salicin daily
—Age 10 to 16: preparations equivalent to 60 to 120 mg salicin (dose is based on weight)
—Not recommended for children younger than 4 years

 Common Questions and Answers

Q: Can willow preparations be used as antithrombotic agents?
A: No. Although aspirin (acetylsalicylic acid) causes irreversible inhibition of platelet aggregation, salicin lacks this effect. White willow extract has a mild inhibiting effect on platelet aggregation, but aspirin is much more potent and has been shown to be effective in clinical trials with cardiovascular disease endpoints.

Q: Can willow be used in salicylate-sensitive individuals?
A: I would avoid this use, although the amount of salicylate is low.

Q: How long has willow been used?
A: The first recorded description of therapeutic use of willow is from Hippocrates, who recommended chewing willow bark for analgesia in childbirth. Dioscorides recommended it as an analgesic, and Galen was the first to describe its antipyretic and anti-inflammatory properties (8). White willow was a folk remedy in England and was studied in about 50 patients with fevers or inflammatory conditions by Reverend Edward Stone of Oxfordshire, England, who was looking for an antipyretic substitute for the expensive cinchona imported from South America (8).

Wormwood

10 Second Take

Wormwood is used to stimulate appetite or bile secretion. Only aqueous solutions or thujone-free extracts should be used; thujone is extremely toxic.

Basics

LATIN NAME

Artemisia absinthium L.

FAMILY

Compositae/Asteraceae

DESCRIPTION

• Wormwood, a gray shrub, has chrysanthemum-like leaves. The leaves and stems are covered with fine silky hairs. Native to the drier areas of Europe and Asia, wormwood was the main ingredient in the liqueur absinthe.

PART USED

Leaf, flowering tops

KNOWN ACTIVE CONSTITUENTS

• *Artemesia absinthium* contains sesquiterpene lactones, especially the guaianolides absinthin (0.2% to 0.28%). The essential oil contains mainly terpenes, including β-thujone, α-thujone, *trans*-sabinyl acetate, and *cis*-epoxyocimene, as well as other monoterpenes and sesquiterpenes. It also contains flavonoids, phenolic carboxylic acids and polyacetylenes (1).

MECHANISM/PHARMACOKINETICS

• Thujone, the highly toxic component of wormwood, appears to be a γ-aminobutyric acid$_A$ (GABA$_A$) receptor chloride channel blocker (2). Alpha-thujone is 2.3 times more active than β-thujone at binding mammalian liver and brain (2). Thujone acts as a central nervous system poison; in cats, the minimal convulsive dose is 0.03 to 0.04 mL of a 1:20 alcohol dilution of essential oil administered intravenously. In rats, 10 mg/kg daily oral administration produced convulsions by Day 38 in 5% of the rats. Oral LD$_{50}$ of mixed α- and β-thujones was 192 mg/kg in rats, 230 mg/kg in mice, and 395 mg/kg in guinea pigs (3).
• No data on pharmacokinetics in humans are available.

Evidence

CLINICAL TRIALS

• Gastrointestinal secretions

—A dried alcohol extract of wormwood suspended in water was given to 15 patients with hepatic conditions. A significant increase in gastrointestinal secretions, including α-amylase, lipase, and bilirubin was demonstrated (3).

ANIMAL/IN VITRO

• Gastrointestinal secretions

—Oral administration of absinthin to dogs results in increased gastric secretory activity and increased acidity. Absinthin administered by gavage did not have this effect. Intravenous administration of wormwood resulted in increased bile secretion in dogs (3).

• Fever

—Several fractions of an ethanolic extract of wormwood have demonstrated antipyretic effects in rabbits (3).

• Analgesia

—(−)-3-isothujone produced antinociceptive effects in mice (3).
—*In vitro* studies have demonstrated activity of two homoditerpene peroxides isolated from wormwood against *Plasmodium falciparum*. Essential oil of wormwood, diluted 1:1,000, exhibited antimicrobial effect against *Staphylococcus aureus* and *Candida albicans* (3).

OTHER CLAIMED BENEFITS/ACTIONS

• Dyspepsia
• Anorexia (illness-associated)
• Antihelminthic (see questions and answers)
• Intestinal spasm
• Biliary disorders
• Immune enhancement

Risks

ADVERSE REACTIONS

• Acute renal failure

—A 31-year-old man, who purchased and consumed 10 mL of essential oil of wormwood (apparently he thought it was absinthe), was hospitalized for disorientation and tonic-clonic seizures with decorticate posturing; rhabdomyolysis and acute renal failure were evident by Day 2 (4).
—Epileptiform seizures have previously been associated with thujone (5).
—The toxic effects of absinthe became known as "absinthism"; symptoms included seizures, gastrointestinal problems, hallucinations, other psychiatric manifestations and increased risk of suicide.

PREGNANCY/LACTATION

This herb should not be used during pregnancy or lactation.

Dose

COMMON DOSAGE FORMS

• Infusion

—1 to 1.5 g of dried herb per 150 mL water up to t.i.d., administered half an hour before meals for anorexia or after meals for dyspepsia or biliary disorders.

Common Questions and Answers

Q: What is absinthe?
A: *Artemisia absinthium* was the primary flavoring ingredient of the liqueur absinthe, which also contained anise (*Pimpinella anisum*), fennel (*Foeniculum vulgare*), Roman wormwood (*A. pontica*), hyssop (*Hyssopus officinalis*), and lemon balm (*Melissa officinalis*). Especially popular in Parisian cafes (some of which were devoted to its consumption), absinthe was usually consumed ritualistically; cold water trickled over a sugar cube held by a slotted spoon caused its emerald-green color to change to an opalescent yellow. Absinthe was the drink of choice among many artists and writers, including Picasso, van Gogh, Gauguin, Toulouse-Lautrec, Rimbaud, and Oscar Wilde. It has been known, however, since 1708, that *A. absinthium* caused deleterious effects on the nervous system. Banned in the United States in 1912 and in France in 1922 (6), absinthe is now illegal in most countries (although it was never formally banned in Spain, Portugal, the Czech Republic, or the United Kingdom) (5). It is still sold today. Analysis of one brand, "Hill's Absinth," made in the Czech Republic and exported to the United Kingdom, found no thujone in the preparation (7) (see next question).

Q: Is it possible to minimize the toxicity of wormwood preparations?
A: Dilute aqueous extracts of dried wormwood contain only trace amounts of the essential oil and, thus, negligible amounts of thujone. Alcohol tinctures or extracts may contain a significant amount. There are, however, extraction procedures for removing thujone from wormwood extracts using water and ethanol 30% (V/V) or supercritical carbon dioxide. The use of the essential oil, very high in thujone, has been banned in most countries.

Q: Is it possible to minimize the bitter taste of wormwood?
A: Unfortunately, the bitter principles are what are therapeutically active, and stimulation of gastrointestinal secretions may not occur if the herb is swallowed in capsules rather than tasted (in dogs, oral administration, but not gavage, stimulated secretions). Although sweetener may be added to tea, it does not really help. A strong distaste for wormwood often develops in patients after a few weeks. Not a bad thing, considering concerns about long-term toxicity.

Q: Is wormwood a good antihelminthic?
A: Wormwood has some activity against worms and is sometimes used as a treatment for threadworm, but it is not particularly impressive. Levant wormseed (*Artemesia cina*) is more effective and shows activity against both threadworms and roundworms (8).

Wormwood, Sweet or Qinghaosu

 10 Second Take

Derivatives of sweet wormwood are safe, effective malaria treatments and also appear to reduce the risk of schistosomiasis.

 Basics

LATIN NAME

Artemisia annua L.

FAMILY

Compositae/Asteraceae

OTHER COMMON NAMES

Sweet Annie, annual wormwood

DESCRIPTION

• An annual, brown-stemmed, green-leafed plant with lacy foliage and a sweet smell, sweet wormwood is a common plant that is sometimes cultivated.
• *Artemisia annua*, used in traditional Chinese medicine, is widely distributed in North America, Europe, India, and Eastern Asia. Sweet wormwood is sometimes used to flavor vermouth.

PART USED

Leaf, flowering top

KNOWN ACTIVE CONSTITUENTS

• *A. annua* contains at least seven sesquiterpenes, one of which, artemisinin (qinghaosu), has dramatic antimalarial properties. Artemisinin is a sesquiterpene lactone; dihydroartemisinin is a reduced lactol derivative; and artesunate and artemether are semisynthetic derivatives (1).

MECHANISM/PHARMACOKINETICS

• Artemisinin and its derivatives are hydrolyzed rapidly to dihydroartemisinin (dihydroqinghaosu). Intravenous artesunate is hydrolyzed rapidly to dihydroartemisinin, which has a half-life of 45 minutes. Oral artesunate appears to be completely hydrolyzed before it enters the systemic circulation. Intramuscular injection of artemether results in peak levels at about 6 hours; elimination half-life is 4 to 11 hours. After suppository administration of 10 mg/kg artemisinin, mean time to peak concentration was 11.3 hours and elimination half-life was 4.1 hours (2).
• Artemisinin derivatives are toxic to malaria parasites at nanomolar concentrations; micromolar concentrations are necessary for mammalian cell toxicity. The killing of parasites is apparently mediated by free radicals, but unlike other oxidant drugs, artemisinin does not react with oxygen to produce superoxide or other free radicals; instead, artemisinin, in an iron-catalyzed reaction, itself becomes a free radical (1).

 Evidence

CLINICAL TRIALS

• Over 2 million patients have been treated with qinghaosu or its derivatives (1).
• A review of 23 treatment-controlled trials (15 randomized, none blinded, with a total of 1,891 patients) before mid-1992 found that qinghaosu shortened fever clearance time by an average of 17% (approximately 7.7 hours) over the comparison drug and shortened parasite clearance time by 32% (approximately 19.8 hours) (2).
• A recent double-blind randomized trial (not included in the previous review) tested the addition of placebo, single-dose artesunate, or triple-dose artesunate (4 mg/kg/day × 3 days) as an adjunct to pyrimethamine-sulphadoxine (25 mg/500 mg) in 600 Gambian children with acute *P. falciparum* malaria (3). Artesunate significantly lowered gametocyte rates over pyrimethamine-sulphadoxine alone.
• A retrospective study of artemisinin in 638 malaria patients in Vietnam showed that parasitemias decreased more than 98% within 24 hours of treatment initiation. Average fever and parasite clearance times were 1.4 to 20 days (4). Total doses ranged from 20 to 60 mg/kg over 2 to 9 days; recrudescence rates were 50% in those receiving less than 5 days treatment and 10% to 23% in those treated for 5 to 10 days. In 21 patients with *P. falciparum* treated with artemisinin for 3 days and tetracycline for 5 days, the recrudescence rate was 9.5%.

• Schistosomiasis

—A randomized controlled trial in 354 children tested placebo against artemether (6 mg/kg orally six times every 3 weeks) as a prophylactic treatment against *Schistosoma mansoni*. The rate of infestation was halved; 31/128 treated children developed schistosomiasis versus 68/140 placebo-treated [relative risk (RR) 0.50, 95% confidence interval (CI) 0.35 to 0.71]. Among infected children, mean egg output was lower in the treated group. A significant reduction was also seen in the prevalence of *P. falciparum*.

ANIMAL/IN VITRO

• Toxicity

—Qinghaosu is much less toxic than quinoline antimalarials, but high doses produce neurotoxicity in large animals, including dogs. Several derivatives have resulted in QT-prolongation on electrocardiogram. In rodents, lethal doses cause multiple system toxicity; sublethal doses cause fetal resorption and depression of reticulocyte counts (2).

• Antimicrobial effects

—Artemisinin derivatives have shown activity against *S. mansoni, Schistosoma japonicum,* and *Pneumocystis carinii, in vitro* and *in vivo.* *In vitro* activity has also been shown against *Leishmania major* and *Toxoplasma gondii* (1).

• Anticancer effects

—Artemisinin derivatives have activity against cancer cells *in vitro*; an effect potentiated by iron loading (5). *In vivo*, a combination of dihydroartemisinin and ferrous sulfate inhibited implanted fibrosarcoma growth in rats. Neither compound individually had an effect. No toxic effects were noted (6).

Risks

ADVERSE REACTIONS

• Significant toxicity has not been seen in the more than 4,000 patients who have been enrolled in clinical trials. However, brief episodes of drug-induced fever have been reported in up to 25% of patients in some studies. There have been occasional reports of transient first-degree heart block and transient reductions in reticulocyte or neutrophil counts. Artemisinin suppositories are generally well tolerated but may result in tenesmus, abdominal pain, or diarrhea (2).

PREGNANCY/LACTATION

There is no evidence of birth defects caused by qinghaosu (see questions and answers).

 Dose

MODE OF ADMINISTRATION

p.o., p.r., i.v., i.m.

COMMON DOSAGE FORMS (7)

Adults and children older than 6 months

• *Uncomplicated malaria*

—Artenusate (available as 50-mg tablets): 5 mg/kg p.o. on Day 1, then 2.5 mg/kg q.d. on Day 2 and Day 3. Mefloquine (15 to 25 mg/kg) should be administered on Day 2.
—Artemisinin (available as 250-mg capsules): 25 mg/kg p.o. on Day 1, then 12.5 mg/kg on Day 2 and Day 3. Mefloquine (15 to 25 mg/kg) should be administered on Day 2.

• *Severe and complicated malaria*

—Artemether (available as solution for injection 80 mg in 1 mL ampoule): 3.2 mg/kg i.m. on Day 1, then 1.6 mg/kg/day until the patient can take p.o. antimalarial therapy or to a maximum of 7 days.
—Artesunate (available as powder for injection): anhydrous artesunic acid 60 mg in 1 mL ampoule is mixed with 5% sodium bicarbonate in 0.6 mL ampoule. 2 mg/kg i.v. is given on Day 1, then 1 mg/kg/day until p.o. therapy is possible. An additional dose of 1 mg/kg may be used 4 to 6 hours after the first dose in hyper-parasitemic cases.

 Common Questions and Answers

Q: Is qinghaosu safe to use in pregnancy?
A: No adverse effects were seen in long-term follow-up of six children exposed to artemisinin or artemether as fetuses (exposure occurred between weeks 17 and 27). Seventeen children exposed at fetal ages 16 to 38 weeks were followed for 3 months to 10 years; no abnormalities were reported (2). No evidence is available on effects of first trimester exposure, but sweet wormwood increases fetal absorption in rats. The World Health Organization (WHO) recommends against its use in the first trimester (7). Although some clinicians avoid the use of the drug in pregnant women with uncomplicated malaria, pregnant women with severe malaria should not be denied this drug on theoretical grounds.

Q: How were the antimalarial properties of sweet wormwood determined?
A: The antimalarial properties of the plant were discovered in 1971 when a low-temperature ethyl ether extraction proved to have antimicrobial activity against a number of organisms, including the rodent malaria parasite *Plasmodium burghei*. In 1972 Chinese scientists isolated seven sesquiterpenes from the plant; one of these, a newly discovered crystalline substance named qinghaosu, proved to be the principal antimalarial compound. In 1979 a landmark paper in the *Chinese Medical Journal* detailed the discovery and evaluation of a group of drugs derived from this plant, which has a long history in Chinese herbal medicine; sweet wormwood has been recommended for fevers since at least 341 AD. More benign and faster-acting than other antimalarials, the use of drugs derived from *A. annua* has had a profound and global beneficial public health impact.

Yam, Wild

 10 Second Take

Wild yams are inedible sources of steroid precursors that cannot be converted endogenously to progesterone. No clinical trials support efficacy for any specific condition.

 Basics

LATIN NAME

Dioscorea villosa L.

FAMILY

Dioscoreaceae

OTHER COMMON NAMES

Wild yam, colic root, rheumatism root, and bitter yam

DESCRIPTION

• Dioscoreas are yams, perennial herbaceous woody climbing plants with tuberous rhizomes. More than 600 species exist. Edible species include *D. alata, D. batatas,* and *D. esculenta.* Species high in saponins are not eaten (1). Inedible species with a steroidal saponin concentration over 2% include yams found in Central America (*D. composita, D. floribunda, D. mexicana, D. spiculiflora*), India (*D. deltoidea*), and China (*D. zingiberensis* and *D. pantaica*) (2). *Diascorea japonica* is used in Chinese herbal medicine; the medicinal use of *Diascorea* species is much more common in Chinese than Western herbal medicine.

PART USED

Tuberous rhizomes

MECHANISM/PHARMACOKINETICS

• Inedible species of *Dioscorea* provides steroidal saponins that can be extracted and hydrolyzed to steroidal aglycones. Dioscin can be hydrolyzed to diosgenin, which can then be converted through a multistep chemical process to sex hormones (estrogens and androgens) and corticosteroids (3). Edible *Dioscorea* species do not contain significant amounts of these saponins.

 Evidence

CLINICAL TRIALS

• Hot flashes

—A double-blind, placebo-controlled crossover trial in 23 menopausal women with hot flashes compared topical wild yam cream with placebo, each given for 3 months (4). There was no difference between treatment and placebo in terms of reducing hot flashes; neither group experienced changes in weight, blood pressure, lipids, FSH, glucose, estradiol, or serum or salivary progesterone.

• Ergogenics

—A diosgenin-containing dietary supplement called SPORT was tested in nine trained athletes (including two women) in a double-blind crossover study; testing sessions were a week apart (5). SPORT, which purportedly decreases recovery time after exercise, contains primarily wild yam; other ingredients include diosgenin, *Smilax* (species not stated), maltodextrin, and "orchic glandular extract" (bull testicles). Participants received a total of eight capsules (two capsules 1 hour before exercise and two capsules immediately after each of three workloads). No effect was seen on time to exhaustion, heart rate, or blood lactate levels.

• Effect on dehydroepiandrosterone (DHEA) and cholesterol

—A preparation containing predominantly wild yam promoted to increase DHEA was tested in seven healthy participants. The products contained wild yam extract 90%; the preparation also contained country mallow, kelp, cayenne, and aloe (6). Placebo was administered for 3 weeks, after which escalating doses of the herb preparation (up to eight pills/day) were administered for 3 weeks, placebo for 1 week, then DHEA 85 mg for 1 week. Wild yam had no effect on DHEA, total cholesterol, or low density lipoprotein (LDL); serum triglycerides and phospholipid levels decreased significantly and high density lipoprotein (HDL)-cholesterol increased significantly after *Dioscorea. Dioscorea* also significantly decreased serum conjugated diene and lipid fluorescence levels (measures of oxidation damage), although not as much as DHEA.
—At the highest dose level, five of seven participants complained of headache, dry mouth, and sleep difficulties; other symptoms noted at the highest dose were fever, vomiting, and upset stomach. No effects were seen at a lower dose level.

ANIMAL/IN VITRO

• Hormonal effects

—In oophorectomized rats, a sustained-release implanted diosgenin capsule for 47 days mitigated increased body weight caused by oophorectomy and increased uterine weights compared with controls. No histologic changes were noted in reproductive tissues or morphologic changes in spleen, kidney, adrenal, heart, liver, or lung (7). DHEA had similar effects.
—In young oophorectomized mice, diosgenin (20 to 40 mg/kg subcutaneously × 15 days) stimulated the growth of mammary epithelium, increasing the number of ducts and terminal end buds and increasing DNA in epithelium (8). When given concurrently with estrogen, augmentation of the estrogenic effect was noted.

• Gastrointestinal tract effects

—Diosgenin apparently protects the hepatobiliary tract and perhaps intestine as well. Dietary diosgenin increases biliary cholesterol output in rats and protects hepatocytes and bile secretory function from cytotoxic doses of the bile salt taurocholate (9). The protective effect was associated with an increased concentration of cholesterol and sphingomyelin in the canalicular membrane. Another study found that in rats fed 0.5% diosgenin, biliary cholesterol increased; after bile duct obstruction, serum hepatic enzyme levels were lower in diosgenin-fed rats (10). Diosgenin apparently increases biliary lipid lamellar secretion. Another rat experiment found that although administration of 17α-ethinylestradiol prevented diosgenin-induced increase of bile cholesterol and lipid lamellae content, diosgenin still prevented some cholestatic effects of 17α-ethinylestradiol (11).
—Dietary diosgenin (more than 80 mg/kg/day) pretreatment significantly reduced indomethacin-induced intestinal inflammation and mitigated weight loss in rats (12). Increased biliary cholesterol output and protection of bile flow and bile acid output were also seen. Diosgenin reduced plasma levels of indomethacin and increased the elimination constant.

OTHER CLAIMED BENEFITS/ACTIONS

• Ergogenics, gastrointestinal problems, gynecologic problems, expectorant, antispasmodic, liver problems, morning sickness, gastrointestinal complaints, childbirth problems, rheumatism, antiinflammatory, and colic. Homeopathic preparations are used for treating gastric disorders.
• *Dioscorea japonica* is used to treat diabetes, menstrual disorders, and infertility.

Risks

ADVERSE REACTIONS

• No information available. However, headache, upset stomach, dry mouth, and other symptoms were noted in a trial of a mixed-herb preparation containing predominately *Dioscorea* (6).

DRUG INTERACTIONS

• No information available on humans. In rats, diosgenin reduced plasma levels of indomethacin and increased the elimination constant (12).

ANIMAL TOXICITY

• No morphologic changes were seen in rat spleen, kidney, adrenal, heart, liver, lung, or reproductive tract after 47 days of diosgenin exposure through a sustained-release implanted capsule (6).

 Dose

COMMON DOSAGE FORMS

• *Decoction:* 1 to 2 teaspoons t.i.d.
• *Tincture:* 2 to 4 mL t.i.d.

 Common Questions and Answers

Q: What about those topical wild yam creams my patients are using for hot flashes, osteoporosis, and premenstrual syndrome (PMS)?
A: Wild yam preparations contain diosgenin, which cannot be converted to progesterone in the body. Some creams sold as wild yam creams, however, actually contain micronized progesterone [derived from precursors in *Diascorea* species or soybeans (*Glycine max*)]. Topical progesterone creams have been promoted for osteoporosis, hot flashes, PMS, fibrocystic breasts, and breast cancer prevention (13). However, a randomized, double-blind, placebo-controlled trial has shown no benefit of transdermal progesterone cream on bone (although it did improve hot flashes). This 1-year long trial in 102 healthy postmenopausal women (90 completed) tested one-fourth teaspoon of cream (containing 20 mg progesterone or placebo) applied to the skin daily; all women received daily multivitamins and 1,200 mg calcium daily (14). The study lasted 1 year and patients were seen every 4 months. There were no significant differences between the treatment and control groups in change from initial bone mineral density (lumbar spine, femoral neck, or total hip), or in the number of participants who showed an increase of bone mineral density of more than 1.2%. Of those who reported vasomotor symptoms initially, 5/26 women in the control group reported improved vasomotor symptoms compared with 25/30 women in the treatment group. No significant changes were seen in lipids or mood ratings between groups or from baseline. Eight women in the treatment group experienced vaginal spotting. Biopsies found proliferative endometrium disorder in one woman; the other seven had tissue insufficient for diagnosis.

Q: Can transdermal progesterone cream replace oral progestins in hormone replacement therapy?
A: No. Although some progesterone is absorbed from transdermal creams, these creams cannot replace oral progestins for preventing estrogen-induced endometrial stimulation. A crossover study of 20 surgically menopausal women found that serum levels of progesterone from transdermal creams (at two to four times the recommended daily dose) were only a third of those obtained from oral micronized progesterone and not considered adequate for endometrial protection (15). Another 12-week randomized clinical trial in 27 postmenopausal women on estrogen that found that transdermal progesterone cream in doses up to 64 mg administered for 14 days to postmenopausal women was insufficient to induce a secretory response in the endometrium (assessed by endometrial biopsy) (16). In concurrence with the Cooper study, progesterone levels rose only to 0.6 to 3.2 nmol/L.

Q: What is the connection between wild yams and oral contraceptives?
A: *Dioscorea* species provided the first inexpensive starting material for steroid synthesis. Although sex steroids were isolated before 1935, they were scarce (4 tons of pig ovaries were necessary to extract 12 mg of estradiol). Russell Marker developed a simple, five-step partial synthesis process to convert diosgenin to progesterone and then surveyed many species of plants to find a good source of diosgenin. He discovered that inedible Mexican *Dioscorea* species were excellent sources of steroid precursors (17). In 1943, after American pharmaceutical companies expressed indifference to his discovery, Marker set up a laboratory and production facility in Mexico. Apparently he showed up at a local drug marketing company, Laboratorios Hormona, with 2 kg progesterone (worth $160,000 at the time) wrapped up in old newspapers; this meeting resulted in the formation of the company Syntex (from the words "synthesis" and "Mexico") (17). Later, another scientist at Syntex, George Rosenkranz, achieved large-scale manufacture of testosterone, also using *Dioscorea* as the starting material (18).

Yarrow

 10 Second Take

Yarrow is a safe herb for those who are not allergic to Asteraceae. There is interesting preliminary work on antitumor effects.

 Basics

LATIN NAME

Achillea millefolium L. and other species

FAMILY

Asteraceae/Compositae

OTHER COMMON NAMES

Milfoil, nosebleed, *plumajillo* (Spanish for *A. lanulosa*)

DESCRIPTION

• An aromatic herb up to 70 cm high, yarrow has feathery, alternate leaves and a white or sometimes pink flower head. There are more than 80 species of yarrow, found in temperate zones around the world.

PART USED

Flowering tops, aerial parts, or whole plant

KNOWN ACTIVE CONSTITUENTS

• Sesquiterpene lactones (including achillicine, achillin, achillifolin, millefin, leukodin, dihydroparthenolide and balchanolide) and polyalkynes (1). Three new sesquiterpenoids, achimillic acids A, B, and C, were recently isolated (2). The essential oil of tetraploid, but not other species, contains significant amounts of proazulenes, which yield azulenes on steam distillation. All species except diploid species contain luteolin, apigenin, and their 7-glucosides, as well as flavones and flavanols (1).
β-Sitosterol is the major sterol; other sterols include stigmasterol, campesterol, and cholesterol (3). The primary triterpene is α-amyrin; other triterpenes include β-amyrin, taraxasterol, and pseudotaraxasterol (3).

 Evidence

CLINICAL TRIALS

• Hyperlipidemia and hypertension

—A randomized, double-blind, placebo-controlled clinical trial of 120 men and women with hyperlipidemia and hypertension tested the effects of a hydroalcoholic extract of 15 to 20 drops twice daily for 6 months of *Achillea wilhelmsii* C. Koch (commonly used in Persian medicine). Triglycerides significantly decreased after 2 months; total cholesterol and low density lipoprotein (LDL)-cholesterol decreased significantly after 4 months. Levels of high density lipoprotein (HDL)-cholesterol significantly increased after 6 months of treatment. Diastolic and systolic blood pressure decreased significantly after 2 and 6 months.
—After a mixture of *A. millefolium*, juniper (*Juniperus communis*), and nettle (*Urtica dioca*) (1:1:1) was found to be active *in vitro* against various oral microorganisms, the mixture was tested in 45 people with moderate gingival inflammation (4). Participants rinsed their mouths twice daily with 10 mL mouthwash for 3 months; the placebo consisted of mouthwash without herbs. At 6 and 8 weeks there was no difference between groups and no improvement from baseline as assessed by plaque index, modified gingival index, or angulated bleeding index.

ANIMAL/IN VITRO

• Anti-fertility effects

—In mice treated with an ethanolic extract (200 mg/kg/day intraperitoneally for 20 days) or a hydroethanolic extract (300 mg/kg/day p.o. × 30 days) of *Achillea millefolium* flowers, antispermatogenic action was noted; alterations included exfoliation of immature germ cells, necrosis of germ cells, and vacuolization of seminiferous tubules (with increased interstitial and leukocytic infiltration) (5). An increased number of metaphases in germ epithelium was seen, resulting from either cytotoxicity or stimulation of cell proliferation. Alterations were not uniform among seminiferous tubules, even within a single testis.

• Anti-cancer effect

—A methanol extract of flowers exhibited activity against P-388 leukemia cells *in vivo*. Three new sesquiterpenoids, achimillic acids A, B, and C, were isolated as methyl esters and tested. In male mice injected intraperitoneally with tumor cells, an increase in lifespan was noted in doses of methyl achimillate A and C (not B). A previously identified compound, secotanapartholide, was also tested; doses below 5 mg/kg increased lifespan, whereas doses above this were toxic (2). Methyl achimillate A and secotanapartholide were both inactive against L-1210 leukemia cells.
—In an anticancer screen, the aqueous extract of *Achillea millefolium* was inactive, whereas the organic extract showed moderate activity (at least 50% of cancer cells killed relative to control in at least 20% of 60 human cell lines tested); the concentration at which this occurred is not stated (the maximum concentration tested was 250 mg/mL) (6).

• Antimicrobial effect

—A screen of various prairie plants showed activity of an aqueous extract of yarrow in an anti-HIV assay (greater than 50% inhibition of infected cells); an organic solvent extraction exhibited less activity (less than 50% inhibition of infected cells) (6).
—An α-peroxyachifolid of *A. millefolium* demonstrated cytotoxic activity against *Plasmodium falciparum* (7).

• Other

—Cirsiliol, a flavone from *A. fragrantissima*, had a concentration-dependent relaxation effect on rat isolated ileum (8).
—A chloroform extract of *Achillea ageratum*, as well as two of its components, stigmasterol and β-sitosterol, were effective topical antiinflammatory agents in the mouse ear model for acute inflammation; there was little effect of any compound tested in chronic edema (9).
—An aqueous extract of *Achillea talagonica* administered intraperitoneally to BALB/c mice in doses up to 2.0 g/kg × 7 days before immunization with sheep red blood cells resulted in a significant dose-dependent decrease in hemagglutinating antibody (HA) titer (10).

OTHER CLAIMED BENEFITS/ACTIONS

- Wounds or skin irritations (topical)
- Gastrointestinal
- Cancer
- Warts
- Styptic
- Analgesic
- Antiviral
- Diuretic, contraceptive
- Fevers
- Rheumatism
- Venous stasis
- Menorrhagia
- Nephritis
- Asthma
- Liver problems
- Loss of appetite
- Dyspepsia

 Risks

ADVERSE REACTIONS

- Allergy

—Allergic contact dermatitis caused by yarrow is not uncommon; cross-reactivity may occur with other members of the Asteraceae family (11,12). The primary sensitizing sesquiterpene lactone is α-peroxyachifolid; other sesquiterpene lactones are less sensitizing. More than 50% of Asteraceae-sensitive individuals reacted to a short ether extract of yarrow (12).

 Dose

COMMON DOSAGE FORMS

- *Dried herb:* 2 to 4 g t.i.d.
- *Infusion:* 1 to 4 g herb t.i.d. between meals.
- *Liquid extract:* (1:1, 25% ethanol) 1 to 2 mL t.i.d. between meals.
- *Tincture:* (1:5, 25% ethanol) 2 to 5 mL t.i.d. between meals.
- *Pressed juice* from fresh herb: 3 to 5 mL t.i.d. between meals.
- Used externally in sitz baths or poultices.
- *Quality note:* Dried aerial parts should contain no less than 0.2% volatile oil.

 Common Questions and Answers

Q: Where does the name come from?
A: "Achillea" comes from Achilles, who was said to use the leaves of yarrow as a styptic for wounded soldiers. This was a common use, reflected in many of its old names, which include Knight's milfoil, staunchweed, bloodwort, and soldier's woundwort. The French name, *herbe aux charpentiers,* apparently refers to the use of this herb by carpenters to deal with wounds. The herb is an effective styptic; I once used it to staunch bleeding from a leg wound sustained in the Idaho mountains by a man who tried to turn his pants into shorts (while he was wearing them) with a pocketknife.

Q: Is yarrow used in foods?
A: Yes, most commonly in alcoholic beverages (including bitters and vermouth). Although it is Food and Drug Administration (FDA)-approved only for use in alcoholic beverages, there is a stipulation that the finished beverage must be free of thujone (13). However, yarrow contains only traces of thujone, which occurs in high concentrations in wormwood, sage, and common tansy. *A. atrata* and musk yarrow [*A. erba-rotta*] are used in the preparations of European alcoholic drinks (including *iva liqueur, esprit d'iva,* iva bitter, and others). In parts of Sweden, *A. millefolium* has sometimes been substituted for hops in the brewing of beer. The young leaves of *A. millefolium* are occasionally used in salads, as a cooked vegetable, in soups or sauces, and in a German dish called *gründonnerstag suppe* (14).

Yohimbe

10 Second Take

Yohimbe contains yohimbine, which is effective for erectile dysfunction and xerostomia, but not weight loss. Yohimbine can cause hypertension and other adverse effects.

Basics

LATIN NAME

Pausinystalia yohimbe (K. Schum.) Pierre ex Beille

FAMILY

Rubiaceae

DESCRIPTION

The yohimbe tree is native to tropical West Africa.

PART USED

Bark

KNOWN ACTIVE CONSTITUENTS

• Alkaloids (up to 6%); yohimbine composes 10 to 15% of total alkaloids (1). Yohimbine (also found in *Rauwolfia serpentina*), an indole alkaloid, is chemically similar to reserpine. Minor alkaloids include ajmaline, alloyohimbine, pseudoyohimbine, corynanthine, corynantheine, α-yohimbane, and β-yohimbane (1).

MECHANISM/PHARMACOKINETICS

• Yohimbine is primarily an α_2-adrenoceptor antagonist, with weak α_1-adrenergic antagonist effects and some dopamine antagonist properties (1). A pharmacokinetic study in 13 men given 0.25 or 0.5 mg/kg intravenously found that the half-life of yohimbine was 0.4 to 18 minutes, and elimination half-life between 0.25 to 2.5 hours. A second, slower elimination phase with a half-life of 13 hours may exist (2).
• An earlier study found that after a 10 mg dose of yohimbine in eight males, the absorption half-life was 0.17 ± 0.11 hours and the elimination half-life was 0.6 ± 0.26 hours (3). Less than 0.5% of the dose was recovered in urine; 20% of yohimbine in blood was in erythrocytes.
• Yohimbine appears to be hepatically cleared; extensive extrahepatic metabolism also occurs. A pharmacokinetic study in 32 volunteers tested doses of yohimbine up to 21.6 mg b.i.d for 6 days. There was substantial inter-patient and intra-patient variability; while most subjects exhibited one-compartment elimination (dose-dependent increases in C_{max} and AUC, with no evidence of drug accumulation), others showed evidence of two-compartment elimination (4).

Evidence

CLINICAL TRIALS

• Erectile dysfunction (ED)

—A systematic review and meta-analysis of yohimbine for ED identified seven placebo-controlled RCTs of yohimbine (5); all found a positive effect, and two (6, 7) were identified as methodologically excellent trials.
—In a double-blind, placebo-controlled crossover RCT of high-dose yohimbine in mixed-type impotence (not included in the meta-analysis above), 29 patients received drug or placebo for 25 day phases (with a 14 day washout) (8). There was no difference between treated and placebo groups (44% vs.48%) in complete or partial response after the first phase. Hypertensive crisis occurred in one patient and severe palpitations in another on yohimbine.
—A double-blind crossover RCT of 62 patients (55 completed) with psychogenic impotence compared placebo to yohimbine 15 mg as an adjunct to trazodone 50 mg/d. After the first 8-week phase, complete or partial response was seen in 71% receiving treatment vs. 22% receiving placebo, a significant difference (9). Those who switched to active drug during the second phase achieved a 74% response rate.

• Aphrodisiac effects

—In a double-blind, controlled study of sexual arousal, intravenous yohimbine (0.3 mg/kg) was compared to apomorphine (0.009 mg/kg subcutaneously) in 10 men. Saline placebo was administered by whichever route not utilized for treatment. Apomorphine, but not yohimbine, induced erection and potentiated visually-induced response to erotica; no subjective increase in sexual excitement was seen (10). Yohimbine significantly decreased sexual excitement, and one subject reported severe anxiety.

• Xerostomia

—Yohimbine appears to have a sialogenic effect (see questions and answers). A double-blind crossover RCT in 10 patients with drug-induced xerostomia compared yohimbine 6 mg t.i.d. to anetholtrithione 25 mg t.i.d., each for 5 days with a 5-day washout. Anetholtrithione increased salivary flow 1.5-fold while yohimbine increased salivary flow 3.5-fold, a significant difference (11). A prior unpublished placebo-controlled study by these researchers showed that yohimbine 4 mg, but not placebo, increased salivary flow for 3 hours.

—In another study, yohimbine (4 mg t.i.d. for 3 weeks) was tested in 11 healthy volunteers and 20 depressed patients on tricyclic antidepressants (12). Yohimbine acutely increased salivary flow within 1 hour in both groups, both at the start and the end of the study. However, yohimbine did not affect resting salivary volume values in either group. Acute administration of yohimbine caused headache in one patient. Chronic treatment caused diarrhea in one patient and palpitations in another. There were no significant changes in heart rate or blood pressure.
—In nine depressed patients on clonipramine or amitriptyline, acute administration of 10-mg yohimbine increased salivary volume and plasma noradrenaline levels for 4 hours; however, side effects included rhinorrhea, facial flush, tachycardia, nausea, tremor, and sweating (13). A second study in the same report assigned ten other depressed patients on clonipramine or amitriptyline and ten normal volunteers to one dose of yohimbine 4 mg or placebo in a double-blind crossover RCT with a 7-day washout period. Compared to placebo, 4-mg yohimbine increased salivary volume for 3 hours in depressed individuals but had no effect on normal individuals. No side effects were noted.

• Weight loss

—A double-blind placebo-controlled study in 19 obese volunteers found no benefit of yohimbine 18 mg/day over placebo as an adjunct to a 1,000 calorie a day diet for 8 weeks (14). There was no difference between the two groups in weight.
—Another double-blind placebo-controlled RCT of 47 men (33 completed) tested high-dose yohimbine (up to 43 mg/day for 6 months); there was no difference between groups in body weight, body mass index (BMI), total cholesterol, high density lipoprotein (HDL), body fat, or fat distribution (15).
—In 10 healthy men, 14 days yohimbine (4 mg t.i.d.) did not significantly modify body weight (5 volunteers lost between 1.4 to 2.2 kg; 5 others experienced no change) (16). One study in 20 obese women found a positive effect of yohimbine as an adjunct to a 1000 kcal/day diet. The group receiving yohimbine (5 mg p.o. q.i.d. for 3 weeks) lost more weight (3.55 ± 0.24 kg) than the placebo-treated group (2.21 ± 0.37 kg) (17).

• Panic attacks

—Yohimbine precipitated panic attacks in six patients with a history of agoraphobia with panic attacks; no attacks were precipitated in seven healthy controls (18).

Risks

WARNING

• Yohimbine or yohimbe products should not be administered with tricyclic or tetracyclic antidepressants, phenothiazines, MAOIs, other sympathomimetics or in patients with hypertension, autonomic failure, renal disease, bipolar disorder, or panic attacks.

ADVERSE REACTIONS

• Yohimbine can cause hypertension, tachycardia, headache, anxiety, diarrhea, palpitations, dizziness, tremor, skin flushing, and increased urinary frequency.
• In patients with autonomic failure, doses of as little as 5 mg/day can cause adverse effects (19).
• In patients with bipolar disorder, yohimbine can induce manic symptoms (19), and yohimbine can induce panic attacks in susceptible patients (18).

• Hypertension

—In 25 hypertensive subjects, yohimbine 21.6 mg increased mean blood pressure (5 mm Hg) and increased plasma norepinephrine levels (20).
—In 25 healthy volunteers and 29 hypertensive patients, 10 mg yohimbine significantly increased blood pressure in hypertensive but not normotensive patients (21). Hypertensive crisis was reported in one patient during a clinical trial (8).

• MAO inhibition

—No cases of MAO inhibition in human have been reported, but yohimbine inhibits MAO in vitro.

• Systemic lupus erythematosus (SLE)

—A 42-year-old hypertensive patient on nifedipine presented with fever, chills, malaise, and pruritic, scaly skin one day after ingesting 16.2 mg yohimbine (22). He was later diagnosed with probable drug-induced systemic lupus erythematosus.

• Overdose

—A 62-year-old diabetic male ingested 200 mg yohimbine with vodka, vomited an hour later, and presented to the emergency room an hour after that. The only symptom that the patient experienced was lightheadedness on standing. His heart rate was 106, and blood pressure was 174/94 supine and 168/88 standing. He was treated with activated charcoal and observed for 19 hours, during which his heart rate decreased to 80 and blood pressure decreased to 128/60 (23). Yohimbine overdose with significant hypertension should probably be treated with sodium nitroprusside or diazoxide rather than clonidine, which has weak α_1-agonist activity (normally overshadowed by its α_2 activity) (23).

DRUG INTERACTIONS

• Tricyclic antidepressants

—Yohimbine, in doses of 15 to 20 mg, may increase blood pressure and induce anxiety, but when combined with tricyclic antidepressants, yohimbine may cause hypertension at 4 mg t.i.d. (19).

• Phenothiazines

—Yohimbine toxicity can be enhanced by phenothiazines (19).

• Opiates and opiate antagonists

—Yohimbine may enhance both opiates and opiate antagonists. A double-blind placebo-controlled study in 30 men tested placebo or yohimbine (5.4 mg t.i.d.) for 3 days prior to dental surgery (24). Yohimbine, which had no analgesic effect on its own, significantly enhanced morphine analgesia.
—In a controlled crossover study, yohimbine (20 mg q.d., 5 mg t.i.d. or 100 mg t.i.d.) was tested in 12 patients (4 in each group) subjected to naloxone-precipitated methadone withdrawal (25). The 20 mg daily dose was poorly tolerated; two of four dropped out after a single dose due to withdrawal-like symptoms, and the other two reported anxiety. Compared to placebo, 20 mg yohimbine increased withdrawal symptoms and increased systolic blood pressure (by 40 mm Hg). Yohimbine 5-10 mg tid was well tolerated and decreased withdrawal symptom scores.

Dose

COMMON DOSAGE FORMS

• Yohimbine HCL 5.4 mg to 6 mg p.o. t.i.d. (dose may be halved if side effects occur).
• The crude herb is not recommended, as it is associated with more adverse effects.

Common Questions and Answers

Q: Is yohimbe better than yohimbine?
A: Probably not. Other alkaloids are present in yohimbe, but there is no evidence that the herb is better than the drug. Also, the amount of alkaloid varies in natural plant material, not to mention marketed products. An analysis of 26 commercial yohimbe products found that concentrations of yohimbine by gas chromatography ranged from <0.1 to 489 ppm, while authentic yohimbe bark contained 7,089 ppm (1). Nine products contained no measurable yohimbine, and eight contained only traces (<1 ppm). Most products contained only yohimbine, not other yohimbe alkaloids, suggesting a synthetic source.

Q: How does yohimbine stimulate salivar?
A: Probably by inhibiting presynaptic α_2 adrenoreceptors on the chorda tympani. Atropine prevents the effect (11). Some sialogenic effects may be due to metabolites; the half-life of yohimbine is too short to justify the 3-hour effect demonstrated in clinical trials.

Q: Does yohimbe work for body-building?
A: No. Yohimbe has been touted as an anabolic agent, and it is claimed that it increases growth hormone, but there is no evidence for either claim (1). One dose of yohimbe (20 mg) did not affect plasma growth hormone levels (26).

Zinc

10 Second Take

Zinc may help diarrhea and dysgeusia; studies are mixed on colds.

Basics

DESCRIPTION

Zinc is an essential trace element.

FOOD SOURCES

Meats, shellfish, whole grains, seeds, nuts, legumes, vegetables, eggs, and milk

MECHANISM/PHARMACOKINETICS

• Zinc is a cofactor for more than 200 enzymes, including alcohol dehydrogenase, carbonic anhydrase, and carboxypeptidase (1). Zinc is needed in biomembranes, for binding transcription factors, and for stabilizing some hormone-receptor complexes (2).
• The human body contains 1.4 to 2.5 g zinc, mostly in bone and muscle; the highest concentrations are in skin, hair, nails, retina, and testes (3). Twenty percent to 30% of dietary zinc is absorbed intestinally, most is excreted via bile; 2% to 10% is found in urine (2). The average American consumes 10 mg zinc/day.

Evidence

CLINICAL TRIALS

• Colds (see questions and answers)

—A meta-analysis of eight placebo-controlled randomized controlled trials (RCTs) found no significant effect of zinc on symptoms at 7 days (4). A review of eight double-blind placebo-controlled trials found trials evenly split; neither of the two small trials that looked at incidence of infection after nasal inoculation of rhinovirus found a benefit (5).
—A double-blind, placebo-controlled trial of 213 participants with cold symptoms found that zinc gluconate nasal gel, applied four times daily until symptoms resolved, significantly shortened duration of symptoms (2.3 ± 0.9 days, compared with 9.0 ± 2.5 days in the placebo group) (6).

• Taste and smell

—A placebo-controlled RCT in 18 patients receiving head and neck radiation tested zinc sulfate (45 mg t.i.d., from the onset of taste alterations to 1 month after radiation ended) (7). Placebo-treated patients had greater worsening of taste acuity and had slower recovery of taste acuity than zinc-treated patients.

—An earlier double-blind crossover trial found no benefit of zinc 100 mg/day for hypogeusia (decreased taste) of various etiologies in 106 patients (8); concurrent medications may have affected results (9).
—A double-blind RCT of 98 patients with taste disorders found no benefit for zinc gluconate (22.6 mg t.i.d. × 4 months) over placebo, although zinc-deficient participants benefited from treatment (10).
—In one study, 426 patients with sensorineural olfactory disorder received topical corticosteroids and oral B complex, zinc sulfate (300 mg/day, for "more than 1 month"), or both (11). Zinc benefited only those with posttraumatic olfactory disorder.

• Diarrhea

—A double-blind RCT of 937 children (age 6 to 35 months) in India found that 20 mg elemental zinc/day as an adjunct to oral rehydration therapy and vitamins reduced the risk of continued diarrhea by 23% [95% confidence interval (CI) 12% to 32%] (12). Another 15-day trial of 684 children (age 6 to 24 months) found that elemental zinc acetate (14.2 mg or 40 mg daily), but not vitamin A [4,500 μg retinol equivalents (RE)], reduced duration of diarrhea 13% and reduced prolonged diarrhea by 43% (13). In 87 hospitalized children (age 6 to 36 months) with persistent diarrhea in Pakistan, 3 mg/kg/day elemental zinc as an adjunct to a rice-lentil and yogurt diet (14) provided no additional benefit in malnourished children with persistent diarrhea. Zinc decreased already low plasma copper levels and may be detrimental in severely malnourished children.

• Head injury

—A double-blind RCT found a benefit for supplemental zinc versus standard zinc therapy in 68 patients with severe closed-head injury on Glasgow coma scale scores and mortality rates (15). More controls underwent craniotomy, possibly skewing results.

• Atopic eczema

—A double-blind placebo-controlled trial found no benefit for oral zinc sulphate (185.4 mg/day × 8 weeks) in 50 children with atopic eczema (16).

• Tinnitus

—A double-blind, placebo-controlled trial found no benefit of oral zinc sulphate (22 mg elemental zinc t.i.d. × 8 weeks) in 48 patients with tinnitus and normal serum zinc levels (17).
—Macular degeneration
—A double-blind, placebo-controlled RCT in 112 patients with age-related, bilateral macular degeneration and unilateral exudative lesions found no benefit of zinc sulfate (200 mg q.d. × 2 years) in preventing progression in the second eye (18).

• Leg ulcers

—A systematic review of six RCTs found no benefit of zinc sulfate for healing chronic venous or arterial ulcers (19).

• Infant/fetal growth

—A placebo-controlled RCT in apparently healthy breast-fed infants (6 to 12 months) in Ethiopia found that zinc sulfate (10 mg q.d. for 6 days a week × 6 months) increased weight and length in stunted and nonstunted infants and decreased morbidity (20).
—A double-blind RCT in 580 healthy African-American pregnant women with low zinc levels tested zinc sulfate (25 mg/day from 19 weeks gestational age until delivery). All received a zinc-free multivitamin/mineral. Zinc-supplemented infants, compared with placebo-treated infants, had significantly greater birthweight and head circumference (21).

• Arthritis

—Three placebo-controlled studies in a total of 86 patients with rheumatoid arthritis (RA) found no benefit of zinc sulphate (up to 220 mg t.i.d.) on clinical criteria (22–24). The longest trial lasted 4 months.
—A double-blind placebo-controlled crossover trial in 24 participants with psoriatic arthritis (220 mg zinc sulphate t.i.d. × 6 weeks) found that zinc significantly benefited joint pains (but not overall condition, morning stiffness, or functional capacity) (25).

Clinical Considerations

DEFICIENCY SIGNS AND SYMPTOMS

• *Factors predisposing to zinc deficiency (3):* Inadequate dietary intake, celiac disease, pancreatic insufficiency, inflammatory bowel disease, malabsorption, starvation, burns, diabetes, ketoacidosis, diuretic treatment, kidney damage, liver disease, sickle cell anemia, porphyria, chelation therapy, chronic blood loss, parasites, dialysis, exfoliative dermatitis, and excessive sweating.
• Zinc deficiency diseases include hypogonadal dwarf syndrome (growth retardation, anemia, altered taste and smell, poor wound healing, and hepatospleno-megaly), and acrodermatitis enteropathica (an inherited disorder characterized by alopecia, hypertrophic, ulcerated skin, chronic diarrhea, and muscle wasting) (1).
• *Symptoms of deficiency (3):* Anorexia, impaired smell and taste, growth retardation, hypogonadism, delayed wound healing, impotence (in renal dialysis patients), depression, intention tremor, nystagmus, dysarthria, jitteriness, photophobia, skin lesions, paronychia, nail abnormalities (growth arrest, loss, Beau's lines), hair growth arrest, diarrhea, decreased cell-mediated immune function, and decreased folic acid availability (because dietary folate is hydrolyzed by the zinc-dependent enzyme pteroylpolyglutamate hydrolase).

FACTORS DECREASING AVAILABILITY/ABSORPTION

• Phytate, fiber, iron (especially ferrous), high calcium intake (especially with a phytate-rich diet), folic acid (may impair zinc status if zinc levels are low; studies are mixed) (2).

LABORATORY TESTS

• Plasma zinc: 70 to 130 μg/dL.
• Levels less than 50 μg/dL or hair concentration less than 70 μg/g may indicate deficiency (3).

 Risks

ADVERSE REACTIONS

• Zinc can cause nausea, vomiting, mouth irritation, dysgeusia, abdominal pain, or diarrhea.
• Excessive zinc interferes with copper absorption (probably by inducing metallothionein, which has a higher affinity for copper than for zinc). A dose of 60 mg zinc daily for several weeks depresses erythrocyte copper-zinc superoxide dismutase. A dose of 50 mg zinc gluconate × 10 weeks reduced hemoglobin and serum ferritin. Elevated zinc concentration reduces high density lipoprotein (HDL)-cholesterol, increases low density lipoprotein (LDL)-cholesterol, and impairs lymphocyte and neutrophil function (1). A 17-year-old who ingested up to 300 mg zinc daily for almost 2 years developed anemia, leukopenia, neutropenia, fatigue, headaches, and reduced serum copper (26). Zinc discontinuation resolved all signs and symptoms in 2 months.
• Exposure to nonsupplemental zinc

—Zinc compounds (especially zinc chloride in concentrations greater than 20%) can erode the gastrointestinal tract and may cause acute tubular necrosis or interstitial nephritis. Gastrointestinal symptoms are more likely after ingesting zinc compounds than elemental zinc (1). Chronic ingestion of more than 425 pennies (97.6% zinc, 2.4% copper) caused diarrhea and gastrointestinal bleeding; the patient died from bacterial and fungal sepsis (1).
—Injected zinc sulfate caused hypotension, diarrhea, vomiting, pulmonary edema, jaundice, elevated amylase concentrations, oliguria, anemia, and thrombocytopenia (1).
—Inhaled zinc chloride can produce chemical pneumonitis and adult respiratory distress syndrome. Zinc oxide fumes can cause metal fume fever, with fatigue, chills, fever, myalgias, cough, dyspnea, leukocytosis, thirst, and metallic taste. Exposed workers can develop tolerance but lose it over a weekend, causing this illness to be termed "Monday morning fever."
—Topical zinc chloride and zinc acetate are more irritating to the skin than zinc sulfite or zinc oxide.

• Minimum risk concentration = 0.3 mg zinc/kg/day.
• Lowest observed adverse effect concentration (LOAEL) = 1 mg zinc/kg/day.
• Maximum contaminant concentration for U.S. drinking water = 5 mg zinc/L.
• Permissible exposure limit-time weighted average (PEL-TWA) zinc oxide fumes 5 mg/m^3, short-term exposure limit (STEL) 10 mg/m^3.

DRUG INTERACTIONS

• Tetracycline: zinc decreases absorption (27)
• Fluoroquinolones: zinc decreases absorption of ciprofloxacin and norfloxacin (28)
• Folic acid (2)
• Iron (2)
• Calcium: may decrease absorption of zinc (2)

PREGNANCY/LACTATION

• Low zinc concentration in breast milk can cause acrodermatitis, irritability, and delayed growth in breast-fed infants (1).

 Dose

RECOMMENDED DIETARY ALLOWANCE

Infants and children

0 to 6 months	2 mg/day (adequate intake)
7 to 12 months	3 mg/day (adequate intake)
1 to 3 years	3 mg/day
4 to 8 years	5 mg/day

Males

9 to 13 years	8 mg/day
14 to 18 years	11 mg/day
19 to 30 years	11 mg/day
31 to 50 years	11 mg/day
51+ years	11 mg/day

Females

9 to 13 years	8 mg/day
14 to 18 years	9 mg/day
19 to 30 years	8 mg/day
31 to 50 years	8 mg/day
51+ years	8 mg/day

Pregnant

≤18 years	13 mg/day
19 to 50 years	11 mg/day

Lactating

≤18 years	14 mg/day
19 to 50 years	12 mg/day

UPPER LIMITS

Infants and children

0 to 6 months	4 mg/day
7 to 12 months	5 mg/day
1 to 3 years	7 mg/day
4 to 8 years	12 mg/day

Males

9 to 13 years	23 mg/day
14 to 18 years	34 mg/day
19 to 50 years	40 mg/day
51+ years	40 mg/day

Females

9 to 13 years	23 mg/day
14 to 18 years	34 mg/day
19 to 50 years	40 mg/day
51+ years	40 mg/day

Pregnant

≤18 years	34 mg/day
19 to 50 years	40 mg/day

Lactating

≤18 years	34 mg/day
19 to 50 years	40 mg/day

• *Quality note:* Zinc gluconate tablets contain 14.3% zinc by weight. Zinc sulfate contains 23% zinc by weight (1).
• Zinc gluconate lozenges: One lozenge (≥ 13.3 mg elemental zinc) every 2 hours while awake. Flavoring compounds, including citric acid and tartaric acid and possibly mannitol and sorbitol, may chelate zinc, diminishing efficacy.

SECTION II
References

References

ACONITE

1. Chan TYK, Tomlinson B, Tse LKK et al. Aconitine poisoning due to Chinese medicine: a review. *Vet Hum Toxicol* 1994;36: 452–455.
2. Ito K, Tanaka S, Funayama M et al. Distribution of aconitum alkaloids in body fluids and tissues in a suicidal case of aconite ingestion. *J Anal Toxicol* 2000;24:348–353.
3. Kimura I, Makino M, Honda R et al. Expression of major histocompatibility complex in mouse peritoneal macrophages increasingly depends on plasma corticosterone levels: stimulation by aconitine. *Biol Pharm Bull* 1995;18:1504–1508.
4. Bisset NG. Arrow poisons in China. Part II. *Aconitum*—botany, chemistry, and pharmacology. *J Ethnopharmacol* 1981;4:247–336.
5. Friese J, Gleitz J, Gutser UT et al. *Aconitum* sp. alkaloids: the modulation of voltage-dependent Na+ channels, toxicity and antinociceptive properties. *Eur J Pharmacol* 1997; 337:165–174.
6. Winslow E. Hemodynamic and arrhythmogenic effects of aconitine applied to the left atria of anesthetized cats: effects of amiodarone and atropine. *J Cardiovasc Pharmacol* 1991;31:611P.
7. Tai Y-T, But PP-H, Young K et al. Cardiotoxicity after accidental herb-induced aconite poisoning. *Lancet* 1992;340: 1254–1256.
8. Tomlinson B, Chan Tyk, Chan JCN et al. Herb-induced aconite poisoning. *Lancet* 1993;341:370–371.
9. Tai Y-T, Lau C-P, But PP-H et al. Bidirectional tachycardia induced by herbal aconite poisoning. *PACE* 1992;15: 831–839.
10. Fatovich DM. Aconite: a lethal Chinese herb. *Ann Emerg Med* 1992;21:309–311.
11. Mori A, Mukaida M, Ishiyama I et al. [Homicidal poisoning by aconite: report of a case from the viewpoint of clinical forensic medicine]. *Nippon Hoigaku Zasshi* 1990;44: 352–357.
12. Yeih DF, Chiang FT, Huang SK. Successful treatment of aconitine induced life threatening ventricular tachyarrhythmia with amiodarone. *Heart* 2000;84:E8.
13. Felgenhauer N, Zilker T, Dorfmann N. Severe intoxication with aconitum. *J Toxicol Clin Toxicol* 1999;37:416(abst).
14. Mann J. *Murder, magic, and medicine* Oxford, England: Oxford University Press, 1994:17.

ALANINE

1. Linder MC. *Nutritional biochemistry and metabolism, with clinical applications,* 2nd ed. East Norwalk CT: Appleton & Lange, 1991.
2. Battezzati A, Haisch M, Brillon DJ et al. Splanchnic utilization of enteral alanine in humans. *Metabolism* 1999;48: 915–921.
3. Weithop BV, Cryer PE. Glycemic actions of alanine and terbutaline in IDDM. *Diabetes Care* 1993;16:1124–1130.
4. Wiethop BV, Cryer PE. Alanine and terbutaline in treatment of hypoglycemia in IDDM. *Diabetes Care* 1993;16: 1131–1136.
5. Saleh TY, Cryer PE. Alanine and terbutaline in the prevention of nocturnal hypoglycemia in IDDM. *Diabetes Care* 1997;20:1231–1236.
6. Patra FC, Sack DA, Islam A et al. Oral rehydration formula containing alanine and glucose for treatment of diarrhea: a controlled trial. *BMJ* 1989;298:1353–1356.
7. Sarker SA, Majid N, Mahalanabis D. Alanine- and glucose-based hypo-osmolar oral rehydration solution in infants with persistent diarrhea: a controlled trial. *Acta Paediatr* 1995;84:775–780.
8. Sazawal S. Bhatnagar S, Bhan MK et al. Alanine-based oral rehydration solution: assessment of efficacy in acute noncholera diarrhea among children. *J Pediatr Gastroenterol Nutr* 1991;12:461–468.
9. Ribeiro H da C Jr, Lifshitz F. Alanine-based oral rehydration therapy for infants with acute diarrhea. *J Pediatr* 1991;118: S86–90.
10. Maezono K, Mawatari K, Kajiwara K et al. Effect of alanine on D-galactosamine-induced acute liver failure in rats. *Hepatology* 1996;24:1211–1216.
11. Hashimoto A, Nishikawa T, Oka T et al. D-alanine inhibits methamphetamine-induced hyperactivity in rats. *Eur J Pharmacol* 1991;202:105–107.

ALFALFA

1. De Smet PAGM. *Medicago sativa. Adverse effects of herbal drugs,* vol 1. Berlin: Springer-Verlag, 1992:161–169.
2. Bruneton J. *Pharmacognosy: phytochemistry medicinal plants,,* 2nd ed. Secaucus NJ: Lavoisier Springer-Verlag, 1999:715–716.
3. Herbert V, Kasdan TS. Alfalfa, vitamin E, and autoimmune disorders. *Am J Clin Nutr* 1994;60:639–642.
4. Malinow MR, Bardana EJ, Pirofsky B et al. Systemic lupus erythematosus-like syndrome in monkeys fed alfalfa sprouts: role of a nonprotein amino acid. *Science* 1982;216: 415–417.
5. Alcocer-Varela J, Iglesias A, Llorente L et al. Effects of L-canavanine on T cells may explain the induction of systemic lupus erythematosus by alfalfa. *Arthritis Rheum* 1985;28: 52–57.
6. Mölgaard J, von Schenck H, Olsson AG. Alfalfa seeds lower low density lipoprotein cholesterol and apolipoprotein B concentrations in patients with Type II hyperlipoproteinemia. *Atherosclerosis* 1987;65:173–179.
7. Malinow MR, McLaughlin P, Kohler GO et al. Prevention of elevated cholesterolemia in monkeys by alfalfa saponins. *Steroids* 1977;29:105–110.
8. Polacheck I, Zehavi U, Naim M et al. Activity of compound G2 isolated from alfalfa roots against medically important yeasts. *Antimicrob Agents Chemother* 1986;30:290–294.
9. Zehavi U, Polacheck I. Saponins as antimycotic agents: glycosides of medicagenic acid. In: Waller GR, Yamasaki K, eds. *Saponins used in traditional and modern medicine.* New York: Plenum, 1996:535–546.
10. Malinow MR, Bardana EJ, Goodnight SH. Pancytopenia during ingestion of alfalfa seeds. *Lancet* 1981;i:615.
11. Roberts JL, Hayashi JA. Exacerbation of SLE associated with alfalfa ingestion. *N Engl J Med* 1983;308:1361.
12. Prete PE. The mechanism of action of L-canavanine in inducing autoimmune phenomena. *Arthritis Rheum* 1985;28: 1198–2000.
13. Malinow MR, McLaughlin P, Bardana EJ et al. Elimination of toxicity from diets containing alfalfa seeds. *Food Chem Toxic* 1984;22:583–587.

ALOE

1. World Health Organization. *WHO monographs on selected medicinal plants,* vol 1. Geneva: WHO, 1999:33–42; 43–49.

2. Reynolds T, Dweck AC. *Aloe vera* leaf gel: a review update. *J Ethnopharmacol* 1999;68:3–37.

3. Joshi SP. Chemical constituents and biological activity of *Aloe barbadensis*—a review. *J Med Aromatic Plant Sci* 1998; 20:768–773.

4. European Scientific Cooperative on Phytotherapy (ESCOP). *Monographs on the medicinal use of plant drugs.* Aloe capensis (Cape Aloes). Exeter, UK, 1997.

5. Fujita K, Ito S, Teradaira R et al. Properties of a carboxypeptidase from aloe. *Biochem Pharmacol* 1979;28:1261–1262.

6. Klein AD, Penneys NS. *Aloe vera. J Am Acad Dermatol* 1988; 18:714–720.

7. Yongchaiyudha S, Rungpitarangsi V, Bunyapraphatsara N et al. Antidiabetic activity of *Aloe vera* juice I. Clinical trial in new cases of diabetes mellitus. *Phytomedicine* 1996;3: 241–243.

8. Bunyapraphatsara N, Yongchaiyudha S, Rungpitarangsi V et al. Antidiabetic activity of *Aloe vera* juice II. Clinical trial in diabetes mellitus patients in combination with glibenclamide. *Phytomedicine* 1996;3:245–248.

9. Fulton JE. The stimulation of postdermabrasion wound healing with stabilized *Aloe vera* gel-polyethylene oxide dressing. *J Dermatol Surg Oncol* 1990;16:460—4-67.

10. Schmidt JM, Greenspoon JS. *Aloe vera* dermal wound gel is associated with a delay in wound healing. *Obstet Gynecol* 1991;78:115–117.

11. Visuthikosol; V. Sukwanarat Y, Chowchuen B et al. Effect of *Aloe vera* gel to healing of burn wound a clinical and histologic study. *J Med Assoc Thai* 1995;78:403–409.

12. Williams MS, Burk M, Loprinzi CL et al. Phase III double-blind evaluation of an *Aloe vera* gel as a prophylactic agent for radiation-induced skin toxicity. *Int J Radiat Oncol Biol Phys* 1996;36:345–349.

13. Plemons JM, Rees TD, Binnie WH et al. Evaluation of acemannan in the treatment of recurrent aphthous stomatitis. *Wounds* 1994;6:40–45.

14. Syed TA, Ahmad SA, Holt AH et al. Management of psoriasis with *Aloe vera* extract in a hydrophilic cream: a placebo-controlled, double-blind study. *Trop Med Int Health* 1996;1: 505–509.

15. Heggers JP, Robson MC, Manavalen K et al. Experimental and clinical observations on frostbite. *Ann Emerg Med* 1987; 16:1056–1062.

16. Pecere T, Gazzola MV, Mucignat C et al. Aloe-emodin is a new type of anticancer agent with selective activity against neuroectodermal tumors. *Cancer Res* 2000;60:2800–2804.

17. Arosio B, Gagliano N, Fusaro LM et al. Aloe-emodin quinone pretreatment reduces acute liver injury induced by carbon tetrachloride. *Pharmacol Toxicol* 2000;87:229–233.

18. Davis RH, Agnew PS, Shapiro E. Antiarthritic activity of anthraquinones found in aloe for podiatric medicine. *J Am Podiatr Med Assoc* 1986;76:61–66.

19. Westendorf J. Anthranoid derivatives—aloe species. *Adverse effects of herbal drugs.* Berlin: Springer-Verlag, 1993: 119–123.

ANGELICA

1. Awang DVC. Dong quai. *Can Pharm J* 1999; 132(April): 38–41.

2. Bisset NG, Wichtl M. *Herbal drugs and phytopharmaceuticals: a handbook for practice on a scientific basis* Boca Raton, FL, CRC Press, 1994:pp.70–72.

3. Hirata JD, Ettinger B, Small R et al. Does dong quai have estrogenic effects in postmenopausal women? A double-blind, placebo-controlled trial. *Fertil Steril* 1997;68: 981–986.

4. Bradley RR, Cunniff PJ, Pereira BJG et al. Hematopoietic effect of Radix Angelicae sinensis in a hemodialysis patient. *Am J Kidney Dis* 1999;34:349–354.

5. Xiaohong Y, Jing-Ping OY, Shuzheng T. Angelica protects the human vascular endothelial cell from the effects of oxidized low-density lipoprotein in vitro. *Clin Hemorheol Microcirc* 2000;22:317–323.

6. Harada M, Suzuki M, Ozaki Y. Effect of Japanese angelica root and peony root on uterine contraction in the rabbit in situ. *J Pharm Dyn* 1984;7:304–311.

7. Mizuno A, Takata M, Okada Y et al. Structures of new coumarins and antitumor-promoting activity of coumarins from Angelica edulis. *Planta Med* 1994;60:333–336.

8. Hann SK, Park YK, Im S et al. Angelica-induced phytophotodermatitis. *Photodermatol Photoimmunol Photomed* 1991; 8:84–85.

9. Page RL, Lawrence JD. Potentiation of warfarin by dong quai. *Pharmacotherapy* 1999;19:870–876.

10. Ellis GR, Stephens MR. Untitled [photograph and brief case report]. In "Minerva." *BMJ* 1999;319:650.

11. Lo AC, Chan K, Yeung YH et al. Danggui (*Angelica sinensis*) affects the pharmacodynamics but not the pharmacokinetics of warfarin in rabbits. *Eur Drug Metab Pharmacokinet* 1995;20:55–60.

12. Ishihara K, Kushida H, Yuzurihara M et al. Interaction of drugs and Chinese herbs: pharmacokinetic changes of tolbutamide and diazepam caused by extracts of Angelica dahurica. *J Pharm Pharmacol* 2000;52:1023–1029.

13. Tisserand R, Balacs T. *Essential oil safety: a guide for health care professionals.* Edinburgh, Scotland, UK: Churchill Livingstone, 1995:p. 116

ANISE

1. European Scientific Cooperative on Phytotherapy (ESCOP). *Monographs on the medicinal use of plant drugs.* Anisi fructus (aniseed). Exeter, UK, 1997.

2. Gershbein LL. Regeneration of rat liver in the presence of essential oils and their components. *Food Cosmet Toxicol* 1977;15:173–181.

3. Rosti L, Nardini A, Bettinelli ME et al. Toxic effects of a herbal tea mixture in two newborns. *Acta Paediatr* 1994;83: 683.

ARGININE

1. Abcouwer SF, Souba WW. Glutamine and arginine. In: Shils ME, Olson JA, Dhike M et al, eds. *Modern nutrition in health and disease,* 9th ed. Baltimore: Williams & Wilkins, 1999.

2. Rector TS, Bank AJ, Mullen KA et al. Randomised, double-blind, placebo-controlled study of supplemental oral L-arginine in patients with heart failure. *Circulation* 1996;93: 2135–2141.

3. Bednarz B, Wolk R, Chamiec T et al. Effects of oral L-arginine supplementation on exercise-induced QT dispersion and exercise tolerance in stable angina pectoris. *Int J Cardiol* 2000;75:205–210.

4. Maxwell AJ, Zapien MP, Pearce GL et al. Randomized trial of a medical food for the dietary management of chronic, stable angina. *J Am Coll Cardiol* 2002;39:37–45.

5. Blum A, Hathaway L, Mincemoyer R et al. Oral L-arginine in

References

patients with coronary artery disease on medical management. *Circulation* 2000;101:2160–2164.

6. Adams MR, McCredie R, Jessup W et al. Oral L-arginine improves endothelium-dependent dilation and reduces monocyte adhesion to endothelial cells in young men with coronary artery disease. *Atherosclerosis* 1997;21;129:261–269.

7. Carrier M, Pellerin M, Page PL et al. Can L-arginine improve myocardial protection during cardioplegic arrest? Results of a phase I pilot study. *Ann Thorac Surg* 1998;66:108–112.

8. Higashi Y, Oshima T, Ono N et al. Intravenous administration of L-arginine inhibits angiotensin-converting enzyme in humans. *J Clin Endocrinol Metab* 1995;80:2198–2202.

9. Clarkson P, Adams MR, Powe AJ et al. Oral L-arginine improves endothelium-dependent dilation in hypercholesterolemic young adults. *J Clin Invest* 1996;97:1989–1994.

10. Wennmalm A, Edlund A, Granstrom EF et al. Acute supplementation with the nitric oxide precursor L-arginine does not improve cardiovascular performance in patients with hypercholesterolemia. *Atherosclerosis* 1995;118:223–231.

11. Wolf A, Zalpour C, Theilmeier G et al. Dietary L-arginine supplementation normalized platelet aggregation in hypercholesterolemic humans. *J Am Coll Cardiol* 1997;219:479–485.

12. Bode-Boger SM, Boger RH, Alfke H et al. L-arginine induces nitric oxide-dependent vasodilation in patients with critical limb ischemia. A randomized, controlled study. *Circulation* 1996;93:85–90.

13. Boger RH, Bod-Boger SM, Thiele W et al. Restoring vascular nitric oxide formation by L-arginine improves the symptoms of intermittent claudication in patients with peripheral arterial occlusive disease. *J Am Coll Cardiol* 1998;32:1336–1344.

14. Klotz T, Mathers MJ, Braun M et al. Effectiveness of oral L-arginine in first-line treatment of erectile dysfunction in a controlled crossover study. *Urology Intl* 1999;63:220–223.

15. Chen J, Wollman Y, Chernichovsky T et al. Effect of oral administration of high-dose nitric oxide donor L-arginine in men with organic erectile dysfunction: results of a double-blind, randomized, placebo-controlled study. *BJU Int* 1999; 83:269–273.

16. Korting GE, Smith SD, Wheeler MA et al. A randomized double-blind trial of oral L-arginine for treatment of interstitial cystitis. *J Urol* 1999;161:558–565.

17. Ehren I, Lundberg JO, Adolfsson J et al. Effects of L-arginine treatment on symptoms and bladder nitric oxide levels in patients with interstitial cystitis. *Urology* 1998;52: 1026–1029.

18. Cartledge JJ, Davies AM, Eardley I. A randomized double-blind placebo-controlled crossover trial of the efficacy of L-arginine in the treatment of interstitial cystitis. *BJU Int* 2000;85:421–426.

19. Battaglia C, Salvatori M, Maxia N. Adjuvant L-arginine treatment for in-vitro fertilization in poor responder patients. *Hum Reprod* 1999;14:1690–1697.

20. Khan F, Litchfield SJ, McLaren M et al. Oral L-arginine supplementation and cutaneous vascular responses in patients with primary Raynaud's phenomenon. *Arthritis Rheum* 1997; 40:352–357.

21. Wascher TC, Graier WF, Dittrich P et al. Effects of low-dose L-arginine on insulin-mediated vasodilatation and insulin sensitivity. *Eur J Clin Invest* 1997;27:690–695.

22. Lubec B, Hayn M, Kitzmuller E et al. L-arginine reduces lipid peroxidation in patients with diabetes mellitus. *Free Radical Biol Med* 1997;22:355–357.

23. Heys SD, Segar A, Payne S et al. Dietary supplementation with L-arginine: modulation of tumour-infiltrating lymphocytes in patients with colorectal cancer. *Br J Surg* 1997;84: 238–241.

24. Loukides S, Kharitonov S, Wodehouse T et al. Effect of arginine on mucociliary function in primary ciliary dyskinesia. *Lancet* 1998;352:371–372.

25. Luiking YC, Weusten BI, Portincasa P. Effects of long-term oral L-arginine on esophageal motility and gallbladder dynamics in healthy humans. *Am J Physiol* 1998;274: G984–991.

26. Bortolotti M, Brunelli F, Sarti P et al. Clinical and manometric effects of L-arginine in patients with chest pain and oesophageal motor disorders. *Ital J Gastroenterol Hepatol* 1997;29:320–324.

27. Ricciardolo FL, Geppeti P, Mistretta A et al. Randomized double-blind placebo-controlled study of the effect of inhibition of nitric oxide synthesis in bradykinin-induced asthma. *Lancet* 1996;348:374–377.

28. McCarter MD, Gentillini OD, Gomez ME et al. Perioperative oral supplement with immunonutrients in cancer patients. *J Parenter Enteral Nutr* 1998;22:206–211.

29. Saffle JR, Wiebke G, Jennings K et al. Randomized trial of immune-enhancing enteral nutrition in burn patients. *J Trauma* 1997;42:793–800.

30. Pichard C, Sudre P, Karsegard V et al. A randomized double-blind controlled study of 6 months of oral nutritional supplementation with arginine and omega-3 fatty acids in HIV-infected patients. Swiss HIV Cohort Study. *AIDS* 1998;12: 53–63.

31. Perera DM, Katz M, Heenbanda SR et al. Nitric oxide synthase inhibitor NG-monomethyl-L-arginine preserves sperm motility after swim-up. *Fertil Steril* 1996;66:830–833.

32. Linder MC. *Nutritional biochemistry and metabolism, with clinical applications,* 2nd ed. East Norwalk, CT: Appleton & Lange, 1991.

33. Christianson G, Mowry J, Kirk M. Hyperkalemia following accidental L-arginine ingestion. Abstract presented at the North American Congress of Clinical Toxicology, September 13–18, 2000. *Clin Tox* 2000;38:523.

34. Gerard JM, Luisiri A. A fatal dose of arginine hydrochloride. *J Tox Clin Tox* 1997;35:621–625.

ARNICA

1. European Scientific Cooperative on Phytotherapy (ESCOP). *Monographs on the medicinal use of plant drugs. Arnicae flos (arnica flower).* Exeter, UK, 1997.

2. Bisset NG, Wichtl M. *Herbal drugs and phytopharmaceuticals: a handbook for practice on a scientific basis with reference to German Commission E monographs.* CRC Press, 1994:83–87.

3. Ernst E, Pittler MH. Efficacy of homeopathic arnica: a systematic review of placebo-controlled clinical trials. *Arch Surg* 1998;133:1187–1190.

4. Hildebrandt G, Eltze C. Über die Wirksamkeit verschiedener Potenzen von Arnica beim experimentell erzeugten Muskelkater. *Erfahrungsheilkunde* 1984;7:430–435.

5. Pinsent RJFM, Baker GPI, Ives G et al. Does arnica reduce pain and bleeding after dental extraction? *Midland Homeopathy Res Group Newslett* 1984;11:71–72.

6. Tveiten D, Bruseth S, Borchgrevink CF et al. Effect of arnica D30 on hard physical exercise: a double-blind controlled trial during the Oslo Marathon. *Tidsskr Nor Loegeforen* 1991; 111:3630–3631.

7. Kaziro GSN. Metronidazole (Flagyl) and *Arnica montana* in the prevention of post-surgical complications: a comparative placebo-controlled clinical trial. *Br J Oral Maxillofac Surg* 1984;22:42–49.

8. Gibson J. Haslam Y, Laurneson L et al. Double-blind trial of arnica in acute trauma patients. *Homeopathy* 1991;41:54–55.

9. Savage RH, Roe PF. A further double-blind trial to assess the benefit of *Arnica montana* in acute stroke illness. *Br Homoeopathic J* 1978;67:211–222.

10. Campbell A. Two pilot controlled trials of *Arnica montana*. *Br Homeopathic J* 1976;65:154–158.

11. Ernst E, Barnes J. Are homeopathic remedies effective for delayed-onset muscle soreness? A systematic review of placebo-controlled trials. *Perfusion* 1998;11:4–8.

12. Jawara N, Lewith GT, Vickers AJ et al. Homeopathic Arnica and Rhus toxicodendron for delayed onset muscle soreness. *Br Homeopathic J* 1997;46:10–15.

13. Hart O, Mule MA, Lewith G et al. Double-blind, placebo-controlled, randomized clinical trial of homoeopathic arnica C30 for pain and infection after total abdominal hysterectomy. *J R Soc Med* 1997;90:73–78.

14. Lüdtke R, Wilkens J. Arnica 30DH after knee surgery—three randomized double-blind clinical trials. FACT: Focus on Alternative and Complementary Therapies 1998;3:190(abst no 38). Presented at the 5th annual symposium on Complementary Health Care, Exeter, UK, December 10–12, 1998.

15. Moog-Schulze JB. Ein medisch experimenteel onderzoek naar de werkzaamheden van een uitwendige toepassing van Arnica-gelei. *Tijdschr Integr Geneeskunde* 1993;9:105–112.

16. Topliff A, Grande G. Significant toxicity after the ingestion of arnica. *J Tox Clin Tox* 2000;38:518

17. Lewis RA. *Lewis' Dictionary of Toxicology*, 1998. CRC Press, Boca Raton.

18. Newall CA, Anderson LA, Phillipson JD. *Herbal medicines: a guide for health care professionals.* London: Pharmaceutical Press, 1996.

19. Hausen BM. Sesquiterpene lactones—*Arnica montana*. In: De Smet PAGM, Keller K, Hänsel R, eds. *Adverse effects of herbal drugs,* vol 1. Berlin: Springer-Verlag, 1992:237–242.

ASHWAGANDHA

1. Duke JA. *CRC handbook of medicinal herbs.* Boca Raton, FL: CRC Press, 1985:514–515.

2. Shohat B, Shaltiel A, Ben-Bassat M et al. The effect of withaferin A, a natural steroidal lactone, on the fine structure of S-180 tumor cells. *Cancer Lett* 1976;2:71–78.

3. Devi PU, Akagi K, Ostapenko V et al. Withaferin A: a new radiosensitizer from the Indian medicinal plant *Withania somnifera*. *Int J Radiat Biol* 1996;69:193–197.

4. Devi PU, Sharada AC, Solomon FE. In vivo growth inhibitory effect of *Withania somnifera* (Ashwagandha) on a transplantable mouse tumor, sarcoma 180. *Indian J Exp Biol* 1992;30:169–172.

5. Sharada AC, Solomon FE, Devi PU et al. Antitumor and radiosensitizing effects of withaferin A on mouse Ehrlich ascites carcinoma in vivo. *Acta Oncol* 1996;35:95–100.

6. Devi PU, Akagi K, Ostapenko V et al. Withaferin A: a new radiosensitizer from the Indian medicinal plant *Withania somnifera*. *Int J Radiat Biol* 1996;69(2):193–197.

7. Das H, Dutta SK, Bhattacharya B et al. Antineoplastic agents from plants antitumor activity of withanolide D. *Indian J Cancer Chemotherapy* 1985;7:59–65.

8. Devi PU, Sharada AC, Solomon FE et al. In vivo growth inhibitory effect of *Withania somnifera* (Ashwagandha) on a transplantable mouse tumor, sarcoma 180. *Indian J Exp Biol* 1992;30:169–172.

9. Singh N, Singh SP, Nath R et al. Prevention of urethane-induced lung adenomas by *Withania somnifera (L.) Dunal* in albino mice. *Int J Crude Drug Res* 1986;24:90–100.

10. Upton R, ed. *Ashwagandha root.* Santa Cruz, CA: American Herbal Pharmacopoeia, 2000.

11. Al-Hindawi MK, Al-Khafaji SH, Abdul-Nabi MH. Anti-granuloma activity of Iraqi *Withania somnifera*. *J Ethnopharmacol* 1992;37:113–116.

12. Choudhary MI, Dur-E-Shahwar, Parveen Z et al. Antifungal steroidal lactones from *Withania somnifera Dunal* coagulance. *Phytochemistry* 1995;40:1243–1246.

13. Dhuley JN. Therapeutic efficacy of Ashwagandha against experimental aspergillosis in mice. *Immunopharmacol Immunotoxicol* 1998;20:191–198.

14. Panda S, Kar A. Changes in thyroid hormone concentrations after administration of ashwagandha root extract to adult male mice. *J Pharm Pharmacol* 1998;50:1065–1068.

15. Panda S, Kar A. Evidence for free radical scavenging activity of Ashwagandha root powder in mice. *Indian J Physiol Pharmacol* 1997;41:424–426.

16. Dhuley JN. Effect of Ashwagandha on lipid peroxidation in stress-induced animals. *J Ethnopharmacol* 1998;60:173–178.

17. Schliebs R, Liebmann A, Bhattacharya SK et al. Systemic administration of defined extracts from *Withania somnifera* (Indian ginseng) and Shilajit differentially affects cholinergic but not glutamatergic and GABAergic markers in rat brain. *Neurochem Int* 1997;30:181–190.

18. Sharada AC, Solomon FE, Devi, PU. Toxicity of *Withania somnifera* root extract in rats and mice. *Int J Pharmacog* 1993; 31:205–212.

ASPARTATE

1. Linder MC. *Nutritional biochemistry and metabolism, with clinical applications,* 2nd ed. East Norwalk, CT: Appleton & Lange, 1991.

2. Martino RL, Fleming TR, Morrell LM et al. Phase II trial of low-dose N-(phosphonacetyl)-disodium L-aspartic acid and high-dose 24-hour infusional 5-fluorouracil in advanced gastric adenocarcinoma: A Southwest Oncology Group study. *Invest New Drugs* 1996;14:419–421.

3. Ardalan B, Ucar A, Reddy R et al. Phase I trial of low dose N-phosphonacetyl-L-aspartic acid and high dose 5-fluorouracil administered concomitantly with radiation therapy for unresectable localized adenocarcinoma of the pancreas. *Cancer* 1994;74:1869–1873.

4. Langer CJ, Schaebler D, Sauter E et al. Phase II study of N-phosphonacetyl-L-aspartate, recombinant interferon-alpha, and fluorouracil infusion in advanced squamous cell carcinoma of the head and neck. *Head Neck* 1998;20: 385–391.

5. Kohne CH, Harstrick A, Hiddemann W et al. Modulation of 5-fluorouracil with methotrexate and low-dose N-(phosphonacetyl)-L-aspartate in patients with advanced colorectal cancer. Results of a phase II study. *Eur J Cancer* 1997;33: 1896–1899.

6. Harstrick A, Kohne CH, Hiddemann W et al. Modulation of 5-flourouracil with methotrexate and low-dose N-(phosphonacetyl)-L-aspartate (PALA) is inactive in advanced pancreatic carcinoma. *Ann Oncol* 1997;8:917–918.

References

7. Jodrell DI, Oster W, Kerr DJ et al. A phase I-II study of N-(phosphonacetyl)-L-aspartic acid (PALA) added to 5-fluorouracil and folinic acid in advanced colorectal cancer. *Eur J Cancer* 1994;30A:950–955.

8. Nassim MA, Rouini MR, Cripps MC et al. Effects of PALA on the pharmacokinetics of 5-fluorouracil. *Oncol Rep* 1998;5:217–221.

9. Steed DL, Ricotta JJ, Prendergast JJ et al. Promotion and acceleration of diabetic ulcer healing by arginine-glycine-aspartic acid (RGD) peptide matrix. RGD Study Group. *Diabetes Care* 1995;18:39–46.

10. Hansbrough JF, Herndon DN, Heimbach DM et al. Accelerated healing and reduced need for grafting in pediatric patients with burns treated with arginine-glycine-aspartic acid peptide matrix. RGD Study Group. *J Burn Care Rehabil* 1995;16:377–387.

11. Sener AI, Ceylan ME, Koyuncuoglu H. Comparison of the suppressive effects of L-aspartic acid and chlorpromazine + diazepam treatments on opiate abstinence syndrome signs in men. *Arzneimittelforschung* 1986;36:1684–1686.

12. Koyuncuoglu H. The treatment with L-aspartic acid of persons addicted to opiates. *Bull Narc* 1983;35:11–15.

13. Kircheis G, Nilius R, Held C et al. Therapeutic efficacy of L-ornithine-L-aspartate infusions in patients with cirrhosis and hepatic encephalopathy: results of a placebo-controlled, double-blind study. *Hepatology* 1997;25:1351–1360.

14. Stauch S, Kircheis G, Adler G et al. Oral L-ornithine-L-aspartate therapy of chronic hepatic encephalopathy: results of a placebo-controlled double-blind study. *J Hepatol* 1998;28:856–864.

15. Baal MG, Gabreels FJ, Renier WO et al. A patient with pyruvate carboxylase deficiency in the liver: treatment with aspartic acid and thiamine. *Dev Med Child Neurol* 1981;23(4):521–530.

16. Mertz PM, Davis SC, Franzen L et al. Effects of an arginine-glycine-aspartic acid peptide-containing artificial matrix on epithelial migration in vitro and experimental second-degree burn wound healing in vivo. *J Burn Care Rehabil* 1996;17:199–206.

17. Cooper ML, Hansbrough JF, Polarek JW. The effect of an arginine-glycine-aspartic acid peptide and hyaluronate synthetic matrix on epithelialization of meshed skin graft interstices. *J Burn Care Rehabil* 1996;17:108–116.

18. Todd JH, Hottendorf GH. Poly-l-aspartic acid protects cultured human proximal tubule cells against aminoglycoside-induced electrophysiological alterations. *Toxicol Lett* 1997;90:217–221.

19. Hulka GF, Prazma J, Brownlee RE et al. Use of poly-l-aspartic acid to inhibit aminoglycoside cochlear ototoxicity. *Am J Otol* 1993;14:352–356.

20. Goligorsky MS, Noiri E, Kessler H et al. Therapeutic effect of arginine-glycine-aspartic acid peptides in acute renal injury. *Clin Exp Pharmacol Physiol* 1998;25:276–279.

21. Leopold CS, Friend DR. In vivo pharmacokinetic study for the assessment of poly(L-aspartic acid) as a drug carrier for colon-specific drug delivery. *J Pharmacokinet Biopharm* 1995;23:397–406.

22. Schieber A, Bruckner H, Rupp-Classen M et al. Evaluation of D-amino acid levels in rat by gas chromatography-selected ion monitoring mass spectrometry: no evidence for subacute toxicity of orally fed D-proline and D-aspartic acid. *J Chromatogr B Biomed Sci Appl* 1997;691:1–12.

23. Stegink LD. Absorption, utilization, and safety of aspartic acid. *J Toxicol Environ Health* 1976;2:215–242.

ASTRAGALUS

1. Qun L, Luo Q, Zhang ZY et al. Effects of astragalus on IL-2/IL-2R system in patients with maintained hemodialysis. *Clin Nephrol* 1999;52:333–334.

2. Upton R (ed.). *Astragalus root.* Santa Cruz, CA: American Herbal Pharmacopoeia, 1999.

3. Hong CY, Ku J, Wu P. *Astragalus membranaceus* stimulates human sperm motility in vitro. *Am J Chin Med* 1992;20:289–294.

4. Zhang R, Qian J, Yang G et al. Medicinal protection with Chinese herb-compound against radiation damage. *Aviat Space Environ Med* 1990;61:729–731.

5. Lau BH, Ruckle HC, Botolazzo T et al. Chinese medicinal herbs inhibit growth of murine renal cell carcinoma. *Cancer Biother* 1994;9:153–161.

6. Chu DT, Lepe-Zuniga J, Wong WL et al. Fractionated extract of *Astragalus membranaceus*, a Chinese medicinal herb, potentiates LAK cell cytotoxicity generated by a low dose of recombinant interleukin-2. *J Clin Lab Immunol* 1988;26:183–187.

7. Chu DT, Wong WL, Mavligit GM. Immunotherapy with Chinese medicinal herbs. I. Immune restoration of local xenogeneic graft-versus-host reaction in cancer patients by fractionated *Astragalus membranaceus* in vitro. *J Clin Lab Immunol* 1988;25:119–123.

8. Chu DT, Wong WL, Mavligit GM. Immunotherapy with Chinese medicinal herbs. II. Reversal of cyclophosphamide-induced immune suppression by administration of fractionated *Astragalus membranaceus* in vivo. *J Clin Lab Immunol* 1988;25:125–129.

9. Li Y, Liu X, Xue SZ. Antidotal effect of glucoside extracted from *Astragalus membranaceus* on dimethoate intoxication in guinea pigs. *Med Lav* 1998;89(Suppl 2):S136–141.

10. Khoo KS, Ang PT. Extract of *Astragalus membranaceus* and Ligustrum lucidum does not prevent cyclophosphamide-induced myelosuppression. *Singapore Med J* 1995;36:387–390.

11. Vickers A, Goyal N, Harland R et al. Do certain countries produce only positive results? A systematic review of controlled trials. *Controlled Clin Trials* 1998;19:159–166.

12. Foster S, Varro I. *Tyler's honest herbal: a sensible guide to the use of herbs and related remedies,* 4th ed. New York: Haworth Herbal Press, 1999.

BEARBERRY

1. Paper DH, Koehler J, Franz G. Bioavailability of drug preparations containing a leaf extract of *Arctostaphylos uva-ursi* (L.) SPRENGL. (Uvae ursi folium). *Pharm Pharmacol Lett* 1993;3:63–66.

2. Schulz V, Hansel R, Tyler VE. *Rational phytotherapy: a physician's guide to herbal medicine,* 3rd ed. Berlin: Springer-Verlag, 1998:66–72.

3. European Scientific Cooperative on Phytotherapy (ESCOP). *Monographs on the medicinal use of plant drugs. Uvae ursi folium (bearberry leaf).* Exeter, UK, 1997.

4. Larsson B, Jonasson A, Fianu S. Prophylactic effect of UVA-E in women with recurrent cystitis: a preliminary report. *Curr Ther Res* 1993;53:441–443.

5. Mills S, Bone K. *Principles and practice of phytotherapy.* Edinburgh, NY: Churchill Livingstone, 2000:280–285.

6. Annuk H, Hirmo S, Turi E et al. Effect on cell surface

hydrophobicity and susceptibility of Helicobacter pylori to medicinal plant extracts. *FEMS Microbiol Lett* 1999;172:41–45.

7. Lewis RA. *Lewis' dictionary of toxicology.* Boca Raton FL: CRC Press, 1998:582.

8. Newall CA, Anderson LA, Phillipson JD. *Herbal medicines: a guide for health care professionals.* London: Pharmaceutical Press, 1996.

9. Matsuda H, Nakamura S, Tanaka T et al. [Pharmacological studies on leaf of *Arctostaphylos uva-ursi (L.) Spreng.* V. Effect of water extract from *Arctostaphylos uva-ursi (L.) Spreng.* (bearberry leaf) on the antiallergic and antiinflammatory activities of dexamethasone ointment]. *Yakugaku Zasshi* 1992;112:673–677.

10. Tilford GL. *Edible and medicinal plants of the west.* Missoula, MT: Mountain Press, 1997.

BETAINE

1. Chambers ST, Lever M. Betaines and urinary tract infections. *Nephron* 1996;74:1–10.

2. Miglio F, Rovati LC, Santoro A et al. Efficacy and safety of oral betaine glucuronate in non-alcoholic steatohepatitis. A double-blind, randomized, parallel-group, placebo-controlled prospective clinical study. *Arzneimittelforschung* 2000;50:722–727.

3. *Taber's encyclopedic medical dictionary,* 18th ed. Philadelphia : FA Davis Company, 1997:214.

4. Walter JH, Wraith JE, White FJ et al. Strategies for the treatment of cystathionine beta-synthase deficiency: the experience of the Willink Biochemical Genetics Unit over the past 30 years. *Eur J Ped* 1998;157(Suppl 2):S71–76.

5. Shils ME, Olson JA, Shike M et al, eds. *Modern nutrition in health and disease,* 9th ed. Philadelphia, PA: Lippincott Williams & Wilkins, 1999:1037.

6. Van Guldener C, Janssen MJ, de Meer K et al. Effect of folic acid and betaine on fasting and postmethionine-loading plasma homocysteine and methionine levels in chronic haemodialysis patients. *J Intern Med* 1999;245:175–183.

7. Bostom AG, Shemin D, Nadeau MR et al. Short term betaine therapy fails to lower elevated fasting total plasma homocysteine concentrations in hemodialysis patients maintained on chronic folic acid supplementation. *Atherosclerosis* 1995;113:129–132.

8. Barak AJ, Beckenhauer HC, Tuma DJ. Betaine, ethanol, and the liver: a review. *Alcohol* 1996;13:395–398.

9. Barak AJ, Beckenhauer HC, Badakhah S et al. The effect of betaine in reversing alcoholic steatosis. *Alcohol Clin Exp Res* 1997;21:1100–1102.

10. Wettstein M, Haussinger D. Cytoprotection by the osmolytes betaine and taurine in ischemia—reoxygenation injury in the perfused rat liver. *Hepatology* 1997;26:1560–1566.

11. Junnila M, Barak AJ, Beckenhauer HC et al. Betaine reduces hepatic lipidosis induced by carbon tetrachloride in Sprague-Dawley rats. *Vet Hum Toxicol* 1998;40:263–266.

12. Murakami T, Nagamura Y, Hirano K. The recovering effect of betaine on carbon tetrachloride-induced liver injury. *J Nutr Sci Vitaminol (Tokyo)* 1998;44:249–255.

13. Peddie BA, Chambers ST. Effects of betaines and urine on the antibacterial activity of aminoglycosides. *J Antimicrob Chemother* 1993;31:481–488.

14. Shulman A. Toxicological problems of traditional remedies and food supplements. *Int J Altern Complement Med* 1997;(Jan):9–10.

15. Fowler JF, Fowler LM, Hunter JE. Allergy to cocamidopropyl betaine may be due to amidoamine: a patch test and product use test study. *Contact Dermatitis* 1997;37:276–281.

16. Herlofson BB, Barkvoll P. Oral mucosal desquamation caused by two toothpaste detergents in an experimental model. *Eur J Oral Sci* 1996;104:21–26.

17. Herlofson BB, Barkvoll P. The effect of two toothpaste detergents on the frequency of recurrent aphthous ulcers. *Acta Odontol Scand* 1996;54:150–153.

18. Soderling E, Le Bell A, Kirstila V et al. Betaine-containing toothpaste relieves subjective symptoms of dry mouth. *Acta Odontol Scand* 1998;56:65–69.

19. Lever M, Sizeland PC, Bason LM et al. Abnormal glycine betaine content of the blood and urine of diabetic and renal patients. *Clin Chim Acta* 1994;230:69–79.

20. Dellow WJ, Chambers ST, Lever M et al. Elevated glycine betaine excretion in diabetes mellitus patients is associated with proximal tubular dysfunction and hyperglycemia. *Diab Res Clin Pract* 1999;43:91–99.

BETEL

1. Morton JF. Widespread tannin intake via stimulants and masticatories, especially guarana, kola nut, betel vine, and accessories. In: Hemingway RW, Laks PE, eds. *Plant polyphenols.* New York: Plenum, 1992:739–765.

2. Trivedy C, Baldwin D, Warnalulasuriya S et al. Copper content in *Areca catechu* (betel nut) products and oral submucous fibrosis. *Lancet* 1997;349:1447–1448.

3. Chu NS. Effects of betel chewing on the central and autonomic nervous systems. *J Biomed Sci* 2001;8:229–236.

4. Chu NS. Neurological aspects of areca and betel chewing. *Addict Biol* 2002;7:111–114.

5. Wyatt TA. Betel nut chewing and selected psychophysiological variables. *Psychol Rep* 1996;79:451–463.

6. Sullivan R, Allen JS, Otto C et al. Effects of chewing betel nut (*Areca catechu*) on the symptoms of people with schizophrenia in Palau, Micronesia. *Br J Psychiatry* 2000;177:174–178.

7. Kapadia GH, Chung EB, Ghosh B et al. Carcinogenicity of some folk medicinal herbs in rats. *J Natl Cancer Inst* 1978;60:683–686.

8. Deng JF, Ger J, Tsai WJ et al. Acute toxicities of betel nut: rare but probably overlooked events. *J Toxicol Clin* 2001;39:355–360.

9. Hung DZ; Deng JF. Acute myocardial infarction temporally related to betel nut chewing. *Vet Hum Toxicol* 1998;40:25–28.

10. Taylor RFH, Al-Jarad N, John LME. Betel-nut chewing and asthma. *Lancet* 1992;339:1134–1136.

11. Tsai JF, Chuang LY, Jeng JE et al. Betel quid chewing as a risk factor for hepatocellular carcinoma: a case-control study. *Br J Cancer* 2001;84:709–713.

12. Thomas SJ, MacLenna R. Slaked lime and betel nut cancer in Papua New Guinea. *Lancet* 1992;340:577–578.

13. Chen CL, Chi CW, Chang KW et al. Safrole-like DNA adducts in oral tissue from oral cancer patients with a betel quid chewing history. *Carcinogenesis* 1999;20:2331–2334.

14. Norton SA. Betel: consumption and consequences. *J Am Acad Dermatol* 1998;38:81–88.

15. Chu NS. Betel chewing increases the skin temperature: effects of atropine and propranolol. *Neurosci Lett* 1995;194:130–132.

16. Deahl M. Betel nut-induced extrapyramidal syndrome: an unusual drug interaction. *Move Disord* 1989;4:330–333.

References

17. Pickwell SM, Schmelpfening, Palinkas LA. Betelmania: betel quid chewing by Cambodian women in the United States and its potential health effects. *West J Med* 1994;160:326–330.
18. Padma PR, Lalitha VS, Amonkar AJ et al. Anticarcinogenic effect of betel leaf extract against tobacco carcinogens. *Cancer Lett* 1989;45:195–202.
19. Liao Y-L, Chiang Y-C, Tsai T-F et al. Contact leukomelanosis induced by the leaves of Piper betle L. (Piperaceae): a clinical and histopathologic survey. *J Am Acad Dermatol* 1999; 40:583–589.

BILBERRY

1. Schulz V, Hansel R, Tyler VE. *Rational phytotherapy: a physician's guide to herbal medicine,* 3rd ed. Berlin: Springer-Verlag, 1998:66–72.
2. Bisset NG, Wichtl M. *Herbal drugs and phytopharmaceuticals: a handbook for practice on a scientific basis with reference to German Commission E monographs,* Boca Raton, FL: CRC Press, 1994.
3. Bailey CJ, Day C. Traditional plant medicines as treatments for diabetes. *Diabetes Care* 1989;12:553–564.
4. Mills S, Bone K. *Principles and practice of phytotherapy.* Edinburgh: Churchill Livingstone, 2000:280–285.
5. Muth ER, Laurent JM, Jasper P. The effect of bilberry nutritional supplementation on night visual acuity and contrast sensitivity. *Altern Med Rev* 2000;5:164–173.
6. Colombo D, Vescovini R. [Studio clinico controllato sull'efficacia degli antocianosidi del mirtillo nel trattamento della dismenorrea esseziale.] *Giorn Ital Ostet Ginecol* 1985;7: 1033–1038.
7. Allen FM. Blueberry leaf extract: physiologic and clinical properties in relation to carbohydrate metabolism. *JAMA* 1927;89:1577–1581.
8. Laplaud PM, Lelubre A, Chapman MJ. Antioxidant action of *Vaccinium myrtillus* extract on human low density lipoproteins in vitro: initial observations. *Fundam Clin Pharmacol* 1997;11:35–40.
9. Cignarella A, Nastasi M, Cavalli E et al. Novel lipid-lowering properties of *Vaccinium myrtillus* L. leaves, a traditional antidiabetic treatment, in several models of rat dyslipidaemia: a comparison with ciprofibrate. *Throm Res* 1996;84: 311–322.
10. Bever BO, Zahnd GR. Plants with oral hypoglycemic action. *Q J Crude Drug Res* 1979;17:139–196.

BIOTIN

1. Dakshinamurti K. Biotin. In: Shils ME, Olson JA, Shike M, eds. *Modern nutrition in health and disease,* 8th ed. Baltimore: Williams & Wilkins, 1994.
2. Weinsier RL, Morgan SL. *Fundamentals of clinical nutrition.* St. Louis: Mosby, 1993.
3. Zempleni J, Mock DM. Bioavailability of biotin given orally to humans in pharmacologic doses. *Am J Clin Nutr* 1999;69: 504–508.
4. Colombo VE, Gerber F, Bronhofer M et al. Treatment of brittle fingernails and onychoschizia with biotin: scanning electron microscopy. *J Am Acad Dermatol* 1990;23: 1127–1132.
5. Zempleni J. Biotin. In: Bowman BA, Russell RM, eds. *Present knowledge in nutrition,* 8th ed. Washington, DC: International Life Sciences Institute Press, 2001:241–252.
6. Linder MC. *Nutritional biochemistry and metabolism, with clinical applications,* 2nd ed. East Norwalk, CT: Appleton & Lange, 1999:122–123.
7. Zempleni J, Mock DM. Marginal biotin deficiency is teratogenic. *Proc Soc Exp Biol Med* 2000;223:14–21.
8. Mock DM. Biotin. In: Ziegler EE, Filer LJ, eds. *Present knowledge in nutrition,* 7th ed. Washington, DC: International Life Sciences Institute Press, 1996.

BLACK COHOSH

1. Beuscher N. *Cimicifuga racemosa.* Die Traubensilberkerze. *Zeitschrift fur Phytoterapie* 1995;16:301–310. Translated in *Q Rev Nat Med* 1996;(Spring):19–27.
2. Kennelly EJ, Baggett S, Nuntanakorn P et al. Formononetin levels in thirteen populations of black cohosh. *Altern Ther* 2001;7:S18(abst).
3. Kruse SO, Lohning A, Pauli GF et al. Fukiic and piscidic acid esters from the rhizome of *Cimicifuga racemosa* and the in vitro estrogenic activity of fukinolic acid. *Planta Med* 1999; 65:763–764.
4. Mills S, Bone K. *Principles and practice of phytotherapy.* Edinburgh, NY: Churchill Livingstone, 2000:303–309.
5. Genazzani E, Sorrentino L. Vascular action of acteina: active constituent of Actaea racemosa L. *Nature* 1962;194:544–545.
6. Jacobson JS, Troxel AB, Evans J et al. Randomized trial of black cohosh for the treatment of hot flashes among women with a history of breast cancer. *J Clin Oncol* 2001;19: 2739–2745.
7. Lehmann-Willenbrock E, Riedel H. Klinische und endokrinologische Untersuchengen zur Therapie ovarieller Ausfallserscheinungen nach Hysterektomie unter Belassung der Adnexe (Clinical and endocrinological examinations concerning therapy of climacteric symptoms following hysterectomy with remaining ovaries). *Zentralblatt fur Gynakologie* 1988;110:611–618.
8. Stoll W. Phytotherapeutikum beeinflusst atrophisches Vaginalepithel: Doppelblindversuch Cimicifuga vs. Östrogenpräparat (Phytotherapy influences atrophic vaginal epithelium—double-blind study—Cimicifuga vs. estrogenic substances). *Therapeutikon* 1987;1:23–31.
9. Warnecke, G. Beeinflussung klimakterischer Beschwerden durch ein Phytotherapeutikum: Erfolgreiche therapie mit Cimicifuga-Monoextrakt (Influence of phytotherapy on menopausal syndrome: successful treatments with monoextract of cimicifuga). *Medizinische Welt* 1985;36:871–874.
10. Liske E. Therapeutic efficacy and safety of *Cimicifuga racemosa* in gynecologic disorders. *Adv Ther* 1998;15:45–53.
11. Liske E, Wüstenberg P. Therapy of climacteric complaints with *Cimicifuga racemosa*: herbal medicine with clinically proven evidence. *Menopause* 1998;5:250(abst)
12. Duker E-M, Kopanski L, Jarry H et al. Effects of extracts from *Cimicifuga racemosa* on gonadotropin release in menopausal women and ovariectomized rats. *Planta Med* 1991;57: 420–424.
13. Gunn TR, Wright IM. The use of black and blue cohosh in labour. *N Z Med J* 1996;109:410–411.
14. Liu Z, Yang Z, Zhu M et al. [Estrogenicity of black cohosh (*Cimicifuga racemosa*) and its effect on estrogen receptor level in human breast cancer MCF-7 cells]. (in Chinese). *Wei Sheng Yan Jiu* 2001;30:77–80.
15. Eagon PK, Swafford DS, Elm MS et al. Estrogenicity of medicinal botanicals. *Proc Am Assoc Cancer Res* 1998;(March): 39(abstr no 2624).

16. Einer-Jensen N, Zhao J, Anderson KP et al. Cimicifuga and Melbrosia lack oestrogenic effects in mice and rats. *Maturitas* 1996;25:149–153.

17. Amato P, Cristophe S, Mellon PL. Estrogenic activity of herbs commonly used as remedies for menopausal symptoms. *Menopause* 2002;9:145–150.

18. Liu J, Burdette JE, Xu H et al. Evaluation of estrogenic activity of plant extracts for the potential treatment of menopausal symptoms. *J Agric Food Chem* 2001;49:2472–2479.

19. Zierau O, Bodinet C, Kolbas et al. Antiestrogenic activities of *Cimicifuga racemosa* extracts. *J Ster Biochem Mol Biol* 2002;80:125–130.

20. Zava DT, Dollbaum CM, Blen M. Estrogen and progestin bioactivity of foods, herbs, and spices. *Proc Soc Exp Biol Med* 1998;217:369–378.

21. Nesselhut T, Schellhas C, Deitrich R et al. [Studies on mammary carcinoma cells regarding the proliferative potential of herbal medications with estrogen-like effects]. (in German). *Arch Gynecol Obstet* 1993;817–818.

22. Dixon-Shanies D, Shaikh N. Growth inhibition of human breast cancer cells by herbs and phytoestrogens. *Oncol Rep* 1999;6(6)1383–1387.

23. Freudenstein J, Bodinet C. *Influence of an isopropanolic aqueous extract of Cimicifugae racemosae rhizoma on the proliferation of MCF-7 cells*. Presentation at International LOF symposium on phytoestrogens, University of Gent, Belgium, January 15, 1999.

24. Löhning A, Verspohl EJ, Winterhoff H. *Cimicifuga racemosa*: in vitro findings using MCF-7 cells. *Phytopharmakaforschung* 2000;1998:72(abst no P07).

25. Freudenstein J, Dasenbrock C, Nissein T. Lack of promotion of estrogen dependent mammary gland tumors in vivo by an isopropanolic black cohosh extract. *Phytomedicine* 2000; Suppl II (7):13.

26. Nesselhut T, Liske E. Pharmacological measures in postmenopausal women with an isopropanolic aqueous extract of Cimicifugae racemosae rhizoma. *Menopause* 1999;6:331(abst P-8).

27. Georgiev DB, Iordanova E. Phytoestrogens—the alternative approach. *Maturitas* 1987;27(Suppl):213(abst P309).

BLACK HAW

1. Upton R, ed. *Cramp bark (Viburnum opulus)*. Santa Cruz, CA: American Herbal Pharmacopeia, 2000.

2. Upton R, ed. *Black haw bark (Viburnum prunifolium)*. Santa Cruz, CA: American Herbal Pharmacopeia, 2000.

3. Evans WC. *Trease and Evans' pharmacognosy*, 14th ed. London: WB Saunders, 1996.

4. Bisset NG, Wichtl M. *Herbal drugs and phytopharmaceuticals: a handbook for practice on a scientific basis with reference to German Commission E monographs*, Boca Raton, FL: CRC Press, 1994.

5. McGuffin M, Hobbs C, Upton R et al. *American Herbal Products Association botanical safety handbook*. Boca Raton, FL: CRC Press, 1997.

BLOODROOT

1. Bruneton J. *Pharmacognosy: phytochemistry medicinal plants*, 2nd ed. Secaucus NJ: Lavoisier Springer-Verlag, 1999:917–918.

2. Lord G, Goldenthal EI, Meyer DL. Sanguinarine and the controversy concerning its relationship to glaucoma in epidemic dropsy. *J Clin Dent* 1989;1:110–115.

3. Cullinan MP, Powell RN, Faddy MJ et al. Efficacy of a dentifrice and oral rinse containing sanguinaria extract in conjunction with initial periodontal therapy. *Aust Dent J* 1997;42:47–51.

4. Kopczyk RA, Abrams H, Brown AT et al. Clinical and microbiological effects of a sanguinaria-containing mouthrinse and dentifrice with and without fluoride during 6 months of use. *J Periodontol* 1991;62:617–622.

5. Tenebaum H, Dahan J, Soell M. Effectiveness of a sanguinarine regimen after scaling and root planing. *J Periodontol* 1999;70:307–311.

6. Polson AM, Garrett S, Stoller NH et al. Multi-center comparative evaluation of subgingivally delivered sanguinarine and doxycycline in the treatment of periodontitis. II. Clinical results. *J Periodontol* 1997;68:119–126.

7. Polson AM, Stoller NH, Hanes PJ et al. 2 Multi-center trials assessing the clinical efficacy of 5% sanguinarine in a biodegradable drug delivery system. *J Clin Periodontol* 1996;23(8)782–788.

8. Harper DS, Mueller LJ, Fine JB et al. Clinical efficacy of a dentifrice and oral rinse containing sanguinaria extract and zinc chloride during 6 months of use. *J Periodontol* 1990;61:352–358.

9. Etemadzadeh H, Ainamo J. Lacking anti-plaque efficacy of 2 sanguinarine mouth rinses. *J Clin Periodontal* 1987;14:176–180.

10. Ahmad N, Gupta S, Husain MM et al. Differential antiproliferative and apoptotic response of sanguinarine for cancer cells versus normal cells. *Clin Cancer Res* 2000;6:1524–1528.

11. Seifen E, Adams RJ, Riemer RK. Sanguinarine: a positive inotropic alkaloid which inhibits cardiac Na+, K+-ATPase. *Eur J Pharmacol* 1979;60:373–377.

12. Agarwal S, Piesco NP, Peterson DE. Effects of sanguinaria, chlorhexidine and tetracycline on neutrophil viability and functions in vitro. *J Periodontal Res* 1997;32:335–344.

13. Godowski KC. Antimicrobial action of sanguinarine. *J Clin Dent* 1989;1:96–101.

14. Keller KA. Reproductive and developmental toxicological evaluation of sanguinaria extract. *J Clin Dent* 1989;1:59–66.

15. Becci PJ. Short-term toxicity studies of sanguinarine and of two alkaloid extracts of *Sanguinaria canadensis* L. *J Toxicol Environ Health* 1987;20:199–208.

16. Lewis WH, Elvin-Lewis MPF. *Medical botany*. New York: John Wiley and Sons, 1977:123–124.

17. Fell JW. *A treatise on cancer, and its treatment*. London: J Churchill, 1857.

18. Phelan JT, Juardo J. Chemosurgical management of carcinoma of the nose. *Surgery* 1963;53:310–314.

BLUE COHOSH

1. Duke JA. *Handbook of medicinal herbs*. Boca Raton: CRC Press, 2001:108.

2. Betz JM et al. Gas chromatographic determination of toxic quinolizidine alkaloids in blue cohosh. *Caulophyllum thalictroides*. *Phytochem Anal* 1998;9:232–236.

3. Tyler VE. *The honest herbal*. Binghamton NY: Haworth Press, 1993.

4. De Smet, PAGM. *Caulophyllum thalictroides*. In: De Smet PAGM,

References

Keller K, Hänsel R, Chandler RF, eds. *Adverse effects of herbal drugs,* vol 2. Berlin: Springer-Verlag, 1993:153–158.

5. Rao RB, Hoffman RS, Desiderio R et al. *Nicotinic toxicity from tincture of blue cohosh (Caulophyllum thalictroides) used as an abortifacient.* North American Congress on Clinical Toxicology, Sept. 9-15, 1998, Orlando, FL. Abstract 68.

6. Jones TK, Lawson BM. Profound neonatal congestive heart failure caused by maternal consumption of blue cohosh herbal medication. *J Pediatr* 1998;132:550–552.

7. Gunn TR, Wright IMR. The use of black and blue cohosh in labor. *N Z Med J* 1996;109:410–411.

8. Lewis WH, Elvin-Lewis MPF. *Medical botany.* New York: John Wiley and Sons, 1977.

9. McFarlin BL et al. A national survey of herbal preparation use by nurse-midwives for labor stimulation. Review of the literature and recommendations for practice. *J Nurse Midwifery* 1999;44:205–216.

10. Ortega JA, Lazerson J. Anagyrine-induced red cell aplasia, vascular anomaly, and skeletal dysplasia. *J Pediatr* 1987; 111:87–89.

BLUE-GREEN ALGAE

1. Carmichael WW. The toxins of cyanobacteria. *Sci Am* 1994; 1:78–86.

2. Thomas P, Stephens M, Wilkie G et al. (+)-Anatoxin-a is a potent agonist at neuronal nicotinic acetylcholine receptors. *J Neurochem* 1993;60:2308–2311.

3. Soliakov L, Gallagher T, Wonnacott S. Anatoxin-a-evoked (3H) dopamine release from rat striatal synaptosomes. *Neuropharmacology* 1995;34:1535–1541.

4. Ostensvik O, Skulberg OM, Underdal B et al. Antibacterial properties of extracts from selected planktonic freshwater cyanobacteria—a comparative study of bacterial bioassays. *J Appl Microbiol* 1998;84:1117–1124.

5. Hitzfeld BC, Höger SJ, Dietrich DR. Cyanobacterial toxins: removal during drinking water treatment, and human risk assessment. *Environ Health Perspect* 2000;108(Suppl 1): 113–122.

6. Elder GH, Hunter PR, Codd GA. Hazardous freshwater cyanobacteria (blue-green algae). *Lancet* 1993;341: 1519–1520.

7. Codd GA, Edwards C, Beattle KA et al. Fatal attraction to cyanobacteria? *Nature* 1992;359:110–111.

8. Papendorf O, Konig GM, Wright AD et al. Mueggelone, a novel inhibitor of fish development from the fresh water cyanobacterium Aphanizomenon flos-aquae. *J Nat Prod* 1997;60:1298–1300.

9. Rapala J, Sivonen K, Lyra C et al. Variation of microcystins, cyanobacterial hepatotoxins, in Anabaena spp. as a function of growth stimuli. *Appl Environ Microbiol* 1997;63: 2206–2212.

BOLDO

1. Speisky H, Cassels BK. Boldo and boldine: an emerging case of natural drug development. *Pharmacol Res* 1994;29:1–12.

2. European Scientific Cooperative on Phytotherapy (ESCOP). *Monographs on the medicinal use of plant drugs. Boldo folium (boldo).* Exeter, UK, 1996.

3. Tisserand R, Balacs T. *Essential oil safety: a guide for health care professionals.* Edinburgh, NY: Churchill Livingstone, 1995:123.

BORAGE

1. De Smet PAGM. *Borago officinalis.* In De Smet PAGM, Keller K, Hänsel R, Chandler RF (eds.) *Adverse effects of herbal drugs,* vol II. Berlin: Springer-Verlag, 1993:147–152.

2. Belch JJF, Ansell D, Madhok R et al. Effects of altering dietary essential fatty acids on requirements for non-steroidal anti-inflammatory drugs in patients with rheumatoid arthritis. *Ann Rheum Dis* 1988;47:96–104.

3. Henz BM, Jablonska S, van de Kerkhof PC et al. Double-blind, multicentre analysis of the efficacy of borage oil in patients with atopic eczema. *Br J Dermatol* 1999;140: 685–688.

4. Leventhal LJ, Boyce EG, Zurier RB. Treatment of rheumatoid arthritis with gamma-linolenic acid. *Ann Int Med* 1993;119: 867–873.

5. Bard JM, Luc G, Jude B et al. A therapeutic dosage (3 g/day) of borage oil supplementation has no effect on platelet aggregation in healthy volunteers. *Fundam Clin Pharmacol* 1997;11:143–144.

6. Betz JM, Eppley RM, Taylor WC et al. Determination of pyrrolizidine alkaloids in commercial comfrey products (Symphytum species). *J Pharm Sci* 1994;83:649–653.

7. Awang DVC. Borage. *Can Pharm J* 1990;123:121–126.

8. Phinney S. Potential risk of prolonged gamma-linolenic acid use. *Ann Int Med* 1994;120:692.

BORON

1. Nielsen FH. Ultratrace minerals. In Shils ME, Olson JA, Shike M et al, eds. *Modern nutrition in health and disease,* 9th ed. Baltimore: Williams & Wilkins 1999:169–192.

2. Nielsen FH. Other trace elements. In Ziegler EE, Filer LJ, eds. *Present knowledge in nutrition,* 7th ed. Washington, DC: International Life Sciences Institute Press, 1996.

3. Linder MC. *Nutritional biochemistry and metabolism, with clinical applications,* 2nd ed. East Norwalk, CT: Appleton & Lange, 1991:162–263.

4. Van Slyke KK, Michel VP, Rein MF. Treatment of vulvovaginal candidiasis with boric acid powder. *Am J Obstet Gynecol* 1981;141:145.

5. Nielsen FH. Biochemical and physiologic consequences of boron deprivation in humans. *Environ Health Perspec* 1994; 102(Suppl 7):59–63.

6. Meacham SL, Taper LJ, Volpe SL. Effects of boron supplementation on blood and urinary calcium, magnesium, and phosphorus, and urinary boron in athletic and sedentary women. *Am J Clin Nutr* 1995;61:341–345.

7. Meacham SL, Taper LJ, Volpe SL. Effects of boron supplementation on bone mineral density and dietary, blood, and urinary calcium, phosphorus, magnesium, and boron in female athletes. *Environ Health Perspect* 1994;102(Suppl 7): 79–82.

8. Hunt CD, Herbel JL, Nielsen FH. Metabolic responses of postmenopausal women to supplemental dietary boron and aluminum during usual and low magnesium intake: boron, calcium, and magnesium absorption and retention and blood mineral concentrations. *Am J Clin Nutr* 1997;65: 803–813.

9. Nielsen FH, Hunt CD, Mullen LM et al. Effect of dietary boron on mineral, estrogen and testosterone metabolism in post-menopausal women. *FASEB J* 1987;1:394–397.

10. Naghii MR, Samman S. The effect of boron supplementation on its urinary excretion and selected cardiovascular risk fac-

tors in healthy male subjects. *Biol Trace Elem Res* 1997;56: 273–286.

11. Newnham RE. Essentiality of boron for healthy bones and joints. *Environ Health Perspect* 1994;102(Suppl 7):83–85.

12. Travers RL, Rennie GC, Newnham RE. Boron and arthritis: the results of a double-blind pilot study. *J Nutr Med* 1990; 1:127–132.

13. Penland JG. Dietary boron, brain function, and cognitive performance. *Environ Health Perspect* 1994;102(Suppl 7): 65–72.

14. Green NR, Ferrando AA. Plasma boron and the effects of boron supplementation in males. *Environ Health Perspect* 1994;102:73–77.

15. Jovanovic R, Congema E, Nguyen HT. Antifungal agents vs. boric acid for treating chronic mycotic vulvovaginitis. *J Reprod Med* 1991;36:593–597.

16. McCoy H, Kenney MA, Montgomery C et al. Relation of boron to the composition and mechanical properties of bone. *Environ Health Perspect* 1994;102(Suppl 7):49–53.

BURDOCK

1. De Smet PAGM. Arctium species. In: De Smet PAGM, Keller K, Hänsel R, et al (eds.). *Adverse effects of herbal drugs*, vol II. Berlin: Springer-Verlag, 1993:141–146.

2. Hirose M, Yamaguchi T, Lin C et al. Effects of arctiin on PhIP-induced mammary, colon, and pnacreatic carcinogenesis in female Sprague-Dawley rats and MeIQx-induced hepatocarcinogenesis in male F344 rats. *Cancer Lett* 2000;155: 79–88.

3. Dombrádi CA, Földeák S. Screening report on the antitumor activity of purified *Arctium lappa* extracts. *Tumori* 1966;52: 173–176.

4. U.S. Congress, Office of Technology Assessment. *Unconventional cancer treatments*. Washington, DC: Superintendent of Documents, US Government Printing Office, September 1990; OTA-H-405.

5. Morita K, Kada T, Namiki M. A desmutagenic factor isolated from burdock (*Arctium lappa*). *Mutat Res* 1984;129:25–31.

6. Swanston-Flatt SK, Day C, Flatt PR et al. Glycaemic effects of traditional European plant treatments for diabetes: Studies in normal and streptozotocin diabetic mice. *Diabetes Res* 1989;10:69–73.

7. Bever BO, Zahnd GR. Plants with oral hypoglycemic action. *Q J Crude Drug Res* 1979;17:139–196.

8. Lin CC, Lu JM, Yang JJ et al. Anti-inflammatory and radical scavenge effects of *Arctium lappa*. *Am J Chin Med* 1996;24: 127–137.

9. Schulte KE, Rücker G, Boehme R. Polyacetylene als Inhaltstoffe der Klettenwurzeln. *Arzneimittelforschung* 1967;17: 829–833.

10. Tyler VE. *The honest herbal*. Binghamton, NY: Pharmaceutical Products Press, 1993.

11. Lin SC, Chung TC, Lin CC et al. Hepatoprotective effects of *Arctium lappa* on carbon tetrachloride- and acetaminophen-induced liver damage. *Am J Chin Med* 2000;28:163–173.

12. Rhoads PM, Tong TG, Banner W et al. Anticholinergic poisoning after the ingestion of burdock root tea. *J Toxicol* 1984–1985;22:581–584.

13. Bryson PD, Watanabe AS, Rumack AS et al. Burdock root tea poisoning: case report involving a commercial preparation. *JAMA* 1978;239:2157. (Also [Letter]. *JAMA* 1978;240: 1586).

14. Rodriguez P, Blanco J, Juste S et al. Allergic contact dermatitis due to burdock (*Arctium lappa*). *Contact Dermatitis* 1995;33:134–135.

CALCIUM

1. Weaver CM, Heaney RP. Calcium. In: Shils ME, Olson JA, Shike M et al, eds. *Modern nutrition in health and disease,* 9th ed. Baltimore: Williams & Wilkins, 1999:141–156.

2. Krall EA, Dawson-Hughes B. Osteoporosis. In: Shils ME, Olson JA, Shike M et al, eds. *Modern nutrition in health and disease,* 9th ed. Baltimore: Williams & Wilkins, 1999: 1353–1364.

3. Dawson-Hughes B, Harris SS, Krall EA et al. Effect of calcium and vitamin D supplementation on bone density in men and women 65 years of age or older. *N Engl J Med* 1997; 337:670–676.

4. Chapuy MC, Arlot ME, Duboeuf F et al. Vitamin D3 and calcium to prevent hip fractures in elderly women. *N Engl J Med* 1992;327:1637–1642.

5. Johnston CC Jr, Miller JZ, Slemenda CW et al. Calcium supplementation and increases in bone mineral density in children. *N Engl J Med* 1992;327:82–87.

6. Baron JA, Beach M, Mandel JS et al. for the Calcium Polyp Prevention Study Group. Calcium supplements for the prevention of colorectal adenomas. *N Engl J Med* 1999;340: 101–107.

7. Holt PR, Atillasoy EO, Gilman J et al. Modulation of abnormal colonic epithelial cell proliferation and differentiation by low-fat dairy foods. *JAMA* 1998;280:1074–1079.

8. Whelan RL, Horvath KD, Gleason NR. Vitamin and calcium supplement use is associated with decreased adenoma recurrence in patients with a previous history of neoplasia. *Dis Colon Rectum* 1999;42:212–217.

9. Hatton DC, McCarron DA. Dietary calcium and blood pressure in experimental models of hypertension. *Hypertension* 1994; 23:513–530.

10. Cutler JA, Brittain E. Calcium and blood pressure: an epidemiologic perspective. *Am J Hypertens* 1990;3:137S–146S.

11. Mikami H, Ogihara T, Tabuchi Y. Blood pressure response to dietary calcium intervention in humans. *Am J Hypertens* 1990;3:147S–151S.

12. Dwyer JH, Dwyer KM, Scribner RA et al. Dietary calcium, calcium supplementation and blood pressure in African American adolescents. *Am J Clin Nutr* 1998;68:648–655.

13. Atallah AN, Hofmeyr GJ, Duley L. Calcium supplementation during pregnancy for preventing hypertensive disorders and related problems. *Cochrane Database Syst Rev* 2000; 3: CD001059.

14. Yabes-Almirante C. Calcium supplementation in pregnancy to prevent pregnancy induced hypertension (PIH). *J Perinat Med* 1998;26:347–353.

15. Bucher HC, Guyatt GH, Cook RJ et al. Effect of calcium supplementation on pregnancy induced by hypertension and pre-eclampsia. *JAMA* 1996;275:1104–1112.

16. Levine RJ, Hauth JC, Curet LB et al. Trial of calcium to prevent preeclampsia. *N Engl J Med* 1997;337:69–76.

17. Herrera J, Arevalo-Herrera M, Herera S. Prevention of preeclampsia by linoleic acid and calcium supplementation: a randomized controlled trial. *Obstet Gynecol* 1998;91: 585–590.

18. Thys-Jacobs S, Starkey P, Bernstein D, Tian J. Calcium carbonate and the premenstrual syndrome: effects on premen-

References

strual and menstrual symptoms. Premenstrual Syndrome Study Group. *Am J Obstet Gynecol* 1998;179:444–452.

19. Vogel GL, Zhang Z, Carey CM et al. Composition of plaque and saliva following a sucrose challenge and use of an alpha-tricalcium-phosphate-containing chewing gum. *J Dent Res* 1998;77:518–524.

20. Singh N, Singh PN, Hershman JM. Effect of calcium carbonate on the absorption of levothyroxine. *JAMA* 2000;283:2822–2825.

21. Bourgoin BP, Evans DR, Cornett JR et al. Lead content in 70 brands of dietary calcium supplements. *Am J Pub Health* 1993;83:1155–1160.

22. Weaver CM, Heaney RP. Calcium. In: Shils ME, Olson JA, Shike M et al, eds. *Modern nutrition in health and disease,* 9th ed. Baltimore: Williams & Wilkins, 1999:141–156.

23. Curhan GC, Willett WC, Speizer FE et al. Comparison of dietary calcium with supplemental calcium and other nutrients as factors affecting the risk for kidney stones in women. *Ann Int Med* 1997;126:497–504.

24. Curhan GC, Willet WC, Rimm EB et al. A prospective study of dietary calcium and other nutrients and the risk of symptomatic kidney stones. *N Engl J Med* 1993;328:833–838.

25. Sowers MR, Jannausch M, Wood C et al. Prevalence of renal stones in a population-based study with dietary calcium, oxalate, and medication exposures. *Am J Epidemiol* 1998;147:914–920.

26. Rodgers AL. Effect of mineral water containing calcium and magnesium on calcium oxalate urolithiasis risk factors. *Urol Int* 1997;58:93–99.

27. Guillemant J, Le H-T, Accarie C et al. Mineral water as a source of dietary calcium: acute effects on parathyroid function and bone resorption in young men. *Am J Clin Nutr* 2000;71:999–1002.

28. Gossel TA. Calcium supplements. *US Pharmacist* 1991; (Apr):26–32.

29. Itoh R, Nishiyama N, Suyama Y. Dietary protein intake and urinary excretion of calcium: a cross-sectional study in a healthy Japanese population. *Am J Clin Nutr* 1998;67:438–444.

30. Matkovic V, Illich JZ, Andon MB, et al. Urinary calcium, sodium, and bone mass of young females. *Am J Clin Nutr* 1995;62:417–425.

CALENDULA

1. European Scientific Cooperative on Phytotherapy (ESCOP). *Monographs on the medicinal use of plant drugs. Calendulae flos (Calendula flower).* Exeter, UK, 1996.

2. Kalvatchev Z, Walder R, Garzaro D. Anti-HIV activity of extracts from *Calendula officinalis* flowers. *Biomed Pharmacother* 1997;51:176–180.

3. Gracza L. Oxygen-containing terpene derivatives from *Calendula officinalis. Planta Med* 1987;53:227.

4. Rawi SM, El-Gindy H, Abd-El-Kader A. New possible molluscicides from *Calendula micrantha officinalis* and Ammi majus. *Ecotox Environ Safety* 1996;35:261–267.

5. Patrick KFM, Kumar S, Edwardson PAD et al. Induction of vascularisation by an aqueous extract of the flowers of *Calendula officinalis* L. the European marigold. *Phytomedicine* 1996;3:11–18.

6. Schmidgall J, Schnetz E, Hensel A. Evidence for bioadhesive effects of polysaccharides and polysaccharide-containing herbs in an ex vivo bioadhesion assay on buccal membranes. *Planta Med* 2000;66:48–53.

7. Mascolo N, Autore G, Capasso F et al. Biological screening of Italian medicinal plants for antiinflammatory activity. *Phytother Res* 1987;1:28–31.

8. Della Loggia R, Becker H, Isaac O et al. Topical anti-inflammatory activity of *Calendula officinalis* extracts. *Planta Med* 1990;56:658.

9. Zitterl-Eglseer K, Sosa S, Jurenitsch J et al. Anti-oedematous activities of the main triterpendiol esters of marigold (*Calendula officinalis* L.). *J Ethnopharmacol* 1997;57:139–144.

10. Della Loggia R, Tubaro A, Sosa S et al. The role of triterpenoids in the topical anti-inflammatory activity of *Calendula officinalis* flowers. *Planta Med* 1994;60:516–520.

11. Newall CA, Anderson LA, Phillipson JD. *Herbal medicine: a guide for health-care professionals.* Pharmaceutical Press, London, 1996:58–59.

CAPSICUM

1. Surh YJ, Lee SS. Capsaicin in hot chili pepper: carcinogen, co-carcinogen or anticarcinogen? *Food Chem Toxicol* 1996;34:313–316.

2. Locock RA. Capsicum. *Can Pharm J* 1985;118:517–519.

3. Hautkappe M, Roizen MF, Toledano A et al. Review of the effectiveness of capsaicin for painful cutaneous disorders and neural dysfunction. *Clin J Pain* 1998;14:97–106.

4. Altman RD, Aven A, Holmburg CE et al. Capsaicin cream 0.025% as monotherapy for osteoarthritis: a double-blind study. *Semin Arthritis Rheum* 1994;23:25–33.

5. McCarthy GM, McCarty DJ. Effect of topical capsaicin in the therapy of painful osteoarthritis of the hands. *J Rheumatol* 1992;19:604–607.

6. McCarty DJ, Csuka M, McCarthy G et al. Treatment of pain due to fibromyalgia with topical capsaicin: a pilot study. *Semin Arthritis Rheum* 1994;23(Suppl 3):41–47.

7. Zycyznski HM, Culbertson S, Gruss J et al. Substance P and the pathophysiology of vulvar vestibulitis. *J Soc Gynecol Invest* 1997;4(Suppl):107A(abst).

8. Capsaicin Study Group. Treatment of painful diabetic neuropathy with topical capsaicin. *Arch Int Med* 1991;151:2225–2229.

9. Watson CPN, Evans RJ, Watt VR. Post-herpetic neuralgia and topical capsaicin. *Pain* 1988;33:333–340.

10. Low PA, Opfer-Gehrking TL, Dyck PJ et al. Double-blind, placebo-controlled study of the application of capsaicin cream in chronic distal painful polyneuropathy. *Pain* 1995;62:163–168.

11. Watson CPN, Evan RJ. The postmastectomy pain syndrome and topical capsaicin: a randomized trial. *Pain* 1992;51:372–379.

12. Ebihara T, Sekizawa K, Nakazawa H et al. Capsaicin and swallowing reflex. *Lancet* 1993;341:432.

13. Wiart L, Joseph PA, Petit H, et al. The effects of capsaicin on the neurogenic hyperreflexic detrusor: a double blind placebo controlled study in patients with spinal cord disease. Preliminary results. *Spinal Cord* 1998;32:95–99.

14. Lim K, Yoshioka M, Kikuzato S et al. Dietary red pepper ingestion increases carbohydrate oxidation at rest and during exercise in runners. *Med Sci Sports Exerc* 1997;29:355–361.

15. Graham DY, Anderson SY, Lang T. Garlic or jalapeno peppers for treatment of Helicobacter pylori infection. *Am J Gastroenterol* 1999;94:1200–1202.

16. Yeoh KG, Kang JY, Yap I et al. Chili protects against aspirin-

induced gastroduodenal mucosal injury in humans. *Dig Dis Sci* 1995;40:580–583.

17. Kawada T, Hagihara K-I, Iwai K. Effects of capsaicin on lipid metabolism in rats fed a high fat diet. *J Nutr* 1968;116: 1272–1278.

18. Surh YJ, Lee E, Lee JM. Chemoprotective properties of some pungent ingredients present in red pepper and ginger. *Mutat Res* 1998;402:259–267.

19. Bouraoui A, Toumi A, Ben Mustapha H et al. Effects of capsicum fruit on theophylline absorption and bioavailability in rabbits. *Drug Nutr Interact* 1998;5:345–350.

20. Cruz L, Castandea-Hernandez G, Navarrete A. Ingestion of chilli pepper (*Capsicum annuum*) reduces salicylate bioavailability after oral aspirin administration in the rat. *Can J Physiol Pharmacol* 1999;77:441–446.

21. Lopez-Carrillo E, Avila MH, Dubrow R. Chili pepper consumption and gastric cancer in Mexico: a case-control study. *Am J Epidemiol* 1994;139:263–271.

CARAWAY

1. European Scientific Cooperative on Phytotherapy (ESCOP). *Monographs on the medicinal use of plant drugs. Carvi fructus (Caraway)*. Exeter, UK, 1997.

2. Micklefield GH, Greving I, May B. Effects of peppermint oil and caraway oil on gastroduodenal motility. *Phytother Res* 2000;14:20–23.

3. Madisch A, Heydenreich, C-J, Wieland V et al. Treatment of functional dyspepsia with a fixed peppermint oil and caraway oil combination preparation as compared to cisapride: a multicenter, reference-controlled double-blind equivalence study. *Arzneim-Forsch/Drug Res* 1999;49;925–932.

4. May B, Kuntz HD, Kieser M et al. Efficacy of a fixed peppermint oil/caraway oil combination in non-ulcer dyspepsia. *Arzneim-Forsch/Drug Res* 1996;46:1149–53. (English summary: Reichert R. Peppermint and caraway oil combination for irritable bowel syndrome. *Q Rev Nat Med* 1997;(Summer): 97–98).

5. May B, Kohler S, Schneider B. Efficacy and tolerability of a fixed combination of peppermint oil and caraway oil in patients suffering from functional dyspepsia. *Aliment Pharmacol Ther* 2000;14:1671–1677.

6. Westphal J, Horning M, Leonhardt K. Phytotherapy in functional upper abdominal complaints. *Phytomedicine* 1996;2: 285–291.

7. Schulz V, Hansel R, Tyler VE. *Rational phytotherapy: a physician's guide to herbal medicine,* 3rd ed. Berlin: Springer-Verlag, 1998:66–72.

8. Shwaireb MH. Caraway oil inhibits skin tumors in female BALB/c mice. *Nutr Cancer* 1993;19:321–325.

9. Wattenberg LW, Sparnins VL, Barany GL. Inhibition of N-nitrosodiethylamine carcinogenesis in mice by naturally-occurring organosulfur compounds and monoterpenes. *Cancer Res* 1989;49:2689–2692.

CARNITINE

1. Linder MC. *Nutritional biochemistry and metabolism, with clinical applications,* 2nd ed. East Norwalk, CT: Appleton 7 Lange, 1991.

2. Rebouche CJ, Paulson DJ. Carnitine metabolism and function in humans. *Ann Rev Nutr* 1986;6:41–66.

3. Rebouche CJ. Carnitine. In: Shils ME, Olson JA, Shike M et al, eds. *Modern nutrition in health and disease,* 9th ed. Baltimore: Williams & Wilkins, 1999:505–512.

4. Jeulin C, Lewin LM. Role of free L-carnitine and acetyl-L-carnitine in post-gonadal maturation of mammalian spermatozoa. *Hum Reprod Update* 1996;2:87–102.

5. Hiatt WR Hiatt WR, Regensteiner JG et al. Propionyl-L-carnitine improves exercise performance and functional status in patients with claudication. *Am J Med* 2001;110:616–622.

6. Dal Lago A, De Martini D, Flore R et al. Effects of propionyl-L-carnitine on peripheral arterial obliterative disease of the lower limbs: a double-blind clinical trial. *Drugs Exp Clin Res* 1999;25(1):29–36.

7. Brevetti G, Diehm C, Lambert D. European multicenter study on propionyl-L-carnitine in intermittent claudication. *J Am Coll Cardiol* 1999;34:1618–1624.

8. Brevetti G, Perna S, Sabba C et al. Propionyl-L-carnitine in intermittent claudication: double-blind, placebo-controlled, dose titration multicenter study. *J Am Coll Cardiol* 1995;26: 1411–1416.

9. Brevetti G, Perna S, Sabba C et al. Effect of propionyl-L-carnitine on quality of life in intermittent claudication. *Am J Cardiol* 1997;79:777–780.

10. Brevetti G, Chiarello M, Ferulano G et al. Increases in walking distance in patients with peripheral vascular disease treated with L-carnitine: a double-blind, cross-over study. *Circulation* 1988;77:767–773.

11. Greco AV, Mingrone G, Bianchi M et al. Effect of propionyl-L-carnitine in the treatment of diabetic angiopathy: controlled double-blind trial versus placebo. *Drugs Exp Clin Res* 1992;18:69–80.

12. Bartels GL, Remme WJ, Hartog FR et al. Additional anti-ischemic effects of long-term L-propionylcarnitine in anginal patients treated with conventional antianginal therapy. *Cardiovasc Drugs Ther* 1995;9:749–753.

13. Bartels GL, Remme WJ, Holwerda KJ et al. Anti-ischaemic efficacy of L-propionylcarnitine—a promising novel metabolic approach to ischaemia? *Eur Heart J* 1996;17:414–420.

14. Cherchi A, Lai C, Angelino F et al. Effects of L-carnitine on exercise tolerance in chronic stable angina: a multicenter, double-blind, randomized, placebo-controlled crossover study. *Int J Clin Pharm Ther Tox* 1985;23:369–372.

15. Rebuzzi AG, Schiavone G, Amico CM et al. Beneficial effects of L-carnitine in the reduction of the necrotic area in acute myocardial infarction. *Drugs Exp Clin Res* 1984;10:219–223.

16. Investigators of the study on propionyl-L-carnitine in chronic heart failure. Study on propionyl-L-carnitine in chronic heart failure. *Eur Heart J* 1999;20:70–76.

17. Caponnetto S, Canale C, Masperone MA et al. Efficacy of L-propionylcarnitine treatment in patients with left ventricular dysfunction. *Eur Heart J* 1994;15:1267–1273.

18. Sano M, Bell K, Cote L et al. Double-blind parallel design pilot study of acetyl levocarnitine in patients with Alzheimer's disease. *Arch Neurol* 1992;49:1137–1141.

19. Spagnoli A, Lucca U, Menasce G et al. Long-term acetyl-L-carnitine treatment in Alzheimer's disease. *Neurology* 1991; 41:1726–1732.

20. Thal LJ, Calvani M, Amato A et al. A 1-year controlled trial of acetyl-L-carnitine in early-onset AD. *Neurology* 2000;55: 805–810.

21. Salvioli G, Neri M. L-acetylcarnitine treatment of mental decline in the elderly. *Drugs Exp Clin Res* 1994;20:169–176.

22. Clarkson PM. Nutrition for improved sports performance: current issues on ergogenic aids. *Sports Med* 1996;6:393–401.

23. Brass EP. Supplemental carnitine and exercise. *Am J Clin Nutr* 2000;72(Suppl 2):618S–623S.

References

24. Villani RG, Gannon J, Self M et al. L-Carnitine supplementation combined with aerobic training does not promote weight loss in moderately obese women. *Int J Sport Nutr Exerc Metab* 2000;10:199–207.
25. Golfer TA, Wolfson M, Ahmad S et al. Multicenter trial of L-carnitine in maintenance hemodialysis patients. I. Carnitine concentrations and lipid effects. *Kidney Int* 1990;38: 904–911.
26. Labonia WD. L-carnitine effects on anemia in hemodialyzed patients treated with erythropoietin. *Am J Kidney Dis* 1995; 26:757–764.
27. Plioplys AV, Plioplys S. Amantadine and L-carnitine treatment of chronic fatigue syndrome. *Neuropsychobiology* 1997;35:16–23.
28. Biagiotti G, Cavallini G. Acetyl-L-carnitine vs tamoxifen in the oral therapy of Peyronie's disease: a preliminary report. *BJU Int* 2001;88:63–67.
29. Serjeant BE, Harris J, Thomas P, Serjeant GR. Propionyl-L-carnitine in chronic leg ulcers of homozygous sickle cell disease: a pilot study. *J Am Acad Dermatol* 1997;37(3PT1): 491–493.
30. Benvenga S, Ruggeri RM, Russo A et al. Usefulness of L-carnitine, a naturally occurring peripheral antagonist of thyroid hormone action, in iatrogenic hyperthyroidism: a randomized, double-blind, placebo-controlled clinical trial. *J Clin Endocrinol Metab* 2001;86:3579–3594.
31. Freeman JM, Vining EPG, Cost S et al. Does carnitine administration improve the symptoms attributed to anticonvulsant medications?: a double-blinded, crossover study. *Pediatrics* 1994;93:893–895.
32. Böhles H, Sewall AC, Wenzel D. The effect of carnitine supplementation to valproate-induced hyperammonaemia. *Acta Paediatr* 1996;85;446–449.
33. Bazzato G, Mezzina C, Ciman M et al. Myasthenia-like syndrome associated with carnitine in patients on long-term dialysis. *Lancet* 1979;i:1041–1042.
34. Lombard KA, Olson AL, Nelson SE et al. Carnitine status of lacto-ovo-vegetarians and strict vegetarian adults and children. *Am J Clin Nutr* 1989;50:301–306.

CAROTENOIDS

1. Olson JA. Carotenoids. In: Shils ME, Olson JA, Shike M et al, eds. Modern nutrition in health and disease, 9th ed. Baltimore: Williams & Wilkins, 1999:525–542.
2. Mayne ST. Beta-carotene, carotenoids, and disease prevention in humans. *FASEB J* 1996;10:690–701.
3. Heinonen OP, Albanes D, for the alpha-tocopherol, beta carotene cancer prevention study group. The effect of vitamin E and beta carotene on the incidence of lung cancer and other cancers in male smokers. *N Engl J Med* 1994;330: 1029–1035.
4. Omen GS, Goodman GE, Thornquist MD et al. Effects of a combination of beta carotene and vitamin A on lung cancer and cardiovascular disease. *N Engl J Med* 1996;334: 1150–1155.
5. Hennekens CH, Buring JE, Manson JE et al. Lack of effect of long-term supplementation with beta carotene on the incidence of malignant neoplasms and cardiovascular disease. *N Engl J Med* 1996;334:1145–1149.
6. Rautalahti MT, Virtamo JR, Taylor PR et al. The effects of supplementation with alpha-tocopherol and beta-carotene on the incidence and mortality of carcinoma of the pancreas in a randomized, controlled trial. *Cancer* 1999;86:37–42.
7. Greenberg ER, Baron JA, Stukel, TA et al. A clinical trial of beta-carotene to prevent basal-cell and squamous-cell cancers of the skin. *N Engl J Med* 1990;323:789–795.
8. Giulano AR, Gapstur S. Can cervical dysplasia and cancer be prevented with nutrients? *Nutr Rev* 1998;56:9–16.
9. Mackerras D, Irwig L, Simpson JM et al. Randomized double-blind trial of beta-carotene and vitamin C in women with minor cervical abnormalities. *Br J Cancer* 1999;79: 1448–1453.
10. Rapola JM, Virtamo J, Ripatti S et al. Randomised trial of α-tocopherol and B-carotene supplements on incidence of major coronary events in men with previous myocardial infarction. *Lancet* 1997;349:1715–1720.
11. Virtamo J, Rapola JM, Ripatti S et al. Effect of vitamin E and beta-carotene on the incidence of primary nonfatal myocardial infarction and fatal coronary heart disease. *Arch Int Med* 1998;158:668–675.
12. Liu S, Ajani U, Chae C et al. Long-term β-carotene supplementation and risk of type 2 diabetes mellitus. *JAMA* 1999; 282:1073–1075.
13. Mathews-Roth MM. Carotenoids in erythropoietic protoporphyria and other photosensitivity diseases. *Ann N Y Acad Sci* 1993;691:127–138.
14. Stahl W, Heinrich U, Jungmann H et al. Carotenoids and carotenoids plus vitamin E protect against ultraviolet light-induced erythema in humans. *Am J Clin Nutr* 2000;71: 795–798.
15. Palozza P. Prooxidant actions of carotenoids in biologic systems. *Nutr Rev* 1998;56:257–265.
16. Leo MA, Lieber CS. Alcohol, vitamin A, and β-carotene: adverse interactions, including hepatotoxicity and carcinogenicity. *Am J Clin Nutr* 1999;69:1071–1085.
17. Leo MA, Kim C-I, Lowe N, Lieber C. Interaction of ethanol with B-carotene: delayed blood clearance and enhanced hepatotoxicity. *Hepatology* 1992;15:883–891.
18. Heywood R, Palmer AK, Gregson RL et al. The toxicity of beta-carotene. *Toxicology* 1985;36:91–100.
19. Van den Berg H. Carotenoid interactions. *Nutr Rev* 1999;157 (1):1–10.
20. Kemmann E, Pasquale SA, Skaf R. Amenorrhea associated with carotenemia. *JAMA* 1983;249:926–929.
21. Mathews-Roth MM. Amenorrhea associated with carotenemia. *JAMA* 1983;250:731.
22. Pan R M-D, Herrmann W. Carrot juice junkies and big bangs. *Fertil Steril* 1998;69:789.
23. Keenan DL, Dharmarajan AM, Zacur HA. Dietary carrot results in diminished ovarian progesterone secretion, whereas a metabolite, retinoic acid, stimulates progesterone secretion in the in vitro perfused rabbit ovary. *Fertil Steril* 1997;68:358–363.
24. Linder MC (personal communication, 2001).

CARTILAGE

1. Physician Data Query. Cartilage (bovine and shark). Physician Data Query. Available at: http://cnetdb.nci.nih.gov/cam/cartilage.htm
2. Berbari P, Thibodeau A, Germain L et al. Antiangiogenic effects of the oral administration of liquid cartilage extract in humans. *J Surg Res* 1999;87:108–113.
3. Miller DR, Anderson GT, Stark JJ et al. Phase I/II trial of the safety and efficacy of shark cartilage in the treatment of advanced cancer. *Clin Oncol* 1998;16:3649–3655.
4. Prudden JF. The treatment of human cancer with agents pre-

pared from bovine cartilage. *J Biol Response Modifiers* 1985; 4:551–584.

5. Romano CF, Lipton A, Harvey HA et al. A phase II study of Catrix-S in solid tumors. *J Biol Response Modifiers* 1985;4: 585–589.

6. Puccio C, Mittelman H, Chun P et al. Treatment of metastatic renal cell carcinoma with Catrix. *Proc Am Soc Clin Oncol* 1994;13:A769(abst).

7. Dupont E, Savard PE, Jourdain C et al. Antiangiogenic properties of a novel shark cartilage extract: potential role in the treatment of psoriasis. *J Cutan Med Surg* 1998;2: 146–152.

8. Prudden JF, Allen J. The clinical acceleration of healing with a cartilage preparation. *JAMA* 1965;192:92–96.

9. Horsman MR, Alsner J, Overgaard J. The effect of shark cartilage extracts on the growth and metastatic spread of the SCCVII carcinoma. *Acta Oncol* 1998;37:441–445.

10. Sheu JR, Fu CC, Tsai ML et al. Effect of U-995, a potent shark cartilage-derived angiogenesis inhibitor, on anti-angiogenesis and anti-tumor activities. *Anticancer Res* 1998;18:4435–4441.

11. McGuire TR, Kazakoff PW, Hoie EB et al. Antiproliferative activity of shark cartilage with and without tumor necrosis factor-α in human umbilical vein endothelium. *Pharmacotherapy* 1996;16:237–244.

12. Golding MR, Oberlander LK, Enquist IF. Cartilage speeds healing in diabetic wounds. *Arch Surg* 1963; 87:131–133.

13. Sabo JC, Oberlander L, Enquist IF. Acceleration of open wound healing by cartilage. *Arch Surg* 1965;90:414–417.

14. Houck JC, Jacob RA, DeAngelo L et al. The inhibition of inflammation and the acceleration of tissue repair by cartilage powder. *Surgery* 1962;51:632–638.

15. Prudden JF, Wolarsky E. The reversal by cartilage of the steroid-induced inhibition of wound healing. *Surg Gynecol Obstet* 1967;125:109–113.

16. Mathews J. Media feeds frenzy over shark cartilage as cancer treatment. *J Natl Cancer Inst* 1993;85:1190–1191.

CASCARA

1. Westendorf J. Anthranoid derivatives-General discussion. In: De Smet PAGM, Keller K, Hänsel R et al. *Adverse effects of herbal drugs,*vol 2. Berlin: Springer-Verlag, 1993:105–118.

2. de Witte P, Lemli L. The metabolism of anthranoid laxatives. *Hepatogastroenterol* 1990;37:601–605.

3. European Scientific Cooperative on Phytotherapy (ESCOP). *Monographs on the medicinal uses of plant drugs. Rhamni purshiana cortex: Cascara. Fascicule 5.* Exeter, UK, 1997:1–7.

4. Silk DBA, Gibson JA, Murray CRH. Reversible finger clubbing in a case of purgative abuse. *Gastroenterology* 1975;68:790–794.

5. Westendorf J. Anthranoid derivatives-General discussion. In: De Smet PAGM, Keller K, Hänsel R et al. *Adverse effects of herbal drugs,* vol 2. Berlin: Springer-Verlag, 1993:105–118.

6. Nadir A, Reddy D, van Thiel DH. Cascara sagrada-induced intrahepatic cholestasis causing portal hypertension: case report and review of herbal hepatotoxicity. *Am J Gastroenterol* 2000;95:3634–3637.

7. Mereto E, Ghia M, Brambilla G. Evaluation of the potential carcinogenic activity of senna and cascara glycosides for the rat colon. *Cancer Lett* 1996;101:79–83.

8. Evans WC. *Trease and Evan's pharmacognosy*, 14th ed. WB Saunders Co., London, 1996:239–241.

9. Hagemann TM. Gastrointestinal medications and breastfeeding. *J Human Lactation* 1998;14:259–262.

10. Blumenthal M, Goldberg A, Brinckmann J. *Herbal Medicine: Expanded Commission E Monographs.* Integrative Medical Communications, Newton MA, 2000:47–51.

11. Mitty RD, Wolfe GRZ, Cosman M. Initial description of gastric melanosis in a laxative-abusing patient. *Am J Gastroenterol* 1997;92:707–708.

12. Siegers CP, von Hertzberg-Lottin E, Otte M et al. Anthranoid laxative abuse—a risk for colorectal cancer? *Gut* 1993;34: 1099–1100.

CATNIP

1. Tucker AO, Tucker SS. Catnip and the catnip response. *Econ Botany* 1988;42:214–231.

2. Tyler VE. *The honest herbal.* Binghamton NY: Haworth Press, 1993.

3. Massoco CO. Behavioral effects of acute and long-term administration of catnip (*Nepeta cataria*) in mice. *Vet Hum Toxicol* 1995;37:530–533.

4. Osterhoudt KC, Lee SK, Callahan JM et al. Catnip and the alteration of human consciousness. *Vet Hum Toxicol* 1997; 39:373–375.

5. Jackson B, Reed A. Catnip and the alteration of consciousness. *JAMA* 1968:207:1349–1350.

CAT'S CLAW

1. Keplinger K, Laus G, Wurm M et al. *Uncaria tomentosa (Willd.) DC.*—Ethnomedicinal use and new pharmacological, toxicological and botanical results. *J Ethnopharmacol* 1999; 64:23–34.

2. Aquino R, De Simone F, Pizza C. Plant metabolites. Structure and in vitro antiviral activity of quinovic acid glycosides from *Uncaria tomentosa* and Guettarda platypoda. *J Nat Prod* 1989;52:679–685.

3. Aquino R, De Feo, V, De Simone F et al. Plant metabolites: New compounds and anti-inflammatory activity of *Uncaria tomentosa. J Nat Prod* 1991;54:453–459.

4. Sandoval M, Charbonnet RM, Okuhama NN et al. Cat's claw inhibits TNF-alpha production and scavenges free radicals: role in cytoprotection. *Free Rad Biol Med* 2000;29:71–78.

5. Piscoya J, Rodriguez Z, Bustamante SA et al. Efficacy and safety of freeze-dried cat's claw in osteoarthritis of the knee: mechanisms of action of the species Uncaria guianensis. *Inflamm Res* 2001;50:442–448.

6. Reinhard K-H. *Uncaria tomentosa (Willd.) DC*: Cat's claw, uña de gato, or saventaro. *J Altern Complement Med* 1999; 5:143–151.

7. Lemaire J, Assinewe V, Cano P et al. Stimulation of interleukin-1 and -6 production in alveolar macrophages by the neotropical liana, *Uncaria tomentosa* (uña de gato). *J Ethnopharmacol* 1999;64:109–115.

8. Stuppner H, Sturm S, Geisen G et al. A differential sensitivity of oxindole alkaloids to normal and leukemic cell lines. *Planta Med* 1993;59(Suppl):A583.

9. D. Awang. Personal communication, 2001.

10. Salazar EL, Jayme V. Depletion of specific binding sites for estrogen receptor by *Uncaria tomentosa. Proc West Pharmacol Soc* 1998;41:123–124.

11. Rizzi R, Re F, Bianchi A et al. Mutagenic and antimutagenic activities of *Uncaria tomentosa. J Ethnopharmacol* 1993;38: 63–77.

12. Sheng Y, Pero RW, Wagner H. Treatment of chemotherapy-induced leukopenia in a rat model with aqueous extract from *Uncaria tomentosa. Phytomedicine* 2000;7:137–143.

References

13. Hilepo JN, Bellucci AG, Mossey RT. Acute renal failure caused by 'cat's claw' herbal remedy in a patient with systemic lupus erythematosus. *Nephron* 1997;77:361.
14. Santa Maria A, Lopez A, Diaz MM et al. Evaluation of the toxicity of *Uncaria tomentosa* by bioassays. *J Ethnopharmacol* 1997;57:183–187.

CHAMOMILE

1. Bisset NG, Wichtl M. *Herbal drugs and phytopharmaceuticals: a handbook for practice on a scientific basis with reference to German Commission E monographs*. Boca Raton, FL: CRC Press, 1994.
2. Ahmad A, Misra LN. Isolation of herniarin and other constituents from Matricaria chamomilla flowers. *Int J Pharmacognosy* 1997;35:121–125.
3. Schulz V, Hansel R, Tyler VE. Rational phytotherapy: a physician's guide to herbal medicine, 3rd ed. Berlin: Springer-Verlag, 1998:253–256.
4. Viola H, Wasowski C, Levi de Stein M et al. Apigenin, a component of *Matricaria recutita* flowers, is a central benzodiazepine receptors-ligand with anxiolytic effects. *Planta Med* 1995;61:213–216.
5. Merfort I, Heilmann J, Hagedorn-Leweke U et al. In vivo skin penetration studies of camomile flavones. *Pharmazie*1994;49:509–511.
6. Patzelt-Wenczler R, Ponce-Pöschl E. Proof of efficacy of Kamillosan ® cream in atopic eczema. *Eur J Med Res* 2000; 5:171–175.
7. Carl W, Emrich LS. Management of oral mucositis during local radiation and systemic chemotherapy: a study of 98 patients. *J Prosthet Dent* 1991;66:361–369.
8. Fidler P, Loprinzi CL, O'Fallon JR et al. Prospective evaluation of a chamomile mouthwash for prevention of 5-FU-induced oral mucositis. *Cancer* 1996;77:522–525.
9. Saller R, Beschorner M, Hellenbrecht D et al. Dose-dependency of symptomatic relief of complaints by chamomile steam inhalation in patients with common cold. *Eur J Pharm* 1990;183:728.
10. Weizman Z, Alkrinawi S, Goldfarb D et al. Efficacy of herbal tea preparation in infantile colic. *J Pediatr* 1993;122:650–652.
11. Maiche AG, Gröhn P, Mäki-Hokkonen. Effect of chamomile cream and almond ointment on acute radiation skin reaction. *Acta Oncol* 1991;30:395–396.
12. Korting HC, Schäfer-Korting M, Hart H et al. Anti-inflammatory activity of hamamelis distillate applied topically to the skin: influence of vehicle and dose. *Eur J Clin Pharmacol* 1993;44:315–318.
13. Miller T, Wittstock U, Lindequest U et al. Effects of some components of the essential oil of chamomile, *Chamomilla recutita*, on histamine release from rat mast cells. *Planta Med* 1996;62:60–61.
14. Jensen-Jarolim E, Reider N, Fritsch R et al. Fatal outcome of anaphylaxis to camomile-containing enema during labor: a case study. *J Allergy Clin Immunol* 1998;1041–1042.
15. Casterline CL. Allergy to chamomile tea. *JAMA* 1980;4: 330–331.
16. Benner MH, Lee HJ. Anaphylactic reaction to chamomile tea. *J Allergy Clin Immunol* 1973;52:307–308.
17. Hausen BM. Sesquiterpene lactones-Chamomilla recutita. In: *Adverse effects of herbal drugs,* vol I. Berlin: Springer-Verlag, 1992:243–248.
18. Hausen BM. A 6-year experience with Compositae mix. *Am J Contact Dermatitis* 1996;7:94–99.

CHAMOMILE, ROMAN

1. Bradley PR (ed.) *British herbal compendium*, vol 1. Dorset, UK: British Herbal Medicine Association, 1992.
2. Schulz V, Hansel R, Tyler VE. *Rational phytotherapy: a physician's guide to herbal medicine,* 3rd ed. Berlin: Springer-Verlag, 1998:253–256.
3. Viola H, Wasowski C, Levi de Stein M et al. Apigenin, a component of Matricaria recutita flowers, is a central benzodiazepine receptors-ligand with anxiolytic effects. *Planta Med* 1995;61:213–216.
4. Merfort I, Heilmann J, Hagedorn-Leweke U et al. In vivo skin penetration studies of camomile flavones. *Pharmazie* 1994;49:509–511.
5. Bisset NG, Wichtl M. *Herbal drugs and phytopharmaceuticals: a handbook for practice on a scientific basis with reference to German Commission E monographs,* Boca Raton, FL: CRC Press, 1994.
6. Newall CA, Anderson LA, Phillipson JD. *Herbal medicines: a guide for health care professionals*. London: Pharmaceutical Press, 1996.

CHAPARRAL

1. Obermeyer WR, Musser SM, Betz JM et al. Chemical studies of phytoestrogens and related compounds in dietary supplements: flax and chaparral. *Proc Soc Exp Biol Med* 1995; 208:6–12.
2. Gardner KD Jr, Reed WP, Evan AP et al. Endotoxin provocation of experimental renal cystic disease. *Kidney Int* 1987; 32:329–334.
3. Sathyamoorthy N, Wang TTY, Phang JM. Stimulation of pS2 expression by diet-derived compounds. *Cancer Res* 1994;54: 957–961.
4. Newton JA, Boodle KM, Dowd PM et al. Topical NDGA (nordihydroguaiaretic acid) in psoriasis. *Br J Dermatol* 1988;199: 404–406.
5. Smart CR, Hogle HH, Robins RK et al. An interesting observation on nordihydroguaiaretic acid (NSC-4291; NDGA) and a patient with malignant melanoma—a preliminary report. *Cancer Chemother Rep Part 1* 1969;53:147–151.
6. US Congress, Office of Technology Assessment. *Unconventional cancer treatments*. Washington, DC: US Government Printing Office, September 1999:70–71; OTA-H-405.
7. Smart CR, Hogle HH, Vogel H et al. Clinical experience with nordihydroguaiaretic acid. *Rocky Mountain Med J* 1970;11: 39–43.
8. Ansar S, Iqbal M, Athar M. Nordihydroguairetic acid is a potent inhibitor of ferric-nitrilotriacetate-mediated hepatic and renal toxicity, and renal tumour promotion, in mice. *Carcinogenesis* 1999;20:599–606.
9. Jordan ML, Hoffman RA, Simmons RL. Prevention of experimental allograft rejection by nordihydroguaiaretic acid. *Transplant Proc* 1987;19:1307.
10. Sheikh NM, Philen RM, Love LA. Chaparral-associated hepatotoxicity. *Arch Intern Med* 1997;157:913–919.
11. Batchelor WB, Heathcote J, Wanless IR. Chaparral-induced hepatic injury. *Am J Gastroenterol* 1995;90:831–833.
12. Alderman S, Kailas S, Goldfarb S et al. Cholestatic hepatitis after ingestion of chaparral leaf: confirmation by endo-

scopic retrograde cholangiopancreatography and liver biopsy. *J Clin Gastroenterol* 1994;19:242–247.

13. Tregellas WM, South SF. Autoimmune syndrome induced by chaparral ingestion. *Transfusion* 1980;20:647–648.

14. Evan AP, Gardner KD Jr. Nephron obstruction in nordihydroguaiaretic acid-induced renal cystic disease. *Kidney Int* 1979;15:7–19.

CHARCOAL

1. Lewis RA. *Lewis' dictionary of toxicology*. Boca Raton, FL: CRC Press, 1998.

2. Jain NK, Patel VP, Pitchumoni CS. Efficacy of activated charcoal in reducing intestinal gas: a double-blind clinical trial. *Am J Gastroenterol* 1986;81:532–535.

3. Jain NK, Patel VP, Pitchumoni CS. Activated charcoal, simethicone, and intestinal gas: a double-blind study. *Ann Int Med* 1986;105:61–62.

4. Pederson JA, Matter BJ et al. Relief of idiopathic generalized pruritus in dialysis patients treated with activated oral charcoal. *Ann Int Med* 1980;93:446–448.

5. Giovannetti S, Barsotti G, Cupisti A et al. Oral activated charcoal in patients with uremic pruritus. *Nephron* 1995;70: 193–196.

6. Kaaja RJ, Kontula KK, Räihä A et al. Treatment of cholestasis of pregnancy with peroral activated charcoal. *Scand J Gastroenterol* 1994;29:178–181.

7. Amitai Y, Regev M, Arad I. Treatment of neonatal hyperbilirubinemia with repetitive oral activated charcoal as an adjunct to phototherapy. *J Perinat Med* 1993;21:189–194.

8. Ziegenhagen DJ, Raedsch R, Kruis W. Traveler's diarrhea in Turkey. Prospective randomized therapeutic comparison of charcoal versus tannin albuminate/ethacridine lactate. (in German). *Medizinische Klinik* 1992;87:637–639.

9. Sebodo T, Sunartini I et al. Carbo-adsorbent (norit) in the treatment of children with diarrhoea. *Southeast Asian J Trop Med Pub Health* 1982;13:424–426.

10. Hoekstra JBL, Erkelens DW. No effect of activated charcoal on hyperlipidemia. *Neth J Med* 1988;33:209–216.

11. Neuvonen PJ, Kuusisto P, Vapaatalo H et al. Activated charcoal in the treatment of hypercholesterolaemia: dose-response relationships and comparison with cholestyramine. *Eur J Clin Pharmacol* 1989;37:225–230.

12. Kuusisto P, Manninen V, Vapaatalo H et al. Effect of activated charcoal on hypercholesterolaemia. *Lancet* 1986;2: 366–367.

13. Gomez HF, Brent JA, Munoz DC et al. Charcoal stercolith with intestinal perforation in a patient treated for amitriptyline ingestion. *J Emerg Med* 1994;12:57–60.

14. Goulbourne KB, Cisek JE. Small-bowel obstruction secondary to activated charcoal and adhesions. *Ann Emerg Med* 1994;24:108–110.

15. Moll J, Kerns W 2nd, Tomaszewski C, Rose R. Incidence of aspiration pneumonia in intubated patients receiving activated charcoal. *J Emerg Med* 1999;17:279–283.

16. Elomaa K, Ranta S, Tuominen J et al. Charcoal treatment and risk of escape ovulation in oral contraception users. *Hum Reprod* 2001;16:76–81.

CHOCOLATE

1. McGee H. *On food and cooking: the science and lore of the kitchen*. New York: Macmillan, 1984.

2. Kondo K, Hirano R, Matsumoto A et al. Inhibition of LDL oxidation by cocoa. *Lancet* 1996;348:1514.

3. Arts ICW, Hollman PCH, Kromhout D. Chocolate as a source of tea flavonoids. *Lancet* 1999;354:488.

4. Bruinsma K, Taren DL. Chocolate: food or drug? *J Am Diet Assoc* 1999;99:1249–1256.

5. Schifano F, Magni G. MDMA ("Ecstasy") abuse: psychopathological features and craving for chocolate: a case series. *Biol Psychiatry* 1994;36:763–767.

6. Di Tomaso E, Beltramo M, Piomelli D. Brain cannabinoids in chocolate. *Nature* 1996;382:677–678.

7. Michener W, Rozin P, Freeman E et al. The role of low progesterone and tension as triggers of perimenstrual chocolate and sweets craving: some negative experimental evidence. *Physiol Behav* 1999;67:417–20.

8. Michener W, Rozin P. Pharmacological versus sensory factors in the satiation of chocolate craving. *Phys Behav* 1994;56: 419–422.

9. Rein D, Lotito S, Holt RR et al. Epicatechin in human plasma: in vivo determination and effect of chocolate consumption on plasma oxidation status. *J Nutr* 2000;130: 2109S–2114S.

10. Schramm DD, Wang JF, Holt RR et al. Chocolate procyanidins decrease the leukotriene-prostacyclin ratio in humans and human aortic endothelial cells. *Am J Clin Nutr* 2001;73: 36–40.

11. Rein D, Paglieroni TG, Wun T et al. Cocoa inhibits platelet activation and function. *Am J Clin Nutr* 2000;72:30–35.

12. Waterhouse AL, Shirley JR, Donovan JL. Antioxidants in chocolate. *Lancet* 1006;348:834.

13. Sanbongi C, Suzuki N, Sakane T. Polyphenols in chocolate, which have antioxidant activity, modulate immune functions in humans in vitro. *Cell Immunol* 1997;177:129–136.

14. Nguyen NU, Heriet MT, Dumoulin G et al. Increase in calciuria and oxaluria after a single chocolate bar load. *Horm Metab Res* 1994;26:383–386.

15. Shahkalili Y, Murset C, Meirim I et al. Calcium supplementation of chocolate: effect on cocoa butter digestability and blood lipids in humans. *Am J Clin Nutr* 2001;73:246–252.

16. Di Marzo V, Sepe N, De Petrocellis L et al. Trick or treat from food endocannabinoids. *Nature* 1998;396:636.

17. Beltramo M, Piomelli D. Trick or treat from food endocannabinoids *Nature* 1998;396:636–637.

18. Tytgat J, Van Boven M, Daenens P. Cannabinoid mimics in chocolate utilized as an argument in court. *Int J Legal Med* 2000;113:137–139.

19. Marcus DA, Scarff L, Turk D et al. A double-blind provocative study of chocolate as a trigger of headache. *Cephalagia* 1997;17:855–862.

CHONDROITIN

1. Towheed TE, Anastassiades TP. Glucosamine and chondroitin for treating symptoms of osteoarthritis. *JAMA* 2000;283: 1483–1484.

2. Conte A, Volpi N, Palmieri L et al. Biochemical and pharmacokinetic aspects of oral treatment with chondroitin sulfate. *Arzneim-Forsch/Drug Res* 1995;45:918–925.

3. Ronca F, Palmieri L, Panicucci P et al. Anti-inflammatory activity of chondroitin sulfate. *Osteoarthritis Cartilage* 1998; 6(Suppl A):14–21.

4. McAlindon TE, LaValley MP, Gulin JP et al. Glucosamine and chondroitin for treatment of osteoarthritis: a systematic

References

quality assessment and meta-analysis. *JAMA* 2000;283: 1469–1475.
5. Morreale P, Manopulo R, Galati M et al. Comparison of the anti-inflammatory efficacy of chondroitin sulfate and diclofenac sodium in patients with knee osteoarthritis. *J Rheumatol* 1996;23:1385–1391.
6. Limberg MB, McCaa C, Kissling GE et al. Topical application of hyaluronic acid and chondroitin sulfate in the treatment of dry eyes. *Am J Ophthalmol* 1987;103:194–197.
7. Lenclud C, Chapelle P, Van Muylem A et al. Effects of chondroitin sulfate on snoring characteristics: a pilot study. *Curr Ther Res* 1998;59:234–243.

CHROMIUM

1. Linder MC. *Nutritional biochemistry and metabolism, with clinical applications,* 2nd ed. East Norwalk, CT: Appleton & Lange, 1991.
2. Stoecker BJ. Chromium. In: Shils ME, Olson JA, Shike M et al, eds. *Modern nutrition in health and disease,* 9th ed. Baltimore: Williams & Wilkins, 1999:277–282.
3. Barceloux DG. Chromium. *Clin Toxicol* 1999;37:173–194.
4. Anderson RA. Chromium, glucose intolerance and diabetes. *J Am Coll Nutr* 1998;17:548–555.
5. Anderson RE, Cheng N, Bryden NA et al. Elevated intakes of supplemental chromium improve glucose and insulin variables in individuals with Type 2 diabetes. *Diabetes* 1997;46: 1786–1791.
6. Mertz W. Chromium in human nutrition: a review. *J Nutr* 1993;123:626–633.
7. Anderson RA, Polansky MM, Bryden NA et al. Supplemental-chromium effects on glucose, insulin, glucagon and urinary chromium losses in subjects consuming controlled low-chromium diets. *Am J Clin Nutr* 1991;54:909–916.
8. Anderson RA. Effects of chromium on body composition and weight loss. *Nutr Rev* 1998;56:266–270.
9. Shils ME, Olson JA, Shike M et al, eds. *Modern nutrition in health and disease,* 9th ed. Baltimore: Williams & Wilkins, 1999.
10. Stoecker BJ. Chromium. In: Shils ME, Olson JA, Shike M et al, eds. *Modern nutrition in health and disease*, 9th ed. Baltimore: Williams & Wilkins, 1999:277–282.
11. Huszonek J. Over-the-counter chromium picolinate. *Am J Psychiatry* 1993;150:1560–1561.

CINNAMON

1. Bisset NG, Wichtl M. *Herbal drugs and phytopharmaceuticals: a handbook for practice on a scientific basis with reference to German Commission E monographs.* Boca Raton, FL: CRC Press, 1994.
2. Quale JM, Landman D, Zaman MM et al. In vitro activity of *Cinnamomum* zeylanicum against azole resistant and sensitive Candida species and a pilot study of cinnamon for oral candidiasis. *Am J Chin Med* 1996;24:103–109.
3. Singh HB, Srivastava M, Singh AB et al. Cinnamon bark oil, a potent fungitoxicant against fungi causing respiratory tract mycoses. *Allergy* 1995;50:995–999.
4. Lima EO, Gompertz OF, Giesbrecht AM et al. In vitro antifungal activity of essential oils obtained from officinal plants against dermatophytes. *Mycoses* 1993;36:333–336.
5. Keller K. *Cinnamomum* species. In: DeSmet PAGM, ed. *Adverse effects of herbal drugs,* vol I. Berlin: Springer-Verlag, 1992:105–114.

6. Yu SM, Wu TS, Teng CM. Pharmacological characterization of cinnamophilin, a novel dual inhibitor of thromboxane synthase and thromboxane A2 receptor. *Br J Pharmacol* 1994; 111:906–912.
7. Yu SM, Ko FN, Wu TS et al. Cinnamophilin, a novel thromboxane A2 receptor antagonist, isolated from *Cinnamomum philippinense. Eur J Pharmacol* 1994;256:85–91.
8. Su MJ, Chen WP, Lo TY et al. Ionic mechanisms for the antiarrhythmic action of cinnamophilin in rat heart. *J Biomed Sci* 1999;6:376–386.
9. Lee CW, Hong DH, Han SB et al. Inhibition of human tumor growth by 2'-hydroxy- and 2'-benzoloxycinnamaldehydes [Letter]. *Planta Med* 1999;65:263–266.
10. Kwon BM, Lee SH, Choi SU et al. Synthesis and in vitro cytotoxicity of cinnamaldehydes to human solid tumor cells. *Arch Pharm Res* 1998;21:147–152.
11. Shan BE, Yoshida Y, Sugiura T et al. Stimulating activity of Chinese medicinal herbs on human lymphocytes in vitro. *Int J Immunopharmacol* 1999;21:149–159.
12. Koh WS, Yoon SY, Kwon BM et al. Cinnamaldehyde inhibits lymphocyte proliferation and modulates T-cell differentiation. *Int J Immunopharmacol* 1998;20:643–660.
13. Mancini-Filho J, Van-Koiij A, Mancini DA et al. Antioxidant activity of cinnamon (*Cinnamomum zeylanicum*, Breyne) extracts. *Boll Chim Farm* 1998;137:443–447.
14. Westra WH, McMurray JS, Califano J. Squamous cell carcinoma of the tongue associated with cinnamon gum use: a case report. *Head Neck* 1998;20:430–433.
15. Sparks T. Cinnamon oil burn. *West J Med* 1985;142:835.
16. Perry PA, Dean BS. Cinnamon oil abuse by adolescents. *Vet Hum Toxicol* 1990;32:162–164.
17. Shah AH, Al-Shareef AH, Ageel Am, et al. Toxicity studies in mice of common spices, *Cinnamomum zeylanicum* bark, and *Piper longum* fruits. *Plants Foods Hum Nutr* 1998;52: 231–239.

COENZYME Q10

1. Artuch R, Vilaseca M-A, Moreno J et al. Decreased serum ubiquinone-10 concentrations in phenylketonuria. *Am J Clin Nutr* 1999;70:892–895.
2. Tran MT, Mitchell TM, Kennedy DT et al. Role of coenzyme A10 in chronic heart failure, angina, and hypertension. *Pharmacotherapy* 2001;21:797–806.
3. Singh RB, Wander GS, Rastogi A et al. Randomized, double-blind placebo-controlled trial of coenzyme Q10 in patients with acute myocardial infarction. *Cardiovasc Drugs Ther* 1998;12:347–353.
4. Kamikawa T, Kobayashi A, Yamashita T et al. Effects of coenzyme Q10 on exercise tolerance in chronic stable angina pectoris. *Am J Cardiol* 1985;56:247–251.
5. Mazzola C, Giffanti EE, Vaccarella A et al. Non-invasive assessment of coenzyme Q10 in patients with chronic stable effort angina and moderate heart failure. *Curr Ther Res* 1987;41:923–932.
6. Soja AM, Mortensen SA. Behandling af kronisk hjerteinsufficiens med coenzyme Q10 belyst ved metaanalyser af klinisk kontrollerede undersogelser. *Ugeskr Laeger* 1997;159: 7302–7308.
7. Watson PS, Scalia GM, Galbraith A et al. Lack of effect of coenzyme Q on left ventricular function in patients with congestive heart failure. *J Am Coll Cardiol* 1999;33: 1549–1552.
8. Khatta M, Alexander BS, Krichten CM et al. The effect of

coenzyme Q10 in patients with congestive heart failure. *Ann Intern Med* 2000;132:636–640.

9. Singh RB, Niaz M, Rastogi SS et al. Effect of hydrosoluble coenzyme Q10 on blood pressure and insulin resistance in hypertensive patients with coronary artery disease. *J Hum Hypertens* 1999;13:203–208.

10. Chello M, Mastroroberto P, Romano R et al. Protection by coenzyme Q10 of tissue reperfusion injury during abdominal aortic cross-clamping. *J Cardiovasc Surg* 1996;37:229–235.

11. Chello M, Mastroroberto P, Romano R et al. Protection by coenzyme Q10 from myocardial reperfusion injury during coronary artery bypass grafting. *Ann Thorac Surg* 1994;58: 1427–1432.

12. Taggart DP, Jenkins M, Hooper J et al. Effects of short-term supplementation with coenzyme Q10 on myocardial protection during cardiac operations. *Ann Thorac Surg* 1996;61: 829–833.

13. Laaksonen R, Fogelholm M, Himberg J-J et al. Ubiquinone supplementation and exercise capacity in trained young and older men. *Eur J Appl Physiol* 1995;72:95–100.

14. Malm C, Svensson M, Ekblom B et al. Effects of ubiquinone-10 supplementation and high intensity training on physical performance in humans. *Acta Physiol Scand* 1997;161: 379–384.

15. Weston SB, Zhou S, Weatherby RP et al. Does exogenous coenzyme Q10 affect aerobic capacity in endurance athletes? *Int J Sport Nutr* 1997;7:197–206.

16. Shults CW, Beal MF, Fontaine D et al. Absorption, tolerability, and effects on mitochondrial activity of oral coenzyme Q10 in Parkinson patients. *Neurology* 1998;50:793–795.

17. Physician Data Query (PDQ)-National Cancer Institute's comprehensive cancer database. Information summary on coenzyme Q10. *http:nci.nih.gov/cancer_information*.

18. Iarussi D, Auricchio U, Agretto A et al. Protective effect of coenzyme Q10 on anthracyclines cardiotoxicity: control study in children with acute lymphoblastic leukemia and non-Hodgkin's lymphoma. *Mol Aspects Med* 1994;15(Suppl): 207–212.

19. Suzuki S, Hinokio Y, Ohtomo M et al. The effects of coenzyme Q10 treatment on maternally inherited diabetes mellitus and deafness, and mitochondrial DNA 3243 (A-G) mutation. *Diabetologia* 1998;41:584–588.

20. Watts TLP. Coenzyme Q-10 and periodontal treatment: is there any beneficial effect? *Br Dent J* 1995;178:209–213.

21. Wilkinson EG, Arnold RM, Folkers K. Bioenergetics in clinical medicine. VI. Adjunctive treatment of periodontal disease with coenzyme Q10. *Res Commun Chem Pathol Pharmacol* 1976;14:715–719.

22. Iwamoto Y, Watanabe T, Okamoto H et al. Clinical effect of coenzyme Q10 on periodontal disease. In: Folkers K, Yamamura Y, eds. *Biomedical and clinical aspects of coenzyme Q,* Vol 3. New York: Elsevier Science, 1981:109–119.

23. Palomaki A, Malminiemi K, Solakivi T et al. Ubiquinone supplementation during lovastatin treatment: effect on LDL oxidation ex vivo. *J Lipid Res* 1998;39:1430–1437.

24. Dlugosz A, Sawicka E. The chemoprotective effect of coenzyme Q on lipids on the paint and lacquer industry workers. *Int J Occup Med Environ Health* 1998;11:153–163.

25. Prieme H, Loft S, Nyyssonen K et al. No effect of supplementation with vitamin E, ascorbic acid, or coenzyme Q10 on oxidative DNA damage estimated by 8-oxo-7, 8-dihydro-2′-deoxyguanosine excretion in smokers. *Am J Clin Nutr* 1997;65:503–507.

26. Laaksonen R, Ojala J-P, Tikkanen MJ et al. Serum ubiquinone concentrations after short- and long-term treatment with HMG-CoA reductase inhibitors. *Eur J Clin Pharm* 1994;46:313–317.

27. Folkers K, Vadhanavikit S, Mortensen SA. Biochemical rationale and myocardial tissue data on the effective therapy of cardiomyopathy with coenzyme Q10. *Proc Natl Acad Sci U S A* 1985;82:901–904.

28. Kontush A, Reich A, Baum K et al. Plasma ubiquinol-10 is decreased in patients with hyperlipidaemia. *Atherosclerosis* 1997;129:119–126.

29. Schiavino D, Nucero E, Zoppi A et al. Rush desensitization with ubiquinone. *Allergy* 1997;52:783–784.

30. Landbo C, Almdal TP. Interaction between warfarin and coenzyme Q10. (In Danish) *Ugeskrift for Laeger* 1998;160: 3226–3227.

COLTSFOOT

1. Bisset NG, Wichtl M. *Herbal drugs and phytopharmaceuticals: a handbook for practice on a scientific basis with reference to German Commission E monographs*. Boca Raton, FL: CRC Press, 1994.

2. Westendorf J. Pyrrolizidine alkaloids—*Tussilago farfara*. In: De Smet PAGM, Keller K, Hänsel R, et al. *Adverse effects of herbal drugs,* vol 1. Berlin: Springer-Verlag, 1992:223–226.

3. Luethy J, Zweifel U, Schlatter C et al. Pyrrolizidine alkaloids in coltsfoot (*Tussilago farfara L. Mitt Geb Lebensmittelunters Hyg* 1980;71:73–80.

4. Li Y-P, Wang Y-M. Evaluation of tussilagone: a cardiovascular-respiratory stimulant isolated from Chinese herbal medicine. *Gen Pharmacol* 1988;19:261–263.

5. Hwang SB, Chang MN, Garcia ML et al. L-652,469—A dual receptor antagonist of platelet activating factor and dihydropyridines from *Tussilago farfara* L. *Eur J Pharmacol* 1987; 141:269–281.

6. Berry M. Coltsfoot. *Pharm J* 1996;256:234–235.

7. Westendorf J. Pyrrolizidine alkaloids—general discussion. In: *Adverse effects of herbal drugs,* vol 1. Berlin: Springer-Verlag, 1992:193–206.

8. Westendorf J. Pyrrolizidine alkaloids—Petasites species. In: *Adverse effects of herbal drugs,* vol 1. Berlin: Springer-Verlag, 1992:211–214.

9. Kopp B, Wawrosch C, Lebada R et al. Pyrrolizidine alkaloid (PA)-free coltsfoot leaves. Part 1. In vitro cultivation and selection culture. *Dtsch Apoth Ztg* 1997;137:44–47.

COMFREY

1. Awang DVC, Dawson BA, Fillion J et al. Echimidine content of commercial comfrey (*Symphytum* spp.-Boraginaceae). *J Herbs Spices Med Plants* 1993;2:21–34.

2. Bisset NG, Wichtl M. In: *Herbal drugs and phytopharmaceuticals: a handbook for practice on a scientific basis with reference to German Commission E monographs*. Boca Raton, FL: CRC Press, 1994:483–485.

3. Awang DVC. Comfrey. *Can Pharm J* 1987;120:101–104.

4. Couet CE, Crews C, Hanley AB. Analysis, separation, and bioassay of pyrrolizidine alkaloids from comfrey (*Symphytum officinale*). *Natural Toxins* 1996;4:163–167.

5. Winship KA. Toxicity of comfrey. *Adverse Drug React Toxicol Rev* 1991;10:47–59.

6. Betz JM, Eppley RM, Taylor WC et al. Determination of pyrrolizidine alkaloids in commercial comfrey products (*Symphytum* sp.). *J Pharmaceutical Sci* 1994;83:649–653.

References

7. Huxtable RJ, Lüthy J, Zweifel U. Toxicity of comfrey-pepsin preparations. *N Engl J Med* 1986;315:1095.
8. Westendorf J. Pyrrolizidine alkaloids—general discussion. In: De Smet PAGM, et al. *Adverse effects of herbal drugs,* vol 1. Berlin: Springer-Verlag, 1992:193–206.
9. Checke PR. Toxicity and metabolism of pyrrolizidine alkaloids. *J Animal Sci* 1988;66:2343–2350.
10. Yeong ML, Swinburn B, Kennedy M et al. Hepatic veno-occlusive disease associated with comfrey ingestion. *J Gastroenterol Hepatol* 1990;5:211–214.
11. US Pharmacopeia. *Comfrey.* Botanical Monograph Series. United States Pharmacopeial Convention Inc., 1998.
12. Yeong ML, Wakefield SJ, Ford HC. Hepatocyte membrane injury and bleb formation following low dose comfrey toxicity in rats. *Int J Exp Pathol* 1993;74:211–217.
13. Awang DVC. Comfrey update. *HerbalGram* 1991;25:20–23.
14. Facciola S. *Cornucopia: a source book of edible plants.* Vista, CA: Kampong Publications, 1990.
15. Westendorf J. *Symphytum.* In: De Smet PAGM et al. *Adverse Effects of Herbal Drugs,* vol 1. Berlin: Springer-Verlag, 1992: 219–221.

COPPER

1. Turnlund JR. Copper. In: Shils ME, Olson JA, Shike M et al, eds. *Modern nutrition in health and disease,* 9th ed. Baltimore: Williams & Wilkins 1999:241–252.
2. Linder MC. Copper. In: Bowman BA, Russell RM, eds. *Present knowledge in nutrition,* 7th ed. Washington, DC: ILSI Press, Human Nutrition Institute, 1996.
3. Baker A, Turley E, Bonham MP et al. No effect of copper supplementation on biochemical markers of bone metabolism in healthy adults. *Br J Nutr* 1999;82:283–290.
4. Walker WR, Keats DM. An investigation of the therapeutic value of the 'copper bracelet'—dermal assimilation of copper in arthritic/rheumatoid conditions. *Agents Actions* 1976;6/4:454–459.
5. Barceloux DG. Copper. *Clin Toxicol* 1999;37:217–230.
6. Pizarro F, Olivares M, Uauy R et al. Acute gastrointestinal effects of graded levels of copper in drinking water. *Environ Health Perspect* 1999;107:117–121.
7. Muller T, Feichtinger H, Berger H et al. Endemic Tyrolean infantile cirrhosis: an ecogenetic disorder. *Lancet* 1996;347:877–880.
8. Wijmenga C, Muller T, Murli IS et al. Endemic Tyrolean infantile cirrhosis is not an allelic variant of Wilson's disease. *Eur J Hum Genet* 1998;6:624–628.
9. Olivares M, Pizarro F, Speisky H et al. Copper in infant nutrition: safety of World Health Organization provisional guideline value for copper content of drinking water. *J Pediatr Gastroenterol Nutr* 1998;26:251–257.
10. Salonen JT, Salonen R, Korpela H et al. Serum copper and the risk of acute myocardial infarction: a prospective population study in men in Eastern Finland. *Am J Epidemiol* 1991;134:268–276.

CRANBERRY

1. Siciliano AA. Cranberry. *HerbalGram* 1995;38:51–54.
2. Kuzminski LN. Cranberry juice and urinary tract infections: is there a beneficial relationship? *Nutr Rev* 1996;54:S87–S90.
3. Sobota AE. Inhibition of bacterial adherence by cranberry juice: potential use for the treatment of urinary tract infections. *J Urol* 1984;131:1013–1016.
4. Schmidt DR, Sobota AE. An examination of the anti-adherence activity of cranberry juice on urinary and non-urinary bacterial isolates. *Microbios* 1988;55:173–181.
5. Ofek I, Goldhar J, Zafriri D et al. Anti-escherichia coli adhesion activity of cranberry and blueberry juices. *N Engl J Med* 1991;324:1599.
6. Howell AB, Vorsa N, Marderosian AD et al. Inhibition of the adherence of P-fimbriated Escherichia coli to uroepithelial-cell surfaces by proanthocyanidin extracts from cranberries. *N Engl J Med* 1998;339:1085–1086.
7. Jepson RG, Mihaljevic L, Craig, J. Cranberries for treating urinary tract infections (Cochrane Review). In: *The Cochrane Library,* issue 4. Oxford, UK: Update Software, 1999.
8. Jepson RG, Mihaljevic L, Craig, J. Cranberries for preventing urinary tract infections (Cochrane Review). In: *The Cochrane Library,* issue 1. Oxford, UK: Update Software, 2000.
9. Avorn J, Monane M, Gurwitz J et al. Reduction of bacteriuria and pyuria with cranberry beverage: a randomized trial. *J Am Geriatr Soc* 1993;41(Suppl):SA13.
10. Haverkorn MJ, Mandigers J. Reduction of bacteriuria and pyuria using cranberry juice. *JAMA* 1994;272(8):590.
11. Walker EB, Barney DP, Mickelsen JN et al. Cranberry concentrate: UTI prophylaxis (letter). *J Fam Pract* 1997;45:167–168.
12. Foda MM, Middlebrook PF, Gatfield CT et al. Efficacy of cranberry in prevention on urinary tract infection in a susceptible pediatric population. *Can J Urol* 1995;2:98–102.
13. Schlager TA, Anderson S, Trudell J et al. Effect of cranberry juice on bacteriuria in children with neurogenic bladder receiving intermittent catheterization. *J Pediatr* 1999;135:698–702.
14. Tsukada K, Tokunaga K, Iwama T et al. Cranberry juice and its impact on peristomal skin conditions for urostomy patients. *Ostomy Wound Manage* 1994;40:60–67.
15. Bomser J, Madhavi DL, Singletary K et al. In vitro anti-cancer activity of fruit extracts from *Vaccinium* species. *Planta Med* 1996;62:212–216.
16. Howell AB, Vorsa N, Marderosian AD, Foo LY. Inhibition of the adherence of P-fimbriated Escherichia coli to unroepithelial-cell surfaces by proanthocyanidin extracts from cranberries. *N Engl J Med* 1998;339:1085–1086.
17. Lee Y-L, Owens J, Thrupp L et al. Does cranberry juice have antibacterial activity? *JAMA* 2000;283:1691.
18. Habash MB, Van der Mei HC, Busscher HJ et al. The effect of water, ascorbic acid, and cranberry derived supplementation on human urine and uropathogen adhesion to silicone rubber. *Can J Microbiol* 1999;45:691–694.
19. Wilson T, Porcari JP, Harbin D. Cranberry extract inhibits low density lipoprotein oxidation. *Life Sci* 1998;62:381–386
20. Terris MK, Issa MM, Tacker JR. Dietary supplementation with cranberry concentrate tablets may increase the risk of nephrolithiasis. *Urology* 2001;57:26–29.

CREATINE

1. Williams MH, Branch JD. Creatine supplementation and exercise performance: an update. *J Am Coll Nutr* 1998;17:216–234.
2. Linder MC. *Nutritional biochemistry and metabolism, with clinical applications,* 2nd ed. East Norwalk, CT: Appleton & Lange, 1991:96.
3. Benzi G. Is there a rationale for the use of creatine either as a nutritional supplementation or drug administration in

humans participating in a sport? *Pharmacol Res* 2000;41: 255–264.

4. Gordon A, Hultman E, Kaijser L et al. Creatine supplementation in chronic heart failure increases skeletal muscle creatine phosphate and muscle performance. *Cardiovasc Res* 1995;30:413–418.

5. Andrews R, Greenhaff P, Curtis S et al. The effect of dietary creatine supplementation on skeletal muscle metabolism in congestive heart failure. *Eur Heart J* 1998;19:617–622.

6. Klopstock T, Querner V, Schmidt F et al. A placebo-controlled crossover trial of creatine in mitochondrial diseases. *Neurology* 2000;55:1748–1751.

7. Walter MC, Lochmuller H, Reilich P et al. Creatine monohydrate in muscular dystrophies: a double-blind, placebo-controlled clinical study. *Neurology* 2000;54:1848–1850.

8. Tarnopolsky M, Martin J. Creatine monohydrate increases strength in patients with neuromuscular disease. *Neurology* 1999;52:854–857.

9. Pritchard NR, Kalra PA. Renal dysfunction accompanying oral creatine supplements. *Lancet* 1998;351:1252–1253.

10. Almada A, Mitchell T, Earnest C. Impact of chronic creatine supplementation on serum enzyme concentrations. *FASEB J* 1006;10:A791(abst).

11. Earnest C, Almada A, Mitchell T. Influence of chronic creatine supplementation on hepatorenal function. *FASEB J* 1006;10:A790(abst).

12. Pepping J. Creatine. *Am J Health Syst Pharm* 1999;56: 1608–1610.

CYSTEINE

1. Shils ME, Olson JA, Shike M et al, eds. *Modern nutrition in health and disease,* 9th ed. Baltimore: Williams & Wilkins, 1999.

2. Linder, MC. *Nutritional biochemistry and metabolism, with clinical applications,* 2nd ed. East Norwalk, CT: Appleton & Lange, 1991:220.

3. Linder MC. *Nutritional biochemistry and metabolism, with clinical applications,* 2nd ed. East Norwalk, CT: Appleton & Lange, 1991:99.

4. Harvey SG, Gibson JR, Burke CA. L-cysteine, glycine and dl-threonine in the treatment of hypostatic leg ulceration: a placebo-controlled study. *Pharmacotherapeutica* 1985;4: 227–230.

5. Linder MC. *Nutritional biochemistry and metabolism, with clinical applications,* 2nd ed. East Norwalk, CT: Appleton & Lange, 1991:98.

DANDELION

1. De Smet PAGM. *Taraxacum officinale.* In: De Smet PAGM, Keller K, Hänsel R, et al. *Adverse effects of herbal drugs,* vol 2. New York: Springer-Verlag, 1993:297–302.

2. Hook I, McGee A, Henman M. Evaluation of dandelion for diuretic activity and variation in potassium content. *Int J Pharmacog* 1993;3:29–34.

3. Racz-Kotilla E, Racz G, Solomon A. The action of *Taraxacum officinale* extracts on the body weight and diuresis of laboratory animals. *Planta Med* 1974;26:212–217.

4. Tita B, Bello U, Faccendini P et al. *Taraxacum officinale W*: pharmacological effect of ethanol extract. *Pharmacol Res* 1993;27(Suppl 1):23–24.

5. European Scientific Cooperative on Phytotherapy (ESCOP). *Monographs of the medicinal use of plant drugs. Taraxaci folium:dandelion leaf and taraxaci radix (dandelion root).* Exeter, UK, 1996.

6. Akhtar MS, Khan QM, Khaliq T. Effects of Portulaca Oleracae (Kulfa) and *Taraxacum officinale* (Dhudhal) in normoglycaemic and alloxan-treated rabbits. *J Pod Med Assoc* 1985; 35:207–10.

7. Swanston-Flatt SK, Day C, Flatt PR, et al. Glycaemic effects of traditional European plant treatments for diabetes: studies in normal and streptozotocin diabetic mice. *Diabetes Res* 1989;10:69–73.

8. Weiss RF. *Herbal medicine.* Translated from the sixth edition of *Lehrbuch der phytotherapie* by AR Meuss. Gothenburg, Sweden: AB Arcanum; Beaconsfield, England: Beaconsfield Publishers, Ltd, 1988.

9. Zhu M, Womg PY, Li RC. Effects of *Taraxacum mongolicum* on the bioavailability and disposition of ciprofloxacin in rats. *J Pharm Sci* 1999;88:632–634.

DANSHEN

1. Huang KC. *The pharmacology of Chinese herbs,* 2nd ed. Boca Raton, FL: CRC Press, 1999:91–94.

2. Colombo G, Agabio R, Lobina C et al. *Salvia miltiorrhiza* extract inhibits alcohol absorption, preference, and discrimination in sP rats. *Alcohol* 1999;18:65–70.

3. Bensky D, Gamble A. *Chinese herbal medicine Materia Medica.* Seattle, WA: Eastland Press, 1986.

4. Yu CM, Chan JCN, Sanderson JE. Chinese herbs and warfarin potentiation by 'Danshen.' *J Int Med* 1997;241:337–339.

5. Tam LS, Chan TYK, Leung WK et al. Warfarin interactions with Chinese traditional medicines: danshen and methyl salicylate medicated oil. *Aust N Z J Med* 1995;25:258.

6. Chan K, Lo AC, Yeung JH et al. The effects of danshen (*Salvia miltiorrhiza*) on warfarin pharmacodynamics and pharmacokinetics of warfarin enantiomers in rats. *J Pharm Pharmacol* 1995;47:402–406.

DEVIL'S CLAW

1. Bisset NG, Wichtl M. *Herbal drugs and phytopharmaceuticals: a handbook for practice on a scientific basis with reference to German Commission E monographs.* Boca Raton, FL: CRC Press, 1994.

2. Chrubasik S, Junck H, Breitschwerdt H et al. Effectiveness of *Harpagophytum* extract WS 1531 in the treatment of exacerbation of low back pain: a randomised, placebo-controlled, double-blind study. *Eur J Anaesth* 1999;16: 118–129.

3. Chrubasik S, Zimpfer CH, Schutt U et al. Effectiveness of *Harpagophytum procumbens* in treatment of acute low back pain. *Phytomedicine*1996;3:1–10.

4. Chantre P, Cappelaere A, Leblan D et al. Efficacy and tolerance of *Harpagophytum procumbens* versus diacerhein in treatment of osteoarthritis. *Phytomedicine* 2000;7: 177–183.

5. Leblan D, Chantre P, Fournie B. *Harpagophytum procumbens* in the treatment of knee and hip osteoarthritis. Four-month results of a prospective, multicenter, double-blind trial versus diacerhein. *Joint Bone Spine* 2000;67:462–467.

6. Grahame R, Robinson BV. Devils claw (*Harpagophytum procumbens*): pharmacological and clinical studies. *Ann Rheum Dis* 1981;40:632.

7. Soulimani R, Younos C. The role of stomachal digestion on the pharmacological activity of plant extracts, using as an

References

example extracts of *Harpagophytum procumbens*. *Can J Phys Pharmacol* 1993;72:1532–1536.

8. Lanhers M-C, Fleurentin J, Mortier F et al. Anti-inflammatory and analgesic effects of an aqueous extract of *Harpagophytum procumbens*. *Planta Med* 1992;58:117.

9. McLeod DW, Revell P, Robinson BV. Investigations of *Harpagophytum procumbens* (Devil's claw) in the treatment of experimental inflammation and arthritis in rats. *Br J Pharmacol* 1979;66:140.

10. Whitehouse LW, Znamirowska M, Paul CJ. Devil's claw (*Harpagophytum procumbens*): no evidence for anti-inflammatory activity in the treatment of arthritic disease. *Can Med Assoc J* 1983;129:249–251.

11. Circosta C, Occiuto F, Ragusa S. A drug used in traditional medicine: *Harpagophytum procumbens* D.C. II. Cardiovascular activity. *J Ethnopharmacol* 1984;11:259–274.

12. Wegener T. Devil's claw: from African traditional remedy to modern analgesic and anti-inflammatory. *HerbalGram* 2000; 50:47–54.

DHEA

1. Kroboth PD, Salek FS, Pittenger AL et al. DHEA and DHEA-S: a review. *J Clin Pharmacol* 1999;39:327–348.

2. Reiter WJ, Pycha A, Schatzl G et al. Dehydroepiandrosterone in the treatment of erectile dysfunction: a prospective, double-blind, randomized, placebo-controlled study. *Urology* 1999;53:590–595.

3. Wolkowitz O, Reus VI, Keebler A et al. Double-blind treatment of major depression with dehydroepiandrosterone. *Am J Psychiatry* 1999;156:646–649.

4. Bloch M. Schmidt PJ, Danaceau MA et al. Dehydroepiandrosterone treatment of midlife dysthymia. *Biol Psychiatry* 1999;45:1533–1541.

5. Barnhart KT, Freeman E, Grisso JA et al. The effect of dehydroepiandrosterone supplementation to symptomatic perimenopausal women on serum endocrine profiles, lipid parameters, and health-related quality of life. *J Clin Endocrinol Metab* 1999;84:3896–3902.

6. Wolf OT, Neumann O, Hellhammer DH et al. Effects of a two-week physiological dehydroepiandrosterone substitution on cognitive performance and well-being in healthy elderly women and men. *J Clin Endocrinol Metab* 1997;82:2363–2367.

7. Wolf OT, Koster B, Kischbaum C et al. A single administration of dehydroepiandrosterone does not enhance memory performance in young healthy adults, but immediately reduces cortisol levels. *Biol Psychiatry* 1997;42:845–848.

8. Stomati M, Rubino S, Spinetti A et al. Endocrine, neuroendocrine and behavioral effects of oral dehydroepiandrosterone sulfate supplementation in postmenopausal women. *Gynecol Endocrinol* 1999;13:15–25.

9. Labrie, F, Diamond P, Cusan L et al. Effect of 12-month dehydroepiandrosterone replacement therapy on bone, vagina, and endometrium in postmenopausal women. *J Clin Endocrinol Metab* 1997;82:3498–3505.

10. Van Vollenhoven RF, Park JL, Genovese MC et al. A double-blind, placebo-controlled, clinical trial of dehydroepiandrosterone in severe systemic lupus erythematosus. *Lupus* 1999; 8:181–87.

11. Grodon CM, Grace E, Emans J et al. Changes in bone turnover markers and menstrual function after short-term oral DHEA in young women with anorexia nervosa. *J Bone Miner Res* 1999;14:136–145.

12. Flynn MA, Weaver-Osterholtz D, Sharpe-Timms KL et al. Dehydroepiandrosterone replacement in aging humans. *J Clin Endocrinol Metab* 1999;84:1527–1533.

13. Morales AJ, Nolan JJ, Nelson JC et al. Effects of replacement dose of dehydroepiandrosterone in men and women of advancing age. *J Clin Endocrinol Metab* 1994;78:1360–1367.

14. Vogiatzi MG, Boeck MA, Vlachopapadopoulou E et al. Dehydroepiandrosterone in morbidly obese adolescents: effects on weight, body composition, lipids, and insulin resistance. *Metabolism* 1996;45:1011–1015.

15. Nestler JE, Barlascini CO, Clore JN et al. Dehydroepiandrosterone reduces serum low density lipoprotein levels and body fat but does not alter insulin sensitivity in normal men. *J Clin Endocrinol Metab* 1988;66:57–61.

16. Diamond P, Cusan L, Gomez JL et al. Metabolic effects of 12-month percutaneous dehydroepiandrosterone replacement therapy in postmenopausal women. *J Endocrinol* 1996; 150(Suppl):S43–50.

17. Van Vollenhoven RF, Engleman EG, McGuire JL. Dehydroepiandrosterone in systemic lupus erythematosus. *Arthritis Rheum* 1995;38:1826–1831.

18. Alexandersen P, Haarbo J, Christiansen C. The relationship of natural androgens to coronary heart disease in males: a review. *Atherosclerosis* 1996;125:1–13.

19. Barrett-Connor E, Khaw K-T. Absence of an inverse relation of dehydroepiandrosterone sulfate with cardiovascular disease mortality in postmenopausal women. *N Engl J Med* 1987;317:711.

20. Zumoff B, Levin J, Rosenfeld RS et al. Abnormal 24-hr mean plasma concentrations of dehydroepiandrosterone and dehydroepiandrosterone sulfate in women with primary operable breast cancer. *Cancer Res* 1981;41:3360–3363.

21. Helzsouer KJ, Alberg AJ, Gordon GB et al. Serum gonadotropins and steroid hormones and the development of ovarian cancer. *JAMA* 1995;274:1926–1930.

22. Gordon GB, Bush TL, Helzsouer KJ et al. Relationship of serum levels of dehydroepiandrosterone and dehydroepiandrosterone sulfate to the risk of developing postmenopausal breast cancer. *Cancer Res* 1990;50:3859–3862.

23. Dorgan JF. Relationship of serum levels of dehydroepiandrosterone (DHEA), DHEA sulfate, and 5-androstene-3 beta, 17 beta-diol to risk of breast cancer in postmenopausal women. *Cancer Epidemiol Biomark Prev* 1997;6:177–181.

24. Helzsouer KJ, Alberg AJ, Gordon GB. Serum gonadotropins and steroid hormones and the development of ovarian cancer. *JAMA* 1995;274(24):1926–1930.

25. Kline MD, Jaggers ED. Mania onset while using dehydroepiandrosterone. *Am J Psychiatry* 1999;156:971.

26. Parasrampuria J, Schwartz K, Petesch R. Quality control of dehydroepiandrosterone dietary supplement products. *JAMA* 1998;280:1565.

ECHINACEA

1. Awang D. Standardization of herbal medicines. *Altern Ther Womens Health* 1999;1:5759.

2. Melchart D, Walther E, Linde K et al. Echinacea root extracts for the prevention of upper respiratory tract infections: a double-blind, placebo-controlled randomized trial. *Arch Fam Med* 1998;7:541–545.

3. Grimm W, Müller H-H. A randomized controlled trial of the effect of fluid extract of *Echinacea purpurea* on the incidence and severity of colds and respiratory infections. *Am J Med* 1999;106:138–143.

4. Schoneberger D. Einfluß der immunstimulierenden Wirkung von Preßsaft aus Herba Echinaceae purpureae auf Verlauf und Schweregrad von Erkaltungskrankheiten. *Forum Immunologie* 1992;2(8):18–22.

5. Turner RB, Riker DK, Gangemi JD. Ineffectiveness of Echinacea for prevention of experimental rhinovirus colds. *Antimicrob Agents Chemother* 2000;44:1708–1709.

6. Braunig B, Knick E. Therapeutische Erfahrungen mit Echinacea pallida bei grippalen Infekten. *Naturheilpraxis mit Naturmedizin* 1993;1:72–75.

7. Dorn M, Knick E, Lewith G. Placebo-controlled, double-blind study of Echinaceae pallidae radix in upper respiratory tract infections. *Complement Ther Med* 1997;3:40–42.

8. Schulten B, Bulitta M, Ballering-Bruhl B et al. Efficacy of *Echinacea purpurea* in patients with a common cold: a placebo-controlled, randomized, double-blind clinical trial. *Arzneimittelforschung* 2001;51:563–568.

9. Hoheisel O, Sandberg M, Bertram S et al. Echinagard treatment shortens the course of the common cold: a double-blind, placebo-controlled clinical trial. *Eur J Clin Res* 1997; 9:261–269.

10. Braunig B, Dorn M, Knick E. Echinaceae purpureae radix: zur Starkung der korpereigenen Abwehr bei grippalen Infekten. *Z Phytother* 1992;13:7–13.

11. Brinkeborn RM, Shah DV, Degenring FH. Echinaforce and other Echinacea fresh plant preparations in the treatment of the common cold. *Phytomedicine* 1999;6:1–5.

12. Lindenmuth GF, Lindenmuth EB. The efficacy of echinacea compound herbal tea preparation on the severity and duration of upper respiratory and flu symptoms: a randomized, double-blind placebo-controlled study. *J Altern Complement Med* 2000;6:327–334.

13. Melchart D, Linde K, Worku F et al. Immunomodulation with Echinacea—a systematic review of controlled clinical trials. *Phytomedicine* 1994;1:245–254.

14. See, DM, Broumand N, Sahl L et al. In vitro effects of echinacea and ginseng on natural killer and antibody-dependent cell cytotoxicity in healthy subjects and chronic fatigue syndrome or acquired immunodeficiency syndrome patients. *Immunopharmacology* 1997;35:229–235.

15. European Scientific Cooperative on Phytotherapy (ESCOP). *Echinaceae pallida radix (pale coneflower root), Echinacea purpureae herba (purple coneflower herb), and Echinacea purpureae radix (purple coneflower root), Fascicule 6.* Exeter, UK, 1999.

16. Currier NL, Miller SC. Natural killer cells from aging mice treated with extracts from *Echinacea purpurea* are quantitatively and functionally rejuvenated. *Exp Gerontol* 2000;35: 627–639.

17. Luettig B, Steinmüller C, Gifford GE et al. Macrophage activation by the polysaccharide arabinogalactan isolated from plant cell cultures of *Echinacea purpurea. J Natl Cancer Inst* 1989;81:669–675.

18. Stimpel M, Proksch A, Wagner H et al. Macrophage activation and induction of macrophage cytotoxicity by purified polysaccharide fractions from the plant *Echinacea purpurea. Infect Immun* 1984;46:845–849.

19. Rehman J, Dillow JM, Carter SM et al. Increased production of antigen-specific immunoglobulins G and M following in vivo treatment with the medicinal plants *Echinacea angustifolia* and *Hydrastis canadensis. Immunol Lett* 1999;68: 391–395.

20. Steinmuller C, Roesler J, Grottrup E et al. Polysaccharides isolated from plant cell cultures of echinacea enhance the resistance of immunosuppressed mice against systemic infections with *Candida albicans* and *Listeria monocytogenes. Int J Immunopharmacol* 1993;15:605–614.

21. Binns SE, Purgina B, Bergeron C et al. Light-mediated antifungal activity of echinacea extracts. *Planta Med* 2000;66: 241–244.

22. Facino RM, Carini M, Aldini G et al. Echinacoside and caffeoyl conjugates protect collagen from free radical-induced degradation: a potential use of Echinacea extracts in the prevention of skin photodamage. *Planta Med* 1995;61: 510–514.

23. Hu C, Kitts DD. Studies on the antioxidant activity of Echinacea root extract. *J Agric Food Chem* 2000;48:1466–1472.

24. Mullins RJ, Heddle R. Adverse reactions associated with echinacea: the Australian experience. *Ann Allergy Asthma Immunol* 2002;88:42–51.

25. Parnham MJ. Benefit-risk assessment of the squeezed sap of the purple coneflower (*Echinacea purpurea*) for long-term oral immunostimulation. *Phytomedicine* 1996;3:95–102.

26. Schwarz S, Knauth M, Schwab S et al. Acute disseminated encephalomyelitis after parenteral therapy with herbal extracts: a report of two cases. *J Neurol Neurosurg Psychiatry* 2000;69:516–518.

27. Gallo M, Au W, Koren G. Pregnancy outcome following gestational exposure to echinacea. *Arch Int Med* 2000;160: 3141–3143.

28. See D, Berman S, Justis J et al. Phase I study on the safety of *Echinacea angustifolia* and its effect on viral load in HIV infected individuals. *J Am Nutraceut Assoc* 1998;1(ISS1): 14–17.

29. Berman S, See DM, See JR et al. Dramatic increase in immune mediated HIV killing activity induced by *Echinacea angustifolia. Int Conf AIDS* 1998;12:582(abst no 32309).

ELDERBERRY

1. Zakay-Rones, Varsanop N, Zlotnick M et al. Inhibition of several strains of influenza virus in vitro and reduction of symptoms by an elderberry extract (*Sambucus nigra L.*) during an outbreak of influenza B Panama. *J Altern Complement Med* 1995;3:361–369.

2. Fischer E, Brossmer R. Sialic acid-binding lectins: submolecular specificity and interaction with sialoglycoproteins and tumour cells. *Glycoconjugate J* 1995;12:707–713.

3. Van Damme EJM, Barre A, Rouge P et al. Isolation and molecular cloning of a novel type 2 ribosome-inactivating protein with an inactive B chain from elderberry (*Sambucus nigra*) bark. *J Biol Chem* 1997;272:8353–8360.

4. Bisset NG, Wichtl M. *Herbal drugs and phytopharmaceuticals: a handbook for practice on a scientific basis with reference to German Commission E monographs.* Boca Raton, FL: CRC Press, 1994.

5. Centers for Disease Control. Poisoning from elderberry juice—California. *MMWR* 1984;33(13):173.

6. Facciola S. *Cornucopia II: a source book of edible plants.* Vista, CA: Kampong Publications, 1998.

ELEUTHERO

1. Sonnenborn U, Hänsel R. *Eleutherococcus senticosus. Adverse effects of herbal drugs,* vol II. Berlin: Springer-Verlag, 1993:159–169.

2. Yat PN, Arnason JT, Awang, DVC. An improved extraction

References

procedure for rapid quantitative HPLC estimation of the main eleutherosides (B and E) in Eleutherococcus senticosus (eleuthero) as used in the American Botanical Council's ginseng evaluation program. American Botanical Council Ginseng Evaluation Program Methodology, *Eleutherococcus senticosus*, July 1998.

3. Pearce PT, Zois I, Wynne KN et al. *Panax ginseng* and *Eleutherococcus senticosus* extracts—in vitro studies on binding to steroid receptors. *Endocrinol Jpn* 1982;29: 567–573.

4. Eschbach LF, Webster MJ, Boyd JC et al. The effect of Siberian ginseng (*Eleutherococcus senticosus*) on substrate utilization and performance. *Int J Sport Nutr Exerc Metab* 2000; 10:444–451.

5. Dowling EA, Redondo DR, Branch JD et al. Effect of *Eleutherococcus senticosus* on submaximal and maximal exercise performance. *Med Sci Sport Exerc* 1996;28:482–489.

6. McNaughton L, Egan LG, Caelli G. A comparison of Chinese and Russian ginseng as ergogenic aids to improve various facets of physical fitness. *Int Clin Nutr Rev* 1989;9:32–35.

7. Asano K, Takahashi T, Myashita M et al. Effect of *Eleutherococcus senticosus* extract on human physical working capacity. *Planta Med* 1986;3:175–177.

8. Szolomicki J, Samochowiec L, Wojcicki J et al. The influence of active components of *Eleutherococcus senticosus* on cellular defense and physical fitness in man. *Phytother Res* 2000;14:30–35.

9. Bohn B, Nebe CT, Birr C. Flow-cytometric studies with *Eleutherococcus senticosus* extract as an immunomodulatory agent. *Arzneim-Forsch/Drug Res* 1987;37:1193–1196.

10. Brekhman II, Dardymov IV. New substances of plant origin which increase nonspecific resistance. *Ann Rev Pharmacol* 1969;9:419–428.

11. Medon PJ, Ferguson PW, Watson CF. Effects of *Eleutherococcus senticosus* extracts on hexobarbital metabolism in vivo and in vitro. *J Ethnopharmacol* 1984;10:235–241.

12. Baldwin CA, Anderson LA, Phillipson JD. What pharmacists should know about ginseng. *Pharm J* 1986;237:583–586.

13. McRae S. Elevated serum digoxin levels in a patient taking digoxin and Siberian ginseng. *Can Med Assoc J* 1996;155: 293–295.

14. Awang DVC. Siberian ginseng toxicity may be case of mistaken identity. *Can Med Assoc J* 1996;155:1237.

15. Koren G, Randor S, Martin S. Maternal ginseng use associated with neonatal androgenization. *JAMA* 1990;264:2866.

16. Awang DVC. Maternal use of ginseng and neonatal androgenization. *JAMA* 1991;266:363.

17. Waller DP, Martin AM, Farnsworth NR et al. Lack of androgenicity of Siberian ginseng. *JAMA* 1992;267:2329.

EPHEDRA

1. Dewick PM. *Medicinal natural products: a biosynthetic approach*. West Sussex, England: John Wiley and Sons, 1997.

2. Jacobs KM, Hirsch KA. Psychiatric complications of Ma-huang. *Psychosomatics* 2000;41:58–75.

3. White LM, Gardner SF, Gurley BJ et al. Pharmacokinetics and cardiovascular effects of Ma-huang (*Ephedra sinica*) in normotensive adults. *J Clin Pharmacol* 1997;37:116–122.

4. Gurley BJ, Gardner SF, White LM et al. Ephedrine pharmacokinetics after the ingestion of nutritional supplements containing *Ephedra sinica* (ma huang). *Ther Drug Monit* 1998; 20:439–445.

5. Boozer CN, Nasser JA, Heymsfield SB et al. An herbal supplement containing Ma Huang-Guarana for weight loss: a randomized, double-blind trial. *Int J Obes Relat Metab Disord* 2001;25(3):316–324.

6. Molnar D, Torok K, Erhardt E et al. Safety and efficacy of treatment with an ephedrine/caffeine mixture. The first double-blind placebo-controlled pilot study in adolescents. *Int J Obes Relat Metab Disord* 2000;24(12);1573–1578.

7. Astrup A, Breum L, Toubro S et al. The effect and safety of an ephedrine/caffeine compound compared to ephedrine, caffeine and placebo in obese subjects on an energy-restricted diet. A double-blind trial. *Int J Obesity* 1992a;16: 269–277.

8. Daly PA, Krieger DR, Dulloo AG et al. Ephedrine, caffeine, and aspirin: safety and efficacy for treatment of human obesity. *Int J Obesity* 1993;17:S73–78.

9. Mancini MC, Marsiaj HI, Hakoyama MM et al. Ephedrine, caffeine and aminophylline preparation (ECA): an alternative in the treatment of obesity. *Int J Obes Rel Metab Disord* 1990;14:141.

10. Buemann B, Marckmann P, Christensen NJ et al. The effect of ephedrine plus caffeine on plasma lipids and lipoproteins during a 4.2 MJ/day diet. *Int J Obes Relat Metab Disord* 1994;18:329–332.

11. Astrup A, Buemann B, Christensen NJ et al. The effect of ephedrine/caffeine mixture on energy expenditure and body composition in obese women. *Metabolism* 1992b;41: 686–688.

12. Pasquali R, Casimirri F. Clinical aspects of ephedrine in the treatment of obesity. *Int J Obesity* 1993;17:S65–S68.

13. Cesari MP. The therapeutic dilemma of ephedrine in obesity and the inefficacy of caffeine. *Int J Obes Rel Metab Disord* 1989;13:152.

14. Breum L, Pedersen J, Ahlstrom F, Frimodt-Moller J. Comparison of an ephedrine/caffeine combination and dexfenfluramine in the treatment of obesity. A double blind multicenter study. *Int J Obesity* 1994;18:99–103.

15. Bell DG, Jacobs I, McLellan TM, et al. Reducing the dose of combined caffeine and ephedrine preserves the ergogenic effect. *Aviat Space Environ Med* 2000;71:415–419.

16. Bell DG, Jacobs I. Combined caffeine and ephedrine ingestion improves run times of Canadian Forces Warrior Test. *Aviat Space Environ Med* 1999;70:325–329.

17. Meston, CM, Heiman JR. Ephedrine-activated physiological sexual arousal in women. *Arch Gen Psychiatry* 1998;55: 652–656.

18. Ling M, Piddlesden SJ, Morgan BP. A component of the medicinal herb ephedra blocks activation in the classical and alternative pathways of complement. *Clin Exp Immunol* 1995;102:582–588.

19. Massachusetts Medical Society. Adverse events associated with ephedrine-containing products—Texas, December 1993–September 1995. *Morb Mortal Wkly Rep* 1996;45: 689–694.

20. Haller CA, Benowitz NL. Adverse cardiovascular and central nervous system events associated with dietary supplements containing ephedra alkaloids. *N Engl J Med* 2000;343: 1833–1838.

21. Powell T, Hsu, FF, Turk J et al. Ma-huang strikes again; ephedrine nephrolithiasis. *Am J Kidney Dis* 1998;32: 153–159.

22. Bruno A, Nolte KB, Chapin J. Stroke associated with ephedrine use. *Neurology* 1993;43:1313–1316.

23. Zaacks SM, Klein L, Tan CD et al. Hypersensitivity myocarditis associated with ephedra use. *J Tox Clin Tox* 1999;37(4):485–489.
24. Whitehouse AM, Duncan JM. Ephedrine psychosis rediscovered. *Br J Psychiatry* 1987;150:258–261.
25. Capwell RR. Ephedrine-induced mania from an herbal diet supplement [Letter]. *Am J Psychiatry* 1995;152:647.
26. Katz JL. A psychotic manic state induced by an herbal preparation. *Psychosomatics* 2000;41:73–74.
27. Nadir A, Agrawal S, King PD et al. Acute hepatitis associated with the use of a Chinese herbal product, ma-huang. *Am J Gastroenterol* 1996;91:1436–1438.
28. Yin P-A. Ephedrine induced intracerebral hemorrhage and central nervous system vasculitis. *Stroke* 1990;11:1641.
29. Tyler VE. *The honest herbal*. Binghamton, NY: Haworth Press, 1993.

ESSIAC

1. Kaegi E. Unconventional therapies for cancer: 1. Essiac. The task force on alternative therapies of the Canadian Breast Cancer Reseach Initiative. *Can Med Assoc J* 1998;158:897–902.
2. US Congress, Office of Technology Assessment. *Unconventional cancer treatments*. Washington DC: Superintendent of Documents, US Government Printing Office, September 1990; OTA-H-405.
3. Canadian Breast Cancer Research Initiative. Essiac: an information package. Toronto: CBCRI, 1996. Available from: Canadian Breast Cancer Research Initiative, Suite 200, 10 Alcorn Avenue, Toronto, Ontario, Canada M4V3B1 or at Web site (http://www.breast.cancer.ca).
4. Lee H, Tsai SJ. Effect of emodin on cooked-food mutagen activation. *Food Chem Toxicol* 1991;29:765–770.
5. Morita K, Kada T, Namiki M. A desmutagenic factor isolated from burdock (*Arctium lappa*). *Mutat Res* 1984;129:25–31.
6. Rhoads PM, Tong TG, Banner W et al. Anticholinergic poisoning after the ingestion of burdock root tea. *J Toxicol* 1984–1985;22:581–584.
7. Bryson PD, Watanabe AS, Rumack AS et al. Burdock root tea poisoning: case report involving a commercial preparation. *JAMA* 1978;239:2157 (Also [Letter] *JAMA* 1978;240:1586).
8. Blumenthal, Mark. Essiac—herbal remedy touted for cancer. In: *HerbClip*. Austin, TX: American Botanical Council, August 2, 1996.

EUCALYPTUS

1. European Scientific Cooperative on Phytotherapy (ESCOP). *Monographs on the medicinal uses of plant drugs. Eucalypti aetheroleum: eucalyptus oil. Fascicule 6*. Exeter, UK, 1999.
2. Corrigan D. Eucalyptus species. In De Smet et al. *Adverse effects of herbal drugs*, vol 1. Berlin: Springer-Verlag, 1992:125–133.
3. Juergens UR, Stober M, Vetter H. Inhibition of cytokine production and arachidonic acid metabolism by eucalyptol (1.8-cineole) in human blood monocytes in vitro. *Eur J Med Res* 1998;3:508–510.
4. Shahi SK, Shukla AC, Bajaj AK et al. Broad spectrum herbal therapy against superficial fungal infections. *Skin Pharmacol Appl Skin Physiol* 2000;13:60–64.
5. Burrow A, Eccles R, Jones AS. The effects of camphor, eucalyptus and menthol vapour on nasal resistance to airflow and nasal sensation. *Acta Oto-Laryngol* 1983;96:157–161.

6. Morice AH, Marshall AE, Higgins KS et al. Effect of inhaled menthol on citric acid induced cough in normal subjects. *Thorax* 1994;49:1024–1026.
7. Göbel H, Schmidt G, Soyka D. Effect of peppermint and eucalyptus oil preparations on neurophysiological and experimental algesimetric headache parameters. *Cephalalgia* 1994;14:228–234.
8. Sato S, Yoshinuma N, Ito K et al. The inhibitory effect of funoran and eucalyptus extract-containing chewing gum on plaque formation. *J Oral Sci* 1998;40:115–117.
9. Trigg JK. Evaluation of a eucalyptus-based repellent against *Culicoides impunctatus* (Diptera: Ceratopogindae) in Scotland. *J Am Mosquito Control Assoc* 1996;12:329–330.
10. Trigg JK. Evaluation of a eucalyptus-based repellent against *Anopheles* spp. in Tanzania. *J Am Mosquito Control Ass* 1996;12:243–246.
11. Palsson K, Jaenson TG. Plant products used as mosquito repellents in Guinea Bissau, West Africa. *Acta Trop* 1999;72:39–52.
12. Braverman Y, Chizov-Ginzburg A, Mullens BA. Mosquito repellent attracts *Culicoides imicola* (Diptera: Ceratopogonidae). *J Med Entomol* 1999;36:113–115.
13. Riechelmann H, Brommer C, Hinni M et al. Response of human ciliated respiratory cells to a mixture of menthol, eucalyptus oil and pine needle oil. *Arzneimittel-Forschung* 1997;47:1035–1039.
14. Tibballis J. Clinical effects and management of eucalyptus oil ingestion in infants and young children. *Med J Aust* 1995;163:177–180.
15. Day LM, Ozanne-Smith J, Parsons BJ et al. Eucalyptus oil poisoning among young children: mechanisms of access and the potential for prevention. *Aust N Z J Public Health* 1997;21:297–302.
16. Webb NJA, Pitt WR. Eucalyptus oil poisoning in childhood: 41 cases in south-east Queensland. *J Paediatr Child Health* 1993;29:368–371.
17. Jori A, Bianchetti A, Prestini PE et al. Effect of eucalyptol (1,8-cineole) on the metabolism of other drugs in rats and in man. *Eur J Pharmacol* 1970;9:362–366.
18. Brummer E. Human defenses against *Cryptococcus neoformans*: an update. *Mycopathologia* 1998–1999;143:121–125.
19. Chen SC, Currie BJ, Campbell HM et al. *Cryptococcus neoformans* var. *gattii* infection in northern Australia: existence of an environmental source other than known host eucalypts. *Trans R Soc Trop Med Hyg* 1997;91:547–550.

EVENING PRIMROSE

1. De Wick PM. *Medicinal natural products: a biosynthetic approach*. West Sussex, England: John Wiley and Sons, 1997:42.
2. Belch JJF, Ansell D, Madhok R et al. Effects of altering dietary essential fatty acids on requirements for nonsteroidal anti-inflammatory drugs in patients with rheumatoid arthritis. *Ann Rheum Dis* 1988;47:96–104.
3. McFarlin BL, Gibson MH, O'Rear J et al. A national survey of herbal preparation use by nurse-midwives for labor stimulation. Review of the literature and recommendations for practice. *J Nurse Midwifery* 1999;44:205–216.
4. Dove D, Johnson P. Oral evening primrose oil: its effect on length of pregnancy and selected intrapartum outcomes in low-risk nulliparous women. *J Nurse Midwifery* 1999;44:320–324.

References

5. Gamma-Linolenic Multicenter Trial Group (Keen H, Payan J, Allawi J et al.). Treatment of diabetic neuropathy with γ-linolenic acid. *Diabetes Care* 1993;16:8–15.
6. Jamal GA, Carmichael H. The effect of gamma-linolenic acid on human diabetic peripheral neuropathy: a double-blind placebo-controlled trial. *Diabet Med* 1990;7:319–323.
7. Leventhal LJ, Boyce EG, Zurier RB. Treatment of rheumatoid arthritis with gammalinolenic acid. *Ann Int Med* 1993;119:867–873.
8. Brzeski M, Madhok R, Capell HA. Evening primrose oil in patients with rheumatoid arthritis and side effects of non-steroidal anti-inflammatory drugs. *Br J Rheumatol* 1991;30:370–372.
9. Budeiri D, Li Wan Po A, Dornan JC. Is evening primrose oil of value in the treatment of premenstrual syndrome? *Control Clin Trials* 1996;17:60–68.
10. Gately CA, Miers M, Mansel RE et al. Drug treatments for mastalgia: 17 years experience in the Cardiff mastalgia clinic. *J R Soc Med* 1992;85:12–15.
11. Pye JK, Mansel RE, Hughes LE. Clinical experience of drug treatments for mastalgia. *Lancet* 1985;2:373–377.
12. Harding C, Harvey J, Kirkman R et al. Hormone replacement therapy-induced mastalgia responds to evening primrose oil. *Br J Surg* 1996;83(Suppl 1):24.
13. Wetzig S, Burton JL. Oral evening-primrose-seed oil improves atopic eczema. *Lancet* 1982;2:1120–1122.
14. Mansel RE, Harrison BJ, Melhuish J et al. A randomized trial of dietary intervention with essential fatty acids in patients with categorized cysts. *Ann N Y Acad Sci* 1990;586:288–294.
15. Chenoy R, Hussain S, Tayob Y et al. Effect of oral gamolenic acid from evening primrose oil on menopausal flushing. *BMJ* 1994;308:501–503.
16. Jenkins AP, Green AT, Thompson RPH. Essential fatty acid supplementation in chronic hepatitis B. *Aliment Pharmacol Ther* 1996;10:665–668.
17. Oliwiecki S, Burton JL. Evening primrose oil and marine oil in the treatment of psoriasis. *Clin Exp Dermatol* 1994;19:127–129.
18. Veale DJ, Torley HI, Richards IM et al. A double-blind placebo controlled trial of Efamol marine on skin and joint symptoms of psoriatic arthritis. *Br J Rheumatol* 1994;33:954–958.
19. Hederos C-A, Berg A. Epogam evening primrose oil treatment in atopic dermatitis and asthma. *Arch Dis Child* 1996;75:494–497.
20. Schalin-Karrila M, Mattila L, Jansen CT et al. Evening primrose oil in the treatment of atopic eczema: affect on clinical status, plasma phospholipid fatty acids and circulating blood prostaglandins. *Br J Dermatol* 1987;117:11–19.
21. Lovell CR, Burton JL, Horrobin DF. Treatment of atopic eczema with evening primrose oil. *Lancet* 1981;1:278.
22. Wright S, Burton JL. Oral evening-primose-seed oil improves atopic eczema. *Lancet* 1982;2:1120–1122.
23. Morse PF, Horrobin DF, Manku MS et al. Meta-analysis of placebo-controlled studies of the efficacy of Epogam in the treatment of atopic eczema. Relationship between plasma essential fatty acid changes and clinical response. *Br J Dermatol* 1989;121:75–90.
24. Whitaker DK, Cilliers J, de Beer C. Evening primrose oil (Epogam) in the treatment of chronic hand dermatitis: disappointing therapeutic results. *Dermatology* 1996;193:115–120.
25. Yoshimoto-Furuie K, Yoshimoto K, Tanaka T et al. Effects of oral supplementation with evening primrose oil for six weeks on plasma essential fatty acids and uremic skin symptoms in hemodialysis patients. *Nephron* 1999;81:151–159.
26. Shuster J. Black cohosh root? Chasteberry tree? Seizures! *Hosp Pharm* 1998;31:1553–1554.
27. Data Sheet Compendium 1994–1995, 1520-1521. Efamast, Epogam (Searle).

EYEBRIGHT

1. Foster S, Varro I. *Tyler's honest herbal: a sensible guide to the use of herbs and related remedies,* 4th ed. New York: Haworth Herbal Press, 1999:307–309.
2. Bisset NG, Wichtl M. *Herbal drugs and phytopharmaceuticals: a handbook for practice on a scientific basis with reference to German commission E monographs.* Boca Raton, FL: CRC Press, 1994.
3. Grieve M. In: Leyel CF, ed. *A modern herbal,* vol I. Twickenham, Great Britain: Tiger Books Intl, 1998:290–293. (First published 1931, Jonathan Cape Ltd).

FENNEL

1. Keller K. *Foeniculum vulgare.* In: De Smet PAGM, Keller K, Hänsel R, Chandler RF, eds. *Adverse effects of herbal drugs,* vol I. Berlin: Springer-Verlag, 1992:135–142.
2. European Scientific Cooperative on Phytotherapy (ESCOP). *Monographs on the medicinal uses of plant drugs. Foeniculi Fructus: fennel. Fascicule 1.* Exeter, UK, 1996.
3. Westphal J, Horning M, Leonhardt K. Phytotherapy in functional upper abdominal complaints. *Phytomedicine* 1996;2:285–291.
4. Tanira MOM, Shah AH, Mohsin A et al. Pharmacological and toxicological investigations on *Foeniculum vulgare* dried fruit extract in experimental animals. *Phytother Res* 1996;10:33–36.
5. Duke JA. *CRC Handbook of medicinal herbs.* Boca Raton, FL: CRC Press, 1985.

FENUGREEK

1. Sauvaire Y, Ribes G, Baccou J-C et al. Implications of steroid saponins and sapogenins in the hypocholesterolemic effect of fenugreek. *Lipids* 1991;26:191–197.
2. Blumenthal M, Goldberg A, Brinckmann J. *Herbal medicine: expanded Commission E monographs.* Newton, MA: Integrative Medicine Consultants, 2000.
3. Sharma RD, Sarkar A, Hazra DK et al. Hypolipidemic effect of fenugreek seeds: a chronic study in non-insulin dependent diabetic patients. *Phytother Res* 1996;16:332–334.
4. Mishkinsky J, Joseph B, Sulman FG et al. Hypoglycaemic effect of trigonelline. *Lancet* 1967;2:1311–1312.
5. Bordia A, Verma SK, Srivastava KC. Effect of ginger (*Zingiber officinale* Rosc.) and fenugreek (*Trigonella foenum-graecum* L.) on blood lipids, blood sugar and platelet aggregation in patients with coronary artery disease. *Prostaglandins Leukot Essent Fatty Acids* 1997;56:379–384.
6. Sowmya P, Rajyalakshmi P. Hypocholesterolemic effect of germinated fenugreek seeds in human subjects. *Plant Foods Hum Nutr* 1999;53:359–365.
7. Valette G, Sauvaire Y, Baccou J-C et al. Hypocholesterolaemic effect of fenugreek seeds in dogs. *Atherosclerosis* 1984;50:105–111.
8. Broca C, Gross R, Petit P et al. 4-Hydroxyisoleucine: exper-

imental evidence of its insulinotropic and antidiabetic properties. *Am J Physiol* 1999;277:E617–623.

9. Broca C, Manteghetti M, Gross R et al. 4-Hydroxyisoleucine: effects of synthetic and natural analogues on insulin secretion. *Eur J Pharmacol* 2000;390:339–345.

10. Panda S, Tahiliani P, Kar A. Inhibition of triiodothyronine production by fenugreek seed extract in mice and rats. *Pharmacol Res* 1999;40:405–409.

11. Muralidhara, Narasimhamurthy K, Viswanatha S et al. Acute and subchronic toxicity assessment of debitterized fenugreek powder in the mouse and rat. *Food Chem Toxicol* 1999; 37:831–838.

12. Sewell AC, Mosandi A, Bohles H. False diagnosis of maple syrup urine disease owing to ingestion of herbal tea. *N Engl J Med* 341:769.

13. Bartley GB, Hilty MD, Anderson BD et al. "Maple-syrup" urine odor due to fenugreek ingestion. *N Engl J Med* 1981; 305:467.

14. Facciola S. *Cornucopia II: a source book of edible plants.* Vista, CA: Kampong Publications, 1998;112.

FEVERFEW

1. Mills S, Bone KO. *Principles and practice of phytotherapy.* Edinburgh, NY: Churchill Livingstone, 2000:385–393.

2. Murch SJ, Simmons CB, Saxena PK. Melatonin in feverfew and other medicinal plants. *Lancet* 1997;350:1598–1599.

3. Awang DVC. Feverfew fever. *HerbalGram* 1993;29;34–36, 66.

4. Awang DVC. Parthenolide content of feverfew (*Tanacetum parthenium*) assessed by HPLC and 1 H-NMR spectroscopy. *J Nat Products* 1991;54:1510–1521.

5. Ernst E, Pittler MH. The efficacy and safety of feverfew (*Tanacetum parthenium L*): an update of a systematic review. *Public Health Nutr* 2000;3:509–514.

6. Murphy JJ, Heptinsall S, Mitchell JRA. Randomized double-blind placebo-controlled trial of feverfew in migraine prevention. *Lancet* 1988;2:189–192.

7. Palevitch, D, Earon G, Carasso R. Feverfew (*Tanacetum parthenium*) as a prophylactic treatment for migraine: a double-blind placebo-controlled study. *Phytother Res* 1997; 11:508–511.

8. Pfaffenrath V, Fischer M, Friede M et al. Clinical dose-response study for the investigation of efficacy and tolerability of *Tanacetum parthenium* in migraine prophylaxis. *Der Schmerz* 1999;13(Suppl 1):1–13.

9. Johnson ES, Kadam NP, Hylands DM et al. Efficacy of feverfew as prophylactic treatment of migraine. *BMJ* 1985;291: 569–573.

10. De Weerdt CJ, Bootsma HPR, Hendriks H. Herbal medicines in migraine prevention: randomized double-blind placebo-controlled crossover trial of a feverfew preparation. *Phytomedicine* 1996;3:225–230.

11. Kuritzky A, Elhacham Y, Yerushalmi Z et al. Feverfew in the treatment of migraine: its effect on serotonin uptake and platelet activity (293P). *Neurology* 1994;44(Suppl 2):A201.

12. Awang DVC. Feverfew for migraine prevention. *Altern Ther Womens Health* 2000;8:62–63.

13. Pattrick M, Heptinstall S, Doherty M. Feverfew in rheumatoid arthritis: a double-blind, placebo-controlled study. *Ann Rheum Dis* 1989;48:547–549.

14. Biggs MJ, Johnson ES, Persaud NP et al. Platelet aggregation in patients using feverfew for migraine [Letter]. *Lancet* 1982;2:776.

15. Awang DVC. Herbal medicine: feverfew. *Can Pharm J* 1989; 122:266–270.

FISH OIL

1. Uauy-Dagach R, Valenzuela A. Marine oils: the health benefits of n-3 fatty acids. *Nutr Rev* 1996;54:S102–S107.

2. Simopoulos AP. Essential fatty acids in health and chronic disease. *Am J Clin Nutr* 1999;70(3:Suppl):560S–569S.

3. Linder MC. *Nutritional biochemistry and metabolism, with clinical applications,* 2nd ed. East Norwalk, CT: Appleton & Lange, 1991.

4. GISSI-Prevenzione Investigators. Dietary supplementation with n-3 polyunsaturated fatty acids and vitamin E after myocardial infarction: results of the GISSI-Prevenzione trial. *Lancet* 1999;354:447–455.

5. Burr ML, Fehily AM, Gilbert JF et al. Effects of changes in fat, fish and fibre intakes on death and myocardial infarction: diet and reinfarction trial. *Lancet* 1989;2:757–761.

6. Von Schacky C, Angerer P, Kothny W et al. The effect of dietary omega-3 fatty acids on coronary atherosclerosis: A randomized, double-blind, placebo-controlled trial. *Ann Int Med* 1999;130:554–562.

7. Singh RB, Niaz MA, Sharma JP et al. Randomized, double-blind, placebo-controlled trial of fish oil and mustard oil in patients with suspected acute myocardial infarction: the Indian experiment of infarct survival—4. *Cardiovasc Drugs Ther* 1997;11:485–491.

8. Harris WS. Omega-3 fatty acids and serum lipoproteins: human studies. *Am J Clin Nutr* 1997;65(Suppl):1645S–1654S

9. Morris MC, Sacks F, Rosner B et al. Does fish oil lower blood pressure? A meta-analysis of controlled trials. *Circulation* 1993;88:523–533.

10. Gapinski JP, VanRuiswyk JV, Heudebert GR et al. Preventing restenosis with fish oils following coronary angioplasty. *Arch Int Med* 1993;153:1595–1601.

11. Sacks FM, Stone PH, Gibson CM et al. Controlled trial of fish oil for regression of human coronary atherosclerosis. HARP Research Group. *J Am Coll Cardiol* 1995;25:1492–1498.

12. Cairns JA, Gill J, Morton B et al. Fish oils and low-molecular-weight heparin for the reduction of restenosis after percutaneous transluminal coronary angioplasty. The EMPAR study. *Circulation* 1996;94:1553–1560.

13. Johansen O, Brekke M, Seljeflot I et al. N-3 fatty acids do not prevent restenosis after coronary angioplasty: results from the CART study. Coronary Angioplasty Restenosis Trial. *J Am Coll Cardiol* 1999;33:1619–1626.

14. Eritsland J, Arnesen H. Gronseth K et al. Effect of dietary supplementation with n-3 fatty acids on coronary bypass graft patency. *Am J Cardiol* 1996;77:31–36.

15. Christensen JH, Christensen MS, Dyerberg J et al. Heart rate variability and fatty acid content of blood cell membranes: a dose-response study with n-3 fatty acids. *Am J Clin Nutr* 1999;70:331–337.

16. Christensen JH, Gustenhoff P, Korup E et al. Effect of fish oil on heart rate variability in survivors of myocardial infarction: a double blind randomized controlled trial. *BMJ* 1996;312:677–678.

17. Sellmayer A, Witzgall H, Lorenz RL et al. Effects of dietary fish oil on ventricular premature complexes. *Am J Cardiol* 1995;76:974–977.

18. Gogos CA, Ginopoulos P, Salsa B et al. Dietary omega-3 polyunsaturated fatty acids plus vitamin E restore immun-

References

odeficiency and prolong survival for severely ill patients with generalized malignancy. *Cancer* 1998;82:395–402.

19. Wigmore SJ, Barber MD, Ross JA et al. Effect of oral eicosapentaenoic acid on weight loss in patients with pancreatic cancer. *Nutr Cancer* 2000;36:177–184.

20. Burns CP, Halabi S, Clamon GH et al. Phase I clinical study of fish oil fatty acid capsules for patients with cancer cachexia: cancer and leukemia group B study 9473. *Clin Cancer Res* 1999;5:3942–3947.

21. Belluzzi A, Boschi S, Brignola C et al. Polyunsaturated fatty acids and inflammatory bowel disease. *Am J Clin Nutr* 2000; 71:339S–342S.

22. Dichi I, Frenhane P, Dichi JB et al. Comparison of omega-3 fatty acids and sulfasalazine in ulcerative colitis. *Nutrition* 2000;16:87–90.

23. Friedberg CE, Janssen MJFM, Heine RJ et al. Fish oil and glycemic control in diabetes. *Diabetes Care* 1998;21:494–500.

24. Fortin PR, Lew RA, Liang MH et al. Validation of a meta-analysis: the effects of fish oil in rheumatoid arthritis. *J Clin Epidemiol* 1995;48:1379–1390.

25. Ilowite NT, Copperman N, Leicht T et al. effects of dietary modification and fish oil supplementation and dyslipoproteinemia in pediatric systemic lupus erythematosus. *J Rheumatol* 1995;22:1347–1351.

26. Clark WF, Parbtani A. Omega-3 fatty acid supplementation in clinical and experimental lupus nephritis. *Am J Kidney Dis* 1994;23:644–647.

27. Bittiner SB, Cartwright I, Tucker WFG et al. A double-blind, randomized, placebo-controlled trial of fish oil in psoriasis. *Lancet* 1988;1:378–380.

28. Maurice PDL, Allen BR, Barkley ASJ et al. The effects of dietary supplementation with fish oil in patients with psoriasis. *Br J Dermatol* 1987;117:599–606.

29. Lassus A, Dahlgren AL, Halpern MJ et al. Effects of dietary supplementation with polyunsaturated ethyl ester lipids (Angiosan) in patients with psoriasis and psoriatic arthritis. *J Int Med Res* 1990;18:68–73.

30. Søyland E, Funk J, Rajka G et al. Effect of dietary supplementation with very-long-chain n-3 fatty acids in patients with psoriasis. *N Engl J Med* 1993;328:1812–1816.

31. Bjorneboe A, Soyland E, Bjorneboe G-EA et al. Effect of dietary supplementation with eicasopentaenoic acid in the treatment of atopic dermatitis. *Br J Dermatol* 1987;117:463–469.

32. Kunz B, Ring J, Braun-Falco O. Eicasopentanoic acid (EPA) treatment in atopic eczema. *J Allergy Clin Immunol* 1989; 83:196.

33. Woods RK, Rhien FC, Abramson MJ. Dietary marine fatty acids (fish oil) for asthma. *Cochrane Database Syst Rev* 2000;(2):CD001283.

34. Lawrence R, Sorrell T. Eicasopentaenoic acid in cystic fibrosis; evidence of a pathogenetic role for leukotriene B4. *Lancet* 1993;342:465–469.

35. Donadio JV Jr. Use of fish oil to treat patients with immunoglobulin a nephropathy. *Am J Clin Nutr* 2000;71(1 Suppl):373S–375S.

36. van der Heide JJH, Bilo HJG, Donker JM et al. Effect of dietary fish oil on renal function and rejection in cyclosporine-treated recipients of renal transplants. *N Engl J Med* 1993;329:769–773.

37. Kooijmans-Coutinho MF, Rischen-Vos J, Hermans J et al. Dietary fish oil in renal transplant recipients treated with cyclosporin-A: no beneficial effects shown. *J Am Soc Nephrol* 1996;7:513–518.

38. Schmitz PG, McCloud LK, Reikes ST, et al. Prophylaxis of hemodialysis graft thrombosis with fish oil: double-blind, randomized, prospective trial. *J Am Soc Nephrol* 2002;13: 184–190.

39. Stoll AL, Severus E, Freeman MP et al. Omega-3 fatty acids in bipolar disorder: a preliminary double-blind, placebo-controlled trial. *Arch Gen Psychiatry* 1999;56:407–412.

40. Joy CB, Mumby-Croft R, Joy LA. Polyunsaturated fatty acid (fish or evening primrose oil) for schizophrenia. *Cochrane Database Syst Rev* 2000(2);CD001257.

41. Harel Z, Biro FM, Kottenhahn RK et al. Supplementation with omega-3 polyunsaturated fatty acids in the management of dysmenorrhea in adolescents. *Am J Obstet Gynecol* 1996;174:1335–1338.

42. Olsen SF, Sorensen JD, Secher NJ et al. Randomised controlled trial of effect of fish-oil supplementation on pregnancy duration. *Lancet* 1992;339:1003–1007.

43. Olsen SF, Secher NJ, Tabor A et al. Randomised clinical trials of fish oil supplementation in high risk pregnancies. Fish Oil Trials In Pregnancy (FOTIP) Team. *BJOG* 2000;107: 382–395.

44. Onwude JL, Lilford RJ, Hjartardottir H et al. A randomised double-blind placebo-controlled trial of fish oil in high risk pregnancy. *Br J Obstet Gynaecol* 1995;102:95–100.

45. Pedersen HS, Mulvad G, Seidelin KN et al. N-3 fatty acids as a risk factor for haemorrhagic stroke. *Lancet* 1999;353:812-13.

46. Dawson JK, Abernethy VE, Graham DR et al. A woman who took cod-liver oil and smoked. *Lancet* 1996;347:1804.

47. Eritsland J. Safety considerations of polyunsaturated fatty acids. *Am J Clin Nutr* 2000;71:197–201.

FLAXSEED

1. Facciola S. *Cornucopia II: a source book of edible plants.* Vista, CA: Kampong Publications, 1998:145.

2. European Scientific Cooperative on Phytotherapy (ESCOP). *Monographs on the medicinal use of plant drugs. Lini semen (Linseed). Fascicule 1.* Exeter, UK, 1996.

3. Jenkins DJA, Kendall CWC, Vidgen E et al. Health aspects of partially defatted flaxseed, including effects on serum lipids, oxidative measures, and ex vivo androgen and progestin activity: a controlled crossover trial. *Am J Clin Nutr* 1999;69:395–402.

4. Lampe JW, Martini MC, Kurzer MS et al. Urinary lignan and isoflavonoid excretion in premenopausal women consuming flaxseed powder. *Am J Clin Nutr* 1994;60:122–128.

5. Cunnane SC, Hamadeh MJ, Leide AC et al. Nutritional attributes of traditional flaxseed in healthy young adults. *Am J Clin Nutr* 1994;61:62–68.

6. Brzezinski A, Adlercreutz H, Shaoul R et al. Short-term effects of phytoestrogen-rich diet on postmenopausal women. *Menopause* 1997;4:89–94.

7. Jenkins DJA, Kendall CWC, Vidgen E et al. Health aspects of partially defatted flaxseed, including effects on serum lipids, oxidative measures, and ex vivo androgen and progestin activity: a controlled crossover trial. *Am J Clin Nutr* 1999;69:395–402.

8. Allman MA, Pena MM, Pang D. Supplementation with flaxseed oil versus sunflower seed oil in healthy young men consuming a low fat diet: effects on platelet composition and function. *Eur J Clin Nutr* 1995;49:169–178.

9. Nestel PJ, Pomeroy SE, Sashara T et al. Arterial compliance in obese subjects is improved with dietary plant n-3 fatty

acide from flaxseed oil despite increased LDL oxidizability. *Arterioscl Thromb Vasc Biol* 1997;17:1163–1170.

10. Nordstrom DC, Honkanen VE, Nasu Y et al. Alpha-linolenic acid in the treatment of rheumatoid arthritis. A double-blind, placebo-controlled and randomized study: flaxseed vs. safflower seed. *Rheumatol Int* 1995;14:231–234.

11. Clark WF, Parbtani A, Huff MW et al. Flaxseed: a potential treatment for lupus nephritis. *Kidney Int* 1995;48:475–480.

12. Phipps WR, Martini MC, Lampe JW et al. Effect of flaxseed ingestion on the menstrual cycle. *J Clin Endocrinol Metab* 1993;77:1215–1219.

13. Haggans CJ, Hutchins AM, Olson BA et al. Effect of flaxseed consumption on urinary estrogen metabolites in post-menopausal women. *Nutr Cancer* 1999;33:188–195.

14. Lezaun A, Fraj J, Colás C et al. Anaphylaxis from linseed. *Allergy* 1998;53:105–106.

15. Rosling H. Cyanide exposure from linseed. *Lancet* 1993;341: 177.

16. Schulz V, Hänsel R, Tyler VE. *Rational phytotherapy*. Berlin: Springer-Verlag, 1998:202–204.

17. Mantzioris E, James MJ, Gibson RA et al. Nutritional attributes of dietary flaxseed oil. *Am J Clin Nutr* 1995;62; 841–844.

FOLIC ACID

1. Herbert V. Folic acid. In: Shils ME, Olson JA, Shike M et al, eds. *Modern nutrition in health and disease,* 9th ed. Baltimore: Williams & Wilkins 1999:433–446.

2. Lumley J, Watson L, Watson M et al. Periconceptional supplementation with folate and/or multivitamins for preventing neural tube defects. *Cochrane Database Syst Rev* 2000; 2:CD001056.

3. Mahomed K. Folate supplementation in pregnancy. *Cochrane Database Syst Rev* 2000;2:CD000183.

4. Ortiz Z, Shea B, Suarez AM et al. Folic acid and folinic acid for reducing side effects in patients receiving methotrexate for rheumatoid arthritis. *Cochrane Database Syst Rev* 2000;2: CD000951.

5. Alpert JE, Fava M. Nutrition and depression: the role of folate. *Nutr Rev* 1997;55:145–149.

6. Fava M, Borus JS, Alpert JE et al. Folate, vitamin B12, and homocysteine in major depressive disorder. *Am J Psychiatry* 1997;154:426–428.

7. Godfrey PS, Toone BK, Carney MW et al. Enhancement of recovery from psychiatric illness by methylfolate. *Lancet* 1990:336:392–395.

8. Coppen A, Bailey J. Enhancement of the antidepressant action of fluoxetine by folic acid: a randomized, placebo-controlled trial. *J Affective Dis* 2000;60:121–130.

9. Snowdon DA, Tully CL, Smith CD et al. Serum folate and the severity of atrophy of the neocortex in Alzheimer disease: findings from the Nun Study. *Am J Clin Nutr* 2000;71: 993–998.

10. Botez MI, Botez T, Ross-Chourinard A et al. Thiamine and folate treatment of chronic epileptic patients: a controlled study with the Wechsler IQ scale. *Epilepsy Res* 1993;16: 157–163.

11. Saito M, Kato H, Tsuchida T et al. Chemoprevention effects on bronchial squamous metaplasia by folate and vitamin B12 in heavy smokers. *Chest* 1994;106:496–499.

12. Butterworth CE, Hatch KD, Soong S-J et al. Oral folic acid supplementation for cervical dysplasia: a clinical intervention trial. *Am J Obstet Gynecol* 1992;166:803–809.

13. Childers et al. Chemoprevention of cervical cancer with folic acid: a phase III. SW Oncology Group intergroup study. *Cancer Epidemiol Biomark Prev* 1995;4:155–159.

14. Zhang S, Hunter DJ, Hankinson SE et al. A prospective study of folate intake and the risk of breast cancer. *JAMA* 1999; 281:1632–1637.

15. Hankey GJ, Eikelboom JW. Homocysteine and vascular disease. *Lancet* 1999;354:407–413.

16. Christen WG, Ajani UA, Glynn RJ et al. Blood levels of homocysteine and increased risks of cardiovascular disease. *Arch Intern Med* 2000;160:422–434.

17. Peterson JD, Spence JD. Vitamins and progression of atherosclerosis in hyperhomocysteinemia. *Lancet* 1998;351:263.

18. Vermeulen EGJ, Stehouwer CDA, Twisk JWR et al. Effect of homocysteine-lowering treatment with folic acid plus vitamin B6 on progression of subclinical atherosclerosis: a randomized, placebo-controlled trial. *Lancet* 2000;355: 517–522.

19. Ashraf H, Rahman MM, Fuchs GJ et al. Folic acid in the treatment of acute watery diarrhoea in children: a double-blind, randomized, controlled trial. *Acta Paediatr* 1998;87: 1113–1115.

20. Brown RS, Di Stanislao PT, Beaver WT et al. The administration of folic acid to institutionalized epileptic adults with phenytoin-induced gingival hyperplasia. A double-blind, randomized, placebo-controlled, parallel study. *Oral Surg Ora Med Oral Pathol* 1991;71:565–568.

21. Backman N, Holm AK, Hanstrom L et al. Folate treatment of diphenylhydantoin-induced gingival hyperplasia. *Scand J Dent Res* 1989;97:222–232.

22. Poppell TD, Keeling SD, Collins JF et al. Effect of folic acid on recurrence of phenytoin-induced gingival overgrowth following gingivectomy. *J Clin Periodontol* 1991;18: 134–139.

23. Selhub J, Rosenberg IH. Folic acid. In: Bowman BA, Russell RM, eds. *Present knowledge in nutrition*, 7th ed. Washington, DC: ILSI Press, 1996:206–219.

24. Butterworth CE, Tamura T. Folic acid safety and toxicity: a brief review. *Am J Clin Nutr* 1989;50:353–358.

25. Recommended levels for individual intake, 1998, B vitamins and choline. Food and Nutrition Board, Institute of Medicine. Dietary reference intakes. Thiamin, riboflavin, niacin, vitamin B12, pantothenic acid, biotin, and choline. Washington, DC: National Academy Press, 1998.

26. Berg MJ, Stumbo PJ, Chenard CA et al. Folic acid improves phenytoin pharmacokinetics. *J Am Diet Assoc* 1995;95: 352–356.

27. Lewis DP, Van Dyke DC, Willhite LA et al. Phenytoin-folic acid interaction. *Ann Pharmacother* 1995;29:726–735.

28. Montes LF, Diaz ML, Lajous J et al. Folic acid and vitamin B12 in vitiligo: a nutritional approach. *Cutis* 1992;50: 39–42.

29. Bentivoglio G, Melica F, Cristoforoni P. Folinic acid in the treatment of human male infertility. *Fertil Steril* 1993;60: 698–701.

30. Bailey LB, Moyers S, Gregory JF. Folate. In: Bowman BA, Russell RM, eds. *Present knowledge in nutrition,* 8th ed. Washington, DC: ILSI Press, 2001:214–229.

FOXGLOVE

1. Lewis WH, Elvin Lewis MPF. *Medical botany*. New York: John Wiley and Sons, 1997:184.

2. Robbers JE, Speedie MF, Tyler VE. *Pharmacognosy and phar-*

References

macobiotechnology. Baltimore: Williams and Wilkins, 1996: 117.

3. Robbers JE, Speedie MF, Tyler VE. Pharmacognosy and pharmacobiotechnology. Baltimore: Williams and Wilkins, 1996: 119.

3a. *Physicians Desk Reference*, 56th ed. Montvale, NJ: Medical Economics, 2002:1588.

4. Dewick PM. *Medicinal natural products: a biosynthetic approach*. Chichester, England: John Wiley and Sons, 199: 232–233.

5. Porter R, Schultz D, Robertson WO. Alternative medicine toxicity: digitalis poisoning! *J Toxicol Clin Toxicol* 1999:37.

6. Colls BM. A salutary lesson: three very unwise men. *BMJ* 1999;318:1729.

7. Bain, RJI. Accidental digitalis poisoning due to drinking herbal tea. *BMJ* 1985;290:1624.

8. Slifman NR, Obermeyer WR, Musser SM et al. Contamination of botanical dietary supplements by *Digitalis lanata*. *N Engl J Med* 1998;339:806–811.

9. Rich SA, Libera JM, Locke RJ. Treatment of foxglove extract poisoning with digoxin-specific Fab fragments. *Ann Emerg Med* 1993;22:1904–1907.

10. Eddleston M, Rajapakse S, Rajakanthan S et al. Anti-digoxin Fab fragments in cardiotoxicity induced by ingestion of yellow oleander: a randomized controlled trial. *Lancet* 2000; 355:967–972.

GARLIC

1. European Scientific Cooperative on Phytotherapy (ESCOP). *Monographs on the medicinal uses of plant drugs. Allii sativi bulbus: garlic. Fascicule 3*. Exeter, UK, 1997.

2. Orekhov AN, Tertov VV, Sobenin IA et al. Direct anti-atherosclerosis-related effects of garlic. *Ann Med* 1995;27:63–65.

3. Agarwal KC. Therapeutic actions of garlic constituents. *Med Res Rev* 1996;16:111–124.

4. Ackermann RT, Mulrow CD, Ramirez G et al. Garlic shows promise for improving some cardiovascular risk factors. *Arch Intern Med* 2001;161:813–824.

5. Stevinson C, Pittler MH, Ernst E. Garlic for treating hypercholesterolemia: a meta-analysis of randomized clinical trials. *Ann Intern Med* 2000;133:420–429.

6. Gardner CD, Chatterjee LM, Carlson JJ. The effect of a garlic preparation on plasma lipid levels in moderately hypercholesterolemic adults. *Atherosclerosis* 2001;154:213–220.

7. Koscielny J, Klüssendorf D, Latza R et al. The antiatherosclerotic effect of *Allium sativum*. *Atherosclerosis* 1999;144: 237–249.

8. Ledezma E, De Sousa L, Jorquera A et al. Efficacy of ajoene, an organosulphur derived from garlic, in the short-term therapy of tinea pedis. *Mycoses* 1996;39:393–395.

9. Stjernberg L, Berglund J. Garlic as an insect repellent. *JAMA* 2000;284:831.

10. Kiesewetter H, Jung F, Jung EM et al. Effects of garlic coated tablets in peripheral arterial occlusive disease. *Clin Invest* 1993;71:383–386.

11. Jepson RG, Kleijnen J, Leng GC. Garlic for peripheral arterial occlusive disease. *Cochrane Database System Rev* 2002(2);CD000095.

12. Kiesewetter H, Jung EM, Mrowietz C et al. Effect of garlic on platelet aggregation in patients with increased juvenile ischemic attack. *Eur J Clin Pharmacol* 1993;45:333–336.

13. Mayeux RR, Agrawal KC, Tou J-SH et al. The pharmacological effects of allicin, a constituent of garlic oil. *Agents Actions* 1998;88:737–744.

14. Fleischauer AT, Poole C, Arab L. Garlic consumption and cancer prevention: meta-analyses of colorectal and stomach cancers. *Am J Clin Nutr* 2000;72:1047–1052.

15. Ernst E. Can Allium vegetables prevent cancer? *Phytomedicine* 1997;4:79–83.

16. You W-C, Blot WJ, Chang Y-S et al. Allium vegetables and reduced risk of stomach cancer. *J Natl Cancer Inst* 1989;81: 162–164.

17. Garty BZ. Garlic burns. *Pediatrics* 1993;91:658–659.

18. Canduela V, Mongil I, Carrascosa M. Garlic: always good for the health? *Br J Dermatol* 1995;1:161–162.

19. Sunter W. Warfarin and garlic. *Pharm J* 1991;246:722.

20. Mennella JA, Beauchamp GK. Maternal diet alters the sensory quantities of human milk and the nursling's behavior. *Pediatrics* 1991;88:737–744.

21. Burden AD, Wilkinson SM, Beck MH et al. Garlic-induced systemic contact dermatitis. *Contact Dermatitis* 1994;30: 299–315.

22. Ruocco V, Brenner S, Lombardi ML. A case of diet-related pemphigus. *Dermatology* 1996;192:373–74.

23. Brenner S, Ruocco V, Wolf R et al. Pemphigus and dietary factors: in vitro acantholysis by allyl compounds of the genus Allium. *Dermatology* 1995;190:197–202.

24. German K, Kumar U, Blackford HN. Garlic and the risk of TURP bleeding. *Br J Urol* 1995;76:518.

25. Burnham BE. Garlic as a possible risk for postoperative bleeding. *Plast Reconstruc Surg* 1995;95:213.

26. Rose KD, Croissant PD, Parliament CF et al. Spontaneous spinal epidural hematoma with associated platelet dysfunction from excessive garlic consumption: a case report. *Neurosurgery* 1990;26:880–882.

27. Añibarro B, Fontela JL, de la Hoz. Occupational asthma induced by garlic dust. *Allergy Clin Immunol* 1997;100: 734–738.

GERMANDER

1. Loeper J, Descatoire V, Letteron P et al. Hepatotoxicity of germander in mice. *Gastroenterology* 1994;106:464–472.

2. Lekehal M, Pessayre D, Lereau JM et al. Hepatotoxicity of the herbal medicine germander: metabolic activation of its furano diterpenoids by cytochrome P450 3A depletes cytoskeleton-associated protein thiols and forms plasma membrane blebs in rat hepatocytes. *Hepatology* 1996;24:212–218.

3. Fau D, Lekehal M, Farrell G et al. Diterpenoids from germander, an herbal medicine, induce apoptosis in isolated rat hepatocytes. *Gastroenetrology* 1997;113:1334–1346.

4. De Smet PAGM. *Teucrium chamaedrys*. In: De Smet PAGM, Keller K, Hänsel R et al, eds. *Adverse effects of herbal drugs*, vol 3. Berlin: Springer Verlag, Berlin, 1997:137–144.

5. Castot A, Larrey D. Hépatites observées au cours d'un traitement par un medicament ou une tisane contenant de la germandrée petit-chene. Bilan des 26 cas rapportés aux Centres Régionaux de Pharmacovigilance. *Gastreoenterol Clin Biol* 1992;16:916–922.

6. Larrey D, Vial T, Pauwels A et al. Hepatitis after germander (*Teucrium chamaedrys*) administration: another instance of herbal medicine hepatotoxicity. *Ann Int Med* 1992;117: 129–132.

7. Mostefa-Kara N, Pauwels A, Pines E et al. Fatal hepatitis after herbal tea. *Lancet* 1992;340:674.

8. Laliberté L, Villeneuve J-P. Hepatitis after the use of germander, a herbal remedy. *Can Med Assoc J* 1996;154: 1689–1692.

GERMANIUM

1. Schauss AG. Nephrotoxicity and neurotoxicity in humans from organogermanium compounds and germanium dioxide. *Biol Trace Element Res* 1991;29:267–280.
2. Tao S-H, Bolger PM. Hazard assessment of germanium supplements. *Regul Toxicol Pharmacol* 1997;25:211–219.
3. Nielson FH. Ultratrace minerals. In Shils ME, Olson JA, Shike M et al; eds. *Modern nutrition in health and disease*, 9th ed. Baltimore: Williams and Wilkins 1999:299.
4. Mainwaring MG, Poor C, Zander DS et al. Complete remission of pulmonary spindle cell carcinoma after treatment with oral germanium sesquioxide. *Chest* 2000;117:591–593.
5. Shils ME, Olson JA, Shike M et al, eds. *Modern nutrition in health and disease,* 9th ed. Baltimore: Williams & Wilkins 1999:299.
6. Linder MC. *Nutritional biochemistry and metabolism, with clinical applications,* 2nd ed. East Norwalk, CT: Appleton & Lange, 1991.
7. Asaka T, Nitta E, Makifuchi T et al. Germanium intoxication with sensory ataxia. *J Neurol Sci* 1995;130:220–223.
8. Becker BN, Greene J, Evanson J et al. Ginseng-induced diuretic resistance. *JAMA* 1996;276:606–607.

GINGER

1. Corrigan D. *Zingiber officinale*. In: De Smet PAGM, Keller K, Hänsel R, Chandler RF. (ed). *Adverse effects of herbal drugs,* vol. 3. Berlin: Springer-Verlag 1997;215–228.
2. European Scientific Cooperative on Phytotherapy (ESCOP). *Monographs on the medicinal uses of plant drugs. Zingiberis rhizoma: ginger. Fascicule 1.* Exeter, UK, 1996.
3. Vutyavanich T, Kraisarin T, Ruangsri R-A. Ginger for nausea and vomiting in pregnancy: randomized, double-masked, placebo-controlled trial. *Obstet Gynecol* 2001;97:577–582.
4. Fischer-Rasmussen W, Kjaer SK, Dahl C et al. Ginger treatment of hyperemesis gravidarum. *Eur J Obstet Gynecol Reprod Biol* 1990;38:19–24.
5. Bone ME, Wilkinson DJ, Young JR et al. Ginger root—a new antiemetic: the effect of ginger root on postoperative nausea and vomiting after major gynaecological surgery. *Anaesthesia* 1990;45:669–667.
6. Phillips S, Hutchinson SE. *Zingiber officinale* (ginger)—an antiemetic for day case surgery. *Anesthesia* 1993;48: 715–717.
7. Arfeen Z, Owen H, Plummer JL et al. A double-blind randomized controlled trial of ginger for the prevention of postoperative nausea and vomiting. *Anaesth Intensive Care* 1995;23:449–452.
8. Meyer K, Schwartz J, Crater D et al. *Zingiber officinale* (ginger) used to prevent 8-MOP associated nausea. *Dermatol Nursing* 1995;7:242–244.
9. Grontved A, Brask T, Kambskard J et al. Ginger root against seasickness: a controlled trial on the open sea. *Acta Otolaryngol* 1988;105:45–49.
10. Schmid R, Schick T, Steffen R et al. Comparison of seven commonly used agents for prophylaxis of seasickness. *J Travel Med* 1994;1:203–206.
11. Mowrey DB. Motion sickness, ginger, and psychophysics. *Lancet* 1982;1(8273):655–657.
12. Grontved A, Hentzer E. Vertigo-reducing effect of ginger root: a controlled clinical study. *J Oto-Rhino-Laryngol* 1986; 48:282–286.
13. Stewart JJ, Wood MJ, Wood, CD et al. Effects of ginger on motion sickness susceptibility and gastric function. *Pharmacology* 1991;42:111–120.
14. Micklefield GH, Redeker Y, Meister V et al. Effects of ginger on gastroduodenal motility. *Int J Clin Pharmacol Ther* 1999; 37:341–346.
15. Bliddal H, Rosetzsky A, Schlichting P et al. A randomized, placebo-controlled, crossover study of ginger extracts and ibuprofen in osteoarthritis. *Osteoarthritis Cartilage* 2000;8: 9–12.
16. Lumb AB. Effect of dried ginger on human platelet function. *Thromb Haemostas* 1994;71:110–111.
17. Bordia A, Verma SK, Srivastava KC. Effect of ginger (*Zingiber officinale* Rosc.) and fenugreek (*Trigonella foenum-graecum L.*) on blood lipids, blood sugar and platelet aggregation in patients with coronary artery disease. *Prostaglandins, Leukotrienes Essential Fatty Acids* 1997;56:379–384.
18. Janssen PLTMK, Meyboom S, van Staveren WA et al. Consumption of ginger (*Zingiber officinale* Roscoe) does not affect ex vivo platelet thromboxane production in humans. *Eur J Clin Nutr* 1996;50:772–774.

GINKGO

1. Fugh-Berman A, Cott JM. Dietary supplements and natural products as psychotherapeutic agents. *Psychosom Med* 1999;61:712–728.
2. Chung KF, McCusker M, Page CP et al. Effect of a ginkgolide mixture (BN 52063) in antagonising skin and platelet responses to platelet activating factor in man. *Lancet* 1987; 1:248–250.
3. Itil T, Martorano D. Natural substances in psychiatry (*Ginkgo biloba* in dementia). *Psychopharm Bull* 1995;31:147–158.
4. Porsolt RD, Roux S, Drieu K. Evaluation of a *Ginkgo biloba* extract (Egb 761) in functional tests for monoamine oxidase inhibition. *Arzneim-Forsch/Drug Res* 2000;50:232–235.
5. Fowler JS, Wang G-J, Volkow ND et al. Evidence that *Ginkgo biloba* extract does not inhibit MAO A and B in living human brain. *Life Sci* 2000;66:141–146.
6. Oken BS, Storzbach DM, Kaye JA. The efficacy of *Ginkgo biloba* on cognitive function in Alzheimer disease. *Arch Neurol* 1998;55:1409–1415.
7. Ernst E, Pittler MH. *Ginkgo biloba* for dementia: a systematic review of double-blind, placebo-controlled trials. *Clin Drug Invest* 1999;17:301–308.
8. Van Dongen MC, van Rossum E, Kessels AG et al. The efficacy of ginkgo for elderly people with dementia and age-associated memory impairment: new results of a randomized clinical trial. *J Am Geriatr Soc* 2000;48:1183–1194.
9. Rai GS, Shovlin C, Wesnes KA. A double-blind, placebo-controlled study of *Ginkgo biloba* extract (`Tanakan') in elderly outpatients with mild to moderate memory impairment. *Curr Med Res Opin* 1991;12:350–355.
10. Mix JA, Crews WD. An examination of the efficacy of *Ginkgo biloba* extract EGb761 on the neuropsychologic functioning of cognitively intact older adults. *J Alt Comp Med* 2000;6: 219–229.
11. Lingaerde O, Foreland AR, Magnusson A. Can winter depression be prevented by *Ginkgo biloba* extract? A placebo-controlled trial. *Acta Psychiatr Scand* 1999;100:62–66.

References

12. Kleijnen J, Knipschild P. *Ginkgo biloba* for cerebral insufficiency. *Br J Clin Pharmacol* 1992;34:352–358.
13. Zhang XY, Zhou DF, Su JM et al. The effect of extract of *Ginkgo biloba* added to haloperidol on superoxide dismutase in inpatients with chronic schizophrenia. *J Clin Psychopharmacol* 2001;21:85–88.
14. Pittler MH, Ernst E. *Ginkgo biloba* extract for the treatment of intermittent claudication: a meta-analysis of randomized trials. *Am J Med* 2000;108:276–281.
15. Kleijnen J, Knipschild P. *Ginkgo biloba*. *Lancet* 1992;340:1136–1139.
16. Schweizer J, Hautmann C. Comparison of two dosages of *Ginkgo biloba* extract EGb 761 in patients with peripheral arterial occlusive disease Fontaine's stage IIb. A randomised, double-blind, multicentric clinical trial. *Arzneimittelforschung* 1999;49:900–904.
17. Ernst E, Stevinson C. *Ginkgo biloba* for tinnitus: a review. *Clin Otolaryngol* 1999;24:164–7.
18. Drew S, Davies E. Effectiveness of *Ginkgo biloba* in treating tinnitus: double-blind, placebo controlled trial. *BMJ* 2001;322:73–75.
19. Plath R, Oliver J. Results of combined low-power laser therapy and extracts of *Ginkgo biloba* in cases of sensorineural hearing loss and tinnitus. *Adv Otorhinolaryngol* 1995;49:101–104.
20. Wedel Hv, Calero L, Walger M et al. Soft-laser/Ginkgo therapy in chronic tinnitus. *Adv Otorhinolaryngol* 1995;49:105–106.
21. Garg RK, Nag D, Agrawal A. A double-blind placebo-controlled trial of *Ginkgo biloba* extract in acute cerebral ischemia. *J Assoc Physicians India* 1995;43:760–763.
22. Cohen AJ, Bartlik B. *Ginkgo biloba* for antidepressant-induced sexual dysfunction. *J Sex Marital Therapy* 1998;24:139–143.
23. Ashton AK, Ahrens K, Gupta S et al. Antidepressant-induced sexual dysfunction in *Ginkgo biloba*. *Am J Psychiatry* 2000;157:836–837.
24. Sikora R, Sohn M, Deutz F-J et al. *Ginkgo biloba* extract in the therapy of erectile dysfunction. *J Urol* 1989;141:188A(abst).
25. Tamborini A, Taurelle R. [Value of standardized *Ginkgo biloba* extract (EGb 761) in the management of congestive symptoms of premenstrual syndrome] (in French). *Rev Fr Gynecol Obstet* 1993;88:447–57.
26. Brochet B, Guinot P, Orgogozo JM et al. Double-blind placebo-controlled multicentre study of ginkgolide B in treatment of acute exacerbations of multiple sclerosis. *J Neurol Neurosurg Psychiatry* 1995;58:360–362.
27. Chung HS, Harris A, Kristinsson JK et al. *Ginkgo biloba* extract increases ocular blood flow velocity. *J Ocul Pharmacol Ther* 1999;15:233–240.
28. Emerit I, Ognanesian N, Sarkisian T et al. Clastogenic factors in the plasma of Chernobyl accident recovery workers: anticlastogenic effect of *Ginkgo biloba* extract. *Radiat Res* 1995;144:198–205.
29. Vale S. Subarachnoid haemorrhage associated with *Ginkgo biloba*. *Lancet* 1998;352:36.
30. Gilbert GJ. *Ginkgo biloba*. *Neurology* 1997;48:1137.
31. Rowin J, Lewis SL. Spontaneous bilateral subdural hematomas associated with chronic *Ginkgo biloba* ingestion. *Neurology* 1996;46:1775–1776.
32. Fessenden JM, Wittenborn W, Clarke L. *Ginkgo biloba*: a case report of herbal medicine and bleeding postoperatively from a laparoscopic cholecystectomy. *Am Surg* 2001;67:33–35.
33. Granger AS. *Ginkgo biloba* precipitating epileptic seizures. *Age Ageing* 2001;30:523–525.
34. Galluzzi S, Zanetti O, Binetti G et al. Coma in a patient with Alzheimer's disease taking low dose trazodone and *Ginkgo biloba*. *J Neurosurg Psychiatry* 2000;68:679–680.
35. Becker LE, Skipworth GB. Ginkgo-tree dermatitis, stomatitis, and proctitis. *JAMA* 1975;231:1162–1163.
36. Arenz A, Klein M, Fiehe K et al. Occurrence of neurotoxic 4'-methylpyridoxine in *Ginkgo biloba* leaves, ginkgo medications and Japanese ginkgo food. *Planta Med* 1996;62:548–551.
37. Kajiyama Y, Fujii K, Takeuchi H, Manabe Y. Ginkgo seed poisoning. *Pediatrics* 2002;109:325–327.
38. Matthews MK. Association of *Ginkgo biloba* with intracerebral hemorrhage. *Neurology* 1998;50:1933.
39. Rosenblatt M, Mindel J. Spontaneous hyphema associated with ingestion of *Ginkgo biloba* extract. *N Engl J Med* 1997;336:1108.

GINSENG

1. Mills S, Bone K. *Principles and practice of phytotherapy*. Edinburgh, NY: Churchill-Livingstone, 2000:418-432.
2. Awang DVC. The neglected ginsenosides of North American ginseng (*Panax quinquefolius* L.). *J Herbs Spices Med Plants* 2000;7:103–109.
3. Pearce PT, Zois I, Wynne KN et al. *Panax ginseng* and *Eleutherococcus senticosus* extracts—in vitro studies on binding to steroid receptors. *Endocrinol Jpn* 1982;29:567–573.
4. Hiai S, Yokoyama H, Oura H et al. Stimulation of pituitary-adrenocortical system by ginseng saponin. *Endocrinol Jpn* 1979;26:661–665.
5. Park H-J, Rhee M-H, Park K-M et al. Effect of non-saponin fraction from *Panax ginseng* on cGMP and thromboxane A2 in human platelet aggregation. *J Ethnopharmacol* 1995;49:157–162.
6. Sonnenborn U, Hänsel R. *Panax ginseng*. In De Smet PAGM, Keller K, Hänsel R et al, eds. *Adverse effects of herbal drugs*, vol 1. Berlin: Springer-Verlag, 1992:179–191.
7. Sotaneimi EA, Haapokoski E, Rautio A. Ginseng therapy in non-insulin-dependent diabetic patients. *Diabetes Care* 1995;18:1373–1375.
8. Vuksan V, Sievenpiper JL, Wong J et al. American ginseng (Panax quinquefolius L.) attenuates postprandial glycemia in a time-dependent but not dose-dependent manner in healthy individuals. *Am J Clin Nutr* 2001;73:753–758.
9. Vuksan V, Sievenpiper JL, Koo VY et al. American ginseng (*Panax quinquefolius* L) reduces postprandial glycemia in nondiabetic subjects and subjects with type 2 diabetes mellitus. *Arch Intern Med* 2000;160:1009–1013.
10. Vuksan V, Stavro MP, Sievenpiper JL et al. Similar postprandial glycemic reductions with escalation of dose and administration time of American ginseng in type 2 diabetes. *Diabetes Care* 2000;23:1221–1226.
11. Wiklund IK, Mattsson LA, Lindgren R et al. Effects of a standardized ginseng extract on quality of life and physiological parameters in symptomatic postmenopausal women: a double-blind, placebo-controlled trial. Swedish Alternative Medicine Group. *Int J Clin Pharmacol Res* 1999;19:89–99.
12. Choi HK, Seong DH, Rha KH. Clinical efficacy of Korean red ginseng for erectile dysfunction. *Int J Impotence Res* 1995;7:181–86.
13. Salvati G, Genovesi G, Marcellini L et al. Effects of *Panax*

ginseng CA Meyer on male fertility. *Panminerva Med* 1996; 38:249–254.

14. Bahrke MS, Morgan WP. Evaluation of the ergogenic properties of ginseng: an update. *Sports Med* 2000;29:113–133.

15. Cardinal BJ, Engels HJ. Ginseng does not enhance psychological well-being in healthy, young adults: results of a double-blind, placebo-controlled, randomized clinical trial. *J Am Diet Assoc* 2001;101:655–660.

16. Sorensen H, Sonne J. A double-masked study of the effects of ginseng on cognitive functions. *Curr Ther Res* 1996;57: 959–968.

17. Thommessen B, Laake K. No identifiable effect of ginseng (Gericomplex) as an adjuvant in the treatment of geriatric patients. *Aging Clin Exp Res* 1996;8:417–420.

18. Marasco C, Ruiz V, Villagomez S et al. Double-blind study of a multivitamin complex supplemented with ginseng extract. *Drugs Exp Clin Res* 1996;22:323–329.

19. Yun TK, Choi SY. A case-control study of ginseng intake and cancer. *Int J Epidemiol* 1990;19:871–876.

20. Yun TK, Choi SY. Preventive effect of ginseng intake against various human cancers: a case-control study on 1987 pairs. *Cancer Epidemiol Biomark Prev* 1995;4:401–408.

21. Yun TK. Experimental and epidemiological evidence of the cancer-preventive effects of *Panax ginseng* CA Meyer. *Nutr Rev* 1996;54;S71–S81.

22. Scaglione F, Cattaneo G, Alessandria M et al. Efficacy and safety of the standardized ginseng extract G115 for potentiating vaccination against common cold and/or influenza syndrome. *Drugs Exp Clin Res* 1996;22:65–72.

23. See DM, Broumand N, Sahl L et al. In vitro effects of echinacea and ginseng on natural killer and antibody-dependent cell cytotoxicity in healthy subjects and chronic fatigue syndrome or acquired immunodeficiency syndrome patients. *Immunopharmacology* 1997;35:229–235.

24. Scaglione F, Weiser K, Alessandria M. Effects of the standardized ginseng extract G115® in patients with chronic bronchitis. *Clin Drug Invest* 2001;21:41–45.

25. Lee FC, Ko JH, Park JK et al. Effects of *Panax ginseng* on blood alcohol clearance in men. *Clin Exp Pharm Physiol* 1987;14:543–546.

26. Ryu S-J, Chien Y-Y. Ginseng-associated cerebral arteritis. *Neurology* 1995;45:829–830.

27. Baldwin CA, Anderson LA, Phillipson JD et al. What pharmacists should know about ginseng. *Pharm J* 1986;237: 583–586.

28. Greenspan EM. Ginseng and vaginal bleeding. *JAMA* 1983; 249:2018.

29. Hopkins MP, Androff L, Bennighoff AS. Ginseng face cream and unexplained vaginal bleeding. *Am J Obstet Gynecol* 1988;159:1121–1122.

30. Punnonen R, Lukola A. Oestrogen-like effect of ginseng. *BMJ* 1980;281:1110.

31. Palmer BV, Montgomery ACV, Monteiro JCMP. Gin Seng and mastalgia. *Br Med J* 1978;1(6122):1284.

32. Gonzalez-Seijo JC, Ramos YM, Lastra I. Manic episode and ginseng: report of a possible case. *J Clin Psychopharmacol* 1995;15:447.

33. Dega H, Laporte J-L, Frances C et al. Ginseng as a cause for Stevens-Johnson syndrome? *Lancet* 1996;347:1344.

34. Hammond TG, Whitworth JA. Adverse reactions to ginseng. *Med J Aust* 1981;1:492.

35. Shader RI, Greenblatt DJ. Phenelzine and the dream machine—ramblings and reflections. *J Clin Psychopharmacol* 1985;5:65.

36. Jones BD, Runikis AM. Interaction of ginseng with phenelzine. *J Clin Pharmacol* 1987;7:201–202.

37. Janetzky K, Morreale AP. Probable interactions between warfarin and ginseng. *Am J Health System Pharm* 1997;54: 692–693.

38. Zhu M, Chan KW, Ng LS et al. Possible influences of ginseng on the pharmacokinetics and pharmacodynamics of warfarin in rats. *J Pharm Pharmacol* 1999;51:175–180.

39. Siegel RK. Ginseng abuse syndrome: problems with the panacea. *JAMA* 1979;241:1614–1615.

40. Cui J, Garle M, Eneroth P, Björkhem I. What do commercial ginseng preparations contain? *Lancet* 1994;344:134.

GLUCOSAMINE

1. Reichelt A, Förster KK, Fischer M et al. Efficacy and safety of intramuscular glucosamine sulfate in osteoarthritis of the knee. *Arzneim-Forsch/Drug Res* 1994;44:75–80.

2. Adams ME. Hype about glucosamine. *Lancet* 1999;354: 353–354.

3. Talent JM, Gracy RW. Pilot study of oral polymeric N-acetyl-ᴅ-glucosamine as a potential treatment for patients with osteoarthritis. *Clin Ther* 1996;18:1184–1190.

4. Barclay TS, Tsourounis C, McCart GM. Glucosamine. *Ann Pharmacother* 1998;32:574–579.

5. McAlindon TE, LaValley MP, Gulin JP et al. Glucosamine and chondroitin for treatment of osteoarthritis: a systematic quality assessment and meta-analysis. *JAMA* 2000;283: 1469–1475.

6. Towheed TE, Anastassiades TP. Glucosamine and chondroitin for treating symptoms of osteoarthritis. *JAMA* 2000;283: 1483–1484.

7. Rindone JP, Hiller D, Collacott E, Nordhaugen N, Arriola G. Randomized, controlled trial of glucosamine for treating osteoarthritis of the knee. *West J Med* 2000;172:91–94.

8. Thie NM, Prasad NG, Major PW. Evaluation of glucosamine sulfate compared to ibuprofen for the treatment of temporomandibular joint osteoarthritis: a randomized double-blind controlled 3 month clinical trial. *J Rheumatol* 2001; 28:1347–1355.

9. Muller-Fassbender H, Bach GL, Haase W et al. Glucosamine sulfate compared to ibuprofen in osteoarthritis of the knee. *Osteoarthritis Cartilage* 1994;2:61–69.

10. Vaz AL. Double-blind clinical evaluation of the relative efficacy of ibuprofen and glucosamine sulphate in the management of osteoarthrosis of the knee in outpatients. *Curr Med Res Opin* 1982;8:145–149.

11. Qiu GX, Gao SH, Giacovelli G et al. Efficacy and safety of glucosamine sulfate versus ibuprofen in patients with knee osteoarthritis. *Arzneim-Forsch/Drug Res* 1998;48:469–474.

12. Reginster JY, Deroisy R, Rovati LC et al. Long-term effects of glucosamine sulphate on osteoarthritis progression: a randomized, placebo-controlled clinical trial. *Lancet* 2001; 357:251–256.

13. Canapp SO Jr, McLaughlin RM Jr, Hoskinson JJ et al. Scintigraphic evaluation of dogs with acute synovitis after treatment with glucosamine hydrochloride and chondroitin sulfate. *Am J Vet Res* 1999;60:1552–1557.

14. Rovati LC, Annefeld M, Giacovelli G et al. Glucosamine in osteoarthritis. *Lancet* 1999;354:1640.

References

15. Matheu V, Gracia Bara MT, Pelta R et al. Immediate hypersensitivity reaction to glucosamine sulfate. *Allergy* 1999;54:643.
16. Pouwels MJ, Jacobs JR, Span PN et al. Short-term glucosamine infusion does not affect insulin sensitivity in humans. *J Clin Endocrinol Metab* 2001;86:2099–2103.
17. Monauni T, Zenti MG, Cretti A et al. Effects of glucosamine infusion on insulin secretion and insulin action in humans. *Diabetes* 2000;49:926–935.
18. Baron AD, Zhu JS, Zhu JH et al. Glucosamine induces insulin resistance in vivo by affecting GLUT 4 translocation in skeletal muscle: implications for glucose toxicity. *J Clin Invest* 1995;96:2792–2801.
19. Patti ME, Virkamaki A, Landaker EJ et al. Activation of the hexosamine pathway by glucosamine in vivo induces insulin resistance of early postreceptor insulin signaling events in skeletal muscle. *Diabetes* 1999;48:1562–1571.
20. Shankar RR, Zhu JS, Baron AD. Glucosamine infusion in rats mimics the beta-cell dysfunction of non-insulin-dependent diabetes mellitus. *Metabolism* 1998;47:573–577.

GLUTAMINE

1. Klimberg VS, McClellan JL. Glutamine, cancer, and its therapy. *Am J Surg* 1996;172:418–424.
2. Shils ME, Olson JA, Shike M et al, eds. *Modern nutrition in health and disease,* 9th ed. Baltimore: Williams & Wilkins, 1999.
3. Powell-Tuck J. Glutamine supplementation in artificial nutritional support. *Lancet* 1997;350:534.
4. Noyer CM, Simon D, Borczuk A et al. A double-blind placebo-controlled pilot study of glutamine therapy for abnormal intestinal permeability in patients with AIDS. *Am J Gastroenterol* 1998;93:972–975.
5. Akobeng AK, Miller V, Stanton J et al. Double-blind randomized controlled trial of glutamine-enriched polymeric diet in the treatment of active Crohn's disease. *J Pediatr Gastroenterol Nutr* 2000;30:78–84.
6. Elia M, Lunn PG. The use of glutamine in the treatment of gastrointestinal disorders in man. *Nutrition* 1997;13:743–747.
7. Decker-Baumann C, Buhl K, Frohmuller S et al. Reduction of chemotherapy-induced side effects by parenteral glutamine supplementation in patients with metastatic colorectal cancer. *Eur J Cancer* 1999;35:202–207.
8. Okuno SH, Woodhouse CO, Loprinzi CL et al. Phase III controlled evaluation of glutamine for decreasing stomatitis in patients receiving fluorouracil (5-FU)-based chemotherapy. *Am J Clin Oncol* 1999;22:258–261.
9. Anderson PM, Ramsay NK, Shu XO et al. Effect of low-dose oral glutamine on painful stomatitis during bone marrow transplantation. *Bone Marrow Transplant* 1998;22:339–344.
10. Anderson PM, Schroeder G, Skubitz KM. Oral glutamine reduces the duration and severity of stomatitis after cytotoxic cancer chemotherapy. *Cancer* 1998;83:1433–1439.
11. Bozzetti F, Biganzoli L, Gavazzi C. Glutamine supplementation in cancer patients receiving chemotherapy: a double-blind randomized study. *Nutrition* 1997;13:748–751.
12. Houdijk, APJ, Rijnsburger ER, Jansen J et al. Randomised trial of glutamine-enriched enteral nutrition on infectious morbidity in patients with multiple trauma. *Lancet* 1998;352:772–776.
13. Haub MD, Potteiger JA, Nau KL et al. Acute L-glutamine ingestion does not improve maximal effort exercise. *J Sports Med Fitness* 1998;38:240–244.

GLYCINE

1. Hall JC. Glycine. *J Parenter Enteral Nutr* 1998;22:393–398.
2. Shils ME, Olson JA, Shike M et al, eds. *Modern nutrition in health and disease,* 9th ed. Baltimore: Williams & Wilkins, 1999.
3. Heresco-Levy U, Javitt DC, Ermilov M et al. Efficacy of high-dose glycine in the treatment of enduring negative symptoms of schizophrenia. *Arch Gen Psychiatry* 1999;56:29–36.
4. Javitt DC, Zylberman I, Zukin SR et al. Amelioration of negative symptoms in schizophrenia with glycine. *Am J Psychiatry* 1994;151:1234–1236.
4a. Potkin SG, Jin Y, Bunney BG et al. Effect of clozapine and adjunctive high-dose glycine in treatment-resistant schizophrenia. *Am J Psych* 1999;156:146–147.
5. Farber NB, Newcomer JW, Olney JW. Glycine agonists: what can they teach us about schizophrenia? *Arch Gen Psychiatry* 1999;56:13–17.
6. Rose ML, Cattley RC, Dunn C et al. Dietary glycine prevents the development of liver tumors caused by the peroxisome proliferator WY-14,643. *Carcinogenesis* 1999;20:2075–2081.
7. Zhong Z, Enomoto N, Connor HD et al. Glycine improves survival after hemorrhagic shock in the rat. *Shock* 1999;12:54–62.
8. Thurman RG, Zhong Z, von Frankenberg M et al. Prevention of cyclosporine-induced nephrotoxicity with dietary glycine. *Transplantation* 1997;63:1661–1667.
9. Zhong Z, Arteel GE, Connor HD et al. Cyclosporin A increases hypoxia and free radical production in rat kidneys: prevention by dietary glycine. *Am J Physiol* 1998;275:F595–604.
10. Yin M, Ikejima K, Arteel GE et al. Glycine accelerates recovery from alcohol-induced liver injury. *J Pharmacol Exp Ther* 1998;286:1014–1019.
11. Linder MC. *Nutritional biochemistry and metabolism, with clinical applications,* 2nd ed. East Norwalk, CT: Appleton & Lange, 1991.

GOLDENSEAL

1. British Herbal Medicine Assn. *British herbal compendium,* vol. 1. Dorset, U.K.: British Herbal Medicine Assoication, 1992:119–120.
2. Lampe KF. Berberine. In: De Smet PAGM, Keller K, Hänsel R, Chandler RF (eds). *Adverse effects of herbal drugs,* vol. 1. Springer-Verlag, Berlin 1992:97–103.
3. Gupte S. Use of berberine in treatment of giardiasis. *Am J Dis Child* 1975;129:866.
4. Mohan M, Pant CR, Angra SK et al. Berberine in trachoma. *Indian J Ophthalmol* 1982;30:69–75.
5. Khin-Maung U, Myo-Khin, Nyunt-Wai et al. Clinical trial of berberine in acute watery diarrhea. *BMJ* 1985;291:1601–1605.
5a. Khin-Mang-U, Myo-Khin, Nyunt-Nyunt-Wai et al. Clinical trial of high-dose berberine and tetracycline in cholera. *J Diarrhoeal Dis Res* 1987;5:184–187.
6. Rabbani GH, Butler T, Knight J et al. Randomized controlled trial of berberine sulfate therapy for diarrhea due to enterotoxigenic *Escherichia coli* and *Vibrio cholerae*. *J Infect Dis* 1987;155:979–984.

7. Marin-Neto JA, Maciel BC, Secches AL et al. Cardiovascular effects of berberine in patients with severe congestive heart failure. *Clin Cardiol* 1988;11:253–260.

8. Wolf S, Mack M. The action of bitters on the stomach in a fistulous patient. *Drug Standards* 1956;24:98–101.

9. Foster S, Varro I. *Tyler's honest herbal: a sensible guide to the use of herbs and related remedies,* 4th ed. New York: Haworth Herbal Press, 1999:195–197.

10. Nishino H, Kitigawa K, Fujiki H et al. Berberine sulfate inhibits tumor-promoting activity of teeocidin in two-stage carcinogenesis on mouse skin. *Oncology* 1986;43:131–134.

11. Ho NK. Traditional Chinese medicine and treatment of neonatal jaundice. *Singapore Med J* 1996;37:645–651.

12. Chan E. Displacement of bilirubin from albumin by berberine. *Biol Neonate* 1993;63:201–208.

13. Scazzocchio F, Cometa MF, Palmery M. Antimicrobial activity of Hydrastis canadensis extract and its major isolated alkaloids. *Fitoterapia* 1998;69(Suppl 5):58–59.

14. Rehman J, Dillow JM, Carter SM et al. Increased production of antigen-specific immunoglobulins G and M following in vivo treatment with the medicinal plants Echinacea angustifolia and Hydrastis canadensis. *Immunol Lett* 1999;68: 391–395.

15. Marinova EK, Nikolova DB, Popova DN et al. Suppression of experimental autoimmune tubulointerstitial nephritis in BALB/c mice by berberine. *Immunopharamcology* 2000;48: 9–16.

16. Fukuda K, Hibiya Y, Mutoh M et al. Inhibition by berberine of cyclooxygenase-2 transcriptional activity in human colon cancer cells. *J Ethnopharmacol* 1999;66:227–233.

17. Chung JG, Wu LT, Chu CB et al. Effects of berberine on arylamine N-acetyltransferase activity in human bladder tumor cells. *Food Chem Toxicol* 1999;37:319–326.

18. Wu HL, Hsu CY, Liu WH et al. Berberine-induced apoptosis of human leukemia HL-60 cells is associated with down-regulation of nucleophosmin/B23 and telomerase activity. *Int J Cancer* 1999;81:923–929.

19. Iizuka N, Miyamoto K, Okita K et al. Inhibitory effect of Coptidis Rhizoma and berberine on the proliferation of human esophageal cancer cell lines. *Cancer Lett* 2000;148: 19–25.

20. Foster S. Goldenseal masking of drug tests. *HerbalGram* 1989;21:7,35.

21. Foster S. *Goldenseal.* Austin, TX: American Botanical Council, 1991.

GOTU KOLA

1. Kartnig T. Clinical applications of *Centella asiatica* (L.) Urb. *Herbs Spices Med Plants* 1988;3:145–173.

2. Rush WR, Murray GR, Graham DJ. The comparative steady-state bioavailability of the active ingredients of Madecassol. *Eur J Drug Metab Pharmacokinet* 1993;18: 323–326.

3. Grimaldi R, De Ponti F, D'Angelo L et al. Pharmacokinetics of the total triterpenic fraction of *Centella asiatica* after single and multiple administrations to healthy volunteers. A new assay for asiatic acid. *J Ethnopharmacol* 1990;28:235–241.

4. Belcaro GV, Rulo A, Grimaldi R. Capillary filtration and ankle edema in patients with venous hypertension treated with TTFCA. *Angiology* 1990;41:12–18.

5. Pointel JP, Boccalon H, Cloaree M et al. Titrated extract of *Centella asiatica* (TECA) in the treatment of venous insufficiency of the lower limbs. *Angiology* 1987;38:46–50.

6. Cesarone MR, Laurora G, De Sanctis MT. The microcirculatory activity of *Centella asiatica* in venous insufficiency. A double-blind study. *Minerva Cardioangiol* 1994;42:299–304.

7. Bradwejn J, Zhou Y, Koszycki D et al. A double-blind, placebo-controlled study on the effects of gotu kola (*Centella asiatica*) on acoustic startle response in healthy subjects. *J Clin Pharmacol* 2000;20:680–684.

8. Herbert D. Paramasivan CN, Prabhakar R et al. In vitro experiments with *Centella asiatica*: investigation to elucidate the effect of an indigenously prepared powder of this plant on the acid-fastness and viability of *M. tuberculosis*. *Indian J Lepr* 1994;66:65–68.

9. Medda S, Das N, Mahato SB. Glycoside-bearing liposomal delivery systems against macrophage-associated disorders involving *Mycobacterium leprae* and *Mycobacterium tuberculosis*. *Indian J Biochem Biophys* 1995;32:147–151.

10. Yoosook C, Bunyapraphatsara N, Boonyakiat Y et al. Anti-herpes simplex virus activities of crude water extracts of Thai medicinal plants. *Phytomedicine* 2000;6:411–419.

11. Shukla A, Rasik AM, Jain GK et al. In vitro and in vivo wound healing activity of asiaticoside isolated from *Centella asiatica*. *J Ethnopharmacol* 1999;65:1–11.

12. Maquart FX, Chastang F, Simeon A et al. Triterpenes from *Centella asiatica* stimulate extracellular matrix accumulation in rat experimental wounds. *Eur J Dermatol* 1999;9: 289–296.

13. Sunilkumar, Parameshwaraiah S, Shivakumar HG. Evaluation of topical formulations of aqueous extract of *Centella asiatica* on open wounds in rats. *Indian J Exp Biol* 1998;36: 569–572.

14. Shukla A, Rasik Am, Dhawan BN. Asiaticoside-induced elevation of antioxidant levels in healing wounds. *Phytother Res* 1999;13:50–54.

15. Chen YJ, Dai YS, Chen BF et al. The effect of tetrandrine and extracts of *Centella asiatica* on acute radiation dermatitis in rats. *Biol Pharm Bull* 1999;22:703–706.

16. Chatterjee TK, Chakraborty A, Pathak M et al. Effects of plant extract *Centella asiatica* (Linn.) on cold restraint stress ulcer in rats. *Indian J Exp Biol* 1992;30:889–891.

17. Sarma DNK, Khosa RL, Chansauria JPN et al. Antistress activity of *Tinospora cordifolia* and *Centella asiatica* extracts. *Phytother Res* 1996;10:181–183.

18. Brinkhaus B, Lindner M, Schuppan D et al. Chemical, pharmacological and clinical profile of the East Asian medical plant *Centella asiatica*. *Phytomedicine* 2000;7:427–448.

19. Babu TD, Kuttan G, Padikkala J. Cytotoxic and anti-tumour properties of certain taxa of Umbelliferae with special reference to *Centella asiatica (L.) Urban*. *J Ethnopharmacol* 1995;48:53–57.

20. Hausen BM. *Centella asiatica* (Indian pennywort), an effective therapeutic but a weak sensitizer. *Contact Dermatitis* 1993;29:175–179.

HAWTHORN

1. Hobbs C, Foster S. Hawthorn: a literature review. *HerbalGram* 1990;22:19–33.

2. Upton R, ed. Hawthorn berry. In: *American herbal pharmacopoeia and therapeutic compendium.* Santa Cruz, CA: American Herbal Pharmacopoeia, June 1999.

References

3. Upton R, ed. *Hawthorn leaf with flower: analytical, quality control, and therapeutic monograph.* Santa Cruz: American Herbal Pharmacopoeia, February 1999.
4. Tauchert M. Efficacy and safety of *Crataegus* extract WS 1442 in comparison with placebo in patients with chronic stable New York Heart Association class III heart failure. *Am Heart J* 2002;143:910–915.
5. Schmidt U, Kuhn U, Ploch M et al. Efficacy of the hawthorn (*Crataegus*) preparation LI 132 in 78 patients with chronic congestive heart failure defined as NYHA functional class II. *Phytomedicine* 1994;1:17–24.
6. Tauchert M, Ploch M, Hübner WD. Wirksamkeit des Weiß-dorn-Extraktes LI 132 in Vergleich mit Captopril. Multizen-trische Doppelblindstudie bei 132 Patienten mit Herzinsuf-fizienz in Stadium II nach NYHA. *Münch Med Wschr* 1994; 136(Suppl 1):27–34.
7. Chen JD, Wu YZ, Tao ZL et al. Hawthorn (Shan Zha) drink and its lowering effect on blood lipid levels in humans and rats. *Plants Hum Nutr* 1995;77:147–154.
8. Schulz V, Hansel R, Tyler VE. *Rational phytotherapy.* Berlin: Springer, 1998:89–128.
9. Della Loggia R. Depressive effect of *Crataegus oxyacantha L* on central nervous system in mice. *Sci Pharm* 1983;51:319–324.
10. Schlegelmilch R, Heywood R. Toxicity of *Crataegus* (hawthorn) extract (WS 1442). *J Am Coll Tox* 1994;13: 103–111.

HISTIDINE

1. Linder MC. *Nutritional biochemistry and metabolism, with clinical applications,* 2nd ed. East Norwalk, CT: Appleton & Lange, 1991.
2. Blumenkrantz MJ, Shapoiro DJ, Swendseid ME et al. Histi-dine supplementation for treatment of anaemia of uraemia. *BMJ* 1975;2:530–533.
3. Gillin JC, Fram DH, Wyatt RJ et al. L-histidine: failure to affect the sleep-waking cycle in man. *Psychopharmacologia* 1975;40:305–311.
4. Steinhauer HB, Kluthe R, Lubrich I et al. Effect of L-histi-dine in vivo on human platelet function and arachidonic acid metabolism. *Prostaglandins Leukotriene Med* 1985;18: 245–254.
5. Schechter PJ, Prakash NJ. Failure of oral L-histidine to influ-ence appetite or affect zinc metabolism in man: a double-blind study. *Am J Clin Nutr* 1979;32:1011–1014.
6. Shils ME, Olson JA, Shike M et al, eds. *Modern nutrition in health and disease,* 9th ed. Baltimore: Williams & Wilkins 1999:1343.
7. Pinals RS, Harris ED, Burnett JB et al. Treatment of rheumatoid arthritis with L-histidine: a randomized, placebo-controlled, double-blind trial. *J Rheumatol* 1977; 4:414–419.
8. Lee JW, Miyawaki H, Bobst EV et al. Improved functional recovery of ischemic rat hearts due to singlet oxygen scav-engers histidine and carnosine. *J Mol Cell Cardiol* 1999;31: 113–121.
9. De Fabo EC, Webber LJ, Ulman EA et al. Dietary L-histidine regulates murine skin levels of trans-urocanic acid, an immune-regulating photoreceptor, with an unanticipated modulation: potential relevance to skin cancer. *J Nutr* 1997; 127:2158–2164.
10. Van Wouwe JP, Veldhuizen M. Growth characteristics in lab-oratory animals fed zinc-deficient, copper-deficient, histi-dine-supplemented diets. *Biol Trace Elem Res* 1996;55: 71–77.
11. Ikezaki S, Nishikawa A, Furukawa F et al. Long-term toxic-ity/carcinogenicity study of L-histidine monohydrochloride in F344 rats. *Food Chem Toxicol* 1996;34:687–691.

HOPS

1. Salvador RL. Hops. *Can Pharm J* 1994;127:203–205.
2. Milligan SR, Kalita JC, Heyerick A et al. Identification of a potent phytoestrogen in hops (*Humulus lupulus L.*) and beer. *J Clin Endo Metab* 1999;83:2249–2252.
3. Tagashira M, Watanabe M, Uemitsu N. Antioxidative activity of hop bitter acids and their analogs. *Biosci Biotech Biochem* 1995;59:740–742.
4. Blumenthal M, Goldberg A, Brinckmann J. *Herbal medicine: expanded Commission E monographs.* Newton, MA: Integra-tive Medicine Consultants, 2000:194.
5. Miranda CL, Stevens JF, Helmrich A et al. Antiproliferative and cytotoxic effects of prenylated flavonoids from hops (*Humulus lupulus*) in human cancer cells. *Food Chem Toxicol* 1999;37:271–285.
6. Yasukawa K, Takeuchi M, Takodo M. Humulon, a bitter in the hop, inhibits tumor promotion by 12-O-tetradecanoylphor-bol-13-acetate in two-stage carcinogenesis in mouse skin. *Oncology* 1995;52:156–158.
7. Henderson MC, Miranda CL, Stevens JF et al. In vitro inhi-bition of human P450 enzymes by prenylated flavonoids from hops, *Humulus lupulus. Xenobiotica* 2000;30:235–251.
8. Mannering GJ, Shoeman JA, Shoeman DW. Effects of colupu-lone, a component of hops and brewers yeast, and chromium on glucose tolerance and hepatic cytochrome P450 in nondiabetic and spontaneously diabetic mice. *Biochem Biophys Res Commun* 1994;200:1455–1462.
9. Mannering GJ, Deloria LB, Shoeman JA et al. Effects of the hop component, colupulone, on the induction of cytochrome P4503A and the replication of human tumor cells. *Food Nutr Chem Toxicol (Int Conf)* 1993;1:311–323.
10. Mannering GJ, Shoeman JA, Deloria LB. Identification of the antibiotic hops component, colupulone, as an inducer of hepatic cytochrome P-450 3A in the mouse. *Drug Metab Dis-pos* 1992;20:142–147.
11. Grieve M. Hops. In: Leyel CF, ed. *A modern herbal,* vol I. Twickenham, Great Britain: Tiger Books Intl, 1998:411–415. (first published 1931, Jonathan Cape Ltd)

HORSE CHESTNUT

1. European Scientific Cooperative on Phytotherapy (ESCOP). *Monographs on the medicinal uses of plant drugs. Hippocas-tani semen: horse-chestnut seed. Fascicule 6.* Exeter, UK, 1999.
2. Pittler MH, Ernst E. Horse-chestnut seed extract for chronic venous insufficiency: a criteria-based systematic review. *Arch Dermatol* 1998;134:1356–1360.
3. Diehm C, Trampisch HJ, Lange S et al. Comparison of leg compression stocking and oral horse-chestnut seed extract therapy in patients with chronic venous insufficiency. *Lancet* 1996;347:292–294.
4. Schulz V, Hansel R, Tyler VE. *Rational phytotherapy: a physi-cian's guide to herbal medicine,* 3rd ed. Berlin: Springer-Ver-lag, 1998:130.
5. Steiner M, Hillemanns HG. Venostatin retard in the man-

agement of venous problems during pregnancy. *Phlebology* 1990;5:41–44.

6. Calabrese C, Preston PA. Report of the results of a double-blind, randomized, single-dose trial of a topical 2% escin gel versus placebo in the acute treatment of experimentally-induced hematoma in volunteers. *Planta Med* 1993;59:394–397.

7. Bombardelli E, Morazzoni P, Griffini A. *Aesculus hippocastanum L. Fitoterapia* 1996;67:483–511.

8. Bougelet C, Roland IH, Ninane N et al. Effect of aescine on hypoxia-induced neutrophil adherence to umbilical vein endothelium. *Eur J Pharmacol* 1998;12;345:89–95.

9. Frick RW. Three treatments for chronic venous insufficiency: escin, hydroxyethylrutoside, and Daflon. *Angiology* 2000;51:197–205.

10. Grases F, Ramis M, Villacampa AI et al. Uric acid urolithiasis and crystallization inhibitors. *Urol Int* 1999;62:210–204.

11. Schulz V, Hansel R, Tyler VE. *Rational phytotherapy: a physician's guide to herbal medicine,* 3rd ed. Berlin: Springer-Verlag, 1998:135.

12. Diehm C. The role of oedema protective drugs in the treatment of chronic venous insufficiency: a review of evidence based on placebo-controlled clinical trials with regard to efficacy and tolerance. *Phlebology* 1996;11:23–29.

13. Blumenthal M, Goldberg E, Brinckmann J. Herbal medicine: expanded Commission E monographs. Newton, MA: American Botanical Council: Integrative Medicine Communications, 2000:201–204.

HYDRAZINE

1. Kaegi E. Unconventional therapies for cancer: 4. Hydrazine sulfate. Task Force on Alternative Therapies of the Canadian Breast Cancer Research Initiative. *Can Med Assoc J* 1998;158:1327–1330.

2. Chlebowski RT, Bulcavage L, Grosvenor M et al. Hydrazine sulfate influence on nutritional status and survival in non-small-cell lung cancer. *J Clin Oncol* 1990;8:9–15.

3. Loprinzi CL, Goldberg RM, Su JQ et al. Placebo-controlled trial of hydrazine sulfate in patients with newly diagnosed non-small-cell lung cancer. *J Clin Oncol* 1994;12:1126–1129.

4. Kosty MP, Fleishman SB, Herndon JE et al. Cisplatin, vinblastine, and hydrazine sulfate in advanced, non-small-cell lung cancer: a randomized placebo-controlled double-blind Phase III study of the Cancer and Leukemia Group B. *J Clin Oncol* 1994;12:1113-1120.

5. Loprinzi CL, Kuross SA, O'Fallon JR et al. Randomized placebo-controlled evaluation of hydrazine sulfate in patients with advanced colorectal cancer. *J Clin Oncol* 1994;12:1121–1125.

6. Chlebowski RT, Heber D, Richardson B et al. Influence of hydrazine sulfate on abnormal carbohydrate metabolism in cancer patients with weight loss. *Cancer Res* 1984;44:857–861.

7. Gold J. Anabolic profiles in late-stage cancer patients responsive to hydrazine sulfate. *Nutr Cancer* 1981;3:13–19.

8. Chlebowski RT, Bulcavage L, Grosvenor M et al. Hydrazine sulfate in cancer patients with weight loss: a placebo-controlled clinical experience. *Cancer* 1987;59:406–410.

9. Gold J. Inhibition by hydrazine sulfate and various hydrazides, of in vivo growth of Walker 256 intramuscular carcinoma, B-16 melanoma, Murphy-Sturm lymphosarcoma

and L-1210 solid leukemia. *Oncology* 1973;27:69–80 (also Ann N Y Acad Sci 1974;230:103–110).

10. Gold J. Enhancement by hydrazine sulfate of antitumor effectiveness of cytoxan, mitomycin C, methotrexate and bleomycin, in Walker 256 carcinosarcoma in rats. *Oncology* 1975;31:44–53.

11. Kamradt JM, Pienta KJ. The effect of hydrazine sulfate on prostate cancer growth. *Oncol Rep* 1998;5:919–921.

12. Silverstein R, Christoffersen CA, Morrison DC. Modulation of endotoxin lethality in mice by hydrazine sulfate. *Infect Immun* 1989;57:2072–2078.

13. Hainer MI, Tsai N, Komura ST et al. Fatal hepatorenal failure associated with hydrazine sulfate. *Ann Int Med* 2000;133:877–880.

14. Tweedie DJ, Erikson JM, Prough RA. Metabolism of hydrazine anti-cancer agents. *Pharmacol Ther* 1987;34:111–127.

HYPERICUM

1. Fugh-Berman A, Cott M. Dietary supplements and natural products as psychotherapeutic agents. *Psychosom Med* 1999;61:712–728.

2. Simmen U, Burkard W, Berger K et al. Extracts and constituents of *Hypericum perforatum* inhibit the binding of various ligands to recombinant receptors expressed with the semiliki forest virus system. *J Receptor Signal Transduction Res* 1999;19:59–74.

3. Schempp CM, Winghofer B, Langheinrich M et al. Hypericin levels in human serum and interstitial skin blister fluid after oral single-dose and steady-state administration of *Hypericum perforatum* extract (St. John's wort). *Skin Pharmacol Appl Skin Physiol* 1999;12:299–304.

4. Fugh-Berman A. Herb-drug interactions. *Lancet* 2000;355:134–138.

5. European Scientific Cooperative on Phytotherapy (ESCOP). *Monographs on the medicinal uses of plant drugs. Hyperici herba: St. John's wort. Fascicule 1.* Exeter, UK, 1996.

6. Linde K, Ramirez G, Mulrow CD et al. St. Johnswort for depression—an overview and meta-analysis of randomized clinical trials. *BMJ* 1996;313:253–258.

7. Shelton RC, Keller MB, Gelenberg A et al. Effectiveness of St. John's wort in major depression. *JAMA* 2001;285:1978–1986.

8. Schrader E. Equivalence of St John's wort extract (Ze 117) and fluoxetine: a randomized, controlled study in mild-moderate depression. *Int Clin Psychopharmacol* 2000;15:61–68.

9. Harrer G, Schmidt U, Kuhn U et al. Comparison of equivalence between the St. John's wort extract LoHyp-57 and fluoxetine. *Arzneim-Forsch/Drug Res* 1999;49:289–296.

10. Philipp M, Kohnen R, Hiller KO. Hypericum extract versus imipramine or placebo in patients with moderate depression: randomised multicentre study of treatment for eight weeks. *BMJ* 1999;319:1534–1538.

11. Woelk H. Comparison of St John's wort and imipramine for treating depression: randomised controlled trial. *BMJ* 2000;321:536–539.

12. Gulick RM, McAuliffe V, Holden-Wiltse J et al. Phase I studies of hypericin, the active compound in St. John's wort, as an antiretroviral agent in HIV-infected adults. *Ann Int Med* 1999;130:510–514.

13. Sindrup SH, Madsen C, Bach FW et al. St. John's wort has no effect on pain in polyneuropathy. *Pain* 2000;91:361–365.

14. Golsch S, Vocks E, Rakoski J et al. [Reversible increase in

References

photosensitivity to UV-B caused by St. John's wort extract]. *Hautartz* 1997;48:249–262.

15. Bove GM. Acute neuropathy after exposure to sun in a patient treated with St. John's wort. *Lancet* 1998;352:1121–1122.

16. Schempp CM, Müller K, Winghofer B et al. Single-dose and steady-state administration of *Hypericum perforatum* extract (St. John's wort) does not influence skin sensitivity to UV radiation, visible light, and solar-simulated radiation. *Arch Dermatol* 2001;137:512–513.

17. Upton R, ed. *St. John's wort*. Santa Cruz, CA: American Herbal Pharmacopoeia, 1997.

18. Lane-Brown MM. Photosensitivity associated with herbal preparations of St. John's wort (*Hypericum perforatum*). *Med J Aust* 2000;172:302.

19. Schempp CM, Ludtke R, Winghofer B et al. Effect of topical application of *Hypericum perforatum* extract (St. John's wort) on skin sensitivity to solar simulated radiation. *Photodermatol Photoimmunol Photomed* 2000;16:125–128.

20. Nierenberg AA, Burt T, Matthews J et al. Mania associated with St. John's wort. *Biol Psychiatry* 1999;46:1707–1708.

21. Moses EL, Mallinger AG. St. John's wort: three cases of possible mania induction. *J Clin Psychopharm* 2000;20:115–117.

22. Brown TM. Acute St. John's wort toxicity. *Am J Emerg Med* 2000;18:231–232.

23. Johne A, Brockmoller J, Bauer S et al. Pharmacokinetic interaction of digoxin with an herbal extract from St John's wort (*Hypericum perforatum*). *Clin Pharmacol Ther* 1999;66:338–345.

24. Maurer A, Johne A, Bauer S et al. Interaction of St. John's wort extract with phenprocoumon. *Eur J Clin Pharmacol* 1999;55:A22.

25. Piscitelli SC, Burstein AH, Chaitt D et al. Indinavir concentrations and St. John's wort. *Lancet* 2000;355:547–548.

26. Roots I, Johne A, Schmider J et al. Interaction of a herbal extract from St. John's wort with amitriptyline and its metabolites. *Clin Pharm Ther* 2000;67:PIII-69(abst).

27. Anonymous. *Altern Ther Womens Health* 2002;4:31. (from Swedish Medical Product Agency Web site http://www.mpa.se/frame_index.html, accessed 3/11/02)

28. Nebel A, Schneider BJ, Baker RK et al. Potential metabolic interaction between St. John's wort and theophylline. *Ann Pharmacother* 1999;33:502.

29. Burstein AH, Horton RL, Dunn T et al. Lack of effect of St. John's wort on carbamazepine pharmacokinetics in healthy volunteers. *Clin Pharmacol Ther* 2000;68:605–612.

30. Waksman JC, Heard K, Joliff H et al. Serotonin syndrome associated with the use of St. John's wort (*Hypericum perforatum*) and paroxetine. *Clin Toxicol* 2000;38:521(abst).

31. Barbanel DM, Yusufi B, O'Shea D et al. Mania in a patient receiving testosterone replacement post-orchidectomy taking St. John's wort and sertraline. *J Psychopharm* 2000;14:84–86.

32. Irefin S, Sprung J. A possible cause of cardiovascular collapse during anesthesia: long term use of St. John's wort. *J Clin Anesthesiol* 2000;12:498–499.

33. Grush LR, Nierenberg A, Keefe B et al. St. John's wort during pregnancy. *JAMA* 1998;280:1566.

34. Rayburn WF, Gonzalez CL, Christensen HD et al. Effect of prenatally administered hypericum (St. John's wort) on growth and physical maturation of mouse offspring. *Am J Obstet Gynecol* 2001;184:191–195.

35. Suzuki O, Katsumata Y, Oya M et al. Inhibition of monamine oxidase by hypericin. *Planta Med* 1984;50:272–274.

36. Raffa RB. Screen of receptor and uptake site activity of hypericin component of St. John's wort reveals σ receptor binding. *Life Sci* 1998;62:265–270.

37. Cott JM. In vitro receptor binding and enzyme inhibition by *Hypericum perforatum* extract. *Pharmacopsychiatry* 1997;30(Suppl II):108–112.

38. Schey KL, Patat S, Chignell CF et al. Photooxidation of lens alpha-crystallin by hypericin. *Photochem Photobiol* 2000;72:200–203.

INOSITOL

1. Linder MC. *Nutritional biochemistry and metabolism, with clinical applications,* 2nd ed. East Norwalk, CT: Appleton & Lange, 1991.

2. Holub BJ. The nutritional importance of inositol and the phosphoinositides. *New Engl J Med* 1992;326:1285–1287.

3. Benjamin J, Agam G, Levine J et al. Inositol treatment in psychiatry. *Psychopharmacol Bull* 1995;31:167–175.

4. Levine J, Rapaport A, Lev L et al. Inositol treatment raises CSF inositol levels. *Brain Res* 1993;627:168–170.

5. Hewlett A, Ohlsson A. Inositol for respiratory distress syndrome in preterm infants (Cochrane review). *Cochrane Database Syst Rev* 2000;4:CD000366.

6. Benjamin J, Levine J, Fux M et al. Double-blind, placebo-controlled, crossover trial of inositol treatment for panic disorder. *Am J Psychiatry* 1995;152:1084–1086.

7. Benjamin J, Nemetz H, Fux M et al. Acute inositol does not attenuate m-CPP-induced anxiety, mydriasis and endocrine effects in panic disorder. *J Psychiatr Res* 1997;31:489–495.

8. Gelber D, Levine J, Belmaker RH. Effect of inositol on bulimia nervosa and binge eating. *Int J Eat Disord* 2001;29:345–348.

9. Fux M, Levine J, Aviv A et al. Inositol treatment of obsessive-compulsive disorder. *Am J Psychiatry* 1996;153:1219–1221.

10. Levine J, Barak Y, Gonzalves M et al. Double-blind, controlled trial of inositol treatment of depression. *Am J Psychiatry* 1995;152:792–794.

11. Levine J, Mishori A, Susnosky M et al. Combination of inositol and serotonin reuptake inhibitors in the treatment of depression. *Biol Psychiatry* 1999;45:270–273.

12. Barak Y, Levine J, Glasman A et al. Inositol treatment of Alzheimer's disease: a double blind, cross-over placebo controlled trial. *Prog Neuropsychopharmacol Biol Psychiatry* 1996;20:729–735.

13. Levine J, Pomerantz T, Stier S et al. Lack of effect of 6 g inositol treatment of post-ECT cognitive function in humans. *J Psychiatric Res* 1995;29:487–489.

14. Levine J, Goldberger I, Rapaport A et al. CSF inositol in schizophrenia and high-dose inositol treatment of schizophrenia. *Eur Neuropsychopharmacol* 1994;4:487–490.

15. Levine J, Aviram A, Holan A et al. Inositol treatment of autism. *J Neural Transm* 1997;104:307–310.

16. Levine J. Controlled trials of inositol in psychiatry. *Eur Neuropsychopharmacol* 1997;7:147–155.

17. Einat H, Belmaker RH. The effects of inositol treatment in animal models of psychiatric disorders. *J Affect Disord* 2001;62:113–121.

18. Shamsudden AM. Inositol phosphates have novel anticancer function. *J Nutr* 1995;125:725S–732S.

19. Souza FG, Mander AJ, Foggo M et al. The effects of lithium discontinuation and the non-effect of oral inositol upon thyroid hormones and cortisol in patients with bipolar affective disorder. *J Affect Disord* 1991;22:165–170.
20. Urbano G, Lopez-Jurado M, Aranda P et al. The role of phytic acid in legumes: antinutrient or beneficial function? *J Physiol Biochem* 2000;56:283–294.
21. Silverstone PH, Hanstock CC, Fabian J et al. Chronic lithium does not alter human myo-inositol or phosphomonoester concentrations as measured by 1H and 31P MRS. *Biol Psychiatry* 1996;40:235–246.

IODINE

1. Stanbury JB. Iodine deficiency and the iodine deficiency disorders. In: Bowman BA, Russell RM, eds. *Present knowledge in nutrition*, 7th ed. Washington, DC: ILSI,1996: 378–383.
2. Hetzel BS, Clugston GA. Iodine. In: Shils ME, Olson JA, Shike M et al, eds. *Modern nutrition in health and disease,* 9th ed. Baltimore: Williams & Wilkins, 1999:253–264.
3. DeLong GR, Leslie PW, Wang S-H et al. Effect on infant mortality of iodination of irrigation water in a severely iodine-deficient area of China. *Lancet* 1997;350:771–773.
4. Ghent WR, Eskin BA, Low DA et al. Iodine replacement in fibrocystic disease of the breast. *Can J Surg* 1993;36:453–460.
5. Linder MC. *Nutritional biochemistry and metabolism, with clinical applications,* 2nd ed. East Norwalk, CT: Appleton & Lange, 1991.
6. Delange F, Lecomte P. Iodine supplementation: benefits outweigh risks. *Drug Safety* 2000;2:89–95.
7. Delange F. Risks and benefits of iodine supplementation. *Lancet* 1998;351:923–924.
8. Khan LK, Li R, Gootnick D. Thyroid abnormalities related to iodine excess from water purification units. *Lancet* 1998; 352:1519.
9. Lewis WH. *Lewis' dictionary of toxicology*. Boca Raton, FL: Lewis Publishers, 1998:617.

IPRIFLAVONE

1. Alexandersen P, Toussaint A, Christiansen C et al. Ipriflavone in the treatment of postmenopausal osteoporosis. *JAMA* 2001;285:1482–1488.
2. Adami S, Bufalino L, Cervetti R, et al. Ipriflavone prevents radial bone loss in postmenopausal women with low bone mass over 2 years. *Osteoporos Int* 1997;7:119–125.
3. Gennari C, Adami S, Agnusdei D et al. Effect of chronic treatment with ipriflavone in postmenopausal women with low bone mass. *Calcif Tissue Int* 1997;61:S19–S22.
4. Gennari C, Agnusdei D, Crepaldi G et al. Effect of ipriflavone—a synthetic derivative of natural isoflavones—on bone mass loss in the early years after menopause. *Menopause* 1998;5:9–15.
5. Ohta H, Komukai S, Makita K et al. Effects of 1-year ipriflavone treatment on lumbar bone mineral density and bone metabolic markers in postmenopausal women with low bone mass. *Horm Res* 1999;51:178–183.
6. Valente M, Bufalino L, Casiglione GN et al. Effects of 1 year treatment with ipriflavone on bone in postmenopausal women with low bone mass. *Calcif Tissue Int* 1994;54:377–380.
7. Passeri M, Biondi M, Costi D et al. Effects of 2-year ipriflavone in elderly women with established osteoporosis. *Ital J Mineral Electrolyte Metab* 1995;9:136–144.

8. Maugeri D, Panebianco P, Russo MS et al. Ipriflavone treatment of senile osteoporosis: results of a multicenter, double-blind clinical trial of 2 years. *Arch Gerentol Geriatr* 1994; 19:253–263.
9. Nozaki M, Hashimoto K, Inoue Y et al. Treatment of bone loss in oophorectomized women with a combination of ipriflavone and conjugated equine estrogen. *Int J Gynecol Obstet* 1998;62:69–75.
10. Agnusdei D, Gennari C, Bufalino L. Prevention of early postmenopausal bone loss using low doses of conjugated estrogens and the non-hormonal, bone active drug ipriflavone. *Osteoporos Int* 1995;5:462–466.
11. De Aloysio D, Gambacciani M, Altieri P. Bone density changes in postmenopausal women with the administration of ipriflavone alone or in association with low-dose ERT. *Gynecol Endocrin* 1997;11:289–293.
12. Gambacciani M, Ciaponi M, Cappagli B et al. Effects of combined low dose of the isoflavone derivative ipriflavone and estrogen replacement on bone mineral density and metabolism in postmenopausal women. *Maturitas* 1997;28: 75–81.
13. Cecchettin M, Bellometti S, Cremonesi G et al. Metabolic and bone effects after administration of ipriflavone and salmon calcitonin in postmenopausal osteoporosis. *Biomed Pharmacother* 1995;49:465–468.
14. Somekawa Y, Chiguchi M, Ishibashi T et al. Efficacy of ipriflavone in preventing adverse effects of leuprolide. *J Clin Endocrinol Metab* 2001;86:3202–3206.
15. Sato Y, Kuno H, Kaji M et al. Effect of ipriflavone on bone in elderly hemiplegic stroke patients with hypovitaminosis D. *Am J Phys Med Rehab* 1999;78:457–463.
16. Agnusdei D, Bufalino L. Efficacy of ipriflavone in established osteoporosis and long-term safety. *Calc Tissue Int* 1997;61:S23–S27.
17. Ceccini MG, Fleisch H, Muhlbauer RC. Ipriflavone inhibits bone resorption in intact and ovariectomized rats. *Calcif Tissue Int* 1997;61:9–11.
18. Yamazaki I. Effect of Ipriflavone on the response of the uterus and thyroid to estrogen. *Life Sci* 1986;38:757–764.
19. Takahashi J, Kawakatsu K, Wakayama T, et al. Elevation of serum theophylline levels by ipriflavone in a patient with chronic obstructive pulmonary disease. *Eur J Clin Pharmacol* 1992;43:207–208.
20. Rondelli I, Acerbi D, Ventura P. Steady-state phamacokinetics of ipriflavone and its metabolites in patients with renal failure. *Int J Clin Pharm Res* 1991;11:183–192.

IRON

1. Linder MC. *Nutritional biochemistry and metabolism, with clinical applications,* 2nd ed. East Norwalk, CT: Appleton & Lange, 1991.
2. Fairbanks VF. Iron in medicine and nutrition. In: Shils ME, Olson JA, Shike M et al, eds. *Modern nutrition in health and disease,* 9th ed. Baltimore: Williams & Wilkins 1999: 193–221.
3. Yip R, Dallman PR. Iron. In: Bowman BA, Russell RM eds. Present knowledge in nutrition, 7th ed. Washington, DC: ILSI, 1996:277–292.
4. O'Keefe ST, Gavin K, Lavan JN. Iron status and restless legs syndrome in the elderly. *Age Ageing* 1994;23:200–203.
5. Sun ER, Chen CA, Ho G et al. Iron and the restless legs syndrome. *Sleep* 1998;21:371–77.

References

6. Davis BJ, Rajput A, Rajput ML et al. A randomized, double-blind placebo-controlled trial of iron in restless legs syndrome. *Eur Neurol* 2000;43:70–75.

7. Mocan H, Yildian A, Orhan F et al. Breath-holding spells in 91 children and response to treatment with iron. *Arch Dis Child* 1999;81:261–262.

8. Daoud AS, Batieha A, Al-Sheyyab M et al. Effectiveness of iron therapy on breath-holding spells. *J Pediatr* 1997;130:547–550.

9. Adish AA, Esrey SA, Gyrokos TW et al. Effect of consumption of food cooked in iron pots on iron status and growth of young children: a randomized trial. *Lancet* 1999;353:712–716.

10. Idjradinata P, Watkins WE, Pollitt E. Adverse effect of iron supplementation on weight gain of iron-replete young children. *Lancet* 1994;343:1252–1254.

11. Bruner AB, Joffe A, Duggan AK. Randomized study of cognitive effects of iron supplementation in non-anaemic iron-deficient adolescent girls. *Lancet* 1996;348:992–996.

12. Hinton PS, Giordano C, Brownlie T et al. Iron supplementation improves endurance after training in iron-depleted, nonanemic women. *J Appl Physiol* 2000;88:1103–1111.

13. Mahomed K. Iron supplementation in pregnancy. *Cochrane Database Syst Rev* 2000;2:CD00017.

14. Salonen JT, Nyyssönen K, Korpela H et al. High stored iron levels are associated with excess risk of myocardial infarction in eastern Finnish men. *Circulation* 1992;86:803–811.

15. Sempos CT, Gillum RF, Looker AC et al. Iron and heart disease: a review of the epidemiologic data. In: Bendich A, Deckelbaum RJ, eds. *Preventive nutrition: the comprehensive guide for health professionals*. Totowa, NJ: Humana Press, 1997:181–192.

16. Morrison HI, Semenciw RM, Mao Y et al. Serum iron and fatal myocardial infarction. *Epidemiology* 1994;5:243–246.

17. Klipstein-Grobusch K, Grobbee DE, den Breeijnen JH et al. Dietary iron and risk of myocardial infarction in the Rotterdam study. *Am J Epidemiol* 1999;149:421–428.

18. Yip R. Iron. In: Bowman BA, Russell RM, eds. *Present knowledge in nutrition*, 8th ed. Washington, DC: ILSI, XXXX:311–328.

19. Miller M, Hutchins GM. Hemachromatosis, multiorgan hemosiderosis, and coronary heart disease. *JAMA* 1994;272:231–233.

20. Danesh J, Appleby P. Coronary heart disease and iron status: meta-analyses of prospective studies. *Circulation* 1999;99:852–854.

21. Sempos CT, Looker AC, Gillum RE et al. Serum ferritin and death from all causes of cardiovascular diseases: the NHANES II mortality study. National Health and Nutrition Examination Survey. *Ann Epidemiol* 2000;10:441–448.

22. Toddler deaths resulting from ingestion of iron supplements—Los Angeles, 1992–1993. *MMWR* 1993;42(6):111–113.

23. Dambro MR. *Griffith's 5-minute clinical consult*. Baltimore, Williams and Wilkins, 1996:576.

24. Weinberg ED. The development of awareness of the carcinogenic hazard of inhaled iron. *Oncol Res* 1999;11:109–113.

ISOLEUCINE

1. Linder MC. *Nutritional biochemistry and metabolism, with clinical applications,* 2nd ed. East Norwalk, CT: Appleton & Lange, 1991.

2. Mero A. Leucine supplementation and intensive training. *Sports Med* 1999;27:347–358.

3. Berry HK, Brunner RL, Hunt MM et al. Valine, isoleucine, and leucine: a new treatment for phenylketonuria. *Am J Dis Child* 1990;144:539–543.

4. Tandan R, Bromberg MB, Forshew D et al. A controlled trial of amino acids therapy in amyotrophic lateral sclerosis. *Neurology* 1996;47:1220–1226.

5. Italian ALS Study Group. Branched-chain amino acids and amyotrophic lateral sclerosis: a treatment failure? The Italian ALS Study Group. *Neurology* 1993;43:2466–2470.

6. Richardson MA, Bevans ML, Weber JB et al. Branched chain amino acids decrease tardive dyskinesia symptoms. *Psychopharmacology (Berl)* 1999;143:358–364.

7. Cangiano C, Laviano A, Meguid MM et al. Effects of administration of oral branched-chain amino acids on anorexia and caloric intake in cancer patients. *J Natl Cancer Inst* 1996;88:550–551.

8. Stein TP, Schluter MD, Leskiw MJ et al. Attenuation of the protein wasting associated with bedrest by branched chain amino acids. *Nutrition* 1999;15:656–660.

9. Shils ME, Olson JA, Shike M et al, eds. *Modern nutrition in health and disease*, 9th ed. Baltimore: Williams & Wilkins, 1999.

KARELA

1. Raman A, Lau C. Anti-diabetic properties and phytochemistry of *Momordica charantia L* (Cucurbitaceae). *Phytomedicine* 1996;2:349–362.

2. Bailey CJ, Day C. Traditional plant medicines as treatments for diabetes. *Diabetes Care* 1989;12:553–564.

3. Ahmad N, Hassan MR, Halder H et al. Effect of *Momordica charantia* (karolla) extracts on fasting and postprandial serum glucose levels in NIDDM patients. *Bangladesh Med Res Counc Bull* 1999;25:11–13.

4. Leatherdale BA, Panesar RK, Singh G et al. Improvement in glucose tolerance due to *Momordica charantia* (karela). *BMJ* 1981;282:1823–1824.

5. Srivastava Y, Ventkatakrishna-Bhatt H, Verma Y et al. Antidiabetic and adaptogenic properties of *Momordica charantia* extract: an experimental and clinical evaluation. *Phytother Res* 1993;7:285–289.

6. Akhtar MS. Trial of *Momordica charantia Linn* (karela) powder in patients with maturity onset diabetes. *J Pak Med Assoc* 1982;32:106–107.

7. Welihinda J, Karunanayake EH, Sheriff MHR et al. Effect of *Momordica charantia* n the glucose tolerance in maturity onset diabetes. *J Ethnopharmacol* 1986;17:277–282.

8. Grover JK, Gupta SR. Hypoglycaemic activity of seeds of *Momordica charantia*. *Eur J Pharmacol* 1990;183:1026–1027.

9. Baldwa VS, Bhandari CM, Pangaria A et al. Clinical trial in patients with diabetes mellitus of an insulin-like compound obtained from plant source. *Ups J Med Sci* 1977;82:39–41.

10. Khanna P, Jain SC, Panagariya A et al. Hypoglycaemic activity of polypeptide-p from a plant source. *J Nat Prod* 1981;44:648–655.

11. Aslam M, Healy MA. Hypoglycaemic properties in traditional medicines with specific reference to karela. *Int Pharm J* 1989;3:226–229.

12. Singh A, Singh SP, Bamezai R et al. *Momordica charantia*

(bitter gourd) peel, pulp, seed, and whole fruit extract inhibits mouse skin papillomagenesis. *Toxicol Lett* 1998;94: 37–46.

13. Lee-Huang S, Huang PL, Sun Y et al. Inhibition of MDA-MB-231 human breast tumor xenografts and HER2 expression by anti-tumor agents GAP31 and MAP30. *Anticancer Res* 2000; 20:653–659.

14. Platel K, Shurpalekar KS, Srinivasan K. Influence of bitter gourd (Momordica charantia) on growth and blood constituents in albino rats. *Die Nahrung* 1993;37:156–160.

15. Bourinbaiar AS, Lee-Huang S. The activity of plant-derived antiretroviral proteins MAP30 and GAP31 against herpes simplex virus in vitro. *Biochem Biophys Res Commun* 1996; 219:923–929.

16. Schreiber CA, Wan L, Sun Y et al. The antiviral agents, MAP30 and GAP31, are not toxic to human spermatozoa and may be useful in preventing the sexual transmission of human immunodeficiency virus type 1. *Fertil Steril* 1999;72: 686–690.

17. Hulin A, Wavelet M, Desbordes JM. Intoxication aiguë par *Momordica charantia* (sorrosi). A propos de deux cas. *Semaine Hopitaux* 1988;64:2847–2848.

18. Patel JC, Dhirawani MK, Doshi JC. "Karela" in the treatment of diabetes mellitus. *Indian J Med Sci* 1968;22:30–32.

19. Bourinbaiar AS, Lee-Huang S. Potentiation of anti-HIV activity of anti-inflammatory drugs, dexamethasone and indomethacin, by MAP30, the antiviral agent from bitter melon. *Biochem Biophys Res Commun* 1995;208:779–785.

KAVA

1. Lopez-Avilla V, Benedicto J. Supercritical fluid extraction of kavalactones from *Piper methysticum* (kava) herb. *J High Resol Chromatogr* 1997;20:555–559.

2. Lechtenberg M, Quandt B, Kohlenberg FJ et al. Qualitative and quantitative micellar electrokinetic chromatography of kavalactones from dry extracts of *Piper methysticum Forst.* and commercial drugs. *J Chromatography A* 1999;848: 457–464.

3. Gleitz J, Friese J, Beile A et al. Anticonvulsive action of (+/-)-kavain estimated from its properties on stimulated synaptosomes and Na+ channel receptor sites. *Eur J Pharmacol* 1996;315:89–97.

4. Jussofie A, Schmiz A, Hiemke C. Kavapyrone enriched extract from *Piper methysticum* as modulator of the GABA binding site in different regions of rat brain. *Psychopharmacology (Berl)* 1994;116:469–474.

5. Davies LP, Drew CA, Duffield P et al. Kavapyrones and resin: studies on $GABA_A$, $GABA_B$ and benzodiazepine binding sites in rodent brain. *Pharmacol Toxicol* 1992;71:120–126.

6. Pittler MH, Ernst E. Efficacy of kava extract for treating anxiety; systematic review and meta-analysis. *J Clin Psychopharmacol* 2000;20:84–89.

7. Woelk H, Kapoula O, Lehrl S et al. Behandlung von Angst-Patienten. *Z Allg Med* 1993;69:271–277.

8. Lindenberg D, Pitule-Schodel H: [D,L-kavain in comparison with oxazepam in anxiety disorders. A double-blind study of clinical effectiveness]. *Fortschr Med* 1990;108:49–50.

9. Münte TF, Heinze HJ, Matzke M et al. Effects of oxazepam and an extract of kava roots (*Piper methysticum*) on event-related potentials in a word recognition task. *Neuropsychobiology* 1993;27:46–53.

10. Warnecke G, Pfaender H, Gerster G et al. Wirksamkeit von Kava-Kava-Extrakt beim klimakterischen Syndrom. *Z Phytother* 1990;11:81–86.

11. Warnecke G. [Psychosomatic dysfunctions in the female climacteric. Clinical effectiveness and tolerance of Kava Extract WS 1490]. *Fortschr Med* 1991;109:119–122.

12. Duffield PH, Jamieson D. Development of tolerance to kava in mice. *Clin Exp Pharmacol Physiol* 1992;18:571–578.

13. Jamieson DD, Duffield PH. Positive interaction of ethanol and kava resin in mice. *Clin Exp Pharmacol Physiol* 1990;17: 509–514.

14. Schulz V, Hansel R, Tyler VE. *Rational phytotherapy: a physician's guide to herbal medicine,* 3rd ed. Berlin: Springer-Verlag, 1998.

15. Mathews JD, Riley MD, Fejo L et al. Effects of the heavy usage of kava on physical health: summary of a pilot survey in an Aboriginal community. *Med J Aust* 1988;148: 548–555.

16. Garner LF, Klinger JD. Some visual effects caused by the beverage kava. *J Ethnopharmacol* 1985;13:307–311.

17. Norton SA, Ruze P. Kava dermopathy. *J Am Acad Dermatol* 1994;31:89–97.

18. Ruze P. Kava-induced dermopathy: a niacin deficiency? *Lancet* 1990;335:1442–1445.

19. Jappe U, Franke I, Reinhold D et al. Sebotropic drug reaction resulting from kava-kava extract therapy: a new entity? *J Am Acad Dermatol* 1998;38:104–106.

20. Schelosky L, Raffauf C, Jendroska K et al. Kava and dopamine antagonism. *J Neurol Neurosurg Psychiatry* 1995; 58:639–640.

21. Escher M, Desmeules J, Giostra E et al. Hepatitis associated with kava, a herbal remedy for anxiety. *BMJ* 2001;322:139.

22. Strahl S, Ehret V, Dahm HH et al. [Necrotizing hepatitis after taking herbal medication] (in German). *Dtsch Med Wschr* 1998;123:1410–1414.

23. Kraft M, Spahn TW, Menzel J et al. [Fulminant liver failure after administration of the herbal antidepressant Kava-Kava] (in German). *Dtsch Med Wochenschr* 2001;126: 970–972.

24. Herberg KW, Winter U. 2nd International Congress on Phytomedicine, Munich, Sept 11–14, 1996.

25. Almeida JC, Grimsley EW. Coma from the health food store: interaction between kava and alprazolam. *Ann Int Med* 1996;125:940.

26. Herberg KW: [Effect of Kava-Special Extract WS 1490 combined with ethyl alcohol on safety-relevant performance parameters]. *Blutalkohol* 1993;30:96–105.

27. Foo H, Lemon J. Acute effects of kava, alone or in combination with alcohol, on subjective measures of impairment and intoxication and on cognitive performance. *Drug Alcohol Rev* 1997;16:147–155.

28. Swensen J. Man convicted of driving under influence of kava. *Deseret News* (Salt Lake City, UT), August 5, 1996.

KELP

1. Foster S, Varro I. *Tyler's honest herbal: a sensible guide to the use of herbs and related remedies,* 4th ed. New York: Haworth Herbal Press, 1999:233–235.

2. Curtis H. *Biology,* 3rd ed. New York: Worth Publishers, 1979.

3. Martinet A, Hostettmann K, Schutz Y. Thermogenic effects of commercially available plant preparations aimed at treating human obesity. *Phytomedicine* 1999;6:231–238.

4. Gong YF, Huang ZJ, Qiang MY et al. Suppression of radioac-

References

tive strontium absorption by sodium alginate in animals and human subjects. *Biomed Environ Sci* 1991;4:273–282.

5. Teas, J, Harbison ML, Gelman RS. Dietary seaweed (*Laminaria*) and mammary carcinogenesis in rats. *Cancer Res* 1984;44:2758–2761.

6. Yamamoto I, Maruyama H. Effect of dietary seaweed preparations on 1,2-dimethylhydrazine-induced intestinal carcinogenesis in rats. *Cancer Lett* 1985;26:241–251.

7. Teas, J. The dietary intake of *Laminaria*, a brown seaweed, and breast cancer prevention. *Nutr Cancer* 1983;4:217–222.

8. Norman JA, Pickford CJ, Sanders TW et al. Human intake of arsenic and iodine from seaweed-based food supplements and health foods available in the UK. *Food Addit Contam* 1987;5:103–109.

9. Chan HM, Kim C, Khoday K et al. Assessment of dietary exposure to trace metals in Baffin Inuit food. *Environ Health Perspect* 1995;103:740–746.

10. Shilo S, Hirsch HJ. Iodine-induced hyperthyroidism in a patient with a normal thyroid gland. *Postgrad Med J* 1986; 62:661–662.

11. de Smet PA, Stricker BH, Wilderink F et al. [Hyperthyroidism during treatment with kelp tablets] (in Dutch). *Nederlands Tijdschrift voor Geneeskunde* 1990;134:1058–1059.

12. Okamura K, Inoue K, Omae T. A case of Hashimoto's thyroiditis with thyroid immunological abnormality manifested after habitual ingestion of seaweed. *Acta Endocrinol* 1978; 88:703–712.

13. Hetzel BS, Clugston GA. Iodine. In: Shils ME, Olson JA, Shike M et al, eds. *Modern nutrition in health and disease,* 9th ed. Baltimore: Williams & Wilkins, 1999:253–264.

14. Nishimura Y, Ishii N, Sugita Y et al. A case of carotenodermia caused by a diet of the dried seaweed called Nori. *J Dermatol* 1998;25:685–687.

15. Harrell BL, Rudolph AH. Kelp diet: a cause of acneiform eruption [Letter]. *Arch Dermatol* 1976;112:560.

16. Facciola S. *Cornucopia II: a source book of edible plants.* Vista CA: Kampong Publications, 1998:258.

17. Rauma AL, Torronen R, Hanninen O et al. Vitamin B-12 status of long-term adherents of a strict uncooked vegan diet ("living food diet") is compromised. *J Nutr* 1995;125: 2511–2515.

KHAT

1. Kalix P. Khat: scientific knowledge and policy issues. *Br J Addict* 1987;82:47–53.

2. Kalix P. Pharmacological properties of the stimulant khat. *Pharm Ther* 1990;48:397–416.

3. Kalix P. The pharmacology of psychoactive alkaloids from ephedra and catha. *J Ethnopharmacol* 1991;32:201–208.

4. Widler P, Mathys K, Brenneisen R et al. Pharmacodynamics and pharmacokinetics of khat: A controlled study. *Clin Pharmacol Ther* 1994;55:556–562.

5. Heymann TD, Bhupulan A, Zureikat EK et al. Khat chewing delays gastric emptying of a semi-solid meal. *Aliment Pharmacol Ther* 1995;9:81–83.

6. Nencini P. *Catha edulis* Forsk: ethnopharmacology of a plant with amphetamine-like properties. *Fitoterapia* 1998;69 (Suppl 5):13–14.

7. el-Shoura SM, Abdel AM, Ali ME et al. Deleterious effects of khat addiction on semen parameters and sperm ultrastructure. *Hum Reprod* 1995;10:2295–2300.

8. Khattab NY, Amer G. Undetected neuropsychophysiological sequelae of khat chewing in standard aviation medical examination. *Aviat Space Environ Med* 1995;66:739–744.

9. Nasher AA, Qirbi AA, Ghafoor MA et al. Khat chewing and bladder neck dysfunction. A randomized controlled trial of alpha 1-adrenergic blockade. *Br J Urol* 1995;75:597–598.

10. Kennedy J, Teague J, Rokaw W et al. A medical evaluation of the use of khat in North Yemen. *Soc Sci Med* 1983;17: 783–793.

11. Pantelis C, Hindler CG, Taylor JC. Use and abuse of khat (*Catha edulis*): a review of the distribution, pharmacology, side effects and a description of psychosis attributed to khat chewing. *Psychol Med* 1989;19:657–668.

12. Giannini AJ, Miller NS, Turner CE. Treatment of khat addiction. *J Subst Abuse Treat* 1992;9:379–382.

13. Attef OA, Ali A-AA, Ali HM. Effect of khat chewing on the bioavailability of ampicillin and amoxicillin. *J Antimicrobial Chemother* 1997;39:523–525.

14. Eriksson M, Ghani NA, Kristiansson B. Khat-chewing during pregnancy—effect upon the offspring and some characteristics of the chewers. *East Afr Med J* 1991;68:106–111.

15. Kristiansson B, Abdul GN, Eriksson M et al. Use of khat in lactating women: a pilot study on breast-milk secretion. *J Ethnopharmacol* 1987;21:85–90.

16. Soufi HE, Kameswaran M, Manatani T. Khat and oral cancer. *J Laryngol Otol* 1991;105:643–45.

17. Kandela P. Women's rights, a tourist boom, and the power of khat in Yemen. *Lancet* 2000;355:1437.

KOMBUCHA

1. Hobbs C. *Medicinal mushrooms: an exploration of tradition, healing, and culture,* 2nd ed. Botanica Press, 1995:178–181.

2. Mayser P, Fromme S, Leitzmann C et al. The yeast spectrum of the `tea fungus Kombucha.' *Mycoses* 1995;38:289–295.

3. Perron AD, Patterson JA, Yanofsky NN. Kombucha "mushroom" hepatotoxicity [Letter]. *Ann Emerg Med* 1995;26: 660–661.

4. Unexplained severe illness possibly associated with consumption of kombucha tea—Iowa, 1995. *MMWR* 1995;44: 892–893, 899–900.

5. Srinivasan R, Smolinske S, Greenbaum D. Probable gastrointestinal toxicity of kombucha tea: is this beverage healthy or harmful? *J Gen Int Med* 1997;12:643–644.

6. Sadjadi J. Cutaneous anthrax associated with the kombucha "mushroom" in Iran. *JAMA* 1998;280:1567–1568.

7. Phan TG, Estell J, Duggin G et al. Lead poisoning from drinking kombucha tea brewed in a ceramic pot. (comments in *Med J Aust* 1999;170:454). *Med J Aust* 1998;169:644–646.

8. Ibrahim ND, Kwanashie HO, Njoku CO et al. Screening of "Kargasok tea." IV: Studies of pathological effects in BALB/C mice and Wistar rats. *Vet Hum Toxicol* 1993;35:399–402.

9. Kwanashie HO, Usman H, Nkim SA. Screening of `kargosok tea' I: anorexia and obesity. *Biochem Soc Transact* 1989;17: 1132–1133.

10. Hauser SP. [Dr. Sklenar's kombucha mushroom infusion—a biological cancer therapy. Documentation No. 18] (in German). *Schweizerische Rundschau Medizin Praxis* 1990;79: 243–246.

LACTOBACILLI

1. Gionchetti P, Fizzello F, Venturi A, Campieri M. Probiotics in infective diarrhea and inflammatory bowel diseases. *J Gastroenterol Hepatol* 2000;15:489–493.

2. Elmer GW, Surawicz CM, McFarland LV. Biotherapeutic agents: a neglected modality for the treatment and prevention of selected intestinal and vaginal infections. *JAMA* 1996;275(11):870–876.

3. Katelaris PH, Salam I, Farthing MJG. Lactobacilli to prevent travelers' diarrhea? *N Engl J Med* 1995;333(20):1360–1361.

4. Oksanen PJ, Salminen S, Saxelin M et al. Prevention of travelers' diarrhea by *Lactobacillus GG*. *Ann Med* 1990;22(1):53–56.

5. De dios Pozo-Olano J, Warram JH Jr, Gomez RG, Cavazos MG. Effect of lactobacilli prevention on travelers' diarrhea. A randomized, double-blind clinical trial. *Gastroenterology* 1978;74(5 Pt 1):829–830.

6. Clements ML, Levine MM, Black RE et al. Lactobacillus prophylaxis for diarrhea due to enterotoxigenic Escherichia coli. *Antimicrob Agents Chemother.* 1981;20(1):104–108.

7. Szajewska H, Kotowska M, Mrukowicz JZ et al. Efficacy of *Lactobacillus GG* in prevention of nosocomial diarrhea in infants. *J Pediatr* 2001;138(3):361–365.

8. Oberhelman RA, Gilman RH, Sheen P et al. A placebo-controlled trial of *Lactobacillus* GG to prevent diarrhea in undernourished Peruvian children. *J Pediatr* 1999;134:15–20.

9. Simakachorn N, Pichaipat V, Rithipornpaisarn P et al. Clinical evaluation of the addition of lyophilized, heat-killed Lactobacillus acidophilus LB to oral rehydration therapy in the treatment of acute diarrhea in children. *J Pediatr Gastroenterol Nutr* 2000;30(1):68–72.

10. Pedone CA, Bernabeu AO, Postaire ER et al. The effect of supplementation with milk fermented by Lactobacillus casei (strain DN-114 001) on acute diarrhea in children attending day care centres. *Int J Clin Pract* 1999;53(3):179–184.

11. Isolauri E, Juntunen M, Rautanen T et al. A human Lactobacillus strain (Lactobacillus GG) promotes recovery from acute diarrhea in children. *Pediatrics* 1991;88:90–97.

12. Shornikova A-V, Casas IA, Mykkänen H et al. Bacteriotherapy with *Lactobacillus reuteri* in rotavirus gastroenteritis. *Pediatr Infect Dis J* 1997;16:1103–1107.

13. Guandalini S, Pensabene L, Zikri MA, et al. Lactobacillus GG administered in oral rehydration solution to children with acute diarrhea: a multicenter European trial. *J Pediatr Gastroenterol Nutr* 2000;30(1):54–60.

14. Pant AR, Graham SM, Allen SJ et al. Lactobacillus GG and acute diarrhea in young children in the tropics. *J Trop Pediatr* 1996;42(3):162–165.

15. Vanderhoof JA, Whitney DB, Antonson DL et al. *Lactobacillus GG* in the prevention of antibiotic-associated diarrhea in children. *J Pediatr* 1999;135(5):564–568.

16. Gotz V, Romankiewicz JA, Moss J et al. Prophylaxis against ampicillin-associated diarrhea with a lactobacillus preparation. *Am J Hosp Pharm* 1979;36(6):754–757.

17. Tankanow RM, Ross MB, Ertel IJ et al. A double-blind, placebo-controlled study of the efficacy of Lactinex in the prophylaxis of amoxicillin-induced diarrhea. *DICP* 1990;24(4):382–384.

18. Gionchetti P, Rizzello F, Venturi A, et al. Oral bacteriotherapy as maintenance treatment in patients with chronic pouchitis: a double-blind, placebo-controlled trial. *Gastroenterology* 2000;119(2):305–309.

19. Dunn SR, Simenhoff ML, Ahmed KE et al. Effect of oral administration of freeze-dried *Lactobacillus acidophilus* on small bowel bacterial overgrowth in patients with end stage kidney disease: reducing uremic toxins and improving nutrition. *Int Dairy J* 1998;8:545–553.

20. Isolauri E, Arvola T, Sutas Y et al. Probiotics in the management of atopic eczema. *Clin Exp Allergy* 2000;30(11):1604–1610.

21. Wheeler JG, Shema SJ, Bogle ML et al. Immune and clinical impact of *Lactobacillus acidophilus* on asthma. *Ann Allergy Asthma Immunol* 1997;79(3):229-233.

22. Hilton E, Isenberg HD, Alperstein P et al. Ingestion of yogurt containing *Lactobacillus acidophilus* as prophylaxis for candidal vaginitis. *Ann Intern Med* 1992;116(5):353–357.

23. Hallén A, Jarstrand C, Påhlson C. Treatment of bacterial vaginosis with lactobacilli. *Sexually Transmitted Diseases* 1992;19:146–148.

24. Shalev E, Battino S, Weiner E et al. Ingestion of yogurt containing *Lactobacillus acidophilus* compared with pasteurized yogurt as prophylaxis for recurrent candidal vaginitis and bacterial vaginosis. *Arch Fam Med* 1996;5:593–596.

25. Bruce AW, Reid G, McGroarty JA et al. Preliminary study on the prevention of recurrent urinary tract infection in adult women using intravaginal lactobacilli. *Int Urogynecol J* 1992;3:22–25.

26. Reid G. Probiotic agents to protect the urogenital tract against infection. *Am J Clin Nutr* 2001;73:437S–443S.

27. Ishibashi N, Yamazaki S. Probiotics and safety. *Am J Clin Nutr* 2001;73(suppl):465S–470S.

28. Patel R, Cockerill FR, Porayko MK et al. Lactobacillemia in liver transplant patients. *Clin Inf Diseases* 1994;18:207–212.

29. Coronado BE, Opal SM, Yoburn DC. Antibiotic-induced D-lactic acidosis. *Ann Intern Med* 1995;122:839–842.

30. Pletincx M, Legein J, Vandenplas Y. Fungemia with Saccharomyces boulardii in a one-year-old girl with protracted diarrhea. *J Pediatr Gastroenterol Nutr* 1995;21:113–115.

LECITHIN

1. Canty DJ, Zeisel SH. Lecithin and choline in human health and disease. *Nutr Rev* 1994;52:327–339.

2. Garrow TA. Choline and carnitine. In: Bowman BA, Russell RM, eds. *Present knowledge of nutrition,* 8th ed. Washington, DC: ILSI Press, 2001:265.

3. Linder MC. *Nutritional biochemistry and metabolism, with clinical applications,* 2nd ed. East Norwalk, CT: Appleton & Lange, 1991.

4. Higgins JP, Flicker L. Lecithin for dementia and cognitive impairment. *Cochrane Database Syst Rev* 2000;2:CD001015.

5. McGrath JJ, Soares KV. Cholinergic medication for neuroleptic-induced tardive dyskinesia. *Cochrane Database Syst Rev* 2000;2:CD000207.

6. Knuiman JT, Beynem AC, Katan MB. Lecithin intake and serum cholesterol. *Am J Clin Nutr* 1989;49:266–268.

7. Buchman AL, Dubin M, Jenden D et al. Lecithin increases plasma free choline and decreases hepatic steatosis in long-term total parenteral nutrition patients. *Gastroenterology* 1992;102:1363–1370.

8. Andrioli G, Carletto A, Guarini P et al. Differential effects of dietary supplementation with fish oil or soy lecithin on human platelet adhesion. *Thromb Haemost* 1999;82:1522–1527.

9. Lieber CS, DeCarli LM, Mak KM et al. Attenuation of alcohol-induced hepatic fibrosis by polyunsaturated lecithin. *Hepatology* 1990;12:1390–1398.

10. Food and Nutrition Board, Institute of Medicine. Dietary reference intakes. Thiamin, riboflavin, niacin, vitamin B12,

References

pantothenic acid, biotin, and choline. Washington, DC: National Academy Press, 1998.

LEMON BALM

1. European Scientific Cooperative on Phytotherapy (ESCOP). *Monographs on the medicinal uses of plant drugs. Melissae folium: Melissa leaf. Fascicule* 2. Exeter, UK, 1996.
2. Wake G, Court J, Pickering A et al. CNS acetylcholine receptor activity in European medicinal plants traditionally used to improve failing memory. *J Ethnopharmacol* 2000;69: 105–114.
3. Peake PW, Pussell BA, Martyn T et al. The inhibitory effect of rosmarinic acid on complement involves the C5 convertase. *Int J Immunopharmacol* 1991;13:853–857.
4. Koytchev R, Alken RG, Dundarov S. Balm mint extract (Lo-701) for topical treatment of recurring *herpes labialis*. *Phytomedicine* 1999;6:225–230.
5. Wölbling RH, Leonhardt K. Local therapy of herpes simplex with dried extract from *Melissa officinalis*. *Phytomedicine* 1994;1:25–31.
6. Soulimani R, Fleurentin J, Mortier F et al. Neurotropic action of the hydroalcoholic extract of *Melissa officinalis* in the mouse. *Planta Med* 1991;57:105–109.
7. Auf'mkolk M, Ingbar JC, Amir SM et al. Inhibition by certain plant extracts of the binding and adenylate cyclase stimulatory effect of bovine thyrotropin in human thyroid membranes. *Endocrinology* 1984;115:527–534.
8. Auf'mkolk M, Ingbar JC, Kubota K et al. Extracts and autooxidized constituents of certain plants inhibit the receptor-binding and the biological activity of Graves' immunoglobulins. *Endocrinology* 1985;116:1687–1693.
9. Larrondo JV, Agut M, Calvo-Torras MA. Antimicrobial activity of essences from labiates. *Microbios* 1995;82:171–172.
10. Yamasaki K, Nakano M, Kawahata T et al. Anti-HIV-1 activity of herbs in Labiatae. *Biol Pharm Bull* 1998;21:829–833.
11. Hohmann J, Zupko I, Redei D et al. Protective effects of the aerial parts of *Salvia officinalis*, *Melissa officinalis* and *Lavandula angustifolia* and their constituents against enzyme-dependent and enzyme-independent lipid peroxidation. *Planta Med* 1999;65:576–578.
12. Hausen BM, Schulze R. Comparative studies of the sensitizing capacity of drugs used in herpes simplex. Dermatosen in Beruf und Umwelt. *Occup Environ Dermatol* 1986;34: 163–170.
13. Burgett M. The use of lemon balm (*Melissa officinalis*) for attracting honeybee swarms. *Bee World* 1980;61:44–46.

LEUCINE

1. Linder MC. *Nutritional biochemistry and metabolism, with clinical applications,* 2nd ed. East Norwalk, CT: Appleton & Lange, 1991.
2. Mero A. Leucine supplementation and intensive training. *Sports Med* 1999;27:347–358.
3. Mero A, Pitkanen H, Oja SS et al. Leucine supplementation and serum amino acids, testosterone, cortisol and growth hormone in male power athletes during training. *J Sports Med Phys Fitness* 1997;37:137–145.
4. Mendell JR, Griggs RC, Moxley RT 3d et al. Clinical investigation in Duchenne muscular dystrophy: IV. Double-blind controlled trial of leucine. *Muscle Nerve* 1984;7:535–541.
5. Berry HK, Brunner RL, Hunt MM et al. Valine, isoleucine, and leucine: a new treatment for phenylketonuria. *Am J Dis Child* 1990;144:539–543.
6. Tandan R, Bromberg MB, Forshew D et al. A controlled trial of amino acids therapy in amyotrophic lateral sclerosis. *Neurology* 1996;47:1220–1226.
7. Italian ALS Study Group. Branched-chain amino acids and amyotrophic lateral sclerosis: a treatment failure? The Italian ALS Study Group. *Neurology* 1993;43:2466–2470.
8. Richardson MA, Bevans ML, Weber JB et al. Branched chain amino acids decrease tardive dyskinesia symptoms. *Psychopharmacology (Berl)* 1999;143:358–364.
9. Cangiano C, Laviano A, Meguid MM et al. Effects of administration of oral branched-chain amino acids on anorexia and caloric intake in cancer patients. *J Natl Cancer Inst* 1996;88:550–551.
10. Stein TP, Schluter MD, Leskiw MJ et al. Attenuation of the protein wasting associated with bedrest by branched chain amino acids. *Nutrition* 1999;656–660.

LICORICE

1. Chandler RF. *Glycyrrhiza glabra*. In: De Smet PAGM, Keller K, Hansel R et al, eds. *Adverse effects of herbal drugs*. Berlin: Springer-Verlag, 1997:67–88.
2. Robbers JE, Speedie MK, Tyler VE. *Pharmacognosy and pharmacobiotechnology*. Baltimore: Williams & Wilkins, 1996.
3. Størmer FC, Reistad R, Alexander J. Glycyrrhizic acid in liquorice—evaluation of health hazard. *Food Chem Toxicol* 1993;31:303–312.
4. van Rossum TGJ, Vulto AG, Hop WCJ et al. Intravenous glycyrrhizin for the treatment of chronic hepatitis C: a double-blind, randomized, placebo-controlled phase I/II trial. *J Gastroenterol Hepatol* 1999;14:1093–1099.
5. Rees WDW, Rhodes J, Wright JE et al. Effect of deglycyrrhizinated liquorice on gastric mucosal damage by aspirin. *Scand J Gastroenterol* 1979;14:605.
6. Schambelan M. Licorice ingestion and blood pressure regulating hormones. *Steroids* 1994;59:127–130.
7. Kassir ZA. Endoscopic controlled trial of four drug regimens in the treatment of chronic duodenal ulcers. *Ir Med J* 1985; 78:153–156.
8. Morgan AG, McAdam WAF, Pacsoo C et al. Comparison between cimetidine and Caved-S in the treatment of gastric ulceration, and subsequent maintenance therapy. *Gut* 1982; 23:545–551.
9. Chamberlain JJ, Abolnik IZ. Pulmonary edema following a licorice binge. *West J Med* 1997;167:184–185.
10. MacKenzie MA, Hoefnagels WHL, Jansen RWMM et al. The influence of glycyrrhetinic acid on plasma cortisol and cortisone in healthy young volunteers. *J Clin Endocrinol Metab* 1990;70:1637–1643.
11. Stewart PM, Wallace A, Valentino R et al. Mineralocorticoid activity of liquorice: 11-beta hydroxysteroid dehydrogenase deficiency comes of age. *Lancet* 1987;2:821–824.
12. Armanini D, Bonanni G, Palermo M. Reduction of serum testosterone in men by licorice. *N Engl J Med* 1999;341: 1158.
13. Josephs RA, Guinn JS, Harper ML. Liquorice consumption and salivary testosterone concentrations. *Lancet* 2001;358: 1613–1614.
14. Werner S, Brismar K, Olsson S. Hyperprolactinaemia and licorice. *Lancet* 1979;1:319.
15. Farese RV, Biglieri EG, Shackleton CHL et al. Licorice-

induced hypermineralocorticoidism. *N Engl J Med* 1991;325: 1223–1227.

16. Epstein MT, Espiner EA, Donald RA et al. Effect of eating liquorice on the renin-angiotensin aldosterone axis in normal subjects. *BMJ* 1977;1:488–490.

17. Eriksson JW, Carlberg B, Hillörn V. Life-threatening ventricular tachycardia due to liquorice-induced hypokalaemia. *J Int Med* 1999;245:307–310.

18. Van der Zwan A. Hypertension encephalopathy after liquorice ingestion. *Clin Neurol Neurosurg* 1993;95:35–37.

19. Hupperets P, de Pauw BE, Holdrinet RSG et al. Reversible coma due to hypokalaemia in a patient treated for acute leukaemia. *Neth J Med*1983;26:21–22.

20. Sigurjonsdottir HA, Ragnarsson J, Franzson L et al. Is blood pressure commonly raised by moderate consumption of liquorice? *J Hum Hypertens* 1995;9:345–348.

21. Shintani S, Murase H, Tsukagoshi H et al. Glycyrrhizin (licorice)-induced hypokalemic myopathy. *Eur Neurol* 1992; 32:44–51.

22. Achar KN, Abduo TJ, Menon NK. Severe hypokalemic rhabdomyolysis due to ingestion of liquorice during Ramadan. *Aust N Z J Med* 1989;19:365–367.

23. Chubachi A, Wakui H, Asakura K et al. Acute renal failure following hypokalemic rhabdomyolysis due to chronic glycyrrhizic acid administration. *Int Med* 1992;31:708–711.

24. Strandberg TE, Järvenpää A-L, Vanhanen H et al. Birth outcome in relation to licorice consumption during pregnancy. *Am J Epidemiol* 2001;153:1085–1088.

25. Teelucksingh S, Mackie ADR, Burt D et al. Potentiation of hydrocortisone activity in skin by glycyrrhetinic acid. *Lancet* 1990;335:1060–1063.

26. De Klerk GJ, Nieuwenhuis G, Beutler JJ. Hypokalaemia and hypertension associated with use of liquorice flavoured chewing gum. *BMJ* 1997;314:731–732.

27. Van Gelderen CE, Bijlsma JA, van Dokkum W et al. Glycyrrhizic acid: the assessment of a no effect level. *Hum Exp Toxicol* 2000;19:434–439.

28. Ibsen KK. Liquorice consumption and its influence on blood pressure in Danish school-children. *Dan Med Bull* 1981;28: 124–126.

29. Bisset NG, Wichtl M. *Herbal drugs and phytopharmaceuticals: a handbook for practice on a scientific basis with reference to German Commission E monographs.* Boca Raton, FL: CRC Press, 1994.

LINDEN

1. Blumenthal M, Goldberg A, Brinckmann J. *Herbal medicine: expanded Commission E monographs.* Newton MA: Integrative Medicine Consultants, 2000.

2. de Smet PAGM. Tilia species. In: de Smet PAGM, ed. *Adverse effects of herbal drugs,* vol 2. Berlin: Springer-Verlag, 1997: 303–306.

3. Medina JH, Peña C, Levi de Stein M, et al. Benzodiazepine-like molecules, as well as other ligands for the brain benzodiazepine receptors, are relatively common constituents of plants. *Biochem Biophys Res Com* 1989;165:547–553.

4. Viola H, Wolfman C, Levi de Stein M et al. Isolation of pharmacologically active benzodiazepine receptor ligands from *Tilia tomentosa. J Ethnopharmacol* 1994;44:47–53.

5. Bradley PR (ed) *British Herbal Compendium,* vol. 1. Dorset, UK: British Herbal Medical Association, 1992:142–144.

6. el-Shobaki FA, Saleh ZA, Saleh N. The effect of some beverage extracts on intestinal iron absorption. *Zeitschrift Ernahrungswissenschaft* 1990;29:264–269.

7. Pahlow M. *Das Grosse Buch der Heilpflanzen.* Munich, Germany: Gräfe und Unzer GmbH, 1979:221–223.

8. Grieve M. Lime tree. In: Leyel CF, ed. *A modern herbal,* vol I. Twickenham, Great Britain: Tiger Books Intl, 1998: 485–486. (First published 1931, Jonathan Cape Ltd)

LOBELIA

1. Bradley PR (ed) *British Herbal Compendium,* vol. 1. Dorset, UK: British Herbal Medical Association, 1992:149–150.

2. Subarnas A, Oshima Y, Sidik O et al. An antidepressant principle of *Lobelia inflata* L. (Campanulaceae). *J Pharm Sci* 1992;81:620–621.

3. Decker MW, Buckley MJ, Brioni JD. Differential effects of pretreatment with nicotine and lobeline on nicotine-induced changes in body temperature and locomotor activity in mice. *Drug Dev Res* 1994;31:52–58.

4. Damaj MI, Patrick GS, Creasy KR et al. Pharmacology of lobeline, a nicotinic receptor ligand. *J Pharmacol Exp Ther* 1997;282:410–419.

5. Teng L, Crooks PA, Dwoskin LP. Lobeline displaces [3H]dihydrotetrabenazine binding and releases [3H]dopamine from rat striatal synaptic vesicles: comparison with d-amphetamine. *J Neurochem* 1998;71:258–265.

6. Subarnas A, Tadano T, Nakahata N et al. A possible mechanism of antidepressant activity of beta-amyrin palmitate isolated from *Lobelia inflata* leaves in the forced swimming test. *Life Sci* 1993;52:289–296.

7. Stead LF, Hughes JR. Lobeline for smoking cessation. *Cochrane Database Syst Rev* 2000;2:CD000124.

8. Wright IS, Littauer D. Lobeline sulfate: its pharmacology and use in the treatment of the tobacco habit. *JAMA* 1937; 109:649–654

9. Rapp GW, Olen AA. A critical evaluation of a lobeline based smoking deterrent. *Am J Med Sci* 1955;230:9–14.

10. Rapp GW, Dusza BT, Blanchet L. Absorption and utility of lobeline as a smoking deterrent. *Am J Med Sci* 1959;237: 287–292.

11. Scott GW, Cox AGC, Maclean KS et al. Buffered lobeline as a smoking deterrent [Letter]. *Lancet* 1962;1:54–55.

12. Kaufmann H, Bensimon L. Le sevrage du tabac [Breaking the tobacco habit] (In French). *Vie Med* 1960;41:1139–1140.

13. London SJ. Clinical evaluation of a new lobeline smoking deterrent. *Curr Ther Res* 1963;5:167–175.

14. Plakun AL, Ambrus J, Bross I et al. Clinical factors in smoking withdrawal: preliminary report. *Am J Public Health* 1966;56:434–441.

15. Decker MW, Majchrzak MJ, Arneric SP. Effects of lobeline, a nicotinic receptor agonist, on learning and memory. *Pharmacol Biochem Behav* 1993;45:571–576.

16. Subarnas A, Tadano T, Oshima Y et al. Pharmacological properties of beta-amyrin palmitate, a novel centrally acting compound, isolated from *Lobelia inflata* leaves. *J Pharm Pharmacol* 1993;45:545–550.

17. Raj H, Singh VK, Anand A et al. Sensory origin of lobeline-induced sensations: a correlative study in man and cat. *J Physiol (London)* 1995;482;235–246.

LYSINE

1. Flodlin NW. The metabolic roles, pharmacology, and toxicology of lysine. *J Am Coll Nutr* 1997;16:7–21.

References

2. Linder MC. *Nutritional biochemistry and metabolism, with clinical applications,* 2nd ed. East Norwalk, CT: Appleton & Lange, 1991.
3. Kagan C. Lysine therapy for herpes simplex. *Lancet* 1974;1:137.
4. Griffith RS, Norins AL, Kagan C. A multicentered study of lysine therapy in herpes simplex infection. *Dermatologica* 1978;156:257–267.
5. Milman N, Scheibel J, Jessen O. Lysine prophylaxis in recurrent herpes simplex labialis. *Lancet* 1978;2(8096):942.
6. Milman N, Scheibel J, Jessen O. Lysine prophylaxis in recurrent herpes labialis: a double-blind, controlled crossover study. *Acta Dermatovener (Stockh)* 1980;60:85–87.
7. DiGiovanna JJ, Blank H. Failure of lysine in frequently recurrent herpes simplex infection. *Arch Dermatol* 1984;120:48–51.
8. Griffith RS, Walsh DE, Myrmel KH et al. Success of L-lysine therapy in frequently recurrent herpes simplex infection. *Dermatologica* 1987;175:183–90.
9. Civitelli R, Villareal DT, Agnusdei D et al. Dietary L-lysine and calcium metabolism in humans. *Nutrition* 1992;8:400–405.
10. Food and Nutrition Board, National Research Council. Recommended dietary allowances, 10th ed. Washington, DC: National Academy Press, 1989.

MAGNESIUM

1. Weisinger JR, Belloín-Font E. Magnesium and phosphorus. *Lancet* 1998;352:391–396.
2. Shils ME. Magnesium. In: Shils ME, Olson JA, Shike M et al, eds. *Modern nutrition in health and disease,* 9th ed. Baltimore: Williams & Wilkins, 1999:169–192.
3. Rowe BH, Bretzlaff JA, Bourdon C et al. Magnesium sulfate for treating exacerbations of acute asthma in the emergency department. *Cochrane Database Syst Rev* 2000;2:CD001490.
4. Mangat HS, D'Souza GA, Jacob MS. Nebulized magnesium sulphate versus nebulized salbutamol in acute bronchial asthma: a clinical trial. *Eur Respir J* 1998;12:341–344.
5. Nannini LJ, Pendino JC, Corna RA et al. Magnesium sulfate as a vehicle for nebulized salbutamol in acute asthma. *Am J Med* 2000;108:193–197.
6. England MR, Gordon G, Salem M et al. Magnesium administration and dysrhythmias after cardiac surgery. *JAMA* 1992;268:2395–2402.
7. Ceremuzynski L, Gebalska J, Wolk R et al. Hypomagnesemia in heart failure with ventricular arrhythmias. Beneficial effects of magnesium supplementation. *J Int Med* 2000;247:78–86.
8. Dorman BH, Sade RM, Burnette JS et al. Magnesium supplementation in the prevention of arrhythmias in pediatric patients undergoing surgery for congenital heart defects. *Am Heart J* 2000;139:522–528.
9. Caspi J, Rudis E, Bar I et al. Effects of magnesium on myocardial function after coronary artery bypass grafting. *Ann Thorac Surg* 1995;59:942–947.
10. Solomon AJ, Berger AK, Trivedi KK et al. The combination of propranolol and magnesium does not prevent postoperative atrial fibrillation. *Ann Thorac Surg* 2000;69:126–129.
11. Frick M, Darpo B, Ostergren J et al. The effect of oral magnesium, alone or as an adjuvant to sotalol, after cardioversion in patients with persistent atrial fibrillation. *Eur Heart J* 2000;21:1177–1185.
12. Woods KL, Fletcher S, Roffe C et al. Intravenous magnesium sulfate in suspected acute myocardial infarction: results of the second Leicester Intravenous Magnesium Intervention Trial (LIMIT-2). *Lancet* 1992;339:1553–1558.
13. Woods KL, Fletcher S. Long-term outcome after intravenous magnesium sulphate in suspected acute myocardial infarction: the second Leicester Intravenous Magnesium Intervention Trial (LIMIT-2). *Lancet* 1994;343:816–819.
14. ISIS-4 (Fourth International Study of Infarct Survival) Collaborative Group. ISIS-4: a randomized factorial trial assessing early oral captopril, oral mononitrate, and intravenous magnesium sulphate in 58,050 patients with suspected acute myocardial infarction. *Lancet* 1995;345:669–685.
15. Santoro GM, Antoniucci D, Bolognese L et al. A randomized study of intravenous magnesium in acute myocardial infarction treated with direct coronary angioplasty. *Am Heart J* 2000;140:891–897.
16. Thel MC, Armstrong AL, McNulty SE et al. Randomised trial of magnesium in in-hospital cardiac arrest. *Lancet* 1997;350:1272–1276.
17. THPCRG. Trials of hypertension prevention collaborative research group. The effects of nonpharmacologic interventions on blood pressure of persons with high normal levels. Results of the trials of hypertension prevention, phase 1. *JAMA* 1992;267:1213–1220.
18. Witteman JCM, Grobbee DE, Derkx FHM et al. Reduction of blood pressure with oral magnesium supplementation in women with mild to moderate hypertension. *Am J Clin Nutr* 1994;60:129–135.
19. Lind L, Lithell H, Pollare T et al. Blood pressure during long-term treatment with magnesium is dependent on magnesium status. *Am J Hypertens* 1991;4:674–679.
20. Yamamoto ME, Applegate WB, Klag MJ et al. Lack of blood pressure effect with calcium and magnesium supplementation in adults with high-normal blood pressure. Results from Phase I of the Trials of Hypertension Prevention (TOHP). Trials of Hypertension Prevention (TOHP) Collaborative Research Group. *Ann Epidemiol* 1995;5:96–107.
21. Kawano Y, Matsuoka H, Takishita S et al. Effects of magnesium supplementation in hypertensive patients: assessment by office, home, and ambulatory blood pressures. *Hypertension* 1998;32:260–265.
22. Attias J, Weisz G, Almog S et al. Oral magnesium intake reduces permanent hearing loss induced by noise exposure. *Am J Otolaryngol* 1994;15:26–32.
23. Frusso R, Zarate M, Augustovski F et al. Magnesium for the treatment of nocturnal leg cramps: a crossover randomized trial. *J Fam Pract* 1999;48:868–871.
24. Dahle LO, Berg G, Hammar M et al. The effect of oral magnesium substitution on pregnancy-induced leg cramps. *Am J Obstet Gynecol* 1995;173:175–180.
25. Gordon D, Groutz A, Ascher-Landsberg J et al. Double-blind, placebo-controlled study of magnesium hydroxide for treatment of sensory urgency and detrusor instability: preliminary results. *Br J Obstet Gynaecol* 1998;105:667–669.
26. Ginder S. Oatman B, Pollack M. A prospective study if i.v. magnesium and i.v. prochlorperazine in the treatment of headaches. *J Emerg Med* 2000;18:311–315.
27. Peikert A, Wilimzig C, Kohne-Volland R. Prophylaxis of migraine with oral magnesium: results from a prospective, multi-center, placebo-controlled and double-blind randomized study. *Cephalagia* 1996;16:257–263.
28. Pfaffenrath V, Wessely P, Meyer C et al. Magnesium in the prophylaxis of migraine: results from a prospective, multi-

center, placebo-controlled and double-blind randomized study. *Cephalagia* 1996;16:257–263.

29. Facchinetti F, Sances G, Borella P et al. Magnesium prophylaxis of menstrual migraine: effects of intracellular magnesium. *Headache* 1991;31:298–301.

30. Facchinetti F, Borella P, Sances G et al. Oral magnesium successfully relieves premenstrual mood changes. *Obstet Gynecol* 1991;78:177–181.

31. Walker AF, De Souza MC, Vickers MF et al. Magnesium supplementation alleviates premenstrual symptoms of fluid retention. *J Womens Health* 1998;7:1157–1165.

32. Whang R, Ryder KW. Frequency of hypomagnesemia and hypermagnesemia: requested vs. routine. *JAMA* 1990;263: 3063–3064.

33. Kulkarni M, Baum C, Krug S. Fatal hypermagnesemia from a dietary supplement. *J Toxicol Clin Toxicol* 1999;37:617–618.

34. Gries A, Bode C, Gross S et al. The effect of intravenously administered magnesium on platelet function in patients after cardiac surgery. *Anesth Analg* 1999;88:1213–1219.

35. Falck G. Lundgaard H, Jareld T et al. Effect of magnesium infusion on bleeding time in healthy male volunteers. *Scand J Clin Lab Invest* 1999;59:425–430.

MANGANESE

1. Barceloux DG. Manganese. *Clin Toxicol* 1999;37:293–307.

2. Linder MC. *Nutritional biochemistry and metabolism, with clinical applications,* 2nd ed. East Norwalk, CT: Appleton & Lange, 1991:237–240.

3. Nielsen FH. In: Shils ME, Olson JA, Shike M et al, eds. *Modern nutrition in health and disease,* 9th ed. Williams & Wilkins, 1999:289–292.

4. Keen CL, Zidenberg-Cherr S. Manganese. In: Ziegler EE, Filer LJ, eds. *Present knowledge in nutrition,* 7th ed. Washington, DC: ILSI Press, 1996:334–343.

5. Pal Kr P, Samii A, Calne DB. Manganese neurotoxicity: a review of clinical features, imaging and pathology. *Neurotoxicology* 1999;20:227–238.

6. de Krom MC, Boreas AM, Hardy EL. Mangaanintoxicatie door het gebruik van Chien Pu Wan-tabletten [Manganese poisoning due to use of Chien Pu Wan tablets]. *Ned Tijdschr Geneeskd* 1994;138:2010–2012.

7. Finley JW. Manganese absorption and retention by young women is associated with serum ferritin concentration. *Am J Clin Nutr* 1999;70:37–43.

MARSHMALLOW

1. European Scientific Cooperative on Phytotherapy (ESCOP). *Monographs on the medicinal uses of plant drugs. Althaeae radix (marshmallow root). Fascicule* 1. Exeter, UK, 1996.

MATE

1. Vázquez A, Moyna P. Studies in mate drinking. *J Ethnopharmacol* 1986;18:267–272.

2. Pizarro F, Olivares M, Hertrampf E et al. [Factors which modify the nutritional state of iron: tannin content of herbal teas.] (in Spanish). *Archivos Latinoamericanos Nutricion* 1994;44:277–280.

3. Blumenthal M, Goldberg A, Brinckmann J. *Herbal medicine: expanded Commission E monographs.* Newton MA: Integrative Medicine Consultants, 2000.

4. Gosmann G, Guillaume D, Taketa AT et al. Triterpenoid saponins from *Ilex paraguariensis. J Nat Prod* 1995;58:438–441.

5. Vera Garcia R, Basualdo I, Peralta J et al. Mineral content of Parguayan yerba mate (*Ilex paraguariensis, S.H.*). *Archivos Latinoamericanos Nutricion* 1997;47:77–80.

6. Ruschenburg U. Benzo[a]pyrene levels in coffee and some other foods. *Colloq Sci Int Café* 1985;11:205–212.

7. Ruschenburg U. Benzo[a]pyrene levels in coffee and some other food products. *Cacao Café* 1986;30:3–10.

8. Martinet A, Hostettmann K, Schutz Y. Thermogenic effects of commercially available plant preparations aimed at treating human obesity. *Phytomedicine* 1999;6:231–238.

9. Schinella GR, Troiani G, Davila V et al. Antioxidant effects of an aqueous extract of *Ilex paraguariensis. Biochem Biophysical Res Comm* 2000;269:357–360.

10. Gugliucci A. Antioxidant effects of *Ilex paraguariensis*: induction of decreased oxidability of human LDL in vivo. *Biochem Biophysical Res Comm* 1996;224:338–344.

11. De Stefani E, Munoz N, Esteve J et al. Mate drinking, alcohol, tobacco, diet, and esophageal cancer in Uruguay. *Cancer Res* 1990;50:426–431.

12. De Stefani E, Correa P, Oreggia F. Black tobacco, wine and mate in oropharyngeal cancer. A case-control study from Uruguay. *Revue Epidemiologie Sante Publique* 1988;36: L38–394.

13. Vassallo A, Correa P, De Stefani E et al. Esophageal cancer in Uruguay: a case-control study. *J Natl Can Inst* 1985;75: 1005–1009.

14. Pintos J, Franco EL, Oliveira BV et al. Mate, coffee, and tea consumption and risk of cancers of the upper aerodigestive tract in southern Brazil. *Epidemiology* 1994;5:583–590.

15. Prudente A. Patologia geographica do cancer no Brasil. *Bol Oncologia* 1963;46:281–287.

16. De Stefani E, Fierro L, Mendilaharsu M et al. Meat intake, 'mate' drinking and renal cell cancer in Uruguay: a case-control study. *Br J Cancer* 1998;78:1239–1243.

17. Munoz SE, Navarro A, Lantieri MJ et al. Alcohol, methylxanthine-containing beverages, and colorectal cancer in Cordoba, Argentina. *Eur J Cancer Prev* 1998;7:207–213.

18. De Stefani E, Fierro L, Correa P et al. Mate drinking and risk of lung cancer in males: a case-control study from Uruguay. *Cancer Epidemiol Biomark Prev* 1996;5:515–519.

19. De Stefani E, Correa P, Fierro L. Black tobacco, mate, and bladder cancer. A case-control study from Uruguay. *Cancer* 1991;67:536–540.

20. Munoz N, Victora CG, Crespi M et al. Hot mate drinking and precancerous lesions of the oesophagus: an endoscopic survey in southern Brazil. *Int J Cancer* 1987;39;708–709.

21. De Stefani E, Correa P, Oreggia F et al. Risk factors for laryngeal cancer. *Cancer* 1987;60:3087–3091.

22. Kusminsky G, Dictar M, Arduino S et al. Do not drink mate. An additional source of infection in South American neutropenic patients [Letter]. *Bone Marrow Transplantation* 1996;17:127.

23. McGee JO'D, Patrick RS, Wood CB et al. A case of veno-occlusive disease of the liver in Britain associated with herbal tea consumption. *J Clin Pathol* 1976;29:788–794.

24. Hsu CK, Leo P, Shastry D et al. Anticholinergic poisoning associated with herbal tea. *Arch Int Med* 1995;155: 2245–2248.

25. Victoria CG, Munoz N, Horta BL et al. Patterns of mate drinking in a Brazilian city. *Cancer Res* 1990;50:7112–7115.

References

26. De Barros SGS, Ghisolfi ES, Luz LP et al. Mate (Chimarrão) é consumido en alta temperatura por população sob risco para o carcinoma epidermóide de esôfago. *Arq Gastroenterol* 2000;37:25–30.
27. Engelke BF, Gentner WA. Determination of cocaine in "mate de coca" herbal tea [Letter]. *J Pharm Sci* 1991;80:96.

MELATONIN

1. Leone M, Bussone G. Melatonin in cluster headache: rationale for use and possible therapeutic potential. *CNS Drugs* 1998;1:7–16.
2. Webb SM, Puig-Domingo M. Role of melatonin in health and disease. *Clin Endocrinol* 1995;42:221–234.
3. Huether G. The contribution of extrapineal sites of melatonin synthesis to circulating melatonin levels in higher vertebrates. *Experientia* 1993;49:665–670.
4. Arendt J, Deacon S, English J et al. Melatonin and adjustment to phase shift. *J Sleep Res* 1995;4(Suppl 2):74–79.
5. Cagnacci A, Zanni AL, Veneri MG. Influence of exogenous melatonin on catecholamine levels in postmenopausal women prior and during oestradiol replacement. *Clin Endocrinol (Oxf)* 2000;53:367–372.
6. Dollins AB, Zhdanova IV, Wurtman RJ et al. Effect of inducing nocturnal serum melatonin concentrations in daytime on sleep, mood, body temperature, and performance. *Proc Natl Acad Sci* 1994;91:1824–1828.
7. Shamir E, Laudon M, Barak Y et al. Melatonin improves sleep quality of patients with chronic schizophrenia. *J Clin Psychiatry* 2000;61:373–377.
8. O'Callaghan FJ, Clarke AA, Hancock E et al. Use of melatonin to treat sleep disorders in tuberous sclerosis. *Develop Med Child Neurol* 1999;41:123–126.
9. Spitzer RL, Terman M, Williams JBW et al. Jet lag: clinical features, validation of a new syndrome-specific scale, and lack of response to melatonin in a randomized, double-blind trial. *Am J Psychiatry* 1999;156:1392–1396.
10. Garfinkel D, Zisapel N, Wainstein J et al. Facilitation of benzodiazepine discontinuation by melatonin. *Arch Intern Med* 1999;159:2456–2460.
11. Jockovich M, Cosentino D, Cosentino L et al. Effect of exogenous melatonin on mood and sleep efficiency in emergency medicine residents working night shifts. *Acad Emerg Med* 2000;7:955–958.
12. Folkard S, Arendt J, Clark M. Can melatonin improve shift workers tolerance of the night shift? Some preliminary findings. *Chronobiol Int* 1993;10:315–320.
13. Naguib M, Samarkandi AH. The comparative dose-response effects of melatonin and midazolam for premedication of adult patients: a double-blinded, placebo-controlled study. *Anesth Analg* 2000;91:473–479.
14. Ghielmini M, Pagani O, de Jong J et al. Double-blind randomized study on the myeloprotective effect of melatonin in combination with carboplatin and etoposide in advanced lung cancer. *Br J Cancer* 1999;80:1058–1061.
15. Lissoni P, Barni S, Mandala M et al. Decreased toxicity and increased efficacy of cancer chemotherapy using the pineal hormone melatonin in metastatic solid tumour patients with poor clinical status. *Eur J Cancer* 1999;35:1688–1692.
16. Dreher F, Gabard B, Schwindt DA et al. Topical melatonin in combination with vitamins E and C protects skin from ultraviolet-induced erythema: a human study in vivo. *Br J Dermatol* 1998;139:332–339.
17. Shamir E, Barak Y, Plopsky I et al. Is melatonin treatment effective for tardive dyskinesia? *J Clin Psychiatry* 2000;61:556–558.
18. Waldhauser F, Lynch HJ, Wurtmann RJ. Melatonin in human body fluids; clinical significance. In: Reiter RJ, ed. *The pineal gland*. New York: Raven Press, 1984:345–369.
19. Sanders DC, Chaturvedi AK, Hordinsky JR. Melatonin: aeromedical, toxicopharmacological, and analytical aspects. *J Anal Toxicol* 1999;23:159–167.
20. Sheldon SH. Pro-convulsant effects of oral melatonin in neurologically disabled children. *Lancet* 1998;351:1254.
21. Force RW, Hansen L, Bedell M. Psychotic episode after melatonin. *Anal Pharmacother* 1997;31:1408.
22. Lehman NL, Johnson LN. Toxic optic neuropathy after concomitant use of melatonin, Zoloft, and a high-protein diet. *J Neuroophthalmol* 1999;19:232–234.
23. Murch SJ, Simmons CB, Saxena PK. Melatonin in feverfew and other medicinal plants. *Lancet* 1997;350:1598–1599.

METHIONINE

1. Shils ME, Olson JA, Shike M et al, eds. *Modern nutrition in health and disease,* 9th ed. Baltimore: Williams & Wilkins, 1999.
2. Friedel HA, Goa KL, Benfield P. S-adenosyl-L-methionine: a review of its pharmacological properties and therapeutic potential in liver dysfunction and affective disorders in relation to its physiological role in cell metabolism. *Drugs* 1989;38:389–416.
3. Frezza M, Centini G, Cammareri G et al. S-adenosylmethionine for the treatment of intrahepatic cholestasis of pregnancy. Results of a controlled clinical trial. *Hepatogastroenterology* 1990;37(Suppl 2):122–125.
4. Frezza M, Tritapepe R, Pozzato G et al. Prevention of S-adenosylmethionine of estrogen-induced hepatobiliary toxicity in susceptible women. *Am J Gastroenterol* 1988;83:1098–1102.
5. Frezza M, Pozzato G, Chiesa L et al. Reversal of intrahepatic cholestasis of pregnancy in women after high dose S-adenosyl-L-methionine administration. *Hepatology* 1984;4:274–278.
6. Ribalta J. Reyes H, Gonzalez MC et al. S-adenosyl-L-methionine in the treatment of patients with intrahepatic cholestasis of pregnancy: a randomized, double-blind, placebo-controlled study with negative results. *Hepatogastroenterology* 1991;13:1084–1089.
7. Mato JM, Camara J, Fernandez de Paz J et al. S-adenosylmethionine in alcoholic liver cirrhosis: a randomized, placebo-controlled, double-blind, multicenter clinical trial. *J Hepatol* 1999;30:1081–1089.
8. Bressa GM. S-adenosyl-L-methionine (SAMe) as antidepressant: meta-analysis of clinical trials. *Acta Neurol Scand* 1994;154(Suppl):7–14.
9. Volkmann H, Norregaard J, Jacobsen S et al. Double-blind, placebo-controlled cross-over study of intravenous S-adenosyl-L-methionine in patients with fibromyalgia. *Scand J Rheumatol* 1997;26:206–211.
10. Ianniello A, Ostuni PA, Sfriso P et al. S-adenosyl-L-methionine in Sjogren's syndrome and fibromyalgia. *Curr Ther Res* 1994;55:699–706.
11. Di Rocco A, Tagliati M, Danisi F et al. A pilot study of L-methionine for the treatment of AIDS-associated myelopathy. *Neurology* 1998;51:266–268.
12. Wright B, Crowe M. Use of oral methionine for overdose below threshold for acetylcysteine. *BMJ* 1998;317:1656.

13. Bellone J, Farello G, Bartolotta E et al. Methionine potentiates both basal and GHRH-induced GH secretion in children. *Clin Endocrinol* 1997;47:61–64.

14. Linder MC. *Nutritional biochemistry and metabolism, with clinical applications*, 2nd ed. East Norwalk, CT: Appleton & Lange, 1991.

15. Food and Nutrition Board, National Research Council. *Recommended dietary allowances*, 10th ed. Washington, DC: National Academy Press, 1989.

16. SAMe for depression. *Med Lett* 1999;41:107–108.

17. McAuley DF, Hanratty CG, McGurk C et al. Effect of methionine supplementation on endothelial function, plasma homocysteine, and lipid peroxidation. *J Toxicol Clin Toxicol* 1999;37:435–440.

18. Bellamy MF, McDowell IF, Ramsey MW et al. Hyperhomocysteinemia after an oral methionine load acutely impairs endothelial function in healthy adults. *Circulation* 1998;98:1848–1852.

19. Constans J, Blann AD, Resplandy F et al. Endothelial dysfunction during acute methionine load in hyperhomocysteinaemic patients. *Atherosclerosis* 1999;147:411–413.

MILK THISTLE

1. Schulz V, Hansel R, Tyler VE. *Rational phytotherapy: a physician's guide to herbal medicine*, 3rd ed. Berlin: Springer-Verlag, 1998:215.

2. Flora K, Hahn M, Rosen H et al. Milk thistle (*Silybum marianum*) for the therapy of liver disease. *Am J Gastroenterol* 1998;93:139–143.

3. Zhao J, Agarwal R. Tissue distribution of silibinin, the major active constituent of silymarin, in mice and its association with enhancement of phase II enzymes: implications in cancer chemoprevention. *Carcinogenesis* 1999;20:2101–2108.

4. Manna SK, Mukhopadhyay A, Van NT et al. Silymarin suppresses TNF-induced activation of NF-kappa B, c-Jun N-terminal kinase, and apoptosis. *J Immunol* 1999;163:6800–6809.

5. Dehmlow C, Erhard J, de Groot H. Inhibition of Kupffer cell function as an explanation for the hepatoprotective properties of silibinin. *Hepatology* 1996;23:749–754.

6. Lawrence V, Jacobs B, Dennehy C et al. *Milk thistle: effects on liver disease and cirrhosis and clinical adverse effects.* Evidence Report/Technology Assessment No. 21. AHRQ Publication No 01-Eo25. Rockville MD: Agency for Healthcare Research and Quality, October 2000.

7. Salmi HA, Sarna S. Effect of silymarin on chemical, functional, and morphological alterations of the liver. *Scand J Gastroenterol* 1982;17:517–521.

8. Bode JC. Silymarin for the therapy of liver disease [Letter]. *Am J Gastroenterol* 1999;94:545–546.

9. Pares A, Planas R, Torres M, et al. Effects of silymarin in alcoholic patients with cirrhosis of the liver: results of a controlled, double-blind, randomized, and multicenter trial. *J Hepatol* 1998;28:615–621.

10. Ferenci P, Dragosics B, Dittrich H et al. Randomized controlled trial of silymarin treatment in patients with cirrhosis of the liver. *J Hepatol* 1989;9:105–113.

11. Palasciano G, Portincasa P, Palmieri V et al. The effect of silymarin on plasma levels of malondialdehyde in patients receiving long-term treatment with psychotropic drugs. *Curr Ther Res* 1994;55:537–545.

12. Allain H, Schuck S, Lebreton S et al. Aminotransferase levels and silymarin in de novo tacrine-treated patients with Alzheimer's disease. *Dement Geriatr Cogn Disord* 1999;10:181–185.

13. Angulo P, Patel T, Jorgensen RA et al. Silymarin in the treatment of patients with primary biliary cirrhosis with a suboptimal response to ursodeoxycholic acid. *Hepatology* 2000;32:897–900.

14. Blumenthal M, Goldberg A, Brinckmann J. *Herbal medicine: expanded Commission E monographs*. Newton MA: Integrative Medicine Consultants, 2000.

15. Jander S, Bischoff J. Treatment of *Amanita phalloides* poisoning: I. Retrospective evaluation of plasmapheresis in 21 patients. *Ther Apher* 2000;4:303–307.

16. Mereish KA, Bunner DL, Ragland DR et al. Protection against microcystin-LR-induced hepatotoxicity by silymarin: biochemistry, histopathology, and lethality. *Pharm Res* 1991;8:273–277.

17. Thamsborg SM, Jørgensen RJ, Brummerstedt E et al. Putative effect of silymarin on sawfly (*Arge pullata*)-induced hepatotoxicosis in sheep. *Vet Hum Toxicol* 1996;38:89–91.

18. Krecǎkottová N, Walterová D et al. Silymarin inhibits the development of diet-induced hypercholesterolemia in rats. *Planta Med* 1998;64:138–142.

19. Skottova N, Krecman V, Simanek V. Activities of silymarin and its flavonolignans upon low density lipoprotein oxidizability in vitro. *Phytother Res* 1999;13:535–537.

20. Locher R, Suter PM, Weyhenmeyer R et al. Inhibitory action of silibinin on low-density lipoprotein oxidation. *Arzneim-Forsch/Drug Res* 1998;48:236–239.

21. Lahiri-Chatterjee M, Katiyar SK, Mohan RR et al. A flavonoid antioxidant, silymarin, affords exceptionally high protection against tumor promotion in the SENCAR mouse skin tumorigenesis model. *Cancer Res* 1999;59(3):622–632.

22. Katiyar SK, Korman NJ, Mukhtar H et al. Protective effects of silymarin against photocarcinogenesis in a mouse skin model. *J Natl Cancer Inst* 1997;89:556–66.

23. Bhatia N, Zhao J, Wolf DM et al. Inhibition of human carcinoma cell growth and DNA synthesis by silibinin, an active constituent of milk thistle: comparison with silymarin. *Cancer Lett* 1999;147:77–84.

24. Zi X, Agarwal R. Silibinin decreases prostate-specific antigen with cell growth inhibition via G1 arrest, leading to differentiation of prostate carcinoma cells: implications for prostate cancer intervention. *Proc Natl Acad Sci U.S.A.* 1999;96:7490–7495.

25. Zi X, Grasso AW, Kung HJ et al. A flavonoid antioxidant, silymarin, inhibits activation of erbB1 signaling and induces cyclin-dependent kinase inhibitors, G1 arrest, and anticarcinogenic effects in human prostate carcinoma DU145 cells. *Cancer Res* 1998;58:1920–1929.

26. Zi X, Feyes DK, Agarwal R. Anticarcinogenic effect of a flavonoid antioxidant, silymarin, in human breast cancer cells MDA-MB 468; induction of G1 arrest through an increase in Cip1/p21 concomitant with a decrease in kinase activity of cyclin-dependent kinases and associated cyclins. *Clin Cancer Res* 4:1055–1064.

27. Gaedeke J, Fels LM, Bokemeyer C et al. Cisplatin nephrotoxicity and protection by silibinin. *Nephrol Dial Transplant* 1996;11:55–62.

28. Von Schonfeld J, Weisbrod B, Muller MK. Silibinin, a plant extract with antioxidant and membrane stabilizing properties, protects exocrine pancreas from cyclosporin A toxicity. *Cell Mol Life Sci* 1997;53:917–920.

References

29. Alarcon de la Lastra AC, Martin MJ, Motilva V et al. Gastro-protection induced by silymarin, the hepatoprotective principle of *Silybum marianum* in ischemia-reperfusion mucosal injury: role of neutrophils. *Planta Med* 1995;61:116–119.
30. Adverse Drug Reactions Advisory Committee (ADRAC). An adverse reaction to the herbal medication milk thistle (*Silybum marianum*). *Med J Aust* 1999;170:218–219.

MOLYBDENUM

1. Barceloux DG. Molybdenum. *Clin Toxicol* 1999;37:231–237.
2. Nielsen FH, Shils ME, Olson JA, et al, eds. Ultratrace minerals. *Modern nutrition in health and disease,* 9th ed. Baltimore: Williams & Wilkins, 1999:292–293.
3. Sardesai VM. Molybdenum: an essential trace element. *Nutr Clin Pract* 1993;8:277–281.
4. Vyskocil A, Viau C. Assessment of molybdenum toxicity in humans. *J Appl Toxicol* 1999;19:185–192.
5. Brewer GJ, Dick RD, Grover DK et al. Treatment of metastatic cancer with tetrathiomolybdate, an anticopper, antiangiogenic agent: phase I study. *Clin Cancer Res* 2000;6:1–10.
6. Blot WJ, Li JY, Taylor PR et al. Nutrition intervention trials in Linxian, China: supplementation with specific vitamin/mineral combinations, cancer incidence, and disease-specific mortality in the general population. *J Natl Cancer Inst* 1993;85:1483–1492.
7. Wang GQ, Dawsey SM, Li JY et al. Effects of vitamin/mineral supplementation on the prevalence of histological dysplasia and early cancer of the esophagus and stomach: results from the general population trial in Linxian, China. *Cancer Epidemiol Biomark Prev* 1994;3:161–166.
8. Brewer GJ, Johnson V, Dick RD et al. Treatment of Wilson disease with ammonium tetrathiomolybdate. II. Initial therapy in 33 neurologically affected patients and follow-up with zinc therapy. *Arch Neurol* 1996;53:1017–1025.
9. Komada H, Kise Y, Nakagawa M et al. Effect of dietary molybdenum on esophageal carcinogenesis in rats induced by N-methyl-N-benzylnitrosamine. *Cancer Res* 1990;50:2418–2422.
10. Koizumi T, Tajima K, Emi H et al. Suppressive effect of molybdenum on hepatotoxicity of N-nitrosodiethylamine in rats. *Biol Pharm Bull* 1995;18:460–462.
11. Flora SJ, Jeevaratnam K, Kumar D. Preventive effects of sodium molybdate in lead intoxication in rats. *Ecotoxicol Environ Safety* 1993;26:133–137.
12. Kambara M, Uemura M, Noshi H et al. Increased remineralization of subsurface enamel lesions with molybdenum treatment. *J Osaka Dent Univ* 1989;23:57–62.
13. Abumrad NN, Schneider AJ, Steel D et al. Amino acid intolerance during prolonged total parenteral nutrition reversed by molybdate therapy. *Am J Clin Nutr* 1981;34:2551–2559.
14. Droste JH, Weyler JJ, Van Meerbeeck JP et al. Occupational risk factors of lung cancer: a hospital based case-control study. *Occup Environ Med* 1999;56:322–327.
15. Federmann M, Morell B, Graetz G, et al. Hypersensitivity to molybdenum as a possible trigger of ANA-negative systemic lupus erythematosus. *Ann Rheum Dis* 1994;53:403–405.
16. Lewis RA. *Lewis' dictionary of toxicology.* Boca Raton, FL: Lewis Publishers, 1998:713.

MOTHERWORT

1. Bradley PR (ed). *British Herbal Compendium*, vol 1. Dorset, UK: British Herbal Medical Association, 1992:161–162.
2. Blumenthal M, Goldberg A, Brinckmann J. *Herbal medicine: expanded Commission E monographs.* Newton MA: Integrative Medicine Consultants, 2000.
3. Nagasawa H, Onoyama T, Suzuki M et al. effects of motherwort (*Leonurus sibiricus* L) on pre-neoplastic and neoplastic mammary gland growth in multiparous GR/A mice. *Anticancer Res* 1990;10:1019–1024.
4. Kong YC, Ng KH. Stimulatory effects of *Leonurus artemisia* (I-Mu Ts'ao) on the contraction of human myometrium in vitro. *Experientia* 1974;30:1281–1282.

MULLEIN

1. Blumenthal M, Goldberg A, Brinckmann J. *Herbal medicine: expanded Commission E monographs.* Newton MA: Integrative Medicine Consultants, 2000.
2. Zgorniak-Nowosielska I, Grzybek J, Manolova N et al. Antiviral activity of Flos verbasci infusion against influenza and Herpes simplex viruses. *Arch Immunol Ther Exp* 1991;39:103–108.
3. McCutcheon AR, Roberts TE, Gibbons E et al. Antiviral screening of British Columbian medicinal plants. *J Ethnopharmacol* 1995;49:101–110.
4. Galasinski W, Chlabicz J, Paszkiewicz-Gadek A et al. The substances of plant origin that inhibit protein biosynthesis. *Acta Poloniae Pharm* 1996;53:311–318.
5. Moore M. *Los remedios: traditional herbal remedies of the Southwest.* Santa Fe: Red Crane Books, 1990:70.
6. Kay M. Poisoning by gordolobo. *HerbalGram* 1994;32:42–57.
7. Huxtable RJ. Herbal teas and toxins: novel aspects of pyrrolizidine poisoning in the United States. *Persp Biol Med* 1980;24:1–14.
8. Lewis WH, Elvin Lewis MPF. *Medical botany.* New York: John Wiley and Sons: 1977:296–297.
9. Grieve M. In Leyel CF, ed. *A modern herbal*, vol I. Twickenham, Great Britain: Tiger Books Intl, 1998:562–566 (first published 1931, Jonathan Cape Ltd).

NEEM

1. Evans WC. *Trease and Evans' Pharmacognosy,* 14th ed. London: WB Saunders, 1996.
2. Upadhyay SN, Dhawan S, Garg S et al. Immunomodulatory effects of neem (*Azadirachta indica*) oil. *Int J Immunopharmacol* 1992;14:1187–1193.
3. van der Nat JM, Klerx JP, van Dijk H et al. Immunomodulatory activity of an aqueous extract of *Azadirachta indica* stem bark. *J Ethnopharmacol* 1987;19:125–31.
4. Kaushic C, Upadhyay S. Mode of long-term antifertility effect of intrauterine neem treatment (IUNT). *Contraception* 1995;51:203–207.
5. Garg GP, Nigam SK, Ogle CW. The gastric antiulcer effects of the leaves of the neem tree. *Planta Med* 1993;59:215–217.
6. Kusamran WR, Ratanavila A, Tepsuwan A. Effects of neem flowers, Thai and Chinese bitter gourd fruits and sweet basil leaves on hepatic monooxygenases and glutathione S-transferase activities, and in vitro metabolic activation of chemical carcinogens in rats. *Food Chem Toxicol* 1998;36:475–484.
7. Mittal A, Kapur S, Garg S et al. Clinical trial with Praneem polyherbal cream in patients with abnormal vaginal discharge due to microbial infections. *Aust N Z J Obstet Gynecol* 1995;35:190–191.
8. Charles V, Charles SX. The use and efficacy of *Azadirachta indica* ADR ('neem') and *Curcuma longa* ('Turmeric') in scabies. A pilot study. *Trop Geogr Med* 1992;44:178–181.

9. Wolinsky LE, Mania S, Nachnani S et al. The inhibiting effect of aqueous *Azadirachta indica* (neem) extract upon bacterial properties influencing in vitro plaque formation. *J Dent Res* 1996;75:816–822.

10. Talwar GP, Raghuvanshi P, Misra R et al. Plant immunomodulators for termination of unwanted pregnancy and for contraception and reproductive health. *Immun Cell Biol* 1997;75:190–192.

11. Dhar R, Zhang K, Talwar GP et al. Inhibition of the growth and development of asexual and sexual stages of drug-sensitive and resistant strains of the human malaria parasite *Plasmodium falciparum* by neem (*Azadirachta indica*) fractions. *J Ethnopharmacol* 1998;61:31–39.

12. Singh K, Singh A, Singh DK. Molluscicidal activity of neem (*Azadirachta indica A. Juss*). *J Ethnopharmacol* 1996;52:35–40.

13. SaiRam M, Ilavazhagan G, Sharma SK et al. Anti-microbial activity of a new vaginal contraceptive NIM-76 from neem oil (*Azadirachta indica*). *J Ethnopharmacol* 2000;71:377–382.

14. Mulla MS, Su T. Activity and biological effects of neem products against arthropods of medical and veterinary importance. *J Am Mosquito Control Assoc* 1999;15:133–152.

15. Sharma SK, Dua VK, Sharma VP. Field studies on the mosquito repellent action of neem oil. *Southeast Asian J Trop Med Public Health* 1995;26:180–182.

16. Sharma VP, Ansari MA. Personal protection from mosquitoes (*Diptera:* Culicidae) by burning neem oil in kerosene. *J Med Entomol* 1994;31:505–507.

17. Cohen E, Quistad GB, Casida JE. Cytotoxicity of nimbolide, epoxyazadiradione and other limonoids from neem insecticide. *Life Sci* 1996;58:1075–1081.

18. Balasenthil S, Arivazhagan S, Ramachandran CR. Chemopreventive potential of neem (*Azadirachta indica*) on 7,12-dimethylbenz[a]anthracene (DMBA) induced hamster buccal pouch carcinogenesis. *J Ethnopharmacol* 1999;67:189–195.

19. Khanna N, Goswami M, Sen P et al. Antinociceptive action of *Azadirachta indica* (neem) in mice: possible mechanisms involved. *Indian J Exp Biol* 1995;33:848–50.

20. Bhanwra S, Singh J, Khosla P. Effect of *Azadirachta indica* (neem) leaf aqueous extract on paracetamol-induced liver damage in rats. *Indian J Physiol Pharm* 2000;44:64—68.

21. Upadhyay S, Dhawan S, Sharma MG et al. Long-term contraceptive effects of intrauterine neem treatment (IUNT) in bonnet monkeys: an alternate to intrauterine contraceptive devices (IUCD). *Contraception* 1994;49:161–169.

22. Upadhyay SN, Dhawan S, Talwar GP. Antifertility effects of neem (*Azadirachta indica*) oil in male rats by single intravas administration: an alternate approach to vasectomy. *J Androl* 1993;14:275–281.

23. Lai SM, Lim KW, Cheng HK. Margosa oil poisoning as a cause of toxic encephalopathy. *Singapore Med J* 1990;31:463–465.

24. Sinniah D, Baskaran G, Looi I et al. Reye-like syndrome due to margosa oil poisoning: report of a case with postmortem findings. *Am J Gastroenterol* 1982;77:158–161.

25. Sivashanmugham R, Bhaskar N, Banumathi N. Ventricular fibrillation and cardiac arrest due to neem leaf poisoning. *J Assoc Physicians India* 1984;32:610–611.

26. Thompsom EB, Anderson CC. Cardiovascular effects of *Azadirachta indica* extract. *J Pharm Sci* 1978;67:1476–1478.

27. Chinnasamy N, Harishankar N, Kumar PU et al. Toxicological studies on debitterized Neem oil (*Azadirachta indica*). *Food Chem Toxicol* 1993;31:297–301.

28. Ali BH. The toxicity of *Azadirachta indica* leaves in goats and guinea pigs. *Vet Hum Toxicol* 1987;29:16–19.

29. Panda S, Kar A. How safe is neem extract with respect to thyroid function in male mice? *Pharm Res* 2000;41:419–422.

NETTLE

1. European Scientific Cooperative on Phytotherapy (ESCOP). *Monographs on the medicinal use of plant drugs. Urticae radixi: nettle root. Fascicule 2*. Exeter, UK, 1996.

2. Hughes RE, Ellery P, Harry T et al. The dietary potential of the common nettle. *J Sci Food Agric* 1980;31:1279–1286.

3. Bombardelli E, Morazzoni P. *Urtica dioica L. Fitoterapia* 1997;48:387–402.

4. Bisset NG, Wichtl M. *Herbal drugs and phytopharmaceuticals: a handbook for practice on a scientific basis with reference to German Commission E monographs*. Boca Raton, FL: CRC Press, 1994.

5. Broekaert WF, Parijs JV, Leyns F et al. A chitin-binding lectin from stinging nettle rhizomes with antifungal properties. *Science* 1989;245:1100–1102.

6. Czarnetzki BM, Thiele T, Rosenbach T. Immunoreactive leukotrienes in nettle plants (*Urtica urens*). *Int Arch Allergy Appl Immunol* 1990;91:43–46.

7. Ganßer D, Spiteller G. Aromatase inhibitors from *Urtica dioica* roots. *Planta Med* 1995;61:138–140.

8. Hryb DJ, Khan MS, Romas NA, Rosner W. The effect of extracts of the roots of the stinging nettle (*Urtica dioica*) on the interaction of SHBG with its receptor on human prostatic membranes. *Planta Med* 1995;61:31–32.

9. Goepel M, Hecker U, Krege S et al. Saw palmetto extracts potently and noncompetitively inhibit human alpha 1-adrenoceptors in vitro. *Prostate* 1999;38:208–215.

10. Van Hees J, Gybels J. C nociceptor activity in human nerve during painful and non painful skin stimulation. *J Neurol Neurosurg Psychiatry* 1981;44:600–607.

11. Oliver F, Amon EU, Breathnach A et al. Contact urticaria due to the common stinging nettle (*Urtica dioica*)—histological, ultrastructural and pharmacological studies. *Clin Exp Dermatol* 1991;16:1–7.

12. Randall C, Randall H, Dobbs F et al. Randomized controlled trial of nettle sting for treatment of base-of-thumb pain. *J R Soc Med* 2000;93:305–309.

13. Chrubasik S, Enderlein W, Bauer R et al. Evidence for antirheumatic effectiveness of herba *Urticae Dioicae* in acute arthritis: A pilot study. *Phytomedicine* 1997;4:105–108.

14. Mittman P. Randomized, double-blind study of freeze-dried *Urtica dioica* in the treatment of allergic rhinitis. *Planta Med* 1990;56:44–46.

15. Vontobel HP, Herzog R, Rutishauser G et al. Ergebnisse einer Doppelblindstudie über die Wirksamkeit von ERU-Kapseln in der konservativen Behandlung der benignen Prostatahyperplasie. *Urologe [A]* 1985;24:49–51.

16. Dathe G, Schmid H. Phytotherapie der benignen Prostatahyperplasie (BPH). Doppelblind studie mit Extraction Radicis Uricae (ERV). *Urologe [B]* 1987;27:223.

17. Sokeland J, Albrecht J. Combination of Sabal and Urtica extract vs. finasteride in benign prostatic hyperplasia (Aiken stages I to II). Comparison of therapeutic effectiveness in a one year double-blind study. *Urologe—Ausgabe A* 1997;36:327–33.

18. Van der Weijden GA, Timmer CJ, Timmerman MF et al. The effect of herbal extracts in an experimental mouthrinse on

References

established plaque and gingivitis. *J Clin Periodontol* 1998; 25:399–403.

19. Lichius JJ, Renneberg H, Blaschek W et al. The inhibiting effects of components of stinging nettle roots on experimentally induced prostatic hyperplasia in mice. *Planta Med* 1999;65:666–668.

20. Hirano T, Homma M, Oka K. Effects of stinging nettle root extracts and their steroidal components on the Na+, K+-ATPase of the benign prostatic hyperplasia. *Planta Med* 1994;60:30–33.

21. Klingelhoefer S, Obertreis B, Quast S et al. Antirheumatic effect of IDS 23, a stinging nettle leaf extract, on in vitro expression of T helper cytokines. *J Rheumatol* 1999;26: 2517–2522.

22. Riehemann K, Behnke B, Schulze-Osthoff K. Plant extracts from stinging nettle (*Urtica dioica*), an antirheumatic remedy, inhibit the proinflammatory transcription factor NF-kappaB. *FEBS Lett* 1999;442:89–94.

23. Tita B, Faccendini P, Bello U et al. *Urtica dioica L.*: pharmacological effect of ethanol extract. *Pharm Res* 1993;27 (Suppl 1):21–22.

24. Konrad L, Muller HH, Lenz C et al. Antiproliferative effect on human prostate cancer cells by a stinging nettle root (*Urtica dioica*) extract. *Planta Med* 2000;66:44–47.

25. Lichius JJ, Lenz C, Lindemann P et al. Antiproliferative effect of a polysaccharide fraction of a 20% methanolic extract of stinging nettle roots upon epithelial cells of the human prostate (LNCaP). *Pharmazie* 1999;54:768–771.

26. Balzarini J, Neyts J, Schols D et al. The mannose-specific plant lectins from *Cymbidium* hybrid and *Epipactis helleborine* and the (N-acetylglucosamine)$_n$-specific plant lectin from *Urtica dioica* are potent and selective inhibitors of human immunodeficiency virus and cytomegalovirus replication in vitro. *Antiviral Res* 1992;18:191–207.

27. Bohm E, Maier RD. Weal-formation by *Urtica dioica*. An intravital reaction? *Zeitschrift fur Rechtsmedizin—J Legal Med* 1975;76:1–9.

NIACIN

1. Cervantes-Laurean D, McElvaney G, Moss J. Niacin. In Shils ME, Olson JA, Shike M et al, eds. *Modern nutrition in health and disease*, 9th ed. Baltimore: Williams and Wilkins, 1999: 401–412.

2. Heimburger DC, Weinsier RL. *Handbook of clinical nutrition.* St. Louis: Mosby, 1997.

3. Elam MB, Hunninghake DB, Davis KB et al. Effect of niacin on lipid and lipoprotein levels and glycemic control in patients with diabetes and peripheral arterial disease: the ADMIT study: a randomized trial. *JAMA* 2000;284:1263–1270.

4. Kelly JJ, Lawson JA, Campbell LV et al. Effects of nicotinic acid on insulin sensitivity and blood pressure in healthy subjects. *J Hum Hypertens* 2000;14:567–572.

5. Chesney CM, Elam MB, Herd JA et al. Effect of niacin, warfarin, and antioxidant therapy on coagulation parameters in patients with peripheral arterial disease in the Arterial Disease Multiple Intervention Trial (ADMIT). *Am Heart J* 2000; 140:631–636.

6. Garg R, Malinow M, Pettinger M et al. Niacin treatment increases plasma homocyst(e)ine levels. *Am Heart J* 1999; 138:1082–1087.

7. Mandrup-Poulsen T, Reimers JI, Andersen HU et al. Nicotinamide treatment in the prevention of insulin-dependent diabetes mellitus. *Diabetes Metab Rev* 1993;9:295–309.

8. Vidal J, Fernandez-Balsells M, Sesmilo G et al. Effects of nicotinamide and intravenous insulin therapy in newly diagnosed type 1 diabetes. *Diabetes Care* 2000;23:360–364.

9. Pozzili P, Visalli N, Cavallo MG et al. Vitamin E and nicotinamide have similar effects in maintaining residual beta cell function in recent onset insulin-dependent diabetes (the IMDIAB IV study). *Eur J Endocrinol* 1997;137:234–239.

10. Visalli N, Cavallo MG, Signore A et al. A multi-centre randomized trial of two different doses of nicotinamide in patients with recent-onset type 1 diabetes (the IMDIAB VI). *Diabetes Metab Res Rev* 1999;15:181–185.

11. Kleijnen J, Knipschild P. Niacin and vitamin B6 in mental functioning: a review of controlled trials in humans. *Biol Psychiatry* 1991;29:931–941.

12. Jacob RA, Swendseid ME. Niacin. In: Ziegler EE, Filer LJ, eds. *Present knowledge in nutrition*, 7th ed. Washington DC: International Life Sciences Institute Press, 1996:184–190.

13. Linder MC. *Nutritional biochemistry and metabolism, with clinical applications.* East Norwalk, CT: Appleton & Lange, 1991.

14. Rader JI, Calvert RJ, Hathcock JN. Hepatic toxicity of unmodified and time-release preparations of niacin. *Am J Med* 1992;92:77–81.

15. McKenney JM, Proctor JD, Harris S et al. A comparison of the efficacy and toxic effects of sustained-release vs. immediate-release niacin in hypercholesterolemic patients. *JAMA* 1994;271:672–677.

16. Henkin Y, Johnson KC, Segrest JP. Rechallenge with crystalline niacin after drug-induced hepatitis from sustained-release niacin. *JAMA* 1990;294:241–243.

17. Garg A, Grundy SM. Nicotinic acid as therapy for dyslipidemia in non-insulin-dependent diabetes mellitus. *JAMA* 1990;264:723–726.

18. Earthman TP, Odom L, Mullins CA. Lactic acidosis associated with high-dose niacin therapy. *South Med J* 1991;84: 496–497.

19. Schwab RA, Bachhuber BH. Delirium and lactic acidosis caused by ethanol and niacin coingestion. *Am J Emerg Med* 1991;9:363.

20. Reaven P, Witztum JL. Lovastatin, nicotinic acid, and rhabdomyolysis. *Ann Int Med* 1988;109:597.

21. Fraunfelder FW, Fraunfelder FT, Illingworth DR. Adverse ocular events associated with niacin therapy. *Br J Ophthalmol* 1995;79:54–56.

22. Bender DA, Earl CJ, Lees AJ. Niacin depletion in Parkinsonian patients treated with L-dopa, benserazide and carbidopa. *Clin Sci* 1979;56(1): 89–93.

23. Black MJ, Brandt RB. Nicotinic acid or N-Methyl nicotinamide prolongs elevated brain dopa and dopamine in L-dopa treatment. Biochemical medicine and metabolic biology. *Biochem Med Metab Biol* 36:244–251.

24. Bourgeois BFD, Dodson WE, Ferrendelli JA. Interactions between primidone, carbamazepine, and nicotinamide. *Neurology* 1982;32:1122–1126.

25. Adrian J, Frangne R. Synthesis and availability of niacin in roasted coffee. *Adv Exp Med Biol* 1991;289:49–50.

26. Urberg M, Benyi J, John R. Hypocholesterolemic effects of nicotinic acid and chromium supplementation. *J Fam Prac* 1988;27:603–606.

27. Kime CE. Bell's palsy: a new syndrome associated with treatment by nicotinic acid. *Arch Otolaryngol* 1958;68:28–32.

NONI

1. Morton JF. The ocean-going noni, or Indian mulberry

(*Morinda citrifolia,* Rubiaceae) and some of its more "color-ful" relatives. *Econ Botany* 1992;46:241–256.

2. Farine JP. Volatile components of ripe fruits of *Morinda citrifolia* and their effects on Drosophila. *Phytochemistry* 1996; 41:433–438.

3. Levand O, Larson HO. Some chemical constituents of *Morinda citrifolia. Planta Med* 1979;36:186–187.

4. Mueller BA, Scott MK, Sowinski KM et al. Noni juice (*Morinda citrifolia*): hidden potential for hyperkalemia? *Am J Kidney Dis* 2000;35:310–312.

5. Hirazumi A, Furusawa E, Chou SC et al. Anticancer activity of *Morinda citrifolia* (noni) on intraperitoneally implanted Lewis lung carcinoma in syngeneic mice. *Proc West Pharmacol Soc* 1994;37:145–146.

6. Hirazumi A, Furusawa E. An immunomodulatory polysaccharide-rich substance from the fruit juice of *Morinda citrifolia* (noni) with antitumour activity. *Phytother Res* 1999;13: 380–387.

7. Hiramatsu T, Imoto M, Koyano T et al. Induction of normal phenotypes in ras-transformed cells by damnacanthal from *Morinda citrifolia. Cancer Lett* 1993;73:161–166.

8. Hiwasa T, Arase Y, Chen Z et al. Stimulation of ultraviolet-induced apoptosis of human fibroblast UVr-1 cells by tyrosine kinase inhibitors. *FEBS Lett* 1999;444:173–176.

9. Younos C, Rolland A, Fleurentin J et al. Analgesic and behavioural effects of *Morinda citrifolia. Planta Med* 1990; 56:430–434.

10. Elkins R. *Hawaiian noni: Morinda citrifolia.* Pleasant Grove, UT: Woodland Publishing, 1998.

11. Heinicke RM. *The pharmacologically active ingredient of noni.* Available at http://www.hmt.com/noni/active.html

12. Anonymous. *Noni: Polynesia's natural pharmacy.* Vineyard, UT: Pride Publishing, 1997.

13. Dixon AR, McMillen H, Etkin NL. Ferment this: the transformation of noni, a traditional Polynesian medicine (*Morinda citrifolia,* Rubiaceae). *Econ Botany* 1999;53:51–68.

OSHA

1. Huang KC. *The pharmacology of Chinese herbs,* 2nd ed. Boca Raton, FL: CRC Press, 1999:94–97.

2. Chang FC, Huang YT, Hong CY et al. Haemodynamic effects of chronic tetramethylpyrazine administration on portal hypertensive rats. *Eur J Gastroenterol Hepatol* 1999;11: 1027–1031.

3. Huang YT, Chang FC, Chen KJ et al. Acute hemodynamic effects of tetramethylpyrazine and tetrandrine on cirrhotic rats. *Planta Med* 1999;65:130–134.

4. Feng J, Wu G, Tan S. The effects of tetramethylpyrazine on the incidence of arrhythmias and the release of PGI2 and TXA2 in the ischemic rat heart. *Planta Med* 1999;65:268–270.

5. Wu BN, Huang YC, Wu HM et al. A highly selective beta-1 adrenergic blocker with partial beta-2 agonist activity derived from ferulic acid, an active component of *Ligusticum wallichii* Franch. *J Cardiovasc Pharm* 1998;31:750–757.

6. Pang PK, Shan JJ, Chiu KW. Tetramethylpyrazine, a calcium antagonist. *Planta Med* 1996;62:431–435.

7. Moore M. *Los remedios: traditional herbal remedies of the Southwest.* Santa Fe, NM: Red Crane Books, 1990.

PANTOTHENIC ACID

1. Plesovsky-Vig N. Pantothenic acid. In: Ziegler EE, Filer LJ, eds. *Present knowledge in nutrition,* 7th ed. Washington DC: ILSI Press, 1997.

2. Loftus EV, Tremaine WJ, Welson RA et al. Dexpanthenol enemas in ulcerative colitis: a pilot study. *Mayo Clin Proc* 1997; 72:616–620.

3. Lokkevik E, Skovlund E, Retan JB et al. Skin treatment with bepanthen cream versus no cream during radiotherapy—a randomized controlled trial. *Acta Oncol* 1997;35:1021–1026.

4. Gaddi A, Descovitch GC, Noseda G et al. Controlled evaluation of pantethine, a natural hypolipidemic compound, in patients with different forms of hyperlipoproteinemia. *Atherosclerosis* 1984;50:73–83.

5. Prisco D, Rogasi PG, Matucci M et al. Effect of oral treatment with pantethine on platelet and plasma phospholipids in IIa hyperlipoproteinemia. *Angiology* 1987:241–247.

6. Coronel F, Tornero F, Torrente J et al. Treatment of hyperlipemia in diabetic patients on dialysis with a physiological substance. *Am J Nephrol* 1991;11:32–36.

7. Donati C, Barbi G, Cairo G et al. Pantethine improves the lipid abnormalities of chronic hemodialysis patients: results of a multicenter clinical trial. *Clin Nephrol* 1986;25:70–74.

8. Arsenio L, Bodria P. Effectiveness of long-term treatment with pantethine in patients with dyslipidemia. *Clin Ther* 1986;8:537–545.

9. Vaxman F, Olender S, Lambert A et al. Effect of pantothenic acid and ascorbic acid supplementation on human skin wound healing process. *Eur Surg Res* 1993;27:158–166.

10. Aprahamian M, Dentinger A, Stock-Damge C et al. Effects of supplemental pantothenic acid on wound healing: experimental study in rabbits. *Am J Clin Nutr* 1985;41:578–589.

11. Jeitner TM, Oliver JR. The depletion of plasma prolactin by pantethine in oestrogen-primed hyperprolactinaemic rats. *J Endocrinol* 1990;124: 397–402.

12. Linder MC. *Nutritional biochemistry and metabolism with clinical applications,* 2nd ed. East Norwalk, CT: Appleton & Lange, 1991.

PASSIONFLOWER

1. Tyler VE. *The honest herbal,* 3rd ed. Binghamton NY: Pharmaceutical Products Press, Haworth Press, 1993.

2. European Scientific Cooperative on Phytotherapy (ESCOP). *Monographs on the medicinal uses of plant drugs. Passiflorae herba (Passiflora). Fascicule 4.* Exeter, UK, 1997.

3. Meier B. *Passiflora incarnata* L.–Passion flower. Portrait of a medicinal plant. *Q Rev Nat Med* 1995;3:191–202.

4. Medina JH, Paladini AC, Wolfman C et al. Chrysin (5,7-di-OH-flavone), a naturally-occurring ligand for benzodiazepine receptors, with anticonvulsant properties. *Biochem Pharmacol* 1990;40:2227–2231.

5. Paladini ACX, Marder M, Viola H et al. Flavonoids and the central nervous system: from forgotten factors to potent anxiolytic compounds. *J Pharm Pharmacol* 1999;51:519–526.

6. Akhondzadeh S, Naghavi HR, Vazirian M et al. Passionflower in the treatment of generalized anxiety: a pilot double-blind randomized controlled trial with oxazepam. *J Clin Pharm Ther* 2001;26:363–367.

7. Maluf E, Barros HMT, Frochtengarten ML et al. Assessment of the hypnotic/sedative effects and toxicity of *Passiflora edulis* aqueous extract in rodents and humans. *Phytother Res* 1991;5:262–266.

8. Bourin M, Bougerol T, Guitton B et al. A combination of plant extracts in the treatment of outpatients with adjustment disorder with anxious mood: controlled study versus placebo. *Fundam Clin Pharmacol* 1997;11:127–132.

9. Akhondzadeh S, Kashani L, Mobaseri M et al. Passionflower in

References

the treatment of opiates withdrawal: a double-blind randomized controlled trial. *J Clin Pharm Ther* 2001;26:369–373.

10. Speroni E, Minghetti A. Neuropharmacological activity of extracts from *Passiflora incarnata*. *Planta Med* 1988;54:488–491.

11. Capasso A, Pinto A. Experimental investigations of the synergistic-sedative effect of Passiflora and Kava. *Acta Ther* 1995:21:127–140.

12. Soulimani R, Younos C, Jamouni S et al. Behavioral effects of *Passiflora incarnata* L and its indole alkaloid and flavonoid derivatives and maltol in the mouse. *J Ethnopharm* 1997;57:11–20.

13. Wolfman C, Viola H, Paladini A et al. Possible anxiolytic effects of chrysin, a central benzodiazepine receptor ligand isolated from *Passiflora coerulea*. *Pharmacol Biochem Behav* 1994;47:1–4.

14. Fisher AA, Purcelli P, Le Couteur DG. Toxicity of *Passiflora incarnata* L. *Clin Tox* 2000;38:63–66.

15. Solbakken AM, Rorbakken G, Gundersen T. [Nature medicine as intoxicant]. *Tidsskrift for Den Norske Nor Laegeforening* 1997;117:1140–1141.

16. Giavina-Bianchi PF Jr, Castro FF, Machado ML et al. Occupational respiratory allergic disease induced by *Passiflora alata* and *Rhamnus purshiana*. *Ann Allergy Asthma Immun* 1997;79:449–454.

17. Smith GW, Chalmers TM, Nuki G. Vasculitis associated with herbal preparation containing passiflora extract. *Br J Rheum* 1993;32:87–88.

P'AU D'ARCO

1. Awang DVC, Dawson BA, Ethier J-C et al. Naphthoquinone constituents of commercial lapacho/pau d'arco/taheebo products. *J Herbs Spices Med Plants* 1994;2(4):27–43.

2. Koyama J, Morita I, Tagahara K et al. Cyclopentene dialdehydes from *Tabebuia impetiginosa*. *Phytochemistry* 2000;53:869–872.

3. Dinnen RD, Ebisuzaki K. The search for novel anticancer agents: a differentiation-based assay and analysis of a folklore product. *Anticancer Res* 1997;17:1027–1033.

4. Boothman DA, Trask DK, Pardee AB. Inhibition of potentially lethal DNA damage repair in human tumor cells by beta-lapachone, an activator of topoisomerase I. *Cancer Res* 1989;49:605–612.

5. U.S. Congress Office of Technology Assessment. Unconventional cancer treatments. OTA-H-405 Washington, D.C.: U.S. Government Printing Office, September 1990:86–87.

6. Houghton PJ, Photiou A, Uddin S et al. Activity of extracts of *Kegelia pinnata* against melanoma and renal carcinoma cell lines. *Planta Med* 1994;60:430–433.

7. Otero R, Nunez V, Jimenez SL et al. Snakebites and ethnobotany in the northwest region of Colombia. Part II: neutralization of lethal and enzymatic effects of Bothrops atrox venom. *J Ethnopharmacol* 2000;71:505–511.

8. Carvalho LH, Rocha EM, Raslan DS et al. In vitro activity of natural and synthetic naphthoquinones against erythrocytic stages of *Plasmodium falciparum*. *Braz J Med Biol Res* 1988;21:485–487.

9. Pinto AV, Pinto MD, Gilbert B et al. *Schistosomiasis mansoni*: blockage of cercarial skin penetration by chemical agents: i. naphthoquinones and derivatives. *Trans R Soc Trop Med Hyg* 1977;71:133–135.

10. Goel RK, Pathak NK, Biswas M et al. Effect of lapachol, a naphthaquinone isolated from *Tectona grandis*, on experimental peptic ulcer and gastric secretion. *J Pharm Pharmacol* 1987;39:138–140.

11. Grazziotin JD, Schapoval EES, Chaves CG et al. Phytochemical and analgesic investigation of *Tabebuia chrysotricha*. *J Ethnopharmacol* 1992;36:249–251.

12. Ferreira de Santana C, Goncalves de Lima O, Leoncio d'Albuquerque I et al. Antitumor and toxicological properties of an extract of wood from the trumpet bush, *Tabebuia avellanedae*. *Rev Inst Antibiot Univ Recife* 1968;8(1–2):89–94.

13. Guerra MO, Mazoni AS, Brandao MA et al. Interceptive effect of lapachol in rats. *Contraception* 1999;60:305–307.

14. Foster S, Tyler VE. *Tyler's Honest Herbal*, 4th ed. Binghamton, NY: Haworth Press, 1999:287–292.

PENNYROYAL

1. Boyd EL. *Hedeoma pulegioides* and *Mentha pulegium*. In: De Smet PAGM, Keller K, Hänsel R, Chandler RF (eds.) *Adverse effects of herbal drugs*. Berlin: Springer-Verlag, 1992;1:151–155.

2. Bakerink JA, Gospe SM, Dimand RJ, Eldridge MW. Multiple organ failure after ingestion of pennyroyal oil from herbal tea in two infants. *Pediatrics* 1996;98:944–947.

3. Anderson IB, Mullen WH, Meeker JE et al. Pennyroyal toxicity: measurement of toxic metabolite levels in two cases and review of the literature. *Ann Int Med* 1996;124:726–734.

4. Khojasteh-Bakht SC, Nelson SD, Atkins WM. Glutathione S-transferase catalyzes the isomerization of (R)-2-hydroxymenthofuran to mintlactones. *Arch Biochem Biophysics* 1999;370:59–65.

5. Carmichael PG. Pennyroyal metabolites in human poisoning [Letter]. *Ann Int Med* 1997;126:250.

6. Sudekum M, Poppenga RH, Raju N et al. Pennyroyal oil toxicosis in a dog. *J Am Vet Med Assoc* 1992;200:817–818.

7. Khojasteh-Bakht SC, Chen W, Koenigs LL et al. Metabolism of (R)-(+) by human liver cytochrome P-450s: evidence for formation of a furan epoxide. *Drug Metab Dispos* 1999;27:574–580.

PEPPERMINT

1. European Scientific Cooperative on Phytotherapy (ESCOP). *Monographs on the medicinal uses of plant drugs. Menthae piperitae folium (peppermint leaf) and Menthae piperitae aetheroliun (peppermint oil). Fascicule 3*. Exeter, UK, 1997.

2. Bowen IH, Cubbin IJ. *Mentha piperita* and *Mentha spicata*. In: De Smet PAGM, Keller K, Hänsel R, Chandler RF (eds.) *Adverse effects of herbal drugs*, vol 1. Berlin: Springer-Verlag, 1992:170–178.

3. De Almeida-Muradian LB, Rios MD, Sasaki R. Determination of provitamin A of green leafy vegetables by high performance liquid chromatography and open column chromatography. *Bollettino Chimico Farmaceutico* 1998;137:290–294.

4. Göbel H, Schmidt G, Dworschak M, et al. Essential plant oils and headache mechanisms. *Phytomedicine* 1995;2:93–102.

5. Pittler MH, Ernst E. Peppermint oil for irritable bowel syndrome: a critical review and metaanalysis. *Am J Gastroenterol* 1998;93:1131–1135.

6. Liu JH, Chen GH, Yeh HZ et al. Enteric-coated peppermint-oil capsules in the treatment of irritable bowel syndrome: a prospective, randomized trial. *J Gastroenterol* 1997;32:765–768.

7. Kline RM, Kline JJ, Di Palma J et al. Enteric-coated, pH-

dependent peppermint oil capsules for the treatment of irritable bowel syndrome in children. *J Pediatr* 2001;138:125–128.

8. Sparks MJ, O'Sullivan P, Herrington AA et al. Does peppermint oil relieve spasm during barium enema? *Br J Radiol* 1995;68:841–843.

9. Göbel H, Fresenius J, Heinze A et al. [Effectiveness of Oleum menthae piperitae and paracetamol in therapy of headache of the tension type]. *Nervenarzt* 1996;67:672–681.

10. Göbel H, Schmidt G, Soyka D. Effect of peppermint and eucalyptus oil preparations on neurophysiological and experimental algesimetric headache parameters. *Cephalalgia* 1994;14:228–234.

11. Tate S. Peppermint oil: a treatment for postoperative nausea. *J Adv Nursing* 1997;26:543–549.

12. Madisch A, Heydenreich C-J, Wieland V et al. Treatment of functional dyspepsia with a fixed peppermint oil and caraway oil combination preparation as compared to cisapride: a multicenter, reference-controlled, double-blind equivalence study. *Arzneim-Forsch/Drug Res* 1999;49:925–932.

13. May B, Kuntz HD, Kieser M et al. Efficacy of a fixed peppermint oil/caraway oil combination in non-ulcer dyspepsia. *Arzneim-Forsch/Drug Res* 1996;46:1149–1153.

14. Westphal J, Horning M, Leonhardt K. Phytotherapy in functional upper abdominal complaints. *Phytomedicine* 1996;2:285–291.

15. Morice AH, Marshall AE, Higgins KS et al. Effect of inhaled menthol on citric acid induced cough in normal subjects. *Thorax* 1994;49:1024–1026.

16. Thomas JG. Peppermint fibrillation [Letter]. *Lancet* 1962;1:222.

17. Luke E. Addiction to mentholated cigarettes [Letter]. *Lancet* 1962;1:110–111.

18. Heng MCY. Local necrosis and interstitial nephritis due to topical methyl salicylate and menthol. *Cutis* 1987;39:442–444.

19. Wacher VJ, Wong S, Wong HT. Peppermint oil enhances cyclosporine oral bioavailability in rats: comparison with D-alpha-tocopheryl poly(ethylene glycol) 1000) succinate (TPGS) and ketoconazole. *J Pharm Sci* 2002;91:77–90.

20. Nair B. Final report on the safety assessment of *Mentha Piperita* (peppermint) oil, *Mentha Piperita* (peppermint) leaf extract, *Mentha Piperita* (peppermint) leaf, and *Mentha Piperita* (peppermint) leaf water. *Int J Toxicol* 2001;20 (Suppl 3):61–73.

PHENYLALANINE

1. Linder MC. *Nutritional biochemistry and metabolism, with clinical applications*, 2nd ed. East Norwalk, CT: Appleton & Lange, 1991.

2. Siddiqui AH, Stolk LML, Bhaggoe R et al. L-Phenylalanine and UVA irradiation in the treatment of vitiligo. *Dermatology* 1994;188:215–218.

3. Camacho F, Mazeucos J. Treatment of vitiligo with oral and topical phenylalanine: 6 years of experience. *Arch Derm* 1999;135:216–217.

4. Elsas and Acosta. Nutritional support of inherited metabolic disease. In: Shils ME, Olson JA, Shike M et al, eds. *Modern nutrition in health and disease*, 9th ed. Baltimore: Williams & Wilkins, 1999:1003–1057.

5. Ravel R. *Clinical laboratory medicine,* 6th ed. New York: Mosby, 1995:597–598.

6. Food and Nutrition Board, National Research Council. *Recommended dietary allowances,* 10th ed. Washington, DC: National Academy Press, 1989.

PHOSPHATIDYLSERINE

1. Pepeu G, Pepeu IM, Amaducci L. A review of phosphatidylserine pharmacological and clinical effects. Is phosphatidylserine a drug for the ageing brain? *Pharmacol Res* 1996;33:73–80.

2. Pepping J. Alternative therapies: phosphatidylserine. *Am J Health Syst Pharm* 1999;56:2038–2044.

3. Heiss W-D, Kessler J, Mielke R et al. Long-term effects of phosphatidylserine, pyritinol, and cognitive training in Alzheimer's disease. *Dementia* 1994;5:88–98.

4. Delwaide PJ, Gyselynck-Mambourg AM, Hurlet A et al. Double-blind randomized controlled study of phosphatidylserine in senile demented patients. *Acta Neurol Scand* 1986;73:136–140.

5. Engel RR, Satzger W, Günther W et al. Double-blind crossover study of phosphatidylserine vs. placebo in patients with early dementia of the Alzheimer type. *Eur Neuropsychopharm* 1992;2:149–155.

6. Crook T, Petrie W, Wells C et al. Effects of phosphatidylserine in Alzheimer's disease. *Psychopharmacol Bull* 1992;28:61–66.

7. Crook TH, Tinklenberg J, Yesavage J et al. Effects of phosphatidylserine in age-associated memory impairment. *Neurology* 1991;41:644–649.

8. Cenacchi T, Bertoldin T, Farina C et al. Cognitive decline in the elderly: a double-blind, placebo-controlled multicenter study on efficacy of phosphatidylserine administration. *Aging Clin Exp Res* 1993;5:123–133.

9. Amaducci L, SMID Group. Phosphatidylserine in the treatment of Alzheimer's disease: results of a multicenter study. *Psychopharmacol Bull* 1988;24:130–134.

PHOSPHORUS

1. Linder MC. *Nutritional biochemistry and metabolism, with clinical applications*, 2nd ed. East Norwalk, CT: Appleton & Lange, 1991.

1a. Kim SH, Morton DJ, Barrett-Connor EL. Carbonated beverage consumption and bone mineral density among older women: the Rancho Bernardo study. *Am J Public Health* 1997;87:276–279.

2. Wyshak G, Frisch RE. Carbonated beverages, dietary calcium, the dietary calcium/phosphorus ratio and bone fractures in girls and boys. *J Adol Health* 1994;15:210–215.

3. Mazariegos-Ramos E, Guerrero-Romero F, Rodriquez-Moran M et al. Consumption of soft drinks with phosphoric acid as a risk factor for the development of hypocalcemia in children: a case-control study. *J Pediatr* 1995;126:940–942.

4. Holland PC, Wilkinson AR, Diez J et al. Prenatal deficiency of phosphate, phosphate supplementation, and rickets in very-low-birthweight infants. *Lancet* 1990;335:697–701.

5. Arnaud CD, Sanchez SD. Calcium and phosphorus. In Ziegler EE, Filer LJ. *Present Knowledge in Nutrition*, 7th ed. ILSI, Washington DC, 1996:245–255.

PSYLLIUM (PLANTAIN)

1. WHO *monographs on selected medicinal plants*, vol. 1., World Health Organization, Geneva, 1999.

2. European Scientific Cooperative on Phytotherapy (ESCOP) *Monographs on the medicinal uses of plant drugs. Psyllii semen (psyllium seed). Fascicule 5.* Exeter, UK, 1997.

3. Schulz V, Hänsel R, Tyler VE. *Rational Phytotherapy*, 3rd ed. Berlin: Springer-Verlag, 1998.

References

4. Marteau P, Flourie B, Cherbut C et al. Digestibility and bulking effect of ispaghula husks in healthy humans. *Gut* 1994; 35:1747–1752.

5. Leng-Peschlow E. Interference of dietary fibres with gastrointestinal enzymes in vitro. *Digestion* 1989;44:200–210.

6. Bisset NG, Wichtl M. *Herbal drugs and phytopharmaceuticals: a handbook for practice on a scientific basis with reference to Commission E monographs.* Boca Raton, FL: CRC Press, 1994:379.

7. Brown L, Rosner B, Willett WW et al. Cholesterol-lowering effects of dietary fiber: a meta-analysis. *Am J Clin Nutr* 1999;69:30–42.

8. Gelissen IC, Brodie B, Eastwoods MA. Effect of *Plantago ovata* (psyllium) husk and seeds on sterol metabolism: studies in normal and ileostomy subjects. *Am J Clin Nutr* 1994; 59:395–400.

9. Turnbull WH, Thomas HG. The effect of a *Plantago ovata* seed containing preparation on appetite variable, nutrient and energy intake. *Int J Obesity* 1995;19:338–342.

10. Uribe M, Dibildox M, Malpica S et al. Beneficial effect of vegetable protein diet supplemented with *psyllium plantago* in patients with hepatic encephalopathy and diabetes mellitus. *Gastroenterology* 1985;88:901–907.

11. Rodriguez-Moran M, Guerrero-Romero F, Lazcano-Burciaga G. Lipid-and glucose-lowering efficacy of *Plantago psyllium* in type II diabetes. *J Diab Complications* 1998;12:273–278.

12. Tomas-Ridocci M, Anon R, Minguez M et al. The efficacy of *Plantago ovata* as a regulator of intestinal transit: a double-blind study compared to placebo (Spanish). *Revista Espanola de Enfermedades Digestivas* 1992;82:17–22.

13. Ewe K, Ueberschaer B, Press AG. Influence of senna, fibre, and fibre + senna on colonic transit in loperamide-induced constipation. *Pharmacology* 1993;47(Suppl 1):242–248.

14. Voderholzer WA, Schatke W, Muhldorfer BE et al. Clinical response to dietary fiber treatment of chronic constipation. *Am J Gastroent* 1997;92:95–98.

15. Perez-Miranda M, Gomez-Cedenilla A, Leon-Colombo T et al. Effect of fiber supplements on internal bleeding hemorrhoids. *Hepato-Gastroenterology* 1996;43:1504–1507.

16. Moesgaard F, Nielsen ML, Hansen JB et al. High-fiber diet reduces bleeding and pain in patients with hemorrhoids: a double-blind trial of Vi-Siblin. *Am Soc Colon Rectal Surg* 1981;454–456.

17. Fernandez-Banares F, Hinojosa J, Sanchez-Lombrana JL et al. Randomized clinical trial of *Plantago ovata* seeds (dietary fiber) as compared with mesalamine in maintaining remission in ulcerative colitis. Spanish Group for the Study of Crohn's Disease and Ulcerative Colitis GETECCU). *Am J Gastroenterol* 1999;94:427–433.

18. Gallagher R. Use of herbal preparations for intractable cough. *J Pain Symptom Manage* [Letter] 1997;14:1–2.

19. Suhonen R, Kantola I, Bjorksten F. Anaphylactic shock due to ingestion of psyllium laxative. *Allergy* 1983;38:363–365.

20. Freeman GL. *Psyllium* hypersensitivity. *Ann Allergy* 1994;73: 490–492.

21. Perlman BB. Interaction between lithium salt and isphagula husk. *Lancet* 1990;335:416.

22. Fernandez N, Diez MF, Teran MT et al. Influence of two commercial fibers in the pharmacokinetics of ethinylestradiol in rabbits. *J Pharmacol Exp Ther* 1998;286:870–874.

23. Slifman NR, Obermeyer WR, Musser SM et al. Contamination of botanical dietary supplements by *Digitalis lanata*. *N Engl J Med* 1998;339:806–811.

POLLEN

1. Leung AY, Foster S. *Encyclopedia of common natural products used in food, drugs, and cosmetics.* New York: John Wiley, 1996:73–75.

2. Habib FK, Ross M, Lewenstein A et al. Identification of a prostate inhibitory substance in a pollen extract. *Prostate* 1995;26:133–139.

3. Iversen T, Kiirgaard KM, Schriver P et al. The effect of NaO Li Su on memory functions and blood chemistry in elderly people. *J Ethnopharmacology* 1997;56:109–116.

4. Szanto E, Gruber D, Sator M et al. Placebo-controlled study of Melbrosia in treatment of climacteric symptoms. *Wein Med Wochenschr* 1994;144:130–133.

5. Wilt T, Mac Donald R, Ishani A et al. Cernilton for benign prostatic hyperplasia. *Cochrane Database Syst Rev* 2000;2: CD001042.

6. MacDonald R, Ishani A, Rutks I et al. A systematic review of Cernilton for the treatment of benign prostatic hyperplasia. *BJU Int* 2000;85:836–841.

7. Buck AC, Rees RW, Ebeling L. Treatment of chronic prostatitis and prostatodynia with pollen extract. *Br J Urol* 1989;64: 496–499.

8. Rugendorff EW, Weidner W, Ebeling L et al. Results of treatment with pollen extract (Cernilton N) in chronic prostatitis and prostatodynia. *Br J Urol* 1993;71:433–438.

9. Buck AC, Cox R, Rees RWM et al. Treatment of outflow tract obstruction due to benign prostatic hyperplasia with the pollen extract, Cernilton: a double-blind, placebo-controlled study. *Br J Urol* 1990;66:398–404.

10. Lowe FC, Ku JC. Phytotherapy in treatment of benign prostatic hyperplasia: a critical review. *Urology* 1996;48:12–20.

11. Habib FK, Ross M, Buck AC et al. In vitro evaluation of the pollen extract, Cernitin T-60, in the regulation of prostate cell growth. *Br J Urol* 1990;66:393–397.

12. Einer-Jensen N, Zhao J, Andersen KP et al. Cimicifuga and Melbrosia lack oestrogenic effects in mice and rats. *Maturitas* 1996;25:149–153.

13. Wojcicki J, Samochowiec L, Bartlomowicz B et al. Effect of pollen extract on the development of experimental atherosclerosis in rabbits. *Atherosclerosis* 1986;62:39–45.

14. Lin FL, Vaughan TR, Vandewalker ML et al. Hypereosinophilia, neurologic, and gastrointestinal symptoms after bee-pollen ingestion. *J Allergy Clin Immunol* 1989;83:793–796.

15. Puente S, Iniguez A, Subirats M et al. Eosinophilic gastroenteritis caused by bee pollen sensitization. *Med Clin (Barc)* 1997;108:698–700.

16. Shad JA, Chinn CG, Brann OS. Acute hepatitis after ingestion of herbs. *South Med J* 1999;92:1095–1097.

PROPOLIS

1. Burdock GA. Review of the biological properties and toxicity of bee propolis (propolis). *Food Chem Toxicol* 1998;36: 347–363.

2. Maichuk IUF, Orlovskaia LE, Andreev VP. The use of ocular drug films of propolis in the sequelae of ophthalmic herpes. *Voen Med Zh* 1995;12:36–39, 80.

3. Murray MC, Worthington HV, Blinkhorn AS. A study to investigate the effect of a propolis-containing mouthrinse on the inhibition of de novo plaque formation. *J Clin Periodontol* 1997;24:796–798.

4. Steinberg D, Kaine G, Gedalia I. Antibacterial effect of propolis and honey on oral bacteria. *Am J Dent* 1996;9:236–239.

5. Huang MT, Ma W, Yen P. Inhibitory effects of caffeic acid phenethyl ester (CAPE) on 12-0-tetradecanoylphorbol-13-acetate-induced tumor promotion in mouse skin and the synthesis of DNA, RNA and protein in HeLa cells. *Carcinogenesis* 1996;17:761–765.

6. Frenkel K, Wei H, Bhimani R et al. Inhibition of tumor-promoter-mediated processes in mouse skin and bovine lens by caffeic acid phenethyl ester. *Cancer Res* 1993;53:1255–1261.

7. Rao CV, Desai D, Kaul B et al. Effect of caffeic acid esters on carcinogen-induced mutagenicity and human colon adenocarcinoma cell growth. *Chem Biol Interact* 1992;84:277–290.

8. Rao CV, Desai D, Simi B et al. Inhibitory effect of caffeic acid esters on azoxymethane-induced biochemical changes and aberrant crypt foci formation in rat colon. *Cancer Res* 1993;53:4182–4188.

9. Rao CV, Desai D, Rivenson A et al. Chemoprevention of colon carcinogenesis by phenylether-3-methyl caffeate. *Cancer Res* 1995;55:2310–2315.

10. Claus R, Kinscherf R, Gehrke C et al. Antiapoptotic effects of propolis extract and propolis on human macrophages exposed to minimally modified low density lipoprotein. *Arzneim-Forsch/Drug Res* 2000;50:373–379.

11. Krol W, Scheller S, Shani J et al. Synergistic effect of ethanolic extract of propolis and antibiotics on the growth of *Staphylococcus aureus. Arzneim-Forsch/Drug Res* 1993;43:607–609.

12. De Castro SL, Higashi KO. Effect of different formulations of propolis on mice infected with *Trypanosoma cruzi. J Ethnopharmacol* 1995;46:55–58.

13. Tosi B, Donini A, Ramagnoli C et al. Antimicrobial activity of some commercial extracts of propolis prepared with different solvents. *Phytotherapy Res* 1996;10:335–336.

14. Harish Z, Rubinstein A, Golodner M et al. Suppression of HIV-1 replication by propolis and its immunoregulatory effect. *Drugs Exp Clin Res* 1997;23:89–96.

15. Dimov V, Ivanovska N, Bankova V et al. Immunomodulatory action of propolis IV. Prophylactic activity against gram-negative infections and adjuvant effect of the water-soluble derivative. *Vaccine* 1992;10:817–823.

16. Rodriguez S, Ancheta O, Ramos ME et al. Effects of Cuban red propolis on galactosamine-induced hepatitis in rats. *Pharmacol Res* 1997;35:1–4.

17. Mahran LG, el-Khatib AS, Agha AM et al. The protective effect of aqueous propolis extract on isolated rat hepatocytes. *Drugs Exp Clin Res* 1996;22:309–316.

18. Merino N. Gonzalez R, Gonzalez A et al. Histopathological evaluation on the effect of red propolis on liver damage induced by CC14 in rats. *Arch Med Res* 1996;27:285–289.

19. Chopra S, Pillai KK, Husain SZ et al. Propolis protects against doxorubicin-induced myocardiopathy in rats. *Exp Molecul Pathol* 1995;62:190–198.

20. Khayyal MT, el-Ghazaly MA, el-Khatib AS. Mechanisms involved in the antiinflammatory effect of propolis extract. *Drugs Exp Clin Res* 1993;19:197–203.

21. El-Ghazaly MA, Khayyal MT. The use of aqueous propolis extract against radiation-induced damage. *Drugs Exp Clin Res* 1995;21:229–236.

22. Mirzoeva OK, Calder PC. The effect of propolis and its components on eicosanoid production during the inflammatory response. *Prostaglandins Leukot Essent Fatty Acids* 1996;55:441–449.

23. Hausen BM, Wollenweber E, Senff H et al. Propolis allergy I. Origin, properties, usage, and literature review. *Contact Dermatitis* 1987:17:163–170.

24. Hausen BM, Wollenweber E, Senff H et al. Propolis allergy II. The sensitizing properties of 1,1-dimethylallyl caffeic acid ester. *Contact Dermatitis* 1987:17:171–177.

PYGEUM

1. Awang DVC. Saw palmetto, African prune and stinging nettle for BPH. *Can Pharm J* 1997;(Nov):37–44, 62.

2. Andro M-C, Riffaud J-P. *Pygeum africanum* extract for the treatment of patients with benign prostatic hyperplasia: a review of 25 years of published experience. *Curr Ther Res* 1995;56:796–817.

3. Yablonsky F, Nicholas V, Riffaud JP et al. Antiproliferative effect of *Pygeum africanum* extract on rat prostatic fibroblasts. *J Urol* 1997;257:2381–2387.

4. Bombardelli E, Morazzoni P. *Prunus africana* (Hook. f.) Kalkm. *Fitoterapia* 1997;68:205–218.

5. Barlet A, Albrecht J, Aubert A et al. Efficacy of *Pygeum africanum* extract in the medical therapy of urination disorders due to benign prostatic hyperplasia: evaluation of objective and subjective parameters. A placebo-controlled double-blind multicenter study. *Weiner Klinische Wochenschrift* 1990;102:667–673.

6. Chatelain C, Autet W, Brackman F. Comparison of once and twice daily dosage forms of *Pygeum africanum* extract in patients with benign prostatic hyperplasia: a randomized, double-blind study, with long-term open label extension. *Urology* 1999;54:473–478.

7. Breza J, Dzurny O, Borowka A et al. Efficacy and acceptability of Tadenan (*Pygeum africanum* extract) in the treatment of benign prostatic hyperplasia (BPH): a multicentre trial in central Europe. *Curr Med Res Opin* 1998;14:127–139.

8. Dutkiewicz S, Kalczak M. Quantitative-comparative histology of prostatic adenomas in medically and surgically treated patients. *Int Urol Nephrol* 1994;26:455–460.

9. Levin RM, Riffaud JP, Bellamy F. Protective effect of Tadenan on bladder function secondary to partial outlet obstruction. *J Urol* 1996:155:1466–1470.

10. Levin RM, Riffaud JP, Bellamy F et al. Effects of Tadenan pretreatment on bladder physiology and biochemistry following partial outlet obstruction. *J Urol* 1996;156:2084–2088.

11. Choo MS, Bellamy F, Constantinou CE. Functional evaluation of tadenan on micturition and experimental prostate growth induced with exogenous dihydrotestosterone. *Urology* 2000;55:292–298.

12. Hartmann RW, Mark M, Soldati F. Inhibition of 5-alpha reductase and aromatase by PHL-00801 (Prostatonin®), a combination of PY102 (*Pygeum africanum*) and UR102 (*Urtica dioica*) extracts. *Phytomedicine* 1996;3:121–128.

13. Mathé G, Orbach-Arbouys S, Bizi E et al. The so-called phyto-estrogenic action of *Pygeum africanum* extract. *Biomed Pharmacother* 1995;49:339–340.

14. Foster S, Varro I. *Tyler's honest herbal: a sensible guide to the use of herbs and related remedies,* 4th ed. New York: Haworth Herbal Press, 1999:307–309.

15. Rhodes L, Porimka RL, Berman C et al. Comparison of finasteride (Proscar), a 5-alpha reductase inhibitor, and various commercial plant extracts in in vitro and in vivo 5-alpha reductase inhibition. *Prostate* 1993;22:43–51.

RASPBERRY

1. Briggs CJ, Briggs K. Raspberry. *Can Pharm J* 1997;41–43.
2. Simpson M, Parsons M, Greenwood J, Wade K. Raspberry leaf

References

in pregnancy: its safety and efficacy in labor. *J Midwifery Womens Health* 2001;46:51–59.

3. McFarlin BL, Bigson MH, O'Rear J et al. A national survey of herbal preparation use by nurse-midwives for labor stimulation. Review of the literature and recommendations for practice. *J Nurse-Midwifery* 1999;44:205–216.

4. Parsons M, Simpson, Ponton T. Raspberry leaf and its effect on labour: safety and efficacy. *J Aust Coll Midwives* 1999; 12(3):20–25.

5. Bamford DS, Percival RC, Tothill AU. Raspberry leaf tea: a new aspect to an old problem. Proc Br Pharm Soc (July 8–10) in *Br J Pharmacol* 1970;40:161P–162P.

6. Beckett AH, Belthle FW, Fell KR. The active constituents of raspberry leaves: a preliminary investigation. *J Pharm Pharmacol* 1954;6:785–796.

7. Wang SY, Lin HS. Antioxidant activity in fruits and leaves of blackberry, raspberry, and strawberry varies with cultivar and development stage. *J Agric Food Chem* 2000;48:140–146.

RED CLOVER

1. Duke JA. *CRC handbook of medicinal herbs.* Boca Raton, FL: CRC Press, 1985.

2. Baber RJ, Templeman C, Morton T et al. Randomized placebo-controlled trial of an isoflavone supplement and menopausal symptoms in women. *Climacteric* 1999;2:85–92.

3. Knight DC, Howes JB, Eden JA. The effect of Promensil, an isoflavone extract, on menopausal symptoms. *Climacteric* 1999;2:79–84.

4. Nestel PJ, Pomeroy S, Kay S et al. Isoflavones from red clover improve systemic arterial compliance but not plasma lipids in menopausal women. *J Clin Endo Metab* 1999;84:895–898.

5. Lewis RA. *Lewis' dictionary of toxicology.* Boca Raton: CRC Press, 1998.

6. Nwannenna AI, Lundh TJ-O, Madej A et al. Clinical changes in ovariectomized ewes exposed to phytoestrogens and 17β-estradiol implants. *Proc Soc Exp Biol Med* 1995;208:92–97.

7. Nachtigal LE, Nachtigal LB. The effects of isoflavones derived from red clover on vasomotor symptoms and endometrial thickness. 9th International World Congress on the Menopause, Oct 1999, Yokohama, Japan (abst P. 128).

8. Zava DT, Dollbaum CM, Blen M. Estrogen and progestin bioactivity of foods, herbs, and spices. *Proc Soc Exp Biol Med* 1998;217:369–378.

9. Facciola S. *Cornucopia II: a source book of edible plants.* Vista CA: Kampong Publications, 1998.

10. Tanaka T. In Nakao S, ed. *Tanaka's cyclopedia of edible plants of the world.* Tokyo: Keigaku, 1976.

11. Uphof JC Th. *Dictionary of economic plants.* New York: Stechert-Hatner Service Agency, 1968.

12. Kloss J. *Back to Eden.* Coalmont, TN: Longview, 1971:301.

RIBOFLAVIN

1. Linder MC. *Nutritional biochemistry and metabolism, with clinical applications.* East Norwalk, CT: Appleton & Lange, 1991.

2. Schoenen J, Jacquy J, Lenaerts M. Effectiveness of high-dose riboflavin in migraine prophylaxis. *Neurology* 1998;50: 466–470.

3. Schoenen J, Lenaerts M, Bastings E. High-dose riboflavin as a prophylactic treatment of migraine: results of an open pilot study. *Cephalalgia* 1994;14:328–329.

4. Ajayi OA, George BO, Ipadeola T. Clinical trial of riboflavin in sickle cell disease. *East Afr Med J* 1993;70:418–421.

5. Fouty B, Frerman F, Reves R. Riboflavin to treat nucleoside analogue-induced lactic acidosis. *Lancet* 1998;352:291–292.

6. Skalka HW, Prchal JT. Cataracts and riboflavin deficiency. *Am J Clin Nutr* 1981;34:861–63.

7. Lopez R, Schwartz JV, Cooperman JM. Riboflavin deficiency in an adolescent population in New York City. *Am J Clin Nutr* 1980;33:1283–86.

8. Kunsman GW, Levine B, Smith ML. Vitamin B2 interference with TDx drugs-of-abuse assays. *J Forensic Sci* 1998;43: 1225–1227.

9. Pinto J, Huang YP, Rivlin RS. Mechanisms underlying the differential effects of ethanol on the bioavailability of riboflavin and flavin adenine dinucleotide. *J Clin Invest* 1987;79:1343–48.

ROSEMARY

1. European Scientific Cooperative on Phytotherapy (ESCOP). *Rosmarini folium cum flore (rosemary). Monographs on the medicinal uses of plant drugs. Fascicule 3.* Exeter, UK, 1997.

2. Offord EA, Mace K, Avanti O et al. Mechanisms involved in the chemoprotective effects of rosemary extract studied in human liver and bronchial cells. *Cancer Lett* 1997;114:275–281.

3. Al-Hader AA, Hasan ZA, Aqel MB. Hyperglycemic and insulin release inhibitory effects of *Rosmarinus officinalis. J Ethnopharmacol* 1994;43:217–221.

4. Hay IC, Jamieson M, Ormerod AD. Randomized trial of aromatherapy: successful treatment for alopecia areata. *Arch Dermatol* 1998;134:1349–1352.

5. Singletary K, MacDonald C. Wallig M. Inhibition by rosemary and carnosol of 7, 12-dimethylbenz[a]anthracene (DMBA)-induced rat mammary tumorigenesis and in vivo DMBA-DNA adduct formation. *Cancer Lett.* 1996 Jun 24;104(1):43–48.

6. Van Dyke TE, Braswell L, Offenbacher S. Inhibition of gingivitis by topical application of ebselen and rosmarinic acid. *Agents Actions* 1986;19:376–377.

7. Zhu BT, Loder DP, Cai MX et al. Dietary administration of an extract from rosemary leaves enhances the liver microsomal metabolism of endogenous estrogens and decreases their uterotropic action in CD-1 mice. *Carcinogenesis* 1998;19: 1821–1827.

8. Navarro MC, Montilla MP, Martin A et al. Free radical scavenger and antihepatotoxic activity of *Rosmarinus tomentosus. Planta Med* 1993;59:312–314.

9. Bisset NG, Wichtl M. *Herbal drugs and phytopharmaceuticals: a handbook for practice on a scientific basis with reference to German Commission E monographs.* Boca Raton, FL: CRC Press, 1994.

ROYAL JELLY

1. Vittek J. Effect of royal jelly on serum lipids in experimental animals and humans with atherosclerosis. *Experientia* 1995;51:927–935.

2. Evans WC. *Trease and Evans' pharmacognosy,* 14th ed. London: WB Saunders, 1996:466.

3. Ishiwata H, Takeda Y, Yamada T et al. Determination and confirmation of methyl p-hydroxybenzoate in royal jelly and other foods produced by the honey bee. *Food Addit Contam* 1995;12:281–285.

4. Fujiwara S, Imai J, Fujiwara M et al. A potent antibacterial protein in royal jelly. Purification and determination of the primary structure of royalisin. *J Biol Chem* 1990;265: 11333–11337.

5. Fujii A, Kobayashi S, Kuboyama N et al. Augmentation of

wound healing by royal jelly (RJ) in streptozotocin-diabetic rats. *Jpn J Pharmacol* 1990;53:331–337.

6. Sver L, Orsolic N, Tadic Z et al. Royal jelly as a new potential immunomodulator in rats and mice. *Comp Immunol Microbiol Infect Dis* 1996;19:31–38.
7. Leung R, Ho A, Chan J et al. Royal jelly consumption and hypersensitivity in the community. *Clin Exp Allergy* 1997;27:333–336.
8. Thien FC, Leung R, Baldo BA. Asthma and anaphylaxis induced by royal jelly. *Clin Exp Allergy* 1996;26:216–222.
9. Yonei Y, Shibagaki K, Tsukada N et al. Case report: haemorrhagic colitis associated with royal jelly intake. *J Gastroenterol Hepatol* 1997;12:495–499.
10. Bloodworth BC, Harn CS, Hock CT et al. Liquid chromatographic determination of trans-10-hydroxy-2-decenoic acid content of commercial products containing royal jelly. *J AOAC Int* 1995;78:1019–1023.

SAGE

1. European Scientific Cooperative on Phytotherapy (ESCOP). *Monographs on the medicinal uses of plant drugs. Salviae folium (sage leaf). Fascicule 2.* Exeter, UK, 1996.
2. Leung AY, Foster S. *Encyclopedia of common natural ingredients used in food, drugs, and cosmetics.* New York: John Wiley and Sons, 1996.
3. Bisset NG, Wichtl M. *Herbal drugs and phytopharmaceuticals: a handbook for practice on a scientific basis with reference to German Commission E monographs.* Boca Raton, FL: CRC Press, 1994.
4. Wang M, Shao Y, Li J et al. Antioxidative phenolic glycosides from sage (*Salvia officinalis*). *J Nat Prod* 1999;62:454–456.
5. Strang J, Arnold WN, Peters T. Absinthe: what's your poison? *BMJ* 1999;319:1590–1592.

SARSAPARILLA

1. Bradley PR (ed). *British Herbal Compendium*, vol. 1. British Herbal Medicine Association. Dorset, UK, 1992. Sarsaparilla 194–195.
2. Jiang J, Wu F, Lu J et al. Anti-inflammatory activity of the aqueous extract from *Rhizoma smilacis glabrae*. *Pharmacol Res* 1997;36:309–314.
3. Ageel AM, Mossa JS, al-Yahya MA, al-Said MS, Tariq M. Experimental studies on antirheumatic crude drugs used in Saudi traditional medicine. Drugs Exp Clin Res 1989;15(8):369–372.
4. Fukunaga T, Miura T, Furuta K et al. Hypoglycemic effect of the rhizomes of *Smilax glabra* in normal and diabetic mice. *Biol Pharm Bull* 1997;20:44–46.
5. Chen T, Li J, Cao J. A new flavanone isolated from *Rhizoma smilacis glabrae* and the structural requirements of its derivatives for preventing immunological hepatocyte damage. *Planta Med* 1999;65:56–59.
6. Vandenplas O, Depelchin S, Toussaint G. Occupational asthma caused by sarsaparilla root dust. *J Allergy Clin Immunol* 1996;97:1416–1418.
7. Hobbs C. Sarsaparilla: a literature review. *HerbalGram* 1988;17:1–15.
8. Alam MI, Gomes A. Adjuvant effects and antiserum action potentiation by a (herbal) compound 2-hydroxy-4-methoxy benzoic acid isolated from the root extract of the Indian medicinal plant sarsaparilla (*Hemidesmus indicus* R. Br). *Toxicon* 1998;36:1423–1431.

SASSAFRAS

1. Kamdem DP, Gage DA. Chemical composition of essential oil from the root bark of *Sassafras albidum*. *Planta Med* 1995;61:574–575.
2. Bisset NG, Wichtl M. *Herbal drugs and phytopharmaceuticals: a handbook for practice on a scientific basis with reference to German Commission E monographs.* Boca Raton, FL: CRC Press, 1994.
3. French LG. The sassafras tree and designer drugs: from herbal tea to ecstasy. *J Chem Ed* 1995;72:484–491.
4. Craig JO. Poisoning by the volatile oils in childhood. *Arch Dis Child* 1953;28:475–483.
5. Grande GA, Dannewitz SR. Symptomatic sassafras oil ingestion. *Vet Hum Toxicol* 1987;29:447.
6. Haines JD. Sassafras tea and diaphoresis. *Postgrad Med* 1991;90:75–76.
7. Lu LJ, Lu LJ, Disher RM, Randerath K. 32-P labeling assay in mice of transplacental DNA damage induced by the environmental carcinogens safrole, aminobiphenyl, and benzo(a) pyrene. *Cancer Res* 1986;46:3046–3054.
8. Lu LJ, Disher RM, Randerath K. Differences in the covalent binding of benzo[a]pyrene, safrole, 1'-hydroxysafrole, and 4-aminobiphenyl to DNA of pregnant and non-pregnant mice. *Cancer Lett* 1986;31:43–52.
9. Kapadia GH, Chung EB, Ghosh B et al. Carcinogenicity of some folk medicinal herbs in rats. *J Natl Cancer Inst* 1978;60:683–686.
10. Heikes DL. SFE with GC and MS determination of safrole and related allylbenzenes in sassafras teas. *J Chromatogr Sci* 1994;32:253–257.
11. Bruneton J. *Pharmacognosy: phytochemistry medicinal plants*, 2nd ed. Secaucus NJ: Lavoisier Springer Verlag, 1999:507.

SAW PALMETTO

1. Bennett BC, Hicklin JR. Uses of saw palmetto (*Serenoa repens*, Arecaceae) in Florida. *Econ Botany* 1998;52;381–393.
2. Awang DVC. Saw palmetto, African prune and stinging nettle for benign prostatic hyperplasia (BPH). *Can Pharm J* 1997;37–44, 62.
3. Lowe FC, Ku JC. Phytotherapy in treatment of benign prostatic hyperplasia: a critical review. *Urology* 1996;48:12–20.
4. Plosker GL, Brogden RN. *Serenoa repens* (Permixon): a review of its pharmacology and therapeutic efficacy in benign prostatic hyperplasia. *Drugs Aging* 1996;9:379–395.
5. Rhodes L, Primka RL, Berman C. Comparison of finasteride (Proscar®), a 5α reductase inhibitor, and various commercial plant extracts in in vitro and in vivo 5α reductase inhibition. *Prostate* 1993;22:43–51.
6. Sultan C, Terraza A, Devillier et al. Inhibition of androgen metabolism and binding by a liposterolic extract of "*Serenoa repens b*" in human foreskin fibroblasts. *J Steroid Biochem* 1984;20:515–519.
7. Strauch G, Perles P, Vergult G. Comparison of finasteride (Proscar) and *Serenoa repens* (Permixon) in the inhibition of 5-alpha reductase in healthy male volunteers. *Eur Urol* 1994;26:247–252.
8. Goepel M, Hecker U, Krege S et al. Saw palmetto extracts potently and noncompetitively inhibit human alpha-1 adrenoreceptors in vitro. *Prostate* 1999;38:208–215.
9. Wilt TJ, Ishani A, Stark G et al. Saw palmetto extracts for treatment of benign prostatic hyperplasia: a systematic review. *JAMA* 1998;280:1604–1609.

References

10. Boyle P, Robertson C, Lowe F et al. Meta-analysis of clinical trials of Permixon in the treatment of symptomatic benign prostatic hyperplasia. *Urology* 2000;55:533–539.
11. Marks LS, Partin AW, Epstein JI et al. Effects of a saw palmetto herbal blend in men with symptomatic benign prostatic hyperplasia. *J Urol* 2000;163:1451–1456.
12. Paubert-Braquet M, Richardson FO, Servent-Saez N et al. Effect of *Serenoa repens* extract on estradiol/testosterone-induced experimental prostate enlargement in the rat. *Pharmacol Res* 1996;34:171–179.
13. Baker VA, Hepburn PA, Kennedy SJ et al. Safety evaluation of phytosterol esters. Part 1. Assessment of oestrogenicity using a combination of in vivo and in vitro assays. *Food Chem Toxicol* 1999;37:13–22.
14. Carraro J-C, Raynaud J-P, Hock G et al. Comparison of phytotherapy (Permixon) with finasteride in the treatment of benign prostate hyperplasia: a randomized international study of 1,098 patients. *Prostate* 1996;29:231–240.
15. Gerber GS, Bales GT, Chodak GW et al. *Serenoa repens* (saw palmetto) in men with benign prostatic hyperplasia (BPH): effects on voiding symptoms, urodynamic parameters and serum prostate specific antigen (PSA). *J Urol* 157:331(abst no 1291).
16. Grasso M, Montesano A, Buonaguidi A et al. Comparative effects of alfuzosin versus *Serenoa repens* in the treatment of symptomatic benign prostatic hyperplasia. *Arch Esp de Urol* 1995;48:97–103.
17. Adriazola Semino M, Lozano OJ, Garcia CE et al. Symptomatic treatment of benign hypertrophy of the prostate: comparative study of prazosin and *Serenoa repens*. *Arch Esp Urol* 1992;45:211–213.

SELENIUM

1. Barceloux DG. Selenium. *Clin Toxicol* 1999;37:145–172.
2. Schrauzer GN. Nutritional selenium supplements: product types, quality, and safety. *J Am Coll Nutr* 2001;20:1–4.
3. Linder MC. *Nutritional biochemistry and metabolism, with clinical applications,* 2nd ed. East Norwalk, CT: Appleton & Lange, 1991:245.
4. Levander OA, Burk RF. Selenium. In: Zeigler EE, Filer LJ (eds). *Present Knowledge in Nutrition,* 7th ed. ILSI, Washington, DC, 1996:320–328.
5. Shils ME, Olson JA, Shike M et al, eds. *Modern nutrition in health and disease,* 9th ed. Baltimore: Williams & Wilkins, 1999.
6. Rayman MP. The importance of selenium to human health. *Lancet* 2000;356:233–241.
7. Clark LC, Combs GF, Turnbull BW. Effects of selenium supplementation for cancer prevention in patients with carcinoma of the skin. *JAMA* 1996;276:1957–1963.
8. Hasselmark L, Malmgren R, Zetterström O et al. Selenium supplementation in intrinsic asthma. *Allergy* 1993;48:30–36.
9. Rosenstein ED, Caldwell JR. Trace elements in the treatment of rheumatic conditions. *Rheum Dis Clin North Am* 1999;25:929–935.
10. Constans J, Pellegrin J-L, Sergeant C et al. Serum selenium predicts outcome in HIV infection (letter). *J AIDS Hum Retroviruses* 1995;10:392.
11. Comstock GW, Helzsouer KJ. Preventive nutrition and lung cancer. In: Bendich A, Deckelbaum RJ, eds. *Preventive nutrition.* Totowa NJ: Humana Press, 1997:109–134.
12. Burk RF. Selenium In: Shils ME, Olson JA, Shike M et al, eds.

Modern nutrition in health and disease, 9th ed. Baltimore: Williams & Wilkins, 1999:265–276.

SENNA

1. Westendorf J. Anthranoid derivatives-Cassia species. In DeSmet PAGM, Keller K, Hänsel R, Chandler RF. *Adverse effects of herbal drugs,* vol 1. Berlin: Springer-Verlag, 1993.
2. de Witte P, Lemli L. The metabolism of anthranoid laxatives. *Hepato-Gastroenterol* 1990;37:601–605.
3. European Scientific Cooperative on Phytotherapy (ESCOP). *Monographs on the medicinal uses of plant drugs.* Sennae folium (senna leaf), *Sennae fructus acutifoliae (Alexandrian senna pods), and Sennae fructus angustifoliae (Tinnevelly senna pods). Fascicule 5.* Exeter, UK, 1997.
4. Krumbiegel G, Schulz HU. Rhein and aloe-emodin kinetics from senna laxatives in man. *Pharmacology* 1993;47:120–124.
5. Agra Y, Sacristán A, Gonzalez M et al. Efficacy of senna versus lactulose in terminal cancer patients treated with opioids. *J Pain Symptom Manage* 1998;15:1–7.
6. Valverde A, Hay JM, Fingerhut A et al for the French Association for Surgical Research. Senna vs polyethylene glycol for mechanical preparation the evening before elective colonic or rectal resection: a multicenter controlled trial. *Arch Surg* 1999;134:514–519.
7. Beuers U, Spengler U, Pape GR. Hepatitis after chronic abuse of senna. *Lancet* 1991;337:372–373.
8. Armstrong RD, Crisp AJ, Grahame R, Woolf DL. Hypertrophic osteoarthropathy and purgative abuse. *Br Med J (Clin Res Ed)*. 1981;282(6279):1836.
9. Brusick D, Mengs U. Assessment of the genotoxic risk from laxative senna products. *Environ Mol Mutagen* 1997;29:1–9.
10. Hagemann TM. Gastrointestinal medications and breastfeeding. *J Hum Lactation* 1998;14:259–262.
11. Mitty RD, Wolfe GRZ, Cosman M. Initial description of gastric melanosis in a laxative-abusing patient. *Am J Gastroenterol* 1997;92:707–708.
12. Siegers CP, von Hertzberg-Lottin E, Otte M et al. Anthranoid laxative abuse—a risk for colorectal cancer? *Gut* 1993;34:1099–1100.
13. Mereto E, Ghia M, Brambilla G. Evaluation of the potential carcinogenic activity of senna and cascara glycosides for the rat colon. *Cancer Lett* 1996;101:79–83.

SERINE

1. Linder MC. *Nutritional biochemistry and metabolism with clinical applications,* 2nd ed. East Norwalk, CT: Applebee & Lange, 1991:93.
2. Tsai G, Yang P, Chung LC et al. D-serine added to antipsychotics for the treatment of schizophrenia. *Biol Psychiatry* 1998;44:1081–1089.
3. Tsai GE, Yang P, Chung LC. D-serine added to clozapine for the treatment of schizophrenia. *Am J Psychiatry* 1999;156:1822–1825.
4. Nilsson M, Carlsson A, Carlsson ML. Glycine and D-serine decrease MK-801-induced hyperactivity in mice. *J Neural Transm* 1997;104:1195–1205.
5. Tariq M, Al Moutaery AR. Gastric anti-ulcer and cytoprotective effect of L-serine in rats. *Res Commun Mol Path Pharmacol* 1997;97:171–184.
6. Sleet RB, Ross WP. Serine-enhanced restoration of 2-methoxyethanol-induced dysmorphogenesis in the rat

embryo and near-term fetus. *Toxicol Appl Pharmacol* 1997; 145:415–424.

SILICA

1. Linder MC. *Nutritional biochemistry and metabolism, with clinical applications,* 2nd ed. East Norwalk, CT: Appleton & Lange, 1991:247–248.
2. Nielsen FH. Other trace elements. In: Ziegler EE, Filer LJ, eds. *Present knowledge in nutrition,* 7th ed. Washington DC: ILSI Press, 1996:353–377.
3. Bellia JP, Birchall JD, Roberts NB. Beer: a dietary source of silicon. *Lancet* 1994;343:235.
4. Nielsen FH. Ultratrace minerals. In: Shils ME, Olson JA, Shike M et al, eds. *Modern nutrition in health and disease,* 9th ed. Baltimore: Williams & Wilkins 1999:295–296.
5. Finkelstein MM. Silica, silicosis, and lung cancer: a risk assessment. *Am J Industr Med* 2000;38:8–18.
6. Haustein UF, Anderegg U. Silica induced scleroderma—clinical and experimental aspects. *J Rheumatol* 1998;25: 1917–1926.

SILVER

1. Fung MC, Bowen DL. Silver products for medical indications: risk-benefit assessment. *Clin Toxicol* 1996;34:119–126.
2. Hanada K. Silver in sugar particles and systemic argyria. *Lancet* 1998;351:960.
3. Kim CS. Argyria secondary to chronic ingestion of colloidal silver. *Clin Toxicol* 2000;38:552(abst no 121).
4. Newman M, Kolecki P. Argyria in the ED. *Am J Emerg Med* 2001;19(6):525–6.
5. Gulbranson SH, Hud JA, Hansen RC. Argyria following the use of dietary supplements containing colloidal silver protein. *Cutis* 2000;66:373–374.
6. Suzuki H, Baba S, Uchigasaki S et al. Localized argyria with chrysiasis caused by implanted acupuncture needles. *J Am Acad Dermatol* 1993;29:833–837.
7. Westhoven M, Schafer H. Generalized argyrosis in man: neurological, ultrastructural and x-ray microanalytical findings. *Arch Otorhinolaryngol* 1986;243:260–264.
8. Ohbo Y. Argyria and convulsive seizures caused by ingestion of silver in a patient with schizophrenia. *Psychiatry Clin Neurosci* 1996;50:89–90.
9. Linder MC, personal communication, 2001.
10. Aschengrau A, Zierler S, Cohen A. Quality of community drinking water and the occurrence of late adverse pregnancy outcomes. *Arch Environ Health* 1993;48:105–113.

SKULLCAP

1. DeSmet, PAGM. *Scutellaria* species. In: DeSmet PAGM, Keller K, Hänsel R, Chandler RF. *Adverse effects of herbal drugs,* vol 2. Berlin: Springer-Verlag, 1992:289–296.
2. Murch SJ, Simmons CB, Saxena PK. Melatonin in feverfew and other medicinal plants. *Lancet* 1997;350:1598–1599.
3. Kim HM, Moon EJ, Li E et al. The nitric oxide-producing activities of *Scutellaria baicalensis*. *Toxicology* 1999;135:109–115.
4. Wakabayashi I. Inhibitory effects of baicalein and wogonin on lipopolysaccharide-induced nitric oxide production in macrophages. *Pharmacol Toxicol* 1999;84:288–291.
5. Hui KM, Wang XH, Xue H. Interaction of flavones from the roots of *Scutellaria baicalensis* with the benzodiazepine site [Letter]. *Planta Med* 2000;66:91–93.
6. Gao Z, Huang K, Yang X et al. Free radical scavenging and antioxidant activities of flavonoids extracted from the radix

of *Scutellaria baicalensis Georgi*. *Biochim Biophys Acta* 1999; 1472:643–650.
7. Liu IX, Durham DG, Richards RM. Baicalin synergy with beta-lactam antibiotics against methicillin-resistant *Staphylococcus aureus* and other beta-lactam-resistant strains of *S. aureus*. *J Pharm Pharmacol* 2000;52:361–366.
8. Li BQ, Fu T, Yan YD et al. Inhibition of HIV infection by baicalin—a flavonoid compound purified from Chinese herbal medicine. *Cell Mol Biol Res* 1993;39:119–124.
9. Baylor NW, Fu T, Yan YD, Ruscetti FW. Inhibition of human T cell leukemia virus by the plant flavonoid baicalin (7-glucuronic acid, 5,6-dihydroxyflavone). *J Infect Dis* 1992;165: 433–437.
10. Konoshima T, Kokumai M, Kozuka M et al. Studies on inhibitors of skin tumor promotion. XI. Inhibitory effects of flavonoids from *Scutellaria baicalensis* on Epstein-Barr virus activation and their anti-tumor-promoting activities. *Chem Pharm Bull* 1992;40:531–533.
11. Franzblau SG, Cross C. Comparative in vitro antimicrobial activity of Chinese medicinal herbs. *J Ethnopharmacol* 1986; 15:279–288.
12. Tsao TF, Newman MG, Kwok YY et al. Effect of Chinese and western antimicrobial agents on selected oral bacteria. *J Dent Res* 1982;61:1103–1106.
13. Yamashiki M, Nishimura A, Suzuki H et al. Effects of the Japanese herbal medicine "Sho-saiko-to" (TJ-9) on in vitro interleukin-10 production by peripheral blood mononuclear cells of patients with chronic hepatitis C. *Hepatology* 1997; 25:1390–1397.
14. Shao ZH, Li CQ, Vanden Hoek TL et al. Extract from *Scutellaria baicalensis* Georgi attenuates oxidant stress in cardiomyocytes. *J Mol Cell Cardiol* 1999;31:1885–1895.
15. Kimura Y, Okuda H, Ogita Z. Effects of flavonoids isolated from scutellariae radix on fibrinolytic system induced by trypsin in human umbilical vein endothelial cells. *J Nat Prod* 1997;60:598–601.
16. Kimura Y, Yokoi K, Matsushita N et al. Effects of flavonoids isolated from scutellariae radix on the production of tissue-type plasminogen activator and plasminogen activator inhibitor-1 induced by thrombin and thrombin receptor agonist peptide in cultured human umbilical vein endothelial cells. *J Pharm Pharmacol* 1997;49:816–822.
17. Chen ZY, Su YL, Lau CW et al. Endothelium-dependent contraction and direct relaxation induced by baicalein in rat mesenteric artery. *Eur J Pharmacol* 1999;374:41–47.
18. Foster S. Scullcap: an herbal enigma. *Business Herbs* 1996; May–June:14–16.
19. MacGregor FB, Abernethy VE, Dahabra S et al. Hepatotoxicity of herbal remedies. *BMJ* 1989;299:1156–1157.
20. Harvey J, Colin-Jones DG. Mistletoe hepatitis. *BMJ Clin Res Ed* 1981;282:186–187.
21. Hullar TE, Sapers BL, Ridker PM et al. Herbal toxicity and fatal hepatic failure [Letter]. *Am J Med* 1999;106:267–268.
22. Huang KC. *Pharmacology of Chinese herbs,* 2nd ed. Boca Raton, FL: CRC Press, 1999:385–386.
23. Yin J, Wennberg RP, Miller M. Induction of hepatic bilirubin and drug metabolizing enzymes by individual herbs present in the traditional Chinese medicine, yin zhi huang. *Dev Pharmacol Ther* 1993;20:186–194.

SLIPPERY ELM

1. Anderson E. The mucilage from slippery elm bark. *J Biol Chem* 1934;104:163–170.

References

2. Beveridge RJ, Stoddart JF, Szarek WA et al. Structural features of the mucilage from the bark of *Ulmus fulva*. *Carbohydr Res* 1969;9:429–439.
3. Beveridge RJ, Szarek WA, Jones JKN. Isolation of three oligosaccharides from the mucilage from the bark of *Ulmus fulva* (slippery-elm mucilage); synthesis of O-(3-)-methyl-B-d-galactopyranosyl)-(1 4)-l-rhamnose. *Carbohydr Res* 1971; 19:107–116.
4. Gallagher R. Use of herbal preparations for intractable cough. *J Pain Symptom Manage* 1997;1:1–2.
5. Castleman M. *The healing herbs: the ultimate guide.* Emmaus, PA: Rodale Press, 1991:342–344.
6. Duke J. *CRC handbook of medicinal herbs.* Boca Raton, FL: CRC Press, 1985:495–496.

SPIRULINA

1. Kuhad RC, Singh A, Tripathi KK, et al. Microorganisms as an alternative source of protein. *Nutr Rev* 1997;55(3): 65–75.
2. Popovich NG. Spirulina. *Am Pharm* 1982;22:8–10.
3. Annapurna VV, Deosthale YG, Bamji MS. Spirulina as a source of vitamin A. *Plant Foods Hum Nutr* 1991;41:125–134.
4. Belay A, Ota Y, Miyakawa K et al. Current knowledge on potential health benefits of *Spirulina*. *J Appl Phycol* 1993;5: 235–241.
5. Mathew B, Sankaranarayanan R, Nair PP et al. Evaluation of chemoprevention of oral cancer with *Spirulina fusiformis*. *Nutr Cancer* 1995;24:197–202.
7. Nakaya N, Homma Y, Goto Y. Cholesterol lowering effect of spirulina. *Nutr Reports Int* 1988;37:1329–1337.
8. Becker EW, Jakover B, Luft D, Schmuelling RM. Clinical and biochemical evaluations of the alga *Spirulina* with regard to its application in the treatment of obesity: a double-blind crossover study. *Nutr Rep Intl* 1986;33:565–574.
9. Mishima T, Murata J, Toyoshima M et al. Inhibition of tumor invasion and metastasis by calcium spirulan (Ca-SP), a novel sulfated polysaccharide derived from a blue-green alga, *Spirulina platensis*. *Clin Exp Metastasis* 1998;16:541–550.
10. Ayehunie S, Belay A, Baba TW, Ruprecht RM. Inhibition of HIV-1 replication by an aqueous extract of *Spirulina platensis* (*Arthrospira platensis*). *J AIDS Hum Retrovirol* 1998;18: 7–12.
11. Hayashi K, Hayashi T, Kojima I. A natural sulfated polysaccharide, calcium spirulan, isolated from *Spirulina platensis*: in vitro and ex vivo evaluation of anti-herpes simplex virus and anti-human immunodeficiency virus activities. *AIDS Res Hum Retroviruses* 1996;12:1463–471.
12. Salazar M, Martinez E, Madrigal E et al. Subchronic toxicity study in mice fed *Spirulina maxima*. *J Ethnopharmacol* 1998; 62:235–241.
13. Salazar M, Chamorro GA, Salazar S et al. Effect of *Spirulina maxima* consumption on reproduction and peri- and post-natal development of rats. *Food Chem Toxicol* 1996;34: 353–359.
14. Chamorro G, Salazar S, Favila-Castillo L. Reproductive and peri-and postnatal evaluation of *Spirulina maxima* in mice. *J Applied Phycol* 1997;9:107–112.
15. Herbert V, Drivas G. Spirulina and vitamin B12. *JAMA* 1982; 248:3096–3097.
16. Johnson PE, Shubert LE. Accumulation of mercury and other elements by *Spirulina* (Cyanophyceae). *Nutr Reports Int* 1986;34:1063–1070.

STEVIA

1. Bruneton J. *Pharmacognosy: phytochemistry medicinal plants,* 2nd ed. Secaucus NJ: Lavoisier Springer Verlag, 1999.
2. Kinghorn AD, Soejarto DD. Current status of stevioside as a sweetening agent for human use. *Econ Med Plant Res* 1985; 1:2–44.
3. Chan P, Tomlinson B, Chen YJ et al. A double-blind placebo-controlled study of the effectiveness and tolerability of oral stevioside in human hypertension. *Br J Clin Pharmacol* 2000; 50:215–220.
4. Curi R, Alvarez M, Bazotte RB et al. Effect of *Stevia rebaudiana* on glucose tolerance in normal adult humans. *Braz J Med Biol Res* 1986;19:771–774.
5. Chan P, Xu D-Y, Liu J-C et al. The effect of stevioside on blood pressure and plasma catecholamines in spontaneously hypertensive rats. *Life Sci* 1998;63:1679–1684.
6. White JR, Kramer J, Campbell RK et al. Oral use of a topical preparation containing an extract of *Stevia rebaudiana* and chrysanthemum flower in the management of hyperglycemia. *Diabetes Care* 1994;17:940.
7. Jeppesen PB, Gregersen S, Poulsen CR et al. Stevioside acts directly on pancreatic beta cells to secrete insulin: actions independent of cyclic adenosine monophosphate and adenosine triphosphate-sensitive K+-channel activity. *Metabolism* 2000;49:208–214.
8. Melis MS. Effects of chronic administration of *Stevia rebaudiana* on fertility in rats. *J Ethnopharmacol* 1999;167:157–161.
9. Das S, Das AK, Murphy RA et al. Evaluation of the cariogenic potential of the intense natural sweeteners stevioside and rebaudioside A. *Caries Res* 1992;26:363–366.
10. Tomita T, Sato N, Arai T et al. Bactericidal activity of a fermented hot-water extract from *Stevia rebaudiana* Bertoni towards enterohemorrhagic *Escherichia coli* O157:H7 and other food-borne pathogenic bacteria. *Microbiol Immunol* 1997;41:1005–1009.
11. Melis MS. Effect of crude extract of *Stevia rebaudiana* on renal water and electrolytes excretion. *Phytomedicine* 1999; 6:247–250.
12. Suttajit M, Vinitketkaumnuen U, Meevatee U et al. Mutagenicity and human chromosomal effect of stevioside, a sweetener from *Stevia rebaudiana* Bertoni. *Environ Health Perspect* 1993;101(Suppl 3):53–56.
13. Yodyingyuad V, Bunyawong S. Effect of stevioside on growth and reproduction. *Hum Reprod* 1991;6:158–165.
14. Wasuntarawat C, Temcharoen P, Toskulkao C et al. Developmental toxicity of steviol, a metabolite of stevioside, in the hamster. *Drug Chem Toxicol* 1998;21:207–222.

TAURINE

1. Shils ME, Olson JA, Shike M et al, eds. *Modern nutrition in health and disease,* 9th ed. Baltimore: Williams & Wilkins, 1999.
2. Zhao X, Jia J, Lin Y. Taurine content in Chinese food and daily intake of Chinese men. *Adv Exp Med Biol* 1998;442: 501–505.
3. Niittynen L, Nurminen M-L, Korpela R et al. Role of arginine, taurine and homocysteine in cardiovascular diseases. *Ann Med* 1999;31:318–326.
4. Linder MC. *Nutritional biochemistry and metabolism, with clinical applications,* 2nd ed. East Norwalk, CT: Appleton & Lange, 1991:195–197.

5. Azuma J, Sawamura A, Nobushisa A et al. Double-blind randomized crossover trial of taurine in congestive heart failure. *Curr Ther Res* 1983;34:543–557.

6. Milei J, Ferreira R, Llesuy S et al. Reduction of reperfusion injury with preoperative rapid intravenous infusion of taurine during myocardial revascularization. *Am Heart J* 1992;123:339–345.

7. Fujita T, Ando K, Noda H et al. Effects of increased adrenomedullary activity and taurine in young patients with borderline hypertension. *Circulation* 1987;75:525–532.

8. Hayes KC, Pronczuk A, Addesa AE et al. Taurine modulates platelet aggregation in cats and humans. *Am J Clin Nutr* 1989;49:1211–1216.

9. Franconi F, Bennardini F, Mattana A et al. Plasma and platelet taurine are reduced in subjects with insulin-dependent diabetes mellitus: effects of taurine supplementation. *Am J Clin Nutr* 1995;61(5):1115–1119.

10. Mizushima S, Nara Y, Sawamura M et al. Effects of oral taurine supplementation on lipids and sympathetic nerve tone. *Adv Exp Med Biol* 1996;403:615–622.

11. Finnegan NM, Redmond HP, Bouchier-Hayes DJ. Taurine attenuates recombinant interleukin-2-activated, lymphocyte-mediated endothelial cell injury. *Cancer* 1998;82:186–189.

12. Wu QD, Wang JH, Fennessy F et al. Taurine prevents high-glucose-induced human vascular endothelial cell apoptosis. *Am J Physiol* 1999;277:C1229–1238.

13. Kerai MD, Waterfield CJ, Kenyon SH et al. Reversal of ethanol-induced hepatic steatosis and lipid peroxidation by taurine: a study in rats. *Alcohol Alcohol* 1999;34:529–541.

14. Stipanuk MH. Homocysteine, cysteine, and taurine. In: Shils ME, Olson JA, Shike M et al, eds. *Modern nutrition in health and disease,* 9th ed. Baltimore: Williams & Wilkins, 1999:543–558.

15. Dhillon SK, Davies WE, Hopkins PC et al. Effects of dietary taurine on auditory function in full-term infants. *Adv Exp Med Biol* 1998;442:507–514.

16. Norberg S, Powell TL, Jansson T. Intrauterine growth restriction is associated with a reduced activity of placental taurine transporters. *Pediatr Res* 1998;44:233–238.

17. Ward RJ, Francaux M, Cuisinier C et al. Changes in plasma taurine levels after different endurance events. *Amino Acids* 1999;16:71–77.

TEA TREE

1. Carson CF, Riley TV. Antimicrobial activity of the major components of the essential oil of *Melaleuca alternifolia*. *J Appl Bacteriol* 1995;78:264–269.

2. Tong MM, Altman PM, Barnetson RS. Tea tree oil in the treatment of tinea pedis. *Australas J Dermatol* 1992;33:145–149.

3. Bassett IB, Pannowitz DL, Barnetson RS. A comparative study of tea tree oil versus benzoylperoxide in the treatment of acne. *Med J Aust* 1990;153:455–458.

4. Jandourek A, Vaishapayan JK, Vazquez JA. Efficacy of melaleuca oral solution for the treatment of fluconazole refractory oral candidiasis in AIDS patients. *AIDS* 1998;12:1033–1037.

5. Buck DS, Nidorf DM, Addino JG. Comparison of two topical preparations for the treatment of onychomycosis: *Melaleuca alternifolia* (tea tree) oil and clotrimazole. *J Fam Pract* 1994;38:601–605.

6. Syed TA, Qureshi ZA, Ali SM et al. Treatment of toenail ony-

chomycosis with 2% butenafine and 4% *Melaleuca alternifolia* (tea tree) oil in cream. *Trop Med Int Health* 1999;4:284–287.

7. Peña EF. *Melaleuca alternifolia* oil. *Obstet Gynecol* 1962;19:793–794.

8. Blackwell AL. Tea tree oil and anaerobic (bacterial) vaginosis. *Lancet* 1991;337:300.

9. Caelli M, Porteous J, Carson CF et al. Tea tree oil as an alternative topical decolonization agent for methicillin-resistant *Staphylococcus aureus*. *J Hosp Infect* 2000;46:236–237.

10. Elsom GKF, Hide D. Susceptibility of methicillin-resistant *Staphylococcus aureus* to tea tree oil and mupirocin. *J Antimicrob Chemother* 1999;43:427–428.

11. Faoagali J, George N, Leditschke JF. Does tea tree oil have a place in the topical treatment of burns? *Burns* 1997;23:349–351.

12. Carson CF, Cookson BD, Farrelly HD et al. Susceptibility of methicillin-resistant *Staphylococcus aureus* to the essential oil of *Melaleuca alternifolia*. *J Antimicrob Chemother* 1995;35:421–424.

13. Veal L. The potential effectiveness of essential oils as a treatment for head lice, *Pediculus humanus capitis*. *Complement Ther Nurse Midwifery* 1996;2:97–101.

14. Hammer KA, Carson CF. In vitro susceptibilities of lactobacilli and organisms associated with bacterial vaginosis to *Melaleuca alternifolia* (tea tree) oil. *Antimicrob Agents Chemother* 1999;43:196.

15. Nenoff P, Haustein UF, Brandt W. Antifungal activity of the essential oil of *Melaleuca alternifolia* (tea tree oil) against pathogenic fungi in vitro. *Skin Pharmacol* 1996;9:388–394.

16. Jacobs MR, Hornfeldt CS. Melaleuca oil poisoning. *Clin Toxicol* 1994;32:461–464.

17. Del Beccaro MA. Melaleuca oil poisoning in a 17 month old. *Vet Hum Toxicol* 1995;37:557–558.

18. Elliott C. Tea tree oil poisoning. *Med J Aust* 1993;159:830–831.

19. Seawright A. Tea tree oil poisoning. *Med J Aust* 1993;159:831.

20. Carson CF, Riley TV, Cookson BD. Efficacy and safety of tea tree oil as a topical antimicrobial agent. *J Hosp Infect* 1998;40:175–178.

21. Hausen BM, Reichling J, Harkenthal M. Degradation products of monoterpenes are the sensitizing agents in tea tree oil. *Am J Contact Dermatitis* 1999;10:68–77.

22. Villar D, Knight MJ, Hansen SR et al. Toxicity of melaleuca oil and related essential oils applied topically on dogs and cats. *Vet Hum Toxicol* 1994;36:139–142.

23. Hammer KA, Carson CF, Riley TV. Susceptibility of transient and commensal skin flora to the essential oil of *Melaleuca alternifolia* (tea tree oil). *Am J Infect Control* 1996;24:186–189.

24. Awang DVC. Personal communication 2001.

THIAMIN

1. Brady JA, Rock CL, Horneffer MR. Thiamin status, diuretic medications, and the management of congestive heart failure. *J Am Diet Assoc* 1995;95:541–544.

2. Shimon I, Almog S, Vered Z et al. Improved left ventricular function after thiamine supplementation in patients with congestive heart failure receiving long-term furosemide therapy. *Am J Med* 1995;98:485–490.

3. Ambrose ML, Bowden SC, Whelan G. Thiamin treatment

References

and working memory function of alcohol-dependent people: preliminary findings. *Alcohol Clin Exp Res* 2001;25: 112–116.

4. Benton D, Griffiths R, Haller J. Thiamine supplementation, mood and cognitive functioning. *Psychopharmacology* 1997; 129:66–71.

5. Meador K, Loring D, Nichols M et al. Preliminary findings of high-dose thiamine in dementia of Alzheimer's type. *J Geriatr Psychiatry Neurol* 1993;6:222–229.

5a. Abbas ZG, Swai AB. Evaluation of the efficacy of thiamine and pyridoxine in the treatment of symptomatic diabetic peripheral neuropathy. *East Afr Med J* 1997;74:803–808.

6. Eisenger J, Ayavou T. Transketolase stimulation in fibromyalgia. *J Am Coll Nutr* 1990;9:56–57.

7. Larrieu AJ. Beneficial effects of cocarboxylase on the treatment of experimental myocardial infarction in dogs. *Am Surg* 1987;53:721–725.

8. Brozek J. Psychological effects of thiamine restriction and deprivation in normal young men. *Am J Clin Nutr* 1957;5: 109–120.

9. Skelton WP, Skelton NK. Thiamine deficiency neuropathy: it's still common today. *Postgrad Med* 1989;85:301–305.

10. Campbell CH. The severe lactic acidosis of thiamine deficiency: acute pernicious or fulminating beriberi. *Lancet* 1984;2(8400):446–449.

11. Centers for Disease Control and Prevention. Deaths associated with thiamine-deficient total parenteral nutrition. *MMWR* 1989;38:43–46.

12. Mandel H, Berant M, Hazani A et al. Thiamine-dependent beriberi in the "thiamine-responsive anemia syndrome." *N Engl J Med* 1984;311:836–838.

13. Older MW, Dickerson JW. Thiamin and the elderly orthopaedic patient. *Age Ageing* 1982;11:101–107.

14. Linder MC. *Nutritional biochemistry and metabolism, with clinical applications.* East Norwalk, CT: Appleton & Lange, 1991.

THREONINE

1. Growden JH, Nader TM, Schoenfeld J et al. L-threonine in the treatment of spasticity. *Clin Neuropharmacol* 1991;14: 403–412.

2. Linder MC. *Nutritional biochemistry and metabolism, with clinical applications,* 2nd ed. East Norwalk, CT: Appleton & Lange, 1991:87–109.

3. Lee A, Patterson V. A double-blind study of L-threonine in patients with spinal spasticity. *Acta Neurol Scand* 1993;88: 334–338.

4. Hauser SL, Dolittle TH, Lopez-Bresnahan M et al. The antispasticity effect of threonine in multiple sclerosis. *Arch Neurol* 1992;49:923–926.

5. Testa D, Caraceni T, Fetoni V et al. Chronic treatment with L-threonine in amyotrophic lateral sclerosis: a pilot study. *Clin Neurol Neurosurg* 1992;94:7–9.

6. Blin O, Pouget J, Aubrespy G et al. A double-blind placebo-controlled trial of L-threonine in amyotrophic lateral sclerosis. *J Neurol* 1992;239:79–81.

7. Food and Nutrition Board, National Research Council. *Recommended dietary allowances,* 10th ed. Washington, DC: National Academy Press, 1989.

THYME

1. Hay IC, Jamieson M, Ormerod AD. Randomized trial of aromatherapy: successful treatment for alopecia areata. *Arch Dermatol* 1998;134:1349–1352.

2. Knols G, Stal PC, Van Ree JW. *Huisart Wetens* 1994;37: 392–394. (Cited in Mills S, Bone K. *Principles and practice of phytotherapy.* Edinburgh: Churchill Livingstone, 2000: 563–568.)

3. Barnard DR. Repellency of essential oils to mosquitoes (*Diptera*: Culicidae). *J Med Entomol* 1999;36:625–629.

4. Cosentino S, Tuberoso CI, Pisano B et al. In-vitro antimicrobial activity and chemical composition of Sardinian *Thymus* essential oils. *Lett Appl Microbiol* 1999;29: 130–135.

5. Hammer KA, Carson CF, Riley TV. Antimicrobial activity of essential oils and other plant extracts. *J Appl Microbiol* 1999;86:985–990.

6. Inouye S, Uchida F, Yamaguchi H. In vitro and in vivo anti-*Trichophyton* activity of essential oils by vapour contact. *Mycoses* 2001;44:99–107.

7. Inouye S, Tsuruoka T, Watanabe M et al. Inhibitory effect of essential oils on apical growth of *Aspergillus fumigatus* by vapour contact. *Mycoses* 2000;43:17–23.

8. Meister A, Bernhardt G, Christoffel V, Buschauer A. Antispasmodic activity of *Thymus vulgaris* extract on the isolated guinea-pig trachea: discrimination between drug and ethanol effects. *Planta Med* 1999;65(6):512–516.

9. Bisset NG, Wichtl M. *Herbal drugs and phytopharmaceuticals: a handbook for practice on a scientific basis with reference to German Commission E monographs.* Boca Raton, FL: CRC Press, 1994.

10. Youdim KA, Deans SG. Beneficial effects of thyme oil on age-related changes in the phospholipid C20 and C22 polyunsaturated fatty acid composition of various rat tissues. *Biochim Biophys Acta* 1999;1438:140–146.

11. Spiewak R, Skorska C, Dutkiewicz J. Occupational airborne contact dermatitis caused by thyme dust. *Contact Dermatitis* 2001;44:235–239.

TRYPTOPHAN

1. Linder MC. *Nutritional biochemistry and metabolism, with clinical applications,* 2nd ed. East Norwalk, CT: Appleton & Lange, 1991:90.

2. Byerley WF, Judd LL, Reimherr FW et al. 5-Hydroxytryptophan: a review of its antidepressant efficacy and adverse effects. *J Clin Psychopharmacol* 1987:7:127–137.

3. Chouinard G, Young SN, Bradwejn J et al. L-Tryptophan in the treatment of depression and mania. *Adv Biol Psychiatry* 1983;10:47–66.

4. Smith KA, Fairburn CG, Cowen PJ. Relapse of depression after rapid depletion of tryptophan. *Lancet* 1997;349: 915–919.

5. Neumeister A, Praschak-Rieder N, Hesselmann B et al. Effects of tryptophan depletion in fully remitted patients with seasonal affective disorder during summer. *Psychol Med* 1998:28:257–264.

6. Neumeister A, Turner EH, Matthews JR et al. Effects of tryptophan depletion vs catecholamine depletion in patients with seasonal affective disorder in remission with light therapy. *Arch Gen Psychiatry* 1998:55:524–530.

7. Smith KA, Fairburn CG, Cowen PJ. Symptomatic relapse in bulimia nervosa following acute tryptophan depletion. *Arch Gen Psychiatry* 1999;56:171–176.

8. Schruers K, Klaassen T, Pols H et al. Effects of tryptophan

depletion on carbon dioxide provoked panic in panic disorder patients. *Psychiatry Res* 2000;93:179–187.

9. Ghadirian AM, Murphy BE, Gendron MJ. Efficacy of light versus tryptophan therapy in seasonal affective disorder. *J Affect Disord* 1998;50:23–27.

10. Steinberg S, Annable L, Young SN et al. A placebo-controlled clinical trial of L-tryptophan in premenstrual dysphoria. *Biol Psychiatry* 1999;45:313–320.

11. Cunliffe A, Obeid OA, Powell-Tuck J. A placebo-controlled investigation of the effects of tryptophan or placebo on subjective and objective measures of fatigue. *Eur J Clin Nutr* 1998;52:425–430.

12. Ribeiro CA. L-5-hydroxytryptophan in the prophylaxis of chronic tension-type headache: a double-blind, randomized, placebo-controlled study. *Headache* 2000;40:451–456

13. Trouillas P, Serratrice G, Laplane D et al. Levorotatory form of 5-hydroxytryptophan in Friedrich's ataxia. Results of a double-blind drug-placebo cooperative study. *Arch Neurol* 1995;52:456–460.

14. Elsas LJ II, Acosta PB. Nutritional support of inherited metabolic disease. In: Shils ME, Olson JA, Shike M et al, eds. *Modern nutrition in health and disease,* 9th ed. Baltimore: Williams & Wilkins, 1999:1003–1056.

15. Hertzman PA, Blevins WL, Mayer J et al. Association of the eosinophilia-myalgia syndrome with the ingestion of tryptophan. *N Engl J Med* 1990:322(13):869–873.

16. Swygert LA, Maes EF, Sewell LE et al. Eosinophilia-myalgia syndrome: results of national surveillance. *JAMA* 1990;264: 1698–1703.

17. Belongia EA, Hedberg CW, Gleich GJ et al. An investigation of the cause of the eosinophilia-myalgia syndrome associated with tryptophan use. *N Engl J Med* 1990;323:357–365.

18. Michelson D, Page SW, Casey R et al. An eosinophilia-myalgia syndrome related disorder associated with exposure to L-5-hydroxytryptophan. *J Rheumatol* 1994;21:2261–2265.

19. Williamson BL, Klarskov K, Tomlinson AJ et al. Problems with over-the-counter 5-hydroxy-L-tryptophan. *Nature Med* 1998;4:5.

20. Klarskov K, Johnson KL, Benson LM et al. Eosinophilia-myalgia syndrome case-associated contaminants in commercially available 5-hydroxytryptophan. *Adv Exp Med Biol* 1999;467:461–468.

21. Ciraulo DA, Shader RI, Greenblatt DJ et al, eds. *Drug interactions in psychiatry,* 2nd ed. Baltimore: Williams & Wilkins, 1995:115.

22. Brennan D, MacManus M, Howe J et al. `Neuroleptic malignant syndrome' without neuroleptics. *Br J Psychiatry* 1988: 152:578–579.

23. Staufenberg EF, Tantam D. Malignant hyperpyrexia syndrome in combined treatment. *Br J Psychiatry* 1989:154:577–578.

24. Steiner W, Fontaine R. Toxic reaction following the combined administration of fluoxetine and L-tryptophan: five case reports. *Biol Psychiatry* 1986:21:1067–1071.

25. Lane R, Baldwin D. Selective serotonin reuptake inhibitor-induced serotonin syndrome: review. *J Clin Psychopharmacol* 199;17:208–221.

26. Welch CA. In: Ciraulo DA, Shader RI, Greenblatt DJ et al, eds. *Drug interactions in psychiatry,* 2nd ed. Baltimore: Williams & Wilkins, 1995:399.

27. Alino JJ, Gutierrez JL, Iglesias ML. 5-Hydroxytryptophan (5-HTP) and a MAOI (nialamide) in the treatment of depressions. A double-blind controlled study. *Int Pharmacopsychiatry* 1976:11:8–15.

28. Nardini M, De Stefano R, Iannuccelli M et al. Treatment of depression with L-5-hydroxytryptophan combined with chlorimipramine, a double-blind study. *Int J Clin Pharmacol* Res 1983:3:239–250.

29. Gwaltney-Brandt SM, Albretsen JC, Khan SA. 5-hydroxytryptophan toxicosis in dogs: 21 cases (1989–1999). *J Am Vet Med Assoc* 2000;216:1937–1940.

30. Gross B, Ronen N, Honigman S et al. Tryptophan toxicity—time and dose response in rats. *Adv Exp Med Biol* 1999;467: 507–516.

31. Love LA, Rader JI, Crofford LJ et al. Pathological and immunological effects of ingesting L-tryptophan and 1, 1′-ethylidenebis (L-tryptophan) in Lewis rats. *J Clin Invest* 1993;91:804–811.

32. Barth H, Berg PA, Klein R. Is there any relationship between eosinophilia myalgia syndrome (EMS) and fibromyalgia syndrome (FMS)? An analysis of clinical and immunological data. *Adv Exp Med Biol* 1999;467:487–496.

TURMERIC

1. Ruby AJ, Kuttan G, Babu KD et al. Anti-tumour and antioxidant activity of natural curcuminoids. *Cancer Lett* 1995;94: 79–83.

2. Srimal RC. Turmeric: a brief review of medicinal properties. *Fitoterapia* 1997;68:483–493.

3. Van Dau N, Ngoc Ham N, Huy Khac DH et al. The effects of a traditional drug, turmeric (*Curcuma longa*), and placebo on the healing of duodenal ulcer. *Phytomedicine* 1998;5: 29–34.

4. Hastak K, Lubri N, Jakhi SD et al. Effect of turmeric oil and turmeric oleoresin on cytogenetic damage in patients suffering from oral submucous fibrosis. *Cancer Lett* 1997;116: 265–269.

5. Satoskar RR, Shah SJ, Shenoy SG. Evaluation of antiinflammatory property of curcumin (diferuloyl methane) in patients with postoperative inflammation. *Int J Clin Pharmacol Ther Toxicol* 1986;24:651–654.

6. Charles V, Charles SC. The use and efficacy of *Azadirachta indica* ADR ('neem') and *Curcuma longa* ('turmeric') in scabies: a pilot study. *Trop Geogr Med* 1992;44:178–181.

7. Ramirez-Bosca A, Soler A, Carrion MA, et al. An hydroalcoholic extract of *Curcuma longa* lowers the apo B/apo A ratio. Implications for atherogenesis prevention. *Mech Ageing Dev* 2000;119(1–2):41–47.

8. Sikka SC, Rajasekaran M, Hellstrom WJG et al. Curcumin (diferuloylmethane) decreases sperm motility without affecting viability or membrane integrity (abstract). *J Androl* 1995;Jan/Feb:P-32.

9. Deshpande SS, Ingle AD, Maru GB. Chemopreventive efficacy of curcumin-free aqueous turmeric extract in 7,12-dimethylbenz(a)anthracene-induced rat mammary tumorigenesis. *Cancer Lett* 1998;123:35–40.

10. Singh SV, Hu X, Srivastava SK et al. Mechanism of inhibition of benzo(a)pyrene-induced forestomach cancer in mice by dietary curcumin. *Carcinogenesis* 1998;19:1357–1360.

11. Pereira MA, Grubbs CJ, Barnes LH et al. Effects of the phytochemicals, curcumin and quercetin, upon azoxymethane-induced colon cancer and 7,12-dimethylbenz(a)anthracene-induced mammary cancer in rats. *Carcinogenesis* 1996;17: 1305–1311.

12. Verma SP, Goldin BR, Lin PS. The inhibition of the estrogenic effects of pesticides and environmental chemicals by

References

curcumin and isoflavonoids. *Environ Health Perspect* 1998; 106:807–812.

13. Liu Y, Chang RL, Cui XX et al. Synergistic effects of curcumin on all-trans retinoic acid- and 1 alpha, 25-dihydroxyvitamin D3-induced differentiation in human promyelocytic leukemia HL-60 cells. *Oncol Res* 1997;9:19–29.

14. Krishnaswamy K, Goud VK, Sesikeran B et al. Retardation of experimental tumorigenesis and reduction in DNA adducts by turmeric and curcumin. *Nutr Cancer* 1998;30:163–166.

15. Dorai T, Gehani N, Katz A. Therapeutic potential of curcumin in human prostate cancer. II. Curcumin inhibits tyrosine kinase activity of epidermal growth factor receptor and depletes the protein. *Mol Urol* 2000;4:1–6.

16. Arbiser JL, Klauber N, Rohan R et al. Curcumin is an in vivo inhibitor of angiogenesis. *Mol Med* 1998;4:376–383.

17. Apisariyakul A, Vanittanakom N, Buddhasukh D. Antifungal activity of turmeric oil extracted from *Curcuma longa* (Zingiberaceae). *J Ethnopharmacol* 1995;49:163–169.

18. Li CJ, Zhang LJ, Dezube BJ et al. Three inhibitors of type 1 human immunodeficiency virus long terminal repeat-directed gene expression and virus replication. *Proc Natl Acad Sci* 1993;90:1839–1842.

19. Awasthi S, Srivatava SK, Piper JT et al. Curcumin protects against 4-hydroxy-2-trans-nonenal-induced cataract formation in rat lenses. *Am J Clin Nutr* 1996;64:761–766.

20. Pandya U, Saini MK, Jin GF et al. Dietary curcumin prevents ocular toxicity of naphthalene in rats. *Toxicol Lett* 2000; 115:195–204.

21. Deshpande UR, Gadre SG, Raste AS et al. Protective effect of turmeric (*Curcuma longa* L) extract on carbon tetrachloride-induced liver damage in rats. *Indian J Exp Biol* 1998; 36:573–577.

22. Chuang S, Cheng A, Lin J et al. Inhibition by curcumin of diethylnitrosamine-induced hepatic hyperplasia, inflammation, cellular gene products and cell-cycle related proteins in rats. *Food Chem Toxicol* 2000;38:991–995.

23. Venkatesan N. Pulmonary protective effects of curcumin against paraquat toxicity. *Life Sci* 2000;66:PL21–28.

24. Rafatullah S, Tariq M, Al-Yahya MA et al. Evaluation of turmeric (*Curcuma longa*) for gastric and duodenal antiulcer activity in rats. *J Ethnopharmacol* 1990;29:25–34.

25. Babu PS, Srinivasan K. Hypolipidemic action of curcumin, the active principle of turmeric (*Curcuma longa*) in streptozotocin induced diabetic rats. *Mol Cell Biochem* 1997;166: 169–175.

26. Kandarkar SV, Sawant SS, Ingle Ad et al. Subchronic oral hepatotoxicity of turmeric in mice—histopathological and ultrastructural studies. *Indian J Exp Biol* 19989;36:675–679.

27. Deshpande SS, Lalitha VS, Ingle AD et al. Subchronic oral toxicity of turmeric and ethanolic turmeric extract in female mice and rats. *Toxicol Lett* 1998;95:183–193.

28. BIBRA working group. Turmeric and curcumin. Toxicity profile. BIBRA Toxicology International, 1991.

TYROSINE

1. Pietz J, Landwehr R, Kutscha A et al. Effect of high-dose tyrosine supplementation on brain function in adults with phenylketonuria. *J Pediatr* 1995;127:936–943.

2. Smith ML, Hanley WB, Clarke JT et al. Randomised controlled trial of tyrosine supplementation on neuropsychological performance in phenylketonuria. *Arch Dis Child* 1998; 78:116–121.

3. Deijen JB, Wientjes CJ, Vullinghs HF et al. Tyrosine improves cognitive performance and reduces blood pressure in cadets after one week of a combat training course. *Brain Res Bull* 1999;48:203–209.

4. Galloway GP, Frederick SL, Thomas S et al. A historically controlled trial of tyrosine for cocaine dependence. *J Psychoactive Drugs* 1996;28:305–309.

5. Neri DF, Wiegmann D, Stanny RR et al. The effects of tyrosine on cognitive performance during extended wakefulness. *Aviat Space Environ Med* 1995;66:313–319.

6. Deijen JB, Orlebeke JF. Effect of tyrosine on cognitive function and blood pressure under stress. *Brain Res Bull* 1994; 33:319–323.

7. Shurtleff D, Thomas JR, Schrot J et al. Tyrosine reverses a cold-induced working memory deficiency in humans. *Pharmacol Biochem Behav* 1994;47:935–941.

8. Deutsch SI, Rosse RB, Schwartz BL et al. L-tyrosine pharmacotherapy of schizophrenia: preliminary data. *Clin Neuropharmacol* 1994;17:53–62.

9. Dollins AB, Krock LP, Storm WF et al. l-tyrosine ameliorates some effects of lower body negative pressure stress. *Physiol Behav* 1995;57:223–230.

10. Shils ME, Olson JA, Shike M et al, eds. *Modern nutrition in health and disease*, 9th ed. Baltimore: Williams & Wilkins, 1999.

11. Linder, personal communication 2001.

12. Linder MC. *Nutritional biochemistry and metabolism, with clinical applications,* 2nd ed. East Norwalk, CT: Appleton & Lange, 1991.

VALERIAN

1. Upton R, ed. *Valerian root monograph*. Santa Cruz, CA: American Herbal Pharmacopeia, 1999.

2. Lindahl O, Lindwall L. Double-blind study of a valerian preparation. *Pharmacol Biochem Behavior* 1989;32: 1065–1066.

3. Bos R, Hendricks H, Scheffer JJC et al. Cytotoxic potential of valerian constituents and valerian tinctures. *Phytomedicine* 1998;5:219–225.

4. European Scientific Cooperative on Phytotherapy (ESCOP). *Monographs on the medicinal uses of plant drugs. Valerianae radix (valerian root). Fascicule 4.* Exeter, UK, 1997.

5. Mennini T, Bernasconi P, Bombardelli E et al. In vitro study on the interaction of extracts and pure compounds from *Valeriana officinalis* roots with GABA, benzodiazepine and barbiturate receptors in rat brain. *Fitotherapia* 1993;64: 291–300.

6. Fauteck J-D, Pietz B, Winterhoff H et al. Interaction of *Valeriana officinalis* with melatonin receptors: a possible explanation of its biological action. *Phytomedicine* 1996/1997; 3(Suppl 1):SL-56.

7. Houghton PJ. The scientific basis for the reputed activity of valerian. *J Pharm Pharmacol* 1999;51:505–512.

8. Donath F, Quispe S, Diefenbach K et al. Critical evaluation of the effect of valerian extract on sleep structure and sleep quality. *Pharmacopsychiatry* 2000;33:47–53.

9. Cerny A, Schmid K. Tolerability and efficacy of valerian/lemon balm in healthy volunteers (a double-blind, placebo-controlled, multicentre study). *Fitoterapia* 1999;70:221–228.

10. Leathwood PD, Chauffard F, Herck E et al. Aqueous extract of valerian root improves sleep quality in man. *Pharmacol Biochem Behavior* 1982;17:65–71.

11. Balderer G, Borbely AA. Effect of valerian on human sleep. *Psychopharmacology* 1985;87:406–409.

12. Schulz H, Stolz C, Muller J. The effect of valerian extract on sleep polygraphy in poor sleepers: a pilot study. *Pharmacopsychiatry* 1994;27:147–151.

13. Bourin M, Bougerol T, Guitton B et al. A combination of plant extracts in the treatment about patients with adjustment disorder with anxious mood: controlled study vs. placebo. *Fundam Clin Pharmacol* 1997;11:127–132.

14. Kohnen R, Oswald W-D. The effects of valerian, propranolol, and their combination on activation, performance, and mood of healthy volunteers under social stress conditions. *Pharmacopsychiatry* 1988;21:447–448.

15. Hiller K-O, Zetler G. Neuropharmacological studies on ethanol extracts of *Valeriana officinalis L.*: behavioral and anticonvulsant properties. *Phytother Res* 1996;10:141–151.

16. Leuschner J, Muller J, Rudmann M. Characterization of the central nervous depressant activity of a commercially available valerian root extract. *Arzneim-Forsch/Drug Res* 1993;43:638–641.

17. Willey LB, Mady SP, Cobaugh DJ et al. Valerian overdose: a case report. *Vet Hum Toxicol* 1995;37:364–365.

18. Chan TYK, Tang CH, Critchley JAJH. Poisoning due to an over-the-counter hypnotic, Sleep-Qik (hyoscine, cyproheptadine, valerian). *Postgrad Med J* 1995;71:227–228.

19. Garges HP. Cardiac complications and delirium associated with valerian root withdrawal [Letter]. *JAMA* 1998;280:1566.

20. MacGregor FB, Abernethy VE, Dahabra S et al. Hepatotoxicity of herbal remedies. *BMJ* 1989;299:1156–1157.

21. Fehri B, Aiache JM, Boukef K et al. [*Valeriana officinalis* and *Crataegus oxyacantha*: toxicity from repeated administration and pharmacologic investigations]. *J Pharm Belg* 1991:46:165–176.

22. Houghton PJ. The biological activity of valerian and related plants. *J Ethnopharmacol* 1988;22:121–142.

VALINE

1. Linder MC. *Nutritional biochemistry and metabolism, with clinical applications,* 2nd ed. East Norwalk, CT: Appleton & Lange, 1991.

2. Mero A. Leucine supplementation and intensive training. *Sports Med* 1999;27:347–358.

3. Williamson DJ, McTavish SF, Park SB et al. The effect of valine on 5HT-mediated prolactin release in healthy volunteers, and on mood in remitted depressed patients. *Br J Psychiatry* 1995;167:238–242.

4. Berry HK, Brunner RL, Hunt MM et al. Valine, isoleucine, and leucine: a new treatment for phenylketonuria. *Am J Disease Child* 1990;144:539–543.

5. Tandan R, Bromberg MB, Forshew D et al. A controlled trial of amino acids therapy in amyotrophic lateral sclerosis. *Neurology* 1996;47:1220–1226.

6. Italian ALS Study Group. Branched-chain amino acids and amyotrophic lateral sclerosis: a treatment failure? The Italian ALS Study Group. *Neurology* 1993;43:2466–2470.

7. Richardson MA, Bevans ML, Weber JB et al. Branched chain amino acids decrease tardive dyskinesia symptoms. *Psychopharmacology (Berl)* 1999;143:358–364.

8. Cangiano C, Laviano A, Meguid MM et al. Effects of administration of oral branched-chain amino acids on anorexia and caloric intake in cancer patients. *J Natl Cancer Inst* 1996;88:550–551.

9. Stein TP, Schluter MD, Leskiw MJ et al. Attenuation of the protein wasting associated with bedrest by branched chain amino acids. *Nutrition* 1999;15:656–660.

10. Shils ME, Olson JA, Shike M et al, eds. *Modern nutrition in health and disease,* 9th ed. Baltimore: Williams & Wilkins, 1999:41.

VANADIUM

1. Barceloux DG. Vanadium. *Clin Toxicol* 1999;37:265–278.

2. Nielsen FH. Ultratrace minerals. In: Shils ME, Olson JA, Shike M et al, eds. *Modern nutrition in health and disease,* 9th ed. Baltimore: Williams & Wilkins, 1999:297–298.

3. Linder MC. *Nutritional biochemistry and metabolism, with clinical applications,* 2nd ed. East Norwalk, CT: Appleton & Lange, 1991:255–256.

4. Goldfine AB, Patti ME, Zuberi L et al. Metabolic effects of vanadyl sulfate in humans with non-insulin-dependent diabetes mellitus: in vivo and in vitro studies. *Metabolism* 2000;49:400–410.

5. Boden G, Chen X, Ruiz J et al. Effects of vanadyl sulfate on carbohydrate and lipid metabolism in patients with non-insulin-dependent diabetes mellitus. *Metabolism* 1996;45:1130–1135.

6. Goldfine AB, Simonson DC, Folli F et al. Metabolic effects of sodium metavanadate in humans with insulin-dependent and non-insulin-dependent diabetes mellitus in vivo and in vitro studies. *J Clin Endo Metab* 1995;80:3311–3320.

7. Cohen N, Halberstam M, Shlimovich P et al. Oral vanadyl sulfate improves hepatic and peripheral insulin sensitivity in patients with non-insulin-dependent diabetes mellitus. *J Clin Invest* 1995;95:2501–2509.

8. Fawcett JP, Farquhar SJ, Walker RJ et al. The effect of oral vanadyl sulfate on body composition and performance in weight-training athletes. *Int J Sport Nutr* 1996;6:382–390.

9. D'Cruz OJ, Vassilev A, Uckun FM. Studies in humans on the mechanism of potent spermicidal and apoptosis-inducing activities of vanadocene complexes. *Biol Reprod* 2000;62:939–949.

10. Ghosh P, D'Cruz OJ, Narla RK et al. Apoptosis-inducing vanadocene compounds against human testicular cancer. *Clin Cancer Res* 2000;6:1536–1545.

11. Verma S, Cam MC, McNeill JH. Nutritional factors that can favorably influence the glucose/insulin system: vanadium. *J Am Coll Nutr* 1998;17:11–18.

12. Sabbioni E, Kueera J, Pietra R et al. A critical review on normal concentrations of vanadium in human blood, serum, and urine. *Sci Total Environ* 1996;188:49–58.

13. Dimond EG, Caravaca J, Benchimol A. Vanadium: excretion, toxicity, lipid effect in man. *Am J Clin Nutr* 1963;12:49–53.

VITAMIN A

1. Linder MC. *Nutritional biochemistry and metabolism, with clinical applications.* East Norwalk, CT: Appleton & Lange, 1991:153–160.

2. Semba RD. Impact of vitamin A on immunity and infection in developing countries. In: Bendich A, Deckelbaum RJ, eds. *Preventive nutrition: the comprehensive guide for health professionals.* Totowa NJ: Humana Press, 1997:337–350.

3. Ross AC. Vitamin A and retinoids. In: Shils ME, Olson JA, Shike M et al, eds. *Modern nutrition in health and disease,* 9th ed. Baltimore: Williams & Wilkins, 1999:305–327.

4. Villamor E, Fawzi WW. Vitamin A supplementation: implica-

References

tions for morbidity and mortality in children. *J Infect Dis* 2000;182(Suppl 1):S122–133.

5. Shils ME, Olson JA, Shike M et al, eds. *Modern nutrition in health and disease,* 9th ed. Baltimore: Williams & Wilkins, 1999.
6. Russell RM. The vitamin A spectrum: from deficiency to toxicity. *Am J Clin Nutr.* 2000;71(4):878–884.
7. Institute of Medicine. Dietary Reference Intakes. National Academy Press, Washington, DC., 2001.
8. Mastroiacova P, Mazzone T, Addis A et al. High vitamin A intake in early pregnancy and major malformations: a multicenter prospective controlled study. *Teratology* 1999;59:7–11.

VITAMIN B6

1. Linder MC. *Nutritional biochemistry and metabolism, with clinical applications,* 2nd ed. East Norwalk, CT: Appleton & Lange, 1991:129–135.
2. Leklem JE, Vitamin B6. In: Shils ME, Olson JA, Shike M et al, eds. *Modern nutrition in health and disease,* 9th ed. Baltimore: Williams & Wilkins, 1999:413–422.
3. Jacobson MD, Plancher KD, Kleinman WB. Vitamin B6 (pyridoxine) therapy for carpal tunnel syndrome. *Hand Clin* 1996; 12:253–257.
4. Wyatt KM, Dimmock PW, Jones PW et al. Efficacy of vitamin B-6 in the treatment of premenstrual syndrome: a systematic review. *BMJ* 1999;318:1375–1381.
5. Vutyavanitch T, Wongtrangan S, Ruangsri R. Pyridoxine for nausea and vomiting of pregnancy: a randomized, double-blind placebo-controlled trial. *Am J Obstet Gynecol* 1995; 173:881–884.
6. Sahakian V, Rouse D, Sipes S et al. Vitamin B6 is effective therapy for nausea and vomiting of pregnancy: a randomized, double-blind placebo-controlled study. *Obstet Gynecol* 1991;78:33–36.
7. Mahajan MK, Singh V J. Assessment of efficacy of pyridoxine in control of radiation induced sickness. *J Indian Med Assoc* 1998;96:82–83.
8. Jiao FY, Gao DY, Takuma Y et al. Randomized, controlled trial of high-dose intravenous pyridoxine in the treatment of recurrent seizures in children. *Pediatr Neurol* 1997;17:54–57.
9. Findling RL, Maxwell K, Scotese-Wojtila L et al. High-dose pyridoxine and magnesium administration in children with autistic disorder: an absence of salutary effects in a double-blind, placebo-controlled study. *J Autism Dev Disord* 1997; 27:467–478.
10. Mabin DC, Hollis S, Lockwood J et al. Pyridoxine in atopic dermatitis. *Br J Dermatol* 1995;133:764–767.
11. Mardel S, Phair I, O'Dwyer F et al. Intravenous pyridoxine in acute ethanol intoxication. *Hum Exp Toxicol* 1994;13: 321–323.
12. Villegas-Salas E, Ponce de Leon R, Juárez MA et al. Effect of vitamin B6 on the side effects of a low-dose combined oral contraceptive. *Contraception* 1997;55:245–248.
13. Bartel PR, Ubbink JB, Delport R, et al. Vitamin B-6 supplementation and theophylline-related effects in humans. *Am J Clin Nutr.*1994 Jul;60(1):93–99.
14. Kleiner MJ, Tate SS, Sullivan JF et al. Vitamin B6 deficiency in maintenance dialysis patients: metabolic effects of repletion. *Am J Clin Nutr* 1980;33:1612–1619.
15. Zempleni J. Pharmacokinetics of vitamin B6 supplements in humans. *J Am Coll Nutr* 1995;14:579–586.
16. Cohen M, Bendich A. Safety of pyridoxine-a review of human and animal studies. *Toxicology Letters*1986:34:129–139.

17. Santucci KA, Shah BR, Linakis JG. Acute isoniazid exposures and antidote availability. *Pediatr Emerg Care* 1999;15: 99–101.
18. Hansson O, Sillanpaa M. Pyridoxine and serum concentration of phenytoin and phenobarbitone. *Lancet* 1976 Jan 31; 1(7953):256.
19. Schaumburg H, Kaplan J, Windebank A et al. Sensory neuropathy from pyridoxine abuse. *N Engl J Med* 1983;309: 445–448.
20. Gordon N. Pyridoxine dependency: an update. *Develop Med Child Neurol* 1997;39:63–65.
21. Baxter P, Aicardi J. Neonatal seizures after pyridoxine use. *Lancet* 1999;354:2082–2083.

VITAMIN B12

1. Flynn MA, Irvin W, Krause G. The effect of folate and cobalamin on osteoarthritic hands. *J Am College Nutr* 1994;13: 351–356.
2. Yaqub BA, Siddique A, Sulimani R. Effects of methylcobalamin on diabetic neuropathy. *Clin Neurol Neurosurg* 1992; 94:105–111.
3. Oren DA, Teicher MH, Schwartz PJ et al. A controlled trial of cyanocobalamin (vitamin B12) in the treatment of winter seasonal affective disorder. *J Affective Disord* 1994;32: 197–200.
4. Rana S, D'Amico F, Merenstein JH. Relationship of vitamin B12 deficiency with incontinence in older people. *J Am Geriatr Soc* 1998;46:931–932.
5. Penninx BWJH, Guralnik JM, Ferrucci L et al. Vitamin B12 deficiency and depression in physically disabled older women: epidemiologic evidence from the Women's Health and Aging study. *Am J Psychiatry* 2000;157:715–721.
6. Houston DK, Johnson MA, Nozza RJ et al. Age-related hearing loss, vitamin B12, and folate in elderly women. *Am J Clin Nutr* 1999;69:564–571.
7. Shemesh Z, Attias J, Ornan M et al. Vitamin B12 deficiency in patients with chronic tinnitus and noise-induced hearing loss. *Am J Otolaryngol* 1993;14:94–99.
8. Weinberg JB, Sauls DL, Misukonis MA et al. Inhibition of productive human immunodeficiency virus-1 infection by cobalamins. *Blood* 1995;86:1281–1287.
9. Heimburger DC, Weinser RL. *Handbook of clinical nutrition,* 3rd Ed. Mosby, St. Louis, 1997:192.
10. Clementz GL, Schade SG. The spectrum of vitamin B12 deficiency. *Am Fam Pract* 1990;41:150–162.
11. Linder MC. *Nutritional biochemistry and metabolism, with clinical applications,* 2nd ed. East Norwalk, CT: Appleton & Lange, 1991.
12. Freeman AG. Sublingual cobalamin for pernicious anaemia. *Lancet* 199;354:2080.
13. Lee P, Smith I, Piesowicz A et al. Spastic paraparesis after anaesthesia. *Lancet* 1999;353:554.
14. Guttormsen AB, Refsum H, Ueland PM. The interaction between nitrous oxide and cobalamin. Biochemical effects and clinical consequences. *Acta Anaesthesiol Scand* 1994; 38:753–756.
15. Rauma A-L, Torronen R, Hanninen O et al. Vitamin B12 status of long-term adherents of a strict vegan diet ("living food diet") is compromised. *J Nutr* 1995;125: 2511–2515.
16. Delpre G, Stark P, Niv Y. Sublingual therapy for cobalamin deficiency as an alternative to oral and parenteral cobalamin supplementation. *Lancet* 1999;354:740–741.

17. Houeto P, Hoffman JR, Imbert M et al. Relation of blood cyanide to plasma cyanocobalamin concentration after a fixed dose of hydroxocobalamin in cyanide poisoning. *Lancet* 1995;346:605–608.
18. Brattstrom L. Vitamins as homocysteine-lowering agents. *J Nutr* 1996;126:1276S–1280S.
19. Perry IJ, Refsum H, Morris RW et al. Prospective study of serum total homocysteine concentration and risk of stroke in middle-aged British men. *Lancet* 1995;346:1395–1398.
20. Den Heijer M, Koster T, Blom HJ et al. Hyperhomocysteinemia as a risk factor for deep-vein thrombosis. *N Engl J Med* 1996;334:759–762.
21. Mills JL, McPartlin JM, Kirke PN et al. Homocysteine metabolism in pregnancies complicated by neural tube defects. *Lancet* 1995;345:149–151.
22. Ubbink JB, Vermaak WJH, van der Merwe A et al. Vitamin requirements for the treatment of hyperhomocysteinemia in humans. *J Nutr* 1994;124:1927–1933.

VITAMIN C

1. Linder MC. *Nutritional biochemistry and metabolism, with clinical applications,* 2nd ed. East Norwalk, CT: Appleton & Lange, 1991.
2. Levine M, Rumsey SC, Daruwala R et al. Criteria and recommendations for vitamin C intake. *JAMA* 1999;281:1415–1423.
3. Shils ME, Olson JA, Shike M et al, eds. *Modern nutrition in health and disease,* 9th ed. Baltimore: Williams & Wilkins, 1999.
4. Simon JA. Vitamin C and cardiovascular disease: a review. *J Am College Nutr* 1992;11:107–125.
5. Blanchard J, Tozer TN, Rowland M. Pharmacokinetic perspectives on megadoses of ascorbic acid. *Am J Clin Nutr* 1997;66:1165–1071.
6. Chalmers TC. Effects of ascorbic acid on the common cold: an evaluation of the evidence. *Am J Med* 1975;58:532–536.
7. Hemilä H. Vitamin C intake and susceptibility to the common cold. *Br J Nutr* 1997;77:59–72.
8. Keller KL, Fenske NA. Uses of vitamins A, C, and E and related compounds in dermatology: a review. *J Am Acad Dermatol* 1998;39:611–625.
9. Eberlein-König B, Fesq H, Abeck D et al. Systemic vitamin C and vitamin E do not prevent photoprovocation test reactions in polymorphous light eruption. *Photodermatol Photoimmunol Photomed* 2000;16:50–52.
10. Eberlein-König B, Placzek M, Przybilla B. Protective effect against sunburn of combined systemic ascorbic acid (vitamin C) and D-α-tocopherol (vitamin E). *J Am Acad Dermatol* 1998;38:45–48.
11. Traikovich SS. Use of topical ascorbic acid and its effects on photodamaged skin topography. *Arch Otolaryngol Head Neck Surg* 1999;125:1091–1098.
12. Halperin EC, Gaspar L, George S et al. A double-blind, randomized, prospective trial to evaluate topical vitamin C solution for the prevention of radiation dermatitis. *Int J Radiat Oncol Biol Phys* 1993;26:413–416.
13. Taylor TV, Rimmer S, Day B et al. Ascorbic acid supplementation in the treatment of pressure-sores. *Lancet* 1974;2:544-546.
14. Hatch GE. Asthma, inhaled oxidants, and dietary antioxidants. *Am J Clin Nutr* 1995;61:625S–30S.
15. Cohen HA, Neuman I, Nahum H. Blocking effect of vitamin C in exercise-induced asthma. *Arch Pediatr Adolesc Med* 1997;151:376–370.
16. Ness A, Sterne J. Hypertension and ascorbic acid. *Lancet* 2000;355:1271.
17. Zollinger PE, Tuinebreijer WE, Kreis RW et al. Effect of vitamin C on frequency of reflex sympathetic dystrophy in wrist fractures: a randomized trial. *Lancet* 1999;354:2025–2028.
18. Chappell LC, Seed PT, Briley AL et al. Effect of antioxidants on the occurrence of pre-clampsia in women at increased risk: a randomised trial. *Lancet* 1999;354:810–816.
19. Creagan ET, Moertel CG, O'Fallon JR et al. Failure of high-dose vitamin C (ascorbic acid) therapy to benefit patients with advanced cancer. *N Engl J Med* 1979;301:687–690.
20. Domingo JL, Gomez M, Llobet JM, et al. Effect of ascorbic acid on gastrointestinal aluminium absorption. *Lancet* 1991 Dec 7;338(8780):1467.
21. Rosenthal G. Interaction of ascorbic acid and warfarin. *JAMA* 1971 Mar 8;215(10):1671.
22. Hume R, Johnstone JM, Weyers E. Interaction of ascorbic acid and warfarin. *JAMA* 1972 Mar 13;219(11):1479.
23. Zamah NM, Humpel M, Kuhnz W, et al. Absence of an effect of high vitamin C dosage on the systemic availability of ethinyl estradiol in women using a combination oral contraceptive. *Contraception* 1993;48(4):377–391.
24. Kuhnz W, Louton T, Humpel M et al. Influence of high doses of vitamin C on the bioavailability and the serum protein binding of levonorgestrel in women using a combination oral contraceptive. *Contraception* 1995;51:111–116.
25. Gonzalez JP, Valdivieso A, Calvo R et al. Influence of vitamin C on the absorption and first pass metabolism of propranolol. *Eur J Clin Pharmacol* 1995;48:295–297.
26. Podmore ID, Griffiths HR, Herbert KE et al. Vitamin C exhibits pro-oxidant properties. *Nature* 1998;392:559.
27. Wandzilak TR, D'Andre SD, Davis PA et al. Effect of high dose vitamin C on urinary oxalate levels. *J Urol* 1994;151:834–837.
28. Curhan GC, Willett WC, Rimm EB et al. A prospective study of the intake of vitamins C and B6, and the risk of kidney stones in men. *J Urol* 1996;155:1847–1851.
29. Curhan GC, Willett WC, Speizer FE et al. Intake of vitamins B6 and C and the risk of kidney stones in women. *J Am Soc Nephrol* 1999;10:840–845.
30. Johnston CS. Comparison of the absorption and excretion of three commercially available sources of vitamin C. *J Am Diet Assoc* 1994;94:779–781.
31. Doyle J, Vreman HJ, Stevenson DK et al. Does vitamin C cause hemolysis in premature newborn infants? Results of a multicenter double-blind, randomized, controlled trial. *J Pediatr* 1997;130:103–109.

VITAMIN D

1. Linder MC (1991). *Nutritional biochemistry and metabolism, with clinical applications.* East Norwalk, CT: Appleton & Lange.
2. Norman AW. Vitamin D. In: Ziegler EE, Filer LJ, eds. *Present knowledge of nutrition,* 7th ed. Washington DC: International Life Sciences Institute, 1996;120–130.
3. Gloth FM 3rd, Alam W, Hollis B. Vitamin D vs broad spectrum phototherapy in the treatment of seasonal affective disorder. *J Nutr Health Aging* 1999;3:5–7.
4. LeBoff MS, Kohlmeier L, Hurwitz S et al. Occult vitamin D deficiency in postmenopausal US women with acute hip fracture. *JAMA* 1999;281:1505–1511.

References

5. Reichel H, Koeffler HP, Norman AW. The role of the vitamin D endocrine system in health and disease. *N Engl J Med* 1989;320:980–991.
6. Vieth R, Chan P-C R, MacFarlane GD. Efficacy and safety of vitamin D3 intake exceeding the lowest observed adverse effect level. *Am J Clin Nutr* 2001;73:288–294.
7. Holick MF. Sunlight "D"ilemma: risk of skin cancer or bone disease and muscle weakness. *Lancet* 2001;357:4–6.
8. Holick MF. Vitamin D. In: Shils ME, Olson JA, Shike M et al, eds. *Modern nutrition in health and disease,* 9th ed. Baltimore: Williams & Wilkins, 1999:329–347.
9. Utiger RD. The need for more vitamin D. *N Engl J Med* 338:828–829.
10. Harris SS, Dawson-Hughes B. The association of oral contraceptive use with plasma 25-hydroxyvitamin D levels. *J Am Coll Nutr* 1998;17:282–284.
11. Welch TR. Vitamin D-deficient rickets: the reemergence of a once-conquered disease. *J Pediatr* 2000;137:143–145.
12. Garland FC, Garland CF, Gorham ED et al. Geographic variation in breast cancer mortality in the United States: a hypothesis involving exposure to solar radiation. *Prev Med* 1990;19:614–622.
13. Jacobus CH, Holick MF, Shao Q et al. Hypervitaminosis D associated with drinking milk. *N Engl J Med* 1992;326:1173–77.
14. Scanlon KS, Blank S, Sinks T et al. Subclinical health effects in a population exposed to excess vitamin D in milk. *Am J Public Health* 1995;85:1418–1422.

VITAMIN E

1. Traber MG. In: Shils ME, Olson JA, Shike M et al, eds. *Modern nutrition in health and disease,* 9th ed. Baltimore: Williams & Wilkins, 1999:347–358.
2. Linder MC. *Nutritional biochemistry and metabolism, with clinical applications,* 2nd ed. East Norwalk, CT: Appleton & Lange, 1991.
3. Christen S, Woodall AA, Shigenaga MK et al. Gamma-tocopherol traps mutagenic electrophiles such as NO(X) and complements alpha-tocopherol: physiological implications. *Proc Natl Acad Sci* 1997;94:3217–322.
4. Soares KV, McGrath. Vitamin E for neuroleptic-induced tardive dyskinesia. *Cochrane Database Syst Rev* 2000;2:CD000209.
5. Shoulson I. DATATOP: a decade of neuroprotective inquiry. Parkinson Study Group. Deprenyl and tocopherol antioxidative therapy of parkinsonism. *Ann Neurol* 1998;44(Suppl 1):S160–66.
6. Sano M, Ernesto C, Thomas RG et al. A controlled trial of selegiline, alpha-tocopherol, or both as treatment for Alzheimer's disease. The Alzheimer's Disease Cooperative Study. *N Engl J Med* 1997;336:1216–1222.
7. Bursell SE, Clermont AC, Aiello LP et al. High-dose vitamin E supplementation normalizes retinal blood flow and creatinine clearance in patients with type 1 diabetes. *Diabetes Care* 1999;22:1245–1251.
8. Paolisso G, Tagliamonte MR, Barbieri M et al. Chronic vitamin E administration improves brachial reactivity and increases intracellular magnesium concentration in type II diabetic patients. *J Clin Endocrinol Metab* 2000;85:109–115.
9. Tutuncu NB, Bayraktar M, Varli K. Reversal of defective nerve conduction with vitamin E supplementation in type 2 diabetes: a preliminary study. *Diabetes Care* 1998;21:1915–1918.

10. Raju TNK, Langenberg P, Bhutani V et al. Vitamin E prophylaxis to reduce retinopathy of prematurity: a reappraisal of published trials. *J Pediatr* 1997;131:844–850.
11. Rimm EB, Stampfer MJ, Ascherio A et al. Vitamin E consumption and the risk of coronary artery disease in men. *N Engl J Med* 1993;328:1450–1456.
12. Stampfer MJ, Hennekens CH, Manson JE et al. Vitamin E consumption and the risk of coronary disease in women. *N Engl J Med* 1993;328:1444–1449.
13. Losonczy KG, Harris TB, Havlik RJ. Vitamin E and vitamin C supplement use and risk of all-cause and coronary heart disease mortality in older persons: the Established Populations for Epidemiologic Studies of the Elderly. *Am J Clin Nutr* 1996;64:190–196.
14. Kushi LH, Folsom AR, Prineas RJ et al. Dietary antioxidant vitamins and death from coronary heart disease in postmenopausal women. *N Engl J Med* 1996;334(18):1156–1162.
15. Heart Outcomes Prevention Evaluation Study Investigators. Vitamin E supplementation and cardiovascular events in high-risk patients. *N Engl J Med* 200;343:154–160.
16. Virtamo J, Rapola JM, Ripatti S et al. Effect of vitamin E and beta carotene on the incidence of primary nonfatal myocardial infarction and fatal coronary heart disease. *Arch Int Med* 1998;158:668–675.
17. Rapola JM, Virtamo J, Ripatti S et al. Randomized trial of alpha-tocopherol and beta-carotene supplements on incidence of major coronary events in men with previous myocardial infarction. *Lancet* 1997;349:1715–1720.
18. Leppala JM, Virtamo J, Fogelholm R et al. Vitamin E and beta-carotene supplementation in high risk for stroke: a subgroup analysis of the Alpha-Tocopherol, Beta-Carotene Cancer Prevention Study. *Arch Neurol* 2000;57:1503–1509.
19. Stephens NG, Parsons A, Schofield PM et al. Randomized controlled trial of vitamin E in patients with coronary disease: Cambridge Heart Antioxidant Study (CHAOS). *Lancet* 1996;347:781–786.
20. GISSI-Prevenzione Investigators. Dietary supplementation with n-3 polyunsaturated fatty acids and vitamin E after myocardial infarction: results of the GISSI-Prevenzione trial. *Lancet* 1999;354:447–455.
21. Keith ME, Jeejeebhoy KN, Langer A et al. A controlled clinical trial of vitamin E supplementation in patients with congestive heart failure. *Am J Clin Nutr* 2001;73:219–224.
22. Rapola JM, Virtamo J, Haukka JK, et al. Effect of vitamin E and beta-carotene on the incidence of angina pectoris. A randomized, double-blind, controlled trial. *JAMA* 1996;275:693–698.
23. Motoyama T, Kawang H, Kugiyama K et al. Vitamin E administration improves impairment of endothelium-dependent vasodilation in patients with coronary spastic angina. *J Am Coll Cardiol* 1998;32:1672–1679.
24. Watanabe H, Kakihana M, Ohtsuka S et al. Randomized, double-blind, placebo-controlled study of supplemental vitamin E on attenuation of the development of nitrate tolerance. *Circulation* 1997;96:2545–2550.
25. Kleijnen J, Mackerras D. Vitamin E for intermittent claudication. *Cochrane Database Syst Rev* 2000;2:CD000987.
26. Rautalahti MT, Virtamo JR, Taylor PR et al. The effects of supplementation with alpha-tocopherol and beta-carotene on the incidence and mortality of carcinoma of the pancreas in a randomized, controlled trial. *Cancer* 1999;86:37–42.
27. Heinonen OP, Albanes D, Virtamo J, et al. Prostate cancer and supplementation with alpha-tocopherol and beta-

carotene: incidence and mortality in a controlled trial. *J Natl Cancer Inst* 1998 Mar 18;90(6):440–446.

28. Barton DL et al. Prospective evaluation of vitamin E for hot flashes in breast cancer survivors. *J Clin Oncol* 1998;16:495–500.

29. Edmonds SE, Winyard PG, Guo R et al. Putative analgesic activity of repeated oral doses of vitamin E in the treatment of rheumatoid arthritis. *J Rheum Dis* 1997;56:649–655.

30. Brand C, Snaddon J, Bailey M, et al. Vitamin E is ineffective for symptomatic relief of knee osteoarthritis: a six-month double-blind, randomized, placebo-controlled study. *Ann Rheum Dis* 2001;60:946–949.

31. Andreone P, Fiorino S, Cursaro C et al. Vitamin E as treatment for chronic hepatitis B: results of a randomized controlled pilot trial. *Antiviral Res* 2001;49:75–81.

32. Ziaei S, Faghihzadeh S, Sohrabrand F et al. A randomized placebo-controlled trial to determine the effect of vitamin E in treatment of primary dysmenorrhea. *Br J Ob Gyn* 2001;108:1181–1183.

33. Suleiman SA, Ali ME, Saki ZMS et al. Lipid peroxidation and human sperm motility: protective role of vitamin E. *J Androl* 1996;17:530–537.

34. Kessopoulou E, Powers HJ, Sharma KK et al. A double-blind randomized placebo cross-over controlled trial using the antioxidant vitamin E to treat reactive oxygen species associated male infertility. *Fertil Steril* 1995;64:825–831.

35. Eberlein-König B, Placzek M, Przybilla B. Protective effect against sunburn of combined systemic ascorbic acid (vitamin C) and D-α-tocopherol (vitamin E). *J Am Acad Dermatol* 1998;38:45–48.

36. Baumann LS, Spencer J. The effects of topical vitamin E on the cosmetic appearance of scars. *Dermatol Surg* 1999;25:311–315.

37. Palmieri B, Gozzi G, Palmieri G. Vitamin E added silicone gel sheets for treatment of hypertrophic scars and keloids. *Int J Dermatol* 1995;34:506–509.

38. Wadleigh RG, Redman RS, Graham ML et al. Vitamin E in the treatment of chemotherapy induced mucositis. *Am J Med* 1992;92:481–484.

39. Shils ME, Olson JA, Shike M et al, eds. *Modern nutrition in health and disease,* 9th ed. Baltimore: Williams & Wilkins, 1999.

40. Corrigan JJ, Marcus FI. Coagulopathy associated with vitamin E ingestion. *JAMA* 1974;230:1300–1301.

41. Liede KE, Haukka JK, Saxén LM et al. Increased tendency towards gingival bleeding caused by joint effect of α-tocopherol supplementation and acetylsalicylic acid. *Ann Med* 1998;30:542–546.

42. Meydani SN, Meydani M, Blumberg JB et al. Assessment of the safety of supplementation with different amounts of vitamin E in healthy older adults. *Am J Clin Nutr* 1998;68:311–318.

43. Kim JM, White RH. Effect of vitamin E on the anticoagulant response to warfarin. *Am J Cardiol* 1996;77:545–546.

VITAMIN K

1. Linder MC. *Nutritional biochemistry and metabolism, with clinical applications,* 2nd ed. East Norwalk, CT: Appleton & Lange, 1991.

2. Olson JA. Vitamin K. In: Shils ME, Olson JA, Shike M et al, eds. *Modern nutrition in health and disease,* 9th ed. Baltimore: Williams & Wilkins, 1999:363–380.

3. Shearer MJ. Vitamin K. *Lancet* 1995;345:229–234.

4. Suttie JW, Binkley NC. Vitamin K nutrition and osteoporosis. *J Nutr* 1995;125:1812–1821.

5. Crowther CA, Henderson-Smart DJ. Vitamin K prior to preterm birth for preventing neonatal periventricular haemorrhage. *Cochrane Database Syst Rev* 2000;4:CD000229.

6. Puckett RM, Offringa M. Prophylactic vitamin K for vitamin K deficiency bleeding in neonates. *Cochrane Database Syst Rev* 2000;4:CD002776.

7. Crowther MA, Julian J, McCarty D et al. Treatment of warfarin-associated coagulopathy with oral vitamin K: a randomised controlled trial. *Lancet* 2000;356;1551–1553.

8. Binkley NC, Suttie JW. Vitamin K nutrition and osteoporosis. *J Nutr* 1995;125:1812–1821.

9. Feskanich D, Weber P, Willett WC et al. Vitamin K intake and hip fractures in women: a prospective study. *Am J Clin Nutr* 1999;69:74–79.

10. Yonemura K, Kimura M, Miyaji T et al. Short-term effect of vitamin K administration on prednisolone-induced loss of bone mineral density in patients with chronic glomerulonephritis. *Calcif Tissue Int* 2000;66:123–128.

11. Sato Y, Honda Y, Kuno H et al. Menatetrenone ameliorates osteopenia in disuse-affected limbs of vitamin D- and K-deficient stroke patients. *Bone* 1998;23:291–296.

VITEX

1. Upton R, ed. Chaste tree fruit (*Vitex agnus-castus*). In: *American herbal pharmacopoeia therapeutic compendium.* Santa Cruz, CA: American Herbal Pharmacopoeia, 2001.

2. Schellenberg R (for the study group). Treatment for the premenstrual syndrome with agnus castus fruit extract: prospective, randomised, placebo controlled study. *BMJ* 2001;322:134–137.

3. Lauritzen C, Reuter HD, Repges R et al. Treatment of premenstrual tension syndrome with *Vitex agnus-castus*; controlled double-blind study versus pyridoxine. *Phytomedicine* 1997;4:183–189.

4. Turner S, Mills S. A double-blind clinical trial on a herbal remedy for premenstrual syndrome: a case study. *Complement Ther Med* 1993;1:73–77.

5. Wuttke W, Solitt G, Gorkow C et al. Behandlung zyklusabhängiger Brustschmerzen mit einem Agnus-castus-haltigen Arzneimittel. Ergebnisse einer randomisierten plazebokontrollierten Doppelblindstudie. *Geb Frauenh* 1997;57:569–574.

6. Halaska M, Beles P, Gorkow C et al. Treatment of cyclical mastalgia with a solution containing an extract of *Vitex agnus-castus*: recent results of a placebo-controlled double-blind study. *Breast* 1999;8:175–181.

7. Kubista E, Müller G, Spona J. Behandlung der mastopathie mit zyklischer mastodynie: klinische ergebnisse und hormonprofile. *Gynäkol Rund* 1986;26:65–79.

8. Blank A, Gerhard I. Agnus castus containing preparation (Mastodynon®, Manufacturer: Bionorica Arzneimittel GmbH) on female sterility. 5th Annual Symposium on Complementary Health Care, December 10–12, 1998, Exeter, UK.

9. Milewicz A, Gejdel E, Sworen H et al. *Vitex agnus-castus*-extrakt zur behandlung von regeltempoanomalien infolge latenter hyperprolaktinämie: ergebnisse einer randomisierten plazbo-kontolllierten doppelblindstudie. *Arzneim Forsch* 1993;43:752–756.

10. Wuttke W, Solitt G, Gorkow C, et al. Behand lung zyklusabhängiger Brustschmerzen mit einem Agnus-castus-haltigen

References

Arzneimittel. Ergebnisse einer randomisierten plazebokontrollierten Doppelblindstudie. *Geb Frauenh* 1997;57(10):569–574.

11. Loew D, Schrodter A, Derick-Tan JSE. Dose dependent tolerability and effects of a special Agnus-castus-extract (BP1095E1) on prolactin secretion in healthy male subjects (abstract). In: 2nd International Congress on Phytomedicine and 7th Congress of the German Society of Phytotherapy, Sept 11–14, 1996, Munich. Abstract no SL-96.

12. Upton R, ed. Chaste tree fruit (*Vitex agnus-castus*). In: *American herbal pharmacopoeia therapeutic compendium*. Santa Cruz, CA: American Herbal Pharmacopoeia, 2001.

13. Jarry H, Leonhardt S, Wuttke W et al. Agnus castus als dopaminerges Wirkprinzip in Mastodynon® (Agnus castus as a dopaminergic active principle in Mastodynon) N. *Zeitschr Phytother* 1991;12:77–82. (English summary in Bohnert K-J. The use of *Vitex agnus castus* for hyperprolactinemia. *Q Rev Nat Med* 1997;(Spring):19–21.

14. Sliutz G, Speiser P, Schultz AM et al. Agnus castus extracts inhibit prolactin secretion of rat pituitary cells. *Horm Metab Res* 1993;25:253–255.

15. Jarry H, Leonardt S, Gorkow C et al. In vitro prolactin but not LH and FSH release is inhibited by compounds in extracts of Agnus castus: direct evidence for a dopaminergic principle by the dopamine receptor assay. *Exp Clin Endocrinol* 1994;102:448–454.

16. Schulz V, Händel R, Tyler VE. *Rational phytotherapy*. Berlin: Springer, 1998:240–243.

17. Cahill DJ, Fox R, Wardle PG et al. Multiple follicular development associated with herbal medicine. *Hum Reprod* 1994; 9:1469–1470.

WILLOW

1. Upton R, ed. Willow Bark. In: American Herbal Pharmacopoeia therapeutic compendium. *Willow bark*. Santa Cruz CA: American Herbal Pharmacopoeia, 1999.

2. European Scientific Cooperative on Phytotherapy (ESCOP). *Salicis cortex: willow bark. Monographs on the medicinal uses of plant drugs*. Exeter, UK, 1997.

3. Chrubasik S, Eisenberg E, Balan E et al. Treatment of low back pain exacerbations with willow bark extract: a randomized double-blind study. *Am J Med* 2000;109:9–14.

4. Chrubasik S, Künzel O, Model A et al. Treatment of low back pain with an herbal or synthetic antirheumatic: a randomized controlled study. Willow bark extract for low back pain. *Rheumatology* 2001;40:1388–1393.

5. Schmid B, Tschirdewahn B, Kötter I et al. Analgesic effects of willow bark extract in osteoarthritis: results of a clinical double-blind trial. *FACT (Focus Altern Complement Ther)* 1998;3:186.

6. Krivoy N, Pavlotzky E, Chrubasik S et al. Effect of Salicis cortex extract on human platelet aggregation. *Planta Med* 2001;67:209–212.

7. Baker S, Thomas PS. Herbal medicine precipitating massive haemolysis. *Lancet* 1987;1:1039–1040.

8. Mueller RL, Scheidt S. History of drugs for thrombotic disease; discovery, development, and directions for the future. *Circulation* 1994;89:432–449.

WORMWOOD, SWEET

1. Meshnick SR, Taylor TE, Kamchonwongpaisan S. Artemisinin and the antimalarial endoperoxides: from herbal remedy to targeted chemotherapy. *Microbiol Rev* 1996;60:301–315.

2. Hien TT, White NJ. Quinghaosu. *Lancet* 1993;341:603–607.

3. Von Seidlein L, Milligan P, Pinder M et al. Efficacy of artesunate plus pyrimethamine-sulphadoxine for uncomplicated malaria in Gambian children: a double-blind, randomised, controlled trial. *Lancet* 2000;355:352–357.

4. Sy ND, Hoan DB, Dung NP et al. Treatment of malaria in Vietnam with oral artemisinin. *Am J Trop Med Hyg* 1993;48: 398–402.

5. Lai H, Singh NP. Selective cancer cell cytotoxicity from exposure to dihydroartemisinin and holotransferrin. *Cancer Lett* 1995;91:41–46.

6. Moore JC, Lai H, Li J-R et al. Oral administration of dihydroartemisinin and ferrous sulfate retarded implanted fibrosarcoma growth in the rat. *Cancer Lett* 1995;98:83–87.

7. World Health Organization. WHO model prescribing information—drugs used in parasitic diseases. *The role of artemisinin and its derivatives in the current treatment of malaria* (1994–1995). Malaria Unit, Division of Control of Tropical Diseases. UNDP/World Bank/WHO Special Programme for Research and Training in Tropical Diseases. World Health Organization, Geneva.

WORMWOOD

1. Bisset NG, Wichtl M. *Herbal drugs and phytopharmaceuticals: a handbook for practice on a scientific basis with reference to German Commission E monographs*. Boca Raton, FL: CRC Press, 1994.

2. Hold KM, Sirisoma NS, Ikeda T et al. Alpha-thujone (the active component of absinthe): gamma-aminobutyric acid type A receptor modulation and metabolic detoxification. *Proc Natl Acad Sci U S A* 2000;97:3826–3831.

3. European Scientific Cooperative on Phytotherapy (ESCOP). *Monographs on the medicinal uses of plant drugs. Absinthiih herba (wormwood) Fascicule 4*. Exeter, UK, 1997.

4. Weisbord SD, Soule JB, Kimmel PL. Poison on line—acute renal failure caused by oil of wormwood purchased through the Internet. *N Engl J Med* 1997;337:825–827.

5. Strang J, Arnold WN, Peters T. Absinthe: what's your poison? *BMJ* 1999;319:1590–1592.

6. Zentner J. Absinthe makes the tart grow fonder. *Herb Q* 1999;6(Spring):40–45.

7. Farrell S, Holston FS. The return of "the green fairy" to London: importation of absinth(e) to the United Kingdom, December, 1998. *J Tox Clin Tox* 1999;37:617(abst 82).

8. Weiss RF. *Herbal Medicine (Lehrbuch der phytotherapie)*. Ab Arcanum, Gothenberg, Sweden, Beaconsfield Publishers, Beaconsfield, England, 1988.

YAM, WILD

1. Duke J. *Handbook of medicinal herbs*. p 168. CRC Press, Boca Raton, 1985.

2. Bruneton J. *Pharmacognosy: phytochemistry medicinal plants*, 2nd ed. Secaucus NJ: Lavoisier Springer Verlag, 1999:685–686.

3. Briggs CJ. Dioscorea: the yams—a traditional source of food and drugs. *Can Pharm J* 1990:413–415.

4. Komesaroff PA, Black CV, Cable V, et al. Effects of wild yam extract on menopausal symptoms, lipids and sex hormones in healthy menopausal women. *Climacteric* 2001;4:144–150.

5. Timmons BW, Newhouse IJ, Thayer RE et al. The efficacy of SPORT as a dietary supplement on performance and recovery in trained athletes. *Can J Appl Physiol* 2000;25:55–67.

6. Araghiniknam M, Chung S, Nelson-White T et al. Antioxidant

activity of dioscorea and dehydroepiandrosterone (DHEA) in older humans. *Life Sci* 1996;59:147–157.

7. Scott A, Higdon K, Benghuzzi H et al. TCPL drug delivery system: the effects of synthetic DHEA and diosgenin using an ovariectomized rat model. *Biomed Sci Instrum* 2000;36; 171–176.

8. Rao A, Rao AR, Kale RK. Diosgenin—a growth stimulator of mammary gland of ovariectomized mouse. *Indian J Exp Biol* 1992;30:367–370.

9. Amigo L, Mendoza H, Zanlungo S et al. Enrichment of canalicular membrane with cholesterol and sphingomyelin prevents bile salt-induced hepatic damage. *J Lipid Res* 1999; 40:533–542.

10. Puglielli L, Amigo L, Arrese M et al. Protective role of biliary cholesterol and phospholipids lamellae against bile acid-induced cell damage. *Gastroenterology* 1994;107:244–254.

11. Accatino L, Pizarro M, Solis N et al. Effects of diosgenin, a plant-derived steroid, on bile secretion and hepatocellular cholestasis induced by estrogens in the rat. *Hepatology* 1998;28:129–140.

12. Yamada T, Hoshino M, Hayakawa T et al. Dietary diosgenin attenuates subacute intestinal inflammation associated with indomethacin in rats. *Am J Physiol* 1997;273:G355–364.

13. Lee JR. *Natural progesterone: the multiple roles of a remarkable hormone.* Sebastopol CA: BLL Publishing, 1993.

14. Leonetti HB, Longo S, Anasti JN. Transdermal progesterone cream for vasomotor symptoms and postmenopausal bone loss. *Obstet Gynecol* 1999;94:225–228.

15. Cooper A, Spencer C, Whitehead MI et al. Systemic absorption of progesterone from Progest cream in postmenopausal women. *Lancet* 1998;351:1255–1256.

16. Wren BG et al. Micronized transdermal progesterone and endometrial response. *Lancet* 1999;354:1447–1448.

17. Mann J. *Murder, magic, and medicine.* Oxford, England: Oxford University Press, 1994.

18. Djerassi C. *The pill, pygmy chimps, and Degas' horse: the remarkable autobiography of the award-winning scientist who synthesized the birth control pill.* Basic Books, 1998: 33–48.

YARROW

1. Bruneton J. *Pharmacognosy: phytochemistry medicinal plants,* 2nd ed. Secaucus NJ: Lavoisier Springer Verlag, 1999:337–339.

2. Tozyo T, Yoshimura Y, Sakurai K et al. Novel antitumor sesquiterpenoids in *Achillea millefolium. Chem Pharm Bull* 1994;42:1096–1100.

3. Chandler RF, Hooper SN, Hooper DL et al. Herbal remedies of the Maritime Indians: sterols and triterpenes of *Achillea millefolium* L. (yarrow). *J Pharm Sci* 1982;71:690–693.

4. Van der Weijden GA, Timmer CJ, Timmerman MF et al. The effect of herbal extracts in an experimental mouthrinse on established plaque and gingivitis. *J Clin Periodontol* 1998; 25:399–403.

5. Montanari T, de Carvalho JE, Dolder H. Antispermatogenic effect of *Achillea millefolium* L in mice. *Contraception* 1998; 58:309–313.

6. Kindscher K, Manfredi KP, Britton M et al. Testing prairie plants with ethnobotanical importance for anti-cancer and anti-AIDS compounds. *J Ethnobiol* 1998;18:229–245.

7. Rücker G, Walter RD, Manns D et al. Antimalarial activity of some natural peroxides. *Planta Med* 1991;57:295–296.

8. Mustafa EH, Abu Zarga M, Abdalla S. Effects of cirsiliol, a flavone isolated from *Achillea fragrantissima,* on rat isolated ileum. *Gen Pharmacol* 1992;23:555–560.

9. Gomez MA, Saenz MT, Garcia MD et al. Study of the topical anti-inflammatory activity of *Achillea ageratum* on chronic and acute inflammation models. *Zeitschrift Naturforschung* 1999;54:937–941.

10. Rezaeipoor R, Saeidnia S, Kamalinejad M. Immunosuppressive activity of *Achillea talagonica* on humoral immune responses in experimental animals. *J Ethnopharmacol* 1999; 65:273–276.

11. Davies MG, Kersey PJ. Contact allergy to yarrow and dandelion. *Contact Dermatitis* 1986;14(4):256–257.

12. Hausen BM, Breuer J, Weglewski J et al. Alpha-peroxyachifolid and other new sensitizing sesquiterpene lactones from yarrow (*Achillea millefolium* L., Compositae). *Contact Dermatitis* 1991;24:274–280.

13. Duke JA. *CRC handbook of medicinal herbs.* Boca Raton, FL: CRC Press, 1985.

14. Facciola S. *Cornucopia II: a source book of edible plants.* Vista CA: Kampong Publications, 1998:32.

YOHIMBE

1. Betz JM, White KD. Gas chromatographic determination of yohimbine in commercial yohimbe products. *J AOAC Int* 1995;78:1189–1194.

2. Hedner T, Edgar B, Edvinsson L. Yohimbine pharmacokinetics and interaction with the sympathetic nervous system in normal volunteers. *Eur J Clin Pharmacol* 1992;43:651–656.

3. Owen JA, Nakatsu SL, Fenemore J et al. The pharmacokinetics of yohimbine in man. *Eur J Clin Pharmacol* 1987;32: 577–582.

4. Sturgill MG, Grasing KW, Rosen RC et al. Yohimbine elimination in normal volunteers is characterized by both one-and two-compartment behavior. *J Cardiovasc Pharm* 1997;29: 697–703.

5. Ernst E, Pittler MH. Yohimbine for erectile dysfunction: a systematic review and meta-analysis of randomized clinical trails. *J Urol* 1998;159:433–436.

6. Riley AJ. Yohimbine in the treatment of erectile disorder. *Br J Clin Pract* 1994;48(3):133–136.

7. Susset JG, Tessier CD, Wincze J et al. Effect of yohimbine hydrochloride on erectile impotence: a double-blind study. *J Urol* 1989;141(6):1360–1363.

8. Kunelius P, Hakkinen J, Lukkarinen O. Is high-dose yohimbine hydrochloride effective in the treatment of mixed-type impotence? A prospective, randomized, controlled double-blind crossover study. *Urology* 1997;49:441–444.

9. Montorsi F, Strambi LF, Guazzoni G et al. Effect of yohimbine-trazodone on psychogenic impotence: a randomized, double-blind, placebo-controlled study. *Urology* 1994;44: 732–736.

10. Danjou P, Alexandre L,Warot D et al. Assessment of erectogenic properties of apomorphine and yohimbine in man. *Br J Clin Pharm* 1988;26:733–739.

11. Bagheri H, Schmitt L, Berlan M et al. A comparative study of the effects of yohimbine and anetholtrithione on salivary secretion in depressed patients treated with psychotropic drugs. *Eur J Clin Pharm* 1997;52:339–342.

12. Bagheri H, Schmitt L, Berlan M et al. Effect of 3 weeks treatment with yohimbine on salivary secretion in healthy volunteers and in depressed patients treated with tricyclic antidepressants. *Br J Clin Pharm* 1992;34:555–558.

References

13. Bagheri H, Picault P, Schmitt L et al. Pharmacokinetic study of yohimbine and its pharmacodynamic effects on salivary secretion in patients treated with tricyclic antidepressants. *Br J Clin Pharm* 1994;37:93–96.
14. Berlin I, Stalla-Bourdillon A, Thuillier Y et al. Lack of efficacy of yohimbine in the treatment of obesity (in French). *J Pharmacologie* 1986;17:343–347.
15. Sax L. Yohimbine does not affect fat distribution in men. *Int J Obesity* 1991;15:561–565.
16. Galitzky J, Rivière D, Tran MA et al. Pharmacodynamic effects of chronic yohimbine treatment in healthy volunteers. *Eur J Clin Pharmacol* 1990;39:447–451.
17. Kucio C, Jonderko K, Piskorska D. Does yohimbine act as a slimming drug? *Israel J Med Sci* 1991;27:550–556.
18. Gurguis GN, Vitton BJ, Uhde TW. Behavioral, sympathetic and adrenocortical responses to yohimbine in panic disorder and normal controls. *Psychiatry Res* 1997;719:27–39.
19. De Smet PAGM, Smeets OSNM. Potential risks of health food products containing yohimbe extracts. *BMJ* 1994;309:958.
20. Grossman E, Rosenthal T, Peleg E et al. Oral yohimbine increases blood pressure and sympathetic nervous outflow in hypertensive patients. *J Cardiovasc Pharm* 1993;22:22–26.
21. Musso NR, Vargassola C, Pende A et al. Yohimbine effects on blood pressure and plasma catecholamines in human hypertension. *Am J Hypertens* 1995;8:565–571.
22. Sandler B, Aronson P. Yohimbine-induced cutaneous drug eruption, progressive renal failure, and lupus-like syndrome. *Urology* 1993;41:343–345.
23. Friesen K, Palatnick W, Tenebein M. Benign course after massive ingestion of yohimbine. *J Emerg Med* 1993;11:287–288.
24. Gear RW, Gordon NC, Heller PH et al. Enhancement of morphine analgesia by the α2-adrenergic antagonist yohimbine. *Neuroscience* 1995;66:5–8.
25. Hameedi FA, Woods SW, Rosen MI et al. Dose dependent effects of yohimbine on methadone maintained patients. *Am J Drug Alcohol Abuse* 1997;23:327–333.
26. Gurguis GNM, Uhde TW. Plasma 3-methoxy-4-hydroxyphenylethylene glycol (MHPG) and growth hormone responses to yohimbine in panic disorder patients and normal controls. *Psychoneuroendocrinology* 1990;15:217–224.

ZINC

1. Barceloux DG. Zinc. *Clin Toxicol* 1999;37:279–292.
2. King JC, Keen CL. Zinc. In Shils ME, Olson JA, Shike M et al, eds. *Modern nutrition in health and disease,* 9th ed. Baltimore: Williams & Wilkins 1999;223–240.
3. Linder MC. *Nutritional biochemistry and metabolism, with clinical applications,* 2nd ed. East Norwalk, CT: Appleton & Lange, 1991.
4. Jackson JL, Lesho E, Peterson C. Zinc and the common cold: a meta-analysis revisited. *J Nutr* 2000;130(5S Suppl):1512S–1515S.
5. Garland ML, Hagmeyer KO. The role of zinc lozenges in treatment of the common cold. *Ann Pharmacother* 1998;32:63–69.
6. Hirt M, Nobel S, Barron E. Zinc nasal gel for the treatment of common cold symptoms: a double-blind, placebo-controlled trial. *Ear Nose Throat J* 2000;778–782.
7. Ripamonti C, Zecca E, Brunelli C et al. A randomized, controlled clinical trial to evaluate the effects of zinc sulfate on cancer patients with taste alterations caused by head and neck irradiation. *Cancer* 1998;82:1938–1945.
8. Henkin RI, Scheicter PJ, Friedewald WT et al. A double-blind study of the effects of zinc sulfate on taste and smell function. *Am J Med Sci* 11976;272:285–299.
9. Heyneman CA. Zinc deficiency and taste disorders. *Ann Pharmacother* 1996;30:186–187.
10. Yoshida S, Endo S, Tomita H. A double-blind study of the therapeutic effect of zinc gluconate on taste disorder. *Auris Nasus Larynx (Tokyo)* 1991;18:153–161.
11. Aiba T, Sugiara M, Mori J et al. Effect of zinc sulfate on sensorineural olfactory disorder. *Acta Otolaryngol Suppl (Stockh)* 1998;538:202–204.
12. Sazawal S, Black RE, Bhan MK et al. Zinc supplementation in young children with acute diarrhea in India. *N Engl J Med* 1995;333:839–844.
13. Faruque AS, Mahalanabis D, Haque SS et al. Double-blind, randomized, controlled trial of zinc or vitamin A supplementation in young children with acute diarrhoea. *Acta Paediatr* 1999;88:154–160.
14. Bhutta ZA, Nizami SQ, Isani Z. Zinc supplementation in malnourished children with persistent diarrhea in Pakistan. *Pediatrics* 1999;103:e42.
15. Young B, Ott L, Kasarskis E et al. Zinc supplementation is associated with improved neurologic recovery rate and visceral protein levels of patients with severe closed head injury. *J Neurotrauma* 1996;13:25–34.
16. Ewing CI, Gibbs AC, Ashcroft C et al. Failure of oral zinc supplementation in atopic eczema. *Eur J Clin Nutr* 1991;45:507–510.
17. Paaske PB, Pedersen CB, Kjems G et al. Zinc in the management of tinnitus: placebo-controlled trial. *Ann Oto Rhino Laryngol* 1991;100:647–49.
18. Stur M, Tittl M, Reitner A et al. Oral zinc and the second eye in age-related macular degeneration. *Invest Ophthalmol Vis Sci* 1996;37:1225–1235.
19. Wilkinson EAJ, Hawke CI. Does oral zinc aid the healing of chronic leg ulcers? *Arch Dermatol* 1998;134:1556–1560.
20. Umeta M, West CE, Haidar J et al. Zinc supplementation and stunted infants in Ethiopia: a randomised controlled trial. *Lancet* 2000;355:2021–2026.
21. Goldenberg RL, Tsunenobu T, Neggers Y et al. The effect of zinc supplementation on pregnancy outcome. *JAMA* 1995;274:463–468.
22. Simkin PA. Oral zinc sulphate in rheumatoid arthritis. *Lancet* 1976;2(7985):539–542.
23. Job C, Menkes CJ, Delbarre F. Zinc sulfate in the treatment of rheumatoid arthritis. *Arthritis Rheum* 1980;23:1408–1409.
24. Mattingley PC, Mowat AG. Zinc sulphate in rheumatoid arthritis. *Ann Rheum Dis* 1982;41:456–457.
25. Clemmensen OJ, Siggaard-Andersen, Worm AM et al. Psoriatic arthritis treated with oral zinc sulphate. *Br J Dermatol* 1980;103:411–415.
26. Porea TJ, Belmont JW, Mahoney DH. Zinc-induced anemia and neutropenia in an adolescent. *J Pediatr* 2000;136:688–690.
27. Tschanz C, Stargel WW, Thomas JA. Interactions between drugs and nutrients. *Adv Pharmacol* 1996;35:1–26.
28. Brouwers JR. Drug interactions with quinolone antibacterials. *Drug Saf* 1992 Jul–Aug;7(4):268–281.

SECTION III
Reference Tables

Tables

Herb Chart

	ENGLISH	LATIN	PHARMACOPOEIAL	SPANISH	FRENCH	GERMAN
1	Aconite—herb	*Aconitum napellus*	Aconiti herba	Acónito	Aconit napel	Blauer Eisenhutkraut Eisenhutkraut
	Aconite—tuber		Aconiti tuber			Blauer Eisenhutwurzel Eisenhutwurzel
2	Alfalfa	*Medicago sativa*	—	Alfalfa	—	—
3	Aloe	*Aloe vera*	Aloe barbadensis	Aloe	Aloès	Curacao-Aloe Venezuela-Aloe Aloe
		Aloe barbadensis				
4	Anise	*Pimpinella anisum*	Anisi fructus	Anís	Anis	Anis Kleiner Anis Süßer Kümmel
5	Arnica	*Arnica montana* *Arnica latifolia*	Arnicae flos	Arnica	Arnica	Arnikablüten Bergwohlverleih Wundkraut Kraftwurz
6	Ashwagandha	*Withania somnifera*	—	—	—	—
7	Astragalus	*Astragalus membranaceus*	—	—	—	—
8	Bearberry	*Arctostaphylos uva-ursi*	Uvae ursi folium	Coralillo Gayuba	Busserole	Bärentraubenblätter Wolfsbeere Wilderbuchs
9	Betel nut	*Areca catechu*	—	—	—	
10	Bilberry—fruit	*Vaccinium myrtillus*	Myrtilli fructus	Mertilo negro	Myrtille fruit frais	Heidelbeeren Blaubeeren Bickbeeren Schwarzbeeren
	Bilberry—leaf		Myrtilli folium		Myrtille	Heidelbeerblätter Blaubeerblätter
11	Bitter melon/karela	*Momordica charantia*	—	—	—	—
12	Black cohosh	*Cimicifuga racemosa*	Cimicifugae racemosae rhizoma	Cimicifuga	Actée américain	Cimicifugawurzelstock Wanzenkrautwurzel
13	Black haw	*Viburnum prunifolium*	Viburni prunifolii cortex	Viburnu	Viburnum	Schneeballbaumrinde
14	Blue cohosh	*Caulophyllum thalictroides*	—	—	—	—
15	Bloodroot	*Sanguinaria canadensis*	—	Sanguinaria	Sanguinaire canadienne	Kanadischeblutwurzel
16	Boldo	*Peumus boldus*	Boldo folium	Boldo	Boldo	Boldoblätter
17	Borage—herb	*Borago officinalis*	Boraginis herba	Borraja	—	Boretsch
18	Burdock	*Arctium lappa*	Bardanae radix	Bardana	Bardane	Klettenwurzel Dollenkrautwurzel Kleberwurzel
19	Calendula (marigold) —flower	*Calendula officinalis*	Calendulae flos	Caléndula	Souci	Ringelblumenblüten Goldblume
20	Caraway—seed	*Carum carvi*	Carvi fructus	Carvi (Comino de Prado)	Carvi	Kümmel Wiesen- or Feldkümmel Kümmich
	Caraway—oil		Carvi aetheroleum			Kümmelöl
21	Cascara	*Rhamnus purshiana*	Rhamni purshiani cortex	Cáscara sagrada	Cascara	Cascararinde Amerikanische Faulbaumrinde
22	Cat's claw	*Uncaria tomentosa*	—	Uña de gato	—	
23	Catnip	*Nepeta cataria*	—	—	Cataire	Katzenminze
24	Cayenne	*Capsicum annuum* *C. frutescens* *Capsicum annuum* var. *annuum*	—	Capsico (Pimentón)	Capsicum	Cayennepfeffer Paprika
25	Chamomile, German	*Matricaria recutita*	Matricariae flos	Manzanilla	Matricaire	Kamillenblüten Kamilenblüten Kleine Kamille Feldkamille

Continued

Herb Chart (continued)

	ENGLISH	LATIN	PHARMACOPOEIAL	SPANISH	FRENCH	GERMAN
26	Chamomile, Roman	*Chamaemelum nobile*	Chomomillae romanae flos	Camomila romana	Camomille romaine	Römische Kamillenblüten Große Kamille
27	Chaparral	*Larrea tridentata*	—	Hediondilla Gobernadora	—	Kreosotstrauch
28	Chaste tree berry	*Vitex agnus-castus*	Agni casti fructus	Sauzgatillo Anocasto	Gattelier	Mönchspfeffer Keuschlammfrüchte
29	Cocoa—seed	*Theobroma cacao*	Cocao semen	Cacao	Cacao	Kakaoschalen Kakaosamen
30	Cinnamon—bark	*Cinnamomum verum*	Cinnamomi ceylanici cortex	Canela	Cannelle dite de Ceylan, Cannelier de Ceylan Canelero de Ceilán	Zimtrinde Echter Kanel
	Chinese cinnamon— bark	*Cinnamomum aromaticum*	Cinnamomi cassiae cortex	Canela de la China Canelero chino	Canelle de Cochinchine, Cannelier casse Cannelier de Chine	Ceylonzimtbaum Zimtblüten Zimtcassie
31	Coltsfoot—leaf	*Tussilago farfara*	Farfarae folium	Tusílago	Tussilage	Huflattichblätter Brandlattich Pferdefuß
32	Comfrey—herb	*Symphytum officinale*	Symphyti herba	Consuelda	Consoude	Beinwellkraut
33	Cranberry	*Vaccinium macrocarpon*	—	—	Ronce d'Amérique	Grosse Moosbeere
34	Dandelion—whole plant	*Taraxacum officinale*	Taraxaci radix cum herba	Chicoria Diente de léon	Dent de lion Pissenlit	Löwenzahn-wurzel-mit Kraut
35	Danshen	*Salvia miltiorrhiza*	—	—	—	—
36	Devil's claw	*Harpagophytum procumbens*	Harpagophyti radix	Harpagofito	Harpagophyton	Teufelskralle Trampelklette Südafrikanische Teufelskrallenwurzel
37	Dong quai	*Angelica sinensis*	—	—	—	—
38	Echinacea	*Echinacea purpurea*	Echinaceae purpurea herba/radix	Echinácea	Echinacée	Purpursonnenhutkraut/ Purpursonnenhutwurzel
39	Elder flower	*Sambucus nigra*	Sambuci flos	Flor sauco Saúco	Sureau noir	Holunderblüten Aalhornblüten Fliedertee Schwitztee
40	Ephedra (Ma huang)	*Ephedra sinica*	Ephedrae herba	—	—	Ephedrakraut
41	Eucalyptus—leaf	*Eucalyptus globulus*	Eucalypti folium	Eucalipto	Eucalyptus	Eucalyptusblätter Eucalyptusöl
42	Evening primrose	*Oenothera biennis*	—	Flor de San Juan	—	
43	Eyebright	*Euphrasia officinalis*	Euphrasiae herba	Eufrasia	Euphraise	Augentrostkraut
44	Fennel—seed	*Foeniculum vulgare*	Foeniculi fructus	Hinojo	Fenouil amer	Fenchel Bitterfenchel Fenchelöl
45	Fenugreek	*Trigonella foenum-graecum*	Foenugraeci semen	Feno-grego	Fenugrec	Bockshornsamen Griechische Heusamen
46	Feverfew	*Tanacetum parthenium*	—	Altamisa mexicana	—	—
47	Flaxseed/linseed	*Linum usitatissimum*	Lini semen	Linaza	Lin (graíne de)	Leinsamen
48	Foxglove	*Digitalis purpurea*	—	—	—	—
49	Garlic	*Allium sativum*	Allii sativi bulbus	Ajo	Ail	Knoblauchzwiebel
50	Germander	*Teucrium chamaedrys*	—	Camedrio Carnesio	Germandrée	Gamanderkraut
51	Ginkgo—leaf	*Ginkgo biloba*	Ginkgo folium	Ginkgo biloba	Ginkgo biloba	Ginkgobaum Ginkgoblätter
52	Ginger	*Zingiber officinale*	Zingiberis rhizoma	Ajenjibre Agenjibre Gengibre	Gingembre	Ingwer Ingberwurzel Ingwerwurzelstock
53	Ginseng—root	*Panax ginseng*	Ginseng radix	Ginseng	Ginseng	Ginsengwurzel Kraftwurzel
54	Ginseng, Siberian	*Eleutherococcus senticosus*	—	—	—	Stachelpanax

Continued

Tables

Herb Chart (continued)

	ENGLISH	LATIN	PHARMACOPOEIAL	SPANISH	FRENCH	GERMAN
55	Goldenseal	Hydrastis canadensis	—	Cáñamo silvestre	Hydrastis	Goldsiegel
56	Gotu kola	Centella asiatica	—			
57	Hawthorn—leaf/flower	Crataegus laevigata	Crataegi folium cum flore	Espino blanco	Aubépine fleur	Weißdornblätter mit Blüten Hagedorn
	Hawthorn—berry		Crataegi fructus		Fruits d'aubépine	Weißdornfrüchte Hagedornbeeren
58	Hops	Humulus lupulus	Lupuli strobulus Lupuli glandula	Lupulo	Houblon	Hopfen Hopfenzapfen Hopfendrüsen
59	Horse chestnut—seed	Aesculus hippocastanum	Hippocastani semen	Castaño de Indias	Marron d'Inde	Roßkastaniensamen Roßkastanienblüten
60	Kava kava	Piper methysticum	Piperis methystici rhizoma	Kava-kava	Kawa kawa	Kawa Kawa Kava-Kava-Wurzelstock
61	Kelp	Laminaria, Macrocystis, Nereocystis, Fucus species	Laminariae stipites	—	—	Laminariastiele
62	Khat	Catha edulis	—	Té de Arabia	—	Katstrauch
63	Lemon balm	Melissa officinalis	Melissae folium	Toronjil Melisa	Melisse	Melissenblätter Zitronenkraut Zitronenmelisse
64	Licorice—root	Glycyrrhiza glabra	Liquiritiae radix	Amolillo Palo Dulce Regalíz	Réglisse	Süßholzwurzel Spanisches or Russisches Süßholz Lakritzenwurzel
65	Limeflower (linden)—flower	Tilia cordata	Tiliae flos	Tilia	Tilleul	Lindenblüten
66	Lobelia	Lobelia inflata	—	Lobelia	Lobélie	Lobelienkraut
67	Marshmallow—leaf	Althaea officinalis	Althaeae folium	Altea Malvavisco	Guimauve	Eibischblätter Altheeblätter
	Marshmallow—root		Althaeae radix		Guimauve racine	Eibischwurzel Schleimwurzel
68	Mate	Ilex paraguariensis	Mate folium	Mate Yerba maté	Thé du Paraguay	Mateblätter
69	Milk thistle—fruit	Silybum marianum	Cardui mariae fructus	Cardo Mariano	Chardon Marie	Mariendistelfrüchte Marienkörner Frauendistelfrüchte
	Milk thistle—herb		Cardui mariae herba			Mariendistelkraut
70	Motherwort	Leonurus cardiaca	Leonuri cardiacae herba	Agripalma cardíaca	Léonure cardiaque	Herzgespannkraut
71	Mullein	Verbascum thapsus	Verbasci flos	Punchon Gordolobo	Bouillon blanc	Wollblumen Königskerzenblumen Windblumen
72	Neem	Azadirachta indica	—	—	—	
73	Nettle (stinging nettle)—herb	Urtica dioica	Urticae herba—herb	Ortiga verde	Ortie	Brennesselkraut Haarnesselkraut Hanfnesselkraut
74	Osha	Ligusticum porteri	—	Oshá Chuchupate	—	
75	Passion flower	Passiflora incarnata	Passiflorae herba	Pasionaria Granadilla	Passiflore	Passionsblumenkraut Fleischfarbige Passionsblume
76	Pau d'arco	Tabebuia impetiginosa	—	—	—	
77	Peppermint—leaf	Mentha x piperita	Menthae piperitae folium	Menta	Menthe poivrée Feuilles de menthe	Pfefferminzblätter Katzenkraut
78	Pennyroyal	Mentha pulegium (European pennyroyal) Hedeoma pulegioides (American pennyroyal)	—	Poleo	Menthe pouliot	Poleiminze

Continued

Herb Chart (continued)

	ENGLISH	LATIN	PHARMACOPOEIAL	SPANISH	FRENCH	GERMAN
79	Plantain	Plantago lanceolata	Plantaginis lanceolatae folium Plantaginis lanceolatae herba	Lantén	Feuilles (Herbe) de plantain Psyllium blond d'Allemagne	Spitzwegerichblätter Heil- or Wundwegerich Spitzwegerichkraut
80	Black psyllium—seed (psyllium, French psyllium)	Plantago psyllium or P. indica	Psyllíí semen	—	Semences (graines) de puces	Flohsamen Heusamen
	Blonde psyllium—seed (ispaghula)	Plantago ovata	Plantaginis ovatae semen		Ispagul	Indische Flohsamen Indisches Psyllium
81	Pygeum	Prunus africana	—	—	—	—
82	Raspberry—leaf	Rubus idaeus R. strigosus	Rubi idaei folium	Zarzamora	Feuille de framboisier	Himbeerblätter
83	Red clover	Trifolium pratense	—	Trébol rojo	Trèfle rouge	Rotklee
84	Rosemary	Rosmarinus officinalis	Rosmarini folium	Romero	Romarin	Rosmarinblätter Krankraut- or Kranzenkrautblätter
85	Sage	Salvia officinalis	Salviae folium	Salvia	Sauge	Salbeiblätter Edelsalbei Gartensalbei
86	Sarsaparilla	Smilax aristolochiifolia	Sarsaparillae radix	Zarzaparilla Zarzaparrilla	Salsepareille	Sarsaparillewurzel Sarsaparillwurzel
87	Sassafras	Sassafras albidum	Sassafras lignum	Sasafras	Bois de Sassafras	Sassafrasholz Fenchelholz
88	Saw palmetto	Serenoa repens	Sabal fructus	Sabal	Serenoa	Sägepalme Sabalfrüchte
89	Senna—leaf Senna—pod	Senna alexandrina	Sennae folium Sennae fructus	Té de Sena Senna hojas	Séné	Sennesblätter Alexandriner-Sennesfrüchte Tinnevelly-Sennesfrüchte Alexandriner-Sennesfrüchte Sennesfrüchte
90	Skullcap	Scutellaria lateriflora	—	—	—	—
91	Slippery elm	Ulmus rubra	—	—	—	—
92	St. John's wort	Hypericum perforatum	Hyperici herba	Corazoncillo	Millepertuis	Johanniskraut Blutkraut Herrgottsblut Walpurgiskraut Hexenkraut
93	Stevia	Stevia rebaudiana	—	—	Stévia	Stevia
94	Tea tree	Melaleuca alternifolia	—	—		
95	Thyme	Thymus vulgaris	Thymi herba	Tomillo	Thym	Garten-Thymian Gemeiner Thymian Thymiankraut
96	Turmeric	Curcuma longa	Curcumae longae rhizoma	Cúrcuma	Curcuma	Kurkumawurzelstock Gelbwurzel Curcumawurzelstock Gelbwürz
97	Valerian	Valeriana officinalis	Valerianae radix	Valeriana	Valériane	Baldrianwurzel Katzenwurzel Balderbrackenwurzel
98	Wild yam	Dioscorea villosa	—	—	—	—
99	White willow	Salix alba	Salicis cortex	Jarita Sauce blanco	Saule blanc	Weidenrinde Fieberweidenrinde Maiholzrinde
100	Wormwood, Bitter	Artemisia absinthium	Absinthii herba	Agenjo/Ajenjo (A. mexicana) Estafiate (A. ludoviciana)	Absinthe	Wermutkraut Bitterer Beifuß Wurmkraut
101	Wormwood, Sweet (Quinghaosu)	Artemisia annua	—	—	—	—

Continued

Tables

Herb Chart   (continued)

	ENGLISH	LATIN	PHARMACOPOEIAL	SPANISH	FRENCH	GERMAN
102	Yarrow—herb	*Achillea millefolium*	Millefolii herba	Plumajillo	Achillée millefeuille	Schafgarbenkraut Achilleskraut Bauchwehkraut Katzenkraut Jungfraukraut
103	Yohimbe	*Pausinystalia yohimbe*	Yohimbehe cortex	—	—	Yohimberinde

Conversion Factors Between Traditional and SI Units

Factors for converting nutrients expressed in metric or milliequivalent units into International System (SI) units.

1. Definitions
   a. Equivalent weight (EW) = atomic weight of element/valence of ionic form. Example with magnesium: atomic wt = 24, valence = 2+; therefore EW = 12
   b. Quantity of an electrolyte in milliequivalents per liter (meq/L) = mg of electrolyte/L/EW.
      Example: 48 mg of magnesium/L/12 = 4 meq/L
   c. Quantity of an electrolyte in mg/dL = (meq/L × EW)/10
   d. To convert mg/dL (= mg%) of an electrolyte to meq/L: mg/dL × 10/EW = meq/L
   e. 1 mol = 1 molecular or atomic weight of element or compound in grams (GMWt). In solutions this is usually expressed as moles per liter; i.e., 1 mol/L = 1 M; 1 mM (mmol) = 1 mol × 10^{-3}, 1 μM (μmol) = 1 mol × 10^{-6}; 1 nM (nmol) = 1 mol × 10^{-9}
   f.
      (1) To convert meq/L of an electrolyte or other ions in solution to mmol/L: meq/L divided by valence = mmol/L; e.g., (a) 2 meq/L of magnesium (Mg^{2+}) = 2/2 = 1 mmol/L; e.g., (b) 140 meq Na^+/L = 140/1 = 140 mmol/L
      (2) To convert mg/dL to mmol/L: (mg/dL × 10/EW) divided by valence = mmol/L; e.g., 2 mg/dL of magnesium = (2 × 10/12) divided by 2 = 0.83 mmol/L
      (3) For organic substances: mmol/L = wt in mg/L/MW (in mg)

2. SI units for expressing clinical laboratory data
   These units are now widely used and are increasingly required for publication of scientific data in physical, biologic, and biomedical publication. Extensive SI conversion tables have been published together with an explanation of the rationale for their use and technical aspects of usage (1–3)

   a. The base units of interest in physical quantities used in clinical chemistry are

Quantity	Base Unit
mass	kilogram
time	second
amount	mole
length	meter

   A derived unit for energy is the kjoule (kJ) 4.18 kJ = 1 kcal
   1 MJ = 239 kcal

   b. Prefixes and symbols for decimal multiples and submultiples include

FACTOR	PREFIX	SYMBOL	FACTOR	PREFIX	SYMBOL
10^9	giga	G	10^{-3}	milli	m
10^6	mega	M	10^{-6}	micro	μ
10^3	kilo	k	10^{-9}	nano	n
10^2	hecto	h	10^{-12}	pico	p
10^1	deca	da	10^{-15}	femto	f
10^{-1}	deci	d	10^{-18}	atto	a
10^{-2}	centi	c			

3. Conversion factors for selected compounds of nutrition interest[a]

COMPONENT	(1) PRESENT UNIT	(2) CONVERSION FACTOR	(3) SI UNIT SYMBOL	(4) MASS CONVERSION FACTOR
Albumin (s)	g/dL	10	g/L	—
Aluminum (s)	μg/L	37.04	nmol/L	μg/27 = mol
Amino acid nitrogen (p)	mg/dL	0.714	mmol/L	mg/14 = mmol
Ascorbic acid (p)	mg/dL	56.78	μmol/L	mg/176 = mmol
Calcium (s)	mg/dL	0.250	mmol/L	mg/40 = mmol
Calcium (s)	meq/dL	0.500	mmol/L	meq/2 = mmol
β-Carotene (s)	μ/dL	0.0186	μmol/L	μg/536.85 μmol
Chloride (s)	meq/L	1.00	mmol/L	meq = mmol
Cholesterol (p)	mg/dL	0.0259	mmol/L	mg/386.6 = mmol
Cobalamin (B_{12})	pg/mL	0.738	pmol/L	pg/1355 = pmol
Copper (s)	μg/dL	0.157	μmol/L	μg/63.5 = μmol
Ethanol (p)	mg/dL	0.217	mmol/L	mg/46 = mmol
Folic acid	ng/mL	2.265	nmol/L	ng/441.4 = nmol
Glucose (p)	mg/dL	0.0555	mmol/L	mg/180.2 = mmol
Iron (s)	μg/dL	0.179	μmol/L	μg/55.9 = μmol
Phosphate (p) (as phosphorus)	mg/dL	0.323	mmol/L	mg/31 = mmol
Potassium (s)	meq/L	1.000	mmol/L	meq = mmol
Potassium	mg/dL	0.256	mmol/L	mg/39.1 = mmol
Magnesium (s)	mg/dL	0.411	mmol/L	mg/24.3 = mmol
Pyridoxal (B)	ng/mL	5.981	nmol/L	ng/167 = nmol
Retinol[b] (p,s)	μg/dL	0.0349	μmol/L	μg/286 = μmol
Riboflavin (s)	μg/dL	26.57	nmol/L	μg/376 = nmol
Sodium (s)	meq/L	1.00	mmol/L	meq = mmol
Thiamin HCl (U)	μg/24 h	0.00298	μmol/d	μg/337 = μmol
α-Tocopherol (p)	mg/dL	23.22	μmol/L	μg/431 = μmol
Vitamin D_3	μg/dL	26.01	nmol/L	μg/384 = nmol
Calcidiol	ng/mL	2.498	nmol/L	ng/400 = nmol
Zinc (s)	μg/dL	0.153	μmol/L	μg/65.4 = μmol

[a]To convert metric or equivalent unit per unit volume (column 1) to SI units per liter (column 3), multiply by the conversion factor in column 2. p, plasma; s, serum; B, blood; U, urine.

References

1. Young DS. *Ann Intern Med* 1987;106:114.

2. Lundberg GD, Iberson C, Radulescu G. *JAMA* 1986;255:2329.

3. Monsen ER. *J Am Diet Assoc* 1987;87:356.

Tables

Dietary Reference Intakes: Vitamins

NUTRIENT	FUNCTION	LIFE STAGE GROUP	RDA/AI*	UL[a]	SELECTED FOOD SOURCES	ADVERSE EFFECTS OF EXCESSIVE CONSUMPTION	SPECIAL CONSIDERATIONS
Biotin	Coenzyme in synthesis of fat, glycogen, and amino acids	Infants	(µg/d)		Liver and smaller amounts in fruits and meats	No adverse effects of biotin in humans or animals were found. This does not mean that there is no potential for adverse effects resulting from high intakes. Because data on the adverse effects of biotin are limited, caution may be warranted.	None
		0–6 mo	5*	ND[b]			
		7–12 mo	6*	ND			
		Children					
		1–3 yr	8*	ND			
		4–8 yr	12*	ND			
		Males					
		9–13 yr	20*	ND			
		14–18 yr	25*	ND			
		19–30 yr	30*	ND			
		31–50 yr	30*	ND			
		50–70 yr	30*	ND			
		>70 yr	30*	ND			
		Females					
		9–13 yr	20*	ND			
		14–18 yr	25*	ND			
		19–30 yr	30*	ND			
		31–50 yr	30*	ND			
		50–70 yr	30*	ND			
		>70 yr	30*	ND			
		Pregnancy					
		≤18 yr	30*	ND			
		19–30 yr	30*	ND			
		31–50 yr	30*	ND			
		Lactation					
		≤18 yr	35*	ND			
		19–30 yr	35*	ND			
		31–50 yr	35*	ND			
Choline	Precursor for acetylcholine, phospholipids and betaine	Infants	(mg/d)	(mg/d)	Milk, liver, eggs, peanuts	Fishy body odor, sweating, salivation, hypotension, hepatotoxicity.	Individuals with trimethylaminuria, renal disease, liver disease, depression and Parkinson's disease may be at risk of adverse effects with choline intakes at the UL. Although AIs have been set for choline, there are few data to assess whether a dietary supply of choline is needed at all stages of the life cycle, and it may be that the choline requirement can be met by endogenous synthesis at some of these stages.
		0–6 mo	125*	ND			
		7–12 mo	150*	ND			
		Children					
		1–3 yr	200*	1,000			
		4–8 yr	250*	1,000			
		Males					
		9–13 yr	375*	2,000			
		14–18 yr	550*	3,000			
		19–30 yr	550*	3,500			
		31–50 yr	550*	3,500			
		50–70 yr	550*	3,500			
		>70 yr					
		Females					
		9–13 yr	375*	2,000			
		14–18 yr	400*	3,000			
		19–30 yr	425*	3,500			
		31–50 yr	425*	3,500			
		31–50 yr	425*	3,500			
		50–70 yr	425*	3,500			
		>70 yr	425*	3,500			
		Pregnancy					
		≤18 yr	450*	3,000			
		19–30 yr	450*	3,500			
		31–50 yr	450*	3,500			
		Lactation					
		≤18 yr	550*	3,000			
		19–30 yr	550*	3,500			
		31–50 yr	550*	3,500			

Continued

Tables

Dietary Reference Intakes: Vitamins (continued)

NUTRIENT	FUNCTION	LIFE STAGE GROUP	RDA/AI*	UL[a]	SELECTED FOOD SOURCES	ADVERSE EFFECTS OF EXCESSIVE CONSUMPTION	SPECIAL CONSIDERATIONS
Folate	Coenzyme in the metabolism of nucleic and amino acids; prevents megaloblastic anemia	Infants	(µg/d)	(µg/d)	Enriched cereal grains, dark leafy vegetables, enriched and whole-grain breads and bread products, fortified ready-to-eat cereals	Masks neurologic complication in people with vitamin B₁₂ deficiency.	In view of evidence linking folate intake with neural tube defects in the fetus, it is recommended that all women capable of becoming pregnant consume 400 µg from supplements or fortified foods in addition to intake of food folate from a varied diet.
Also known as:		0–6 mo	65*	ND[b]			
Folic acid		7–12 mo	80*	ND		No adverse effects associated with folate from food or supplements have been reported. This does not mean that there is no potential for adverse effects resulting from high intakes. Because data on the adverse effects of folate are limited, caution may be warranted.	
Folacin		Children					
Pteroylpolyglutamates		1–3 yr	150	300			
Note: Given as dietary folate equivalents (DFE).		4–8 yr	200	400			
		Males					
1 DFE = 1 µg		9–13 yr	300	600			
food folate = 0.6 µg		14–18 yr	400	800			
of folate from		19–30 yr	400	1,000			
fortified food or as		31–50 yr	400	1,000			
a supplement		50–70 yr	400	1,000			
consumed with		>70 yr	400	1,000			
food = 0.5 µg of a		Females				The UL for folate applies to synthetic forms obtained from supplements and/or fortified foods.	It is assumed that women will continue consuming 400 µg from supplements or fortified food until their pregnancy is confirmed and they enter prenatal care, which ordinarily occurs after the end of the periconceptional period—the critical time for formation of the neural tube.
supplement taken		9–13 yr	300	600			
on an empty		14–18 yr	400	800			
stomach		19–30 yr	400	1,000			
		31–50 yr	400	1,000			
		50–70 yr	400	1,000			
		>70 yr	400	1,000			
		Pregnancy					
		≤18 yr	600	800			
		19–30 yr	600	1,000			
		31–50 yr	600	1,000			
		Lactation					
		≤18 yr	500	800			
		19–30 yr	500	1,000			
		31–50 yr	500	1,000			
Niacin	Coenzyme or cosubstrate in many biologic reduction and oxidation reactions—thus required for energy metabolism	Infants	(mg/d)	(mg/d)	Meat, fish, poultry, enriched and whole-grain breads and bread products, fortified ready-to-eat cereals	There is no evidence of adverse effects from the consumption of naturally occurring niacin in foods.	Extra niacin may be required by persons treated with hemodialysis or peritoneal dialysis, or those with malabsorption syndrome.
Includes nicotinic acid amide, nicotinic acid (pyridine-3-carboxylic acid), and derivatives that exhibit the biologic activity of nicotinamide.		0–6 mo	2*	ND			
		7–12 mo	4*	ND			
		Children					
		1–3 yr	6	10			
		4–8 yr	8	15		Adverse effects from niacin containing supplements may include flushing and gastrointestinal distress.	
		Males					
		9–13 yr	12	20			
		14–18 yr	16	30			
		19–30 yr	16	35			
Note: Given as niacin equivalents (NE).		31–50 yr	16	35			
		50–70 yr	16	35			
1 mg of niacin = 60 mg of tryptophan;		>70 yr	16	35			
		Females				The UL for niacin applies to synthetic forms obtained from supplements, fortified foods, or a combination of the two.	
0–6 months = preformed niacin (not NE).		9–13 yr	12	20			
		14–18 yr	14	30			
		19–30 yr	14	35			
		31–50 yr	14	35			
		50–70 yr	14	35			
		>70 yr	14	35			
		Pregnancy					
		≤18 yr	18	30			
		19–30 yr	18	35			
		31–50 yr	18	35			
		Lactation					
		≤18 yr	17	30			
		19–30 yr	17	35			
		31–50 yr	17	35			

Continued

Tables

Dietary Reference Intakes: Vitamins (continued)

NUTRIENT	FUNCTION	LIFE STAGE GROUP	RDA/AI*	ULa	SELECTED FOOD SOURCES	ADVERSE EFFECTS OF EXCESSIVE CONSUMPTION	SPECIAL CONSIDERATIONS
Pantothenic acid	Coenzyme in fatty acid metabolism	Infants	(mg/d)	(mg/d)	Chicken, beef, potatoes, oats, cereals, tomato products, liver, kidney, yeast, egg yolk, broccoli, whole grains	No adverse effects associated with pantothenic acid from food or supplements have been reported. This does not mean that there is no potential for adverse effects resulting from high intakes. Because data on the adverse effects of pantothenic acid are limited, caution may be warranted.	None
		0–6 mo	1.7*	NDb			
		7–12 mo	1.8*	ND			
		Children					
		1–3 yr	2*	ND			
		4–8 yr	3*	ND			
		Males					
		9–13 yr	4*	ND			
		14–18 yr	5*	ND			
		19–30 yr	5*	ND			
		31–50 yr	5*	ND			
		50–70 yr	5*	ND			
		>70 yr	5*	ND			
		Females					
		9–13 yr	4*	ND			
		14–18 yr	5*	ND			
		19–30 yr	5*	ND			
		31–50 yr	5*	ND			
		50–70 yr	5*	ND			
		>70 yr	5*	ND			
		Pregnancy					
		≤18 yr	6*	ND			
		19–30 yr	6*	ND			
		31–50 yr	6*	ND			
		Lactation					
		≤18 yr	7*	ND			
		19–30 yr	7*	ND			
		31–50 yr	7*	ND			
Riboflavin *Also known as:* Vitamin B₂	Coenzyme in numerous redox reactions	Infants	(mg/d)	(mg/d)	Organ meats, milk, bread products, and fortified cereals	No adverse effects associated with riboflavin consumption from food or supplements have been reported. This does not mean that there is no potential for adverse effects resulting from high intakes. Because data on the adverse effects of riboflavin are limited, caution may be warranted.	None
		0–6 mo	0.3*	ND			
		7–12 mo	0.4*	ND			
		Children					
		1–3 yr	**0.5**	ND			
		4–8 yr	**0.6**	ND			
		Males					
		9–13 yr	**0.9**	ND			
		14–18 yr	**1.3**	ND			
		19–30 yr	**1.3**	ND			
		31–50 yr	**1.3**	ND			
		50–70 yr	**1.3**	ND			
		>70 yr	**1.3**	ND			
		Females					
		9–13 yr	**0.9**	ND			
		14–18 yr	**1.0**	ND			
		19–30 yr	**1.1**	ND			
		31–50 yr	**1.1**	ND			
		50–70 yr	**1.1**	ND			
		>70 yr	**1.1**	ND			
		Pregnancy					
		≤18 yr	**1.4**	ND			
		19–30 yr	**1.4**	ND			
		31–50 yr	**1.4**	ND			
		Lactation					
		≤18 yr	**1.6**	ND			
		19–30 yr	**1.6**	ND			
		31–50 yr	**1.6**	ND			

Continued

Dietary Reference Intakes: Vitamins (continued)

NUTRIENT	FUNCTION	LIFE STAGE GROUP	RDA/AI*	UL[a]	SELECTED FOOD SOURCES	ADVERSE EFFECTS OF EXCESSIVE CONSUMPTION	SPECIAL CONSIDERATIONS
Thiamin *Also known as:* Vitamin B$_1$ Aneurin	Coenzyme in the metabolism of carbohydrates and branched-chain amino acids	Infants 0–6 mo 7–12 mo Children 1–3 yr 4–8 yr Males 9–13 yr 14–18 yr 19–30 yr 31–50 yr 50–70 yr >70 yr Females 9–13 yr 14–18 yr 19–30 yr 31–50 yr 50–70 yr >70 yr Pregnancy ≤18 yr 19–30 yr 31–50 yr Lactation ≤18 yr 19–30 yr 31–50 yr	(mg/d) 0.2* 0.8* 0.5 0.6 0.9 1.2 1.2 1.2 1.2 1.2 0.9 1.0 1.1 1.1 1.1 1.1 1.4 1.4 1.4 1.4 1.4 1.4	(mg/d) ND[b] ND ND ND ND ND ND ND ND ND ND ND ND ND ND ND ND ND ND ND ND ND	Enriched, fortified, or whole-grain products; bread, and bread products; mixed foods whose main ingredient is grain; and ready-to-eat cereals	No adverse effects associated with thiamin from food or supplements have been reported. This does not mean that there is no potential for adverse effects resulting from high intakes. Because data on the adverse effects of thiamin are limited, caution may be warranted.	Persons who may have increased needs for thiamin include those being treated with hemodialysis or peritoneal dialysis, or individuals with malabsorption syndrome.
Vitamin A Includes provitamin A carotenoids that are dietary precursors of retinol. Note: Given as retinol activity equivalents (RAEs). 1 RAE = 1 µg retinol, 12 µg β-carotene, 24 µg α-carotene, or 24 µg β-cryptoxanthin. To calculate RAEs from REs of provitamin A carotenoids in foods, divide the REs by 2. For preformed vitamin A in foods or supplements and for provitamin A carotenoids in supplements 1 RE = 1 RAE.	Required for normal vision, gene expression, reproduction, embryonic development, and immune function	Infants 0–6 mo 7–12 mo Children 1–3 yr 4–8 yr Males 9–13 yr 14–18 yr 19–30 yr 31–50 yr 50–70 yr >70 yr Females 9–13 yr 14–18 yr 19–30 yr 31–50 yr 50–70 yr >70 yr Pregnancy ≤18 yr 19–30 yr 31–50 yr Lactation ≤18 yr 19–30 yr 31–50 yr	(µg/d) 400* 500* 300 400 600 900 900 900 900 900 600 700 700 700 700 700 750 770 770 1,200 1,300 1,300	(µg/d) 600 600 600 900 1,700 2,800 3,000 3,000 3,000 3,000 1,700 2,800 3,000 3,000 3,000 3,000 2,800 3,000 3,000 2,800 3,000 3,000	Liver, dairy products, fish	Teratological effects, liver toxicity. Note: From preformed Vitamin A only.	Individuals with high alcohol intake, pre-existing liver disease, hyperlipidemia or severe protein malnutrition may be distinctly susceptible to the adverse effects of excess preformed vitamin A intake. β-carotene supplements are advised only to serve as a provitamin A source for individuals at risk of vitamin A deficiency.

Continued

Tables

Dietary Reference Intakes: Vitamins   (continued)

NUTRIENT	FUNCTION	LIFE STAGE GROUP	RDA/AI*	ULᵃ	SELECTED FOOD SOURCES	ADVERSE EFFECTS OF EXCESSIVE CONSUMPTION	SPECIAL CONSIDERATIONS
Vitamin B$_6$	Coenzyme in the	Infants	(mg/d)	(mg/d)	Fortified cereals,	No adverse effects	None
Vitamin B$_6$	metabolism of	0–6 mo	0.1*	ND^b	organ meats,	associated with	
comprises a group	amino acids,	7–12 mo	0.3*	ND	fortified soy-based	vitamin B$_6$ from	
of six related	glycogen, and	Children			meat substitutes	food have been	
compounds:	sphingoid bases	1–3 yr	0.5	30		reported. This does	
pyridoxal, pyridoxine,		4–8 yr	0.6	40		not mean that	
pyridoxamine, and		Males				there is no	
5'-phosphates (PLP,		9–13 yr	1.0	60		potential for	
PNP, PMP)		14–18 yr	1.3	80		adverse effects	
		19–30 yr	1.3	100		resulting from high	
		31–50 yr	1.3	100		intakes. Because	
		50–70 yr	1.7	100		data on the adverse	
		>70 yr	1.7	100		effects of vitamin	
		Females				B$_6$ are limited,	
		9–13 yr	1.0	60		caution may be	
		14–18 yr	1.2	80		warranted.	
		19–30 yr	1.3	100		Sensory neuropathy	
		31–50 yr	1.3	100		has occurred from	
		50–70 yr	1.5	100		high intakes of	
		>70 yr	1.5	100		supplemental forms.	
		Pregnancy					
		≤18 yr	1.9	80			
		19–30 yr	1.9	100			
		31–50 yr	1.9	100			
		Lactation					
		≤18 yr	2.0	80			
		19–30 yr	2.0	100			
		31–50 yr	2.0	100			
Vitamin B$_{12}$	Coenzyme in nucleic	Infants	(μg/d)		Fortified cereals,	No adverse effects	Because 10% to
Also known as:	acid metabolism;	0–6 mo	0.4*	ND	meat, fish, poultry	have been	30% of older
Cobalamin	prevents	7–12 mo	0.5*	ND		associated with	people may
	megaloblastic	Children				the consumption	malabsorb food-
	anemia	1–3 yr	0.9	ND		of the amounts of	bound vitamin B$_{12}$,
		4–8 yr	1.2	ND		vitamin B$_{12}$ normally	it is advisable for
		Males				found in foods or	those older than 50
		9–13 yr	1.8	ND		supplements. This	years to meet their
		14–18 yr	2.4	ND		does not mean that	RDA mainly by
		19–30 yr	2.4	ND		there is no	consuming foods
		31–50 yr	2.4	ND		potential for	fortified with
		50–70 yr	2.4	ND		adverse effects	vitamin B$_{12}$ or a
		>70 yr	2.4	ND		resulting from high	supplement
		Females				intakes. Because	containing vitamin
		9–13 yr	1.8	ND		data on the adverse	B$_{12}$.
		14–18 yr	2.4	ND		effects of vitamin	
		19–30 yr	2.4	ND		B$_{12}$ are limited,	
		31–50 yr	2.4	ND		caution may be	
		50–70 yr	2.4	ND		warranted.	
		>70 yr	2.4	ND			
		Pregnancy					
		≤18 yr	2.6	ND			
		19–30 yr	2.6	ND			
		31–50 yr	2.6	ND			
		Lactation					
		≤18 yr	2.8	ND			
		19–30 yr	2.8	ND			
		31–50 yr	2.8	ND			

Continued

Dietary Reference Intakes: Vitamins   (continued)

NUTRIENT	FUNCTION	LIFE STAGE GROUP	RDA/AI*	UL[a]	SELECTED FOOD SOURCES	ADVERSE EFFECTS OF EXCESSIVE CONSUMPTION	SPECIAL CONSIDERATIONS
Vitamin C	Cofactor for reactions	Infants	(mg/d)	(mg/d)	Citrus fruits,	Gastrointestinal	Individuals who
Also known as:	requiring reduced	0–6 mo	40*	ND[b]	tomatoes, tomato	disturbances,	smoke require an
Ascorbic acid	copper or iron	7–12 mo	50*	ND	juice, potatoes,	kidney stones,	additional 35 mg/d
Dehydroascorbic acid	metalloenzyme and	Children			Brussels sprouts,	excess iron	of vitamin C over
(DHA)	as a protective	1–3 yr	15	400	cauliflower, broccoli,	absorption	that needed by
	antioxidant	4–8 yr	25	650	strawberries,		nonsmokers.
		Males			cabbage, and		Nonsmokers
		9–13 yr	45	1,200	spinach		regularly exposed
		14–18 yr	75	1,800			to tobacco smoke
		19–30 yr	90	2,000			are encouraged
		31–50 yr	90	2,000			to ensure they
		50–70 yr	90	2,000			meet the RDA for
		>70 yr	90	2,000			vitamin C.
		Females					
		9–13 yr	45	1,200			
		14–18 yr	65	1,800			
		19–30 yr	75	2,000			
		31–50 yr	75	2,000			
		50–70 yr	75	2,000			
		>70 yr	75	2,000			
		Pregnancy					
		≤18 yr	80	1,800			
		19–30 yr	85	2,000			
		31–50 yr	85	2,000			
		Lactation					
		≤18 yr	115	1,800			
		19–30 yr	120	2,000			
		31–50 yr	120	2,000			
Vitamin D	Maintain serum	Infants	(µg/d)	(µg/d)	Fish liver oils, flesh	Elevated plasma	Patients on
Also known as:	calcium and	0–6 mo	5*	25	of fatty fish, liver	25 (OH) D	glucocorticoid
Calciferol	phosphorus	7–12 mo	5*	25	and fat from seals	concentration	therapy may
Note: 1 µg calciferol	concentrations	Children			and polar bears,	causing	require additional
= 40 IU vitamin D		4–8 yr	5*	50	eggs from hens	hypercalcemia	vitamin D.
The DRI values are		Males			that have been fed		
based on the		9–13 yr	5*	50	vitamin D, fortified		
absence of adequate		14–18 yr	5*	50	milk products, and		
exposure to sunlight.		19–30 yr	5*	50	fortified cereals		
		31–50 yr	5*	50			
		1–3 yr	5*	50			
		50–70 yr	10*	50			
		>70 yr	15*	50			
		Females					
		9–13 yr	5*	50			
		14–18 yr	5*	50			
		19–30 yr	5*	50			
		31–50 yr	5*	50			
		50–70 yr	10*	50			
		>70 yr	15*	50			
		Pregnancy					
		≤18 yr	5*	50			
		19–30 yr	5*	50			
		31–50 yr	5*	50			
		Lactation					
		≤18 yr	5*	50			
		19–30 yr	5*	50			
		31–50 yr	5*	50			

Continued

Tables

Dietary Reference Intakes: Vitamins   (continued)

NUTRIENT	FUNCTION	LIFE STAGE GROUP	RDA/AI*	UL^a	SELECTED FOOD SOURCES	ADVERSE EFFECTS OF EXCESSIVE CONSUMPTION	SPECIAL CONSIDERATIONS
Vitamin E	A metabolic function has not yet been identified. Vitamin E's major function appears to be as a non-specific chain-breaking antioxidant.	Infants	(mg/d)	(mg/d)	Vegetable oils, unprocessed cereal grains, nuts, fruits, vegetables, meats	There is no evidence of adverse effects from the consumption of vitamin E naturally occurring in foods. Adverse effects from vitamin E containing supplements may include hemorrhagic toxicity.† The UL for vitamin E applies to any form of α-tocopherol obtained from supplements, fortified foods, or a combination of the two.	Patients on anticoagulant therapy should be monitored when taking vitamin E supplements.†
Also known as: α-tocopherol Note: As α-tocopherol. α-Tocopherol includes *RRR*-α-tocopherol, the only form of α-tocopherol that occurs naturally in foods, and the *2R*-stereoisomeric forms of α-tocopherol (*RRR-, RSR-, RRS-,* and *RSS*-α-tocopherol) that occur in fortified foods and supplements. It does not include the 2S-stereoisomeric forms of α-tocopherol (*SRR-, SSR-, SRS-,* and *SSS*-α-tocopherol), also found in fortified foods and supplements.		0–6 mo	4*	ND^b			
		7–12 mo	5*	ND			
		Children					
		1–3 yr	6	200			
		4–8 yr	7	300			
		Males					
		9–13 yr	11	600			
		14–18 yr	15	800			
		19–30 yr	15	1,000			
		31–50 yr	15	1,000			
		50–70 yr	15	1,000			
		>70 yr	15	1,000			
		Females					
		9–13 yr	11	600			
		14–18 yr	15	800			
		19–30 yr	15	1,000			
		31–50 yr	15	1,000			
		50–70 yr	15	1,000			
		>70 yr	15	1,000			
		Pregnancy					
		≤18 yr	15	800			
		19–30 yr	15	1,000			
		31–50 yr	15	1,000			
		Lactation					
		≤18 yr	19	800			
		19–30 yr	19	1,000			
		31–50 yr	19	1,000			
Vitamin K	Coenzyme during the synthesis of many proteins involved in blood clotting and bone metabolism	Infants	(µg/d)		Green vegetables (collards, spinach, salad greens, broccoli), Brussels sprouts, cabbage, plant oils, and margarine	No adverse effects associated with vitamin K consumption from food or supplements have been reported in humans or animals. This does not mean that there is no potential for adverse effects resulting from high intakes. Because data on the adverse effects of vitamin K are limited, caution may be warranted.	Patients on anticoagulant therapy should monitor vitamin K intake.
		0–6 mo	2.0*	ND			
		7–12 mo	2.5*	ND			
		Children					
		1–3 yr	30*	ND			
		4–8 yr	55*	ND			
		Males					
		9–13 yr	60*	ND			
		14–18 yr	75*	ND			
		19–30 yr	120*	ND			
		31–50 yr	120*	ND			
		50–70 yr	120*	ND			
		>70 yr	120*	ND			
		Females					
		9–13 yr	60*	ND			
		14–18 yr	75*	ND			
		19–30 yr	90*	ND			
		31–50 yr	90*	ND			
		50–70 yr	90*	ND			
		>70 yr	90*	ND			

Continued

440

Dietary Reference Intakes: Vitamins   (continued)

NUTRIENT	FUNCTION	LIFE STAGE GROUP	RDA/AI*	UL[a]	SELECTED FOOD SOURCES	ADVERSE EFFECTS OF EXCESSIVE CONSUMPTION	SPECIAL CONSIDERATIONS
Vitamin K		Pregnancy					
(continued)		≤18 yr	75*	ND			
		19–30 yr	90*	ND			
		31–50 yr	90*	ND			
		Lactation					
		≤18 yr	75*	ND			
		19–30 yr	90*	ND			
		31–50 yr	90*	ND			

NOTE: The table is reprinted with permission from the website of the Institute of Medicine, National Academy of Sciences. The table is adapted from the DRI reports (see *www.nap.edu*). It represents recommended dietary allowances (RDAs) in **bold type**, adequate intakes (AIs) in ordinary type followed by an asterisk (*), and upper limits (ULs)[a]. RDAs and AIs may both be used as goals for individual intake. RDAs are set to meet the needs of almost all 97% to 98% individuals in a group. For healthy breastfed infants, the AI is the mean intake. The AI for other life stage and gender groups is believed to cover the needs of all individuals in the group, but lack of data prevent being able to specify with confidence the percentage of individuals covered by this intake.

[a]UL, The maximum level of daily nutrient intake that is likely to pose no risk of adverse effects. Unless otherwise specified, the UL represents total intake from food, water, and supplements. Due to lack of suitable data, ULs could not be established for vitamin K, thiamin, riboflavin, vitamin B_{12}, pantothenic acid, biotin, or carotenoids. In the absence of ULs, extra caution may be warranted in consuming levels above recommended intakes.

[b]ND, Not determinable due to lack of data of adverse effects in this age group and concern with regard to lack of ability to handle excess amounts. Source of intake should be from food only to prevent high levels of intake.

[†]Author's note: Recent research indicates that vitamin E does not increase bleeding risk. See vitamin E entry.

SOURCES: *Dietary Reference Intakes for Calcium, Phosphorous, Magnesium, Vitamin D, and Fluoride* (1997); *Dietary Reference Intakes for Thiamin, Riboflavin, Niacin, Vitamin B₆, Folate, Vitamin B₁₂, Pantothenic Acid, Biotin, and Choline* (1998); *Dietary Reference Intakes for Vitamin C, Vitamin E, Selenium, and Carotenoids* (2000); and *Dietary Reference Intakes for Vitamin A, Vitamin K, Arsenic, Boron, Chromium, Copper, Iodine, Iron, Manganese, Molybdenum, Nickel, Silicon, Vanadium, and Zinc* (2001). These reports may be accessed via www.nap.edu.

Dietary Reference Intakes: Elements

NUTRIENT	FUNCTION	LIFE STAGE GROUP	RDA/AI*	UL[a]	SELECTED FOOD SOURCES	ADVERSE EFFECTS OF EXCESSIVE CONSUMPTION	SPECIAL CONSIDERATIONS
Arsenic	No biological function in humans although animal data indicate a requirement	Infants	ND[b]	ND	Dairy products, meat, poultry, fish, grains,and cereal	No data on the possible adverse effects of organic arsenic compounds in food were found. Inorganic arsenic is a known toxic substance.	None
		0–6 mo	ND	ND			
		7–12 mo	ND	ND			
		Children					
		1–3 yr	ND	ND			
		4–8 yr	ND	ND		Although the UL was not determined for arsenic, there is no justification for adding arsenic to food or supplements.	
		Males					
		9–13 yr	ND	ND			
		14–18 yr	ND	ND			
		19–30 yr	ND	ND			
		31–50 yr	ND	ND			
		50–70 yr	ND	ND			
		>70 yr	ND	ND			
		Females					
		9–13 yr	ND	ND			
		14–18 yr	ND	ND			
		19–30 yr	ND	ND			
		31–50 yr	ND	ND			
		50–70 yr	ND	ND			
		>70 yr	ND	ND			
		Pregnancy					
		≤18 yr	ND	ND			
		19–30 yr	ND	ND			
		31–50 yr	ND	ND			
		Lactation					
		≤18 yr	ND	ND			
		19–30 yr	ND	ND			
		31–50 yr	ND	ND			

Continued

441

Tables

Dietary Reference Intakes: Elements (continued)

NUTRIENT	FUNCTION	LIFE STAGE GROUP	RDA/AI*	ULᵃ	SELECTED FOOD SOURCES	ADVERSE EFFECTS OF EXCESSIVE CONSUMPTION	SPECIAL CONSIDERATIONS
Boron	No clear biological function in humans although animal data indicate a functional role	Infants		(mg/d)	Fruit-based beverages and products, potatoes, legumes, milk, avocado, peanut butter, peanuts	Reproductive and developmental effects as observed in animal studies	None
		0–6 mo	ND	ND			
		7–12 mo	ND	ND			
		Children					
		1–3 yr	ND	3			
		4–8 yr	ND	6			
		Males					
		9–13 yr	ND	11			
		14–18 yr	ND	17			
		19–30 yr	ND	20			
		31–50 yr	ND	20			
		50–70 yr	ND	20			
		>70 yr	ND	20			
		Females					
		9–13 yr	ND	11			
		14–18 yr	ND	17			
		19–30 yr	ND	20			
		31–50 yr	ND	20			
		50–70 yr	ND	20			
		>70 yr	ND	20			
		Pregnancy					
		≤18 yr	ND	17			
		19–30 yr	ND	20			
		31–50 yr	ND	20			
		Lactation					
		≤18 yr	ND	17			
		19–30 yr	ND	20			
		31–50 yr	ND	20			
Calcium	Essential role in blood clotting, muscle contraction, nerve transmission, and bone and tooth formation	Infants	(mg/d)	(mg/d)	Milk, cheese, yogurt, corn tortillas, calcium-set tofu, Chinese cabbage, kale, broccoli	Kidney stones, hypercalcemia, milk alkali syndrome, and renal insufficiency	Amenorrheic women (exercise- or anorexia nervosa-induced) have reduced net calcium absorption.
		0–6 mo	210*	NDᵇ			
		7–12 mo	270*	ND			
		Children					
		1–3 yr	500*	2,500			
		4–8 yr	800*	2,500			There are no consistent data to support that a high protein intake increases calcium requirement.
		Males					
		9–13 yr	1,300*	2,500			
		14–18 yr	1,300*	2,500			
		19–30 yr	1,000*	2,500			
		31–50 yr	1,000*	2,500			
		50–70 yr	1,200*	2,500			
		>70 yr	1,200*	2,500			
		Females					
		9–13 yr	1,300*	2,500			
		14–18 yr	1,300*	2,500			
		19–30 yr	1,000*	2,500			
		31–50 yr	1,000*	2,500			
		50–70 yr	1,200*	2,500			
		>70 yr	1,200*	2,500			
		Pregnancy					
		≤18 yr	1,300*	2,500			
		19–30 yr	1,000*	2,500			
		31–50 yr	1,000*	2,500			
		Lactation					
		≤18 yr	1,300*	2,500			
		19–30 yr	1,000*	2,500			
		31–50 yr	1,000*	2,500			

Continued

Dietary Reference Intakes: Elements (continued)

NUTRIENT	FUNCTION	LIFE STAGE GROUP	RDA/AI*	UL[a]	SELECTED FOOD SOURCES	ADVERSE EFFECTS OF EXCESSIVE CONSUMPTION	SPECIAL CONSIDERATIONS
Chromium	Helps to maintain normal blood glucose levels	Infants	(µg/d)		Some cereals, meats, poultry, fish, beer	Chronic renal failure	Individuals with Wilson's disease, Indian childhood cirrhosis and idiopathic copper toxicosis may be at increased risk of adverse effects from excess copper intake.
		0–6 mo	0.2*	ND			
		7–12 mo	5.5*	ND			
		Children					
		1–3 yr	11*	ND			
		4–8 yr	15*	ND			
		Males					
		9–13 yr	25*	ND			
		14–18 yr	35*	ND			
		19–30 yr	35*	ND			
		31–50 yr	35*	ND			
		50–70 yr	30*	ND			
		>70 yr	30*	ND			
		Females					
		9–13 yr	21*	ND			
		14–18 yr	24*	ND			
		19–30 yr	25*	ND			
		31–50 yr	25*	ND			
		50–70 yr	20*	ND			
		>70 yr	20*	ND			
		Pregnancy					
		≤18 yr	29*	ND			
		19–30 yr	30*	ND			
		31–50 yr	30*	ND			
		Lactation					
		≤18 yr	44*	ND			
		19–30 yr	45*	ND			
		31–50 yr	45*	ND			
Copper	Component of enzymes in iron metabolism	Infants	(µg/d)	(µg/d)	Organ meats, seafood, nuts, seeds, wheat bran cereals, whole grain products, cocoa products	Gastrointestinal distress, liver damage	None
		0–6 mo	200*	ND[b]			
		7–12 mo	220*	ND			
		Children					
		1–3 yr	340	1,000			
		4–8 yr	440	3,000			
		Males					
		9–13 yr	700	5,000			
		14–18 yr	890	8,000			
		19–30 yr	900	10,000			
		31–50 yr	900	10,000			
		50–70 yr	900	10,000			
		>70 yr	900	10,000			
		Females					
		9–13 yr	700	5,000			
		14–18 yr	890	8,000			
		19–30 yr	900	10,000			
		31–50 yr	900	10,000			
		50–70 yr	900	10,000			
		>70 yr	900	10,000			
		Pregnancy					
		≤18 yr	1,000	8,000			
		19–30 yr	1,000	10,000			
		31–50 yr	1,000	10,000			
		Lactation					
		≤18 yr	1,300	8,000			
		19–30 yr	1,300	10,000			
		31–50 yr	1,300	10,000			

Continued

Tables

Dietary Reference Intakes: Elements   (continued)

NUTRIENT	FUNCTION	LIFE STAGE GROUP	RDA/AI*	UL[a]	SELECTED FOOD SOURCES	ADVERSE EFFECTS OF EXCESSIVE CONSUMPTION	SPECIAL CONSIDERATIONS
Fluoride	Inhibits the initiation and progression of dental caries and stimulates new bone formation	Infants	(mg/d)	(mg/d)	Fluoridated water, teas, marine fish, fluoridated dental products	Enamel and skeletal fluorosis	None
		0–6 mo	0.01*	0.7			
		7–12 mo	0.5*	0.9			
		Children					
		1–3 yr	0.7*	1.3			
		4–8 yr	1*	2.2			
		Males					
		9–13 yr	2*	10			
		14–18 yr	3*	10			
		19–30 yr	4*	10			
		31–50 yr	4*	10			
		50–70 yr	4*	10			
		>70 yr	4*	10			
		Females					
		9–13 yr	2*	10			
		14–18 yr	3*	10			
		19–30 yr	3*	10			
		31–50 yr	3*	10			
		50–70 yr	3*	10			
		>70 yr	3*	10			
		Pregnancy					
		≤18 yr	3*	10			
		19–30 yr	3*	10			
		31–50 yr	3*	10			
		Lactation					
		≤18 yr	3*	10			
		19–30 yr	3*	10			
		31–50 yr	3*	10			
Iodine	Component of the thyroid hormones; prevents goiter and cretinism	Infants	(µg/d)	(µg/d)	Marine origin, processed foods, iodized salt	Elevated thyroid stimulating hormone (TSH) concentration	Individuals with autoimmune thyroid disease, previous iodine deficiency, or nodular goiter are distinctly susceptible to the adverse effect of excess iodine intake. Therefore, individuals with these conditions may not be protected by the UL for iodine intake for the general population.
		0–6 mo	110*	ND[b]			
		7–12 mo	130*	ND			
		Children					
		1–3 yr	90	200			
		4–8 yr	90	300			
		Males					
		9–13 yr	120	600			
		14–18 yr	150	900			
		19–30 yr	150	1,100			
		31–50 yr	150	1,100			
		50–70 yr	150	1,100			
		>70 yr	150	1,100			
		Females					
		9–13 yr	120	600			
		14–18 yr	150	900			
		19–30 yr	150	1,100			
		31–50 yr	150	1,100			
		50–70 yr	150	1,100			
		>70 yr	150	1,100			
		Pregnancy					
		≤18 yr	220	900			
		19–30 yr	220	1,100			
		31–50 yr	220	1,100			
		Lactation					
		≤18 yr	290	900			
		19–30 yr	290	1,100			
		31–50 yr	290	1,100			

Continued

Dietary Reference Intakes: Elements   (continued)

NUTRIENT	FUNCTION	LIFE STAGE GROUP	RDA/AI*	UL[a]	SELECTED FOOD SOURCES	ADVERSE EFFECTS OF EXCESSIVE CONSUMPTION	SPECIAL CONSIDERATIONS
Iron (mg/d)	Component of hemoglobin and numerous enzymes; prevents microcytic hypochromic anemia	Infants	(mg/d)	(mg/d)	Fruits, vegetables and fortified bread and grain products such as cereal (non-heme iron sources), meat and poultry (heme iron sources)	Gastrointestinal distress	Non-heme iron absorption is lower for those consuming vegetarian diets than for those eating nonvegetarian diets. Therefore, it has been suggested that the iron requirement for those consuming a vegetarian diet is approximately 2-fold greater than for those consuming a nonvegetarian diet.
		0–6 mo	0.27*	40			
		7–12 mo	11	40			
		Children					
		1–3 yr	7	40			
		4–8 yr	10	40			
		Males					
		9–13 yr	8	40			
		14–18 yr	11	45			
		19–30 yr	8	45			
		31–50 yr	8	45			
		50–70 yr	8	45			
		>70 yr	8	45			
		Females					
		9–13 yr	8	40			
		14–18 yr	15	45			
		19–30 yr	18	45			
		31–50 yr	18	45			
		50–70 yr	8	45			
		>70 yr	8	45			Recommended intake assumes 75% of iron is from heme iron sources.
		Pregnancy					
		≤18 yr	27	45			
		19–30 yr	27	45			
		31–50 yr	27	45			
		Lactation					
		≤18 yr	10	45			
		19–30 yr	9	45			
		31–50 yr	9	45			
Magnesium	Cofactor for enzyme systems	Infants	(mg/d)	(mg/d)	Green leafy vegetables, unpolished grains, nuts, meat, starches, milk	There is no evidence of adverse effects from the consumption of naturally occurring magnesium in foods	None
		0–6 mo	30*	ND[b]			
		7–12 mo	75*	ND			
		Children					
		1–3 yr	80	65			
		4–8 yr	130	110			
		Males					
		9–13 yr	240	350		Adverse effects from magnesium containing supplements may include osmotic diarrhea	
		14–18 yr	410	350			
		19–30 yr	400	350			
		31–50 yr	420	350			
		50–70 yr	420	350			
		>70 yr	420	350			
		Females					
		9–13 yr	240	350		The UL for magnesium represents intake from a pharmacologic agent only and does not include intake from food and water	
		14–18 yr	360	350			
		19–30 yr	310	350			
		31–50 yr	320	350			
		50–70 yr	320	350			
		>70 yr	320	350			
		Pregnancy					
		≤18 yr	400	350			
		19–30 yr	350	350			
		31–50 yr	360	350			
		Lactation					
		≤18 yr	360	350			
		19–30 yr	310	350			
		31–50 yr	320	350			

Continued

Tables

Dietary Reference Intakes: Elements   (continued)

NUTRIENT	FUNCTION	LIFE STAGE GROUP	RDA/AI*	UL[a]	SELECTED FOOD SOURCES	ADVERSE EFFECTS OF EXCESSIVE CONSUMPTION	SPECIAL CONSIDERATIONS
Manganese	Involved in the formation of bone, as well as in enzymes involved in amino acid, cholesterol, and carbohydrate metabolism	Infants	(mg/d)	(mg/d)	Nuts, legumes, tea, and whole grains	Elevated blood concentration and neurotoxicity	Because manganese in drinking water and supplements may be more bioavailable than manganese from food, caution should be taken when using manganese supplements, especially among those persons already consuming large amounts of manganese from diets high in plant products.
		0–6 mo	0.003*	ND			
		7–12 mo	0.6*	ND			
		Children					
		1–3 yr	1.2*	2			
		4–8 yr	1.5*	3			
		Males					
		9–13 yr	1.9*	6			
		14–18 yr	2.2*	9			
		19–30 yr	2.3*	11			
		31–50 yr	2.3*	11			
		50–70 yr	2.3*	11			
		>70 yr	2.3*	11			
		Females					
		9–13 yr	1.6*	6			
		14–18 yr	1.6*	9			
		19–30 yr	1.8*	11			
		31–50 yr	1.8*	11			
		50–70 yr	1.8*	11			
		>70 yr	1.8*	11			In addition, individuals with liver disease may be distinctly susceptible to the adverse effects of excess manganese intake.
		Pregnancy					
		≤18 yr	2.0*	9			
		19–30 yr	2.0*	11			
		31–50 yr	2.0*	11			
		Lactation					
		≤18 yr	2.6*	9			
		19–30 yr	2.6*	11			
		31–50 yr	2.6*	11			
Molybdenum	Cofactor for enzymes involved in catabolism of sulfur amino acids, purines and pyridines	Infants	(µg/d)	(µg/d)	Legumes, grain products, and nuts	Reproductive effects as observed in animal studies	Individuals who are deficient in dietary copper intake or have some dysfunction in copper metabolism that makes them copper-deficient could be at increased risk of molybdenum toxicity.
		0–6 mo	2*	ND[b]			
		7–12 mo	3*	ND			
		Children					
		1–3 yr	17	300			
		4–8 yr	22	600			
		Males					
		9–13 yr	34	1,100			
		14–18 yr	43	1,700			
		19–30 yr	45	2,000			
		31–50 yr	45	2,000			
		50–70 yr	45	2,000			
		>70 yr	45	2,000			
		Females					
		9–13 yr	34	1,100			
		14–18 yr	43	1,700			
		19–30 yr	45	2,000			
		31–50 yr	45	2,000			
		50–70 yr	45	2,000			
		>70 yr	45	2,000			
		Pregnancy					
		≤18 yr	50	1,700			
		19–30 yr	50	2,000			
		31–50 yr	50	2,000			
		Lactation					
		≤18 yr	50	1,700			
		19–30 yr	50	2,000			
		31–50 yr	50	2,000			

Continued

Dietary Reference Intakes: Elements (continued)

NUTRIENT	FUNCTION	LIFE STAGE GROUP	RDA/AI*	UL[a]	SELECTED FOOD SOURCES	ADVERSE EFFECTS OF EXCESSIVE CONSUMPTION	SPECIAL CONSIDERATIONS
Nickel	No clear biological function in humans has been identified. May serve as a cofactor of metalloenzymes and facilitate iron absorption or metabolism in microorganisms	Infants		(mg/d)	Nuts, legumes, cereals, sweeteners, chocolate milk powder, chocolate candy	Decreased body weight gain	Individuals with preexisting nickel hypersensitivity (from previous dermal exposure) and kidney dysfunction are distinctly susceptible to the adverse effects of excess nickel intake.
		0–6 mo	ND	ND			
		7–12 mo	ND	ND		Note: As observed in animal studies	
		Children					
		1–3 yr	ND	0.2			
		4–8 yr	ND	0.3			
		Males					
		9–13 yr	ND	0.6			
		14–18 yr	ND	1.0			
		19–30 yr	ND	1.0			
		31–50 yr	ND	1.0			
		50–70 yr	ND	1.0			
		>70 yr	ND	1.0			
		Females					
		9–13 yr	ND	0.6			
		14–18 yr	ND	1.0			
		19–30 yr	ND	1.0			
		31–50 yr	ND	1.0			
		50–70 yr	ND	1.0			
		>70 yr	ND	1.0			
		Pregnancy					
		≤18 yr	ND	1.0			
		19–30 yr	ND	1.0			
		31–50 yr	ND	1.0			
		Lactation					
		≤18 yr	ND	1.0			
		19–30 yr	ND	1.0			
		31–50 yr	ND	1.0			
Phosphorus	Maintenance of pH, storage and transfer of energy and nucleotide synthesis	Infants	(mg/d)	(mg/d)	Milk, yogurt, ice cream, cheese, peas, meat, eggs, some cereals and breads	Metastatic calcification, skeletal porosity, interference with calcium absorption	Athletes and others with high energy expenditure frequently consume amounts from food greater than the UL without apparent effect.
		0–6 mo	100*	ND[b]			
		7–12 mo	275*	ND			
		Children					
		1–3 yr	460	3,000			
		4–8 yr	500	3,000			
		Males					
		9–13 yr	1,250	4,000			
		14–18 yr	1,250	4,000			
		19–30 yr	700	4,000			
		31–50 yr	700	4,000			
		50–70 yr	700	4,000			
		>70 yr	700	3,000			
		Females					
		9–13 yr	1,250	4,000			
		14–18 yr	1,250	4,000			
		19–30 yr	700	4,000			
		31–50 yr	700	4,000			
		50–70 yr	700	4,000			
		>70 yr	700	3,000			
		Pregnancy					
		≤18 yr	1,250	3,500			
		19–30 yr	700	3,500			
		31–50 yr	700	3,500			
		Lactation					
		≤18 yr	1,250	4,000			
		19–30 yr	700	4,000			
		31–50 yr	700	4,000			

Continued

Tables

Dietary Reference Intakes: Elements   (continued)

NUTRIENT	FUNCTION	LIFE STAGE GROUP	RDA/AI*	UL[a]	SELECTED FOOD SOURCES	ADVERSE EFFECTS OF EXCESSIVE CONSUMPTION	SPECIAL CONSIDERATIONS
Selenium	Defense against oxidative stress, regulation of thyroid hormone action, and the reduction and oxidation status of vitamin C and other molecules	Infants	(µg/d)	(µg/d)	Organ meats, seafood, plants (depending on soil selenium content)	Hair and nail brittleness and loss	None
		0–6 mo	15*	45			
		7–12 mo	20*	60			
		Children					
		1–3 yr	20	90			
		4–8 yr	30	150			
		Males					
		9–13 yr	40	280			
		14–18 yr	55	400			
		19–30 yr	55	400			
		31–50 yr	55	400			
		50–70 yr	55	400			
		>70 yr	55	400			
		Females					
		9–13 yr	40	280			
		14–18 yr	55	400			
		19–30 yr	55	400			
		31–50 yr	55	400			
		50–70 yr	55	400			
		>70 yr	55	400			
		Pregnancy					
		≤18 yr	60	400			
		19–30 yr	60	400			
		31–50 yr	60	400			
		Lactation					
		≤18 yr	70	400			
		19–30 yr	70	400			
		31–50 yr	70	400			
Silicon	No biological function in humans has been identified	Infants			Plant-based foods	There is no evidence that silicon that occurs naturally in food and water produces adverse health effects	None
		0–6 mo	ND[b]	ND			
		7–12 mo	ND	ND			
		Children					
	Involved in bone function in animal studies	1–3 yr	ND	ND			
		4–8 yr	ND	ND			
		Males					
		9–13 yr	ND	ND			
		14–18 yr	ND	ND			
		19–30 yr	ND	ND			
		31–50 yr	ND	ND			
		50–70 yr	ND	ND			
		>70 yr	ND	ND			
		Females					
		9–13 yr	ND	ND			
		14–18 yr	ND	ND			
		19–30 yr	ND	ND			
		31–50 yr	ND	ND			
		50–70 yr	ND	ND			
		>70 yr	ND	ND			
		Pregnancy					
		≤18 yr	ND	ND			
		19–30 yr	ND	ND			
		31–50 yr	ND	ND			
		Lactation					
		≤18 yr	ND	ND			
		19–30 yr	ND	ND			
		31–50 yr	ND	ND			

Continued

Dietary Reference Intakes: Elements   (continued)

NUTRIENT	FUNCTION	LIFE STAGE GROUP	RDA/AI*	ULᵃ	SELECTED FOOD SOURCES	ADVERSE EFFECTS OF EXCESSIVE CONSUMPTION	SPECIAL CONSIDERATIONS
Vanadium	No biological function in humans has been identified	Infants		(mg/d)	Mushrooms, shellfish, black pepper, parsley, and dill seed	Renal lesions as observed in animal studies	None
		0–6 mo	ND	ND			
		7–12 mo	ND	ND			
		Children					
		1–3 yr	ND	ND			
		4–8 yr	ND	ND			
		Males					
		9–13 yr	ND	ND			
		14–18 yr	ND	ND			
		19–30 yr	ND	1.8			
		31–50 yr	ND	1.8			
		50–70 yr	ND	1.8			
		>70 yr	ND	1.8			
		Females					
		9–13 yr	ND	ND			
		14–18 yr	ND	ND			
		19–30 yr	ND	1.8			
		31–50 yr	ND	1.8			
		50–70 yr	ND	1.8			
		>70 yr	ND	1.8			
		Pregnancy					
		≤18 yr	ND	ND			
		19–30 yr	ND	ND			
		31–50 yr	ND	ND			
		Lactation					
		≤18 yr	ND	ND			
		19–30 yr	ND	ND			
		31–50 yr	ND	ND			
Zinc	Component of multiple enzymes and proteins; involved in the regulation of gene expression	Infants	(mg/d)	(mg/d)	Fortified cereals, red meats, certain seafood	Reduced copper status	Zinc absorption is lower for those consuming vegetarian diets than for those eating nonvegetarian diets. Therefore, it has been suggested that the zinc requirement for those consuming a vegetarian diet is approximately 2-fold greater than for those consuming a nonvegetarian diet.
		0–6 mo	2*	4			
		7–12 mo	3	5			
		Children					
		1–3 yr	3	7			
		4–8 yr	5	12			
		Males					
		9–13 yr	8	23			
		14–18 yr	11	34			
		19–30 yr	11	40			
		31–50 yr	11	40			
		50–70 yr	11	40			
		>70 yr	11	40			
		Females					
		9–13 yr	8	23			
		14–18 yr	9	34			
		19–30 yr	8	40			
		31–50 yr	8	40			
		50–70 yr	8	40			
		>70 yr	8	40			

Continued

Tables

Dietary Reference Intakes: Elements   (continued)

NUTRIENT	FUNCTION	LIFE STAGE GROUP	RDA/AI*	UL[a]	SELECTED FOOD SOURCES	ADVERSE EFFECTS OF EXCESSIVE CONSUMPTION	SPECIAL CONSIDERATIONS
Zinc		Pregnancy					
(continued)		≤18 yr	**13**	34			
		19–30 yr	**11**	40			
		31–50 yr	**11**	40			
		Lactation					
		≤18 yr	**14**	34			
		19–30 yr	**12**	40			
		31–50 yr	**12**	40			

NOTE: This table is reprinted with permission from the website of the Institute of Medicine, National Academy of Sciences. The table is adapted from the DRI reports (see *www.nap.edu*). It represents recommended dietary allowances (RDAs) in **bold type,** adequate intakes (AIs) in ordinary type followed by an asterisk (*), and upper limits (ULs)[a]. RDAs and AIs may both be used as goals for individual intake. RDAs are set to meet the needs of almost all (97% to 98%) individuals in a group. For healthy breastfed infants, the AI is the mean intake. The AI for other life stage and gender groups is believed to cover the needs of all individuals in the group, but lack of data prevent being able to specify with confidence the percentage of individuals covered by this intake.

[a]UL, The maximum level of daily nutrient intake that is likely to pose no risk of adverse effects. Unless otherwise specified, the UL represents total intake from food, water, and supplements. Due to lack of suitable data, ULs could not be established for vitamin K, thiamin, riboflavin, vitamin B_{12}, pantothenic acid, biotin, or carotenoids. In the absence of ULs, extra caution may be warranted in consuming levels above recommended intakes.

[b]ND, Not determinable due to lack of data of adverse effects in this age group and concern with regard to lack of ability to handle excess amounts. Source of intake should be from food only to prevent high levels of intake.

SOURCES: *Dietary Reference Intakes for Calcium, Phosphorous, Magnesium, Vitamin D, and Fluoride* (1997); *Dietary Reference Intakes for Thiamin, Riboflavin, Niacin, Vitamin B_6, Folate, Vitamin B_{12}, Pantothenic Acid, Biotin, and Choline* (1998); *Dietary Reference Intakes for Vitamin C, Vitamin E, Selenium, and Carotenoids* (2000); and *Dietary Reference Intakes for Vitamin A, Vitamin K, Arsenic, Boron, Chromium, Copper, Iodine, Iron, Manganese, Molybdenum, Nickel, Silicon, Vanadium, and Zinc* (2001). These reports may be accessed via www.nap.edu.

Reference Nutrient Intakes (RNI) for Vitamins, United Kingdom[a]

AGE	THIAMIN (MG/DAY)	RIBOFLAVIN (MG/DAY)	NIACIN (NICOTINIC ACID EQUIVALENT) (MG/DAY)	VITAMIN B_6 (MG/DAY)[b]	VITAMIN B_{12} (μG/DAY)	FOLATE (μG/DAY)	VITAMIN C (MG/DAY)	VITAMIN A (μG/DAY)	VITAMIN D (μG/DAY)
0–3 months	0.2	0.4	3	0.2	0.3	50	25	350	8.5
4–6 months	0.2	0.4	3	0.2	0.3	50	25	350	8.5
7–9 months	0.2	0.4	4	0.3	0.4	50	25	350	7
10–12 months	0.3	0.4	5	0.4	0.4	50	25	350	7
1–3 years	0.5	0.6	8	0.7	0.5	70	30	400	7
4–6 years	0.7	0.8	11	0.9	0.8	100	30	400	—
7–10 years	0.7	1.0	12	1.0	1.0	150	30	500	—
Males									
11–14 years	0.9	1.2	15	1.2	1.2	200	35	600	—
15–18 years	1.1	1.3	18	1.5	1.5	200	40	700	—
19–50 years	1.0	1.3	17	1.4	1.5	200	40	700	—
50+ years	0.9	1.3	16	1.4	1.5	200	40	700	—[c]
Females									
11–14 years	0.7	1.1	12	1.0	1.2	200	35	600	—
15–18 years	0.8	1.1	14	1.2	1.5	200	40	600	—
19–50 years	0.8	1.1	13	1.2	1.5	200	40	600	—
50+ years	0.8	1.1	12	1.2	1.5	200	40	600	—[c]
Pregnancy	+0.1[d]	+0.3	—[e]	—[e]	—[e]	+100	+10[d]	+100	10
Lactation									
0–4 months	+0.2	+0.5	+2	—[e]	+0.5	+60	+30	+350	10
4+ months	+0.2	+0.5	+2	—[e]	+0.5	+60	+30	+350	10

From Report on Health and Social Subjects: no. 41. Dietary reference values for food energy and nutrients for the United Kingdom. Report of the Panel on Dietary Reference Values of the Committee on Medical Aspects of Food Policy. London: Her Majesty's Stationery Office, 1991. This is the U.K.'s Report Table 1-4.

[a]The Reference Nutrient Intake is a point in the distribution that is two notional standard deviations above the Estimated Average Requirement (EAR). Intakes above this amount will almost certainly be adequate.

[b]Based on protein providing 14.7% of EAR for energy.

[c]After age 65 the RNI is 10 μg/day for men and women.

[d]For last trimester only.

[e]No increment.

Average Values for Triglycerides, Fatty Acids (FA) (Including Omega-3 Fatty Acids)[a] and Cholesterol of Marine Foods and Oils

FISH (100 G)	FAT (G)	CHOL (MG)	SFA (G)	MFA (G)	PFA (G)	M18:1 (G)	P18:2 (G)	P18:3 (G)	P20:5 (G)	P22:5 (G)	P22:6 (G)
Anchovy, European, raw	4.84	60.00	1.28	1.18	1.64	0.62	0.10	—[b]	0.54	0.03	0.91
Bass, striped, raw	2.33	80.00	0.51	0.66	0.78	0.45	0.02	0.02	0.17	0.00	0.58
Bluefish, raw	4.24	59.00	0.92	1.79	1.06	0.68	0.06	0.00	0.25	0.06	0.52
Burbot, raw	0.81	60.00	0.16	0.13	0.30	0.10	0.01	—[b]	0.07	0.03	0.10
Carp, raw	5.60	66.00	1.08	2.33	1.43	1.15	0.52	0.27	0.24	0.08	0.11
Catfish, wild, raw	2.82	58.00	0.72	0.84	0.86	0.59	0.10	0.07	0.13	0.10	0.23
Catfish, farmed, raw	7.59	47.00	1.77	3.59	1.57	3.17	0.88	0.10	0.07	0.09	0.21
Cod, Atlantic, raw	0.67	43.00	0.13	0.09	0.23	0.06	trace[c]	trace[c]	0.06	0.01	0.12
Eel, all varieties, raw	11.66	126.00	2.36	7.19	0.95	2.77	0.20	0.43	0.08	0.07	0.06
Flounder, unspecified, raw	1.19	48.00	0.28	0.23	0.33	0.12	0.01	0.01	0.09	0.05	0.11
Haddock, raw	0.72	57.00	0.13	0.12	0.24	0.07	0.01	trace[c]	0.06	0.02	0.13
Halibut, raw	2.29	32.00	0.32	0.75	0.73	0.36	0.03	0.06	0.07	0.09	0.29
Herring, Atlantic, raw	9.04	60.00	2.04	3.74	2.13	1.52	0.13	0.10	0.71	0.06	0.86
Mackerel, Atlantic, raw	13.89	70.00	3.26	5.46	3.35	2.28	0.22	0.16	0.90	0.21	1.40
Mussel, blue, raw	2.24	28.00	0.42	0.51	0.61	0.20	0.02	0.02	0.19	0.02	0.25
Octopus, raw	1.04	48.00	0.23	0.16	0.24	0.06	0.01	0.00	0.08	0.01	0.08
Oyster, Eastern, wild, raw	2.46	53.00	0.77	0.31	0.97	0.12	0.06	0.05	0.27	0.06	0.29
Oyster, Eastern, farmed, raw	1.55	25.00	0.44	0.15	0.59	0.07	0.03	0.04	0.19	—[b]	0.20
Perch, all varieties, raw	0.92	90.00	0.18	0.15	0.37	0.07	0.01	0.10	0.08	0.03	0.17
Pike, walleye, raw	1.22	86.00	0.25	0.29	0.45	0.20	0.03	0.01	0.09	0.04	0.22
Pollock, Atlantic, raw	0.98	71.00	0.14	0.11	0.48	0.07	0.01	0.00	0.07	0.02	0.35
Sablefish, raw	15.30	49.00	3.20	8.06	2.04	4.07	0.16	0.10	0.68	0.17	0.72
Salmon, Chinook, raw	10.44	66.00	2.51	4.48	2.08	2.80	0.11	0.09	0.79	0.23	0.57
Salmon, coho, wild, raw	5.93	45.00	1.26	2.13	1.99	1.20	0.21	0.16	0.43	0.23	0.66
Salmon, coho, farmed, raw	7.67	51.00	1.82	3.33	1.86	1.72	0.35	0.08	0.38	—[b]	0.82
Sea bass, all varieties, raw	2.00	41.00	0.51	0.42	0.74	0.29	0.02	0.00	0.16	0.08	0.43
Smelt, rainbow, raw	2.42	70.00	0.45	0.64	0.88	0.41	0.04	0.05	0.28	0.02	0.42
Squid, all varieties, raw	1.38	233.00	0.36	0.11	0.52	0.05	trace[c]	trace[c]	0.15	trace[c]	0.34
Red snapper, all varieties, raw	1.34	37.00	0.28	0.25	0.46	0.16	0.02	trace[c]	0.05	0.06	0.26
Sole, raw	1.19	48.00	0.28	0.23	0.33	0.12	0.01	0.01	0.09	0.05	0.11
Sturgeon, all varieties, raw	4.04	60.00	0.92	1.94	0.69	1.43	0.07	0.10	0.19	0.04	0.09
Swordfish, raw	4.01	39.00	1.10	1.54	0.92	1.09	0.03	0.19	0.11	0.00	0.53
Trout, rainbow, wild, raw	3.46	59.00	0.72	1.13	1.24	0.61	0.24	0.12	0.17	0.11	0.42
Trout, rainbow, farmed, raw	5.40	59.00	1.55	1.54	1.80	1.06	0.71	0.06	0.26	0.00	0.67
Tuna, bluefin, fresh, raw	4.90	38.00	1.26	1.60	1.43	0.92	0.05	0.00	0.28	0.12	0.89
Whitefish, all varieties, raw	5.86	60.00	0.91	2.00	2.15	1.35	0.27	0.18	0.32	0.16	0.94
Cod liver oil	100.00	570.00	22.61	46.71	22.54	20.65	0.94	0.94	6.90	0.94	10.97
Herring oil	100.00	766.00	21.29	56.56	15.60	11.96	1.15	0.76	6.27	0.62	4.21
Menhaden oil	100.00	521.00	30.43	26.69	34.20	14.53	2.15	1.49	13.17	4.92	8.56
Max EPA conc fish body oil	100.00	600.00	25.00	28.00	41.00	7.00	2.00	5.00	18.00	0.00	12.00
Salmon oil	100.00	485.00	19.87	29.04	40.32	16.98	1.54	1.06	13.02	2.99	18.23

Data compiled from U.S. Department of Agriculture nutrient database for standard reference, release 11-1 and the Nutrition Coordinating Center, University of Minnesota, Nutrient database, version 28. Table compiled by the Nutrition Coordinating Center, University of Minnesota, 1997, with permission.

[a]CHOL, cholesterol; SFA, saturated fatty acid; MFA, monounsaturated fatty acid; PFA, polyunsaturated fatty acid; M18:1, oleic acid; P18:2, linoleic acid; P18:3, linolenic acid; P20:5, eicosapentaenoic acid (EPA); P22:5, docosapentaenoic acid (DPA); P22:6, docosahexaenoic acid (DHA). The omega-3 fatty acids are P20:5, P22:5, and P22:6.

[b]Denotes lack of reliable data for nutrient.

[c]Trace is ≤0.005 g/100 g food.

Tables

Caffeine Content of Selected Common Foods per Serving Portion

FOOD NAME	SERVING PORTION	CAFFEINE (MG)
Candy, milk chocolate	1.0 oz	7.24
Candy, semisweet chocolate	1.0 oz	17.58
Candy, sweet chocolate	1.0 oz	18.71
Chocolate, unsweetened, baking type	1.0 oz	57.83
Chocolate beverage mix, prepared	8.0 fl oz	7.98
Cocoa mix, prepared	6.0 fl oz	4.12
Cocoa powder, unsweetened	1.0 tbsp	12.42
Coffee, brewed, regular	6.0 fl oz	103.24
Coffee, brewed, espresso	6.0 fl oz	377.54
Coffee, instant, regular, prepared	6.0 fl oz	57.28
Coffee, instant, decaffeinated, prepared	6.0 fl oz	1.79
Coffee, instant, cappuccino flavor, prepared	6.0 fl oz	74.88
Coffee, instant, french flavor, prepared	6.0 fl oz	51.03
Coffee, instant, mocha flavor, prepared	6.0 fl oz	33.84
Cola beverage, regular	12.0 fl oz	37.00
Cola beverage, diet	12.0 fl oz	49.70
Ice cream, chocolate	0.5 cup	40.92
Milk, chocolate	8.0 fl oz	5.00
Pudding, chocolate	0.5 cup	5.65
Tea, brewed	6.0 fl oz	35.60
Tea, instant, unsweetened, prepared	6.0 fl oz	23.14
Tea, instant, unsweetened, lemon flavored, prepared	6.0 fl oz	19.64
Topping, chocolate, fudge type	1.0 tbsp	1.89
Topping, chocolate, syrup	1.0 tbsp	2.63

Data compiled from U.S. Department of Agriculture Nutrient database for standard reference, release 11-1, and the Nutrition Coordinating Center, University of Minnesota, Nutrient database, version 28. Table compiled by the Nutrition Coordinating Center, University of Minnesota, 1997, with permission.

Carnitine Content of Selected Foods

FOOD ITEM	CARNITINE CONTENT[a]	FOOD ITEM	CARNITINE CONTENT[a]
Meat products		*Fruits*	
Beef steak	592 ± 260 (4)	Bananas	0.0056
Ground beef	582 ± 32 (3)	Apples	0.0002
Pork	172 ± 32 (3)	Strawberries	ND
Canadian bacon	146 ± 52 (3)	Peaches	0.0060
Bacon	145 ± 24 (3)	Pineapple	0.0063
Fish (cod)	34.6 ± 11.7 (3)	Pears	0.0107
Chicken breast	24.3 ± 8.0 (3)	*Grains*	
Dairy products		White bread	0.912
Whole milk	20.4	Whole-wheat bread	2.26
American cheese	23.2	Rice (cooked)	0.090
Ice cream	23.0	Macaroni	0.780
Butter	3.07	Corn flakes	0.078
Cottage cheese	6.96	*Nondairy beverages*	
Vegetables		Grapefruit juice	ND
Broccoli (fresh)	0.0228	Orange juice	0.012
(cooked)	0.0111	Tomato juice	0.030
Carrots (fresh)	0.0408	Coffee	0.009
(cooked)	0.0393	Cola	ND
Green beans (cooked)	0.0369	Grape juice	0.093
Asparagus (cooked)	1.21	*Miscellaneous*	
Beets (cooked)	0.0195	Eggs	0.075
Potato (cooked)	0.0800	Peanut butter	0.51
Lettuce	0.0066		

Adapted from Rebouche CJ, Engel AG. *J Clin Invest* 1984;73:857–867.

[a]Units are μmol/100 g (solid foods) or μmol/100 mL (liquids). ND, not detectable. Values for meat products are mean ± SD (number of observations in parentheses) and are based on precooked weight. Values reported are for total (nonesterified plus esterified) carnitine.

Choline Content of Some Common Foods

| FOOD | CONCENTRATION (μMOL/KG)[a] | | |
	CHOLINE	PHOSPHATIDYLCHOLINE	SPHINGOMYELIN
Apple	27	280	15
Banana	240	37	20
Beef liver	5831	43500	1850
Beef steak	75	6030	506
Butter	42	1760	460
Cauliflower	1306	2770	183
Corn oil	3	12	5
Coffee	90	34	23
Cucumber	218	76	27
Egg	42	52000	2250
Ginger ale	2	4	3
Grape juice	475	15	5
Iceberg lettuce	2930	132	50
Margarine	30	450	15
Milk (bovine, whole)	150	148	82
Orange	200	490	24
Peanut butter	3895	3937	9
Peanuts	4546	4960	78
Potato	511	300	26
Tomato	430	52	32
Whole wheat bread	968	340	11

Modified from Zeisel SH. Biological consequences of choline deficiency. In: Wurtman R, Wurtman J, eds. Choline metabolism and Brain Function. New York: Raven Press, 1990:75–99.

[a]Choline, phosphatidylcholine, and sphingomyelin were measured using a gas chromatography/mass spectrometry assay in foods prepared in the form in which they would normally be consumed.

Tables

Oxalate Content by Food Group

FOODS	LITTLE OR NO OXALATE <2 MG OXALATE/SERVING EAT AS DESIRED	MODERATE-OXALATE CONTENT 2–10 MG OXALATE/SERVING LIMIT: TWO (½ CUP) SERVINGS/DAY OR TWO SERVINGS OF THE STATED SERVING SIZE	HIGH-OXALATE FOODS >10 MG OXALATE/SERVING AVOID COMPLETELY
Beverages/juices	Apple juice	Beer, Budweiser (12 fl oz)	Beer; Stout, Guinness, Draft, Lager, Tuborg, Pilsner
	Beer, bottled	Coffee, any kind (8 oz serving)	
	Black coffee (brewed 5 min)	Cranberry juice (4 oz serving)	Juices containing berries not allowed
	Cranberry juice	Cocoa, Carnation dry	Ovaltine and other beverage mixes
	Diet Coke	Nescafe powder (1 tsp)	Tea, cocoa
	Grapefruit juice	Tomato juice (4 oz serving)	
	Lemonade or limeade	Lipton tea (steeped 5 min)	
	Wine, red, rosé		
	Pineapple juice		
	Tap water (preferred for extra calcium)		
	Orange soda (12 fl oz Minute Maid)		
	Ginger ale (Schweppes)		
	Root beer (Borg's and A&W)		
	Aloe vera juice		
Milk (2 or more cups)	Buttermilk	Yogurt plain, nonfat (1 cup)	
	Low-fat milk		
	Low-fat yogurt with allowed fruit		
	Skim milk		
	Whole milk		
Meat group	Eggs	Sardines	Baked beans canned in tomato sauce
	Cheese, cheddar		Peanut butter
	Lean lamb, beef, or pork		Soybean curd (tofu)
	Poultry		
	Seafood		
Vegetables	Avocado	Asparagus	Beans, boiled or raw: green, wax, dried
	Broccoli, boiled	Carrots, canned	Beets, boiled; tops, roots, and green
	Brussels sprouts, boiled	Cauliflower, boiled	Celery
	Cabbage, boiled	Corn, sweet white and yellow	Chard, Swiss
	Chive	Cucumbers, peeled raw	Collards
	Potatoes, white, boiled	Onions, raw, boiled	Dandelion greens
	Radishes	Green peas, boiled, canned	Eggplant, raw
	Turnips, boiled	Lettuce, iceberg, fresh	Leeks
	Waterchestnuts	Lima beans, cooked	Mustard greens
		Parsnips	Okra
		Tomato, fresh, 1 small	Parsley, raw
		Mushrooms, fresh	Peppers, green
		Escarole	Pokeweed
		Kale, raw	Potatoes, sweet
			Rutabagas
			Spinach
			Summer squash
			Watercress
Fruits	Avocado	Apple	Berries
	Banana	Apricots	Concord grapes
	Cherries, Bing or sour	Black currants	Red currants
	Cranberries, canned	Cranberries, dried	Fruit cocktail
	Grapes, Thompson seedless	Grapefruit	Gooseberries
	Mangoes	Orange	Lemon peel
	Melons: cantaloupe	Peaches, Alberta	Lime peel
	casaba	Pears, raw	Orange peel
	honeydew	Plums, stewed	Raspberries
	watermelon	Prunes, Italian	Rhubarb, canned, stewed
	Nectarines	Pineapple, Dole's	Strawberries, canned
	Peaches, Hiley, canned	Coconut	Tangerine
	Pineapple, canned, stewed	Kiwi	Plums, Damson
	Plums, green or Golden age		
	Pear, Bartlett, canned		
	Orange juice fresh		

Continued

Oxalate Content by Food Group   (continued)

FOODS	LITTLE OR NO OXALATE <2 MG OXALATE/SERVING EAT AS DESIRED	MODERATE-OXALATE CONTENT 2–10 MG OXALATE/SERVING LIMIT: TWO (½ CUP) SERVINGS/DAY OR TWO SERVINGS OF THE STATED SERVING SIZE	HIGH-OXALATE FOODS >10 MG OXALATE/SERVING AVOID COMPLETELY
	Papaya, Hawaiian		
	Strawberries, fresh		
Breadstarches	Cornflakes	Cornbread	Fruit cake
	Macaroni, boiled	Sponge cake	Grits, white corn
	Noodles, egg boiled	Spaghetti, canned in tomato sauce	Soybean crackers
	Oatmeal, porridge	Cornmeal, yellow, dry	Wheat germ
	Rice, boiled	Cheerios (1 cup)	Fig Newtons
	Wild rice, cooked	Bagel (1 medium; 2 oz)	Graham crackers
	Bread, white	Brown rice, cooked	Popcorn (4 cups popped)
	Barley, cooked	Garbanzo beans, canned	Whole wheat flour
		Lentils, cooked	
		Split peas, cooked	
		Macaroni, cooked	
		Spaghetti, cooked	
		Corn tortilla (1 medium; 1.5 oz)	
		English muffin (1 medium; 2 oz)	
		Bread, whole wheat	
Fats & oils	Mayonnaise	Bacon	Nuts: Peanuts and pecans
	Salad dressing		Sunflower seeds
	Vegetable oils		Mayonnaise (Heinz)
	Butter		
	Margarine		
Miscellaneous	Jelly or preserves, made with allowable fruits	Vegetable soup	Chocolate, plain
	Lemon/lime juice, fresh	Tomato soup	Dry cocoa, plain
	Salt, pepper (1 tsp/day)	Tofu (firm)	Pepper (in excess of 1 tsp/day)
	Soups with allowed ingredients	Malt (1 tbsp)	Cinnamon, ground (1 tsp)
	Sugar	Basil, fresh (1 tbsp)	
	Honey (1 tbsp)	Mustard, Dijon style (1 tbsp)	
	Corn syrup (Karo)	Ginger, raw (1 tbsp sliced)	
	Unflavored gelatin (Knox), 1 pkt		
	Maple syrup, pure		
	Vanilla extract		
	Oregano, dried (1 tsp)		
	Apple cider vinegar (1 tsp. Ralph's Supermarket)		
	Nutmeg, dry (1 tsp)		
	Cornstarch (1 tbsp)		

From Brzezinski E, Durning AM, Grasse B, Fusselman E, Ciaraldi T. Oxalate content of selected foods. The General Clinical Research Center, University of California, San Diego Medical Center, 1996:1–53, with permission. There is now a 1998 edition available.

Tables

Foods to Use and Avoid

THESE CONTAIN SMALL AMOUNTS OF OXALATE: 0–2 MG OXALATE PER SERVING (½ CUP)

VEGETABLES	*FRUITS*	*BEVERAGES*	*MISCELLANEOUS*
Broccoli	Avocado	Apple juice	Butter
Brussels sprouts	Banana	Barley water	Cheese, cheddar
Cabbage	Cherries	Beer, bottled	Chicken noodle soup
Cauliflower	Grapes, seedless	Cider	Cornflakes
Chives	Mangoes	Coca-cola	Eggs
Cucumber	Melons	Grapefruit juice	Egg noodle (chow mein)
Lettuce	Peaches, canned	Lemonade	Fish (except sardines)
Mushrooms	Hiley	Lucozade, bottled	Jelly with allowed fruit
Onions	Stokes	Milk	Lemon juice
Peas	Pineapple	Orange juice	Lime juice
Potato, white	Plums:	Pepsi-Cola	Macaroni
Radishes	Golden Gage	Pineapple juice	Margarine

THESE ARE HIGH IN OXALATE: >15 MG OXALATE PER SERVING (½ CUP)

VEGETABLES	*FRUITS*	*BEVERAGES*	*MISCELLANEOUS*
Beans in tomato sauce	Berries;	Chocolate	Cocoa, dry
Beets	Black	Tuborg, Pilsner	Grits, white corn
Celery	Blue	Ovaltine (24 mg/8 oz)	Peanuts
Chard, Swiss	Green goose	Tea (132–181.2 mg/8 oz)	Pecans
Collards	Raspberries		Soybean crackers
Dandelion greens	Currants, red		Wheat germ
Eggplant	Grapes, concord		
Escarole	Lemon peel		
Leeks			
Okra			
Parsley			
Pepper, green			
Pokeweed			
Potato, sweet			
Rutabagas			
Spinach			
Squash, summer			

From Brezinski E, Durning AM, Grasse B, Fusselman E, Ciaraldi T. Oxalate content of selected foods. The General Clinical Research Center, University of California, San Diego Medical Center, 1996:1–52, with permission. There is now a 1998 edition available.

Oxalate Content of Foods per 100 Grams (~ ½ Cup) and per Portion

FOOD	PORTION	MG/100 G	MG/PORTION
Cereals, grains, and ceral products			
Bagel, plain	1 medium; 55 g	12.37	6.804
Barley, cooked	1 cup; 156.25 g	3.46	5.404
Bread, white	1 slice; 25 g	4.9	1.225
Bread, whole wheat	1 slice; 25 g	20.9	5.225
Cake, fruit	1 slice; 15 g	11.8	1.77
Cake, sponge	1 slice; 66 g	7.4	4.884
Cheerios	1 cup; 22.6 g	20.66	4.67
Corn tortilla	1 medium; 21.3 g	11.51	2.45
Cornflakes	1 cup; 22.7 g	2	0.454
Cornmeal, yellow	1 cup dry; 138 g	6.25	8.624
Cornstarch	1 Tbsp; 8 g	14.51	1.61
Crackers, soybean	1 ounce; 28.35 g	204	58.685
Egg noodle (chow mein)	1 cup; 45 g	1	0.45
English muffin, white	1 each; 58 g	10.22	5.93
Graham crackers (Keebler)	2 crackers; 14 g	12.41	1.74
Fig Newtons	1 each; 14.7 g	14.05	2.07
Garbanzo beans, canned	1 cup; 164 g	11.18	18.34
Grits, white corn	1 cup cooked; 242 g	41	99.22
Grits, white corn	1 cup dry; 156 g	41	63.96
Lentils, cooked	1 cup; 198 g	8.48	16.795
Macaroni, boiled	1 cup boil tender; 140 g	1	1.4
Macaroni, cooked soft	1 cup; 140 g	5.44	7.62
Oatmeal porridge	1 cup; 234 g	1	2.34
Popcorn, Orville Redenbacker, popped	Single-serving bag; 4 cups = 50.39 g	33.29	16.777
Rice, brown, cooked	1 cup; 195 g	6.54	12.76
Rice, boiled	1 cup; 175 g	0	0
Spaghetti, boiled	1 cup boil tender; 140 g	1.5	2.1
Spaghetti, cooked soft	1 cup; 140 g	6.24	8.73
Spaghetti in tomato sauce	1 cup; 250 g	4	10
Split peas, cooked	1 cup; 196 g	4.83	9.48
Wheat germ	1 Tbsp; 7.2 g	299	19.37
Wild rice, cooked	1 cup; 164 g	1.65	2.71
Whole wheat flour	1 cup; 120 g	25.03	30.031
Milk and milk products			
Butter	1 Tbsp; 14 g	0	0
Cheddar cheese	1 ounce; 28.35 g	0	0
Margarine	1 Tbsp; 14.1 g	0	0
Milk	1 cup; 244 g	0.15	0.366
Milk, whole	1 cup; 244 g	0.54	1.31
Yogurt, natural, nonfat plain	1 cup; 227 g	1	2.266
Meats, eggs, and meat alternates			
Bacon, streaky, fried	1 strip; 6.3 g	3.3	0.21
Beef, canned, corned	3 oz; 85 g	0	0
Beef, topside roast	4 oz; 113.4 g	0	0
Chicken roast	4 oz; 113.4 g	0	0
Egg, boiled	1 medium; 50 g	0	0
Fish: haddock	4 oz; 113.4 g	0.2	0.23
plaice	4 oz; 113.4 g	0.3	0.34
sardines	4 oz; 113.4 g	4.8	5.42
Ham	4 oz; 113.4 g	1.6	1.81
Hamburger, grilled	4 oz; 113.4 g	0	0
Lamb; roast	4 oz; 113.4 g	trace	trace
Liver	4 oz; 113.4 g	7.1	8.02
Pork, roast	4 oz; 113.4 g	1.7	1.92
Tofu, raw firm	125 g	5.08	6.35
Vegetables			
Asparagus	1 cup; 180 g	5.2	9.36
Green beans, boiled	1 cup; 135 g	15	20.25
Beans in tomato sauce	1 cup	19	
Beetroot, boiled	1 cup; 170 g	675	1147.5

Continued

Tables

Oxalate Content of Foods per 100 Grams (~½ Cup) and per Portion   (continued)

FOOD	PORTION	MG/100 G	MG/PORTION
Beetroot, pickled	1 cup; 227 g	500	1135
Broccoli, boiled	1 cup; 155 g	trace	trace
Brussels sprouts, boiled	1 cup; 156 g	0	0
Cabbage, boiled	1 cup common; 70 g	0	0
Carrots, canned	1 cup; 146 g	4	5.84
Cauliflower, boiled	1 cup; 124 g	1	1.24
Celery	1 cup diced; 120 g	20	24
Chard, Swiss	1 cup raw; 36 g	645	232.2
Chard, Swiss	1 cup boiled; 175 g	645	1128.75
Chive	1 cup raw; 48 g	1.1	0.53
Collards	1 cup raw/boil; 128 g	74	94.72
Corn, yellow	1 cup; 165 g	5.2	8.58
Cucumber, raw	1 med whole; 301 g	1	3.01
Dandelion greens	1 cup raw; 55 g	24.6	13.53
Dandelion greens	1 cup boiled; 105 g	24.6	25.83
Eggplant	1 cup boiled; 96 g	18	17.28
Escarole	1 cup raw; 28 g	31	8.68
Kale	1 cup raw/boil; 130 g	13	16.9
Leek	1 cup raw/boil; 124 g	89	110.36
Lettuce	1 cup; 55 g	3	1.65
Lima beans	1 cup canned; 248 g	4.3	10.66
Mushrooms	1 cup raw/chopped; 70 g	2	1.4
Okra	1 cup boiled; 160 g	146	233.6
Onion, boiled	1 cup; 210 g	3	6.3
Parsley, raw	1 cup; 64 g	100	64
Parsnips	1 cup sliced/boil; 156 g	10	15.6
Peas, canned	1 cup; 170 g	1	1.7
Pepper, green	1 item; 74 g	16	11.84
Pokeweed	1 item; 136 g	476	
Potatoes, white boiled	1 item; 136 g	0	0
Potato, sweet	1 cup boil/mashed; 238 g	56	183.68
Radishes	1 each; 4.5 g	0.3	0.014
Rutabagas	1 cup boil; 170 g	19	32.3
Spinach, boiled	1 cup; 56 g	750	420
Spinach, frozen	1 cup frozen/boil; 250 g	600	1230
Squash, summer	1 cup sliced; 180 g	22	39.6
Tomato, raw	1 cup diced; 240 g	2	4.8
Turnips, boiled	1 cup; 156 g	1	1.56
Waterchestnut canned, whole slices	1/2 cup; 70 g	1.22	0.86
Watercress early, fine curled	1 cup raw; 34 g	10	3.4
Fruits			
Apple, raw	1 medium; 138 g	3	4.14
Apricot, w/o pit	1 each; 35.3 g	2.8	0.99
Avocado	1 California; 173 g	0	0
Avocado	1 Florida; 173 g	0	0
Banana, raw	1 medium peeled; 114 g	trace	trace
Berries: black	1 cup; 144 g	18	25.92
blue	1 cup; 145 g	15	21.75
Berries: dew	1 cup; 144 g	14	20.16
Berries: green goose	1 cup; 150 g	88	132
raspberries, black	1 cup; 123 g	53	65.19
raspberries, red	1 cup; 123 g	15	18.45
Coconut fresh (flesh only)	45 g; 1.5 oz	2.14	0.96
Cranberries, dried	1/2 cup; 25 g	3.07	0.77
Cranberries, canned Ocean Spray	1/2 cup; 138 g	0.71	0.98
Cherries: Bing	1 cup; 150 g	0	0
Cherries: sour	1 cup; 155 g	1.1	1.705
Currants: black	1 cup; 112 g	4.3	4.82
red	1 cup; 122 g	19	21.28
Fruit salad, canned	1 cup; 249 g	12	29.88
Grapes, red, fresh	1 cup; 92 g	0.52	0.475

Continued

Oxalate Content of Foods per 100 Grams (~ ½ Cup) and per Portion   (continued)

FOOD	PORTION	MG/100 G	MG/PORTION
Grapes: concord	1 cup; 160 g	25	40
Grapes: Thompson seedless	1 cup; 160 g	0	0
Kiwi, fresh	1 medium; 76 g	2.6	1.97
Lemon, peel	1 Tbsp; 6 g	83	4.98
Lime, peel	1 Tbsp; 6 g	100	6
Melons: cantaloupe	1 cup; 160 g	0	0
casaba	1 cup; 170 g	0	0
honeydew	1 cup; 170 g	0	0
Mangoes	1 medium; 207 g	0	0
Mango, fresh	1 medium; 207 g	1.06	2.19
Nectarines	1 medium; 136 g	0	0
Orange, raw	1 medium; 131 g	4	5.24
Orange, navel	1 medium; 140 g	2.18	3.06
Papaya, Hawaiian, fresh	1 medium; 304 g	1.99	6.065
Peaches: Alberta	1 medium; 87 g	5	4.35
canned	1 cup; 250 g	1.2	3
Hiley	1 medium; 87 g	0	0
Stokes	1 medium; 87 g	1.2	1.044
Pears, Bartlett, canned	1 cup; 248 g	1.7	4.22
Pineapple, canned	1 cup; 252 g	1	2.52
Pineapple, Dole's (chunks, canned)	1/2 cup; 125 g	3.07	4.86
Plums: Damson	1 medium; 66 g	10	6.6
Golden Gage	1 medium; 66 g	1.1	0.73
Green Gage	1 medium; 66 g	0	0
Preserves: red plum, jam	1 Tbsp; 20 g	0.5	0.1
strawberry, jam	1 Tbsp; 20 g	9.4	1.88
Rhubarb: canned	1 cup; 240 g	600	1440
stewed, no sugar	1 cup; 242 g	860	2081.2
Strawberries, fresh	1 cup; 149 g	0.7	1.04
Strawberries, canned	1 cup; 254 g	15	38.1
Strawberries, raw	1 cup whole; 149 g	10	14.9
Watermelon	1 cup; 160 g	0	0
Nuts			
Peanuts, roasted	1 cup; 146 g	187	273
Pecans	1 cup; 110 g	202	222.2
Sunflower seeds, hulled, dry roasted, unsalted	1 oz; 28 g	18.9	5.29
Confectionery			
Chocolate, plain	1 oz; 28.35 g	117	33.17
Jelly with allowed fruit	1 Tbsp; 20 g	0	0
Marmalade	1 Tbsp; 20 g	10.8	2.16
Preserves: red plum jam	1 Tbsp; 20 g	0.5	0.1
strawberry jam	1 Tbsp; 20 g	9.4	1.88
Sweets, boiled (plain candies)	Hard candy 1 oz	0	—
Beverages			
Barley water, bottled	1 cup; 237 g	0	0
Beer:	12 fl oz; 356 g		
bottled	12 fl oz	0	0
draft	12 fl oz	1	3.56
lager, draft, Tuborg, Pisner	12 fl oz	4	14.24
stout, Guinness draft	12 fl oz	2	7.12
Beer, Budweiser	12 fl oz; 355 g	1.05	3.73
Cider	1 cup; 248 g	0	0
Coca-Cola	12 fl oz; 370 g	trace	trace
Coke	12 fl oz; 370 g	0.12	0.444
Coke, diet	12 fl oz; 354 g	0.1	0.35
Coffee (0.5 g Nescafe/100 mL)	1 tsp powder; 1.8 g	3.2	11.52
Coffee, black, brewed (brewed 4 min)	1 cup; 236 g	0.61	1.44
Coffee infusion:			
2 g per 100 mL infused 5 min		1	
4.4 g (1 tsp) per 100 mL infused 13 min		7.3	
Cocoa, Carnation Dry	1 pkt; 1 oz	7.69	2.184

Continued

Tables

Oxalate Content of Foods per 100 Grams (~½ Cup) and per Portion   (continued)

FOOD	PORTION	MG/100 G	MG/PORTION
Ginger Ale (Schweppes)	12 fl oz; 366 g	0.05	0.196
Lemon squash drink (lemonade)	12 fl oz; 349 g	1	3.49
Lucozade, bottled (soda)	12 fl oz; 350 g	0	0
Orange soda (Minute Maid)	12 fl oz; 372 g	0.24	0.91
Orange squash drink (orangeade)	12 fl oz; 372 g	2.5	9.3
Ovaltine drink, 2 g in 100 mL	1 tsp powder; 2.67 g	10	13.35
Pepsi Cola	12 fl oz; 370 g	trace	trace
Ribena concentrate (black currant drink)	12 fl oz; 360 g	2	7.2
Root beer (Borgs and A&W)	12 fl oz; 370 g	0.19	0.696
Sherry dry	1 cup; 240 g	trace	trace
Tea Indian:			
2-min infusion	1 cup; 237 g	55	130.35
4-min infusion	1 cup; 237 g	72	170.64
6-min infusion	1 cup; 237 g	78	184.86
Tea rosehip	1 cup; 237 g	4	9.48
Tea Lipton, steeped 5 min	1 cup; 237 g	3.74	8.86
Teas (steeped for 5 min w/o stirring, the tea bag then removed)			
Celestial Seasoning teas	1 cup; 250 mL		
Sleepytime	250 mL	0.99	—
Peppermint	250 mL	1.71	—
Wild Forest Blackberry	250 mL	0.9	—
Mandarin Orange Spice	250 mL	0.9	—
Cinnamon Apple Spice	250 mL	1.17	—
R.C. Bigelow			
Cranberry Apple	250 mL	0.9	—
Red Raspberry	250 mL	0.72	—
I Love Lemon	250 mL	0.81	—
Orange and Spice	250 mL	0.81	—
Mint Medley	250 mL	1.71	—
Sweet Dreams	250 mL	1.53	—
Thomas J. Lipton			
Gentle Orange	250 mL	1.08	—
Lemon Soother	250 mL	0.63	—
Chamomile Flowers	250 mL	1.26	—
Lyons Tetley Black Tea			
Tetley Tea (5-min steep)	250 mL	20.79	—
Tetley Tea (1-min steep)	250 mL	10.8	—
Tetley Tea (1-min steep with stirring)	250 mL	19.26	—
Thomas J. Lipton			
Red Rose Classic Tea (5-min steep)	250 mL	11.97	—
Red Rose Classic Tea (1-min steep)	250 mL	10.8	—
Red Rose Classic Tea (1-min steep with stirring)	250 mL	15.75	—
Green Tea R. Twining & Co.			
China Oolong Tea	250 mL	6.84	—
Coffee			
Maxwell House (extra fine) coffee	250 mL	1.44	—
Tomato juice	1 cup; 244 g	5	12.2
Wine:	1 cup; 236 g		
port	1 cup	trace	trace
rose	1 cup	1.5	3.54
white	1 cup	0	0
Fruit juices			
Aloe vera juice	1 cup; 250 g	0.83	2.07
Apple juice from concentrate	1 cup; 248 g	0.51	1.26
Apple juice	1 cup; 248 g	trace	trace
Cranberry juice	1 cup; 253 g	6.6	16.7
Cranberry juice from concentrate	1 cup; 252 g	0.31	0.78
Grapefruit juice	1 cup; 247 g	0	0
Orange juice	1 cup; 249 g	0.5	1.245
Pineapple juice	1 cup; 250 g	0	0

Continued

Oxalate Content of Foods per 100 Grams (~ ½ Cup) and per Portion   (continued)

FOOD	PORTION	MG/100 G	MG/PORTION
Miscellaneous			
Basil, fresh	1 Tbsp; 2.5 g	115.6	2.89
Cinnamon, ground	1 tsp; 2 g	362.74	7.255
Cocoa, dry powder	1 cup; 86 g	623	535.78
Coffee, powder (Nescafe)	1 tsp; 1.8 g	33	11.52
Corn syrup, Karo	1 Tbsp; 21 g	0.32	0.07
Chicken noodle soup	1 cup; 241 g	1	2.41
Gelatin, unflavored Knox	1 pkt; 7 g	11.73	0.82
Ginger, raw	1 Tbsp sliced; 6 g	115.03	6.902
Honey (clover)	1 Tbsp; 21 g	1.51	0.32
Lemon juice	1 cup; 244 g	1	2.44
Lime juice	1 cup; 246 g	0	0
Malt, powder	1 Tbsp; 12.25 g	19.97	2.447
Maple syrup, pure	1 Tbsp; 20 g	0.7	0.14
Mayonnaise, Heinz	1 Tbsp; 14 g	11.98	1.677
Mustard, Dijon style	1 Tbsp; 15 g	6.57	0.985
Nutmeg, dry	1 tsp; 2 g	63.76	1.275
Oregano, dried	1 tsp; 1.5 g	8.58	0.13
Ovaltine powder, canned	1 tsp; 2.67 g	10	13.35
Oxtail soup	1 cup; 376 g	1	3.76
Pepper	1 tsp; 2.1 g	419	8.8
Tomato soup	1 cup; 244 g	3	7.32
Vanilla extract, imitation	1 tsp; 5 g	0.42	0.021
Vegetable soup	1 cup; 241 g	5	12.05
Vinegar, apple cider Ralph's brand	1 tsp; 5 g	1.31	0.066

From Brzezinski E, Durning AM, Grasse B, Fusselman E, Ciaraldi T. Oxalate content of selected foods. The General Clinical Research Center, University of California, San Diego Medical Center, 1996:1–53, with permission. There is now a 1998 edition available.

Index

Page numbers preceded by a "t" denote tables.

Index

Index

Index

Index

Index

Index